Essential
Pathology
for Dental Students

The photographs on the cover of the textbook depict images of diseases as follows:

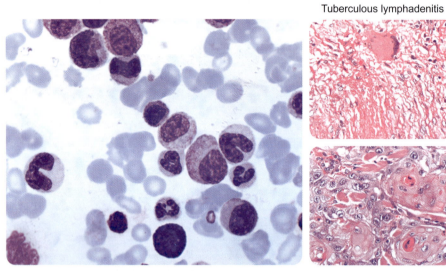

Myeloma cells in bone marrow aspirate

Tuberculous lymphadenitis

Squamous cell carcinoma

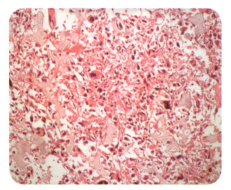

Osteosarcoma

Essential Pathology
for Dental Students

Fifth Edition

Harsh Mohan
MD, FAMS, FICPath, FUICC
Ex-Professor and Head
Department of Pathology
Government Medical College and Hospital
Chandigarh-160 031
INDIA
E-mail: *drharshmohan@gmail.com*

Sugandha Mohan
BDS, DDS (NYUCD, NY, USA)
E-mail: *sugandha1987@gmail.com*

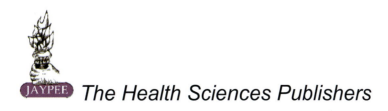

The Health Sciences Publishers

New Delhi | London | Philadelphia | Panama

Jaypee Brothers Medical Publishers (P) Ltd.

Headquarters
Jaypee Brothers Medical Publishers (P) Ltd.
4838/24, Ansari Road, Daryaganj
New Delhi 110 002, India
Phone: +91-11-43574357
Fax: +91-11-43574314
E-mail: jaypee@jaypeebrothers.com

Overseas Offices

J.P. Medical Ltd.
83, Victoria Street, London
SW1H 0HW (UK)
Phone: +44-20 3170 8910
Fax: +44(0) 20 3008 6180
E-mail: info@jpmedpub.com

Jaypee-Highlights Medical Publishers Inc.
City of Knowledge, Building 235, 2nd Floor
Clayton, Panama City, Panama
Phone: +1 507-301-0496
Fax: +1 507-301-0499
E-mail: cservice@jphmedical.com

Jaypee Medical Inc.
325, Chestnut Street
Suite 412, Philadelphia, PA 19106
USA
Phone: +1 267-519-9789
E-mail: support@jpmedus.com

Jaypee Brothers Medical Publishers (P) Ltd.
17/1-B, Babar Road, Block-B
Shaymali, Mohammadpur
Dhaka-1207, Bangladesh
Mobile: +08801912003485
E-mail: jaypeedhaka@gmail.com

Jaypee Brothers Medical Publishers (P) Ltd.
Bhotahity, Kathmandu, Nepal
Phone: +977-9741283608
E-mail: kathmandu@jaypeebrothers.com

Website: www.jaypeebrothers.com
Website: www.jaypeedigital.com

© 2017, Jaypee Brothers Medical Publishers

The views and opinions expressed in this book are solely those of the original contributor(s)/author(s) and do not necessarily represent those of editor(s) of the book.

All rights reserved. No part of this publication may be reproduced, stored or transmitted in any form or by any means, electronic, mechanical, photocopying, recording or otherwise, without the prior permission in writing of the publishers.

All brand names and product names used in this book are trade names, service marks, trademarks or registered trademarks of their respective owners. The publisher is not associated with any product or vendor mentioned in this book.

Medical knowledge and practice change constantly. This book is designed to provide accurate, authoritative information about the subject matter in question. However, readers are advised to check the most current information available on procedures included and check information from the manufacturer of each product to be administered, to verify the recommended dose, formula, method and duration of administration, adverse effects and contraindications. It is the responsibility of the practitioner to take all appropriate safety precautions. Neither the publisher nor the author(s)/editor(s) assume any liability for any injury and/or damage to persons or property arising from or related to use of material in this book.

This book is sold on the understanding that the publisher is not engaged in providing professional medical services. If such advice or services are required, the services of a competent medical professional should be sought.

Every effort has been made where necessary to contact holders of copyright to obtain permission to reproduce copyright material. If any have been inadvertently overlooked, the publisher will be pleased to make the necessary arrangements at the first opportunity.

Inquiries for bulk sales may be solicited at: jaypee@jaypeebrothers.com

Assistant Editor: Praveen Mohan

Essential Pathology for Dental Students

First Edition : 1995
Second Edition : 2002
Third Edition : 2005
Fourth Edition : 2011

Fifth Edition : **2017**

ISBN 978-93-86107-74-9

Printed at Replika Press Pvt. Ltd.

Preface

तस्मात् असक्तः राततम् कार्यम् कर्म समाचर।
असक्तः हि आचरन् कर्म परम् आप्नोति पुरूषः।।

**Thus do your duty without attachment
Perform the work that has to be done,
Since the person attains supreme form
By doing duty in a spirit of sacrifice.**

(The Bhagvatgita: Ch III, Verse 19)

In keeping pace with newer developments in the field of pathology and in order to cater to the contemporary needs of users, the fifth edition of *Essential Pathology for Dental Students* is presented after a gap of six years since the last edition of this book. The new edition has been thoroughly updated and contains newer contents and it is expected to be highly useful and more appealing. In fact, for eager learners, the revised edition has more material than the current syllabus recommended by the Dental Council of India (DCI). The revised edition has a large number of new illustrations, line drawings, schematic drawings and newer tables, in an attempt to enhance understanding and learning of the subject readily, besides being a visual treat. A new feature incorporated in this edition is placing of Gist Boxes at the end of each topic presenting summary of the topic just covered so that the learner can quickly revise it in a short time. In addition, the present edition has been redesigned in illustrations, lay-out and in printing for a more aesthetic look as well. In doing all this, I used my discretion as a teacher in including many newer examples of diseases, especially in infections and neoplasms, and had the help of a more modern approach of my co-author (SM).

In recent years, there have been widespread advancements in molecular, immunologic and genetic basis of several diseases which have heightened our understanding of the mechanisms of diseases. As a result, mention of 'idiopathic' in etiology and pathogenesis of many diseases in the literature is slowly disappearing. Surely, the students of 21st century need to be enlightened on these modern advances in diseases; these aspects have been dealt with in the revised edition with a simple and lucid approach.

Key Features of the fifth edition are as follows:

Thorough updating: All the chapters and topics have undergone thorough revision and updating of various aspects. While most of the newer information has been inserted between the lines, a few topics have been rewritten. In doing so, the basic accepted style of the book—simple, easy-to-understand and reproducibility of the subject matter, and emphasis on clarity and accuracy, has not been changed.

Reorganised contents: The revised edition has 30 chapters divided into two parts: *Part A: General Pathology* (4 sections) and *Part B: Systemic Pathology* (2 sections). This has been done in conformity with the revised recommendations in the syllabus prescribed by the DCI; however, a few additional topics have been added for an inquisitive learner. Topics such as Techniques in Pathology and Normal Values have been shifted to *Practical Pathology for Dental Students* where these topics belong.

More and new figures/tables: There are several newer figures and tables in the revised edition. All free-hand labelled sketches of gross specimens and line-drawings of microscopic features of an entity have been placed alongside the corresponding specimen photograph and photomicrograph, respectively, enhancing the understanding of the subject for the beginners in pathology.

Gist Boxes: Throughout the book, at the end of every topic, a uniquely coloured box containing summary of the topic just covered has been placed. These Gist Boxes are meant for quick revision of the topics in a short time. Since these boxes have a distinct colour scheme throughout the book, the student can revise the entire subject by quickly turning pages of the book and these boxes become readily visible without having to search for them, making the book truly user-friendly.

Free! Practical Pathology (Second Edition): Introduction of *Practical Pathology for Dental Students* in the previous edition of this book was widely welcomed, and that too free with the book! Second edition of *Practical Pathology for Dental Students* is also available free with the fifth revised edition of *Essential Pathology for Dental Students* and has now 27 Practical Exercises (instead of 25 in previous edition) on the pattern of practical classes of students. A newer feature of the second edition of this companion book is addition of a few *Key Questions for Viva Voce* at the end of each practical exercise. This is likely to benefit the students greatly in quick revision of the practical subject and also an exercise in self-assessment. This book has a few additional exercises than the practicals recommended by the DCI for those desirous of learning more.

Thus, the revised edition is a comprehensive twin package covering updated text of theory and practical exercises along with questions for viva voce in pathology for students of dentistry. It is anticipated that with such a complete coverage of the subject, the users will not have to refer to any other book during their routine learning of pathology. It is also hoped that practicing clinicians and students of other branches of medicine such as pharmacy, physiotherapy, laboratory medicine, nursing and alternate systems of medicine, would also find it useful.

ACKNOWLEDGEMENTS

In preparing the revised fifth edition, suggestions and corrections received from my colleagues at different places and students have been carefully taken into consideration which is gratefully acknowledged. As in my other books, liberal and skilful technical assistance rendered by Ms Agam Verma, MSc (MLT), Senior Laboratory Technician, is thankfully acknowledged.

My special thanks to the team of dedicated staff of M/s Jaypee Brothers Medical Publishers (P) Ltd, New Delhi, India, in general, and Mrs Y Kapoor (Senior Desktop Operator), in particular for acceding to my requests for amendments and insertions till the very last minute, and Mr Manoj Pahuja (Senior Graphic Designer), for all his help in skilful and appealing art work. All the team members at Jaypee who have contributed in a variety of ways deserve my gratitude—for meticulous proof-reading, for designing of cover, and for promotion of sales and marketing, etc. Finally, my gratitude to the motivating and inspiring leadership of Shri Jitendar P Vij (Group Chairman) and Mr Ankit Vij (Group President) of the M/s Jaypee Brothers Medical Publishers (P) Ltd, New Delhi, India, who have been always conscious of quality of the final product and the results show it.

In spite of my best efforts, element of human error is still likely. As in the previous editions, the readers are welcome to point out all such mistakes and render valuable suggestions for further improvements which will be gratefully acknowledged.

Harsh Mohan MD, FAMS, FICPath, FUICC
E-mail: *drharshmohan@gmail.com*

Sugandha Mohan BDS, DDS (NYUCD, NY, USA)
E-mail: *sugandha1987@gmail.com*

Contents

Revised Syllabus in Pathology for BDS Students as per Recommendations of the Dental Council of India

Part A: General Pathology

Section I: The Cell in Health and Disease

1. Introduction to Pathology — 1
2. Cell Structure and Function, Cellular Ageing — 9
3. Cellular Adaptations — 18
4. Cell Injury: Etiology and Pathogenesis — 27
5. Morphology of Cell Injury: Degenerations and Cell Death — 36
6. Intracellular Accumulations — 52
7. Amyloidosis — 61
8. Genetic and Paediatric Diseases — 73
9. Environmental, Nutritional and Vitamin Deficiency Disorders — 85

Section II: Inflammation and Healing, Immunity and Hypersensitivity, Infections and Infestations

10. Inflammation: Acute — 107
11. Inflammation: Chronic and Granulomatous — 129
12. Healing of Tissues — 155
13. Infectious and Parasitic Diseases — 166
14. Diseases of Immunity including AIDS — 195

Section III: Fluid and Haemodynamic Disorders

15. Derangements of Body Fluids — 222
16. Blood Flow Volume Disorders — 235
17. Obstructive Haemodynamic Derangements — 247

Section IV: Neoplasia

18. General Aspects of Neoplasia — 265
19. Etiology and Pathogenesis of Neoplasia — 282
20. Host-Tumour Relationship and Diagnosis of Neoplasms — 311
21. Common Specific Tumours — 321

Part B: Systemic Pathology

Section V: Haematology and Lymphoreticular Tissues

22.	Disorders of Erythroid Series: Anaemias	357
23.	Platelets and Bleeding Disorders	400
24.	Diseases of Leucocytes and Lymphoid Tissues	415

Section VI: Selected Topics from Systemic Pathology

25.	Diseases of Cardiovascular System	467
26.	Diseases of Oral Cavity and Salivary Glands	514
27.	Jaundice, Hepatitis and Cirrhosis	532
28.	Hypertension and its Consequences	559
29.	Diabetes Mellitus and its Complications	569
30.	Common Diseases of Bones, Cartilage and Joints	584

Index   *615*

Revised Syllabus in Pathology for BDS Students as per Recommendations of the Dental Council of India

COURSE CONTENTS IN THEORY

A. GENERAL PATHOLOGY

Introduction to Pathology: Terminologies, the cell in health, the normal cell structure, the cellular functions.

Etiology and Pathogenesis of Disease: Cell injury, types—congenital, acquired, mainly acquired causes of disease (hypoxic injury, chemical injury, physical injury, immunological injury).

Degenerations: Amyloidosis, fatty change, cloudy swelling, hyaline change, mucoid degeneration.

Cell Death and Necrosis: Apoptosis; definition, causes, features and types of necrosis; gangrene—dry, wet, gas; pathological calcifications (dystrophic and metastatic).

Inflammation: Definition, causes, types and features; acute inflammation—the vascular response, the cellular response, chemical mediators, the inflammatory cells, fate; chronic inflammation; granulomatous inflammation.

Healing: Regeneration, repair—mechanisms, healing by primary intention, healing by secondary intention, fracture healing, factors influencing healing process, complications.

Tuberculosis: Epidemiology, pathogenesis (formation of tubercle), pathological features of primary and secondary TB, complications and fate.

Syphilis: Epidemiology, types and stages of syphilis, pathological features, diagnostic criteria, oral lesions.

Typhoid: Epidemiology, pathogenesis, pathological features, diagnostic criteria.

Thrombosis: Definition, pathophysiology, formation, complications and fate of a thrombus.

Embolism: Definition, types, effects.

Ischaemia and Infarction: Definition, etiology, types; infarction of various organs.

Derangements of Body Fluids: Oedema—pathogenesis, different types.

Disorders of Circulation: Hyperaemia, shock.

Nutritional Disorders: Common vitamin deficiencies.

Immunological Mechanisms in Disease: Humoral and cellular immunity, hypersensitivity and autoimmunity, AIDS

Adaptive Disorders of Growth: Atrophy and hypertrophy, hyperplasia, metaplasia and dysplasia.

General Aspects of Neoplasia: Definition, terminology, classification; differences between benign and malignant neoplasms; the neoplastic cell; metastasis; etiology and pathogenesis of neoplasia, carcinogenesis; tumour biology; oncogenes and anti-oncogenes; precancerous lesions; common specific tumours—squamous papilloma and carcinoma, basal cell carcinoma, adenoma and adenocarcinoma, fibroma and fibrosarcoma, lipoma and liposarcoma.

B. SYSTEMIC PATHOLOGY

Anaemias: Iron deficiency anaemia, megaloblastic anaemia.

Leukaemias: Acute and chronic leukaemias, diagnosis and clinical features.

Diseases of Lymph Nodes: Hodgkin's disease, non-Hodgkin's lymphoma, metastatic carcinoma.

Diseases of Oral Cavity: Lichen planus, stomatitis, leukoplakia, squamous cell carcinoma, dental caries, dentigereous cyst, ameloblastoma.

Diseases of Salivary Glands: Normal structure, sialadenitis, tumours.

Hepatitis

Hypertension: Definition, classification; pathophysiology, effects in various organs.

Diabetes Mellitus: Definition, classification, pathogenesis, pathology in different organs.

Common Diseases of Bone: Osteomyelitis, metabolic bone diseases, bone tumours—osteosarcoma, osteoclastoma (giant cell tumour), Ewing's sarcoma, fibrous dysplasia, aneurysmal bone cyst.

Diseases of Cardiovascular System: Cardiac failure, congenital heart disease—ASD, VSD, PDA, Fallot's tetralogy, infective endocarditis, atherosclerosis, ischaemic heart disease.

Haemorrhagic Disorders: Coagulation cascade, coagulation disorder, platelet function, platelet disorders.

Section I ▶ The Cell in Health and Disease

▶ SECTION CONTENTS

Chapter 1: Introduction to Pathology
Chapter 2: Cell Structure and Function, Cellular Ageing
Chapter 3: Cellular Adaptations
Chapter 4: Cell Injury: Etiology and Pathogenesis
Chapter 5: Morphology of Cell Injury: Degenerations and Cell Death
Chapter 6: Intracellular Accumulations
Chapter 7: Amyloidosis
Chapter 8: Genetic and Paediatric Diseases
Chapter 9: Environmental, Nutritional and Vitamin Deficiency Disorders

1 Introduction to Pathology

STUDY OF PATHOLOGY

The word *'Pathology'* is derived from two Greek words—*pathos* (meaning suffering) and *logos* (meaning study). Pathology is, thus, scientific study of changes in the structure and function of the body in disease. In other words, pathology consists of the abnormalities in normal anatomy (including histology) and normal physiology owing to disease. Another commonly used term with reference to study of diseases is *'pathophysiology'* (*patho*=suffering, *physiology*=study of normal function). Pathophysiology, thus, includes study of disordered function (i.e. physiological changes) and breakdown of homeostasis in diseases (i.e. biochemical changes). Pathologists contribute in patient management by providing final diagnosis of disease. Therefore, knowledge and understanding of pathology is essential for all would-be practitioners of art of healing and science because unless they have knowledge and understanding of the language and pathologic basis of diseases, they would not be able to institute appropriate treatment or suggest preventive measures to the patient.

For the student of any stream of medical science, the discipline of pathology forms a vital bridge between initial learning phase of preclinical sciences and the final phase of clinical subjects. The role and significance of learning of pathology in clinical medicine is quite well summed up by *Sir William Osler* (1849-1919), acclaimed physician and teacher in medicine considered as 'Father of Modern Medicine', by his famous quote "your practice of medicine will be as good as is your understanding of pathology" **(Fig. 1.1)**.

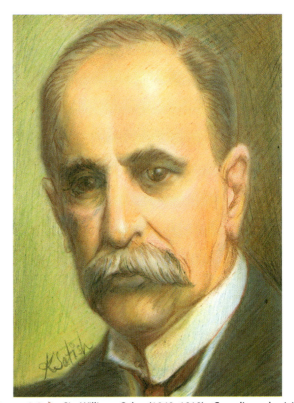

Figure 1.1 ▶ Sir William Osler (1849–1919). Canadian physician and one of the four founding Professors of Johns Hopkins Hospital, Baltimore, US, is regarded as *'Father of Modern Medicine'*, Sir Osler had keen interest in pathology, was an acclaimed teacher and is also remembered for his famous quotations.

HEALTH AND DISEASE

Before there were humans on earth, there was disease, albeit in early animals. Since pathology is the study of disease, then what is *disease*? In simple language, disease is opposite of health i.e. what is not healthy is disease. *Health* may be defined as a condition when the individual is in complete accord with the surroundings, while *disease* is loss of ease (or comfort) to the body (i.e. dis+ease). However, it must be borne in mind that in health there is a wide range of 'normality' in various parameters e.g. in height, weight, blood and tissue chemical composition etc. It also needs to be appreciated that at cellular level, the cells display wide range of activities within the broad area of health similar to what is seen in diseased cells. Thus, a disease or an illness means a condition marked by pronounced deviation from the normal healthy state. The term *syndrome* (meaning running together) is used for a combination of several clinical features caused by altered physiologic processes.

COMMON TERMS IN PATHOLOGY

It is important for a beginner in pathology to be familiar with the language used in pathology **(Fig.1.2)**:
- *Patient* is the person affected by disease.
- *Lesions* are the characteristic changes in tissues and cells produced by disease in an individual or an experimental animal.
- *Pathologic changes* or *morphology* consist of examination of diseased tissues. These can be recognised with the naked eye *(gross or macroscopic changes)* or studied by *microscopic examination* of tissues.
- Causal factors responsible for the lesions are included in *etiology* of disease (i.e. 'why' of disease).
- Mechanism by which the lesions are produced is termed *pathogenesis* of disease (i.e. 'how' of disease).
- Functional implications of the lesion felt by the patient are *symptoms*, and those discovered by the clinician by examination are the *physical signs*.
- Clinical significance of the morphologic and functional changes together with results of other investigations help to arrive at an answer to what is wrong *(diagnosis)*, what is going to happen *(prognosis)*, what can be done about it *(treatment)*, and finally what should be done to avoid complications and spread *(prevention)* (i.e. 'what' of disease).

EVOLUTION OF PATHOLOGY

Pathology as the scientific study of disease processes has its deep roots in medical history. Since the beginning of mankind, there has been desire as well as need to know more about the causes, mechanisms and nature of diseases. The answers to these questions have evolved over the centuries—from supernatural beliefs to the present state of our knowledge of modern pathology. However, pathology owes its development to interaction and interdependence on advances in diverse neighbouring branches of science, in addition to the strides made in medical technology. As we

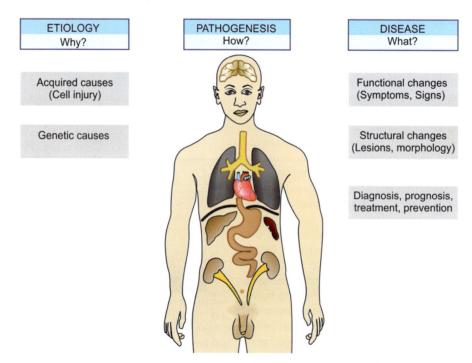

Figure 1.2 ▶ Diagrammatic depiction of disease and various terms used in pathology.

shall see in the pages that follow, pathology has evolved over the years as a distinct discipline from anatomy, medicine and surgery, in that sequence.

PREHISTORIC TIMES TO MEDIEVAL PERIOD

Present-day knowledge of primitive culture which was prevalent in the world in prehistoric times reveals that religion, magic and medical treatment were quite linked to each other in those times. The earliest concept of disease understood by the patient and the healer was the religious belief that disease was the outcome of 'curse from God' or the belief in magic that the affliction had supernatural origin from 'evil eye of spirits.' To ward them off, priests through prayers and sacrifices, and magicians by magic power, used to act as faith-healers and invoke supernatural powers and please the gods. Remnants of ancient superstitions still exist in some parts of the world. The link between medicine and religion became so firmly established throughout the world that different societies had their gods and goddesses of healing; for example: mythological Greeks had *Aesculapius* and *Apollo* as the principal gods of healing, *Dhanvantri* as the deity of medicine in India.

The insignia of healing, the Caduceus, having snake and staff, is believed to represent the god Hermes or Mercury, which according to Greek mythology has power of healing since snake has regenerative powers expressed by its periodic sloughing of its skin. God of Greek medicine, *Aesculapius*, performed his functions with a staff having a single serpent wound around it. Later (around AD 1800), however, the Caduceus got replaced with twin-serpents wound around a staff topped by a round knob and flanked by two wings and now represents the symbol of medicine **(Fig. 1.3)**.

The period of ancient religious and magical beliefs was followed by the philosophical and rational approach to disease by the methods of observations. This happened at the time when great Greek philosophers—*Socrates, Plato* and *Aristotle,* introduced philosophical concepts to all natural phenomena.

But the real practice of medicine began with *Hippocrates* (460–370 BC), the great Greek clinical genius of all times and regarded as 'the father of medicine' **(Fig. 1.4)**. Hippocrates dissociated medicine from religion and magic. Instead, he firmly believed in study of patient's symptoms and described methods of diagnosis. He recorded his observations on cases in the form of collections of writings called Hippocratic Corpus which remained the mainstay of learning of medicine for nearly two thousand years. Hippocrates followed rational and ethical attitudes in practice and teaching of medicine and is revered by the medical profession by taking *'Hippocratic oath'* at the time of entry into practice of medicine.

After Hippocrates, Greek medicine reached Rome (Italy) which controlled Greek world after 146 BC and, therefore, it dominated the field of development of medicine in ancient Europe then. In fact, since old times, many tongue-twisting terminologies in medicine have their origin from

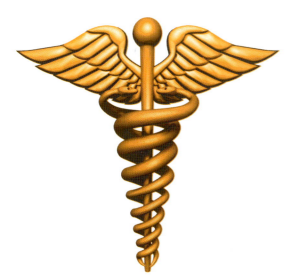

Figure 1.3 ▶ The Caduceus, representing symbol of medicine, is the traditional symbol of god Hermes or Mercury. It features twin serpents winding around a winged staff.

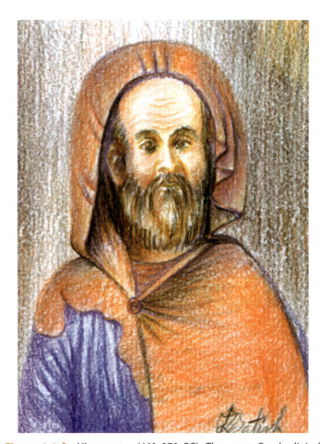

Figure 1.4 ▶ Hippocrates (460–370 BC). The great Greek clinical genius and regarded as *'the Father of Medicine'*. He introduced ethical aspects to medicine.

Latin language which was the official language of countries included in ancient Roman Empire (Spanish, Portuguese, Italian, French and Greek languages have their origin from Latin).

In Rome, Hippocratic teaching was propagated by Roman physicians, notably by *Cornelius Celsus* (53 BC-7 AD) and *Claudius Galen* (130-200 AD). Celsus first described four cardinal signs of inflammation—rubor (redness), tumor (swelling), calor (heat), and dolor (pain). Galen postulated humoral theory, later called Galenic theory. This theory suggested that the illness resulted from imbalance between *four humors* (or body fluids): blood, lymph, black bile (believed at that time to be from the spleen), and biliary secretion from the liver.

The hypothesis of disequilibrium of four elements constituting the body *(Dhatus)* similar to Hippocratic doctrine finds mention in ancient Indian medicine books compiled about 200 AD—*Charaka Samhita*, a finest document by *Charaka* on medicine listing 500 remedies, and *Sushruta Samhita,* similar book of surgical sciences by *Sushruta,* and includes about 700 plant-derived medicines.

The end of Medieval period was marked by backward steps in medicine. There were widespread and devastating epidemics which reversed the process of rational thinking again to supernatural concepts and divine punishment for 'sins.' The dominant belief during this period was that life was due to influence of vital substance under the control of soul *(theory of vitalism)*.

HUMAN ANATOMY AND ERA OF GROSS PATHOLOGY

The backwardness of Medieval period was followed by the Renaissance period, i.e. revival of learning. The Renaissance began from Italy in late 15th century and spread to whole of Europe. During this period, there was quest for advances in art and science.

The beginning of the development of human anatomy took place during this period with the art works and drawings of human muscles and embryos by famous Italian painter *Leonardo da Vinci* (1452-1519). Dissection of human body was started by *Vesalius* (1514-1564) on freshly executed criminals. His pupils further popularised the practice of human anatomic dissection for which special postmortem amphitheatres came in to existence in various parts of ancient Europe.

Antony van Leeuwenhoek (1632-1723), a cloth merchant by profession in Holland, during his spare time invented the first ever microscope by grinding the lenses himself through which he recognised male spermatozoa and also introduced histological staining in 1714 using saffron to examine muscle fibres.

Marcello Malpighi (1624-1694) used microscope extensively and observed the presence of capillaries and described the malpighian layer of the skin, and lymphoid tissue in the spleen (malpighian corpuscles). Malpighi is known as 'the father of histology.'

The credit for beginning of the study of morbid anatomy (pathologic anatomy) goes to Italian anatomist-pathologist, *Giovanni B. Morgagni* (1682-1771). By his work, Morgagni demolished the ancient humoral theory of disease and published his life-time experiences based on 700 postmortems and their corresponding clinical findings. He, thus, laid the foundations of clinicopathologic methodology in the study of disease and introduced the concept of clinicopathologic correlation (CPC), establishing a coherent sequence of cause, lesions, symptoms, and outcome of disease.

Sir Percivall Pott (1714-1788), famous surgeon in England, described arthritic tuberculosis of the spine (Pott's disease) and identified the first ever occupational cancer (cancer of scrotal skin) in the chimney sweeps in 1775 and discovered chimney soot as the first carcinogenic agent. The study of anatomy in England during the latter part of 18th Century was dominated by the two Hunter brothers. These were *John Hunter* (1728-1793), a student of Sir Percivall Pott, who rose to become the greatest surgeon-anatomist of all times and his elder brother *William Hunter* (1718-1788) who was a reputed anatomist-obstetrician. These brothers together started the first ever museum by collection of surgical specimens from their flourishing practice, which came to be known as the Hunterian Museum, now housed in Royal College of Surgeons of London. Among many pupils of John Hunter was *Edward Jenner* (1749-1823) whose work on inoculation in smallpox is well known. The era of gross pathology had three more illustrious and brilliant physician-pathologists in England who were colleagues at Guy's Hospital in London:

◆ *Richard Bright* (1789-1858) who described non-suppurative nephritis, later termed glomerulonephritis or Bright's disease;
◆ *Thomas Addison* (1793-1860) who gave an account of chronic adrenocortical insufficiency termed Addison's disease; and
◆ *Thomas Hodgkin* (1798-1866), who observed the complex of chronic enlargement of lymph nodes, often with enlargement of the liver and spleen, later called Hodgkin's disease.

R.T.H. Laennec (1781-1826), a French physician, dominated the early part of 19th century by his numerous discoveries. He described several lung diseases (tubercles, caseous lesions, miliary lesions, pleural effusion, and bronchiectasis), chronic sclerotic liver disease (later called Laennec's cirrhosis) and invented stethoscope.

Morbid anatomy attained its zenith with appearance of *Carl F. von Rokitansky* (1804-1878), self-taught German pathologist who performed nearly 30,000 autopsies himself and described acute yellow atrophy of the liver, wrote an outstanding monograph on diseases of arteries and congenital heart defects.

ERA OF TECHNOLOGY DEVELOPMENT AND CELLULAR PATHOLOGY

Up to middle of the 19th century, correlation of clinical manifestations of disease with gross pathological findings at autopsy became the major method of study of disease. Sophistication in surgery led to advancement in pathology. The anatomist-surgeons of earlier centuries got replaced largely with surgeon-pathologists in the 19th century.

Pathology started developing as a diagnostic discipline in later half of the 19th century with the evolution of cellular pathology which was closely linked to technological advancements in machinery manufacture for cutting thin sections of tissue, improvement in microscope, and development of chemical industry and dyes for staining.

The discovery of existence of disease-causing microorganisms was made by French chemist *Louis Pasteur* (1822–1895), thus demolishing the prevailing theory of spontaneous generation of disease and firmly established germ theory of disease. Subsequently, *G.H.A. Hansen* (1841–1912) in Germany identified Hansen's bacillus in 1873 as the first microbe causative for leprosy (Hansen's disease). While the study of infectious diseases was being made, the concept of immune tolerance and allergy emerged which formed the basis of immunisation initiated by Edward Jenner.

Developments in chemical industry helped in switch over from earlier dyes of plant and animal origin to synthetic dyes; aniline violet being the first such synthetic dye in 1856. This led to emergence of a viable dye industry for histological and bacteriological purposes. The impetus for the flourishing and successful dye industry came from the works of numerous pioneers as under:

◈ *Paul Ehrlich* (1854–1915), German physician, conferred Nobel Prize in 1908 for his work in immunology, described Ehrlich's test for urobilinogen using Ehrlich's aldehyde reagent, staining techniques of cells and bacteria, and laid the foundations of clinical pathology.
◈ *Christian Gram* (1853–1938), Danish physician, developed bacteriologic staining by crystal violet.
◈ *D.L. Romanowsky* (1861–1921), Russian physician, developed stain for peripheral blood film using eosin and methylene blue derivatives.
◈ *Robert Koch* (1843–1910), German bacteriologist, besides Koch's postulate and Koch's phenomena, developed techniques of fixation and staining for identification of bacteria, discovered tubercle bacilli in 1882 and cholera vibrio organism in 1883.
◈ *May-Grünwald* in 1902 and *Giemsa* in 1914 developed blood stains and applied them for classification of blood cells and bone marrow cells.
◈ *Sir William Leishman* (1865–1926) described Leishman's stain for blood films in 1914 and observed Leishman-Donovan bodies (LD bodies) in leishmaniasis.

Simultaneous technological advances in machinery manufacture led to development and upgrading of microtomes for obtaining thin sections of organs and tissues for staining by dyes for enhancing detailed study of sections.

Rudolf Virchow (1821–1905) in Germany is credited with the beginning of microscopic examination of diseased tissue at cellular level and thus began histopathology as a method of investigation. Virchow hypothesised cellular theory having following two components:
◈ All cells come from other cells.
◈ Disease is an alteration of normal structure and function of these cells.

Virchow was revered as the Pope of pathology in Europe and is aptly known as the 'father of cellular pathology' **(Fig. 1.5)**. Thus, sound foundation of diagnostic pathology based on microscopy had been laid which was followed and promoted by numerous brilliant successive workers. This gave birth to biopsy pathology and thus emerged the discipline of surgical pathology. Virchow also described etiology of embolism (Virchow's triad—slowing of blood-stream, changes in the vessel wall, changes in the blood itself), metastatic spread of tumours (Virchow's lymph node), and components and diseases of blood (fibrinogen, leukocytosis, leukaemia).

A few other landmarks in further evolution of modern pathology in this era are as follows:
◈ *Karl Landsteiner* (1863–1943) described the existence of major human blood groups in 1900 and is considered "father of blood transfusion"; he was awarded Nobel Prize in 1930.

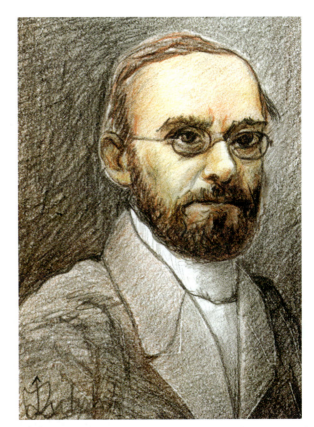

Figure 1.5 ▶ Rudolf Virchow (1821–1905). German pathologist who proposed cellular theory of disease and initiated biopsy pathology for diagnosis of diseases and is known as 'the *Father of Cellular Pathology*'.

- *Ruska* and *Lorries* in 1933 developed electron microscope which aided the pathologist to view ultrastructure of cell and its organelles.
- The development of exfoliative cytology for early detection of cervical cancer began with *George N. Papanicolaou* (1883–1962), a Greek-born, American pathologist, in 1930s and is known as 'father of exfoliative cytology' **(Fig. 1.6)**.

Another pioneering contribution in pathology in the 20th century was by an eminent teacher-author, *William Boyd* (1885–1979), psychiatrist-turned pathologist, whose textbooks—'Pathology for Surgeons' (first edition 1925) and 'Textbook of Pathology' (first edition 1932), dominated and inspired the students of pathology all over the world for a few generations due to his flowery language and lucid style.

MODERN PATHOLOGY

The strides made in the latter half of 20th century until recent times in 21st century have made it possible to study diseases at genetic and molecular level, and provide an evidence-based and objective diagnosis that may enable the physician to institute targeted therapy. The major impact of advances in molecular biology are in the field of diagnosis and treatment of genetic disorders, immunology and in cancer. Some of the revolutionary discoveries during this time are as under **(Fig. 1.7)**:

- Description of *the structure of DNA* of the cell by Watson and Crick in 1953.
- Identification of *chromosomes and their correct number* in humans (46) by *Tijo* and *Levan* in 1956.
- Identification of *Philadelphia chromosome* in chronic myeloid leukaemia by Nowell and Hagerford in 1960 as the first chromosomal abnormality in any cancer.
- *In Situ hybridization* (ISH) introduced in 1969 in which a labelled probe is employed to detect and localise specific RNA or DNA sequences *'in situ'* (i.e. in the original place). Its later modification employs use of fluorescence microscopy (FISH) to detect specific localisation of the defect on chromosomes.
- *Recombinant DNA technique* developed in 1972 using restriction enzymes to cut and paste bits of DNA.
- Introduction of *polymerase chain reaction* (PCR) i.e. "xeroxing" of DNA fragments by Kary Mullis in 1983 has revolutionised the diagnostic molecular genetics. PCR analysis is more rapid than ISH, can be automated by thermal cyclers and requires much lower amount of starting DNA.
- Invention of *flexibility and dynamism of DNA* by Barbara McClintock for which she was awarded Nobel Prize in 1983.
- *Mammalian cloning* started in 1997 by *Ian Wilmut* and his colleagues at Roslin Institute in Edinburgh, by successfully using a technique of somatic cell nuclear transfer to create the clone of a sheep named Dolly. Human reproductive cloning, however, is very risky, besides being absolutely unethical.
- The era of *stem cell research* started in 21st century by harvesting these primitive cells isolated from embryos and maintaining their growth in the laboratory. There are 2 types of sources of stem cells in humans: embryonic stem cells and adult stem cells, the former being more numerous. Stem cells are seen by many researchers as having virtually unlimited applications in the treatment of many human diseases such as Alzheimer's disease, diabetes, cancer, strokes, etc. At some point of time, stem cell therapy may be able to replace whole organ transplant and instead stem cells 'harvested' from the embryo may be used.
- *Human Genome Project (HGP)* consisting of a consortium of countries was completed in April 2003 coinciding with 50 years of description of DNA double helix by Watson and Crick in April 1953. The sequencing of human genome reveals that human genome contains approximately 3 billion base pairs of amino acids, which are located in the 23 pairs of chromosomes within the nucleus of each human cell. Each chromosome contains an estimated 30,000 genes in the human genome which carry the instructions for making proteins. The HGP has given us the ability to read nature's complete genetic blueprint used in making of each human being (i.e. gene mapping). Clinical trials by gene therapy on treatment of some single gene defects have resulted in some

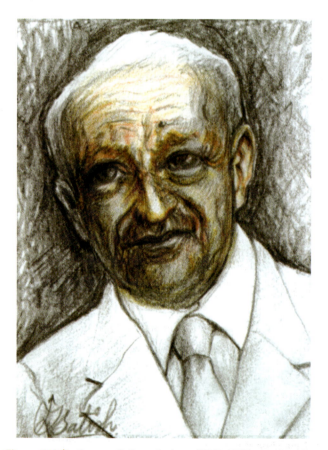

Figure 1.6 ▶ George N Papanicolaou (1883–1962). An American pathologist, who developed Pap test for diagnosis of cancer of uterine cervix and is known as 'the *Father of Exfoliative Cytology*'.

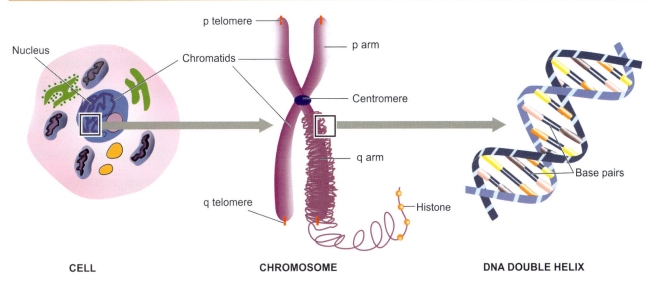

Figure 1.7 ▶ Molecular structure of human chromosome

success, especially in haematological and immunological diseases. Future developments in genetic engineering may result in designing new and highly effective individualised treatment options for genetic diseases as well as suggest prevention against diseases.

TELEPATHOLOGY

Telepathology is defined as the practice of diagnostic pathology by a remote pathologist utilising images of tissue specimens transmitted over a telecommunication network. Depending upon need and budget, telepathology system is of two *types*:

Static (store-and-forward, passive telepathology) In this, selected images are captured, stored and then transmitted over the internet via e-mail attachment, file transfer protocol, web page or CD-ROM. It is quite inexpensive and is more common but suffers from disadvantage of having sender's bias in selection of transmitted images.

Dynamic (Robotic interactive telepathology) Here, the images are transmitted in real-time from a remote microscope. Robotic movement of stage of microscope is controlled remotely and the desired images and fields are accessioned from a remote/local server. Thus, it almost duplicates to perfection the examination of actual slides under the microscope, hence is referred to as *Virtual Microscopy*. However, image quality and speed of internet can be major hurdles.

SUBDIVISIONS OF PATHOLOGY

Human pathology is conventionally studied under two broad divisions: *General Pathology* dealing with general principles of disease, and *Systemic Pathology* that includes study of diseases pertaining to the specific organs and body systems. Diagnostic pathology, however, involves morphological and non-morphological disciplines of laboratory sciences as follows:

MORPHOLOGICAL BRANCHES

These branches essentially involve application of microscope as an essential tool for the study and include histopathology, cytopathology and haematology.

A. HISTOPATHOLOGY Histopathology, used synonymously with anatomic pathology, pathologic anatomy, morbid anatomy, or tissue pathology, is the classic method of study and still the most useful one which has stood the test of time. The study includes structural changes observed by naked eye examination referred to as gross or macroscopic changes, and the changes detected by microscopy, which may be further supported by numerous special staining methods such as histochemistry and immunohistochemistry to arrive at the most accurate diagnosis. In modern times, anatomic pathology includes sub-specialities such as cardiac pathology, pulmonary pathology, neuropathology, renal pathology, gynaecologic pathology, breast pathology, dermatopathology, gastrointestinal pathology, oral pathology, and so on. Anatomic pathology includes the following subdivisions:

1. ***Surgical pathology*** It deals with the study of tissues removed from the living body by biopsy or surgical resection. Surgical pathology constitutes the bulk of work for the pathologist and includes study of tissue by conventional *paraffin embedding* technique; intraoperative *frozen section* may be employed for rapid diagnosis.

2. ***Experimental pathology*** This is defined as production of disease in the experimental animal and study of morphological changes in organs after sacrificing the animal.

3. *Forensic pathology and autopsy work* This includes the study of organs and tissues removed at postmortem for medicolegal work and for determining the underlying sequence and cause of death. By this, the pathologist attempts to reconstruct the course of events how they may have happened in the patient during life which culminated in his death. Postmortem anatomical diagnosis is helpful to the clinician to enhance his knowledge about the disease and his judgement while forensic autopsy is helpful for medicolegal purposes. The significance of a careful postmortem examination is appropriately summed up in the old saying 'the dead teach the living'.

B. CYTOPATHOLOGY Though a branch of anatomic pathology, cytopathology has developed as a distinct subspeciality in recent times. It includes study of cells shed off from the lesions (exfoliative cytology) and fine-needle aspiration cytology (FNAC) of superficial and deep-seated lesions for diagnosis.

C. HAEMATOLOGY Haematology deals with the diseases of blood. It includes laboratory haematology and clinical haematology; the latter covers the management of patient as well.

NON-MORPHOLOGICAL BRANCHES

These include clinical pathology, clinical biochemistry, microbiology, immunology, genetics and molecular pathology. In these diagnostic branches, qualitative, semi-quantitative or quantitative determinations are carried out in the laboratory, while microscope may be required for only some of these lab tests.

A. CLINICAL PATHOLOGY Analysis of various fluids including blood, urine, semen, CSF and other body fluids is included in this branch of pathology. Such analysis may be qualitative, semi-quantitative or quantitative.

B. CLINICAL BIOCHEMISTRY Quantitative determination of various biochemical constituents in serum and plasma, and in other body fluids is included in clinical biochemistry.

C. MICROBIOLOGY This is study of disease-causing microbes implicated in human diseases. Depending upon the type of microorganims studied, it has further developed into such as bacteriology, parasitology, mycology, virology etc.

D. IMMUNOLOGY Detection of abnormalities in the immune system of the body comprises immunology and immunopathology.

E. MEDICAL GENETICS This is the branch of human genetics that deals with the relationship between heredity and disease. There have been important developments in the field of medical genetics e.g. in blood groups, inborn errors of metabolism, chromosomal aberrations in congenital malformations and neoplasms etc.

F. MOLECULAR PATHOLOGY The detection and diagnosis of abnormalities at the level of DNA of the cell is included in molecular pathology such as in situ hybridisation, PCR etc. These methods are now not only used for research purposes but are also being used as a part of diagnostic pathology reports.

The above divisions of pathology into several subspecialities are quite artificial since overlapping of disciplines is likely, ultimate aim of pathologist being to establish the final diagnosis and learn the causes and mechanisms of disease.

> ### GIST BOX 1.1 — Introduction to Pathology
>
> - Pathology is the study of structural and functional changes in disease.
> - Pathologic changes present with clinical features (symptoms, signs) in the patient.
> - In pathology, we study causes (etiology), mechanisms (pathogenesis) and arrive at final diagnosis by various laboratory methods; gross and microscopic examination of tissues is the major method.
> - The Caduceus representing ancient Greek gods is symbol of medicine.
> - 'Father of medicine' is Hippocrates; 'Father of modern medicine' is Sir William Osler.
> - 'Father of pathology' is Rudolf Virchow; 'Father of CPCs' is Giovanni B. Morgagni; 'Father of museum' is John Hunter; 'Father of clinical pathology' is Paul Ehrlich; 'Father of blood transfusion' is Karl Landsteiner; 'Father of cytology' is George N. Papanicolaou.
> - Morphologic branches of diagnostic pathology are histopathology, cytopathology and haematology.
> - Important ancillary diagnostic techniques in pathology are immunohistochemistry, cytogenetics and molecular methods such as ISH and PCR.

2 Cell Structure and Function, Cellular Ageing

Cells are the basic units of tissues, which form organs and systems in the human body. Traditionally, body cells are divided into two main types: epithelial and mesenchymal cells. In health, the cells remain in accord with each other. In 1859, Virchow first published cellular theory of disease, bringing in the concept that diseases occur due to abnormalities at the cellular level. Since then, study of changes in structure and function of cells in disease has remained the focus of attention in understanding of diseases. But before doing that, a quick overview of basic knowledge of normal structure and functions of cell is considered essential.

NORMAL CELL STRUCTURE AND FUNCTION

Different types of cells of the body possess features which distinguish one type from another. However, most mammalian cells have a basic plan of common structure and function outlined below.

CELL STRUCTURE

Under normal conditions, cells are dynamic structures existing in fluid environment. A cell is enclosed by cell membrane that extends internally to enclose nucleus and various subcellular organelles suspended in cytosol (Fig. 2.1).

Cell Membrane

Electron microscopy has shown that cell membrane or plasma membrane has a trilaminar structure having a total thickness of about 7.5 nm and is known as *unit membrane*. The three layers consist of two electron-dense layers separated by an electron-lucent layer. Biochemically, the cell membrane is composed of complex mixture of phospholipids, glycolipids, cholesterol, proteins and carbohydrates. These layers are in a gel-like arrangement and are in a constant state of flux. The outer surface of some types of cells shows a coat of mucopolysaccharide forming a fuzzy layer called *glycocalyx*. Proteins and glycoproteins of the cell membrane may act as antigens (e.g. blood group antigens), or may form receptors (e.g. for viruses, bacterial products, hormones, immunoglobulins and many enzymes). The cell receptors are related to the cytoskeleton (microtubules and microfilaments) of the underlying cytoplasm.

The cell membrane performs following important functions:

i) Selective permeability that includes diffusion, membrane pump (sodium pump) and pinocytosis (cell drinking).
ii) Bears membrane antigens (e.g. blood group antigens, transplantation antigen).
iii) Possesses cell receptors for cell—cell recognition and communication.

Nucleus

The nucleus consists of an outer nuclear membrane enclosing nuclear chromatin and nucleoli.

NUCLEAR MEMBRANE The nuclear membrane is the outer envelop consisting of 2 layers of the unit membrane which are separated by a 40-70 nm wide space. The outer layer of the nuclear membrane is studded with ribosomes and is continuous with endoplasmic reticulum. The two layers of nuclear membrane at places are fused together forming circular nuclear pores which are about 50 nm in diameter. The nuclear membrane is crossed by several factors which regulate the gene expression and repair the DNA damage soon after it occurs.

NUCLEAR CHROMATIN The main substance of the nucleus is comprised by the nuclear chromatin which is in the form of shorter pieces of thread-like structures called *chromosomes* of which there are 23 pairs (46 chromosomes) together measuring about a metre in length in a human diploid cell. Of these, there are 22 pairs (44 chromosomes) of *autosomes* and one pair of *sex chromosomes,* either XX (female) or XY (male). Each chromosome is composed of two chromatids connected at the centromere to form 'X' configuration having variation in location of the centromere. Depending upon the length of chromosomes and centromeric location, 46 chromosomes are categorised into 7 groups from A to G according to *Denver classification* (adopted at a meeting in Denver, USA).

Chromosomes are composed of 3 components, each with distinctive function. These are: deoxyribonucleic acid (DNA) comprising about 20%, ribonucleic acid (RNA) about 10%, and the remaining 70% consists of nuclear proteins that include a number of basic proteins (histones), neutral proteins, and acid proteins. DNA of the cell is largely contained in the nucleus. The only other place in the cell that contains small amount of DNA is mitochondria. Nuclear DNA along with histone nuclear proteins forms bead-like structures called nucleosomes which are studded along the coils of DNA.

Section I: The Cell in Health and Disease

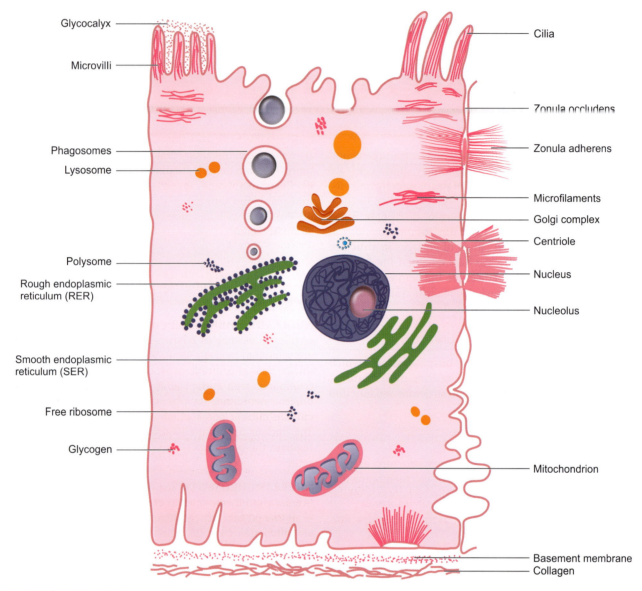

Figure 2.1 ▶ Schematic diagram of the structure of an epithelial cell.

Nuclear DNA carries the genetic information that is passed via messenger RNA into the cytoplasm for manufacture of proteins of similar composition. During cell division, one half of DNA molecule acts as a template for the manufacture of the other half by the enzyme, DNA polymerase, so that the genetic characteristics are transmitted to the next progeny of cells *(replication)*.

The **DNA molecule** as proposed by Watson and Crick in 1953 consists of two complementary polypeptide chains forming a double helical strand which is wound spirally around an axis composed of pentose sugar-phosphoric acid chains. The molecule is spirally twisted in a ladder-like pattern, the steps of which are composed of 4 *nucleotide bases: two purines* (adenine and guanine, i.e. A and G) and *two pyrimidines* (cytosine and thymine, i.e. C and T); however, A pairs specifically with T while G pairs with C **(Fig. 2.2)**. The sequence of these nucleotide base pairs in the chain, determines the information contained in the DNA molecule or constitutes the genetic code.

In the interphase nucleus (i.e. between mitosis), part of the chromatin that remains relatively inert metabolically and appears deeply basophilic due to condensation of chromosomes is called *heterochromatin,* while the part of chromatin that is lightly stained (i.e. vesicular) due to dispersed chromatin is called *euchromatin.* For example, in lymphocytes there is predominance of heterochromatin while the nucleus of a hepatocyte is mostly euchromatin.

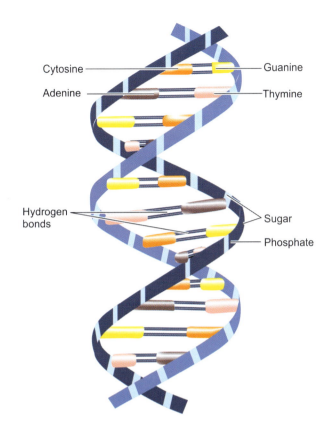

Figure 2.2 ▶ Diagrammatic structure of portion of helical structure of DNA molecule.

NUCLEOLUS The nucleus may contain one or more rounded bodies called nucleoli. Nucleolus is the site of synthesis of ribosomal RNA. Nucleolus is composed of granules and fibrils representing newly synthesised ribosomal RNA.

Cytosol and Organelles

The cytosol or the cytoplasm is the gel-like ground substance in which the organelles (meaning *little organs*) of the cells are suspended. These organelles are the site of major enzymatic activities of the cell which are possibly mediated by enzymes in the cytosol. The major organelles are the cytoskeleton, mitochondria, ribosomes, endoplasmic reticulum, Golgi apparatus, lysosomes, and microbodies or peroxisomes.

CYTOSKELETON Microfilaments, intermediate filaments, and microtubules are responsible for maintaining cellular form and movement and are collectively referred to as cytoskeleton.

i) **Microfilaments** are long filamentous structures having a diameter of 6-8 nm. They are composed of contractile proteins, actin and myosin, and diverse materials like parts of microtubules and ribonucleoprotein fibres. Bundles of microfilaments are especially prominent close to the plasma membrane and form terminal web. Extension of these bundles of microfilaments along with part of plasma membrane on the surface of the cell form microvilli which increase the absorptive surface of secretory cells (e.g. small intestinal mucosa) increasing their surface area.

ii) **Intermediate filaments** are filamentous structures, 10 nm in diameter, and are cytoplasmic constituent of a number of cell types. They are composed of proteins. A few principal types of intermediate filaments are as under:
a) *Cytokeratin* (found in epithelial cells).
b) *Desmin* (found in skeletal, smooth and cardiac muscle).
c) *Vimentin* (found in cells of mesenchymal origin).
d) *Glial fibrillary acidic protein* (present in astrocytes and ependymal cells).
e) *Neurofilaments* (seen in neurons of central and peripheral nervous system).

Their main function is to mechanically integrate the cell organelles within the cytoplasm.

iii) **Microtubules** are long hollow tubular structures about 25 nm in diameter. They are composed of a protein called tubulin. *Cilia* and *flagella* which project from the surface of cell are composed of microtubules enclosed by plasma membrane and are active in locomotion of the cells. *Basal bodies* present at the base of each cilium or flagellum and *centriole* located at the mitotic spindle of cells are the two other morphologically similar structures composed of microtubules.

MITOCHONDRIA Mitochondria are oval structures and are more numerous in metabolically active cells. They are enveloped by two layers of membrane—the outer smooth and the inner folded into incomplete septa or sheaf-like ridges called *cristae*. Chemically and structurally, membranes of mitochondria are similar to cell membrane. The inner membrane, in addition, contains lollipop-shaped globular structures projecting into the matrix present between the layers of membrane. The matrix of the mitochondria contains enzymes required in the Krebs' cycle by which the products of carbohydrate, fat and protein metabolism are oxidised to produce energy which is stored in the form of ATP in the lollipop-like globular structures. In addition, mitochondria also have some DNA and ribosomes. Mitochondria are not static structures but undergo changes in their configuration during energised state by alteration in the matrix and intercristal space; outer membrane is, however, less elastic.

Mitochondria perform following important metabolic function:
a) Oxidative phosphorylation, and in the process generate free radicals injurious to membranes.
b) They also have role in apoptosis.
c) Protein synthesis by mitochondria; they contain 37 genes out of which 13 encode for synthesising proteins.

RIBOSOMES Ribosomes are spherical particles which contain 80-85% of the cell's RNA. They may be present in the cytosol in 'free' unattached form, or in 'bound' form attached to membrane of endoplasmic reticulum. They may lie as 'monomeric units' or as 'polyribosomes' when many monomeric ribosomes are attached to a linear molecule of messenger RNA.

Ribosomes synthesise proteins by translation of messenger RNA into peptide sequences followed by packaging of proteins for the endoplasmic reticulum.

ENDOPLASMIC RETICULUM Endoplasmic reticulum is composed of vesicles and intercommunicating canals. It is composed of unit membrane which is continuous with both nuclear membrane and the Golgi apparatus, and possibly with the cell membrane. The main function of endoplasmic reticulum is the manufacture of protein. Morphologically, there are 2 forms of endoplasmic reticulum: rough (or granular) and smooth (or agranular).

i) *Rough endoplasmic reticulum (RER)* is so-called because its outer surface is rough or granular due to attached ribosomes on it. RER is especially well-developed in cells active in protein synthesis e.g. Russell bodies of plasma cells, Nissl granules of nerve cells.

ii) *Smooth endoplasmic reticulum (SER)* is devoid of ribosomes on its surface. SER and RER are generally continuous with each other. SER contains many enzymes which metabolise drugs, steroids, cholesterol, and carbohydrates and partake in muscle contraction.

GOLGI APPARATUS Golgi apparatus or Golgi complex is generally located close to the nucleus. Morphologically, it appears as vesicles, sacs or lamellae composed of unit membrane and is continuous with the endoplasmic reticulum. The Golgi apparatus is particularly well-developed in exocrine glandular cells.

Its main functions are synthesis of carbohydrates and complex proteins and packaging of proteins synthesised in the RER into vesicles. Some of these vesicles may contain lysosomal enzymes and specific granules such as in neutrophils and in beta cells of the pancreatic islets.

LYSOSOMES Lysosomes are rounded to oval membrane-bound organelles containing powerful lysosomal digestive (hydrolytic) enzymes. There are 3 forms of lysosomes:

i) *Primary lysosomes or storage vacuoles* are formed from the various hydrolytic enzymes synthesised by the RER and packaged in the Golgi apparatus.

ii) *Secondary lysosomes or autophagic vacuoles* are formed by fusion of primary lysosomes with the parts of damaged or worn-out cell components.

iii) *Residual bodies* are indigestible materials in the lysosomes e.g. lipofuscin.

CENTRIOLE OR CENTROSOME Each cell contains a pair of centrioles in the cytoplasm close to nucleus in the area called centrosome. Centrioles are cylindrical structures composed of electron-dense evenly-shaped microtubules.

They perform the function of formation of cilia and flagellae and constitute the mitotic spindle of fibrillary protein during mitosis.

| GIST BOX 2.1 | Normal Cell Structure and Function |

- ❖ A cell is enclosed by cell membrane that extends internally to enclose nucleus and various subcellular organelles suspended in cytosol.
- ❖ Cell membrane or plasma membrane has a trilaminar structure having selective permeability and bearing surface antigens.
- ❖ Nucleus consists of an outer nuclear membrane enclosing nuclear chromatin and nucleoli. Most of the DNA of the cell is contained in the nucleus.
- ❖ Cytosol has various suspended cell organelles. These are:
  - Cytoskeleton (microfilaments, intermediate filaments, and microtubules) responsible for maintaining cellular form and movement.
  - Mitochondria contain enzymes for cell metabolism and produce energy which is stored as ATP.
  - Ribosomes contain RNA and may be 'free' or as 'bound' form.
  - Endoplasmic reticulum may be 'rough' (granular) due to attached ribosomes, or 'smooth' devoid of ribosomes and instead has enzymes for metabolism.
  - Golgi apparatus has function of synthesis and storage of carbohydrates and proteins.
  - Lysosomes have hydrolytic enzymes.

INTERCELLULAR COMMUNICATIONS

All cells in the body constantly exchange information with each other to perform their functions properly. This process is accomplished in the cells by direct cell-to-cell contact (*intercellular junctions*), and by chemical agents, also called as molecular agents or factors (*molecular interactions between cells*) as under.

INTERCELLULAR JUNCTIONS

Plasma membranes of epithelial and endothelial cells, though closely apposed physically, are separated from each other by 20 nm wide space. These cells communicate across this space through intercellular junctions or junctional complexes visible under electron microscope and are of 4 types **(Fig. 2.3)**:

1. Occluding junctions (Zonula occludens) These are tight junctions situated just below the luminal margin of adjacent cells. As a result, the regions of occluding zones are impermeable to macromolecules. The examples of occluding zones are seen in renal tubular epithelial cells, intestinal epithelium, and vascular endothelium in the brain constituting blood-brain barrier.

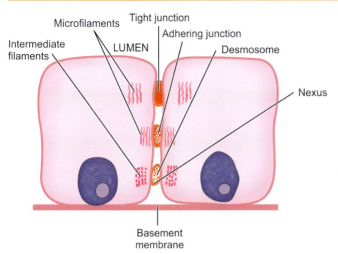

Figure 2.3 ▶ Diagrammatic representation of the intercellular junctions.

2. Adhering junctions (Zonula adherens) These are located just below the occluding zones between the adjacent cells and are permeable to tracer particles. These zones are in contact with actin microfilaments e.g. in small cell carcinoma of the lung.

3. Desmosomes (Macula densa) These are tiny adhesion plates present focally between the adjacent epithelial cells, especially numerous in the epidermis. Bundles of intermediate filaments (termed tonofilaments in the case of epidermis) project from the intercellular desmosomes and radiate into the cytoplasm. Hemidesmosomes are a variant of desmosomes, occurring at the basal region of epithelial cells between plasma membrane and the basement membrane.

4. Gap junctions (Nexus) Gap junctions or nexus are the regions on the lateral surfaces of epithelial cells where the gap between the adjoining plasma membranes is reduced from 20 nm to about 2 nm in width. Pits or holes are present in the regions of gap junctions so that these regions are permeable to small tracer particles.

MOLECULAR INTERACTIONS BETWEEN CELLS

Besides having intercellular junctions, most cells communicate at molecular level by the following:
1. Cell adhesion molecules (CAMs)
2. Cytokines
3. Membrane receptors

CELL ADHESION MOLECULES (CAMs) These are chemicals which mediate the interaction between cells (cell-cell interaction) as well as between cells and extracellular matrix (cell-ECM interaction). The *ECM* is the ground substance or matrix of connective tissue which provides environment to the cells and consists of 3 components:
i) fibrillar structural proteins (collagen, elastin);
ii) adhesion proteins (fibronectin, laminin, fibrillin, osteonectin, tenacin); and
iii) molecules of proteoglycans and glycosaminoglycans (heparan sulphate, chondroitin sulphate, dermatan sulphate, keratan sulphate, hyaluronic acid).

CAMs participate in fertilisation, embryogenesis, tissue repair, haemostasis, cell death by apoptosis and in inflammation. CAMs may be detected on the surface of cells as well as free in circulation. There are 5 groups of CAMs:

i) Integrins They have alpha (or CD11*) and beta (CD18) subunits and have a role in cell-ECM interactions and in leucocyte-endothelial cell interaction.

ii) Cadherins These are calcium-dependent adhesion molecules which bind adjacent cells together and prevent invasion of ECM by cancer cells. Various types of cadherins include: E-cadherin (epithelial cell), N-cadherin (nerve cell), M-cadherin (muscle cell), and P-cadherin (placenta).

iii) Selectins Also called as lectins, these CAMs contain lectins or lectin-like protein molecules which bind to glycoproteins and glycolipids on the cell surface. Their major role is in movement of leucocytes and platelets and develop contact with endothelial cells. Selectins are of 3 types: *P-selectin* (from platelets, also called CD62), *E-selectin* (from endothelial cells, also named ECAM), and *L-selectin* (from leucocytes, also called LCAM).

iv) Immunoglobulin superfamily This group consists of a variety of immunoglobulin molecules present on most cells of the body. These partake in cell-to-cell contact through various other CAMs and cytokines. They have a major role in recognition and binding of immunocompetent cells. This group includes ICAM-1,2 (intercellular adhesion molecule, also called CD54), VCAM (vascular cell adhesion molecule, also named CD106), NCAM (neural cell adhesion molecule).

v) CD44 The last group of adhesion molecules is a break away from immunoglobulin superfamily. CD44 molecule binds to hyaluronic acid and is expressed on leucocytes. It is involved in leucocyte-endothelial interactions as well as in cell-ECM interactions.

CYTOKINES Another way the cells may communicate with each other is by release of peptides and other molecules acting as paracrine function. Cytokines are soluble proteins secreted by haemopoietic and non-haemopoietic cells in response to various stimuli. Their main role is in activation of immune system. Presently, about 200 cytokines have been identified which are grouped in 6 categories:
i)   Interferons (IFN)
ii) Interleukins (IL)
iii) Tumour necrosis factor group (TNF, cachectin)

---

*CD number (for Cluster of Differentiation) is the nomenclature given to the clone of cells which carry these molecules on their cell surface or in their cytoplasm.

iv) Transforming growth factor (TGF)
v) Colony stimulating factor (CSF)
vi) Growth factors (e.g. platelet-derived growth factor–PDGF, epidermal growth factor–EGF, fibroblast growth factor–FGF, endothelial-derived growth factor–EDGF, transforming growth factor–TGF).

Many of these cytokines have further subtypes as alpha, beta, or are identified by numbers. Cytokines involved in leucocyte-endothelial cell interaction are called *chemokines* while growth factors and other cytokines are named *crinopectins*.

CELL MEMBRANE RECEPTORS Cell receptors are molecules consisting of proteins, glycoproteins or lipoproteins and may be located on the outer cell membrane, inside the cell, or may be trans-membranous. These receptor molecules are synthesised by the cell itself depending upon their requirement, and thus there may be upregulation or downregulation of number of receptors. There are 3 main types of receptors:

i) Enzyme-linked receptors These receptors are involved in control of cell growth e.g. tyrosine kinase associated receptors take part in activation of synthesis and secretion of various hormones.

ii) Ion channels The activated receptor for ion exchange such as for sodium, potassium and calcium and certain peptide hormones, determines inward or outward movement of these molecules.

iii) G-protein receptors These are trans-membranous receptors and activate phosphorylating enzymes for metabolic and synthetic functions of cells. The activation of adenosine monophosphate-phosphatase (AMP) by the G-proteins (guanosine nucleotide binding regulatory proteins) is the most important signal system, also known as 'second messenger' activation. The activated second messenger (cyclic-AMP) then regulates other intracellular activities.

STRESS PROTEINS
(HEAT SHOCK PROTEINS AND UBIQUITIN)

When cells are exposed to stress of any type, a protective response by the cell is by release of proteins that move molecules within the cell cytoplasm. There are two types of stress-related proteins: *heat shock proteins (HSP)* and *ubiquitin* (so named due to its universal presence in the cells of the body).

HSPs These are a variety of intracellular carrier proteins present in most cells of the body, especially in renal tubular epithelial cells. They normally perform the role of *chaperones* (house-keeping) i.e. they direct and guide metabolic molecules to the sites of metabolic activity e.g. protein folding, disaggregation of protein-protein complexes and transport of proteins into various intracellular organelles (*protein kinesis*). However, in response to stresses of various types (e.g. toxins, drugs, poisons, ischaemia), their level goes up both inside the cell and their leakage out into the plasma, and hence the name stress proteins.

In experimental studies, HSPs have been shown to limit tissue necrosis in ischaemic reperfusion injury in myocardial infarcts. In addition, they have also been shown to have a central role in protein aggregation in amyloidosis.

Ubiquitin This is another related stress protein which has ubiquitous presence in human body cells. Like HSPs, ubiquitin too directs intracellular molecules for either degradation or for synthesis. Ubiquitin has been found to be involved in a variety of human degenerative diseases, especially in the nervous system in ageing e.g. activation of genes for protein synthesis in neurodegenerative diseases such as in Alzheimer's disease, Creutzfeldt-Jakob disease, Parkinson's disease.

| GIST BOX 2.2 | Intercellular Communications |

- Intercellular junctions are the sites of direct cell-to-cell contact. These are occluding junctions, adhering junctions, desmosomes, and gap junctions.
- Molecular interactions between cells takes place by cell adhesion molecules (namely integrins, cadherins, selectins, immunoglobulin superfamily, CD34) various cytokines and membrane receptors.
- Stress proteins (heat shock proteins and ubiquitins) are intracellular proteins released as a form of protective response to environmental stresses and carry molecules within the cell cytoplasm.

CELL CYCLE

Multiplication of the somatic (mitosis) and germ (meiosis) cells is the most complex of all cell functions. Period between the mitosis is called *interphase*. The *cell cycle* is the phase between two consecutive divisions **(Fig. 2.4)**. There are 4 sequential phases in the cell cycle: G1 (gap 1) phase, S (synthesis) phase, G2 (gap 2) phase, and M (mitotic) phase.

G1 (Pre-mitotic gap) phase is the stage when messenger RNAs for the proteins and the proteins themselves required for DNA synthesis (e.g. DNA polymerase) are synthesised. The process is under control of cyclin E and CDKs.

S phase involves replication of nuclear DNA. Cyclin A and CDKs control it.

G2 (Pre-mitotic gap) phase is the short gap phase in which correctness of DNA synthesised is assessed. This stage is promoted by cyclin B and CDKs.

M phase is the stage in which process of mitosis to form two daughter cells is completed. This occurs in 4 sequential stages: *prophase, metaphase, anaphase,* and *telophase* (acronym= PMAT).

- *Prophase* Each chromosome divides into 2 chromatids which are held together by centromere. The centriole divides and the two daughter centrioles move towards

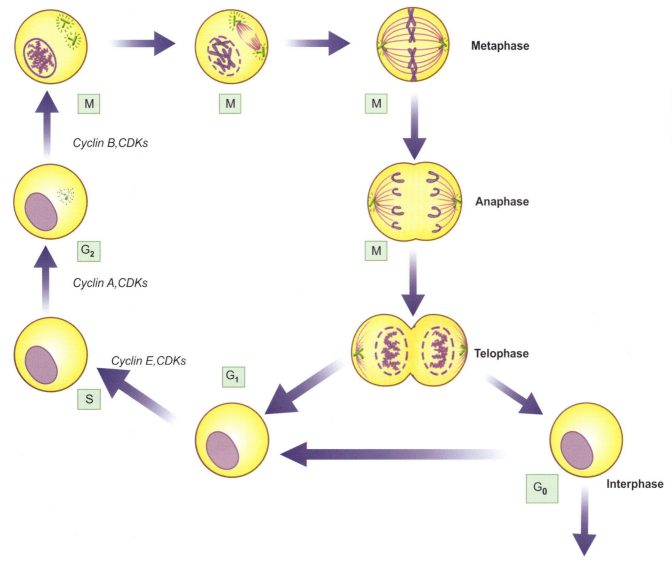

Figure 2.4 ▶ The cell cycle in mitosis. Premitotic phases are the G_1, S and G_2 phase while M (mitotic) phase is accomplished in 4 sequential stages: prophase, metaphase, anaphase, and telophase. On completion of cell division, two daughter cells are formed which may continue to remain in the cell cycle or go out of it in resting phase (interphase), the G_0 phase. Two checkpoints for DNA damage are G_1-S and G_2-M phase. (CDK = *cyclin dependent kinase*).

opposite poles of the nucleus and the nuclear membrane disintegrates.
- *Metaphase* The microtubules become arranged between the two centrioles forming spindle, while the chromosomes line up at the equatorial plate of the spindle.
- *Anaphase* The centromeres divide and each set of separated chromosomes moves towards the opposite poles of the spindle. Cell membrane also begins to divide.
- *Telophase* There is formation of nuclear membrane around each set of chromosomes and reconstitution of the nucleus. The cytoplasm of the two daughter cells completely separates.

G0 phase is the phase when the daughter cells rather than continuing to remain in the cell cycle and divide further, instead goes out of the cell cycle into resting phase.

Mitosis is controlled by genes which encode for release of specific proteins molecules that promote or inhibit the process of mitosis at different steps. Mitosis-promoting protein molecules are *cyclins* which are over 15 types. However, cyclin D, E, A and B appear in sequence, and each of them take up the function from preceding one. These cyclins bind to *cyclin-dependent kinases (CDKs)* which are enzymes forming complexes with cyclins. After the mitosis is complete, cyclins and CDKs are degraded and the residues of used molecules are taken up by cytoplasmic caretaker proteins, *ubiquitin*, to the peroxisome for further degradation.

Inbuilt into the cell cycle are certain 'checkpoints' which check DNA for any defects or damage before the cell proceeds to DNA replication. These checkpoints are G1-S and G2-M checkpoint gaps. During these gaps at checkpoints, CDK-inhibitors (CDKI) alter the cyclin-CDK complex activity as per requirement. Depending upon the extent of DNA damage, cell replication is either delayed allowing the damaged DNA to be repaired by intrinsic mechanisms, or the cell is directed to apoptosis when the DNA is irreparably damaged.

| GIST BOX 2.3 | Cell Cycle |

- Cell cycle is the phase between two consecutive divisions and as 4 sequential phases: G1 (gap 1) phase, S (synthesis) phase, G2 (gap 2) phase, and M (mitotic) phase.
- M phase results into two daughter cells and occurs in 4 sequential stages: prophase, metaphase, anaphase, and telophase (acronym= PMAT).
- Mitosis is controlled by genes; promoter genes are cyclins (D, E, A, B in sequence), which are activated by CDKs, while CDK-inhibitors alter the cyclin-CDK activity depending upon the report of checkpoints at G1-S and G2-M phase.

CELLULAR AGEING

Old age is a concept of longevity in human beings. The consequences of ageing appear after reproductive life when evolutionary role of the individual has been accomplished. However, ageing is distinct from mortality and disease although aged individuals are more vulnerable to disease. With ageing, the mechanism of homeostasis is slow; hence the response to various stresses takes longer to revert back to normal structure and function.

The average age of death of primitive man was barely 20-25 years. However, currently average life-expectancy in the West is about 80 years. In India, due to improved health care, it has gone up from an average of 26 years at the time of independence in 1947 to 64 years at present. In general, survival is longer in women than men (3: 2). About a century ago, the main causes of death were accidents and infections. But now with greater safety and sanitation, the mortality in the middle years has sufficiently declined. However, the maximum human lifespan has remained stable at about 110 years. Higher life expectancy in women is not due to difference in the response of somatic cells of the two sexes but higher mortality rate in men is attributed to violent causes and greater susceptibility to cardiovascular disease, cancer, cirrhosis and respiratory diseases, for which cigarette smoking and alcohol consumption are two most important contributory factors.

In general, the life expectancy of an individual depends upon the following factors:

1. *Intrinsic genetic process* i.e. the genes controlling response to endogenous and exogenous factors initiating apoptosis in senility. It has been seen that long life runs in families and high concordance in lifespan of identical twins has been observed. Studies in centenarians have shown that they lack carrier of apolipoprotein E4 allele which is associated with risk for both heart disease and Alzheimer's disease.

2. *Environmental factors* e.g. consumption and inhalation of harmful substances, type of diet, role of antioxidants etc.

3. *Lifestyle of the individual* such as diseases due to alcoholism (e.g. cirrhosis, hepatocellular carcinoma), smoking (e.g. bronchogenic carcinoma and other respiratory diseases), drug addiction.

4. *Age-related diseases* e.g. atherosclerosis and ischaemic heart disease, diabetes mellitus, hypertension, osteoporosis, Alzheimer's disease, Parkinson's disease etc.

THEORIES OF AGEING

With age, structural and functional changes occur in different organs and systems of the human body. Although no definitive biologic basis of ageing is established, most acceptable theory is the functional decline of non-dividing cells such as neurons and myocytes. The following hypotheses based on investigations mostly in other species explain the cellular basis of ageing:

1. **Experimental cellular senescence** By *in vitro* studies of tissue culture, it has been observed that cultured human fibroblasts replicate for up to 50 population doublings and then the culture dies out. It means that *in vitro* there is reduced functional capacity to proliferate with age. Studies have shown that there is either loss of chromosome 1 or deletion of its long arm (1q). It has also been observed that with every cell division there is progressive shortening of *telomere* present at the tips of chromosomes, which in normal cell is repaired by the presence of RNA enzyme, *telomerase*. However, due to ageing there is inadequate presence of telomerase enzyme; therefore lost telomere is not repaired resulting in interference in viability of cell **(Fig. 2.5)**.

2. **Genetic control in invertebrates** Clock *(clk)* genes responsible for controlling the rate and time of ageing have been identified in lower invertebrates e.g. *clk-1* gene mutation in the metazoa, *Caenorhabditis elegans*, results in prolonging the lifespan of the worm and slowing of some metabolic functions.

3. **Diseases of accelerated ageing** A heritable condition associated with signs of accelerated ageing process, *progeria*, seen in children is characterised by baldness, cataracts, and coronary artery disease. Another example is Werner's syndrome, a rare autosomal recessive disease, characterised by similar features of premature ageing, atherosclerosis and risk for development of various cancers.

Chapter 2: Cell Structure and Function, Cellular Ageing

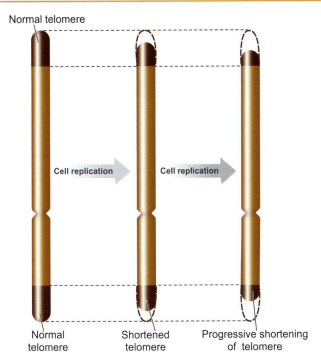

Figure 2.5 ▶ Telomeres on chromosomes. In ageing, the end components of chromosome are progressively shortened.

4. Oxidative stress hypothesis (Free radical-mediated injury) Ageing is partly caused by progressive and reversible molecular oxidative damage due to persistent oxidative stress on the human cells. In normal cells, very small amount (3%) of total oxygen consumption by the cell is converted into reactive oxygen species. The rate of generation of reactive oxygen species is directly correlated with metabolic rate of the organisms. With ageing, there is low metabolic rate with generation of toxic oxygen radicals, which fail to get eliminated causing their accumulation and hence cell damage due to mitochondrial injury. The role of antioxidants in retarding the oxidant damage has been reported in some studies.

5. Hormonal decline With age, there is loss of secretion of some hormones resulting in their functional decline.

6. Defective host defenses Ageing causes impaired immune function and hence reduced ability to respond to microbes and environmental agents.

7. Failure to renew Ageing causes accumulation of senescent cells without corresponding renewal of lost cells.

ORGAN CHANGES IN AGEING

Although all organs start showing deterioration with ageing, following organs show evident morphologic and functional decline:

1. *Cardiovascular system:* Atherosclerosis, arteriosclerosis with calcification, Mönckeberg's medial calcification, brown atrophy of the heart, loss of elastic tissue from aorta and major arterial trunks causing their dilatation.

2. *Nervous system:* Atrophy of gyri and sulci, Alzheimer's disease, Parkinson's disease.

3. *Musculoskeletal system*: Degenerative bone diseases, frequent fractures due to loss of bone density, age-related muscular degeneration.

4. *Eyes:* Deterioration of vision due to cataract and vascular changes in retina.

5. *Hearing:* Disability in hearing due to senility is related to otosclerosis.

6. *Immune system:* Reduced IgG response to antigens, frequent and more severe infections.

7. *Skin:* Laxity of skin due to loss of elastic tissue.

8. *Cancers:* As discussed later in Chapter 19, 80% of cancers occur in the age range of 50-80 years.

 GIST BOX 2.4 | **Cellular Ageing**

- Life expectancy of an individual depends upon certain factors: genetic, environmental, life style and some age-related diseases.
- There are several hypothesis of ageing. These are: shortening of telomere without replacement of damaged ends, persistent oxidative stress (accumulation of free radicals), hormonal decline, defective host defenses and failure to renew old cells.
- Ageing causes decline in morphology and function of multiple organs: cardiovascular system, nervous system, muscles, bones, eyes, ears, immune system and skin. About 80% of cancers are seen in the age range of 50-80 years.

3 Cellular Adaptations

The concept of cellular basis of disease propagated first by Virchow means that most forms of diseases begin with cell injury followed by consequent loss of cellular function. However, when body cells are exposed to injurious agents, they have inbuilt mechanism to deal with changes in environment to an extent without undergoing cellular injury. The cellular response to stress may, therefore, vary depending upon following two types of factors:

i) Host factors i.e. the type of cell and tissue involved.
ii) Factors pertaining to injurious agent i.e. extent and type of cell injury.

Accordingly, various forms of cellular responses to injurious agents may be as follows *(Fig. 3.1)*:

1. When there is altered functional demand (increased or decreased), the cell may adapt to the changes which are expressed morphologically, which then revert back to normal after the stress is removed; these are termed *cellular adaptations*.
2. When the stress is mild to moderate, the injured cell may recover *(reversible cell injury)*, while persistent and severe form of cell injury may cause cell death *(irreversible cell injury)*.
3. The residual effects of reversible cell injury may persist in the cell as evidence of cell injury at subcellular level *(subcellular changes)*, or metabolites may accumulate within the cell *(intracellular accumulations)*.

Cellular adaptations are, thus, the adjustments which the cells make in response to stresses which may be for physiologic needs *(physiologic adaptation)* or a response to non-lethal pathologic injury *(pathologic adaptation)*.

Broadly speaking, such physiologic and pathologic adaptations occur by following processes **(Fig. 3.2)**:

◆ Decreasing or increasing their size i.e. *atrophy* and *hypertrophy* respectively, or by increasing their number i.e. *hyperplasia* (postfix word *-trophy* means nourishment).
◆ Changing the pathway of phenotypic differentiation of cells i.e. *metaplasia* and *dysplasia* (postfix word *-plasia* means growth of new cells; prefix word *meta-* means transformation; *dys-* means bad development).

In general, adaptive responses are reversible on withdrawal of stimulus. However, if the irritant stimulus persists for long time, the cells may not be able to survive and may either die or progress further e.g. cell death may occur in sustained atrophy; dysplasia may progress into carcinoma *in situ*. Thus, the concept of evolution 'survival of the fittest' holds true for adaptation as *'survival of the adaptable'*.

Various mechanisms which may be involved in adaptive cellular responses include the following:
1. Altered cell surface receptor binding.
2. Alterations in signal for protein synthesis.
3. Synthesis of new proteins by the target cell such as heat-shock proteins (HSPs).

Common forms of cellular adaptive responses along with examples of physiologic and pathologic adaptations are briefly discussed here.

ATROPHY

Reduction of the number and size of parenchymal cells of an organ or its parts which was once normal is called atrophy

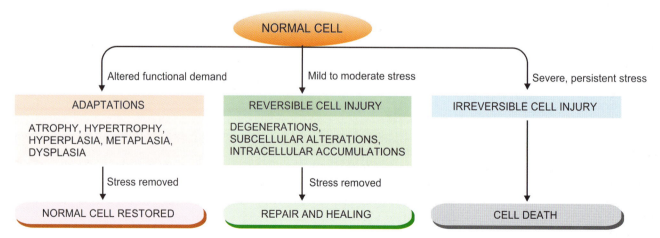

Figure 3.1 ▶ Cellular responses to cell injury.

Chapter 3: Cellular Adaptations

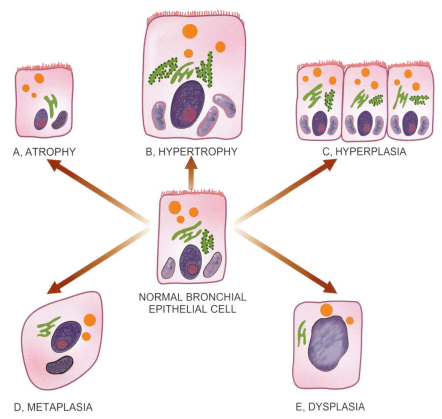

Figure 3.2 ▶ Adaptive disorders of growth.

(compared from *hypoplasia* which is the term used for developmentally small size, and *aplasia* for extreme failure of development leaving only rudimentary tissue).

CAUSES Atrophy may occur from physiologic or pathologic causes:

A. Physiologic atrophy Atrophy is a normal process of ageing in some tissues, which could be due to loss of endocrine stimulation or arteriosclerosis. For example:
i) Atrophy of lymphoid tissue with age.
ii) Atrophy of thymus in adult life.
iii) Atrophy of gonads after menopause.
iv) Atrophy of brain with ageing.
v) Osteoporosis with reduction in size of bony trabeculae due to ageing.

B. Pathologic atrophy It includes following causes:

1. *Starvation atrophy* In starvation, there is first depletion of carbohydrate and fat stores followed by protein catabolism. There is general weakness, emaciation and anaemia referred to as cachexia seen in cancer and in severely ill patients.

2. *Ischaemic atrophy* Gradual diminution of blood supply due to atherosclerosis may result in shrinkage of the affected organ e.g.

i) Small atrophic kidney in atherosclerosis of renal artery.
ii) Atrophy of the brain in cerebral atherosclerosis.

3. *Disuse atrophy* Prolonged diminished functional activity is associated with disuse atrophy of the organ e.g.
i) Wasting of muscles of limb immobilised in cast.
ii) Myopathies
iii) Atrophy of the pancreas in obstruction of pancreatic duct.
iv) Senile testicular atrophy **(Fig. 3.3)**.

4. *Neuropathic atrophy* Interruption in nerve supply leads to wasting of muscles e.g.
i) Poliomyelitis
ii) Motor neuron disease
iii) Nerve section

5. *Endocrine atrophy* Loss of endocrine regulatory mechanism results in reduced metabolic activity of tissues and hence atrophy e.g.
i) Hypopituitarism may lead to atrophy of thyroid, adrenal and gonads.
ii) Hypothyroidism may cause atrophy of the skin and its adnexal structures.

6. *Pressure atrophy* Prolonged pressure from benign tumours or cyst or aneurysm may cause compression and atrophy of the tissues e.g.

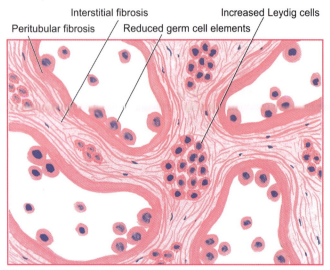
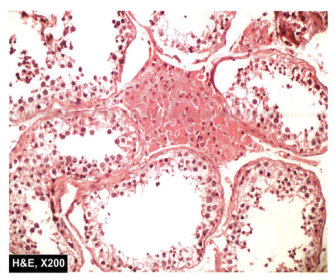

Figure 3.3 ▶ Microscopic appearance of senile testicular atrophy.

i) Erosion of the spine by tumour in nerve root.
ii) Erosion of the skull by meningioma arising from pia-arachnoid.
iii) Erosion of the sternum by aneurysm of arch of aorta.

> ***MORPHOLOGIC FEATURES*** Irrespective of the underlying cause for atrophy, the pathologic changes are similar. The organ is small, often shrunken. The cells become smaller in size but are not dead cells. Shrinkage in cell size is due to reduction in cell organelles, chiefly mitochondria, myofilaments and endoplasmic reticulum. There is often increase in the number of autophagic vacuoles containing cell debris. These autophagic vacuoles may persist to form 'residual bodies' in the cell cytoplasm e.g. lipofuscin pigment granules in brown atrophy.

HYPERTROPHY

Hypertrophy is an increase in the size of parenchymal cells resulting in enlargement of the organ or tissue, without any change in the number of cells.

CAUSES Hypertrophy may be physiologic or pathologic. In either case, it is caused by increased functional demand or by hormonal stimulation. Hypertrophy without accompanying hyperplasia affects mainly muscles. In non-dividing cells too, only hypertrophy occurs.

A. Physiologic hypertrophy Enlarged size of the uterus in pregnancy is an example of physiologic hypertrophy as well as hyperplasia of myometrium.

B. Pathologic hypertrophy Examples of certain diseases associated with hypertrophy are as under:

1. *Hypertrophy of cardiac muscle* may occur in a number of cardiovascular diseases. A few conditions producing left ventricular hypertrophy are as under:
i) Systemic hypertension
ii) Aortic valve disease (stenosis and insufficiency)
iii) Mitral insufficiency

2. *Hypertrophy of smooth muscle* e.g.
i) Cardiac achalasia (in oesophagus)
ii) Pyloric stenosis (in stomach)
iii) Intestinal strictures
iv) Muscular arteries in hypertension.

3. *Hypertrophy of skeletal muscle* e.g. hypertrophied muscles in athletes and manual labourers.

4. *Compensatory hypertrophy* may occur in an organ when the contralateral organ is removed e.g.
i) Following nephrectomy on one side in a young patient, there is compensatory hypertrophy as well as hyperplasia of the nephrons of the other kidney.
ii) Adrenal hyperplasia following removal of one adrenal gland.

> ***MORPHOLOGIC FEATURES*** Affected organ is enlarged and heavy. For example, a hypertrophied heart of a patient with systemic hypertension may weigh as high as 700-800 g as compared to average normal adult weight of 350 g **(Fig. 3.4)**. There is enlargement of muscle fibres as well as of nuclei. At ultrastructural level, there is increased synthesis of DNA and RNA, increased protein synthesis and increased number of organelles such as mitochondria, endoplasmic reticulum and myofibrils **(Fig. 3.5)**.

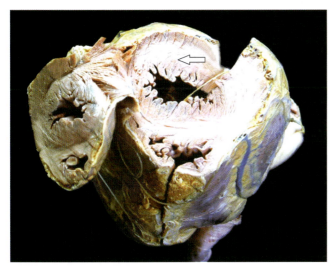

Figure 3.4 ▶ Cardiac hypertrophy. Weight of the heart is increased. The chambers opened up at the apex show concentric thickening of left ventricular wall (white arrow) with obliterated lumen (hypertrophy without dilatation).

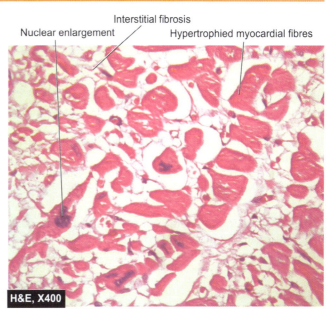

Figure 3.5 ▶ Cardiac hypertrophy. The myocardial fibres are thick with abundance of eosinophilic cytoplasm. Nuclei are also enlarged with irregular outlines.

HYPERPLASIA

Hyperplasia is an increase in the number of parenchymal cells resulting in enlargement of the organ or tissue. Quite often, both hyperplasia and hypertrophy occur together. Hyperplasia occurs due to increased recruitment of cells from G0 (resting) phase of the cell cycle to undergo mitosis, when stimulated. All body cells do not possess hyperplastic growth potential. Labile cells (e.g. epithelial cells of the skin and mucous membranes, cells of the bone marrow and lymph nodes) and stable cells (e.g. parenchymal cells of the liver, pancreas, kidney, adrenal, and thyroid) can undergo hyperplasia, while permanent cells (e.g. neurons, cardiac and skeletal muscle) have little or no capacity for regenerative hyperplastic growth (page 155). Neoplasia differs from hyperplasia in having hyperplastic growth with loss of growth-regulatory mechanism due to change in genetic composition of the cell, while hyperplasia persists so long as stimulus is present.

CAUSES Hyperplasia may also be physiologic and pathologic.

A. Physiologic hyperplasia Two most common types are hormonal and compensatory:

1. *Hormonal hyperplasia* i.e. hyperplasia occurring under the influence of hormonal stimulation e.g.
i)   Hyperplasia of female breast at puberty, during pregnancy and lactation.
ii) Hyperplasia (as well as hypertrophy) of myometrium in pregnancy.
iii) Proliferative activity of normal endometrium after a normal menstrual cycle.
iv) Prostatic hyperplasia in old age (Fig. 3.6).

2. *Compensatory hyperplasia* i.e. hyperplasia occurring following removal of part of an organ or in the contralateral organ in paired organ e.g.
i)   Regeneration of the liver following partial hepatectomy.
ii) Regeneration of epidermis after skin abrasion.
iii) Following nephrectomy on one side, there is hyperplasia (as well as hypertrophy) of nephrons of the other kidney.

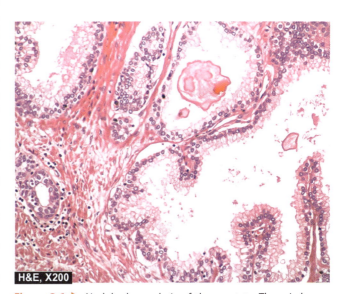

Figure 3.6 ▶ Nodular hyperplasia of the prostate. There is hyperplasia of both fibromuscular elements and epithelium seen as areas of intra-acinar papillary infoldings (convolutions) lined by two layers of epithelium with basal polarity of nuclei.

B. Pathologic hyperplasia Most examples of pathologic hyperplasia are due to excessive stimulation of hormones or growth factors e.g.
i) Endometrial hyperplasia following oestrogen excess.
ii) In wound healing, there is formation of granulation tissue due to proliferation of fibroblasts and endothelial cells.
iii) Formation of skin warts from hyperplasia of epidermis due to human papilloma virus.
iv) Pseudocarcinomatous hyperplasia of the skin occurring at the margin of a non-healing ulcer.
v) Intraductal epithelial hyperplasia in fibrocystic change in the breast.

> *MORPHOLOGIC FEATURES* There is enlargement of the affected organ or tissue and increase in the number of cells. This is due to increased rate of DNA synthesis and hence increased mitoses of the cells.

METAPLASIA

Metaplasia is defined as a reversible change of one type of epithelial or mesenchymal adult cells to another type of adult epithelial or mesenchymal cells, usually in response to abnormal stimuli, and often *reverts back to normal on removal of stimulus*. However, if the stimulus persists for a long time, epithelial metaplasia may progress to dysplasia and further into cancer (Fig. 3.7).

Metaplasia is broadly divided into 2 types: epithelial and mesenchymal.

A. EPITHELIAL METAPLASIA It is the more common than mesenchymal metaplasia. The metaplastic change may be patchy or diffuse and usually results in replacement by stronger but less well-specialised epithelium. However, the metaplastic epithelium, being less well-specialised such as squamous type, results in deprivation of protective mucus secretion and hence more prone to infection. Depending upon the type of epithelium transformed, two types of epithelial metaplasia are seen: squamous and columnar.

1. Squamous metaplasia This is more common. Various types of specialised epithelia are capable of undergoing squamous metaplastic change due to chronic irritation that may be initiated by mechanical, chemical or infective causes. Some common examples of squamous metaplasia are seen at following sites:
i) In *bronchus* (normally lined by pseudostratified columnar ciliated epithelium), in chronic smokers.
ii) In *uterine endocervix* (normally lined by simple columnar epithelium), in prolapse of the uterus and in old age (Fig. 3.8).
iii) In *gallbladder* (normally lined by simple columnar epithelium), in chronic cholecystitis with cholelithiasis.
iv) In *prostate* (ducts normally lined by simple columnar epithelium), in chronic prostatitis and oestrogen therapy.
v) In *renal pelvis* and *urinary bladder* (normally lined by transitional epithelium), in chronic infection and stones.
vi) In *vitamin A deficiency*, apart from xerophthalmia, there is squamous metaplasia in the nose, bronchi, urinary tract, lacrimal and salivary glands.

2. Columnar metaplasia A few examples having transformation to columnar epithelium are as under:
i) Intestinal metaplasia in healed chronic gastric ulcer.
ii) Columnar metaplasia in Barrett's oesophagus, in which there is change of normal squamous epithelium to columnar epithelium (Fig. 3.9).
iii) Transformation of pseudostratified ciliated columnar epithelium in chronic bronchitis and bronchiectasis to columnar type.

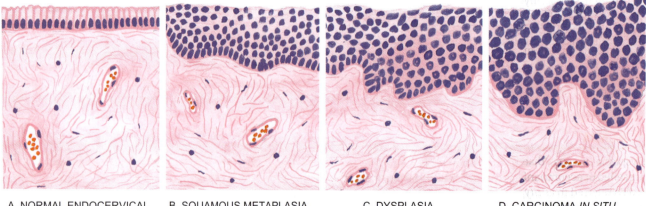

A, NORMAL ENDOCERVICAL EPITHELIUM B, SQUAMOUS METAPLASIA C, DYSPLASIA D, CARCINOMA *IN SITU*

Figure 3.7 ▶ Schematic diagram showing sequential changes in uterine cervix from normal epithelium to development of carcinoma *in situ*. A, Normal mucus-secreting endocervical epithelium. B, Squamous metaplasia. C, Dysplastic change. D, Carcinoma *in situ*.

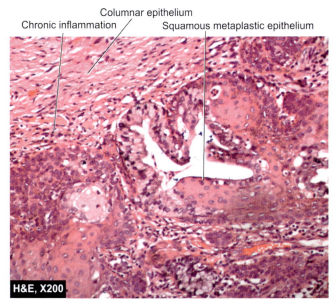

Figure 3.8 ▶ Squamous metaplasia of the uterine cervix. Part of the endocervical mucosa is lined by normal columnar epithelium while foci of metaplastic squamous epithelium are seen at other places.

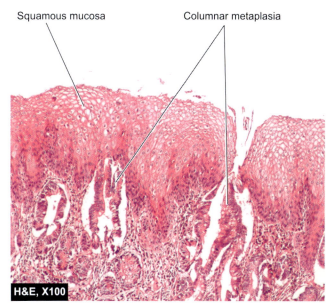

Figure 3.9 ▶ Columnar metaplasia oesophagus (Barrett's oesophagus). Part of the oesophagus which is normally lined by squamous epithelium undergoes metaplastic change to columnar epithelium of intestinal type.

iv) In cervical erosion (congenital and adult type), variable area of endocervical glandular mucosa everted into the vagina.

B. MESENCHYMAL METAPLASIA Less often, there is transformation of one adult type of mesenchymal tissue to another. Some examples are as under:

1. Osseous metaplasia Osseous metaplasia is formation of bone in fibrous tissue, cartilage and myxoid tissue e.g.
i) In arterial wall in old age (Mönckeberg's medial calcific sclerosis)
ii) In soft tissues in myositis ossificans
iii) In cartilage of larynx and bronchi in elderly people
iv) In scar of chronic inflammation of prolonged duration
v) In the fibrous stroma of tumour e.g. in leiomyoma.

2. Cartilaginous metaplasia In healing of fractures, rarely cartilaginous metaplasia may occur where there is undue mobility.

DYSPLASIA

Dysplasia means 'disordered cellular development', often preceded or accompanied with metaplasia and hyperplasia; it is also referred to as *atypical hyperplasia*. The term 'dysplasia' has been commonly used for atypical cytologic changes in the layers of squamous epithelium, the changes being progressive. The two most common examples of dysplastic changes are the *uterine cervix* and *respiratory tract*.

Dysplastic changes often occur due to chronic irritation or prolonged inflammation. On removal of the inciting stimulus, the changes may disappear. In a proportion of cases, however, dysplasia may progress into carcinoma *in situ* (cancer confined to layers superficial to basement membrane) or invasive cancer. The differences between dysplasia and metaplasia are contrasted in **Table 3.1**.

Presently, following concept has emerged in use of terms dysplasia, CIN, carcinoma *in situ*, and SIL, especially with regard to uterine cervical epithelium.

Grades of dysplasia Depending upon the thickness of squamous epithelium involved by atypical cells, dysplasia is conventionally graded as *mild*, *moderate* and *severe*. Carcinoma *in situ* is the full-thickness involvement by atypical cells, or in other words carcinoma confined to layers above the basement membrane. At times, severe dysplasia may not be clearly demarcated from carcinoma *in situ*. It is well accepted that invasive cervical cancer evolves through progressive stages of dysplasia and carcinoma *in situ*.

CIN An alternative classification is to group various grades of dysplasia and carcinoma *in situ* together into cervical intraepithelial neoplasia (CIN) which is similarly graded from grade I to III. According to this concept, the criteria are as under:

◆ *CIN-1* represents less than one-third involvement of the thickness of epithelium (mild dysplasia).
◆ *CIN-2* is one-third to two-third involvement (moderate dysplasia).

Table 3.1	Differences between metaplasia and dysplasia.		
	FEATURE	METAPLASIA	DYSPLASIA
i)	Definition	Change of one type of epithelial or mesenchymal cell to another type of adult epithelial or mesenchymal cell	Disordered cellular development, may be accompanied with hyperplasia or metaplasia
ii)	Types	Epithelial (squamous, columnar) and mesenchymal (osseous, cartilaginous)	Epithelial only
iii)	Tissues affected	Most commonly affects bronchial mucosa, uterine endocervix; others mesenchymal tissues (cartilage, arteries)	Uterine cervix, bronchial mucosa
iv)	Cellular changes	Mature cellular development	Disordered cellular development (pleomorphism, nuclear hyperchromasia, mitosis, loss of polarity)
v)	Natural history	Reversible on withdrawal of stimulus	May regress on removal of inciting stimulus, or may progress to higher grades of dysplasia or carcinoma *in situ*

◆ CIN-3 is full-thickness involvement or equivalent to carcinoma *in situ* (severe dysplasia and carcinoma *in situ*).

SIL Currently, the National Cancer Institute (NCI) of the US has proposed *The Bethesda System (TBS)* for reporting cervical and vaginal cytopathology. Besides cytomorphology, TBS takes into consideration important etiologic role of *low-risk* and *high-risk types of human papilloma viruses (HPV)*. According to TBS, three grades of CIN are readjusted into two grades of squamous intraepithelial lesions (SIL)—low-grade SIL (L-SIL) and high-grade SIL (H-SIL) as under:

◆ L-SIL corresponds to CIN-1 and is a flat condyloma, having koilocytic atypia, usually related to low-risk HPV 6 and 11 infection (i.e. it includes mild dysplasia and HPV infection). About 10% cases of L-SIL may progress to H-SIL.

◆ H-SIL corresponds to CIN-2 and 3 and has abnormal pleomorphic atypical squamous cells. High-risk HPV 16 and 18 are implicated in the etiology of H-SIL (i.e. it includes moderate dysplasia, severe dysplasia, and carcinoma *in situ*). Approximately, 10% cases of H-SIL may progress to invasive cervical cancer over a period of about two years.

A comparison of these classifications is shown in **Table 3.2**.

Progressive grades of dysplasia/CIN/SIL is a classical example of progression of malignancy through stepwise epithelial changes and that it can be detected early by simple Papanicolaou cytologic test ('Pap smear'). The use of Pap smear followed by colposcopy-directed biopsy confirms the diagnosis which has helped greatly in instituting early effective therapy and thus has reduced the incidence of cervical cancer in many developed countries.

CIN or SIL can develop at any age though it is rare before puberty. Low-grade reversible changes arise in young women between 25 and 30 years of age, whereas progressively higher grades of epithelial changes develop a decade later. Hence, the desirability of periodic Pap smears on all women after they become sexually active.

MORPHOLOGIC FEATURES **Grossly,** no specific picture is associated with cellular atypia found in dysplasias or carcinoma *in situ* except that the changes begin at the squamocolumnar junction or transitional zone of the uterine cervix. The diagnosis can be suspected clinically on the basis of Schiller's test done on bedside.

Histologically, distinction between various grades of CIN is quite subjective, but, in general dysplastic cells are distributed in the layers of squamous epithelium for varying thickness, and accordingly graded as mild, moderate and severe dysplasia, and carcinoma *in situ* **(Fig. 3.10,B)**.

◆ In *mild dysplasia (CIN-1)*, the abnormal cells extend up to one-third thickness from the basal to the surface layer;

◆ In *moderate dysplasia (CIN-2)* up to two-thirds;

◆ In *severe dysplasia (CIN-3)*, these cells extend from 75-90% thickness of epithelium; and

Table 3.2	Classification of cervical intraepithelial neoplasia/squamous intraepithelial lesion (CIN/SIL).				
BETHESDA SYSTEM	HPV TYPES	MORPHOLOGY		CIN	DYSPLASIA
L-SIL	6, 11	Koilocytic atypia, flat condyloma		CIN-1	Mild
H-SIL	16, 18	Progressive cellular atypia, loss of maturation		CIN-2, CIN-3	Moderate, severe, carcinoma *in situ*

(L-SIL = Low-grade squamous intraepithelial lesions; H-SIL = High-grade squamous intraepithelial lesion; CIN = Cervical intraepithelial neoplasia)

Chapter 3: Cellular Adaptations

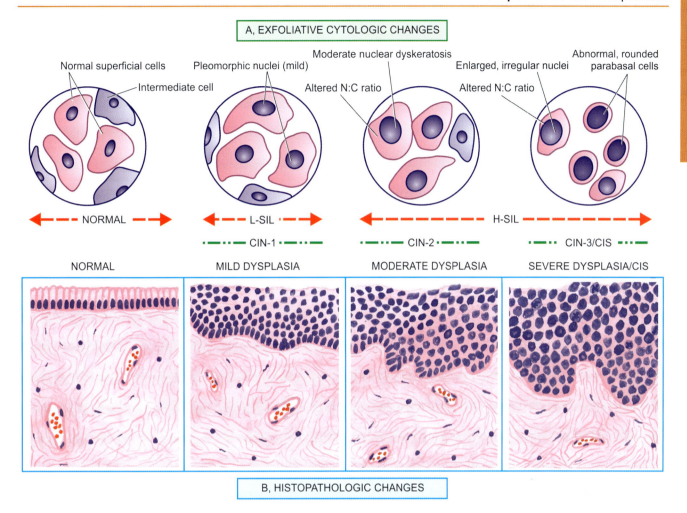

Figure 3.10 ▶ Uterine cervical dysplasia, cervical intraepithelial neoplasia (CIN) and squamous intraepithelial lesions (SIL). A, Exfoliative cytologic studies in various grades of cellular changes (upper part of figure). B, Schematic representation of histologic changes (lower part of figure). The grades of CIN-1 or mild dysplasia (L-SIL), CIN-2 (moderate dysplasia) and CIN-3 (severe dysplasia and carcinoma *in situ*) (together grouped as H-SIL) show progressive increase in the number of abnormal cells parallel to the increasing severity of grades.

◆ In *carcinoma in situ* (included in *CIN-3)*, the entire thickness from the basement membrane to the surface shows dysplastic cells.

The atypical cells migrate to the surface layers from where they are shed off (exfoliated) into vaginal secretions in Pap smear. The individual dysplastic or abnormal cells in these grades of atypia show various cytologic changes such as: crowding of cells, pleomorphism, high nucleocytoplasmic ratio, coarse and irregular nuclear chromatin, numerous mitoses and scattered dyskaryotic cells.

The diagnosis of dysplasia and carcinoma *in situ* or CIN/SIL is best made by *exfoliative cytologic studies*. The degree of atypicality in the exfoliated surface epithelial cells can be objectively graded on the basis of 3 principal features **(Fig. 3.10, A)**:

1. More severe nuclear dyskaryotic changes such as increased hyperchromasia and nuclear membrane folding.

2. Decreased cytoplasmic maturation i.e. less cytoplasm as the surface cells show less maturation.

3. In lower grades of dysplasia (CIN-1/L-SIL) predominantly superficial and intermediate cells are shed off whereas in severe dysplasia and in carcinoma *in situ* (CIN-3/H-SIL) the desquamated cells are mainly small, dark basal cells. The lesions of SIL in cytology have histologic correlation with colposcopy-directed cervical biopsy in 70-90% cases.

GIST BOX 3.1 — Cellular Adaptations

- *Atrophy* is reduction of the number and size of parenchymal cells of an organ or its parts which was once normal.
- *Hypertrophy* is an increase in the size of parenchymal cells resulting in enlargement of the organ or tissue, without any change in the number of cells.
- *Hyperplasia* is an increase in the number of parenchymal cells resulting in enlargement of the organ or tissue.
- *Metaplasia* is defined as a reversible change of one type of epithelial or mesenchymal adult cells to another type of adult epithelial or mesenchymal cells, usually in response to abnormal stimuli, and often reverts back to normal on removal of stimulus.
- *Dysplasia* is 'disordered cellular development', often preceded or accompanied with metaplasia and hyperplasia; most common sites being uterine cervix and bronchus. The cellular changes may range from mild (low grade) to moderate and severe (high grade). Carcinoma in situ refers to epithelial changes in all the layers above the basement membrane.

4 Cell Injury: Etiology and Pathogenesis

Cell injury is defined as the functional and morphologic effects of a variety of stresses due to etiologic agents a cell encounters resulting in changes in its internal and external environment. As already discussed, the cellular response depends upon factors pertaining to the host and the injurious agent. Accordingly, initially there may be cellular adaptive response, and later there may be reversible or irreversible cell injury (see Fig. 3.1).

In order to learn the fundamentals of disease processes at cellular level, it is essential to have an understanding of the causes (etiology) and mechanisms (pathogenesis) of cell injury, leading to deranged cell function.

ETIOLOGY OF CELL INJURY

The cells may be broadly injured by two major groups of causes:
A. Genetic causes
B. Acquired causes

The genetic causes of various diseases are discussed in Chapter 8. The acquired causes of disease comprise vast majority of common diseases afflicting mankind. Based on underlying agent, the acquired causes of cell injury can be further categorised as under:
1. Hypoxia and ischaemia
2. Physical agents
3. Chemical agents and drugs
4. Microbial agents
5. Immunologic agents
6. Nutritional derangements
7. Ageing
8. Psychogenic diseases
9. Iatrogenic factors
10. Idiopathic diseases.

In a given situation, more than one of the above etiologic factors may be involved. These factors are briefly outlined below.

HYPOXIA AND ISCHAEMIA Cells of different tissues essentially require oxygen to generate energy and perform metabolic functions. Deficiency of oxygen or hypoxia results in failure to carry out these activities by the cells. Hypoxia is the most common cause of cell injury. Hypoxia may result from the following 2 ways:
◆ The most common mechanism of hypoxic cell injury is by reduced supply of blood to cells due to interruption i.e. ischaemia.

◆ Hypoxia may also result from impaired blood supply from causes other than interruption e.g. disorders of oxygen-carrying RBCs (e.g. anaemia, carbon monoxide poisoning), heart diseases, lung diseases and increased demand of tissues.

PHYSICAL AGENTS Physical agents in causation of disease are as under:
i) mechanical trauma (e.g. road accidents);
ii) thermal trauma (e.g. by heat and cold);
iii) electricity;
iv) radiation (e.g. ultraviolet and ionising); and
v) rapid changes in atmospheric pressure.

CHEMICALS AND DRUGS An ever-increasing list of chemical agents and drugs may cause cell injury. Important examples include the following:
i) chemical poisons such as cyanide, arsenic, mercury;
ii) strong acids and alkalis;
iii) environmental pollutants;
iv) insecticides and pesticides;
v) oxygen at high concentrations;
vi) hypertonic glucose and salt;
vii) social agents such as alcohol and narcotic drugs; and
viii) therapeutic administration of drugs.

MICROBIAL AGENTS Injuries by microbes include infections caused by bacteria, rickettsiae, viruses, fungi, protozoa, metazoa, and other parasites.

Diseases caused by biologic agents are discussed in Chapter 13.

IMMUNOLOGIC AGENTS Immunity is a 'double-edged sword'—it protects the host against various injurious agents but it may also turn lethal and cause cell injury e.g.
i) hypersensitivity reactions;
ii) anaphylactic reactions; and
iii) autoimmune diseases.

Immunologic tissue injury is discussed in Chapter 14.

NUTRITIONAL DERANGEMENTS A deficiency or an excess of nutrients may result in nutritional imbalances.
◆ Nutritional deficiency diseases may be due to overall deficiency of nutrients (e.g. starvation), of protein calorie (e.g. marasmus, kwashiorkor), of minerals (e.g. anaemia), or of trace elements.
◆ Nutritional excess is a problem of affluent societies resulting in obesity, atherosclerosis, heart disease and hypertension.

Nutritional diseases are discussed in Chapter 9.

AGEING Cellular ageing or senescence leads to impaired ability of the cells to undergo replication and repair, and ultimately lead to cell death culminating in death of the individual (page 16).

PSYCHOGENIC DISEASES There are no specific biochemical or morphologic changes in common acquired mental diseases due to mental stress, strain, anxiety, overwork and frustration e.g. depression, schizophrenia. However, problems of drug addiction, alcoholism, and smoking result in various organic diseases such as liver damage, chronic bronchitis, lung cancer, peptic ulcer, hypertension, ischaemic heart disease etc.

IATROGENIC CAUSES Although as per Hippocratic oath, every physician is bound not to do or administer anything that causes harm to the patient, there are some diseases as well as deaths attributed to iatrogenic causes (owing to physician). Examples include occurrence of disease or death due to error in judgement by the physician and untoward effects of administered therapy (drugs, radiation).

IDIOPATHIC DISEASES Idiopathic means "of unknown cause". Finally, although so much is known about the etiology of diseases, there still remain many diseases for which exact cause is undetermined. For example, most common form of hypertension (90%) is idiopathic (or essential) hypertension. Similarly, exact etiology of many cancers is still incompletely known.

> **GIST BOX 4.1** — **Etiology of Cell Injury**
>
> - Cell injury is the effect of a variety of stresses due to etiologic agents a cell encounters resulting in changes in its internal and external environment.
> - Cellular response to stress depends upon the type of cell and tissue involved, and the extent and type of cell injury.
> - Initially, cells adapt to the changes due to injurious agent and may revert back to normal.
> - Mild to moderate stress for shorter duration causes reversible cell injury; severe and persistent stress causes cell death.
> - Among various etiologic factors, hypoxia-ischaemia is most important; others are chemical and physical agents, microbes, immunity, ageing etc.

PATHOGENESIS OF CELL INJURY

Injury to the normal cell by one or more of the above listed etiologic agents may result in a state of reversible or irreversible cell injury. The underlying alterations in biochemical systems of cells for reversible and irreversible cell injury by various agents are complex and varied. However, in general, irrespective of the type, following features apply to most forms of cell injury by different agents:

1. Factors pertaining to etiologic agent and host As mentioned above, factors pertaining to host cells and etiologic agent determine the outcome of cell injury:

i) Type, duration and severity of injurious agent: The extent of cellular injury depends upon type, duration and severity of the stimulus e.g. small dose of chemical toxin or short duration of ischaemia causes reversible cell injury while large dose of the same chemical agent or persistent ischaemia causes cell death.

ii) Type, status and adaptability of target cell: The type of cell as regards its susceptibility to injury, its nutritional and metabolic status, and adaptation of the cell to hostile environment determine the extent of cell injury e.g. skeletal muscle can withstand hypoxic injury for a long time while cardiac muscle suffers irreversible cell injury after persistent ischaemia due to total coronary occlusion for ≥ 20 minutes.

2. Common underlying mechanisms Irrespective of other factors, following essential intracellular biochemical phenomena underlie all forms of cell injury:
i) Mitochondrial damage causing ATP depletion.
ii) Cell membrane damage disturbing the metabolic and trans-membrane exchanges.
iii) Release of toxic free radicals.

3. Usual morphologic changes Biochemical and molecular changes underlying cell injury from various agents become apparent first, and are associated with appearance of ultrastructural changes in the injured cell. However, eventually, gross and light microscopic changes in morphology of organ and cells appear. The morphologic changes of reversible cell injury (e.g. hydropic swelling) appear earlier while later morphologic alterations of cell death are seen (e.g. in myocardial infarction).

4. Functional implications and disease outcome Eventually, cell injury affects cellular function adversely which has bearing on the body. Consequently, clinical features in the form of symptoms and signs would appear. Further course or prognosis will depend upon the response to treatment versus the biologic behaviour of disease.

The interruption of blood supply (i.e. ischaemia) and impaired oxygen supply to the tissues (i.e. hypoxia) are most common form of cell injury in human beings. Pathogenesis of hypoxic and ischaemic cell injury is, therefore, described in detail below followed by brief discussion on pathogenesis of chemical and physical (principally ionising radiation) agents.

PATHOGENESIS OF ISCHAEMIC AND HYPOXIC INJURY

Ischaemia and hypoxia are the most common forms of cell injury. Although underlying intracellular mechanisms and ultrastructural changes seen in reversible and irreversible

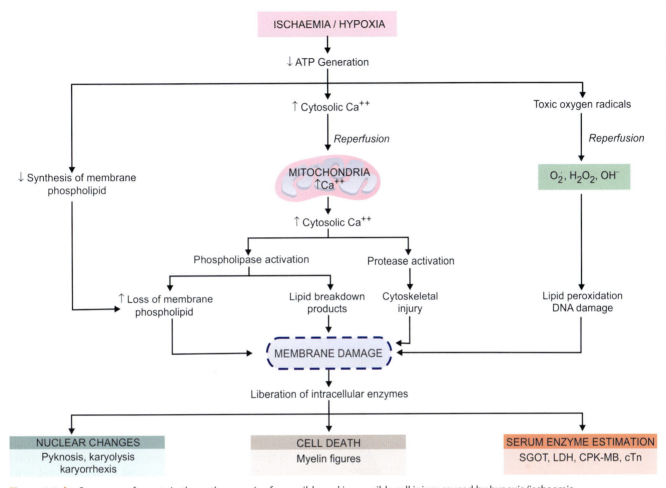

Figure 4.1 ▶ Sequence of events in the pathogenesis of reversible and irreversible cell injury caused by hypoxia/ischaemia.

cell injury by hypoxia-ischaemia (depending upon extent of hypoxia and type of cells involved) are a continuation of the process, these mechanisms are discussed separately below and illustrated diagrammatically in **Figs. 4.1 and 4.2**:

REVERSIBLE CELL INJURY If the ischaemia or hypoxia is of short duration, the effects may be reversible on rapid restoration of circulation e.g. in coronary artery occlusion, myocardial contractility, metabolism and ultrastructure are reversed if the circulation is quickly restored. The sequential biochemical and ultrastructural changes in reversible cell injury are as under **(Fig. 4.2, A)**:

1. Decreased generation of cellular ATP: Damage by ischaemia from interruption versus **hypoxia from other causes** All living cells require continuous supply of oxygen to produce ATP which is essentially required for a variety of cellular functions (e.g. membrane transport, protein synthesis, lipid synthesis and phospholipid metabolism). ATP in human cell is derived from 2 sources:

◆ *Firstly*, by aerobic respiration or oxidative phosphorylation (which requires oxygen) in the mitochondria.

◆ *Secondly*, cells may subsequently switch over to anaerobic glycolytic oxidation to maintain constant supply of ATP (in which ATP is generated from glucose/glycogen in the absence of oxygen).

Ischaemia due to interruption in blood supply as well as hypoxia from other causes limit the supply of oxygen to the cells, thus causing decreased ATP generation from ADP:

◆ In *ischaemia* from interruption of blood supply, aerobic respiration as well as glucose availability are both compromised resulting in more severe and faster effects of cell injury. Ischaemic cell injury also causes accumulation of metabolic waste products in the cells.

◆ On the other hand, in *hypoxia from other causes* (RBC disorders, heart disease, lung disease), anaerobic glycolytic ATP generation continues, and thus cell injury is less severe.

However, highly specialised cells such as myocardium, proximal tubular cells of the kidney, and neurons of the CNS are dependent solely on aerobic respiration for ATP generation and thus these tissues suffer from ill-effects of ischaemia more severely and rapidly.

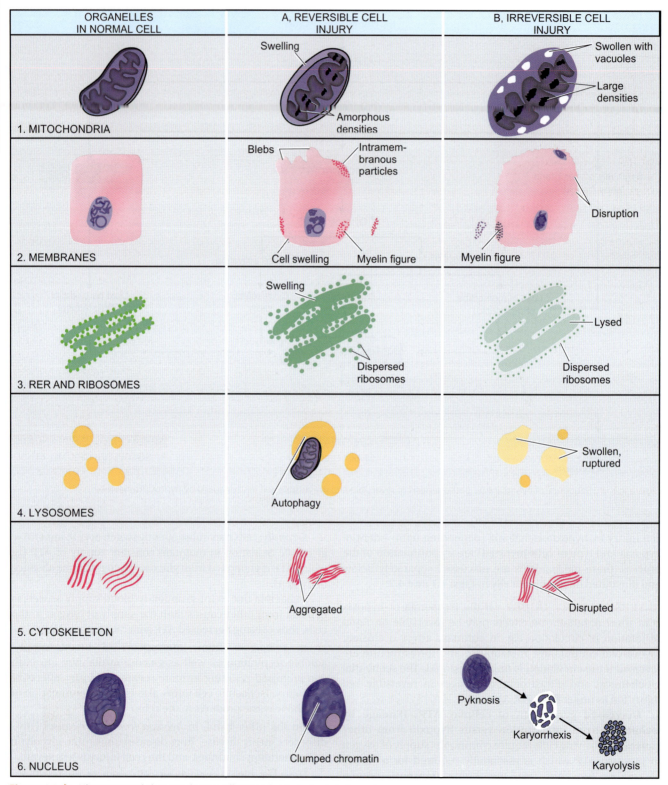

Figure 4.2 ▶ Ultrastructural changes during cell injury due to hypoxia-ischaemia.

2. **Intracellular lactic acidosis: Nuclear clumping** Due to low oxygen supply to the cell, aerobic respiration by mitochondria fails first. This is followed by switch to anaerobic glycolytic pathway for the requirement of energy (i.e. ATP). This results in rapid depletion of glycogen and accumulation of lactic acid lowering the intracellular pH. Early fall in intracellular pH (i.e. intracellular lactic acidosis) results in clumping of nuclear chromatin.

3. **Damage to plasma membrane pumps: Hydropic swelling and other membrane changes** Lack of ATP interferes in generation of phospholipids from the cellular fatty acids which are required for continuous repair of membranes. This results in damage to membrane pumps operating for regulation of sodium-potassium and calcium as under:

i) Failure of sodium-potassium pump Normally, the energy (ATP)-dependent sodium pump (also called Na^+-K^+ ATPase) operating at the plasma membrane allows active transport of sodium out of the cell and diffusion of potassium into the cell. Lowered ATP in the cell lowers the activity of sodium pump and consequently interferes with this membrane-regulated process. This results in intracellular accumulation of sodium and diffusion of potassium out of the cell. The accumulation of sodium in the cell leads to increase in intracellular water to maintain iso-osmotic conditions (i.e. hydropic swelling occurs, page 36).

ii) Failure of calcium pump Membrane damage causes disturbance in the calcium ion exchange across the cell membrane. Excess of calcium moves into the cell (i.e. calcium influx), particularly in the mitochondria, causing its swelling and deposition of phospholipid-rich amorphous densities.

4. **Reduced protein synthesis: Dispersed ribosomes** As a result of continued hypoxia, membranes of endoplasmic reticulum and Golgi apparatus swell up. Ribosomes are detached from granular (rough) endoplasmic reticulum and polysomes are degraded to monosomes, thus dispersing ribosomes in the cytoplasm and inactivating their function. Similar reduced protein synthesis occurs in Golgi apparatus.

Ultrastructural evidence of reversible cell membrane damage is seen in the form of loss of microvilli, intramembranous particles and focal projections of the cytoplasm (blebs). *Myelin figures* may be seen lying in the cytoplasm or present outside the cell; these are derived from membranes (plasma or organellar) enclosing water and dissociated lipoproteins between the lamellae of injured membranes.

Up to this point, withdrawal of acute stress can restore the cell to normal state i.e. a state of reversible cell injury.

IRREVERSIBLE CELL INJURY Persistence of ischaemia or hypoxia results in irreversible damage to the structure and function of the cell (cell death). The stage at which this *point of no return or irreversibility* is reached from reversible cell injury is unclear but the sequence of events is a continuation of reversibly injured cell. Two essential phenomena always distinguish irreversible from reversible cell injury **(Fig. 4.1)**:

◆ Inability of the cell to reverse *mitochondrial dysfunction* on reperfusion or reoxygenation.

◆ *Disturbance in cell membrane function* in general, and in plasma membrane in particular.

In addition, there is further reduction in ATP, continued depletion of proteins, reduced intracellular pH, and leakage of lysosomal enzymes into the plasma. These biochemical changes have effects on the ultrastructural components of the cell **(Fig. 4.2, B)**:

1. **Calcium influx: Mitochondrial damage** As a result of continued hypoxia, a large cytosolic influx of calcium ions occurs, especially after reperfusion of irreversibly injured cell. Excess intracellular calcium collects in the mitochondria disabling its function. Morphological changes are in the form of vacuoles in the mitochondria and deposits of amorphous calcium salts in the mitochondrial matrix.

2. **Activated phospholipases: Membrane damage** Damage to membrane function in general, and plasma membrane in particular, is the most important event in irreversible cell injury. Increased cytosolic influx of calcium in the cell activates endogenous *phospholipases*. These, in turn, degrade membrane phospholipids progressively which are the main constituent of the lipid bilayer membrane. Besides, there is also decreased replacement-synthesis of membrane phospholipids due to reduced ATP. Other lytic enzyme which is activated is *ATPase* which causes further depletion of ATP.

3. **Intracellular proteases: Cytoskeletal damage** Normal cytoskeleton of the cell (microfilaments, microtubules and intermediate filaments) which anchors the cell membrane is damaged due to degradation by activated intracellular proteases or by physical effect of cell swelling producing irreversible cell membrane injury.

4. **Activated endonucleases: Nuclear damage** DNA or nucleoproteins are damaged by the activated lysosomal enzymes such as proteases and endonucleases. Irreversible damage to the nucleus can be in three forms:
i) *Pyknosis:* Condensation and clumping of nucleus which becomes dark basophilic.
ii) *Karyorrhexis:* Nuclear fragmentation in to small bits dispersed in the cytoplasm.
iii) *Karyolysis:* Dissolution of the nucleus.

Damaged DNA activates proapoptotic proteins leading the cell to death.

5. **Lysosomal hydrolytic enzymes: Lysosomal damage, cell death and phagocytosis** Lysosomal membranes are damaged and that results in escape of lysosomal hydrolytic enzymes. These enzymes are activated due to lack of oxygen in the cell and acidic pH. These hydrolytic enzymes (e.g. hydrolase, RNAase, DNAase, protease, glycosidase, phosphatase, lipase, amylase, cathepsin etc) on activation bring about enzymatic digestion of cellular components and hence cell death. The dead cell is eventually replaced by

Section I: The Cell in Health and Disease

Table 4.1 Common enzyme markers of cell death.

ENZYME	DISEASE
1. *Aspartate aminotransferase (AST, SGOT)*	Diffuse liver cell necrosis e.g. viral hepatitis, alcoholic liver disease; Acute myocardial infarction
2. *Alanine aminotransferase (ALT, SGPT)*	More specific for diffuse liver cell damage than AST e.g. viral hepatitis
3. *Creatine kinase-MB (CK-MB)*	Acute myocardial infarction, myocarditis; Skeletal muscle injury
4. *Lipase*	More specific for acute pancreatitis
5. *Amylase*	Acute pancreatitis; Sialadenitis
6. *Lactic dehydrogenase (LDH)*	Acute myocardial infarction; Myocarditis; Skeletal muscle injury
7. *Cardiac troponin (CTn)*	Specific for acute myocardial infarction

masses of phospholipids called *myelin figures* which are either phagocytosed by macrophages or there may be formation of calcium soaps.

Liberated enzymes just mentioned leak across the abnormally permeable cell membrane into the serum, estimation of which may be used as clinical parameters of cell death. For example, in myocardial infarction, estimation of elevated serum glutamic oxaloacetic transaminase (SGOT), lactic dehydrogenase (LDH), isoenzyme of creatine kinase (CK-MB), and cardiac troponins (cTn) are useful guides for death of heart muscle. Some of the common enzyme markers for different forms of cell death are given in **Table 4.1**.

While cell damage from oxygen deprivation by above mechanisms develops slowly, taking several minutes to hours, cell injury may be accentuated after restoration of blood supply and subsequent events termed *ischaemic-reperfusion injury* by liberation of toxic free radicals (or reactive oxygen species), discussed below.

ISCHAEMIA-REPERFUSION INJURY AND FREE RADICAL-MEDIATED CELL INJURY

Depending upon the duration of ischaemia/hypoxia, restoration of blood flow may result in the following 3 different consequences:

1. From ischaemia to reversible injury When the period *of ischaemia is of short duration,* reperfusion with resupply of oxygen restores the structural and functional state of the injured cell i.e. reversible cell injury.

2. From ischaemia to irreversible injury Another extreme is when much longer period of ischaemia has resulted in irreversible cell injury *during ischaemia itself* i.e. when so much time has elapsed that neither blood flow restoration is helpful nor reperfusion injury can develop. Cell death in such cases is not attributed to formation of activated oxygen species. But instead, on reperfusion there is further marked intracellular excess of sodium and calcium ions due to persistent cell membrane damage.

3. From ischaemia to reperfusion injury When ischaemia *is for somewhat longer duration,* then restoration of blood supply to injured but viable cells (i.e. reperfusion), rather than restoring structure and function of the cell, paradoxically deteriorates the already injured cell and leads to its cell death. This is termed ischaemia-reperfusion injury. The examples of such forms of cell injury are irreversible cell injury in myocardial and cerebral ischaemia.

Ischaemia-reperfusion injury occurs due to excessive accumulation of free radicals or reactive oxygen species. The mechanism of reperfusion injury by free radicals is complex and evolves through following mechanisms:
1. Calcium overload.
2. Excessive generation of free radicals (superoxide, H_2O_2, hydroxyl radical, pernitrite).
3. Subsequent inflammatory reaction.

These are discussed below:

1. CALCIUM OVERLOAD Upon restoration of blood supply, the ischaemic cell is further bathed by the blood fluid that has more calcium ions at a time when the ATP stores of the cell are low. This results in further calcium overload on the already injured cells, triggering lipid peroxidation of the membrane causing further membrane damage.

2. EXCESSIVE GENERATION OF FREE RADICALS Although oxygen is the lifeline of all cells and tissues, its molecular forms as reactive oxygen radicals or reactive oxygen species can be most devastating for the cells. Free radical-mediated cell injury has been extensively studied and a brief account is given below.

Oxygen free radical generation Normally, reduction-oxidation (redox) reaction in the metabolism of the cell involves generation of ATP by oxidative process in which biradical oxygen (O_2) combines with hydrogen atom (H), and in the process, water (H_2O) is formed. This normal reaction of O_2 to H_2O involves 'four electron donation' in four steps involving transfer of one electron at each step. Free radicals are intermediate chemical species having a single unpaired electron in its outer orbit. These are generated within mitochondrial inner membrane where cytochrome oxidase catalyses O_2 to H_2O reaction. Three intermediate molecules of partially reduced species of oxygen are generated depending upon the number of electrons transferred **(Fig. 4.3)**:

i) Superoxide oxygen (O'_2): one electron
ii) Hydrogen peroxide (H_2O_2): two electrons
iii) Hydroxyl radical (OH^-): three electrons

These are generated from enzymatic and non-enzymatic reaction as under:

Chapter 4: Cell Injury: Etiology and Pathogenesis

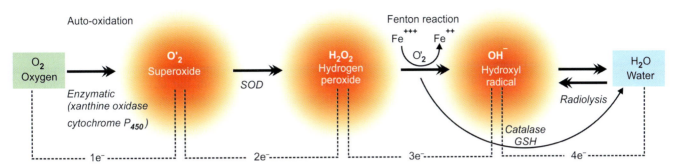

Figure 4.3 ▶ Mechanisms of generation of free radicals by four electron step reduction of oxygen. (SOD = *superoxide dismutase*; GSH = *glutathione peroxidase*).

i) Superoxide (O'_2): Superoxide anion O'_2 may be generated by direct auto-oxidation of O_2 during mitochondrial electron transport reaction. Alternatively, O'_2 is produced enzymatically by xanthine oxidase and cytochrome P_{450} in the mitochondria or cytosol.

ii) Hydrogen peroxide (H_2O_2): O'_2 so formed as above is catabolised to produce H_2O_2 by superoxide dismutase (SOD). H_2O_2 is reduced to water enzymatically by catalase (in the peroxisomes) and glutathione peroxidase, GSH (both in the cytosol and mitochondria).

iii) Hydroxyl radical (OH^-): OH^- radical is formed by 2 ways in biologic processes—by radiolysis of water and by reaction of H_2O_2 with ferrous (Fe^{++}) ions; the latter process is termed as Fenton reaction. Fenton reaction involves reduction of normal intracellular ferric (Fe^{+++}) to ferrous (Fe^{++}) form, a reaction facilitated by O'_2.

Other free radicals In addition to superoxide, H_2O_2 and hydroxyl radicals generated during conversion of O_2 to H_2O reaction, a few other free radicals active in the body are as follows:

i) *Nitric oxide (NO) and peroxynitrite (ONOO):* NO is a chemical mediator formed by various body cells (endothelial cells, neurons, macrophages etc), and is also a free radical. NO can combine with superoxide and forms ONOO which is a highly reactive free radical.

ii) *Halide reagent* (chlorine or chloride) released in the leucocytes reacts with superoxide and forms *hypochlorous acid (HOCl)* which is a cytotoxic free radical.

iii) *Exogenous sources* of free radicals include some environmental agents such as tobacco and industrial pollutants.

Cytotoxicity of free radicals Free radicals are formed in physiologic as well as pathologic processes. Basically, oxygen radicals are unstable and are destroyed spontaneously. The rate of spontaneous destruction is determined by catalytic action of certain enzymes such as superoxide dismutase (SOD), catalase and glutathione peroxidase (GSH). The net effect of free radical injury in physiologic and disease states, therefore, depends upon the rate of their formation and rate of their elimination.

However, if not degraded, then free radicals are highly destructive to the cell since they have electron-free residue and thus bind to all molecules of the cell; this is termed *oxidative stress*. Out of various free radicals, hydroxyl radical is the most reactive species. Free radicals may produce membrane damage by the following mechanisms **(Fig. 4.4)**:

i) *Lipid peroxidation* Polyunsaturated fatty acids (PUFA) of membrane are attacked repeatedly and severely by oxygen-derived free radicals to yield highly destructive PUFA radicals—lipid hydroperoxy radicals and lipid hypoperoxides. This reaction is termed lipid peroxidation. The lipid peroxides are decomposed by transition metals such as iron. Lipid peroxidation is propagated to other sites causing widespread membrane damage and destruction of organelles.

ii) *Oxidation of proteins* Oxygen-derived free radicals cause cell injury by oxidation of protein macromolecules of the cells,

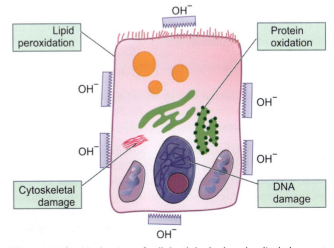

Figure 4.4 ▶ Mechanism of cell death by hydroxyl radical, the most reactive oxygen species.

cross-linkages of labile amino acids as well as by fragmentation of polypeptides directly. The end-result is degradation of cytosolic neutral proteases and cell destruction.

iii) *DNA damage* Free radicals cause breaks in the single strands of the nuclear and mitochondrial DNA. This results in cell injury; it may also cause malignant transformation of cells.

iv) *Cytoskeletal damage* Reactive oxygen species are also known to interact with cytoskeletal elements and interfere in mitochondrial aerobic phosphorylation and thus cause ATP depletion.

Conditions with free radical injury Currently, oxygen-derived free radicals have been known to play an important role in many forms of cell injury:
i) Ischaemic reperfusion injury
ii) Ionising radiation by causing radiolysis of water
iii) Chemical toxicity
iv) Chemical carcinogenesis
v) Hyperoxia (toxicity due to oxygen therapy)
vi) Cellular ageing
vii) Killing of microbial agents
viii) Inflammatory damage
ix) Destruction of tumour cells
x) Atherosclerosis.

Antioxidants Antioxidants are endogenous or exogenous substances which inactivate the free radicals. These substances include the following:
i) Vitamins E, A and C (ascorbic acid)
ii) Sulfhydryl-containing compounds e.g. cysteine and glutathione.
iii) Serum proteins e.g. ceruloplasmin and transferrin.

3. SUBSEQUENT INFLAMMATORY REACTION Ischaemia-reperfusion event is followed by inflammatory reaction. Incoming activated neutrophils utilise oxygen quickly (*oxygen burst*) and release large excess of oxygen free radicals. Ischaemia is also associated with accumulation of precursors of ATP, namely ADP and pyruvate, which further build-up generation of free radicals.

PATHOGENESIS OF CHEMICAL INJURY

Chemicals induce cell injury by one of the two mechanisms: by direct cytotoxicity, or by conversion of chemical into reactive metabolites.

DIRECT CYTOTOXIC EFFECTS Some chemicals combine with components of the cell and produce direct cytotoxicity without requiring metabolic activation. The cytotoxic damage is usually greatest to cells which are involved in the metabolism of such chemicals e.g. in mercuric chloride poisoning, the greatest damage occurs to cells of the alimentary tract where it is absorbed and the kidney where it is excreted. Cyanide kills the cell by poisoning mitochondrial cytochrome oxidase thus blocking oxidative phosphorylation.

Other examples of directly cytotoxic chemicals include chemotherapeutic agents used in treatment of cancer, toxic heavy metals such as mercury, lead and iron.

CONVERSION TO REACTIVE TOXIC METABOLITES This mechanism involves metabolic activation to yield ultimate toxin that interacts with the target cells. The target cells in this group of chemicals may not be the same cell that metabolised the toxin. Example of cell injury by conversion of reactive metabolites is toxic liver necrosis caused by carbon tetrachloride (CCl_4), acetaminophen (commonly used analgesic and antipyretic) and bromobenzene. Cell injury by CCl_4 is classic example of an industrial toxin (earlier used in dry-cleaning industry) that produces cell injury by conversion to a highly toxic free radical, CCl_3, in the body's drug-metabolising P_{450} enzyme system in the liver cells. Thus, it produces profound liver cell injury by free radical generation. Other mechanism of cell injury includes direct toxic effect on cell membrane and nucleus.

PATHOGENESIS OF PHYSICAL INJURY

Injuries caused by mechanical force are of medicolegal significance. But they may lead to a state of shock. Injuries by changes in atmospheric pressure (e.g. decompression sickness) are detailed in Chapter 17. Radiation injury to human by accidental or therapeutic exposure is of importance in treatment of persons with malignant tumours as well as may have carcinogenic influences (Chapter 19).

Killing of cells by *ionising radiation* is the result of direct formation of hydroxyl radicals from radiolysis of

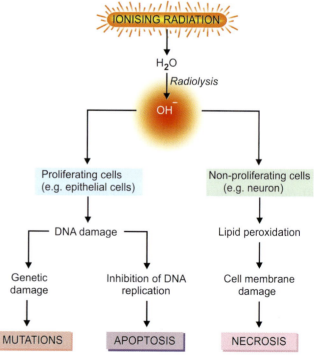

Figure 4.5 ▶ Mechanisms of cell injury by ionising radiation.

water **(Fig. 4.5)**. These hydroxyl radicals damage the cell membrane as well as may interact with DNA of the target cell. In proliferating cells, there is inhibition of DNA replication and eventual cell death by apoptosis (e.g. epithelial cells). In non-proliferating cells, there is no effect of inhibition of DNA synthesis and in these cells there is cell membrane damage followed by cell death by necrosis (e.g. neurons).

> **GIST BOX 4.2** — **Pathogenesis of Cell Injury**
>
> - Irrespective of the type of cell injury, common underlying mechanism involves mitochondrial damage and cell membrane damage.
> - Hypoxic-ischaemic cell injury is the prototype. It may be reversible or irreversible.
> - Reversible cell injury occurs due to decreased cellular ATP causing initially impaired aerobic respiration, followed by anaerobic glycolytic oxidation. Other changes are intracellular lactic acidosis, damage to membrane pumps (Na^+-K^+, and Ca^{++}), and dispersal of ribosomes.
> - Irreversible cell injury is due to continuation of earlier changes and includes further calcium influx in the mitochondria, and further damage to membranes, cytoskeleton and nucleus.
> - Lysosomal damage causes release of hydrolytic enzymes which can be estimated in the blood as indictors of cell death e.g. SGOT, SGPT, LDH, CK-MB, cardiac troponins etc.
> - Ischaemia-reperfusion injury is due to release of reactive oxygen species or free radicals. These include OH^- as the most potent radical; others are O_2^- and H_2O_2.
> - Free radical injury occurs when their generation exceeds their elimination and is implicated in mechanism of cell injury from various etiologies.

5 Morphology of Cell Injury: Degenerations and Cell Death

Morphologic changes of cell injury from various etiologic agents become apparent after molecular events. Depending upon the extent and severity of cell injury, various terms used for morphologic effects of reversible and irreversible cell injury (or cell death) are given in **Table 5.1**.

MORPHOLOGY OF REVERSIBLE CELL INJURY

In older literature, the term degeneration was commonly used to denote morphology of reversible cell injury. However, since this term does not provide any information on the nature of underlying changes, currently the term *retrogressive changes* or simply reversible cell injury are applied to non-lethal cell injury. Common examples of morphologic forms of reversible cell injury are discussed below.

HYDROPIC CHANGE

Hydropic change means accumulation of water within the cytoplasm of the cell. Other synonyms used are *cloudy swelling* (for gross appearance of the affected organ) and *vacuolar degeneration* (due to cytoplasmic vacuolation). Hydropic swelling is an entirely reversible change upon removal of the injurious agent.

ETIOLOGY This is the commonest and earliest form of cell injury from almost all causes. The common causes include acute and subacute cell injury from various etiologic agents such as bacterial toxins, chemicals, poisons, burns, high fever, intravenous administration of hypertonic glucose or saline etc.

PATHOGENESIS Cloudy swelling results from impaired regulation of sodium and potassium at the level of cell membrane. This results in intracellular accumulation of sodium and escape of potassium. This, in turn, is accompanied with rapid inflow of water in the cell to maintain iso-osmotic conditions and hence cellular swelling occurs. In addition, influx of calcium too occurs.

MORPHOLOGIC FEATURES *Grossly,* the affected organ such as kidney, liver, pancreas, or heart muscle is enlarged due to swelling. The cut surface bulges outwards and is slightly opaque.

Microscopically, the features of hydropic swelling of kidney are as under **(Fig. 5.1)**:

i) The tubular epithelial cells are swollen and their cytoplasm contains small clear vacuoles and hence the term vacuolar degeneration. These vacuoles represent distended cisternae of the endoplasmic reticulum.
ii) Small cytoplasmic blebs may be seen.
iii) The nucleus may appear pale.
iv) The microvasculature of the interstitium is compressed due to swollen tubular cells.

HYALINE CHANGE

The word 'hyaline' or 'hyalin' means glassy (*hyalos* = glass). Hyalinisation is a common descriptive histologic term for glassy, homogeneous, eosinophilic appearance of proteinaceous material in haematoxylin and eosin-stained sections and does not refer to any specific substance. Though fibrin and amyloid have hyaline appearance, they have distinctive features and staining reactions and can be distinguished from non-specific hyaline material. Hyaline change is seen in heterogeneous pathologic conditions and may be intracellular or extracellular.

INTRACELLULAR HYALINE Intracellular hyaline is mainly seen in epithelial cells. A few examples are as follows:
1. *Hyaline droplets* in the proximal tubular epithelial cells due to excessive reabsorption of plasma proteins in proteinuria.
2. *Hyaline degeneration* of rectus abdominalis muscle called Zenker's degeneration, occurring in typhoid fever. The muscle loses its fibrillar staining and becomes glassy and hyaline.
3. *Mallory's hyaline* represents aggregates of intermediate filaments in the hepatocytes in alcoholic liver cell injury.
4. Nuclear or cytoplasmic *hyaline inclusions* seen in some viral infections.

Table 5.1 Classification of morphologic forms of cell injury.

MECHANISM OF CELL INJURY	NOMENCLATURE
1. Reversible cell injury	Retrogressive changes (older term: degenerations)
2. Irreversible cell injury	Cell death—necrosis
3. Programmed cell death	Apoptosis
4. Deranged cell metabolism	Intracellular accumulation of lipid, protein, carbohydrate
5. After-effects of necrosis	Gangrene, pathologic calcification

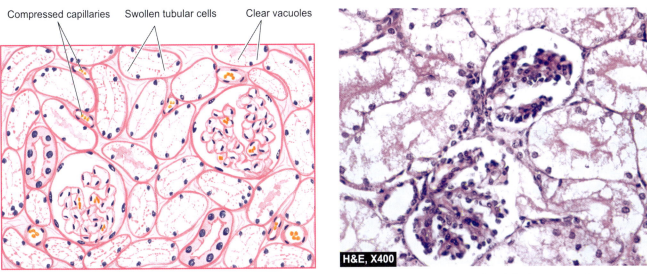

Figure 5.1 ▶ Hydropic change kidney. The tubular epithelial cells are distended with cytoplasmic vacuoles while the interstitial vasculature is compressed. The nuclei of affected tubules are pale.

5. *Russell's bodies* representing excessive immunoglobulins in the rough endoplasmic reticulum of the plasma cells (Fig. 5.2).

EXTRACELLULAR HYALINE Extracellular hyaline commonly termed hyalinisation is seen in connective tissues. A few examples of extracellular hyaline change are as under:
1. Hyaline degeneration in *leiomyomas* of the uterus (Fig. 5.3).
2. Hyalinised *old scar* of fibrocollagenous tissues.
3. *Hyaline arteriolosclerosis* in renal vessels in hypertension and diabetes mellitus.
4. Hyalinised glomeruli in *chronic glomerulonephritis*.
5. *Corpora amylacea* seen as rounded masses of concentric hyaline laminae in the enlarged prostate in the elderly, in the brain and in the spinal cord in old age, and in old infarcts of the lung.

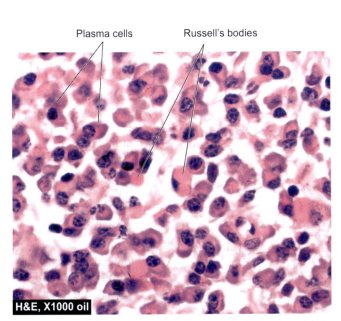

Figure 5.2 ▶ Intracellular hyaline as Russell's bodies in the plasma cells. The cytoplasm shows pink homogeneous globular material due to accumulated immunoglobulins.

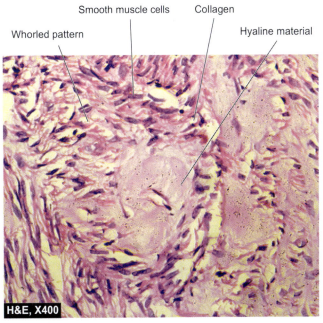

Figure 5.3 ▶ Extracellular hyaline deposit in leiomyoma uterus. The centres of whorls of smooth muscle and connective tissue show pink homogeneous hyaline material (connective tissue hyaline).

MUCOID CHANGE

Mucoid means mucus-like. Mucus is the secretory product of mucous glands and is a combination of proteins complexed with mucopolysaccharides. *Mucin*, a glycoprotein, is its chief constituent. Mucin is normally produced by epithelial cells of mucous membranes and mucous glands, as well as by some connective tissues such as ground substance in the umbilical cord. By convention, connective tissue mucin is termed myxoid. Epithelial and connective tissue mucin are both stained by alcian blue. However, the two can be distinguished by periodic acid-Schiff (PAS) stain: epithelial mucin stains PAS positive, while connective tissue mucin is PAS negative; the latter can, however, be stained positively with colloidal iron.

EPITHELIAL MUCIN Following are some examples of functional excess of epithelial mucin:
1. Catarrhal inflammation of mucous membrane (e.g. of respiratory tract, alimentary tract, uterus).
2. Obstruction of duct leading to mucocele in the oral cavity and gallbladder.
3. Cystic fibrosis of the pancreas.
4. Mucin-secreting tumours (e.g. of ovary, stomach, large bowel etc.) **(Fig. 5.4)**.

CONNECTIVE TISSUE MUCIN A few examples of disturbances of connective tissue mucin or myxoid change are as under:
1. Mucoid or myxoid change in some tumours e.g. myxomas, neurofibromas, fibroadenoma, soft tissue sarcomas etc **(Fig. 5.5)**.

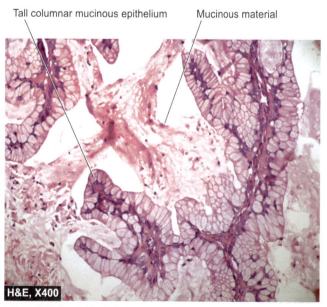

Figure 5.4 ▶ Epithelial mucin. Mucinous cystadenoma of the ovary showing intracytoplasmic mucinous material in the epithelial cells lining the cyst.

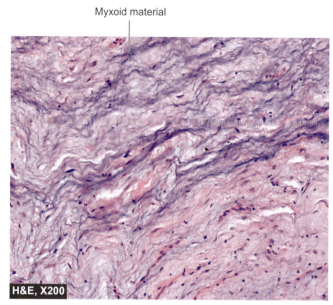

Figure 5.5 ▶ Connective tissue mucin (myxoid change) in neurofibroma.

2. Dissecting aneurysm of the aorta due to Erdheim's medial degeneration and Marfan's syndrome.
3. Myxomatous change in the dermis in myxoedema.
4. Myxoid change in the synovium in ganglion on the wrist.

 GIST BOX 5.1 | **Morphology of Reversible Cell Injury**

- Degenerations or reversible cell injury depict light microscopic changes occurring at ultrastructural level.
- Hydropic swelling is the earliest form of cell injury from various etiologies and its main features are cellular swelling due to cytoplasmic vacuoles.
- Hyaline change is intra- and extracellular deposition of pink, proteinaceous material.
- Mucoid change is deposition of mucinous material in epithelial and connective tissues in excessive amounts.

MORPHOLOGY OF IRREVERSIBLE CELL INJURY (CELL DEATH)

Cell death is a state of irreversible injury. It may occur in the living tissues as a local or focal change caused by external factors (i.e. *necrosis*), or mediated by intracellular programmes (i.e. *programmed cell death*). While prototype of programmed cell death is *apoptosis*, a few other types are *necroptosis, pyroptosis, ferroptosis and autophagy*. Necrosis may be followed by some pathologic changes (i.e. *gangrene and pathologic calcification*), or may result in end of the life (*somatic death*).

The term *autolysis* (i.e. self-digestion) is used for disintegration of the cell by its own hydrolytic enzymes liberated from lysosomes and is generally used for post-

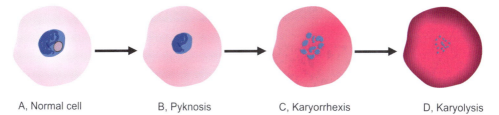

Figure 5.6 ▶ Nuclear and cytoplasmic changes in necrosis. A, Normal cell. B, Cytoplasm is more pink and nucleus is shrunken (pyknosis). C, Cytoplasm is more pink and the nucleus is fragmented (karyorrhexis). D, The cytoplasm is intensely pink and nuclear material has disappeared (karyolysis).

mortem change, and is therefore devoid of surrounding inflammatory response. Autolysis is *rapid* in some tissues rich in hydrolytic enzymes such as in the pancreas, and gastric mucosa; *intermediate* in tissues like the heart, liver and kidney; and *slow* in fibrous tissue.

Major forms of cell death in living tissues is discussed below.

NECROSIS

Necrosis is defined as a localised area of death of tissue followed later by degradation of tissue by hydrolytic enzymes liberated from dead cells; it is invariably accompanied by inflammatory reaction. Necrosis can be caused by various agents such as hypoxia, chemical and physical agents, microbial agents, immunological injury, etc.

Based on etiology and morphologic appearance, there are 5 types of necrosis: coagulative, liquefaction (colliquative), caseous, fat, and fibrinoid necrosis.

1. COAGULATIVE NECROSIS This is the most common type of necrosis caused by irreversible focal injury, mostly from sudden cessation of blood flow (ischaemic necrosis), and less often from bacterial and chemical agents. The organs commonly affected are the heart, kidney, and spleen.

Grossly, focus of coagulative necrosis in the early stage is pale, firm, and slightly swollen and is called infarct. With progression, the affected area becomes more yellowish, softer, and shrunken.

Microscopically, hallmark of coagulative necrosis is the conversion of normal cells into their 'tombstones' i.e. outlines of the cells are retained and the cell type can still be recognised but their cytoplasmic and nuclear details are lost. The necrosed cells are swollen and have more eosinophilic cytoplasm than the normal. These cells show nuclear changes of pyknosis, karyorrhexis and karyolysis **(Fig. 5.6)**. However, cell digestion and liquefaction fail to occur (*c.f.* liquefaction necrosis). Eventually, the necrosed focus is infiltrated by inflammatory cells and the dead cells are phagocytosed leaving granular debris and fragments of cells **(Fig. 5.7)**.

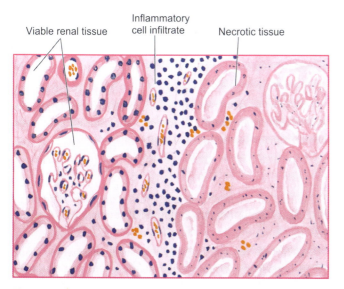
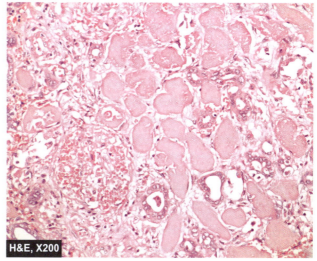

Figure 5.7 ▶ Coagulative necrosis in infarct kidney. The affected area on right shows cells with intensely eosinophilic cytoplasm of tubular cells but the outlines of tubules are still maintained. The nuclei show granular debris. The interface between viable and non-viable area shows non-specific chronic inflammation and proliferating vessels.

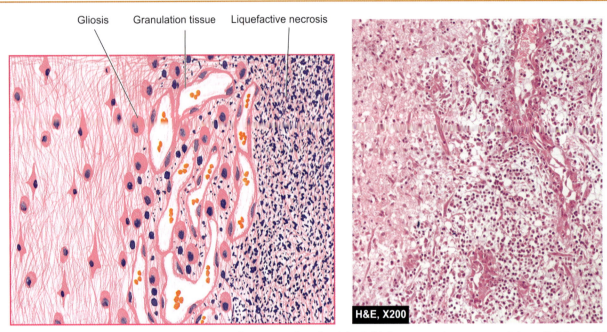

Figure 5.8 ▶ Liquefactive necrosis brain. The necrosed area on right side of the field shows a cystic space containing cell debris, while the surrounding zone shows granulation tissue and gliosis.

2. LIQUEFACTION (COLLIQUATIVE) NECROSIS Liquefaction or colliquative necrosis also occurs commonly due to ischaemic injury and bacterial or fungal infections but hydrolytic enzymes in tissue degradation have a dominant role in causing semi-fluid material. The common examples are infarct brain and abscess cavity.

Grossly, the affected area is soft with liquefied centre containing necrotic debris. Later, a cyst wall is formed.

Microscopically, the cystic space contains necrotic cell debris and macrophages filled with phagocytosed material. The cyst wall is formed by proliferating capillaries, inflammatory cells, and gliosis (proliferating glial cells) in the case of brain, and proliferating fibroblasts in the case of abscess cavity **(Fig. 5.8)**.

3. CASEOUS NECROSIS Caseous (caseous=cheese-like) necrosis is found in the centre of foci of tuberculous infections. It combines features of both coagulative and liquefactive necrosis.

Grossly, foci of caseous necrosis resemble dry cheese and are soft, granular and yellowish. This appearance is partly attributed to the histotoxic effects of lipopolysaccharides present in the capsule of the tubercle bacilli, *Mycobacterium tuberculosis*.

Microscopically, centre of the necrosed focus contain structureless, eosinophilic material having scattered granular debris of disintegrated nuclei **(Fig. 5.9)**. The surrounding tissue shows characteristic granulomatous inflammatory reaction consisting of epithelioid cells (modified macrophages having slipper-shaped vesicular nuclei), interspersed giant cells of Langhans' and foreign body type and peripheral mantle of lymphocytes (page 130).

4. FAT NECROSIS Fat necrosis is a special form of cell death occurring at mainly fat-rich anatomic locations in the body. The examples are: traumatic fat necrosis of the breast, especially in heavy and pendulous breasts, and mesenteric fat necrosis due to acute pancreatitis.

In the case of acute pancreatitis, there is liberation of pancreatic lipases from injured or inflamed tissue that results in necrosis of the pancreas as well as of the fat depots throughout the peritoneal cavity, and sometimes, even affecting the extra-abdominal adipose tissue.

In fat necrosis, there is hydrolysis and rupture of adipocytes, causing release of neutral fat which changes into glycerol and free fatty acids. The leaked out free fatty acids complex with calcium to form calcium soaps (saponification) discussed later under dystrophic calcification.

Grossly, fat necrosis appears as yellowish-white and firm deposits. Formation of calcium soaps imparts the necrosed foci firmer and chalky white appearance.

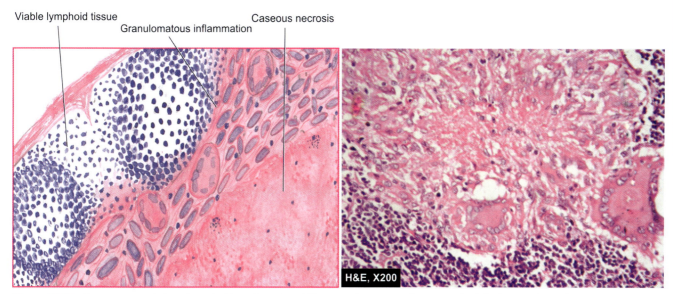

Figure 5.9 ▶ Caseous necrosis lymph node. There is eosinophilic, amorphous, granular material, while the periphery shows granulomatous inflammation.

Microscopically, the necrosed fat cells have cloudy appearance and are surrounded by an inflammatory reaction. Formation of calcium soaps is identified in the tissue sections as amorphous, granular and basophilic material **(Fig. 5.10)**.

5. FIBRINOID NECROSIS Fibrinoid necrosis is characterised by deposition of fibrin-like material which has the staining properties of fibrin such as phosphotungstic acid haematoxylin (PTAH) stain. It is encountered in various examples of immunologic tissue injury (e.g. in immune complex vasculitis, autoimmune diseases, Arthus reaction etc), arterioles in hypertension, peptic ulcer etc.

Microscopically, fibrinoid necrosis is identified by brightly eosinophilic, hyaline-like deposition in the vessel wall. Necrotic focus is surrounded by nuclear debris of neutrophils (leucocytoclasis) **(Fig. 5.11)**. Local haemorrhage may occur due to rupture of the blood vessel.

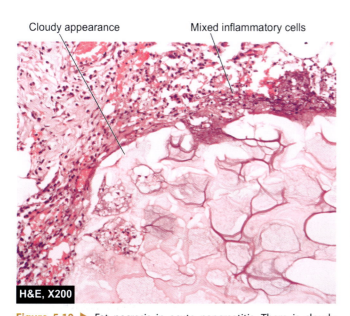

Figure 5.10 ▶ Fat necrosis in acute pancreatitis. There is cloudy appearance of adipocytes, coarse basophilic granular debris while the periphery shows a few mixed inflammatory cells.

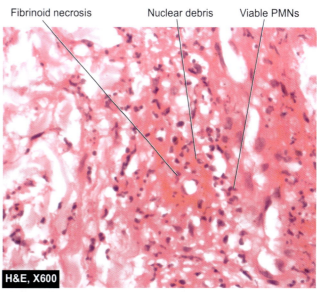

Figure 5.11 ▶ Fibrinoid necrosis in autoimmune vasculitis. The vessel wall shows brightly pink amorphous material and nuclear fragments of necrosed neutrophils.

Section I: The Cell in Health and Disease

APOPTOSIS

Apoptosis is a form of 'coordinated and internally programmed cell death' having significance in a variety of physiologic and pathologic conditions (*apoptosis*=falling off or dropping off, as that of leaves or petals). The term was first introduced in 1972 distinct from necrosis by being controlled and regulated cell death, and opposed to that of mitosis by having regulated size of the cell turn over. When the cell is not needed, pathway of cell death is activated ('cell suicide'). Unlike necrosis, apoptosis is not accompanied by any inflammation and collateral tissue damage.

APOPTOSIS IN BIOLOGIC PROCESSES Apoptosis is responsible for mediating cell death in a wide variety of physiologic and pathologic processes as under:

Physiologic Processes:

1. Organised cell destruction in sculpting of tissues during *development of embryo*.

2. Physiologic involution of cells in *hormone-dependent tissues* e.g. endometrial shedding, regression of lactating breast after withdrawal of breast-feeding.

3. Normal cell destruction followed by *replacement proliferation* such as in intestinal epithelium.

4. *Involution of the thymus* in early age.

Pathologic Processes:

1. Cell death in tumours exposed to *chemotherapeutic agents*.

2. *Cell death by cytotoxic T cells* in immune mechanisms such as in graft-versus-host disease and rejection reactions.

3. Progressive *depletion of CD4+T cells* in the pathogenesis of AIDS.

4. *Cell death in viral infections* e.g. formation of Councilman bodies in viral hepatitis.

5. *Pathologic atrophy* of organs and tissues on withdrawal of stimuli e.g. prostatic atrophy after orchiectomy, atrophy of kidney or salivary gland on obstruction of ureter or ducts, respectively.

6. Cell death in response to low dose of *injurious agents* involved in causation of necrosis e.g. radiation, hypoxia and mild thermal injury.

7. In *degenerative diseases of CNS* e.g. in Alzheimer's disease, Parkinson's disease, and chronic infective dementias.

8. *Heart diseases* e.g. in acute myocardial infarction (20% necrosis and 80% apoptosis).

MORPHOLOGIC FEATURES The characteristic morphologic changes in apoptosis by light microscopy and electron microscopy are as under:
1. Involvement of *single cells or small clusters of cells* in the background of viable cells.

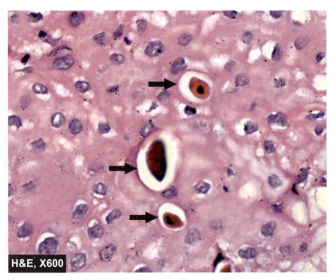

Figure 5.12 ▶ Apoptotic bodies in the layer of squamous mucosa (shown by arrows). The dead cell seen in singles, is shrunken, the nucleus has clumped chromatin, while the cytoplasms in intensely eosinophilic. There is no inflammation, unlike necrosis.

2. Apoptotic cells are round to oval *shrunken masses* of intensely eosinophilic cytoplasm (mummified cell) containing shrunken or almost-normal organelles (Fig. 5.12).
3. Nuclear chromatin is condensed under the nuclear membrane i.e. *pyknosis*.
4. The cell membrane may show *blebs or projections* on the surface.
5. There may be formation of membrane-bound near-spherical bodies containing condensed organelles around the cell called *apoptotic bodies*.
6. Characteristically, unlike necrosis, there is *no acute inflammatory reaction* around apoptosis.
7. *Phagocytosis* of apoptotic bodies by macrophages takes place at varying speed. There may be swift phagocytosis, or loosely floating apoptotic cells after losing contact with each other and basement membrane as single cells, or may result in major cell loss in the tissue without significant change in the overall tissue structure.

Techniques to identify and count apoptotic cells Apoptotic cells can be identified and counted by following methods:
1. Staining of chromatin condensation by haematoxylin, Feulgen stain.
2. Fluorescent stain with acridine orange dye.
3. Flow cytometry to visualise rapid cell shrinkage.
4. DNA changes detected by *in situ* techniques or by gel electrophoresis.
5. Immunohistochemical stain with annexin V for plasma membrane of apoptotic cell having phosphatidylserine on the cell exterior.

BIOCHEMICAL CHANGES Biochemical processes underlying the morphologic changes are as under:
1. Proteolysis of cytoskeletal proteins.
2. Protein-protein cross linkages.
3. After initial pyknosis of nucleus, there is fragmentation of chromatin by activation of nuclease.
4. Appearance of phosphatidylserine on the outer surface of cell membrane.
5. In some forms of apoptosis, appearance of an adhesive glycoprotein thrombospondin on the outer surface of apoptotic bodies.
6. Appearance of phosphatidylserine and thrombospondin on the outer surface of apoptotic cell facilitates early recognition by macrophages for phagocytosis prior to appearance of inflammatory cells.

MOLECULAR MECHANISMS OF APOPTOSIS Several physiologic and pathologic processes activate apoptosis in a variety of ways. However, in general, the following molecular events sum up the sequence involved in apoptosis (Fig. 5.13):

1. Initiators of apoptosis All cells have inbuilt effector mechanisms for cell survival and signals of cell death; it is the loss of this balance that determines survival or death of a cell. Accordingly, a cell may be initiated to programmed cell death as follows:

i) Withdrawal of normal cell survival signals e.g. absence of certain hormones, growth factors, cytokines.

ii) Agents of cell injury e.g. heat, radiation, hypoxia, toxins, free radicals.

2. Initial steps in apoptosis After the cell has been initiated into self-destruct mode, cell death signaling mechanisms get activated from *intrinsic (mitochondrial)* and *extrinsic (cell death receptor initiated)* pathways as outlined below. However, finally mediators of cell death are activated caspases. Caspases are a series of proteolytic or protein-splitting enzymes which act on nuclear proteins and organelles containing protein components. The term 'caspase' is derived from: *c* for cystein protease; *asp* for aspartic acid; and *ase* is used for naming an enzyme.

i) Intrinsic (mitochondrial) pathway: This pathway of cell death signaling is due to increased mitochondrial permeability and is a major mechanism. Mitochondria contain a protein called cytochrome c which is its lifeline in an intact mitochondria. But release of this protein from mitochondria into the cytoplasm of the cell triggers the cell into apoptosis. The major mechanism of regulation of this mitochondrial protein is by pro- and anti-apoptotic members of Bcl proteins. Bcl-2 oncogene was first detected on B-cell lymphoma and hence its name. Bcl-2 gene located on the mitochondrial inner membrane is a human counterpart of *CED-9* (*cell d*eath) gene regulating cell growth and cell death of nematode worm *Caenorhabditis elegans* which has been studied in detail. Among about 20 members of Bcl family of oncogenes, the growth promoter (anti-apoptotic) proteins

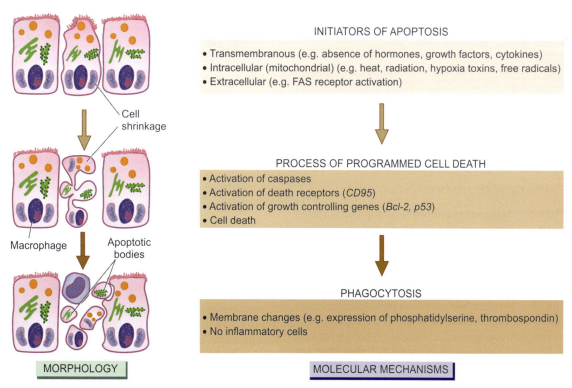

Figure 5.13 ▶ Molecular mechanism of apoptosis contrasted with sequence of morphologic changes.

are Bcl-2, Bcl-x and Mcl-1, while pro-apoptotic proteins are Bim, Bid and Bad which contain single Bcl-2 homology domain (also called BH-only proteins). The net effect on the mitochondrial membrane is based on the pro-apoptotic and anti-apoptotic actions of Bcl-2 gene family. Pro-apoptotic mechanism in turn activates Bcl-2 family effectors, Bax and Bak, which damage mitochondrial membrane and allow leakage of cytochrome c protein into cytoplasm. This, in turn, activates caspase cascade.

ii) Extrinsic (cell death receptor initiated) pathway: This signaling pathway of cell death is by activation of death receptors on the cell membrane. An important cell death receptor is type 1 tumour necrosis factor receptor (TNF-R1) and a related transmembrane protein called Fas (CD95) and its ligand (FasL). Fas is present on cytotoxic (CD 8+) T cells. Binding of Fas and FasL activates Fas-associated death domain (FADD) in the cytoplasm of the cell that activates caspases.

3. Final phase of apoptosis The final culmination of either of the above two mechanisms is activation of caspases. Mitochondrial pathway activates caspase-9 and death receptor pathway activates caspases-8 and 10. Other caspases which actively partake in the apoptotic process are caspases-3 and 6. These caspases act on various components of the cell such as DNAase and nuclear matrix proteins and lead to proteolytic actions on nucleus, chromatin clumping, cytoskeletal damage, disruption of endoplasmic reticulum, mitochondrial damage, and disturbed cell membrane.

4. Phagocytosis Dead apoptotic cells develop membrane changes which promote their phagocytosis. Phosphatidylserine and thrombospondin molecules which are normally present on the inside of the cell membrane, appear on the outer surface of the cells in apoptosis, which facilitate their identification by adjacent phagocytes and promotes phagocytosis. The phagocytosis is rapid and is unaccompanied by any inflammatory cells.

The contrasting features of apoptosis and necrosis are illustrated in **Fig. 5.14** and summarised in **Table 5.2**.

OTHER FORMS OF PROGRAMMED CELL DEATH

NECROPTOSIS
As the name indicates, necroptosis is a cross between necrosis and apoptosis; in other words it is a form of programmed necrosis. In usual forms of necrosis, there is leakage of cell's contents into extracellular compartment after cell death, while in necroptosis the process of leaking of the membrane is internally regulated or programmed.

Necroptosis is biochemically and morphologically similar to necrosis. However, at molecular level, necroptosis has some similarity with apoptosis in being triggered by ligation of TNFR1, FAS, and by proteins of viral DNA and RNA but differs from apoptosis in not involving caspase activation.

The examples of necroptosis are in following conditions:
1. Physiologic conditions such as in formation of bony growth plate

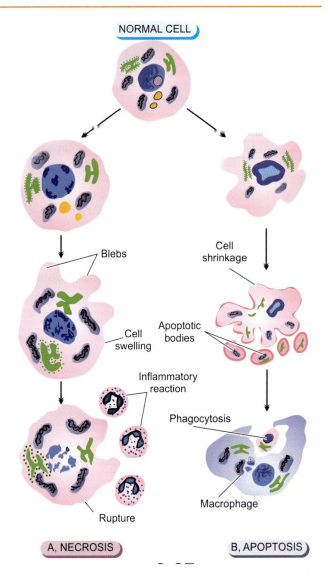

Figure 5.14 ▶ Necrosis and apoptosis. A, Cell necrosis is identified by homogeneous, eosinophilic cytoplasm and nuclear changes of pyknosis, karyolysis, and karyorrhexis. B, Apoptosis consists of condensation of nuclear chromatin and fragmentation of the cell into membrane-bound apoptotic bodies which are engulfed by macrophages.

2. Viral defense mechanism
3. Steatohepatitis
4. Inflammatory diseases e.g. Crohn's disease, pancreatitis.

PYROPTOSIS
Pyroptosis is a form of apoptosis in which there is release of fever-producing cytokine IL-1 (pyro=fever). Pyroptosis is triggered by cytoplasmic entry of microbial products which activates inflammasomes (inflammasomes are innate immune receptors that regulate the activation of caspases and induce inflammation when exposed to microbes). In pyroptosis, cell death is brought about by activation of caspase 1 and 11 which also generate IL-1.

Chapter 5: Morphology of Cell Injury: Degenerations and Cell Death

Table 5.2 Contrasting features of apoptosis and necrosis.

	FEATURE	APOPTOSIS	NECROSIS
1.	Definition	Programmed and coordinated cell death	Cell death along with degradation of tissue by hydrolytic enzymes
2.	Causative agents	Physiologic and pathologic processes	Hypoxia, toxins
3.	Morphology	i) No inflammatory reaction ii) Death of single cells iii) Cell shrinkage iv) Cytoplasmic blebs on membrane v) Apoptotic bodies vi) Chromatin condensation vii) Phagocytosis of apoptotic bodies by macrophages	i) Inflammatory reaction always present ii) Death of many adjacent cells iii) Cell swelling initially iv) Membrane disruption v) Damaged organelles vi) Nuclear disruption vii) Phagocytosis of cell debris by macrophages
4.	Molecular changes	i) Lysosomes and other organelles intact ii) Initiation of apoptosis by loss of signals of normal cell survival and by action of agents injurious to the cell iii) Triggered by intrinsic (mitochondrial) pathway (pro- and anti-apoptotic members of Bcl-2 family), extrinsic (cell death receptor initiated) pathway (TNF-R1, Fas, Fas-L) and finally by activated capases	i) Lysosomal breakdown with liberation of hydrolytic enzymes ii) Initiated by various etiologies (ischaemia hypoxia, chemicals, physical agents, microbes etc). iii) Cell death by ATP depletion, membrane damage, free radical injury

FERROPTOSIS Ferroptosis is cell death triggered by iron-dependent (i.e. by Fenton reaction) accumulation of reactive oxygen species in the cell. Cell death in these cases can be suppressed by iron-chelating agent, dysferroxamine.

AUTOPHAGY Autophagy (auto=self, phagy=eating) is a form of catabolic mechanism by which the cell degrades its own dysfunctional and worm out components by way of cannabilism. Autophagy is mediated by lysosomes.

Autophagy involves formation of a double membrane around organelle to be engulfed and degraded, generating autophagosome. Autophagosome moves through the cytosol of the cell and eventually fuses with lysosome, forming autolysosome which may be degraded by cell's own lysosomal hydrolases, or may even bring about cell death. The entire process of autophagy is induced by genes such as phosphoinositide-3-kinase, autophagy-related gene 6 and ubiquitin.

Besides being a mechanism of self-eating, autophagy has a role in following processes:
1. Promotes cell survival by providing energy during starvation and nutrient deprivation.
2. Role of accelerated autophagy in Alzheimer's disease.
3. In degradation of mycobacteria.
4. In causing lesions in inflammatory bowel disease (ulcerative colitis and Crohn's disease).

GIST BOX 5.2 Morphology of Irreversible Cell Injury (Cell Death)

- *Cell death* is a state of irreversible injury. Examples are autolysis, necrosis, and programmed cell death.
- Necrosis is a localised area of death in living tissue and is accompanied by inflammatory reaction.
- *Coagulative necrosis* is caused by sudden cessation of blood flow (ischaemic necrosis) e.g. infarcts of the heart, kidney, and spleen, or occurs by reduced supply of blood from other causes.
- *Liquefaction necrosis* also occurs due to ischaemic injury and bacterial or fungal infections but the hydrolytic enzymes in tissue degradation have a dominant role in causing semi-fluid material e.g. infarct brain and abscess cavity.
- *Caseous necrosis* combines features of both coagulative and liquefactive necrosis. It is found in the centres of foci of tuberculous infections and is accompanied by granulomatous inflammation.
- *Fat necrosis* is seen in the breast and acute pancreatitis; *fibrinoid necrosis* occurs due to immunologic tissue injury.
- *Programmed cell death* is coordinated and internally programmed cell death. Its classic form is apoptosis which has significance in a variety of physiologic (e.g. endometrial shedding) and pathologic conditions (e.g. viral infections).
- Morphologically, apoptotic cells appear as round to oval shrunken masses of intensely eosinophilic cytoplasm (*mummified cell*) containing pyknotic nucleus; it is not accompanied by any inflammation.
- Pathogenetically, apoptosis is triggered by loss of signals of normal cell survival and by action of agents injurious to the cell.
- Molecular mechanism of apoptosis is under genetic control which may be by intrinsic (mitochondrial) pathway (pro- and anti-apoptotic members of Bcl-2 family), extrinsic (cell death receptor initiated) pathway

(TNF-R1, Fas, Fas-L) and finally by activated capases. This is followed by phagocytosis of apoptotic bodies.
- ❖ A few other forms of programmed cell death are *necroptosis* (programmed necrosis), *pyroptosis* (associated with fever-producing cytokine IL-1), *ferroptosis* (iron-dependent reactive oxygen species) and *autophagy* (self-eating).

CHANGES AFTER CELL DEATH

Two types of pathologic changes may superimpose following cell injury: gangrene (after necrosis) and pathologic calcification (after degenerations as well as necrosis).

GANGRENE

Gangrene is necrosis of tissue associated with superadded putrefaction, most often following coagulative necrosis due to ischaemia (e.g. in gangrene of the bowel, gangrene of limb). On the other hand, *gangrenous or necrotising inflammation* is characterised primarily by inflammation provoked by virulent bacteria resulting in massive tissue necrosis. Thus, the end-result of necrotising inflammation and gangrene is the same but the way the two are produced, is different. The examples of necrotising inflammation are: gangrenous appendicitis, gangrenous stomatitis (noma, cancrumoris).

There are 2 main types of gangrene—dry and wet, and a variant of wet gangrene called gas gangrene. In all types of gangrene, necrosis undergoes liquefaction by the action of putrefactive bacteria.

Dry Gangrene

This form of gangrene begins in the distal part of a limb due to ischaemia. The typical example is the dry gangrene in the toes and feet of an old patient due to severe atherosclerosis. Other causes of dry gangrene foot include thromboangiitis obliterans (Buerger's disease), Raynaud's disease, trauma, ergot poisoning. It is usually initiated in one of the toes which is farthest from the blood supply, containing so little blood that even the invading bacteria find it hard to grow in the necrosed tissue. The gangrene spreads slowly upwards until it reaches a point where the blood supply is adequate to keep the tissue viable. A *line of separation* is formed at this point between the gangrenous part and the viable part.

MORPHOLOGIC FEATURES Grossly, the affected part is dry, shrunken and dark black, resembling the foot of a mummy. It is black due to liberation of haemoglobin from haemolysed red blood cells which is acted upon by hydrogen disulfide (H_2S) produced by bacteria resulting in formation of black iron sulfide. The line of separation usually brings about complete separation with eventual falling off of the gangrenous tissue if it is not removed surgically (*i.e. spontaneous amputation*) **(Fig. 5.15)**.

Histologically, there is necrosis with smudging of the tissue. The line of separation consists of inflammatory granulation tissue **(Fig. 5.16)**.

Wet Gangrene

Wet gangrene occurs in naturally moist tissues and organs such as the bowel, lung, mouth, cervix, vulva etc. Two other

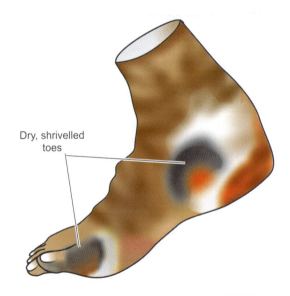
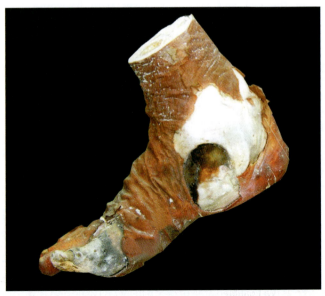

Figure 5.15 ▶ Dry gangrene of the foot. The gangrenous area is dry, shrunken and dark and is separated from the viable tissue by clear line of separation.

Chapter 5: Morphology of Cell Injury: Degenerations and Cell Death

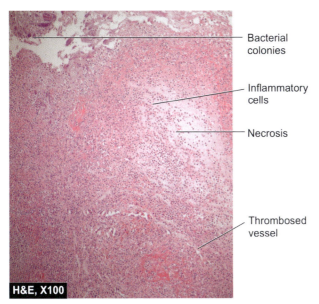

Figure 5.16 ▶ Dry gangrene of the foot. Microscopy shows coagulative necrosis of the skin, muscle and other soft tissue, and thrombosed vessels.

examples of wet gangrene having clinical significance are as follows:

◈ *Diabetic foot* which is due to high glucose content in the necrosed tissue which favours growth of bacteria.

◈ *Bed sores* occurring in a bed-ridden patient due to pressure on sites like the sacrum, buttocks and heel.

Wet gangrene usually develops due to blockage of both venous as well as arterial blood flow and is more rapid. The affected part is stuffed with blood which favours the rapid growth of putrefactive bacteria. The toxic products formed by bacteria are absorbed causing profound systemic manifestations of septicaemia, and finally death. The spreading wet gangrene generally lacks clear-cut line of demarcation and may spread to peritoneal cavity causing peritonitis.

MORPHOLOGIC FEATURES **Grossly,** the affected part is soft, swollen, putrid, rotten and dark. The classic example is gangrene of the bowel, commonly due to strangulated hernia, volvulus or intussusception. The part is stained dark black due to the same mechanism as in dry gangrene (Fig. 5.17).

Histologically, there is coagulative necrosis with stuffing of affected part with blood. The mucosa is ulcerated and sloughed. Lumen of the bowel contains mucus and blood. There is intense acute inflammatory exudates and thrombosed vessels. The line of demarcation between gangrenous segment and viable bowel is generally not clear-cut (Fig. 5.18).

Contrasting features of two main forms of gangrene are summarised in Table 5.3.

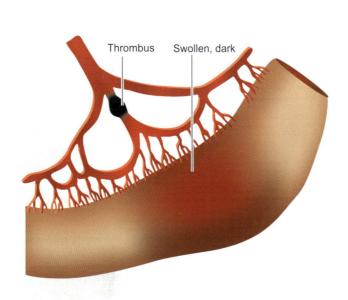

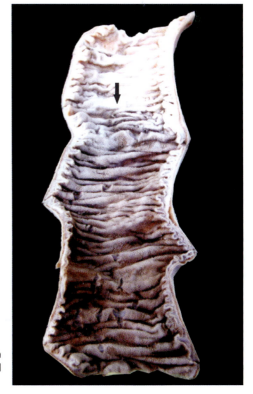

Figure 5.17 ▶ Wet gangrene of the small bowel. The affected part is soft, swollen and dark. Line of demarcation between gangrenous segment and the viable bowel is not clear-cut.

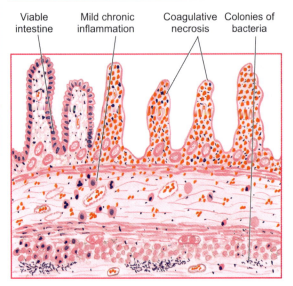
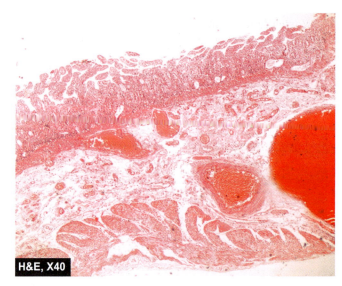

Figure 5.18 ▶ Wet gangrene of the small bowel. Microscopy shows coagulative necrosis of the affected bowel wall and thrombosed vessels while the junction with normal intestine is indistinct and shows an inflammatory infiltrate.

GAS GANGRENE It is a special form of wet gangrene caused by gas-forming clostridia (gram-positive anaerobic bacteria) which gain entry into the tissues through open contaminated wounds, especially in the muscles, or as a complication of operation on colon which normally contains clostridia. Clostridia produce various toxins which produce necrosis and oedema locally and are also absorbed producing profound systemic manifestations.

MORPHOLOGIC FEATURES *Grossly*, the affected area is swollen, oedematous, painful and crepitant due to accumulation of gas bubbles of carbon dioxide within the tissues formed by fermentation of sugars by bacterial toxins. Subsequently, the affected tissue becomes dark black and is foul smelling.
Microscopically, the muscle fibres undergo coagulative necrosis with liquefaction. Large number of gram-positive bacilli can be identified. At the periphery, a zone of leucocytic infiltration, oedema and congestion are found. Capillary and venous thrombi are common.

PATHOLOGIC CALCIFICATION

Deposition of calcium salts in tissues other than osteoid or enamel is called pathologic or heterotopic calcification. Two distinct types of pathologic calcification are recognised:
◈ *Dystrophic calcification* is characterised by deposition of calcium salts in dead or degenerated tissues with normal calcium metabolism and normal serum calcium level.
◈ *Metastatic calcification*, on the other hand, occurs in apparently normal tissues and is associated with deranged calcium metabolism and hypercalcaemia.
Etiology and pathogenesis of the two are different but morphologically the deposits in both resemble normal minerals of the bone.

Table 5.3 Contrasting features of dry and wet gangrene.

	FEATURE	DRY GANGRENE	WET GANGRENE
1.	Site	Commonly limbs	More common in bowel
2.	Mechanisms	Arterial occlusion	Blockage of both venous drainage and arterial obstruction
3.	Macroscopy	Organ dry, shrunken and black	Part moist, soft, swollen, rotten and dark
4.	Putrefaction	Limited due to very little blood supply	Marked due to stuffing of organ with blood
5.	Line of demarcation	Present at the junction between healthy and gangrenous part	No clear line of demarcation
6.	Bacteria	Bacteria fail to survive	Numerous present
7.	Prognosis	Generally better due to little septicaemia	Generally poor due to profound toxaemia

Histologically, in routine H and E stained sections, calcium salts appear as deeply basophilic, irregular and granular clumps. The deposits may be intracellular, extracellular, or at both locations. Occasionally, heterotopic bone formation (ossification) may occur. Calcium deposits can be confirmed by special stains like silver impregnation method of *von-Kossa* producing black colour, and *alizarin red S* that produces red staining. Pathologic calcification is often accompanied by diffuse or granular deposits of iron giving positive Prussian blue reaction in Perl's stain.

Etiopathogenesis

These two types of pathologic calcification result from distinctly different etiologies and mechanisms.

DYSTROPHIC CALCIFICATION As apparent from definition, dystrophic calcification may occur due to 2 types of causes:
- Calcification in dead tissue.
- Calcification of degenerated tissue.

Calcification in dead tissue
1. *Caseous necrosis* in tuberculosis is the most common site for dystrophic calcification. Living bacilli may be present even in calcified tuberculous lesions, lymph nodes, lungs, etc (Fig. 5.19).
2. *Liquefaction necrosis* in chronic abscesses may get calcified.
3. *Fat necrosis* following acute pancreatitis or traumatic fat necrosis in the breast results in deposition of calcium soaps.
4. *Gamna-Gandy bodies* in chronic venous congestion (CVC) of the spleen is characterised by calcific deposits admixed with haemosiderin on fibrous tissue.
5. *Infarcts* may sometimes undergo dystrophic calcification.
6. *Thrombi,* especially in the veins, may produce phleboliths.
7. *Haematomas* in the vicinity of bones may undergo dystrophic calcification.
8. *Dead parasites* like in hydatid cyst, Schistosoma eggs, and cysticercosis are some of the examples showing dystrophic calcification.
9. Microcalcification in *breast cancer* detected by mammography.
10. *Congenital toxoplasmosis* involving the central nervous system visualised by calcification in the infant brain.

Calcification in degenerated tissues
1. *Dense old scars* may undergo hyaline degeneration and subsequent calcification.
2. *Atheromas* in the aorta and coronaries frequently undergo calcification.
3. *Mönckeberg's sclerosis* shows calcification in the degenerated tunica media of muscular arteries in elderly people (Fig. 5.20).
4. *Stroma of tumours* such as uterine fibroids, breast cancer, thyroid adenoma, goitre etc show calcification.
5. *Goitre* of the thyroid may show presence of calcification in areas of degeneration.
6. Some tumours show characteristic spherules of calcification called *psammoma bodies* or calcospherites such as in meningioma, papillary serous cystadenocarcinoma of the ovary and papillary carcinoma of the thyroid.
7. *Cysts* which have been present for a long time may show calcification of their walls e.g. epidermal and pilar cysts.

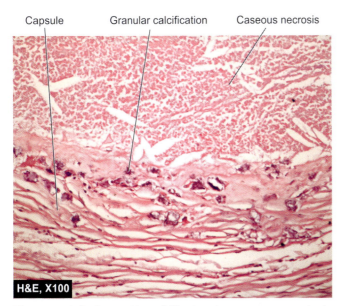

Figure 5.19 ▶ Dystrophic calcification in caseous necrosis in tuberculous lymph node. In H and E, the deposits are basophilic granular while the periphery shows healed granulomas.

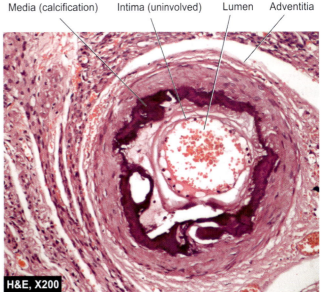

Figure 5.20 ▶ Dystrophic calcification in degenerated tunica media of muscular artery of uterine myometrium in Mönckeberg's arteriosclerosis.

8. *Calcinosis cutis* is a condition of unknown cause in which there are irregular nodular deposits of calcium salts in the skin and subcutaneous tissue.
9. *Senile degenerative changes* may be accompanied by dystrophic calcification such as in costal cartilages, tracheal or bronchial cartilages, and pineal gland in the brain etc.

Pathogenesis of dystrophic calcification Process of dystrophic calcification has been likened to the formation of normal hydroxyapatite of bone i.e. binding of phosphate ions with calcium ions to form precipitates of calcium phosphate. It involves phases of initiation and propagation as follows:

❖ *Initiation:* Following cell injury (i.e. degeneration or necrosis), there is membrane damage and release of membrane phospholipids. Phosphatases associated with phospholipids generate phosphate ions. It is also known that there is excess uptake of calcium by injured mitochondria in degeneration and necrosis. Thus, calcium and phosphate so generated from these mechanisms form precipitates of calcium phosphate.

❖ *Propagation:* Simultaneously, some structural changes occur in calcium and phosphate groups which result in further propagation of deposits and form mineral crystals.

METASTATIC CALCIFICATION Since metastatic calcification occurs in normal tissues due to hypercalcaemia, its causes would include either of the following two groups of causes:
❖ Excessive mobilisation of calcium from the bone.
❖ Excessive absorption of calcium from the gut.

Excessive mobilisation of calcium from the bone These causes are more common and include the following:
1. *Hyperparathyroidism* which may be primary such as due to parathyroid adenoma, or secondary such as from parathyroid hyperplasia, chronic renal failure etc.
2. *Bony destructive lesions* such as multiple myeloma, metastatic carcinoma.
3. *Hypercalcaemia* as a part of paraneoplastic syndrome e.g. in breast cancer.
4. *Prolonged immobilisation* of a patient results in disuse atrophy of the bones and hypercalcaemia.

Excessive absorption of calcium from the gut Less often, excess calcium may be absorbed from the gut causing hypercalcaemia and metastatic calcification. These causes are as under:
1. *Hypervitaminosis D* from excessive intake or in sarcoidosis.
2. *Milk-alkali syndrome* caused by excessive oral intake of calcium in the form of milk and administration of calcium carbonate in the treatment of peptic ulcer.
3. *Idiopathic hypercalcaemia of infancy* (William's syndrome).
4. *Renal causes* such as in renal tubular acidosis.

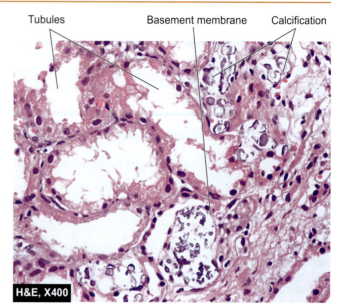

Figure 5.21 ▶ Metastatic calcification in tubular basement membrane in nephrocalcinosis due to hypercalcaemia.

Sites of metastatic calcification Metastatic calcification may occur in any normal tissue of the body but preferentially affects the following organs and tissues:
1. *Kidneys*, especially at the basement membrane of tubular epithelium and in the tubular lumina, causing nephrocalcinosis **(Fig. 5.21)**.
2. *Lungs*, especially in the alveolar walls.
3. *Stomach*, on the acid-secreting fundal glands.
4. *Blood vessels*, especially on the internal elastic lamina.
5. *Cornea* is another site affected by metastatic calcification.
6. *Synovium* of the joint causing pain and dysfunction.

Pathogenesis of metastatic calcification Metastatic calcification occurs due to excessive binding of inorganic phosphate ions with elevated calcium ions due to underlying metabolic derangement. This leads to precipitates of calcium phosphate at the preferential sites, due to presence of acid secretions or rapid changes in pH levels at these sites. Metastatic calcification is reversible upon correction of underlying metabolic disorder.

The distinguishing features between the two types of pathologic calcification are summarised in **Table 5.4**.

 GIST BOX 5.3 | **Changes after Cell Death**

❖ *Gangrene* is necrosis of tissue associated with superadded putrefaction, most often following coagulative necrosis due to ischaemia. There are 2 main types of gangrene—dry and wet.
❖ *Dry gangrene* begins in the distal part of a limb due to ischaemia e.g. due to severe atherosclerosis and

Chapter 5: Morphology of Cell Injury: Degenerations and Cell Death

Table 5.4	Differences between dystrophic and metastatic calcification.	
FEATURE	DYSTROPHIC CALCIFICATION	METASTATIC CALCIFICATION
1. Definition	Deposits of calcium salts in dead and degenerated tissues	Deposits of calcium salts in normal tissues
2. Calcium metabolism	Normal	Deranged
3. Serum calcium level	Normal	Hypercalcaemia
4. Reversibility	Generally irreversible	Reversible upon correction of metabolic disorder
5. Causes	Necrosis (caseous, liquefactive, fat), infarcts, thrombi, haematomas, dead parasites, old scars, atheromas, Mönckeberg's sclerosis, certain tumours, cysts, calcinosis cutis	Hyperparathyroidism (due to adenoma, hyperplasia, CRF), bony destructive lesions (e.g. myeloma, metastatic carcinoma), prolonged immobilisation, hypervitaminosis D, milk-alkali syndrome, hypercalcaemia of infancy
6. Pathogenesis	Increased binding of phosphates with necrotic and degenerative tissue, which in turn binds to calcium forming calcium phosphate precipitates	Increased precipitates of calcium phosphate due to hypercalcaemia at certain sites e.g. in lungs, stomach, blood vessels and cornea

Buerger's disease. A line of separation generally marks the junction of viable and gangrenous tissue e.g. gangrene foot.
❖ *Wet gangrene* occurs in naturally moist tissues and organs e.g. gangrene bowel, lungs. A line of separation between viable and non-viable tissue is not distinct.
❖ *Diabetic foot* and *bed sores* are also examples of wet gangrene. *Gas gangrene* is a special form of wet gangrene caused by gas-forming clostridia.

❖ **Pathologic or heterotopic calcification** is deposition of calcium salts in tissues other than osteoid or enamel. It is of 2 types: dystrophic and metastatic calcification.
❖ **Dystrophic calcification** is characterised by deposition of calcium salts in necrotic or degenerated tissues with normal calcium metabolism and normal serum calcium level e.g. in caseous necrosis in tuberculosis, severe atherosclerosis.
❖ **Metastatic calcification** occurs in normal tissues and is associated with deranged calcium metabolism and hypercalcaemia e.g. from excessive mobilisation of calcium from bones, and excessive intestinal absorption.

6 Intracellular Accumulations

Intracellular accumulation of substances in abnormal amounts can occur within the cytoplasm (especially lysosomes) or nucleus of the cell. This phenomenon was previously referred to as *infiltration*, meaning thereby that something unusual has infiltrated the cell from outside which is not always the case. Intracellular accumulation of the substance in mild degree causes reversible cell injury while more severe damage results in irreversible cell injury.

Abnormal intracellular accumulations can be divided into 3 groups:

i) *Accumulation of constituents of normal cell metabolism produced in excess* e.g. accumulations of lipids (fatty change, cholesterol deposits), proteins and carbohydrates.

ii) *Accumulation of abnormal substances* produced as a result of abnormal metabolism due to lack of some enzymes e.g. storage diseases or inborn errors of metabolism (Chapter 8).

iii) *Accumulation of pigments* e.g. endogenous pigments under special circumstances, and exogenous pigments due to lack of enzymatic mechanisms to degrade the substances or transport them to other sites.

It may be mentioned here that amyloid is extracellular deposition of abnormal proteinaceous substance discussed in Chapter 7.

Various examples of these conditions are discussed below.

EXCESSIVE INTRACELLULAR ACCUMULATION OF NORMAL CONSTITUENTS

These substances accumulate inside the cell when they are produced in excess e.g. fats, proteins and carbohydrates.

FATTY CHANGE (STEATOSIS)

Fatty change, steatosis or fatty metamorphosis is the intracellular accumulation of neutral fat within parenchymal cells. It includes the older, now abandoned, terms of *fatty degeneration* and *fatty infiltration* because fatty change neither necessarily involves degeneration nor an infiltration. The deposit is in the cytosol and represents an absolute increase in the intracellular lipids. Fatty change is particularly common in the liver but may occur in other non-fatty tissues as well e.g. in the heart, skeletal muscle, kidneys (lipoid nephrosis or minimum change disease) and other organs.

Fatty Liver

Liver is the commonest site for accumulation of fat because it plays central role in fat metabolism. Depending upon the cause and amount of accumulation, fatty change may be mild and reversible, or severe producing irreversible cell injury and cell death.

ETIOLOGY Fatty change in the liver may result from one of the two types of causes:

1. **Conditions with excess fat** i.e. conditions in which the capacity of the liver to metabolise fat is exceeded e.g.
i) Obesity
ii) Diabetes mellitus
iii) Congenital hyperlipidaemia

2. **Liver cell damage** i.e. conditions in which fat cannot be metabolised due to liver cell injury e.g.
i) Alcoholic liver disease (most common)
ii) Starvation
iii) Protein calorie malnutrition
iv) Chronic illnesses (e.g. tuberculosis)
v) Acute fatty liver in late pregnancy
vi) Hypoxia (e.g. anaemia, cardiac failure)
vii) Hepatotoxins (e.g. carbon tetrachloride, chloroform, ether, aflatoxins and other poisons)
viii) Drug-induced liver cell injury (e.g. administration of methotrexate, steroids, CCl_4, halothane anaesthetic, tetracycline etc)
ix) Reye's syndrome

PATHOGENESIS Mechanism of fatty liver depends upon the stage at which the etiologic agent acts in the normal fat transport and metabolism. Hence, pathogenesis of fatty liver is best understood in the light of normal fat metabolism in the liver **(Fig. 6.1)**.

Lipids as free fatty acids enter the liver cell from either of the following 2 sources:

◆ *From diet* as chylomicrons (containing triglycerides and phospholipids) and as free fatty acids.

◆ *From adipose tissue* as free fatty acids.

Normally, besides above two sources, a small part of fatty acids is also synthesised from acetate in the liver cells. Most of free fatty acid is esterified to triglycerides by the action of α-glycerophosphate and only a small part is changed

Chapter 6: Intracellular Accumulations

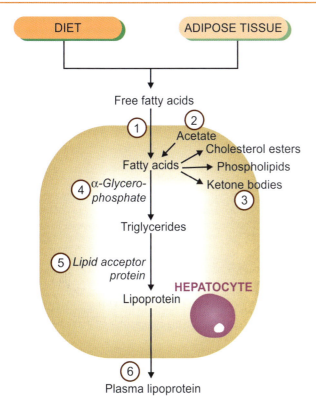

Figure 6.1 ▶ Lipid metabolism in the pathogenesis of fatty liver. Defects in any of the six numbered steps (corresponding to the description in the text) can produce fatty liver by different etiologic agents.

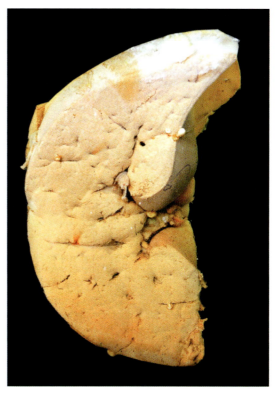

Figure 6.2 ▶ Fatty liver. Sectioned slice of the liver shows pale yellow parenchyma with rounded borders.

into cholesterol, phospholipids and ketone bodies. While cholesterol, phospholipids and ketones are used in the body, intracellular triglycerides are converted into lipoproteins, which require 'lipid acceptor protein'. Lipoproteins are released from the liver cells into circulation as plasma lipoproteins (LDL, VLDL).

In fatty liver, intracellular accumulation of triglycerides occurs due to defect at one or more of the following *6 steps* in the normal fat metabolism shown in **Fig. 6.1**:
1. Increased entry of free fatty acids into the liver.
2. Increased synthesis of fatty acids by the liver.
3. Decreased conversion of fatty acids into ketone bodies resulting in increased esterification of fatty acids to triglycerides.
4. Increased α-glycerophosphate causing increased esterification of fatty acids to triglycerides.
5. Decreased synthesis of 'lipid acceptor protein' resulting in decreased formation of lipoprotein from triglycerides.
6. Block in the excretion of lipoprotein from the liver into plasma.

In fatty liver from many causes, one of the above mechanisms is operating, but liver cell injury from chronic alcoholism is multifactorial which includes following:
i) Increased lipolysis
ii) Increased free fatty acid synthesis
iii) Decreased triglyceride utilisation
iv) Decreased fatty acid oxidation to ketone bodies
v) Block in lipoprotein excretion

Even a severe form of fatty liver may be reversible if the liver is given time to regenerate and progressive fibrosis has not developed. For example, intermittent drinking is less harmful because the liver cells get time to recover; similarly a chronic alcoholic who becomes teetotaler the enlarged fatty liver may return to normal if fibrosis has not developed. This subject is discussed in detail in Chapter 27.

MORPHOLOGIC FEATURES **Grossly**, the liver in fatty change is enlarged with a tense, glistening capsule and rounded margins. The cut surface bulges slightly and is pale-yellow to yellow and is greasy to touch (**Fig. 6.2**).

Microscopically, characteristic feature is the presence of numerous lipid vacuoles in the cytoplasm of hepatocytes. Fat in H & E stained section prepared by paraffin-embedding technique appear as non-staining vacuoles because it is dissolved in organic solvents used (**Fig. 6.3**):
i) The vacuoles are initially small and are present around the nucleus *(microvesicular)*.
ii) With progression of the process, the vacuoles become larger pushing the nucleus to the periphery of the cells *(macrovesicular)*.

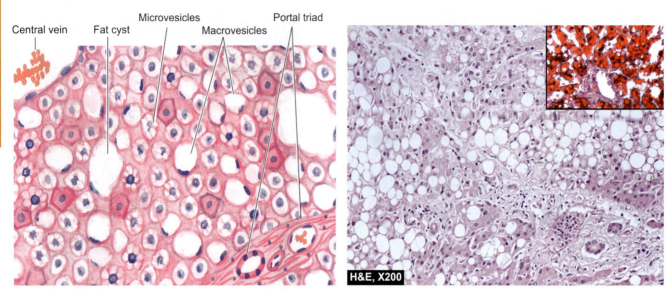

Figure 6.3 ▶ Fatty liver. Many of the hepatocytes are distended with large fat vacuoles pushing the nuclei to the periphery (macrovesicles), while others show multiple small vacuoles in the cytoplasm (microvesicles). Inbox shows red colour in the cytoplasmic fat in the hepatocytes in Oil Red O stain in frozen section.

iii) At times, the hepatocytes laden with large lipid vacuoles may rupture and lipid vacuoles coalesce to form fatty cysts.
iv) Infrequently, *lipogranulomas* may appear as a reaction to extravasated fat and consist of collections of lymphocytes, macrophages, and some multinucleated giant cells.
v) Fat can be demonstrated in fresh unfixed tissue by frozen section by *fat stains* e.g. Sudan dyes (Sudan III, IV, Sudan black) and oil red O. Alternatively, osmic acid which is a fixative as well as a stain can be used to demonstrate fat in the tissue.

Cholesterol Deposits

Intracellular deposits of cholesterol and its esters in macrophages may occur when there is hypercholesterolaemia. This turns macrophages into foam cells. The examples are as follows:
1. *Fibrofatty plaques* of atherosclerosis (Chapter 25).
2. Clusters of foam cells in tumour-like masses called *xanthomas* and *xanthelasma*.

Stromal Fatty Infiltration

This form of lipid accumulation is quite different from parenchymal fatty change just described. Stromal fatty infiltration is the deposition of mature adipose cells in the stromal connective tissue in contrast to intracellular deposition of fat in the parenchymal cells in fatty change. The condition occurs most often in patients with obesity. The two commonly affected organs are the heart and the pancreas. Thus, heart can be the site for intramyocardial fatty change as well as epicardial (stromal) fatty infiltration. The presence of mature adipose cells in the stroma generally does not produce any dysfunction.

INTRACELLULAR ACCUMULATION OF PROTEINS

Pathologic accumulation of proteins in the cytoplasm of cells may occur in the following conditions:
1. In *proteinuria*, there is excessive renal tubular reabsorption of proteins by the proximal tubular epithelial cells which show pink hyaline droplets in their cytoplasm. The change is reversible; with control of proteinuria the protein droplets disappear.
2. The cytoplasm of actively functioning plasma cells shows pink hyaline inclusions called *Russell's bodies* representing synthesised immunoglobulins.
3. In α1-*antitrypsin deficiency*, the cytoplasm of hepatocytes shows eosinophilic globular deposits of a mutant protein.
4. *Mallory's body* or alcoholic hyaline in the hepatocytes is intracellular accumulation of intermediate filaments of cytokeratin and appear as amorphous pink masses.

INTRACELLULAR ACCUMULATION OF GLYCOGEN

Conditions associated with excessive accumulation of intracellular glycogen are as under:
1. In *diabetes mellitus*, there is intracellular accumulation of glycogen in different tissues because normal cellular uptake of glucose is impaired. Glycogen deposits in diabetes mellitus are seen in epithelium of distal portion of proximal convoluted tubule and descending loop of Henle, in the hepatocytes, in beta cells of pancreatic islets, and in cardiac muscle cells. In routine H & E stained sections, deposits of glycogen produce clear vacuoles in the cytoplasm of

the affected cells. Best's carmine and periodic acid-Schiff (PAS) staining may be employed to confirm the presence of glycogen in the cells.

2. In *glycogen storage diseases or glycogenosis*, there is defective metabolism of glycogen due to genetic disorders. These conditions along with other similar genetic disorders are discussed in Chapter 8.

> **GIST BOX 6.1   Intracellular Accumulations**
>
> ❖ Intracellular accumulations may occur from normal constituents of cell metabolism (e.g. fats, proteins, carbohydrates), or accumulation of abnormal substances due to either absence of some metabolic enzymes or due to pigments.
> ❖ Fatty change is deposition of fat in the parenchymal cells or organs such as liver, kidneys, muscle, pancreas etc.
> ❖ Fatty liver is more common and occurs from various etiologies, most often from alcoholic liver disease; others are obesity, diabetes, starvation, pregnancy, drugs etc.
> ❖ Mechanism for fatty liver is due to excess of free fatty acids, either from diet or from adipose tissues, resulting in intracellular accumulation of triglycerides in the hepatocytes.
> ❖ Fatty liver is characterised by enlarged pale-yellow liver, having cytoplasmic vacuoles (microvesicles or macrovesicles) in the hepatocytes.
> ❖ Fat in the sections can be stained by fat stains e.g. Sudan black, Sudan II, IV, Oil Red O and osmic acid.
> ❖ Stromal fatty infiltration is extracellular accumulation of adipocytes.
> ❖ Intracellular accumulation of proteins may occur in tubular epithelial cells in diabetes, alcoholic hyaline in liver cells, Russells's bodies in the plasma cells.
> ❖ Intracellular glycogen accumulates in tubular cells in diabetes and in parenchymal cells in glycogen storage diseases.

PIGMENTS

Pigments are coloured substances present in most living beings including humans. There are 2 broad categories of pigments: endogenous and exogenous **(Table 6.1)**.

A. ENDOGENOUS PIGMENTS

Endogenous pigments are either normal constituents of cells or accumulate under special circumstances e.g. melanin, alkaptonuria, haemoprotein-derived pigments, and lipofuscin.

Melanin

Melanin is the brown-black, non-haemoglobin-derived pigment normally present in the hair, skin, mucosa at some places, choroid of the eye, meninges and adrenal medulla.

Table 6.1	Pigments of the body.

A. ENDOGENOUS PIGMENTS
  1. Melanin
  2. Melanin-like pigment
     a. Alkaptonuria
     b. Dubin-Johnson syndrome
  3. Haemoprotein-derived pigments
     i)   Haemosiderin
     ii) Acid haematin (Haemozoin)
     iii) Bilirubin
     iv) Porphyrins
  4. Lipofuscin (Wear and tear pigment)

B. EXOGENOUS PIGMENTS
  1. Inhaled pigments
  2. Ingested pigments
  3. Injected pigments (Tattooing)

In skin, it is synthesised in the melanocytes and dendritic cells, both of which are present in the basal cells of the epidermis and is stored in the form of cytoplasmic granules in the phagocytic cells called the melanophores, present in the underlying dermis. Melanocytes possess the enzyme tyrosinase necessary for synthesis of melanin from tyrosine. However, sometimes tyrosinase is present but is not active and hence no melanin pigment is visible. In such cases, the presence of tyrosinase can be detected by incubation of tissue section in the solution of dihydroxy phenyl alanine (DOPA). If the enzyme is present, dark pigment is identified in pigment cells. This test is called as *DOPA reaction* and may be used for differentiating amelanotic melanoma from other anaplastic tumours.

Various disorders of melanin pigmentation cause generalised and localised hyperpigmentation and hypo-pigmentation:

i) Generalised hyperpigmentation:

a) In *Addison's disease*, there is generalised hyperpigmentation of the skin, especially in areas exposed to light, and of buccal mucosa.

b) *Chloasma* observed during pregnancy is the hyperpigmentation on the skin of face, nipples, and genitalia and occurs under the influence of oestrogen. A similar appearance may be observed in women taking oral contraceptives.

c) In *chronic arsenical poisoning*, there is characteristic raindrop pigmentation of the skin.

ii) Focal hyperpigmentation:

a) *Cäfe-au-lait spots* are pigmented patches seen in neurofibromatosis and Albright's syndrome.

b) *Peutz-Jeghers syndrome* is characterised by focal peri-oral pigmentation.

c) *Melanosis coli* is pigmentation of the mucosa of the colon.

d) *Melanotic tumours*, both benign such as pigmented naevi **(Fig. 6.4)**, and malignant such as melanoma, are associated with increased melanogenesis.

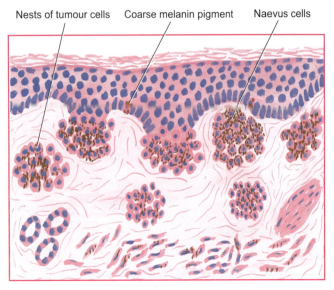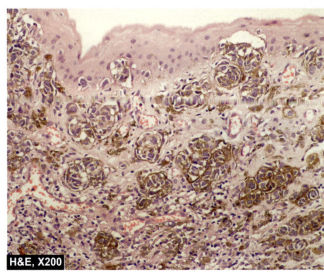

Figure 6.4 ▶ Compound naevus showing clusters of benign naevus cells in the dermis as well as in lower epidermis. These cells contain coarse, granular, brown-black melanin pigment.

e) *Lentigo* is a pre-malignant condition in which there is focal hyperpigmentation on the skin of hands, face, neck, and arms.

f) *Dermatopathic lymphadenitis* is an example of deposition of melanin pigment in macrophages of the lymph nodes draining skin lesions.

iii) **Generalised hypopigmentation** *Albinism* is an extreme degree of generalised hypopigmentation in which tyrosinase enzyme is genetically defective and no melanin is formed in the melanocytes. Oculocutaneous albinos have no pigment in the skin and have blond hair, poor vision and severe photophobia. They are highly sensitive to sunlight. Chronic sun exposure may lead to precancerous lesions and squamous and basal cell cancers of the skin in such individuals.

iv) **Localised hypopigmentation**

a) *Leucoderma* is an autoimmune condition with localised loss of pigmentation of the skin.

b) *Vitiligo* is also local hypopigmentation of the skin and is more common. It may have familial tendency.

c) *Acquired focal hypopigmentation* can result from various causes such as leprosy, healing of wounds, DLE, radiation dermatitis etc.

Melanin-like Pigments

ALKAPTONURIA This is a rare autosomal recessive disorder in which there is deficiency of an oxidase enzyme required for breakdown of homogentisic acid; the latter then accumulates in the tissues and is excreted in the urine (homogentisicaciduria). The urine of patients of alkaptonuria, if allowed to stand for some hours in air, turns black due to oxidation of homogentisic acid. The pigment is melanin-like and is termed *ochronosis*, first described by Virchow. It is deposited both intracellularly and intercellularly, most often in the periarticular tissues such as cartilages, capsules of joints, ligaments and tendons.

DUBIN-JOHNSON SYNDROME Hepatocytes in patients of Dubin-Johnson syndrome, an autosomal recessive form of hereditary conjugated hyperbilirubinaemia, contain melanin-like pigment in the cytoplasm (page 536).

Haemoprotein-derived Pigments

Haemoproteins are the most important endogenous pigments derived from haemoglobin, cytochromes and their break-down products. For an understanding of disorders of haemoproteins, it is essential to have knowledge of normal iron metabolism and its transport which is described in Chapter 22. In disordered iron metabolism and transport, haemoprotein-derived pigments accumulate in the body. These pigments are haemosiderin, acid haematin (haemozoin), bilirubin, and porphyrins.

1. **HAEMOSIDERIN** Iron is stored in the tissues in 2 forms:
◆ *Ferritin*, which is iron complexed to apoferritin and can be identified by electron microscopy.
◆ *Haemosiderin*, which is formed by aggregates of ferritin and is identifiable by light microscopy as golden-yellow to brown, granular pigment, especially within the mononuclear phagocytes of the bone marrow, spleen and liver where break-down of senescent red cells takes place (**Fig. 6.5, A**). Haemosiderin is ferric iron that can be demonstrated by

Chapter 6: Intracellular Accumulations

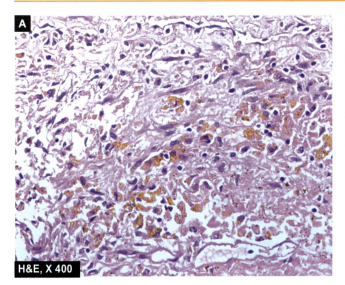
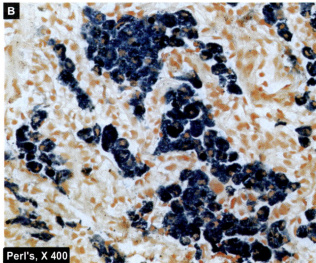

Figure 6.5 ▶ Haemosiderin pigment in the cytoplasm. H & E stain shows golden brown granules in the cytoplasm of macrophages (A) which stain positive in Perl's stain as Prussian blue granules (B).

Perl's stain that produces Prussian blue reaction. In this reaction, colourless potassium ferrocyanide reacts with ferric ions of haemosiderin to form deep blue *ferric-ferrocyanide* (**Fig. 6.5, B**).

Excessive storage of haemosiderin occurs in conditions when there is increased break-down of red cells causing systemic overload of iron. This may occur due to primary (idiopathic, hereditary) haemochromatosis, and secondary (acquired) causes such as in chronic haemolytic anaemias (e.g. thalassaemia), sideroblastic anaemia, alcoholic cirrhosis, multiple blood transfusions etc.

Accordingly, the effects of haemosiderin excess are as under (**Fig. 6.6**):

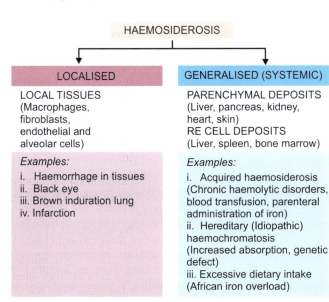

Figure 6.6 ▶ Effects of haemosiderosis.

a) Localised haemosiderosis This develops whenever there is haemorrhage into the tissues. With lysis of red cells, haemoglobin is liberated which is taken up by macrophages where it is degraded and stored as haemosiderin. A few examples are as under:

◈ Changing colours of a bruise or a *black eye* are caused by the pigments like biliverdin and bilirubin which are formed during transformation of haemoglobin into haemosiderin.

◈ *Brown induration* of the lungs as a result of small haemorrhages occurring in mitral stenosis and left ventricular failure. Microscopy reveals the presence of 'heart failure cells' in the alveoli which are haemosiderin-laden alveolar macrophages.

b) Generalised (Systemic or Diffuse) haemosiderosis Systemic overload with iron may result in generalised haemosiderosis. There can be two types of patterns:

◈ *Parenchymatous deposition* occurs in the parenchymal cells of the liver, pancreas, kidney, and heart.

◈ *Reticuloendothelial (RE) deposition* occurs in the RE cells of the liver, spleen, and bone marrow.

Causes for generalised or systemic overload of iron may be as under:

i) Increased erythropoietic activity In various forms of chronic haemolytic anaemia, there is excessive break-down of haemoglobin and hence iron overload. The problem is further compounded by treating the condition with blood transfusions (transfusional haemosiderosis) or by parenteral iron therapy. The deposits of iron in these cases, termed as *acquired haemosiderosis,* are initially in reticuloendothelial tissues but may eventually affect the parenchymal cells of the organs.

ii) Excessive intestinal absorption of iron A form of haemosiderosis in which there is excessive intestinal absorption of iron even when the intake is normal, is known as *idiopathic or hereditary haemochromatosis*. It is an autosomal dominant disease associated with much more deposits of iron than in cases of acquired haemosiderosis. Haemochromatosis is characterised by *triad* of features: pigmentary liver cirrhosis, pancreatic damage resulting in diabetes mellitus, and skin pigmentation. On the basis of the last two features, the condition has come to be termed as *bronze diabetes*.

iii) Excessive dietary intake of iron An example of excessive iron absorption is *African iron overload* (earlier called *Bantu siderosis*) seen in blacks in South Africa. Initially, it was observed in those rural South African communities who consumed alcohol brewed in ungalvanised iron vessels that served as a rich source of additional dietary iron. However, subsequently it was found that this type of siderosis also occurred in other individuals of African descent who had no history of such alcohol consumption. This led to identification of a gene, ferroportin, which predisposes iron overload in such people of African descent and hence the name. The excess iron gets deposited in various organs including the liver causing pigment cirrhosis.

2. ACID HAEMATIN (HAEMOZOIN) Acid haematin or haemozoin, also called malarial pigment, is a haemoprotein-derived brown-black pigment containing haem iron in ferric form in acidic medium. But it differs from haemosiderin because it cannot be stained by Prussian blue (Perl's) reaction, probably because of formation of complex with a protein so that it is unable to react in the stain. Haematin pigment is seen most commonly in chronic malaria and in mismatched blood transfusions. Besides, the *malarial pigment* can also be deposited in macrophages and in the hepatocytes. Another variety of haematin pigment is *formalin pigment* formed in blood-rich tissues which have been preserved in acidic formalin solution.

3. BILIRUBIN Bilirubin is the normal non-iron containing pigment present in the bile. It is derived from porphyrin ring of the haem moiety of haemoglobin. Normal level of bilirubin in blood is less than 1 mg/dl. Excess of bilirubin or hyperbilirubinaemia causes an important clinical condition called jaundice. Normal bilirubin metabolism and pathogenesis of jaundice are described in Chapter 27. Hyperbilirubinaemia may be unconjugated or conjugated; accordingly jaundice may appear in one of the following 3 ways:
i) An increase in the rate of bilirubin production due to excessive destruction of red cells (predominantly unconjugated hyperbilirubinaemia).
ii) A defect in handling of bilirubin due to hepatocellular injury (biphasic jaundice).
iii) Some defect in bilirubin transport within intrahepatic or extrahepatic biliary system (predominantly conjugated hyperbilirubinaemia).

Excessive accumulation of bilirubin pigment can be seen in different tissues and fluids of the body, especially in the hepatocytes, Kupffer cells and bile sinusoids. Skin and sclerae become distinctly yellow. In infants, rise in unconjugated bilirubin may produce toxic brain injury called *kernicterus*.

4. PORPHYRINS Porphyrins are normal pigment present in haemoglobin, myoglobin and cytochrome. Porphyria refers to an uncommon disorder of inborn abnormality of porphyrin metabolism. It results from genetic deficiency of one of the enzymes required for the synthesis of haem, resulting in excessive production of porphyrins. Often, the genetic deficiency is precipitated by intake of some drugs. Porphyrias are associated with excretion of intermediate products in the urine—delta-aminolaevulinic acid, porphobilinogen, uroporphyrin, coproporphyrin, and protoporphyrin. Porphyrias are broadly of 2 types—erythropoietic and hepatic.

(a) Erythropoietic porphyrias These have defective synthesis of haem in the red cell precursors in the bone marrow. These may be further of 2 subtypes:

i) *Congenital erythropoietic porphyria*, in which the urine is red due to the presence of uroporphyrin and coproporphyrin. The skin of these infants is highly photosensitive. Bones and skin show red brown discolouration.

ii) *Erythropoietic protoporphyria*, in which there is excess of protoporphyrin but no excess of porphyrin in the urine.

(b) Hepatic porphyrias These are more common and have a normal erythroid precursors but have a defect in synthesis of haem in the liver. Its further subtypes include the following:

i) *Acute intermittent porphyria* is characterised by acute episodes of 3 patterns: abdominal, neurological, and psychotic. These patients do not have photosensitivity. There is excessive delta aminolaevulinic acid and porphobilinogen in the urine.

ii) *Porphyria cutanea tarda* is the most common of all porphyrias. Porphyrins collect in the liver and small quantity is excreted in the urine. Skin lesions are similar to those in variegate porphyria. Most of the patients have associated haemosiderosis with cirrhosis which may eventually develop into hepatocellular carcinoma.

iii) *Mixed (Variegate) porphyrias* It is rare and combines skin photosensitivity with acute abdominal and neurological manifestations.

Lipofuscin (Wear and Tear Pigment)

Lipofuscin or lipochrome is yellowish-brown intracellular lipid pigment (*lipo* = fat, *fuscus* = brown). The pigment is often found in atrophied cells of old age and hence the name 'wear and tear pigment'. It is seen in the myocardial fibres, hepatocytes, Leydig cells of the testes and in neurons in senile dementia. However, the pigment may, at times, accumulate rapidly in different cells in wasting diseases unrelated to ageing.

Chapter 6: Intracellular Accumulations 59

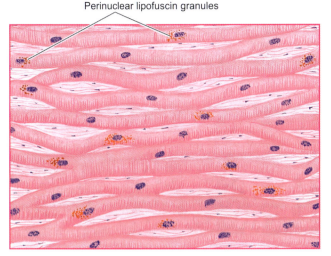
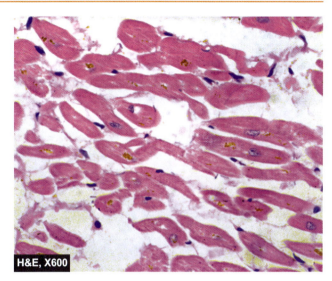

Figure 6.7 ▶ Brown atrophy of the heart. The lipofuscin pigment granules are seen in the cytoplasm of the myocardial fibres, especially around the nuclei.

Microscopically, the pigment is coarse, golden-brown granular and often accumulates in the central part of the cells around the nuclei. In the heart muscle, the change is associated with wasting of the muscle and is commonly referred to as 'brown atrophy' (Fig. 6.7). The pigment can be stained by fat stains but differs from other lipids in being fluorescent and having positive acid-fast staining.

By *electron microscopy*, lipofuscin appears as intra-lysosomal electron-dense granules in perinuclear location.

Lipofuscin granules are composed of lipid-protein complexes. Unlike in normal cells, in ageing or debilitating diseases the phospholipid end-products of membrane damage mediated by oxygen free radicals fail to get eliminated by intracellular lipid peroxidation. These, therefore, persist as collections of indigestible material in the lysosomes; thus lipofuscin is an example of residual bodies.

B. EXOGENOUS PIGMENTS

Exogenous pigments are the pigments introduced into the body from outside such as by inhalation, ingestion or inoculation.

Inhaled Pigments

The lungs of most individuals, especially of those living in urban areas due to atmospheric pollutants and of smokers, show a large number of inhaled pigmented materials. The most commonly inhaled substances are carbon or coal dust; others are silica or stone dust, iron or iron oxide, asbestos and various other organic substances. These substances may produce occupational lung diseases called pneumoconiosis.

The pigment particles after inhalation are taken up by alveolar macrophages. Some of the pigment-laden macrophages are coughed out via bronchi, while some settle in the interstitial tissue of the lung and in the respiratory bronchioles and pass into lymphatics to be deposited in the hilar lymph nodes. *Anthracosis* (i.e. deposition of carbon particles) is seen in almost every adult lung and generally provokes no reaction of tissue injury (Fig. 6.8). However, extensive deposition of particulate material over many years in coal-miners' pneumoconiosis, silicosis, asbestosis etc. provoke low grade inflammation, fibrosis and impaired respiratory function.

Ingested Pigments

Chronic ingestion of certain metals may produce pigmentation. The examples are as under:

i) *Argyria* is chronic ingestion of silver compounds and results in brownish pigmentation in the skin, bowel, and kidney.

ii) *Chronic lead poisoning* may produce the characteristic blue lines on teeth at the gumline.

iii) *Melanosis coli* results from prolonged ingestion of certain cathartics.

iv) *Carotenaemia* is yellowish-red colouration of the skin caused by excessive ingestion of carrots which contain carotene.

Injected Pigments (Tattooing)

Pigments like India ink, cinnabar and carbon are introduced into the dermis in the process of tattooing where the pigment is taken up by macrophages and lies permanently in the

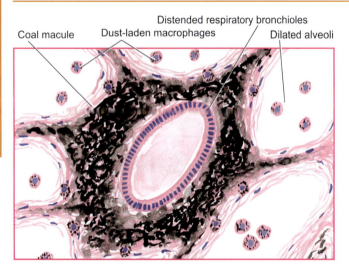
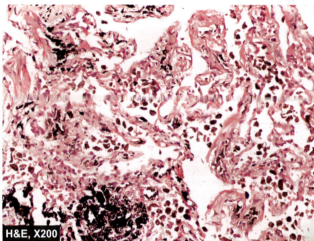

Figure 6.8 ▶ Anthracosis lung. There is presence of abundant coarse black carbon pigment in the septal walls and around the bronchiole.

connective tissue. The examples of injected pigments are prolonged use of ointments containing mercury, dirt left accidentally in a wound, and tattooing by pricking the skin with dyes.

 GIST BOX 6.2 | **Pigments**

- Pigments may be endogenous in origin or exogenously introduced in the body.
- The most common endogenous pigment is melanin. Disorders of melanin are due to defect in tyrosine metabolism and may give rise to hyper- and hypopigmentation, each of which may be generalised or localised.
- Haem-derived pigments are haemosiderin, acid haematin, bilirubin and porphyrin.
- Excess of haemosiderin may get deposited in local tissues, or as generalised deposits in the reticuloendothelial tissues and in parenchymal cells. Haemosiderin in tissues stains positive for Perl's Prussian blue stain.
- Haemozoin is an acid haematin or malarial pigment which is negative for Perl's Prussian blue stain.
- Bilirubin is non-iron containing pigment; its increase (conjugated or unconjugated) in the blood causes jaundice. Bilirubin in blood may rise from its increased production, hepatocellular disease or due to obstruction in its excretion.
- Porphyrias are due to inborn errors in porphyrin metabolism for haem synthesis.
- Lipofuscin is a golden brown intralysosomal pigment seen in ageing and in debilitating diseases; it is an expression of residual bodies or wear and tear pigment.
- Exogenous pigments may appear in the body from inhalation (e.g. carbon dust), ingestion (e.g. argyria) and by tattooing.

7 Amyloidosis

Amyloidosis is the term used for a group of diseases characterised by *extracellular deposition* of fibrillar insoluble proteinaceous substance called amyloid having common morphological appearance, staining properties and physical structure but with variable protein (or biochemical) composition.

First described by Rokitansky in 1842, the substance was subsequently named by Virchow as 'amyloid' under the mistaken belief that the material was starch-like (*amylon* = starch). This property was demonstrable *grossly* on the cut surface of an organ containing amyloid which stained brown with iodine and turned violet on addition of dilute sulfuric acid. By H&E staining under *light microscopy,* amyloid appears as extracellular, homogeneous, structureless and eosinophilic hyaline material; it stains *positive with Congo red* staining and shows apple-green birefringence on *polarising microscopy.*

The nomenclature of different forms of amyloid is done by putting the alphabet A (A for amyloid), followed by the suffix derived from the name of specific protein constituting amyloid of that type e.g. AL (A for amyloid, L for light chain-derived), AA, ATTR etc.

PHYSICAL AND CHEMICAL NATURE OF AMYLOID

Ultrastructural examination and chemical analysis reveal the complex nature of amyloid. It emerges that on the basis of morphology and physical characteristics, all forms of amyloid are similar in appearance, but they are chemically heterogeneous. Based on analysis, amyloid is composed of 2 main types of complex proteins (Fig. 7.1):
I. *Fibril proteins* comprise about 95% of amyloid.
II. *Non-fibrillar components* which include *P-component* predominantly; and there are several other different proteins which together constitute the remaining 5% of amyloid.

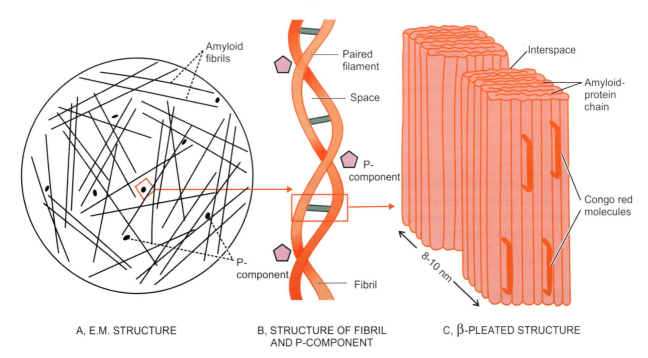

Figure 7.1 ▶ Diagrammatic representation of the ultrastructure of amyloid. A, Electron microscopy shows major part consisting of amyloid fibrils (95%) randomly oriented, while the minor part is essentially P-component (5%). B, Each fibril is further composed of double helix of two pleated sheets in the form of *twin filaments* separated by a clear space. P-component has a pentagonal or doughnut profile. C, X-ray crystallography and infra-red spectroscopy shows fibrils having *cross-β-pleated* sheet configuration which produces periodicity that gives the characteristic staining properties of amyloid with Congo red and birefringence under polarising microscopy.

I. FIBRIL PROTEINS

By electron microscopy, it became apparent that major component of all forms of amyloid (about 95%) consists of meshwork of fibril proteins. These consist of delicate, randomly dispersed, non-branching amyloid fibres having 4-6 *fibrils*, each measuring 7.5-10 nm in diameter and having indefinite length. These fibrils are wound on each other and are separated by a clear space which contains regularly placed binding sites for Congo red dye. By X-ray crystallography and infra-red spectroscopy, the fibrils are shown to have *cross-β-pleated* sheet configuration which produces 1000 A° periodicity. These properties give amyloid its characteristic staining properties with Congo red dye and birefringence under polarising microscopy. Based on these features, amyloid is given an alternate name of *β-fibrillosis*.

Chemical analysis of fibril proteins of amyloid reveals heterogeneous nature of amyloid. Chemically, following two major forms of amyloid fibril proteins were first identified in 1970s. However, currently in different clinicopathologic settings in humans, over 20 other biochemically different proteins have been identified which form amyloid fibrils. Thus, these proteins can be categorised as under:
i) AL (amyloid light chain) protein
ii) AA (amyloid associated) protein
iii) Other proteins

AL PROTEIN AL amyloid fibril protein is derived from immunoglobulin light chain, which may be complete light chain, or may include amino-terminal segment and part of C region of the immunoglobulin light chain. AL fibril protein is more frequently derived from the lambda (λ) light chain (twice more common) than kappa (κ). However, in any given case, there is amino acid sequence homology.

AL type of fibril protein is produced by immunoglobulin-secreting cells and is therefore seen in association with plasma cell dyscrasias and is included in primary systemic amyloidosis.

AA PROTEIN AA fibril protein is composed of protein with molecular weight of 8.5-kDa which is derived from larger precursor protein in the serum called SAA (serum amyloid-associated protein) with a molecular weight of 12.5-kDA. Unlike AL amyloid, the deposits of AA amyloid do not have sequence homology. In the plasma, SAA circulates in association with HDL3 (high-density lipoprotein). SAA is an acute phase reactant protein synthesised in the liver, in response to chronic inflammatory and traumatic conditions, and thus the level of SAA is high in these conditions.

AA fibril protein is found in secondary amyloidosis which is seen in association with several examples of chronic infectious and autoimmune inflammatory diseases and disseminated malignancies.

OTHER PROTEINS Apart from the two major forms of amyloid fibril proteins, a few other forms of proteins are found in different clinical states:

1. **Transthyretin (TTR)** It is a serum protein synthesised in the liver and normally *trans*ports *thy*roxine and *retin*ol (trans-thy-retin). Single amino acid substitution mutations in the structure of TTR results in variant form of protein which is responsible for this form of amyloidosis termed as ATTR.

ATTR is the most common form of heredofamilial amyloidosis seen in familial amyloid polyneuropathies. However, the deposits of ATTR in the elderly in the heart (senile cardiac amyloidosis) consists of normal TTR without any mutation. Another interesting aspect in ATTR is that despite being inherited, the disease appears in middle age or elderly.

2. **Aβ2-microglobulin (Aβ2M)** This form of amyloid is seen in cases of long-term haemodialysis (for 10-12 years). As the name suggests, β2M is a small protein which is a normal component of major histocompatibility complex (MHC) class I and has β-pleated sheet structure. β2M is 11.8 kDa protein that is not filtered by the haemodialysis membrane and thus there is high serum concentration of β2M protein in these patients. Although the deposit due to Aβ2M may be systemic in distribution, it has predilection for bones and joints.

3. **Amyloid β-peptide (Aβ)** Aβ is distinct from Aβ2M and is deposited in cerebral amyloid angiopathy and neurofibrillary tangles in Alzheimer's disease. Aβ is derived from amyloid beta precursor protein (AβPP). The latter is a cell surface protein having a single transmembranous domain that functions as a receptor. The Aβ portion of this protein is seen extending into extracellular region. Out of three intramembranous cleavage sites—secretase-α, -β and -γ, partial proteolysis of AβPP due to cleavage of β-secretase and γ-secretase sites generates Aβ i.e. amylyoidogenic protein in Alzheimer's disease (Fig. 7.2).

4. **Endocrine amyloid from hormone precursor proteins** It includes examples such as amyloid derived from pro-calcitonin (ACal), islet amyloid polypeptide (AIAPP, amylin), pro-insulin (AIns), prolactin (APro) etc.

5. **Amyloid of prion protein (APrP)** It is derived from precursor prion protein which is a plasma membrane glycoprotein. Prion proteins are proteinaceous infectious particles lacking in RNA or DNA. Amyloid in prionosis occurs due to abnormally folded isoform of the PrP.

II. NON-FIBRILLAR COMPONENTS

Non-fibrillar components comprise about 5% of the amyloid material. These components include the following:

1. **Amyloid P (AP)-component** It is synthesised in the liver and is present in all types of amyloid. It is derived from circulating serum amyloid P-component, a glycoprotein resembling the normal serum α1-glycoprotein and is PAS-positive. It is structurally related to C-reactive protein, an acute phase reactant, but is not similar to it. By electron microscopy, it has a pentagonal profile (P-component) or doughnut-shape with an external diameter of 9 nm and internal diameter of 4 nm.

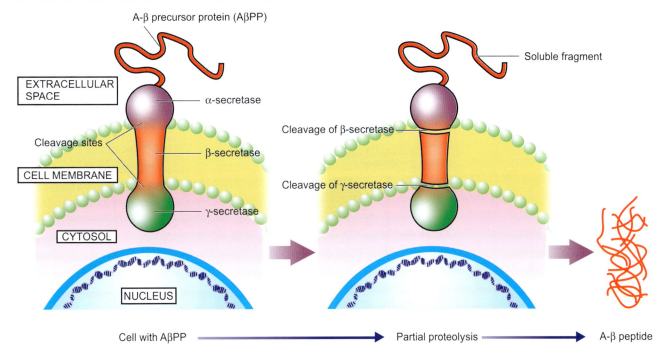

Figure 7.2 ▶ Mechanism of amyloid deposits in Alzheimer's disease.

2. Apolipoprotein-E (apoE) It is a regulator of lipoprotein metabolism and is found in all types of amyloid. One allele, apoE4, increases the risk of Alzheimer precursor protein (APP) deposition in Alzheimer's disease but not in all other types of amyloid deposits.

3. Sulfated glycosaminoglycans (GAGs) These are constituents of matrix proteins; particularly associated is heparin sulfate in all types of tissue amyloid.

4. Other components Besides above, other components such as α-1 anti-chymotrypsin, protein X, components of complement, proteases, and membrane constituents may be seen in the amyloid deposits.

PATHOGENESIS OF AMYLOIDOSIS

The earliest observation that amyloidosis developed in experimental animals who were injected repeatedly with antigen to raise antisera for human use led to the concept that amyloidogenesis was the result of immunologic mechanisms. Thus, AL variety of amyloid protein was isolated first. It is now appreciated that amyloidosis or fibrillogenesis is multifactorial and that different mechanisms are involved in various types of amyloid.

Irrespective of the type of amyloid, amyloidogenesis in general *in vivo*, occurs in the following sequence **(Fig. 7.3)**:

1. *Pool of amyloidogenic precursor protein* is present in circulation in different clinical settings and in response to stimuli e.g. increased hepatic synthesis of AA or ATTR, increased synthesis of AL etc.

2. *A nidus for fibrillogenesis*, meaning thereby an alteration in microenvironment, to stimulate deposition of amyloid protein is formed. This alteration involves changes and interaction between basement membrane proteins and amyloidogenic protein.

3. *Partial degradation or proteolysis* occurs prior to deposition of fibrillar protein which may occur in macrophages or reticuloendothelial cells. However, there are exceptions to this generalisation when there is no degradation of proteins such as in ATTR (heredofamilial type in which there are amino acid mutations in most cases), Aβ2M (in which there are elevated levels of normal β2M protein which remain unfiltered during haemodialysis) and prionosis (in which β-pleated sheet is formed *de novo*).

4. The role of *non-fibrillar components* (e.g. AP, apoE and GAGs) in amyloidosis is fibril stabilisation by protein aggregation and protein folding in a way that it is protected from soublisation or degradation.

Based on this general pathogenesis, deposition of AL and AA amyloid is briefly outlined below:

DEPOSITION OF AL AMYLOID

1. The stimulus for production of AL amyloid is some disorder of *immunoglobulin synthesis* e.g. multiple myeloma, B cell lymphoma, other plasma cell dyscrasias.

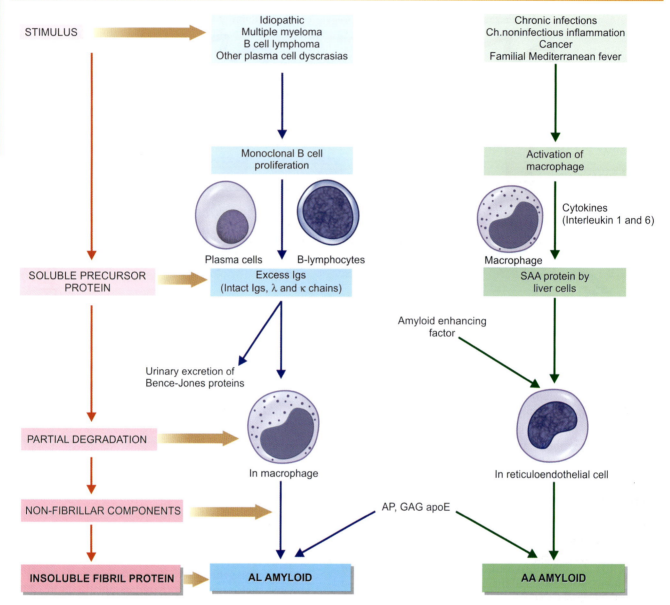

Figure 7.3 ▶ Pathogenesis of two main forms of amyloid deposition (AL = Amyloid light chain; AA = Amyloid-associated protein; GAG = Glycosaminoglycan; AP = Amyloid P component). The sequence on left shows general schematic representation common to both major forms of amyloidogenesis.

2. Excessive immunoglobulin production is in the form of *monoclonal gammopathy* i.e. there is production of either intact immunoglobulin, or λ light chain, or κ light chain, or rarely heavy chains. This takes place by monoclonal proliferation of plasma cells, B lymphocytes, or their precursors.

3. *Partial degradation* in the form of limited proteolysis of larger protein molecules occurs in macrophages that are anatomically closely associated with AL amyloid.

4. *Non-fibrillar components* like AP and GAGs play role in folding and aggregation of fibril proteins.

DEPOSITION OF AA AMYLOID

1. AA amyloid is directly related to *SAA levels,* a high-density lipoprotein. SAA is synthesised by the liver in response to *cytokines*, notably interleukin 1 and 6, released from activated macrophages.

2. The levels of SAA are elevated in *long-standing tissue destruction* e.g. in chronic inflammation, cancers. However, SAA levels in isolation do not always lead to AA amyloid.

3. As in AL amyloid, *partial degradation* in the form of limited proteolysis takes place in reticuloendothelial cells.

4. In AA amyloid, a significant role is played by another glycoprotein, *amyloid enhancing factor (AEF)*. AEF is elaborated in chronic inflammation, cancer and familial Mediterranean fever. AEF acts as a nidus and accelerates AA amyloid deposition.

5. As in AL amyloid, there is a role of *AP component* and *glycosaminoglycans* in the fibril protein aggregation and its protection from disaggregation again.

CLASSIFICATION OF AMYLOIDOSIS

Over the years, amyloidosis has been classified in a number of ways:

- **Based on cause**, into *primary* (with unknown cause and the deposition is in the disease itself) and *secondary* (as a complication of some underlying known disease) amyloidosis.
- **Based on extent of amyloid deposition**, into *systemic (generalised)* involving multiple organs and *localised-amyloidosis* involving one or two organs or sites.
- **Based on clinical location**, into *pattern I* (involving tongue, heart, bowel, skeletal and smooth muscle, skin and nerves), *pattern II* (principally involving liver, spleen, kidney and adrenals) and *mixed pattern* (involving sites of both pattern I and II).
- **Based on precursor biochemical proteins**, into specific type of serum amyloid proteins.

With availability of biochemical composition of various forms of amyloid and diverse clinical settings in which these specific biochemical forms of amyloid are deposited, a *clinicopathologic classification* has been proposed which is widely accepted (Table 7.1). According to this classification, amyloidosis can be divided into 2 major categories and their subtypes depending upon clinical settings:

A. *Systemic (generalised) amyloidosis:*
1. Primary (AL)
2. Secondary/reactive/inflammatory (AA)
3. Haemodialysis-associated (Aβ_2M)
4. Heredofamilial (ATTR, AA, Others)

B. *Localised amyloidosis:*
1. Senile cardiac (ATTR)
2. Senile cerebral (Aβ, APrP)
3. Endocrine (Hormone precursors)
4. Tumour-forming (AL)

A. SYSTEMIC AMYLOIDOSIS

1. Primary Systemic (AL) Amyloidosis

Primary amyloidosis consisting of AL fibril proteins is systemic or generalised in distribution. About 30% cases of AL amyloid have some form of plasma cell dyscrasias, most commonly multiple myeloma (in about 15-20% cases), and less often other monoclonal gammopathies such as

Table 7.1 Classification of amyloidosis.

CATEGORY		ASSOCIATED DISEASE	BIOCHEMICAL TYPE	ORGANS COMMONLY INVOLVED
A.	SYSTEMIC (GENERALISED) AMYLOIDOSIS			
	1. Primary	Plasma cell dyscrasias	AL type	Heart, bowel, skin, nerves, kidney
	2. Secondary (Reactive)	Chronic inflammation, cancers	AA type	Liver, spleen, kidneys, adrenals
	3. Haemodialysis-associated	Chronic renal failure	Aβ_2M	Synovium, joints, tendon sheaths
	4. Heredofamilial			
	i. Hereditary polyneuropathies	—	ATTR	Peripheral and autonomic nerves, heart
	ii. Familial Mediterranean fever	—	AA type	Liver, spleen, kidneys, adrenals
	iii. Rare hereditary forms	—	AApoAI, AGel ALys, AFib, ACys	Systemic amyloidosis
B.	LOCALISED AMYLOIDOSIS			
	1. Senile cardiac	Senility	ATTR	Heart
	2. Senile cerebral	Alzheimer's, transmissible encephalopathy	Aβ, APrP	Cerebral vessels, plaques, neurofibrillary tangles
	3. Endocrine	Medullary carcinoma Type 2 diabetes mellitus	Procalcitonin Proinsulin	Thyroid Islets of Langerhans
	4. Tumour-forming	Lungs, larynx, skin, urinary bladder, tongue, eye	AL	Respective anatomic location

(AL= Amyloid light chain; AA= Amyloid-associated protein; Aβ_2M= Amyloid β_2-microglobulin; ATTR= Amyloid transthyretin; APrP=Amyloid of prion proteins, Aβ= β-amyloid protein).

Waldenström's macroglobulinaemia, heavy chain disease, solitary plasmacytoma and B cell lymphoma. The neoplastic plasma cells usually are a single clone and, therefore, produce the same type of immunoglobulin light chain or part of light chain. Almost all cases of multiple myeloma have either λ or κ light chains (Bence Jones proteins) in the serum and are excreted in the urine. However, in contrast to normal or myeloma light chains, AL is twice more frequently derived from λ light chains.

The remaining 70% cases of AL amyloid do not have evident B-cell proliferative disorder or any other associated diseases and thus are cases of true 'primary' (idiopathic) amyloidosis. However, by more sensitive methods, some plasma cell dyscrasias are detectable in virtually all patients with AL. Majority of these cases too have a single type of abnormal immunoglobulin in their serum (monoclonal) and that these patients have some degree of plasmacytosis in the bone marrow, suggesting the origin of AL amyloid from precursor plasma cells.

AL amyloid is most prevalent type of systemic amyloidosis in North America and Europe and is seen in individuals past the age of 40 years and is rapidly progressive disease if not treated. Primary amyloidosis is often severe in the heart, kidney, bowel, skin, peripheral nerves, respiratory tract, skeletal muscle and tongue (macroglossia).

Treatment of AL amyloid is targeted at reducing the underlying clonal expansion of plasma cells. Median survival with no treatment after diagnosis is about one year.

2. Secondary/Reactive (AA) Systemic Amyloidosis

The second form of systemic or generalised amyloidosis is reactive or inflammatory or secondary in which the fibril proteins contain AA amyloid. Secondary or reactive amyloidosis occurs typically as a complication of chronic infectious (e.g. tuberculosis, bronchiectasis, chronic osteomyelitis, chronic pyelonephritis, leprosy, chronic skin infections), non-infectious chronic inflammatory conditions associated with tissue destruction (e.g. autoimmune disorders such as rheumatoid arthritis, lupus, inflammatory bowel disease), some tumours (e.g. renal cell carcinoma, Hodgkin's disease) and in familial Mediterranean fever, an inherited disorder (discussed below).

Secondary amyloidosis is typically distributed in solid abdominal viscera like the kidney, liver, spleen and adrenals. Secondary reactive amyloidosis is seen less frequently in developed countries due to containment of infections before they become chronic but this is the more common type of amyloidosis in underdeveloped and developing countries of the world.

Secondary systemic amyloidosis can occur at any age and is the only form of amyloid which can also occur in children. Treatment lies in treating the underlying infectious or inflammatory disorder resulting in lowering of SAA protein in blood.

The contrasting features of the two main forms of systemic amyloidosis are given in **Table 7.2**.

3. Haemodialysis-Associated (Aβ2M) Amyloidosis

Patients on long-term dialysis for more than 10 years for chronic renal failure may develop systemic amyloidosis derived from β2-microglobulin which is normal component of MHC. The amyloid deposits are preferentially found in the vessel walls at the synovium, joints, tendon sheaths and subchondral bones. Carpal tunnel syndrome is common

Table 7.2 Contrasting features of primary and secondary amyloidosis.

FEATURE	PRIMARY AMYLOID	SECONDARY AMYLOID
1. Biochemical composition	AL (Light chain proteins); lambda chains more common than kappa; sequence homology of chains	AA (Amyloid associated proteins); derived from larger precursor protein SAA; no sequence homology of polypeptide chain
2. Associated diseases	Plasma cell dyscrasias e.g. multiple myeloma, B cell lymphomas, others	Chronic inflammation e.g. infections (TB, leprosy, osteomyelitis, bronchiectasis), autoimmune diseases (rheumatoid arthritis, IBD), cancers (RCC, Hodgkin's disease), FMF
3. Pathogenesis	Stimulus → Monoclonal B cell proliferation → Excess of Igs and light chains → Partial degradation → Insoluble AL fibril	Stimulus → Chronic inflammation → Activation of macrophages → Cytokines (IL1,6) → Partial degradation → AEF → Insoluble AA fibril
4. Incidence	Most common in US and other developed countries	Most common worldwide, particularly in developing countries
5. Age	>40 years	Any age including children
6. Course and prognosis	Rapidly progressive, dismal	Better, treat the underlying cause
7. Organ distribution	Kidney, heart, bowel, nerves	Kidney, liver, spleen, adrenals
8. Stains to distinguish	Congophilia persists after permanganate treatment of section; specific immunostains anti-λ, anti-κ	Congophilia disappears after permanganate treatment of section; specific immunostain anti-AA

presentation. However, systemic distribution has also been observed in these cases showing bulky visceral deposits of amyloid. Cessation of dialysis after renal transplant causes symptomatic improvement.

4. Heredofamilial Amyloidosis

A few rare examples of genetically-determined amyloidosis having familial occurrence and seen in certain geographic regions have been described. These are as under:

i) Hereditary polyneuropathic (ATTR) amyloidosis This is an autosomal dominant disorder in which amyloid is deposited in the peripheral and autonomic nerves resulting in muscular weakness, pain and paraesthesia, or may have cardiomyopathy. This type of amyloid is derived from transthyretin (ATTR) with single amino acid substitution in the structure of TTR; about 60 types of such mutations have been described. Though hereditary, the condition appears well past middle life.

ii) Amyloid in familial Mediterranean fever (AA) This is an autosomal recessive disease and is seen in the Mediterranean region (i.e. people residing in the countries surrounding the Mediterranean sea e.g. Sephardic Jews, Armenians, Arabs and Turks). The condition is characterised by periodic attacks of fever and polyserositis i.e. inflammatory involvement of the pleura, peritoneum, and synovium causing pain in the chest, abdomen and joints respectively. Amyloidosis occurring in these cases is AA type, suggesting relationship to secondary amyloidosis due to chronic inflammation. The distribution of this form of heredofamilial amyloidosis is similar to that of secondary amyloidosis.

iii) Rare hereditary forms Heredofamilial mutations of several normal proteins have been reported e.g. apolipo-protein I (AApoAI), gelsolin (AGel), lysozyme (ALys), fibrinogen α-chain (AFib), cystatin C (ACys) and amyloid of familial dementia etc. These types may also result in systemic amyloidosis.

B. LOCALISED AMYLOIDOSIS

1. Senile cardiac amyloidosis (ATTR) Senile cardiac amyloidosis is seen in 50% of people above the age of 70 years. The deposits are seen in the heart and aorta. The type of amyloid in these cases is ATTR but without any change in the protein structure of TTR.

2. Senile cerebral amyloidosis (Aβ, APrP) Senile cerebral amyloidosis is heterogeneous group of amyloid deposition of varying etiologies that includes sporadic, familial, hereditary and infectious. Some of the important diseases associated with cerebral amyloidosis and the corresponding amyloid proteins are: Alzheimer's disease (Aβ), Down's syndrome (Aβ) and transmissible spongiform encephalopathies (APrP) such as in Creutzfeldt-Jakob disease, fatal familial insomnia, mad cow disease, kuru.

In Alzheimer's disease, deposit of amyloid is seen as Congophilic angiopathy (amyloid material in the walls of cerebral blood vessels), neurofibrillary tangles and in senile plaques.

3. Endocrine amyloidosis (Hormone precursors) Some endocrine lesions are associated with microscopic deposits of amyloid. The examples are as follows:

i) Medullary carcinoma of the thyroid (from procalcitonin i.e. ACal).

ii) Islet cell tumour of the pancreas (from islet amyloid polypeptide i.e. AIAPP or amylin).

iii) Type 2 diabetes mellitus (from pro-insulin, i.e. AIns).

iv) Pituitary amyloid (from prolactin i.e. APro).

v) Isolated atrial amyloid deposits (from atrial natriuretic factor i.e. AANF).

vi) Familial corneal amyloidosis (from lactoferrin i.e. ALac).

4. Localised tumour forming amyloid (AL) Sometimes, isolated tumour like formation of amyloid deposits are seen e.g. in lungs, larynx, skin, urinary bladder, tongue, eye, isolated atrial amyloid. In most of these cases, the amyloid type is AL.

> **GIST BOX 7.1 — Amyloidosis: Characteristics, Classification, Pathogenesis**
>
> ❖ By H&E staining under light microscopy, all forms of amyloid appear as extracellular, homogeneous, structureless and eosinophilic hyaline material; it stains positive with Congo red staining and shows apple-green birefringence on polarising microscopy.
>
> ❖ Biochemically, fibril proteins comprise about 95% of amyloid while non-fibrillar components constitute the remaining 5% of amyloid.
>
> ❖ Fibrils proteins are predominantly are of two types: AL (primary amyloid in association with plasma cell and B cell proliferative disorders) and AA (secondary amyoid seen in chronic infections and chronic inflammatory diseases); others are transthyretin or ATTR (in heredo-familial forms), Aβ2-microglobulin or Aβ2M (seen in patients on long-term haemodialysis), amyloid β-peptide or Aβ (seen in Alzheimer's disease), endocrine amyloid from hormone precursor proteins (seen in type 2 diabetes, medullary carcinoma thyroid etc.) and amyloid of prion protein or APrP.
>
> ❖ Non-fibrillar components consist mainly of P component seen in all forms of amyloid; others are apolipoprotein-E, sulphated glycosaminoglycans etc.
>
> ❖ Pathogenesis of amyloid includes rise in level of precursor of fibrillary protein (AL in primary and SAA in secondary form) followed by its partial degradation by reticuloendothelial cells. Non-fibrillary components facilitate protein aggregation and protection against solubilisation.

STAINING CHARACTERISTICS OF AMYLOID

1. STAIN ON GROSS The oldest method since the time of Virchow for demonstrating amyloid on cut surface of a gross specimen, or on the frozen/paraffin section is iodine stain. Lugol's iodine imparts *mahogany brown* colour to the amyloid-containing area which on addition of dilute sulfuric acid turns blue. This starch-like property of amyloid is due to AP component, a glycoprotein, present in all forms of amyloid.

Various stains and techniques employed to distinguish and confirm amyloid deposits in sections are given in Table 7.3.

2. H & E Amyloid by light microscopy with haematoxylin and eosin staining appears as extracellular, homogeneous, structureless and eosinophilic hyaline material, especially in relation to blood vessels. However, if the deposits are small, they are difficult to detect by routine H and E stains. Besides, a few other hyaline deposits may also take pink colour (page 36).

3. METACHROMATIC STAINS (ROSANILINE DYES) Amyloid has the property of metachromasia i.e. the dye reacts with amyloid and undergoes a colour change. Metachromatic stains employed are rosaniline dyes such as methyl violet and crystal violet which impart *rose-pink* colouration to amyloid deposits. However, small amounts of amyloid are missed, mucins also have metachromasia; moreover, aqueous mountants are required for seeing the preparation. Therefore, this method has low sensitivity and lacks specificity.

4. CONGO RED AND POLARISED LIGHT All types of amyloid have affinity for Congo red stain; therefore this method is used for confirmation of amyloid of all types. The stain may be used on both gross specimens and microscopic sections; amyloid of all types stains *pink red colour*. If the stained section is viewed in polarised light, the amyloid characteristically shows *apple-green birefringence* due to cross-β-pleated sheet configuration of amyloid fibrils. The stain can also be used to distinguish between AL and AA amyloid (primary and secondary amyloid respectively). After prior treatment with permanganate or trypsin on the section, Congo red stain is repeated—in the case of primary amyloid (AL amyloid), the Congo red positivity (congophilia) persists,* while it turns negative for Congo red in secondary amyloid (AA amyloid). Congo red dye can also be used as an *in vivo* test (described below).

5. FLUORESCENT STAINS Fluorescent stain thioflavin-T binds to amyloid and fluoresces *yellow* under ultraviolet light i.e. amyloid emits secondary fluorescence. Thioflavin-S is less specific.

6. IMMUNOHISTOCHEMISTRY Type of amyloid can be classified by immunohistochemical stains in which corresponding antibody stain is used against the specific amyloid protein acting as antigen. However, for mere confirmation of any type of amyloid, most useful stain is *anti-AP stain* since P component is present in all forms of amyloid. But for determining the biochemical type of amyloid, various antibody stains against the specific antigenic protein types of amyloid are commercially available such as *anti-AA, anti-lambda (λ), anti-kappa (κ,), transthyretin* antibody stains etc.

MORPHOLOGIC FEATURES OF AMYLOIDOSIS OF ORGANS

Although amyloidosis of different organs shows variation in morphologic pattern, some features are applicable in general to most of the involved organs.

Locations of amyloid deposit In general, amyloid proteins get filtered from blood across the basement membrane of vascular capillaries into extravascular spaces. Thus, most commonly amyloid deposits appear at the contacts between the vascular spaces and parenchymal cells, in the extracellular matrix and within the basement membranes of blood vessels.

> *Grossly*, the affected organ is usually enlarged, pale and rubbery. Cut surface shows firm, waxy and translucent parenchyma which takes positive staining with the iodine test.
>
> *Microscopically*, the deposits of amyloid are found in the extracellular locations, initially in the walls of small blood vessels producing microscopic changes and effects, while later the deposits are in large amounts causing pressure atrophy of parenchymal cells.

Based on these general features of amyloidosis, the salient pathologic findings of major organ involvements are described here.

AMYLOIDOSIS OF KIDNEYS

Amyloidosis of the kidneys is most common and most serious because of ill-effects on renal function. The deposits in the kidneys are found in most cases of secondary amyloidosis and

Table 7.3	Staining characteristics of amyloid.
STAIN	APPEARANCE
1. H & E	Pink, hyaline, homogeneous
2. Methyl violet/Crystal violet	Metachromasia: rose-pink
3. Congo red	Light microscopy: pink-red Polarising light: red-green birefringence
4. Thioflavin-T/Thioflavin-S	Ultraviolet light: fluorescence
5. Immunohistochemistry (antibody against fibril protein)	Immunoreactivity: Positive

---

*Easy way to remember: Three *p*s i.e. there is *p*ersistence of congophilia after *p*ermanganate treatment in *p*rimary amyloid

Chapter 7: Amyloidosis

in about one-third cases of primary amyloidosis. Amyloidosis of the kidney accounts for about 20% of deaths from amyloidosis. Even small quantities of amyloid deposits in the glomeruli can cause proteinuria and nephrotic syndrome.

Grossly, the kidneys may be normal-sized, enlarged or terminally contracted due to ischaemic effect of narrowing of vascular lumina. Cut surface is pale, waxy and translucent **(Fig. 7.4)**.

Microscopically, amyloid deposition occurs primarily in the glomeruli, though it may involve peritubular interstitial tissue and the walls of arterioles as well **(Fig. 7.5)**:

◆ *In the glomeruli,* the deposits initially appear on the basement membrane of the glomerular capillaries, but later extend to produce luminal narrowing and distortion of the glomerular capillary tuft. This results in abnormal increase in permeability of the glomerular capillaries to macromolecules with consequent proteinuria and nephrotic syndrome.

◆ *In the tubules,* the amyloid deposits likewise begin close to the tubular epithelial basement membrane. Subsequently, the deposits may extend further outwards into the intertubular connective tissue, and inwards to produce degenerative changes in the tubular epithelial cells and amyloid casts in the tubular lumina.

◆ *Vascular involvement* affects chiefly the walls of small arterioles and venules, producing narrowing of their lumina and consequent ischaemic effects.

◆ *Congo red staining* imparts red pink colour and polarising microscopy shows apple-green birefringence which confirms the presence of amyloid **(Fig. 7.6)**.

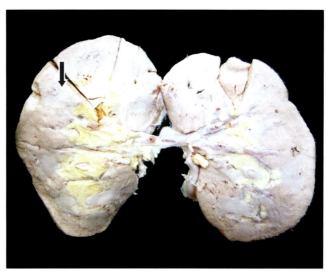

Figure 7.4 ▶ Amyloidosis of kidney. The kidney is small and pale in colour. Sectioned surface shows loss of cortico-medullary distinction (arrow) and pale, waxy translucency.

AMYLOIDOSIS OF SPLEEN

Amyloid deposition in the spleen, for some unknown reasons, may have one of the following two patterns **(Fig. 7.7)**:

1. SAGO SPLEEN ***Grossly,*** splenic enlargement is not marked and cut surface shows characteristic translucent pale and waxy nodules resembling sago grains and hence the name.

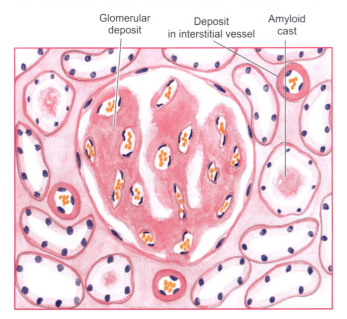

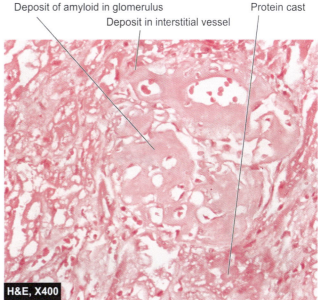

Figure 7.5 ▶ Amyloidosis of kidney. The amyloid deposits are seen mainly in the glomerular capillary tuft. The deposits are also present in peritubular connective tissue producing atrophic tubules and amyloid casts in the tubular lumina, and in the arterial wall producing luminal narrowing.

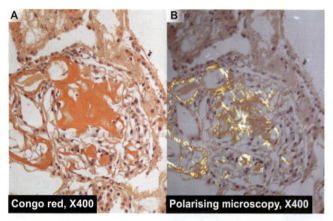

Figure 7.6 ▶ Amyloidosis kidney, Congo red stain. A, The amyloid deposits are seen mainly in the glomerular capillary tuft stained red-pink (Congophilia). B, Viewing the same under polarising microscopy, the congophilic areas show apple-green birefringence.

Microscopically, the amyloid deposits begin in the walls of the arterioles of the white pulp and may subsequently extend out and replace the follicles.

2. LARDACEOUS SPLEEN *Grossly,* there is generally moderate to marked splenomegaly (weight up to 1 kg). Cut surface of the spleen shows map-like areas of amyloid (lardaceous-lard-like; *lard* means fat of pigs) **(Fig. 7.8)**.

Microscopically, the deposits involve the red pulp in the walls of splenic sinuses and the small arteries and in the connective tissue **(Fig. 7.9)**. Confirmation is by observing

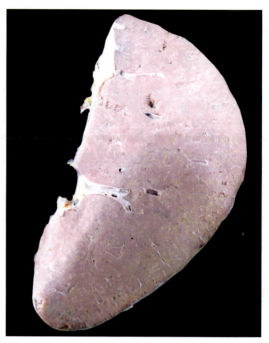

Figure 7.8 ▶ Lardaceous amyloidosis of the spleen. The sectioned surface shows presence of pale waxy translucency in a map-like pattern.

Congophilia in Congo red staining and demonstration of apple-green birefringence under polarising microscopy in the corresponding positive areas.

AMYLOIDOSIS OF LIVER

In about half the cases of systemic amyloidosis, liver is involved by amyloidosis.

Grossly, the liver is often enlarged, pale, waxy and firm.

Histologically, the features are as under **(Fig. 7.10)**:

◆ The amyloid initially appears in the space of Disse (the space between the hepatocytes and sinusoidal endothelial cells).

◆ Later, as the deposits increases, they compress the cords of hepatocytes so that eventually the liver cells are shrunken and atrophic and replaced by amyloid. However, hepatic function remains normal even at an advanced stage of the disease.

◆ To a lesser extent, portal tracts and Kupffer cells are involved in amyloidosis.

AMYLOIDOSIS OF HEART

Heart is involved in systemic amyloidosis quite commonly, more so in the primary than in secondary systemic amyloidosis. It may also be involved in localised form of amyloidosis (senile

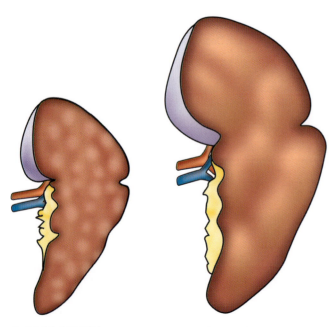

A, SAGO SPLEEN   B, LARDACEOUS SPLEEN

Figure 7.7 ▶ Gross patterns of amyloidosis of the spleen.

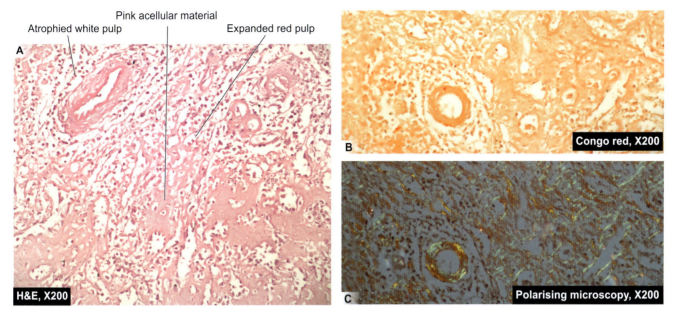

Figure 7.9 ► Amyloidosis spleen. A, The pink acellular amyloid material is seen in the red pulp causing atrophy of while pulp. B, Congo red staining shows Congophilia as seen by red-pink colour. C, When viewed under polarising microscopy the corresponding area shows apple-green birefringence.

cardiac). In advanced cases, there may be a pressure atrophy of the myocardial fibres and impaired ventricular function which may produce restrictive cardiomyopathy. Amyloidosis of the heart may produce arrhythmias due to deposition in the conduction system.

Grossly, the heart may be enlarged. The external surface is pale, translucent and waxy. The epicardium, endocardium and valves show tiny nodular deposits or raised plaques of amyloid.

Microscopically, the changes are as under:

◈ Amyloid deposits are seen in and around the coronaries and their small branches.

◈ In cases of primary amyloidosis of the heart, the deposits of AL amyloid are seen around the myocardial fibres in ring-like formations (ring fibres).

◈ In localised form of amyloid of the heart, the deposits are seen in the left atrium and in the interatrial septum.

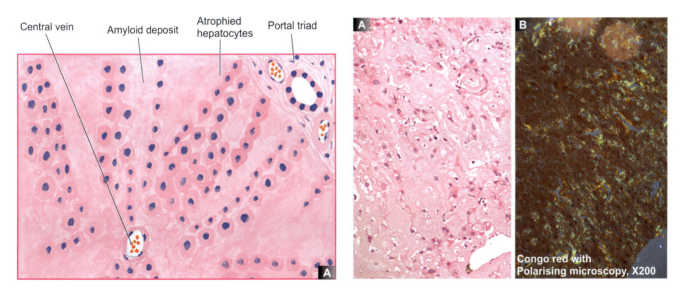

Figure 7.10 ► Amyloidosis of the liver. A, The deposition is extensive in the space of Disse causing compression and pressure atrophy of hepatocytes. B, Congo red staining shows congophilia which under polarising microscopy shows apple-green birefringence.

AMYLOIDOSIS OF ALIMENTARY TRACT

Involvement of the gastrointestinal tract by amyloidosis may occur at any level from the oral cavity to the anus. Rectal and gingival biopsies are the common sites for diagnosis of systemic amyloidosis. The deposits are initially located around the small blood vessels but later may involve adjacent layers of the bowel wall. Tongue may be the site for tumour-forming amyloid, producing macroglossia.

OTHER ORGANS

The deposits of amyloid may also occur in various other tissues such as pituitary, thyroid, adrenals, skin, lymph nodes, respiratory tract and peripheral and autonomic nerves.

DIAGNOSIS AND PROGNOSIS

DIAGNOSIS

Amyloidosis may be detected as an unsuspected morphologic finding in a case, or the changes may be severe so as to produce symptoms and may even cause death. The diagnosis of amyloid disease can be made from the following investigations:

1. **TISSUE DIAGNOSIS** Routine examination of biopsy or fine needle aspiration, followed by Congo red staining and examination under polarizing microscopy, are the two confirmatory methods of tissue diagnosis of amyloidosis:

❖ **Histologic examination** of biopsy material is the commonest and confirmatory method for diagnosis in a suspected case of amyloidosis. Biopsy of an obviously *affected organ* is likely to offer the best results e.g. *kidney biopsy* in a case on dialysis, sural nerve biopsy in familial polyneuropathy. In systemic amyloidosis, renal biopsy provides the best detection rate, but *rectal biopsy* also has a good pick up rate. However, *gingiva* and *skin biopsy* have poor result.

❖ **Fine needle aspiration** of abdominal *subcutaneous fat* followed by Congo red staining and polarising microscopic examination for confirmation has become an acceptable simple and useful technique with excellent result.

2. **IN VIVO CONGO RED TEST** A known quantity of Congo red dye may be injected intravenously in living patient. If amyloidosis is present, the dye gets bound to amyloid deposits and its levels in blood rapidly decline. The test is, however, not popular due to the risk of anaphylaxis to the injected dye.

3. **OTHER TESTS** Besides tissue diagnosis, a few other tests which are supportive but not confirmatory of amyloidosis include protein electrophoresis, immunoelectrophoresis of urine and serum, and bone marrow aspiration.

PROGNOSIS

Amyloidosis may be an incidental finding at autopsy, or in symptomatic cases diagnosis can be made from the methods given above, biopsy examination being the most important method. The prognosis of patients with generalised amyloidosis is generally poor. Primary amyloidosis, if left untreated, is rapidly progressive and fatal. Therapy in these cases is directed at reducing the clonal marrow plasma cells as is done for treatment of multiple myeloma. For secondary reactive amyloidosis, control of inflammation or infection is the mainstay of treatment. Secondary amyloidosis has somewhat better outcome due to controllable underlying condition.

Renal failure and cardiac arrhythmias are the most common causes of death in most cases of systemic amyloidosis.

GIST BOX 7.2 — Amyloidosis: Stains, Morphology, Diagnosis, Prognosis

- Amyloid deposition causes morphologic and functional disturbance of the affected organ. The affected organ is enlarged, waxy and translucent.
- Confirmation of amyloid in tissue is done by special stains, most commonly Congo red staining (pink red colour) followed by its examination under polarising microscope (apple-green birefringence).
- Primary amyloidosis is rapidly progressive with poor prognosis. Secondary form can occur at any age including children and has better outlook by control of the underlying chronic infection or autoimmune disease.

8 Genetic and Paediatric Diseases

This chapter deals with the group of disorders affecting the foetus during intrauterine life (genetic as well as developmental) and paediatric age group. In the western countries, developmental and genetic birth defects constitute about 50% of total mortality in infancy and childhood, while in the developing and underdeveloped countries 95% of infant mortality is attributed to environmental factors such as poor sanitation and undernutrition.

GENETIC DISEASES

It is estimated that genetic disorders account for 10 per 1000 population globally. However, this incidence is based on lifetime risk of genetic diseases in live births while about 50% of spontaneous abortions, particularly in first trimester, are also due to severe chromosomal abnormalities incompatible with life. In view of advancements in DNA sequencing, it is now possible to determine even minor genetic aberrations in human genome. Before describing this group of diseases, it is important to be familiar with a few commonly used terms:

◈ *Hereditary* means derived from parents while *familial* means transmitted through germ line. Thus, hereditary diseases are familial.

◈ *Congenital* means born with. Not all congenital diseases are genetic e.g. a newborn may be born with congenital syphilis (which is not a genetic disease), nor do all genetic diseases make their appearance at birth e.g. Alzheimer's disease.

In this chapter, following groups of genetic diseases have been discussed:
1. Developmental defects
2. Cytogenetic (Karyotypic) abnormalities
3. Single-gene defects (Mendelian disorders)
4. Multifactorial inheritance disorders
5. Storage diseases (Inborn errors of metabolism)

DEVELOPMENTAL DEFECTS

Developmental defects are a group of abnormalities during foetal life due to errors in morphogenesis. The branch of science dealing with the study of developmental anomalies is called *teratology*. Certain chemicals, drugs, physical and biologic agents are known to induce such birth defects and are called *teratogens*. The morphologic abnormality or defect in an organ or anatomic region of the body so produced is called *malformation*.

Pathogenesis

The teratogens may result in one of the following outcomes:
i) Intrauterine death
ii) Intrauterine growth retardation (IUGR)
iii) Functional defects
iv) Malformation

The effects of teratogens in inducing developmental defects are related to the following factors:

i) *Variable individual susceptibility to teratogen:* All patients exposed to the same teratogen do not develop birth defect.
ii) *Intrauterine stage at which patient is exposed to teratogen:* Most teratogens induce birth defects during the first trimester of pregnancy.
iii) *Dose of teratogen:* Higher the exposure dose of teratogen, greater the chances of inducing birth defects.
iv) *Specificity of developmental defect for specific teratogen:* A particular teratogen acts in a particular way and induces the same specific developmental defect.

Classification

Various developmental anomalies resulting from teratogenic effects are categorised as under:

Agenesis means the complete absence of an organ e.g. unilateral or bilateral agenesis of kidney.

Aplasia is the absence of development of an organ with presence of rudiment or anlage e.g. aplasia of lung with rudimentary bronchus.

Hypoplasia is incomplete development of an organ not reaching the normal adult size e.g. microglossia.

Atresia refers to incomplete formation of lumen in hollow viscus e.g. oesophageal atresia.

Developmental dysplasia is defective development of cells and tissues resulting in abnormal or primitive histogenetic structures e.g. renal dysplasia (*Developmental dysplasia* is quite different from *cellular dysplasia* in relation to precancerous lesions discussed earlier on page 23).

Dysraphic anomalies are the defects resulting from failure of fusion e.g. spina bifida.

Ectopia or heterotopia refers to abnormal location of tissue at ectopic site e.g. pancreatic heterotopia in the wall of stomach.

Examples of Developmental Defects

A few clinically important common examples are given below:

1. **Anencephaly-spina bifida complex** This is the group of anomalies resulting from failure to fuse (dysraphy). While anencephaly results from failure of neural tube closure, spina bifida occurs from incomplete closure of the spinal cord and vertebral column, often in the lumbar region. The latter results in meningocele or meningomyelocele, depending upon whether the content of the sac contains meninges alone or also includes neural tissue.

2. **Thalidomide malformations** Thalidomide is the best known example of teratogenic drug which was used as a sedative by pregnant women in 1960s in England and Germany and resulted in high incidence of limb-reduction anomalies (phocomelia) in the newborns.

3. **Foetal hydantoin syndrome** Babies born to mothers on anti-epileptic treatment with hydantoin have characteristic facial features and congenital heart defects.

4. **Foetal alcohol syndrome** Ethanol is another potent teratogen. Consumption of alcohol by pregnant mother in first trimester increases the risk of miscarriages, stillbirths, growth retardation and mental retardation in the newborn.

5. **TORCH complex** Infection with TORCH group of organisms (*T*oxoplasma, *O*thers, *R*ubella, *C*ytomegalovirus, and *H*erpes simplex) during pregnancy is associated with multisystem anomalies and TORCH syndrome in the newborn (page 193).

6. **Congenital syphilis** As discussed in Chapter 11, vertical transmission of syphilis from mother to foetus is characterised by Hutchinson's triad: interstitial keratitis, sensorineural deafness and deformed Hutchinson's teeth, along with saddle-nose deformity.

GIST BOX 8.1 | **Developmental Defects**

- Developmental defects are errors in morphogenesis during foetal life which occur from use of teratogens.
- Effects of teratogens are intrauterine death and growth retardation, defects in functions or malformations.
- Developmental defects may be of varying grades that include agenesis, aplasia, hypoplasia, atresia, developmental dysplasia, failure of fusion and ectopia.
- A few common examples are anencephaly, spina bifida, thalidomide malformations, foetal hydantoin and alcohol syndrome, TORCH complex, and lesions of congenital syphilis.

CYTOGENETIC (KARYOTYPIC) ABNORMALITIES

Human germ cells (ova and sperms) contain 23 chromosomes (haploid or 1N) while all the nucleated somatic cells of the human body contain 23 pairs of chromosomes (diploid or 2N)—44 autosomes and 2 sex chromosomes, being XX in females (46, XX) and XY in males (46, XY). The branch of science dealing with the study of human chromosomal abnormalities is called cytogenetics.

In a female, one of the two X chromosomes (paternal or maternal derived) is inactivated during embryogenesis as stated in *Lyon hypothesis*. This inactivation is passed to all the somatic cells while the germ cells in the female remain unaffected i.e. ovary will always have active X chromosome. Such an inactive X chromosome in the somatic cells in a female lies condensed in the nucleus and is called as *sex chromatin* seen specifically in the somatic cells in females. *Nuclear sexing* can be done for genetic female testing by preparing and staining the smears of squamous cells scraped from oral cavity, or by identifying the *Barr body* in the circulating neutrophils as drumstick appendage attached to one of the nuclear lobes **(Fig. 8.1)**. A minimum of 30% cells positive for sex chromatin is indicative of genetically female composition.

Though chromosomes can be studied in any human nucleated cells, circulating lymphocytes are more often used for this purpose. The study is done by arresting the dividing cells in metaphase by colchicine and then spreading them on glass slide and staining them with Giemsa stain.

Karyotype is the photographic representation of the stained preparation of chromosomes.

Each chromosome is composed of a pair of identical double helix of chromosomal DNA called *chromatids*. The chromosomes are classified based on their length and location of the *centromere;* centromere is the point where the two chromatids cross each other **(Fig. 8.2)**. The distal end of each chromosome is called telomere.

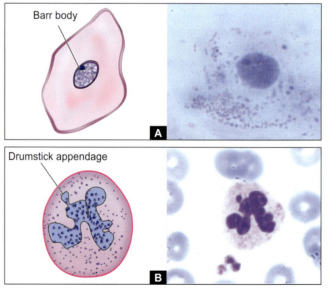

Figure 8.1 ▶ Nuclear sexing. A, Sex chromatin as seen in scraped squamous cells from oral cavity. B, Barr body seen as drumstick appendage attached to a lobe of a circulating neutrophil.

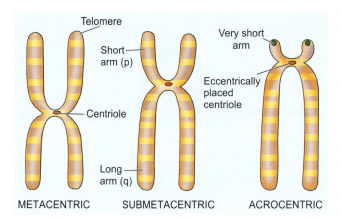

Figure 8.2 ▶ Classification of chromosomes based on size and location of centromere.

Based on centromeric location, they are classified into 3 groups:

1. *Metacentric chromosomes* (numbers 1-3, 16, 19, 20) are those in which the centromere is exactly in the middle.
2. *Submetacentric chromosomes* (numbers 4, 5, 17, 18, 6-12, X) in which the centromere divides the chromosomes into short arm (*p* arm; *petit* means short in French) and long arm (*q* arm; for alphabet next to p).
3. *Acrocentric chromosomes* (numbers 13-15, 21, 22, Y) have very short arm and the centromere is eccentrically located.

Based on length of chromosomes, they are divided into 7 groups—A to G, called *Denver classification* adopted at a meeting in Denver, Colorado in US.

Chromosomal banding techniques are employed for study of classes of chromosomes. Chromosomal bands are unique alternate dark and light staining patterns. Banding techniques include:
i) G-banding (Giemsa stain);
ii) Q-banding (quinacrine fluorescence stain);
iii) R-banding (reverse Giemsa staining); and
iv) C-banding (constitutive heterochromatin demonstration).

With these brief introductory comments, we now turn to abnormalities of chromosomes which can be divided into 2 types:
1. Numerical abnormalities; and
2. Structural abnormalities.

Numerical Abnormalities

As mentioned above, normal karyotype of a human nucleated somatic cell is diploid or 2N (46 chromosomes) while the germ cells have haploid or 1N (23 chromosomes).

1. Polyploidy is the term used for the number of chromosomes which is a multiple of haploid number e.g. triploid or 3N (69 chromosomes), tetraploid or 4N (92 chromosomes). Polyploidy occurs normally in megakaryocytes and dividing liver cells. Polyploidy in somatic cells of conceptus results in spontaneous abortions.

2. Aneuploidy is the number of chromosomes which is not an exact multiple of haploid number e.g. hypodiploid or 2N-1 (45 chromosomes) monosomy, hyperdiploid or 2 N+1 (47 chromosomes) trisomy.

The most common mechanism of aneuploidy is **nondisjunction.** Nondisjunction is the failure of chromosomes to separate normally during cell division during first or second anaphase meiosis, or in mitosis, resulting in too few or too many chromosome in divided cells.

i) In *nondisjunction during first anaphase meiotic division* stage, one pair of homologous chromosomes do not separate. This results in two cells having an extra copy of one chromosome (N+1) and two cells lack that chromosomes (N-1)(nullisomic).

ii) In *Nondisjunction during second anaphase meiotic division* stage, one pair of chromatids do not separate. This will result in two cells with normal haploid number of chromosomes, while one cell will have one extra chromosome (N+1) and one cell will have one less chromosome (N-1).

iii) *Nondisjunction during mitosis* results in mosaicism, meaning thereby that the individual has two or more types of cell lines derived from the same zygote. Mosaicism of mitotic nondisjunction of chromosomes occurs in cancers.

iv) *Anaphase lag* is a form of nondisjunction involving single pair of chromosomes in which one chromosome in meiosis or a chromatid in mitosis fails to reach the pole of dividing cell at the same time (i.e. it lags behind) and is left out of the nucleus of daughter cell. This results in one normal daughter cell and the other monosomic for the missing chromosome.

Three clinically important syndromes resulting from numerical aberrations of chromosomes due to nondisjunction are as under and their main clinical features are illustrated in **Fig. 8.3**:

◆ **Down's syndrome** There is trisomy 21 in about 95% cases of Down's syndrome due to nondisjunction during meiosis in one of the parents. Down's syndrome is the most common chromosomal disorder and is the commonest cause of mental retardation. The incidence of producing offspring with Down's syndrome rises in mothers over 35 years of age.

◆ **Klinefelter's syndrome** Klinefelter's syndrome is the most important example of sex chromosome trisomy. About 80% cases have 47, XXY karyotype while others are mosaics. Typically, these patients have testicular dysgenesis. In general, sex chromosome trisomies are more common than trisomies of autosomes.

◆ **Turner's syndrome** Turner's syndrome is an example of monosomy (45, X0) most often due to loss of X chromosome in paternal meiosis.

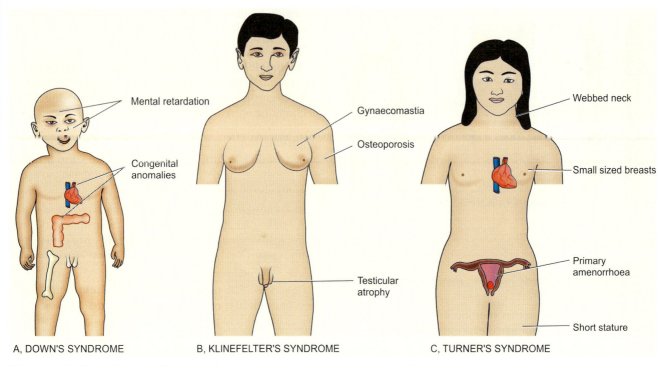

Figure 8.3 ▶ Clinical features of important forms of numerical chromosomal abnormalities.

Structural Abnormalities

During cell division (meiosis as well as mitosis), certain structural abnormalities of chromosomes may appear. These may occur during gametogenesis and then transmitted to all somatic cells and cause hereditary transmissible disorders, or may produce somatic cell mutations and result in changes varying from no effect to some forms of cancers. Structural abnormalities may be balanced or unbalanced.

i) *Balanced structural alteration* means no change in total number of genes or genetic material.

ii) *Unbalanced structural alteration* refers to gene rearrangement resulting in loss or gain of genetic material.

Some common forms of structural abnormalities are as under **(Fig. 8.4)**:

1. TRANSLOCATIONS Translocation means crossing over or exchange of fragment of chromosome which may occur between non-homologous or homologous chromosomes. There are two main types of translocations: reciprocal in about two-third and Robertsonian in one-third cases:

◆ **Reciprocal translocation** is the exchange of genetic material between two non-homologous (heterologous) chromosomes without involving centromere (acentric). Such translocations occur due to single breaks in both the chromosomes and the exchange is detected by banding techniques. Reciprocal translocation may be balanced (without any loss of genetic material during the exchange) or unbalanced (with some loss of genetic material).

i) *Balanced reciprocal translocation* is more common and the individual is phenotypically normal e.g. translocation between long arm (q) of chromosomes 22 and long arm (q) of chromosome 9 written as t (9;22). This translocation is termed Philadelphia chromosome seen in most cases of chronic myeloid leukaemia (page 430).

ii) *Unbalanced reciprocal translocations* are less common and account for repeated abortions and malformed children.

◆ **Robertsonian translocation** is less common than reciprocal translocation. In this, there is fusion of two acrocentric chromosomes (having very short arms) at the centromere (centric fusion) with loss of short arms. The result of this fusion is one very large chromosome and the other very small one. Individuals born with Robertsonian translocation may be phenotypically normal but suffer from infertility and are at higher risk of producing malformed children in the next progeny.

2. DELETIONS Loss of genetic material from the chromosome is called deletion. Deletion may be from the terminal or middle portion of the chromosome. The examples of deletion are: *cri du chat* (cry of infant like that of a cat) syndrome (deletion of short arm of chromosome 5) and several cancers with hereditary basis (e.g. retinoblastoma with deletion of long arm of chromosome 13, Wilms' tumour with deletion of short arm of chromosome 11).

3. INVERSION Inversion is a form of rearrangement involving breaks of a single chromosome at two points.

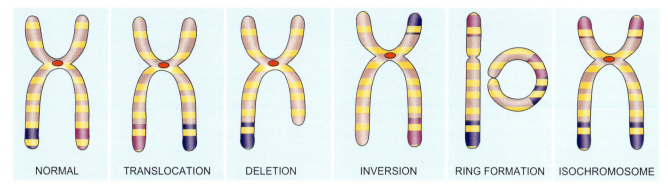

Figure 8.4 ▶ Common structural abnormalities of human chromosomes.

Inversion may be pericentric or paracentric, depending upon whether the rotation occurs at the centromere or at the acentric portion of the arm of chromosome. Inversions are not associated with any abnormality.

4. RING CHROMOSOME A ring of chromosome is formed by a break at both the telomeric (terminal) ends of a chromosome followed by deletion of the broken fragment and then end-to-end fusion. The consequences of ring chromosome depend upon the amount of genetic material lost due to break.

5. ISOCHROMOSOME When centromere, rather than dividing parallel to the long axis, instead divides transverse to the long axis of chromosome, it results in either two short arms only or two long arms only called isochromosomes. The example involving isochromosome of X-chromosome is seen in some cases (15%) of Turner's syndrome.

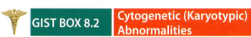

| GIST BOX 8.2 | Cytogenetic (Karyotypic) Abnormalities |

- Abnormalities of chromosomes may be numerical or structural.
- Numerical abnormalities may be due to polyploidy (i.e. multiple of haploid number) or aneuploidy (i.e. which is not a multiple of haploid number).
- A few common examples of numerical aberrations of chromosomes due to nondisjunction are Down's syndrome (trisomy 21), Klinefelter's syndrome (47,XXY) and Turner's syndrome (45,XO).
- Common structural abnormalities are translocations (reciprocal or Robertsonian) and deletions; others are inversion, ring chromosome, and isochromosome.

SINGLE-GENE DEFECTS (MENDELIAN DISORDERS)

The classic laws of inheritance of characteristics or traits were outlined by Austrian monk Gregor Mendel in 1866 based on his observations of cross-breeding of red and white garden peas. Single-gene defects follow the classic mendelian patterns of inheritance and are also called mendelian disorders. These disorders are the result of mutation of a single gene of large effect.

MUTATIONS Term mutation is applied to permanent change in the DNA of the cell. Mutations affecting germ cells are transmitted to the next progeny producing *inherited diseases*, while the mutations affecting somatic cells produce developmental diseases and congenital malformations. Presently, following types of mutations have been described:

i) **Point mutation** is the result of substitution of a single nucleotide base by a different base i.e. replacement of an amino acid by another e.g. in sickle cell anaemia there is point mutation by substitution of glutamic acid by valine in the polypeptide chain.

ii) **Stop codon or nonsense mutation** refers to a type of mutation in which the protein chain is prematurely terminated or truncated.

iii) **Frameshift mutation** occurs when there is insertion or deletion of one or two base pairs in the DNA sequence e.g. in cystic fibrosis of pancreas.

iv) **Trinucleotide repeat mutation** is characterised by amplification of a sequence of three nucleotides.

Thus, it can be summed up from above that single-gene defects are synonymous with various types of heritable mutations. Currently, approximately 5000 single-gene defects have been described—some major and others of minor consequence. While most of these disorders are discussed in relevant chapters later, the group of storage diseases (inborn errors of metabolism) is considered below.

INHERITANCE PATTERN The inheritance pattern of genetic abnormalities may be *dominant or recessive, autosomal or sex-linked:*

A dominant gene* produces its effects, whether combined with similar dominant or recessive gene. *Recessive genes* are

---

*A particular characteristic of an individual is determined by a pair of single *genes,* located at the same specific site termed *locus,* on a pair of homologous chromosomes. These paired genes are called *alleles* which may be *homozygous* when alike, and *heterozygous* if dissimilar. *Genotype* is the genetic composition of an individual while *phenotype* is the effect of genes produced.

effective only if both genes are similar. However, when both alleles of a gene pair are expressed in heterozygous state, it is called *codominant inheritance*. A single gene may express in multiple allelic forms known as *polymorphism*. *Autosomal diseases* are due to defect in any of 1 to 22 autosomes while *sex-linked disorders* are mostly X-linked.

◆ **Autosomal dominant inheritance** pattern is characterised by one faulty copy of gene (i.e. mutant allele) in any autosome and one copy of normal allele; disease phenotype is seen in all such individuals. Patients having autosomal dominant inheritance disease have 50% chance of passing on the disease to the next generation.

◆ In **autosomal recessive inheritance**, both copies of genes are mutated. Usually, it occurs when both parents are carriers of the defective gene, i.e. having one normal allele and one defective allele in each parent, and each parent passes on their defective gene to the next progeny causing disease. There is 25% chance of transmission of autosomal recessive disease when both parents are carriers.

◆ **X-linked disorders** are caused by mutations in genes on X-chromosome, derived from either one of the two X-chromosomes in females, or from the single X-chromosome of the male.

◆ There are much fewer genes on Y-chromosome and are determinant for testis. **Y-linked diseases** are rare and include male infertility, excessive hair on pinna, retinitis pigmentosa and XYY syndrome.

Table 8.1 lists important examples of groups of genetic disorders: *autosomal* recessive (the largest group), co-dominant (intermediate), and dominant, and *sex-(X-) linked* recessive and dominant disorders.

MULTIFACTORIAL INHERITANCE

Some normal phenotypic characteristics have also multifactorial inheritance e.g. colour of hair, eye, skin, height and intelligence. Multifactorial disorders are those disorders which result from the combined effect of genetic composition and environmental influences. Some common examples of such disorders in which environmental influences express the mutant genes are as under:
1. Cleft lip and cleft palate
2. Pyloric stenosis
3. Diabetes mellitus
4. Hypertension
5. Congenital heart disease
6. Coronary heart disease.

GIST BOX 8.3 — Single Gene Defects and Multifactorial Inheritance

❖ Mutation is permanent change in the DNA of the cell. Mutations are of different types: point, stop codon (nonsense), frameshift and trinucleotide repeat.

Table 8.1: Important examples of Mendelian disorders (single gene defects).

I. AUTOSOMAL RECESSIVE INHERITANCE
1. β-thalassaemia
2. Sickle cell anaemia
3. Haemochromatosis
4. Cystic fibrosis of pancreas
5. Albinism
6. Wilson's disease
7. Xeroderma pigmentosum
8. Inborn errors of metabolism (Lysosomal storage diseases, glycogenosis, alkaptonuria, phenylketonuria)

II. AUTOSOMAL CODOMINANT INHERITANCE
1. ABO blood group antigens
2. α 1-antitrypsin deficiency
3. HLA antigens

III. AUTOSOMAL DOMINANT INHERITANCE
1. Familial polyposis coli
2. Adult polycystic kidney
3. Hereditary spherocytosis
4. Neurofibromatosis (von Recklinghausen's disease)
5. Marfan's syndrome
6. von Willebrand's disease
7. Hereditary haemorrhagic telangiectasia
8. Acute intermittent porphyria
9. Familial hypercholesterolaemia
10. Osteogenesis imperfecta

IV. SEX-(X-) LINKED RECESSIVE INHERITANCE
1. Haemophilia A
2. G6PD deficiency
3. Diabetes insipidus
4. Chronic granulomatous disease
5. Colour blindness
6. Bruton's agammaglobulinaemia
7. Muscular dystrophies

V. SEX-(X-) LINKED DOMINANT INHERITANCE
1. Hypophosphataemic rickets
2. Incontinentia pigmenti

❖ The inheritance pattern of genetic abnormalities may be dominant or recessive, autosomal or sex-linked. Most sex-linked diseases are actually X-linked since Y chromosome has very few functional genes.

❖ Multifactorial inheritance is responsible for several normal phenotypic characters. Hypertension and pyloic stenosis are common examples.

STORAGE DISEASES (INBORN ERRORS OF METABOLISM)

Storage diseases or inborn errors of metabolism are biochemically distinct groups of disorders occurring due to genetic defect in the metabolism of carbohydrates, lipids, and proteins resulting in intracellular accumulation of metabolites. These substances may collect within the cells throughout the body but most commonly affected organ or site is the one where the stored material is normally found and degraded. Since lysosomes comprise the chief site of intracellular digestion (autophagy as well as heterophagy), the material is naturally stored in the lysosomes, and hence the generic name 'lysosomal storage diseases'. Cells of mononuclear-phagocyte system are particularly rich in lysosomes; therefore, reticuloendothelial organs containing numerous phagocytic cells like the liver and spleen are most commonly involved in storage disease.

Based on the biochemical composition of the accumulated material within the cells, storage diseases are classified into distinct groups, each group containing a number of diseases depending upon the specific enzyme deficiency. A summary of major groups of storage diseases along with their respective enzyme deficiencies, major accumulating metabolites and the organs involved is presented in **Table 8.2**. A few general comments can be made about all storage diseases:

◆ All the storage diseases occur either as a result of autosomal recessive, or sex-(X-) linked recessive genetic transmission.

◆ Most, but not all, of the storage diseases are lysosomal storage diseases. However, out of the glycogen storage diseases, type II (Pompe's disease) is the only example of lysosomal storage disease.

A few important forms of storage diseases are described below:

Glycogen Storage Diseases (Glycogenoses)

These are a group of inherited disorders in which there is defective glucose metabolism resulting in excessive intracellular accumulation of glycogen in various tissues. Based on specific enzyme deficiencies, glycogen storage diseases are divided into 8 main types designated by Roman numerals I to VIII. However, based on pathophysiology, glycogen storage diseases can be divided into 3 main subgroups:

Table 8.2 Storage diseases (inborn errors of metabolism).

DISEASE	ENZYME DEFICIENCY	ACCUMULATING METABOLITE	ORGANS INVOLVED
GLYCOGEN STORAGE DISEASE			
Type I (von Gierke's disease)	Glucose-6-phosphatase	Glycogen	Liver, kidney
Type II (Pompe's disease)	Acid-α-glucosidase (acid maltase)	Glycogen	Heart, skeletal muscle
Type III (Forbes'/Cori's disease)	Amyloglucosidase (debrancher)	Limit dextrin	Heart, skeletal muscle
Type IV (Anderson's disease)	Amylotransglucosidase (brancher)	Amylopectin	Liver, brain, heart, muscle
Type V (McArdle's disease)	Muscle phosphorylase	Glycogen	Skeletal muscle
Type VI (Hers' disease)	Liver phosphorylase	Glycogen	Brain, heart, liver, muscle
Type VII	Phosphofructokinase	Glycogen	Muscle
Type VIII	Phosphorylase kinase	Glycogen	Liver
MUCOPOLYSACCHARIDOSES (MPS)			
Type I to type VI MPS syndromes	Different lysosomal enzymes	Chondroitin sulphate, dermatan sulphate, heparan sulphate, keratan sulphate	Connective tissue, liver, spleen, bone marrow, lymph nodes, kidneys, heart, brain
SPHINGOLIPIDOSES (GANGLIOSIDOSES)			
GM1-gangliosidosis (infantile and juvenile types)	GM1 ganglioside-galactose	GM1-ganglioside	Liver, kidney, spleen, heart, brain
GM2-gangliosidosis (Tay-Sachs, Sandhoff's disease)	Hexosaminidase	GM2-ganglioside	Liver, kidney, spleen, heart, brain
SULFATIDOSES			
Metachromatic leucodystrophy	Aryl sulfatase A	Sulfatide	Brain, liver, spleen, heart, kidney
Krabbe's disease	Galactocerebrosidase	Galactocerebroside	Nervous system, kidney
Fabry's disease	α-Galactosidase	Ceramide	Skin, kidney, heart, spleen
Gaucher's disease	Glucocerebrosidase	Glucocerebroside	Spleen, liver, bone marrow
Niemann-Pick disease	Sphingomyelinase	Sphingomyelin	Spleen, liver, bone marrow, lymph nodes, lung

1. **Hepatic forms** are characterised by inherited deficiency of hepatic enzymes required for synthesis of glycogen for storage (e.g. von Gierke's disease or type I glycogenosis) or due to lack of hepatic enzymes necessary for breakdown of glycogen into glucose (e.g. type VI glycogenosis).

2. **Myopathic forms** on the other hand, are those disorders in which there is genetic deficiency of glycolysis to form lactate in the striated muscle resulting in accumulation of glycogen in the muscles (e.g. McArdle's disease or type V glycogenosis, type VII disease).

3. **Other forms** are those in which glycogen storage does not occur by either hepatic or myopathic mechanisms. In Pompe's disease or type II glycogenosis, there is lysosomal storage of glycogen, while in type IV there is deposition of abnormal metabolites of glycogen in the brain, heart, liver and muscles.

The prototypes of these three forms are briefly considered below.

VON GIERKE'S DISEASE (TYPE I GLYCOGENOSIS)
This condition is inherited as an autosomal recessive disorder due to deficiency of enzyme, glucose-6-phosphatase. In the absence of glucose-6-phosphatase, excess of normal type of glycogen accumulates in the liver and also results in hypoglycaemia due to reduced formation of free glucose from glycogen. As a result, fat is metabolised for energy requirement leading to hyperlipoproteinaemia and ketosis. Other changes due to deranged glucose metabolism are hyperuricaemia and accumulation of pyruvate and lactate.

The disease manifests clinically in infancy with failure to thrive and stunted growth. Most prominent feature is enormous hepatomegaly with intracytoplasmic and intranuclear glycogen. The kidneys are also enlarged and show intracytoplasmic glycogen in tubular epithelial cells. Other features include gout, skin xanthomas and bleeding tendencies due to platelet dysfunction.

POMPE'S DISEASE (TYPE II GLYCOGENOSIS)
This is also an autosomal recessive disorder due to deficiency of a lysosomal enzyme, acid maltase, and is the only example of *lysosomal* storage disease amongst the various types of glycogenoses. Acid maltase is normally present in most cell types and is responsible for the degradation of glycogen. Its deficiency, therefore, results in accumulation of glycogen in many tissues, most often in the heart and skeletal muscle, leading to cardiomegaly and hypotonia.

McARDLE'S DISEASE (TYPE V GLYCOGENOSIS)
The condition occurs due to deficiency of muscle phosphorylase resulting in accumulation of glycogen in the muscle (deficiency of liver phosphorylase results in type VI glycogenosis). The disease is common in 2nd to 4th decades of life and is characterised by painful muscle cramps, especially after exercise, and detection of myoglobinuria in half the cases.

Mucopolysaccharidoses (MPS)

Mucopolysaccharidoses are a group of six inherited syndromes numbered from MPS I to MPS VI. Each of these result from deficiency of specific lysosomal enzyme involved in the degradation of mucopolysaccharides or glycosaminoglycans, and are, therefore, a form of lysosomal storage diseases. Mucopolysaccharides which accumulate in the MPS are: chondroitin sulphate, dermatan sulphate, heparan sulphate and keratan sulphate. All these syndromes are autosomal recessive disorders except MPS II (Hunter's syndrome) which has X-linked recessive transmission.

Syndrome of MPS manifests in infancy or early childhood and involves multiple organs and tissues, chiefly connective tissues, liver, spleen, bone marrow, lymph nodes, kidneys, heart and brain. The mucopolysaccharides accumulate in mononuclear phagocytic cells, endothelial cells, intimal smooth muscle cells and fibroblasts. The material is finely granular and PAS-positive by light microscopy. By electron microscopy, it appears in the swollen lysosomes and can be identified biochemically as mucopolysaccharide.

Gaucher's Disease

This is an autosomal recessive disorder in which there is mutation in lysosomal enzyme, acid β-glucosidase (earlier called glucocerebrosidase), which normally cleaves glucose from ceramide. This results in lysosomal accumulation of glucocerebroside (ceramide-glucose) in phagocytic cells of the body and sometimes in the neurons. The main sources of glucocerebroside in phagocytic cells are the membrane glycolipids of old leucocytes and erythrocytes, while the deposits in the neurons consist of gangliosides.

Clinically, 3 subtypes of Gaucher's disease are identified based on neuronopathic involvement:

◈ **Type I or classic form** is the adult form of disease in which there is storage of glucocerebrosides in the phagocytic cells of the body, principally involving the spleen, liver, bone marrow, and lymph nodes. This is the most common type comprising 80% of all cases of Gaucher's disease.

◈ **Type II** is the infantile form in which there is progressive involvement of the central nervous system.

◈ **Type III** is the juvenile form of the disease having features in between type I and type II i.e. they have systemic involvement like in type I and progressive involvement of the CNS as in type II.

Clinical features depend upon the clinical subtype of Gaucher's disease. In addition to involvement of different organs and systems (splenomegaly, hepatomegaly, lymphadenopathy, bone marrow and cerebral involvement), a few other features include pancytopenia, or thrombocytopenia secondary to hypersplenism, bone pains and pathologic fractures.

Chapter 8: Genetic and Paediatric Diseases

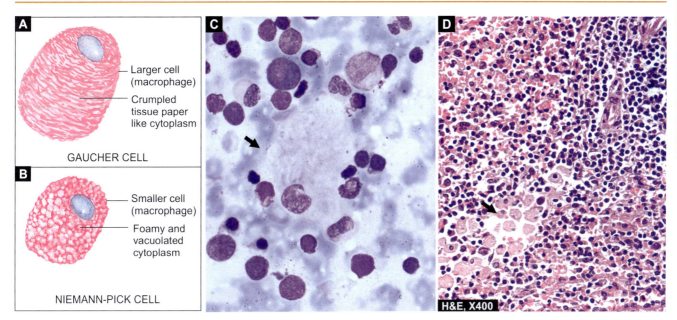

Figure 8.5 ▶ Diagrammatic view of comparative features of typical Gaucher cell (A) and typical macrophage in Niemann-Pick disease (B). C, A Gaucher cell (arrow) in bone marrow aspirate smear. D, Infiltration by Gaucher cells in red pulp of splenic parenchyma.

Microscopy shows large number of characteristically distended and enlarged macrophages called *Gaucher cells* which are found in the spleen, liver, bone marrow and lymph nodes, and in the case of neuronal involvement, in the Virchow-Robin space. The cytoplasm of these cells is abundant, granular and fibrillar resembling crumpled tissue paper. They have mostly a single nucleus but occasionally may have two or three nuclei **(Fig. 8.5, A, C, D)**. Gaucher cells are positive with PAS, oil red O, and Prussian-blue reaction indicating the nature of accumulated material as glycolipids admixed with haemosiderin. These cells often show erythrophagocytosis and are rich in acid phosphatase.

Niemann-Pick Disease

This is also an autosomal recessive disorder characterised by accumulation of sphingomyelin and cholesterol due to defect in acid sphingomyelinase.

Two types have been described: type A and B.

◆ **Type A** is more common and typically presents in infancy and is characterised by hepatosplenomegaly, lymphadenopathy, rapidly progressive deterioration of CNS and physical underdevelopment. About a quarter of patients present with familial amaurotic idiocy with characteristic cherry-red spots in the macula of the retina (*amaurosis* = loss of vision without apparent lesion of the eye).

◆ **Type B** develops later and has a progressive hepatosplenomegaly with development of cirrhosis due to replacement of the liver by foam cells, and impaired lung function due to infiltration in lung alveoli.

Microscopy shows storage of sphingomyelin and cholesterol within the lysosomes, particularly in the cells of mononuclear phagocyte system. The cells of Niemann-Pick disease are somewhat smaller than Gaucher cells and their cytoplasm is not wrinkled but is instead foamy and vacuolated which stains positively with fat stains **(Fig. 8.5, B)**. These cells are widely distributed in the spleen, liver, lymph nodes, bone marrow, lungs, bowel and brain.

GIST BOX 8.4 Storage Diseases

- Storage diseases or inborn errors of metabolism are biochemically distinct disorders occurring due to genetic defect in the metabolism of carbohydrates, lipids, and proteins resulting in intracellular accumulation of metabolites.
- Most of the storage diseases are lysosomal storage diseases. Out of the glycogen storage diseases, type II (Pompe's disease) is the only example of lysosomal storage disease.
- Mucopolysaccharidoses are inherited syndromes resulting from deficiency of specific lysosomal enzyme involved in the degradation of mucopolysaccharides or glycosaminoglycans.
- Gaucher's disease is an autosomal recessive disorder due to mutation in lysosomal enzyme, acid β-glucosidase (earlier called glucocerebrosidase), which normally cleaves glucose from ceramide.
- Niemann-Pick disease is also an autosomal recessive disorder characterised by accumulation of sphingomyelin and cholesterol due to defect in acid sphingomyelinase.

OTHER PAEDIATRIC DISEASES

As mentioned in the foregoing discussion, many diseases affecting infancy and childhood are genetic or developmental in origin. Here, other diseases affecting the period from birth to puberty are discussed under the heading of paediatric diseases. This period is conventionally subdivided into 4 stages:

i) *Neonatal period:* birth to first 4 weeks
ii) *Infancy:* first year of life
iii) *Early childhood:* 1-4 years
iv) *Late childhood:* 5-14 years

Each of these four stages has distinct anatomic, physiologic and immunologic development compared to adults and, therefore, has different groups of diseases unique to particular age groups. Before discussing these diseases affecting different age groups, a few general comments about these stages can be made:

1. Neonatal period is the period of continuation of dependent intrauterine foetal life to independent postnatal period. Therefore, this is the period of maximum risk to life due to perinatal causes (e.g. prematurity, low birth weight, perinatal infections, respiratory distress syndrome, birth asphyxia, birth trauma etc) and congenital anomalies. If adequate postnatal medical care is not provided, neonatal mortality is high. Neonatal mortality in first week after birth is about 10-times higher compared to second week, and shows improvement with every passing week at this stage.

2. In infancy, the major health problems are related to congenital anomalies, infections of lungs and bowel, and sudden infant death syndrome (often during sleep).

3. Young children from 1-4 years are exposed to higher risk of sustaining injuries, and manifest certain congenital anomalies. Some malignant tumours are peculiar to this age group.

4. Older children from 5-14 years too have higher risk of injuries from accidents and have other problems related to congenital anomalies and certain malignant tumours at this age.

Thus, hazardous effects of congenital anomalies are a common denominator for all age groups from birth to adolescence. Specific tumours peculiar to infants and children are discussed along with discussion in related chapters later. However, a short note on general aspects of this subject is given below.

TUMOURS OF INFANCY AND CHILDHOOD

Tumours of infancy and childhood comprise 2% of all malignant tumours but they are the leading cause of death in this age group exceeded only by accidents. Benign tumours are more common than malignant neoplasms but they are generally of little immediate consequence. Another aspect requiring consideration here is the difficulty in differentiating benign tumours from tumour-like lesions.

HISTOGENESIS Histogenetic evolution of tumours at different age groups takes place as under:

1. Some tumours have probably evolved *in utero* and are apparent at birth or in immediate postnatal period. Such tumours are termed *developmental tumours.*

2. Many other tumours originate in abnormally developed organs and organ rests; they become apparent subsequently and are termed *embryonic tumours.*

3. In embryonic tumours, proliferation of embryonic cells occurs which *have not reached the differentiation stage* essential for specialised functions i.e. the cells proliferate as *undifferentiated or as partially differentiated* stem cells and an embryonal tumour (embryoma or blastoma) is formed.

4. Tumours of infancy and childhood have *some features of normal embryonic or foetal cells* in them which proliferate under growth promoting influence of oncogenes and suffer from mutations which make them appear morphologically malignant.

5. Under appropriate conditions, these malignant embryonal cells may *cease to proliferate* and transform into non-proliferating mature differentiated cells e.g. a neonatal neuroblastoma may mature and differentiate into benign ganglioneuroma; tissues in foetal sacrococcygeal teratoma may mature with age to adult tissues and is assigned better prognosis.

Thus, normal somatic cell maturation and neoplastic development in embryonal tumours represent two opposite ends of *ontogenesis,* with capability of some such tumours to mature and differentiate to turn benign from malignant.

Benign Tumours and Tumour-like Conditions

Many of the benign tumours seen in infancy and childhood are actually growth of displaced cells and masses of tissues and their proliferation takes place along with the growth of the child. Some of these tumours undergo a phase of spontaneous regression subsequently—a feature usually not seen in true benign tumours. While some consider such lesions as mere *'tumour-like lesions or malformations'*, others call them benign tumours. A few such examples are as under:

1. Hamartomas Hamartomas are focal accumulations of cells normally present in that tissue but are arranged in an abnormal manner i.e. though present at normal site they do not reproduce normal architecture identical to adjacent tissues (page 266).

2. Choristoma (heterotopia) Choristoma or heterotopia is collection of normal cells and tissues at aberrant locations e.g. heterotopic pancreatic tissue in the wall of small bowel or stomach.

A list of common benign tumours and tumour-like lesions is presented in Table 8.3.

Table 8.3: Common paediatric benign tumours and tumour-like lesions.

NOMENCLATURE	MAIN FEATURES
BENIGN TUMOURS	
i. *Haemangioma*	• Most common in infancy • Commonly on skin (e.g. port-wine stain) • May regress spontaneously
ii. *Lymphangioma*	• Cystic and cavernous type common • Located in skin or deeper tissues • Tends to increase in size after birth
iii. *Sacrococcygeal teratoma*	• Often accompanied with other congenital malformations • Majority (75%) are benign; rest are immature or malignant
iv. *Fibromatosis*	• Solitary (which generally behaves as benign) to multifocal (aggressive lesions)
TUMOUR-LIKE LESIONS/BENIGN TUMOURS	
i. *Naevocellular naevi*	• Very common lesion on the skin
ii. *Liver cell adenoma*	• Most common benign tumour of liver
iii. *Rhabdomyoma*	• Rare foetal and cardiac tumour

Malignant Tumours

Cancers of infancy and childhood differ from those in adults in the following respects:

1. **Sites** Cancers of this age group more commonly pertain to haematopoietic system, neural tissue and soft tissues compared to malignant tumours in adults at sites such as the lung, breast, prostate, colon and skin.

2. **Genetic basis** Many of paediatric malignant tumours have underlying genetic abnormalities.

3. **Regression** Foetal and neonatal malignancies have a tendency to regress spontaneously or to mature.

4. **Histologic features** These tumours have unique histologic features in having primitive or embryonal appearance rather than pleomorphic-anaplastic histologic appearance.

5. **Management** Many of paediatric malignant tumours are curable by chemotherapy and/or radiotherapy but may develop second malignancy.

A few *generalisations* can be drawn about paediatric cancers:

◆ In infants and children under 4 years of age: the most common malignant tumours are various types of *blastomas*.

◆ Children between 5 and 9 years of age: *haematopoietic malignancies* are more common.

◆ In the age range of 10-14 years (prepubertal age): *soft tissue and bony sarcomas* are the prominent tumours.

Based on these broad guidelines, classification of common paediatric malignant tumours at different age groups is presented in **Table 8.4**. These have been discussed in related chapters later.

Table 8.4: Common paediatric malignant tumours.

	SYSTEM	AGE < 4 YRS	AGE 5-9 YRS	AGE 10-14 YRS
1.	Haematopoietic	Acute leukaemia	Acute leukaemia Lymphoma	Hodgkin's
2.	Blastomas	Neuroblastoma Hepatoblastoma Retinoblastoma Nephroblastoma (Wilms' tumour) Pleuropulmonary blastoma	Neuroblastoma Hepatocellular carcinoma	Hepatocellular carcinoma
3.	Soft tissues	Rhabdomyosarcoma	Soft tissue sarcoma	Soft tissue sarcoma
4.	Bony	—	Ewing's sarcoma	Osteogenic sarcoma
5.	Neural	CNS tumours	CNS tumours	—
6.	Others	Teratoma	—	Thyroid cancer

GIST BOX 8.5 — Other Paediatric Diseases

- Tumours of infancy and childhood may evolve during intrauterine life (developmental tumours), or may be embryonic tumours arising from fully or partially differentiated stage or undifferentiated stem cells.
- Common examples of benign paediatric tumours are haemangioma, lymphangioma, sacrococcygeal teratoma and fibromatosis, besides a few possible tumours (naevi, liver cell adenoma).
- Common malignant tumours in children under 4 years of age are acute leukaemias, blastomas/embryomas (neuroblastoma, hepatoblastoma, retinoblastoma, nephroblastoma or Wilms' tumour), gliomas and teratomas.
- Common malignant tumours in older children (beyond 4 and under 14 years of age) are lymphomas, soft tissue sarcomas, osteogenic sarcoma, Ewing's sarcoma and thyroid cancer.

9 Environmental, Nutritional and Vitamin Deficiency Disorders

The subject of environmental hazards to health has assumed great significance in the modern world. In olden times, the discipline of 'tropical medicine' was of interest to the physician, largely due to contamination of air, food and water by infectious and parasitic organisms. Subsequently, the interest got focussed on 'geographic pathology' due to occurrence of certain environment-related diseases confined to geographic boundaries. Then emerged the knowledge of 'occupational diseases' caused by overexposure to a pollutant by virtue of an individual's occupation. Currently, the field of 'environmental pathology' encompasses all such diseases caused by progressive deterioration in the environment, most of which is man-made. In addition, there is the related problem of over- and under-nutrition.

Some of the important factors which have led to the alarming environmental degradation are as under:
1. Population explosion
2. Urbanisation of rural and forest land to accommodate the increasing numbers
3. Accumulation of wastes
4. Unsatisfactory disposal of radioactive and electronic waste
5. Industrial effluents and automobile exhausts.

But the above atmospheric pollutants appear relatively minor compared with *voluntary intake of three pollutants*—use of tobacco, consumption of alcohol and intoxicant drugs. The WHO estimates that 80% cases of cardiovascular disease and type 2 diabetes mellitus, and 40% of all cancers are preventable through 'three pillars of prevention': avoidance of tobacco, healthy diet and physical activity. The WHO has further determined that about a quarter of global burden of diseases and 23% of all deaths are related to modifiable environmental factors. Infant mortality related to environmental factors in developing countries is 12 times higher than in the developed countries.

Attempts at prohibition of alcohol in some states in India have not been quite effective due to difficulty in implementation. Instead, prohibition has only resulted in off and on catastrophe of 'hooch tragedies' in some parts of this country due to illicit liquor consumption.

The subject of environmental and nutritional diseases is covered under the following headings:

A. ENVIRONMENTAL DISEASES
1. *Environmental pollution:*
    i. Air pollution
    ii. Environmental chemicals
    iii. Tobacco smoking
2. *Chemical and drug injury:*
    i. Therapeutic (iatrogenic) drug injury
    ii. Non-therapeutic toxic agents (e.g. alcohol, lead, carbon monoxide, drug abuse)
    iii. Environmental chemicals
3. *Injury by physical agents:*
    i. Thermal and electrical injury
    ii. Injury by ionising radiation

B. NUTRITIONAL DISEASES
1. Overnutrition (obesity)
2. Undernutrition (starvation, protein energy malnutrition)
3. Vitamin deficiencies

ENVIRONMENTAL DISEASES

ENVIRONMENTAL POLLUTION

Environment is air we collectively breathe and share with others at all places—outside, inside homes and at work place. *Pollution* is the contamination of the natural environment which determines adverse effects on health. Any agent—chemical, physical or microbial, that alters the composition of environment is called pollutant. In addition, our personal environment gets affected by smoking of tobacco, water we drink and food we eat. Thus, the subject of environmental pollution is briefly reviewed below under 3 headings: air pollution, environmental chemicals and tobacco smoking.

Air Pollution

For survival of mankind, it is important to prevent depletion of ozone layer (O_3) in the outer space from pollutants such as chlorofluorocarbons and nitrogen dioxide produced in abundance by day-to-day activities on our planet earth due to industrial effluent and automobile exhausts.

A vast variety of pollutants are inhaled daily, some of which may cause trivial irritation to the upper respiratory pathways, while others may lead to acute or chronic injury to the lungs, and some are implicated in causation of lung cancer. Whereas some pollutants are prevalent in certain industries (such as coal dust, silica, asbestos), others are general pollutants present widespread in the ambient atmosphere (e.g. sulphur dioxide, nitrogen dioxide, carbon monoxide). The latter group of environmental pollutants is acted upon by sunlight to produce secondary pollutants such as ozone and free radicals capable of oxidant cell injury to respiratory passages. In highly polluted cities where coal consumption and automobile exhaust accumulate in the atmosphere, the air pollutants become visible as 'smog'. It has been reported that 6 out of 10 largest cities in India have such severe air pollution problem that the annual level of suspended particles is about three times higher than the WHO standards. An estimated 50,000 persons die prematurely every year due to high level of pollution in these cities.

The adverse effects of air pollutants on lung depend upon a few variables that include:
i) longer duration of exposure;
ii) total dose of exposure;
iii) impaired ability of the host to clear inhaled particles; and
iv) particle size of 1-5 μm capable of getting impacted in the distal airways to produce tissue injury.

Pneumoconioses or dust diseases of the lung are the group of lung diseases due to occupational over-exposure to pollutants.

Environmental Chemicals

Our environment gets affected by long-term or accidental exposure to certain man-made or naturally-occurring chemicals. A large number of chemicals are found as contaminants in the ecosystem, food and water supply and find their way into the food chain of man. These substances exert their toxic effects depending upon their mode of absorption, distribution, metabolism and excretion. Some of the substances are directly toxic while others cause ill-effects via their metabolites. Environmental chemicals may have slow damaging effect or there may be sudden accidental exposure such as the Bhopal gas tragedy in India due to accidental leakage of methyl isocyanate (MIC) gas in December 1984.

Some of the common examples of environmental chemicals are given below:

1. Agriculture chemicals Modern agriculture thrives on pesticides, fungicides, herbicides and organic fertilisers which may pose a potential acute poisoning as well as long-term hazard. The problem is particularly alarming in developing countries like India, China and Mexico where farmers and their families are unknowingly exposed to these hazardous chemicals during aerial spraying of crops.

◆ Acute poisoning by organophosphate insecticides is quite well known in India as accidental or suicidal poison by inhibiting acetyl cholinesterase and sudden death.

◆ Chronic human exposure to low level agricultural chemicals is implicated in cancer, chronic degenerative diseases, congenital malformations and impotence but the exact cause-and-effect relationship is lacking.

According to the WHO estimates, about 7.5 lakh people are taken ill every year worldwide with pesticide poisoning, half of which occur in the developing countries due to ready availability and indiscriminate use of hazardous pesticides which are otherwise banned in developed countries. Pesticide residues in food items such as in fruits, vegetables, cereals, grains, pulses etc. is of greatest concern.

2. Volatile organic solvents Volatile organic solvents and vapours are used in industry quite commonly and their exposure may cause acute toxicity or chronic hazard, often by inhalation than by ingestion. Such substances include methanol, chloroform, petrol, kerosene, benzene, ethylene glycol, toluene etc.

3. Metals Pollution by occupational exposure to toxic metals such as mercury, arsenic, cadmium, iron, nickel and aluminium are important hazardous environmental chemicals.

4. Aromatic hydrocarbons Halogenated aromatic hydrocarbons containing polychlorinated biphenyl which are contaminant in several preservatives, herbicides and antibacterial agents are a chronic health hazard.

5. Cyanide Cyanide in the environment is released by combustion of plastic, silk and is also present in cassava and the seeds of apricots and wild cherries. Cyanide is a very toxic chemical and kills by blocking cellular respiration by binding to mitochondrial cytochrome oxidase.

6. Environmental dusts These substances cause pneumoconioses while others are implicated in cancer.

Tobacco Smoking

Habits

Tobacco smoking is the most prevalent and preventable cause of disease and death. The harmful effects of smoking pipe and cigar are somewhat less. Long-term smokers of filter-tipped cigarettes appear to have 30-50% lower risk of development of cancer due to reduced inhalation of tobacco smoke constituents.

Cigarette smoking is a major health problem all over the world. In India, a country of 1.25 billion people, a quarter (300 million) are tobacco users in one form or the other **(Fig. 9.1)**. Smoking *bidis* and chewing *pan masala*, *zarda* and *gutka* are more widely practiced than cigarettes. Habit of smoking *chutta* (a kind of indigenous cigar) in which the lighted end is put in mouth is practiced in the Indian state of Andhra Pradesh and is associated with higher incidence of squamous cell carcinoma of hard palate. Another habit prevalent in Indian states of Uttar Pradesh and Bihar is

Chapter 9: Environmental, Nutritional and Vitamin Deficiency Disorders

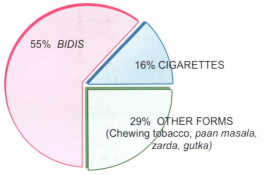

Figure 9.1 ▶ Consumption of tobacco in India as estimated by weight (*Source:* National Council of Applied Economic Research, New Delhi).

Table 9.1	Major constituents of tobacco smoke with adverse effects.	
	ADVERSE EFFECTS	CONSTITUENTS
1.	Carcinogenesis	• Tar • Polycyclic aromatic hydrocarbons • Nitrosamines
2.	Tumour promoters	• Nicotine • Phenol
3.	Irritation and toxicity to respiratory mucosa	• Formaldehyde • Nitrogen oxide
4.	Reduced oxygen transport	• Carbon monoxide

chewing of tabacco alone or mixed with slaked lime as a bolus of *paan* kept in mouth for long hours which is the major cause of cancer of upper aerodigestive tract and oral cavity. *Hookah* smoking, in which tobacco smoke passes through a water-filled chamber which cools the smoke before it is inhaled by the smoker, is believed by some reports to deliver less tar and nicotine than cigarettes and hence fewer tobacco-related health consequences.

In view of serious health hazards of tobacco, the WHO launched Tobacco Free Initiative in 2002. India enacted a law in 2008 banning smoking at all public places, imposing world's biggest smoking ban which is showing favourable results. In US, Canada and most European countries, health awareness by people has resulted in decline in tobacco smoking by about 20%.

Besides the harmful effects of smoking on active smokers themselves, involuntary exposure of smoke to bystanders (passive smoking) is also injurious to health, particularly to infants and children.

Dose and Duration

Tobacco contains several harmful constituents which include nicotine, many carcinogens, carbon monoxide and other toxins **(Table 9.1)**.

The harmful effects of smoking are related to a variety of factors, the most important of which is dose of exposure expressed in terms of pack years. For example, one pack of cigarettes daily for 5 years means 5 pack years. It is estimated that a person who smokes 2 packs of cigarettes daily at the age of 30 years reduces his life by 8 years than a non-smoker. On cessation of smoking, the higher mortality slowly declines and the beneficial effect reaches the level of non-smokers after 20 or more of smoke-free years.

Tobacco-Related Diseases

Tobacco contains numerous toxic chemicals having adverse effects varying from minor throat irritation to carcinogenesis.

Some of the important constituents of tobacco smoke with adverse effects are given in **Table 9.1**.

The relative risk of major diseases in tobacco smokers compared from non-smokers and accounting for higher mortality include the following **(Fig. 9.2)** (in descending order of frequency):

i) Cancer of the lung: 12 to 23 times
ii) Chronic obstructive pulmonary disease (COPD): 10-13 times

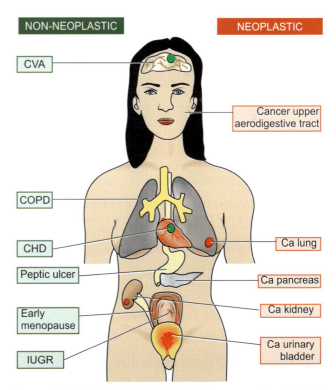

Figure 9.2 ▶ Major adverse effects of tobacco smoking. *Right side* shows smoking-related neoplastic diseases while *left side* indicates non-neoplastic diseases associated with smoking, numbered serially in order of frequency of occurrence.

iii) Cancers of upper aerodigestive tract (larynx, pharynx, lip, oral cavity, oesophagus): 6 to 14 times
iv) Aortic aneurysm: 6-7 times
v) Other cancers by systemic effects (kidneys, pancreas, urinary bladder, stomach, cervix): 2-3 times
vi) Cerebrovascular accidents (CVA): 2-4 times
vii) Coronary heart disease: 2 to 3 times relative risk
viii) Sudden infant death syndrome: 2 times
ix) Buerger's disease (thromboangiitis obliterans)
x) Peptic ulcer disease: 70% higher risk
xi) Early menopause in smoker women
xii) In smoking pregnant women, higher risk of lower birth weight of foetus, higher perinatal mortality and intellectual deterioration of newborn.

GIST BOX 9.1 — Environmental Pollution

- The adverse effects of air pollutants on lung depend upon duration of exposure, total dose of exposure, impaired ability of the host to clear inhaled particles and particle size of 1-5 μm. The effects may range from trivial upper respiratory irritation to pneumoconiosis.
- Our environment gets affected by long-term or accidental exposure to certain man-made or naturally-occurring chemicals e.g. pesticides, volatile organic solvents, toxic metals, aromatic hydrocarbons, cyanide and several environmental dusts.
- Cigarette smoking is a major health problem all over the world. Its effects depend upon the dose and duration.
- Smoking is strongly implicated in many cancers (lung, upper aerodigestive tract, kidneys, pancreas, urinary bladder, cervix) and there is increased incidence of certain non-neoplastic diseases (coronary artery disease, cerebrovascular accidents, Buerger's disease, COPD, peptic ulcer).

CHEMICAL AND DRUG INJURY

During life, each one of us is exposed to a variety of chemicals and drugs. These are broadly divided into the following two categories:
1. *Therapeutic (iatrogenic) agents* e.g. drugs, which when administered indiscriminately are associated with adverse effects.
2. *Non-therapeutic agents* e.g. alcohol, lead, carbon monoxide, drug abuse.

THERAPEUTIC (IATROGENIC) DRUG INJURY

Though the basis of patient management is rational drug therapy, nevertheless adverse drug reactions do occur in 2-5% of patients. In general, the risk of adverse drug reaction increases with increasing number of drugs administered. Adverse effects of drugs may appear due to:
i) overdose;
ii) genetic predisposition;
iii) exaggerated pharmacologic response;
iv) interaction with other drugs; and
v) unknown factors.

It is beyond the scope of this book to delve into the list of drugs with their harmful effects which forms a separate subject of study. However, some of the common forms of iatrogenic drug injury and the offending drugs are listed in **Table 9.2**.

NON-THERAPEUTIC TOXIC AGENTS

Alcoholism

Chronic alcoholism is defined as the regular imbibing of an amount of ethyl alcohol (ethanol) that is sufficient to harm an individual socially, psychologically or physically. It is difficult to give the number of 'drinks' after which the diagnosis of alcoholism can be made because of differences in individual susceptibility. However, adverse effects—acute as well as chronic, are related to the quantity of alcohol content imbibed and duration of consumption. Generally, 10 gm of ethanol is present in:

- one can of beer (or half a bottle of beer);
- 120 ml of neat wine; or
- 30 ml of 43% liquor (small peg).

A daily consumption of 40 gm of ethanol (4 small pegs or 2 large pegs) is likely to be harmful; intake of 100 gm or more daily is certainly dangerous. Daily and heavy consumption of alcohol is more harmful than moderate social drinking having gap periods, since the liver where ethanol is metabolised, gets time to heal.

Metabolism

Absorption of alcohol begins in the stomach and small intestine and appears in blood shortly after ingestion. Alcohol is then distributed to different organs and body fluids proportionate to the blood levels of alcohol. About 2-10% of absorbed alcohol is excreted via urine, sweat and exhaled through breath, the last one being the basis of breath test employed by law-enforcement agencies for alcohol abuse. Metabolism of alcohol is discussed in detail in Chapter 27 (page 549); in brief alcohol is metabolised in the liver by the following 3 pathways **(Fig. 9.3)**:

1. By the major rate-limiting pathway of alcohol dehydrogenase (ADH) in the cytosol, which is then quickly destroyed by aldehyde dehydrogenase (ALDH), especially with low blood alcohol levels.
2. Via microsomal P-450 system (microsomal ethanol oxidising system, MEOS) when the blood alcohol level is high.
3. Minor pathway via catalase from peroxisomes.

In any of the three pathways, ethanol is biotransformed to toxic acetaldehyde in the liver and finally to carbon dioxide and water by acetyl coenzyme A.

Chapter 9: Environmental, Nutritional and Vitamin Deficiency Disorders

Table 9.2	Iatrogenic drug injury.
	ADVERSE EFFECT	OFFENDING DRUG
1.	**GASTROINTESTINAL TRACT**	
	Gastritis, peptic ulcer	Aspirin, nonsteroidal anti-inflammatory drugs (NSAIDs)
	Jejunal ulcer	Enteric-coated potassium tablets
	Pancreatitis	Thiazide diuretics
2.	**LIVER**	
	Cholestatic jaundice	Phenothiazines, tranquilisers, oral contraceptives
	Hepatitis	Halothane, isoniazid
	Fatty change	Tetracycline
3.	**NERVOUS SYSTEM**	
	Cerebrovascular accidents	Anticoagulants
	Peripheral neuropathy	Oral contraceptives
	8th nerve deafness	Vincristine, antimalarials Streptomycin
4.	**SKIN**	
	Acne	Corticosteroids
	Urticaria	Penicillin, sulfonamides
	Exfoliative dermatitis	Penicillin, sulfonamides, phenyl butazone
	Stevens-Johnson syndrome	
	Fixed drug eruptions	Chemotherapeutic agents
5.	**HEART**	
	Arrhythmias	Digitalis, propranalol
	Congestive heart failure	Corticosteroids
	Cardiomyopathy	Adriamycin
6.	**BLOOD**	
	Aplastic anaemia	Chloramphenicol
	Agranulocytosis, thrombocytopenia	Antineoplastic drugs
	Immune haemolytic anaemia	Penicillin
	Megaloblastic anaemia	Methotrexate
7.	**LUNGS**	
	Alveolitis, interstitial pulmonary fibrosis	Anti-neoplastic drugs
	Asthma	Aspirin, indomethacin
8.	**KIDNEYS**	
	Acute tubular necrosis	Gentamycin, kanamycin
	Nephrotic syndrome	Gold salts
	Chronic interstitial nephritis, papillary necrosis	Phenacetin, salicylates
9.	**METABOLIC EFFECTS**	
	Hypercalcaemia	Hypervitaminosis D, thiazide diuretics
	Hepatic porphyria	Barbiturates
	Hyperuricaemia	Anti-cancer chemotherapy
10.	**FEMALE REPRODUCTIVE TRACT**	
	Cholelithiasis, thrombophlebitis, thromboembolism, benign liver cell adenomas	Long-term use of oral contraceptives
	Vaginal adenosis, adenocarcinoma in daughters	Diethylstilbesterol by pregnant women
	Foetal congenital anomalies	Thalidomide in pregnancy

Ill-Effects of Alcoholism

Alcohol consumption in moderation and socially acceptable limits is practiced mainly for its mood-altering effects. Heavy alcohol consumption in unhabituated person is likely to cause acute ill-effects on different organs. Though the diseases associated with alcoholism are discussed in respective chapters later, the spectrum of ill-effects is outlined below.

A. ACUTE ALCOHOLISM Acute effects of inebriation are most prominent on the central nervous system but it also injures the stomach and liver.

1. Central nervous system Alcohol acts as a CNS depressant; the intensity of effects of alcohol on the CNS is related to the quantity consumed and duration over which consumed, which are reflected by the blood levels of alcohol:

i) Initial effect of alcohol is on subcortical structures which is followed by disordered cortical function, motor ataxia and behavioural changes. These changes are apparent when blood alcohol level does not exceed *100 mg/dl* which is the upper limit of sobriety in drinking as defined by law-enforcing agencies in most Western countries while dealing with cases of driving in drunken state.

ii) Blood level of *100-200 mg/dl* is associated with depression of cortical centres, lack of coordination, impaired judgement and drowsiness.

iii) Stupor and coma supervene when blood alcohol level is *about 300 mg/dl*.

iv) Blood level of alcohol *above 400 mg/dl* can cause anaesthesia, depression of medullary centre and death from respiratory arrest.

However, chronic alcoholics develop CNS tolerance and adaptation and, therefore, can withstand higher blood levels of alcohol without such serious effects.

2. Stomach Acute alcohol intoxication may cause vomiting, acute gastritis and peptic ulceration.

3. Liver Acute alcoholic injury to the liver leads to alcoholic hepatitis and its consequences.

B. CHRONIC ALCOHOLISM Chronic alcoholism produces widespread injury to organs and systems. Contrary to the earlier belief that chronic alcoholic injury results from nutritional deficiencies, it is now known that most of the alcohol-related injury to different organs is due to toxic effects of alcohol and accumulation of its main toxic metabolite, acetaldehyde, in the blood. Other proposed mechanisms of tissue injury in chronic alcoholism are free-radical mediated injury and genetic susceptibility to alcohol-dependence and tissue damage.

Some of the more important organ effects in chronic alcoholism are as under **(Fig. 9.4)**:

1. Liver Alcoholic liver disease and cirrhosis are the most common and important effects of chronic alcoholism.

2. Pancreas Chronic calcifying pancreatitis and acute pancreatitis are serious complications of chronic alcoholism.

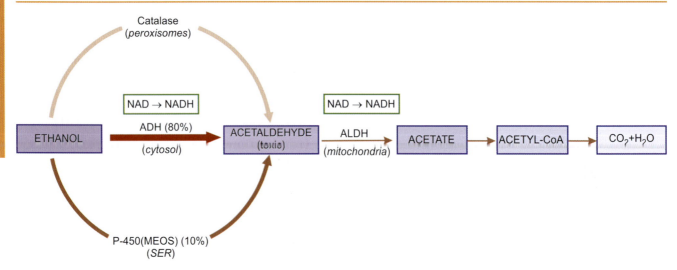

Figure 9.3 ▶ Metabolism of ethanol in the liver. Thickness and intensity of colour of arrow on left side of figure corresponds to extent of metabolic pathway followed (MEOS = microsomal ethanol oxidizing system; ADH = alcohol dehydrogenase; ALDH = aldehyde dehydrogenase; NAD = nicotinamide adenine dinucleotide; NADH = reduced NAD; NADP = nicotinamide adenine dinucleotide phosphate; NADPH = reduced NADP).

3. **Gastrointestinal tract** Gastritis, peptic ulcer and oesophageal varices associated with fatal massive bleeding may occur.

4. **Central nervous system** Peripheral neuropathies and Wernicke-Korsakoff syndrome, cerebral atrophy, cerebellar degeneration and amblyopia (impaired vision) are seen in chronic alcoholics.

5. **Cardiovascular system** Alcoholic cardiomyopathy and beer-drinkers' myocardiosis with consequent dilated cardiomyopathy may occur. Level of HDL (atherosclerosis-protective lipoprotein), however, has been shown to increase with moderate consumption of alcohol.

6. **Endocrine system** In men, testicular atrophy, feminisation, loss of libido and potency, and gynaecomastia may develop. These effects appear to be due to lowering of testosterone levels.

7. **Blood** Haematopoietic dysfunction with secondary megaloblastic anaemia and increased red blood cell volume may occur.

8. **Immune system** Alcoholics are more susceptible to various infections.

9. **Cancer** There is higher incidence of cancers of upper aerodigestive tract in chronic alcoholics but the mechanism is not clear.

Lead Poisoning

Lead poisoning may occur in children or adults due to accidental or occupational ingestion.

In children, following are the main sources of lead poisoning:
i) Chewing of lead-containing furniture items, toys or pencils.
ii) Eating of lead paint flakes from walls.

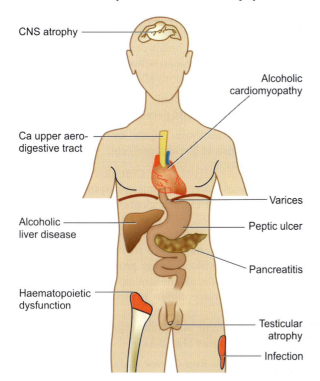

Figure 9.4 ▶ Complications of chronic alcoholism.

Chapter 9: Environmental, Nutritional and Vitamin Deficiency Disorders

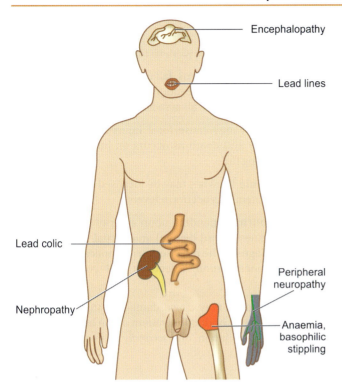

Figure 9.5 ▶ Complications of lead poisoning.

In adults, the sources are as follows:
1. Occupational exposure to lead during spray painting, recycling of automobile batteries (lead oxide fumes), mining, and extraction of lead.
2. Accidental exposure by contaminated water supply, house freshly coated with lead paint, and sniffing of lead-containing petrol (hence unleaded petrol introduced as fuel).

Lead is absorbed through the gastrointestinal tract or lungs. The absorbed lead is distributed in two types of tissues (Fig. 9.5):

a) *Bones, teeth, nails and hair* representing relatively harmless pool of lead. About 90% of absorbed lead accumulates in the developing metaphysis of bones in children and appears as areas of increased bone densities ('lead lines') on X-ray. Lead lines are also seen in the gingiva.

b) *Brain, liver, kidneys and bone marrow* accumulate the remaining 10% lead which is directly toxic to these organs. It is excreted via kidneys.

Lead toxicity occurs in the following organs predominantly:

1. **Nervous system** Following changes are seen:
i) *In children,* lead encephalopathy; oedema of brain, flattening of gyri and compression of ventricles.
ii) *In adults,* demyelinating peripheral motor neuropathy which typically affects radial and peroneal nerves resulting in wrist-drop and foot-drop respectively.

2. **Haematopoietic system** Changes in the blood are quite characteristic:
i) *Microcytic hypochromic anaemia* due to inhibition of two enzymes: delta-aminolevulinic acid dehydrogenase required for haem synthesis, and through inhibition of ferroketolase required for incorporation of ferrous iron into the porphyrin ring.
ii) Prominent basophilic stippling of erythrocytes.

3. **Kidneys** Lead is toxic to proximal tubular cells of the kidney and produces *lead nephropathy* characterised by accumulation of intranuclear inclusion bodies consisting of lead-protein complex in the proximal tubular cells.

4. **Gastrointestinal tract** Lead toxicity in the bowel manifests as acute abdomen presenting as lead colic.

Carbon Monoxide Poisoning

Carbon monoxide (CO) is a colourless and odourless gas produced by incomplete combustion of carbon. Sources of CO gas are:
i) automobile exhaust;
ii) burning of fossil fuel in industries or at home; and
iii) tobacco smoke.

CO is an important cause of accidental death due to systemic oxygen deprivation of tissues. This is because haemoglobin has about 200-times higher affinity for CO than for O_2 and thus varying amount of carboxyhaemoglobin is formed depending upon the extent of CO poisoning. Besides, carboxyhaemoglobin interferes with the release of O_2 from oxyhaemoglobin causing further aggravation of tissue hypoxia. Diagnosis of CO poisoning is, therefore, best confirmed by carboxyhaemoglobin levels in the blood.

CO poisoning may present in 2 ways:
◈ **Acute CO poisoning** in which there is sudden development of brain hypoxia characterised by oedema and petechial haemorrhages.
◈ **Chronic CO poisoning** presents with nonspecific changes of slowly developing hypoxia of the brain.

Drug Abuse

Drug abuse is defined as the use of certain drugs for the purpose of 'mood alteration' or 'euphoria' or 'kick' but subsequently leading to habit-forming, dependence and eventually addiction. Some of the commonly abused drugs and substances are as under:

1. **Marijuana or 'pot'** is psychoactive substance most widely used. It is obtained from the leaves of the plant *Cannabis sativa* and contains tetrahydrocannabinol (THC). It may be smoked or ingested.

2. **Derivatives of opium** that includes heroin and morphine. Opioids are derived from the poppy plant.

Heroin and morphine are self-administered intravenously or subcutaneously.

3. **CNS depressants** include barbiturates, tranquilisers and alcohol.

4. **CNS stimulants** e.g. cocaine and amphetamines.

5. **Psychedelic drugs** (meaning enjoyable perception-giving) e.g. LSD.

6. **Inhalants** e.g. glue, paint thinner, nail polish remover, aerosols, amyl nitrite.

It is beyond the scope of the present discussion to go into the pharmacologic actions of all these substances. However, apart from pharmacologic and physiologic actions of these street drugs, the most common complication is introduction of infection by parenteral use of many of these drugs. Sharing of needles by the drug-addicts accounts for high risk of most feared viral infections in them, AIDS and viral hepatitis (HBV and HCV). Following are a few common drug abuse-related infectious complications:

1. At the site of injection—cellulitis, abscesses, ulcers, thrombosed veins
2. Thrombophlebitis
3. Bacterial endocarditis
4. High risk for AIDS
5. Viral hepatitis and its complications
6. Focal glomerulonephritis
7. Talc (foreign body) granuloma formation in the lungs.

| GIST BOX 9.2 | Chemical and Drug Injury |

- Harmful chemicals and drugs can be broadly divided into 2 groups: therapeutic (iatrogenic) agents (e.g. drugs, which when administered indiscriminately are associated with adverse effects) and non-therapeutic agents (e.g. alcohol, lead, carbon monoxide, drug abuse).
- Alcoholism may produce acute and chronic effects on the body. Most prominent ill-effect of acute alcoholism is on the central nervous system; other acute effects are on the stomach and liver. Chronic alcoholism causes alcoholic liver disease, pancreatitis, and other systemic adverse manifestations pertaining to CNS, CVS, endocrines, blood, and immune system.
- Lead poisoning may occur in children by eating lead-contaminated items and in adults from occupational or accidental exposure. The adverse effects pertain to nervous system and blood.
- Carbon monoxide poisoning may cause accidental death or may produce chronic effects.
- Drug abuse from marijuana, opium, barbiturates, cocaine, inhalants etc may cause a variety of local and systemic effects.

INJURY BY PHYSICAL AGENTS

THERMAL AND ELECTRICAL INJURY

Thermal and electrical burns, fall in body temperature below 35°C (hypothermia) and elevation of body temperature above 41°C (hyperthermia), are all associated with tissue injury.

1. **Hypothermia** may cause focal injury as in frostbite, or systemic injury and death as occurs on immersion in cold water for varying time.

2. **Hyperthermia** likewise, may be localised as in cutaneous burns, and systemic as occurs in fevers.

3. **Thermal burns** depending upon severity are categorised into full thickness (third degree) and partial thickness (first and second degree). The most serious complications of burns are haemoconcentration, infections and contractures on healing.

4. **Electrical burns** may cause damage *firstly,* by electrical dysfunction of the conduction system of the heart and death by ventricular fibrillation, and *secondly* by heat produced by electrical energy.

INJURY BY RADIATION

The most important form of radiation injury is ionising radiation which has three types of effects on cells:
i) Somatic effects which cause acute cell killing.
ii) Genetic damage by mutations and therefore, passes genetic defects in the next progeny of cells.
iii) Malignant transformation of cells (Chapter 19).

Ionising radiation is widely employed for diagnostic purpose as well as for radiotherapy of malignant tumours. Radiation-induced cell death is mediated by radiolysis of water in the cell with generation of toxic hydroxyl radicals (page 34). During radiotherapy, some normal cells coming in the field of radiation are also damaged. In general, radiation-induced tissue injury predominantly affects endothelial cells of small arteries and arterioles, causing necrosis and ischaemia.

Ionising radiation causes damage to the following major organs:
1. *Skin:* radiation dermatitis, cancer.
2. *Lungs:* interstitial pulmonary fibrosis.
3. *Heart:* myocardial fibrosis, constrictive pericarditis.
4. *Kidney:* radiation nephritis.
5. *Gastrointestinal tract:* strictures of small bowel and oesophagus.
6. *Gonads:* testicular atrophy in males and destruction of ovaries.
7. *Haematopoietic tissue:* pancytopenia due to bone marrow depression.
8. *Eyes:* cataract.

Besides ionising radiation, other form of harmful radiation is *solar (u.v.) radiation* which may cause acute skin injury as sunburns, chronic conditions such as solar keratosis and early onset of cataracts in the eyes. It may, however, be mentioned in passing here that electromagnetic radiation produced by microwaves (ovens, radars, diathermy) or ultrasound waves used for diagnostic purposes do not produce ionisation and thus are not known to cause any tissue injury.

GIST BOX 9.3 — Injury by Physical Agents

- Physical agents causing tissue injury are thermal and electrical burns, fall in body temperature below 35°C (hypothermia) and elevation of body temperature above 41°C (hyperthermia).
- Ionising radiation and solar radiation cause damage to somatic cells, genetic damage and malignant transformation.

NUTRITIONAL DISORDERS

NUTRITIONAL REQUIREMENT

Nutritional status of a society varies according to the socioeconomic conditions. In the Western world, nutritional imbalance is more often a problem accounting for increased frequency of obesity, while in developing countries of Africa, Asia and South America, chronic malnutrition is a serious health problem, particularly in children.

Before describing the nutritional diseases, it is essential to know the components of normal and adequate nutrition. For good health, humans require energy-providing nutrients (proteins, fats and carbohydrates), vitamins, minerals, water and some non-essential nutrients.

1. Energy The requirement of energy by the body is calculated in Kcal per day. In order to retain stable weight and undertake day-to-day activities, the energy intake must match the energy output. The average requirement of energy for an individual is estimated by the formula: 900+10w for males, and 700+7w for females (where w stands for the weight of the individual in kilograms). Since the requirement of energy varies according to the level of physical activities performed by the person, the figure arrived at by the above formula is multiplied by: 1.2 for sedentary person, 1.4 for moderately active person and 1.8 for very active person.

2. Proteins Dietary proteins provide the body with amino acids for endogenous protein synthesis and are also a metabolic fuel for energy (1 g of protein provides 4 Kcal). *Nine essential amino acids* (histidine, isoleucine, leucine, lysine, methionine/cystine, phenylalanine/tyrosine, theonine, tryptophan and valine) must be supplied by dietary intake as these cannot be synthesised in the body. The recommended average requirement of proteins for an adult is 0.6 g/kg of the desired weight per day. For a healthy person, 10-14% of caloric requirement should come from proteins.

3. Fats Fats and fatty acids (in particular linolenic, linoleic and arachidonic acid) should comprise about 35% of diet. In order to minimise the risk of atherosclerosis, poly-unsaturated fats should be limited to <10% of calories and saturated fats and trans-fats should comprise <10% of calories while monounsaturated fats to constitute the remainder of fat intake (1 g of fat yields 9 Kcal).

4. Carbohydrates Dietary carbohydrates, are the major source of dietary calories, especially for the brain, RBCs and muscles (1 g of carbohydrate provides 4 Kcal). At least 55% of total caloric requirement should be derived from carbohydrates.

5. Vitamins These are mainly derived from exogenous dietary sources and are essential for maintaining the normal structure and function of cells. A healthy individual requires 4 fat-soluble vitamins (A, D, E and K) and 11 water-soluble vitamins (C, B_1 or thiamine, B_2 or riboflavin, B_3 or niacin or nicotinic acid, B_5 or pantothenic acid, B_6 or pyridoxine, folate or folic acid, B_{12} or cyanocobalamin, choline, biotin, and flavonoids). Vitamin deficiencies result in individual deficiency syndromes, or may be part of a multiple deficiency state.

6. Minerals A number of minerals like iron, calcium, phosphorus and certain trace elements (e.g. zinc, copper, selenium, iodine, chlorine, sodium, potassium, magnesium, manganese, cobalt, molybdenum etc) are essential for health. Their deficiencies result in a variety of lesions and deficiency syndromes.

7. Water Water intake is essential to cover the losses in faeces, urine, exhalation and insensible loss so as to avoid under- or over-hydration. Although body's water needs vary according to physical activities and weather conditions, average requirement of water is 1.0-1.5 ml water/Kcal of energy spent. Infants and pregnant women have relatively higher requirements of water.

8. Non-essential nutrients Dietary fibre composed of cellulose, hemicellulose and pectin, though considered non-essential, are important due to their beneficial effects in lowering the risk of colonic cancer, diabetes and coronary artery disease.

Pathogenesis of Deficiency Diseases

The nutritional deficiency disease develops when the essential nutrients are not provided to the cells adequately. The nutritional deficiency may be of 2 types:

1. Primary deficiency This is due to either the lack or decreased amount of essential nutrients in diet.

2. Secondary or conditioned deficiency Secondary or conditioned deficiency is malnutrition occurring as a result of the various factors. These are as under:

i) *Interference with ingestion* e.g. in gastrointestinal disorders such as malabsorption syndrome, chronic alcoholism, neuropsychiatric illness, anorexia, food allergy, pregnancy.

ii) *Interference with absorption* e.g. in hypermotility of the gut, achlorhydria, biliary disease.

iii) *Interference with utilisation* e.g. in liver dysfunction, malignancy, hypothyroidism.

iv) *Increased excretion* e.g. in lactation, perspiration, polyuria.

v) *Increased nutritional demand* e.g. in fever, pregnancy, lactation, hyperthyroidism.

Irrespective of the type of nutritional deficiency (primary or secondary), nutrient reserves in the tissues begin to get depleted, which initially result in biochemical alterations and eventually lead to functional and morphological changes in tissues and organs.

In the following pages, a brief account of nutritional imbalance (viz. *obesity*) is followed by description of multiple or mixed deficiencies (e.g. *starvation, protein-energy malnutrition*) and individual nutrient deficiencies (e.g. *vitamin deficiencies*).

OBESITY

Dietary imbalance and overnutrition may lead to obesity. *Obesity is defined as an excess of adipose tissue that imparts health risk; a body weight of 20% excess over ideal weight for age, sex and height is considered a health risk.* The most widely used method to gauge obesity is body mass index (BMI) which is equal to weight in kg/height in m^2. A cut-off BMI value of 30 is used for obesity in both men and women.

ETIOLOGY *Obesity results when caloric intake exceeds utilisation.* The imbalance of these two components can occur in the following situations:

1. *Inadequate pushing of oneself away from the dining table* causing overeating.
2. *Insufficient pushing of oneself out of the chair* leading to inactivity and sedentary life style.
3. *Genetic predisposition* to develop obesity.
4. *Diets largely derived from carbohydrates* and fats than protein-rich diet.
5. *Secondary obesity* may result following a number of underlying diseases such as hypothyroidism, Cushing's disease, insulinoma and hypothalamic disorders.

PATHOGENESIS The lipid storing cells, adipocytes comprise the adipose tissue, and are present in vascular and stromal compartment in the body. Besides the generally, accepted role of adipocytes for fat storage, these cells also release endocrine-regulating molecules. These molecules include: energy regulatory hormone (leptin), cytokines (TNF-α and interleukin-6), insulin sensitivity regulating agents (adiponectin, resistin and RBP4), prothrombotic factors (plasminogen activator inhibitor), and blood pressure regulating agent (angiotensinogen).

Adipose mass is increased due to enlargement of adipose cells due to excess of intracellular lipid deposition as well as due to increase in the number of adipocytes. The most important environmental factor is excess consumption of nutrients which can lead to obesity. However, underlying molecular mechanisms of obesity are beginning to unfold based on observations that obesity is familial and is seen in identical twins. Recently, two obesity genes have been found: *ob* gene and its protein product leptin, and *db* gene and its protein product leptin receptor.

SEQUELAE OF OBESITY Marked obesity is a serious health hazard and may predispose to a number of clinical disorders and pathological changes described below and illustrated in **Fig. 9.6**.

> **MORPHOLOGIC FEATURES** Obesity is associated with increased adipose stores in the subcutaneous tissues, skeletal muscles, internal organs such as the kidneys, heart, liver and omentum; fatty liver is also more common in obese individuals. There is increase in both size and number of adipocytes i.e. there is hypertrophy as well as hyperplasia.

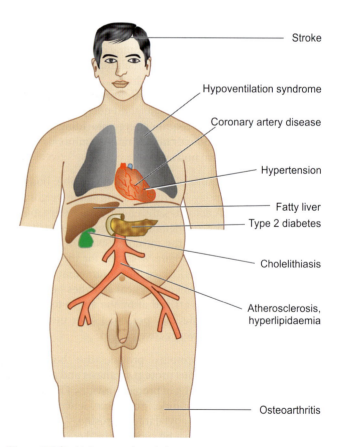

Figure 9.6 ▶ Major sequelae of obesity.

EFFECTS OF OBESITY Obesity may cause following ill-effects:

1. **Hyperinsulinaemia** Increased insulin secretion is a feature of obesity. Many obese individuals exhibit hyperglycaemia or frank diabetes despite hyperinsulinaemia. This is due to a state of insulin-resistance consequent to tissue insensitivity.

2. **Type 2 diabetes mellitus** There is a strong association of type 2 diabetes mellitus with obesity. Obesity often exacerbates the diabetic state and in many cases weight reduction often leads to amelioration of diabetes.

3. **Hypertension** A strong association between hypertension and obesity is observed which is perhaps due to increased blood volume. Weight reduction leads to significant reduction in systolic blood pressure.

4. **Hyperlipoproteinaemia** The plasma cholesterol circulates in the blood as low-density lipoprotein (LDL) containing most of the circulating triglycerides. Obesity is strongly associated with VLDL and mildly with LDL. Total blood cholesterol levels are also elevated in obesity.

5. **Atherosclerosis** Obesity predisposes to development of atherosclerosis. As a result of atherosclerosis and hypertension, there is increased risk of myocardial infarction and stroke in obese individuals.

6. **Nonalcoholic fatty liver disease (NAFLD)** Obesity contributes to development of NAFLD which may progress further to cirrhosis of the liver.

7. **Cholelithiasis** There is six times higher incidence of gallstones in obese persons, mainly due to increased total body cholesterol.

8. **Hypoventilation syndrome (Pickwickian syndrome)** This is characterised by hypersomnolence, both at night and during day in obese individuals along with carbon dioxide retention, hypoxia, polycythaemia and eventually right-sided heart failure (Mr Pickwick was a character, the fat boy, in Charles Dickens' *Pickwick Papers*. The term pickwickian syndrome was first used by Sir William Osler for the sleep-apnoea syndrome).

9. **Osteoarthritis** These individuals are more prone to develop degenerative joint disease due to wear and tear following trauma to joints as a result of large body weight.

10. **Cancer** Diet rich in fats, particularly derived from animal fats and meats, is associated with higher incidence of cancers of colon, breast, endometrium and prostate.

STARVATION

Starvation is a state of overall deprivation of nutrients. Its causes may be the following:
i) deliberate fasting—religious or political;
ii) famine conditions in a country or community; or
iii) secondary under nutrition such as due to chronic wasting diseases (infections, inflammatory conditions, liver disease), cancer etc. Cancer results in malignant cachexia as a result of which cytokines are elaborated e.g. tumour necrosis factor-α, elastases, proteases etc.

A starved individual has lax, dry skin, wasted muscles and atrophy of internal organs.

METABOLIC CHANGES The following metabolic changes take place in starvation:

1. **Glucose** *Glucose stores* of the body are sufficient for one day's metabolic needs only. During fasting state, insulin-independent tissues such as the brain, blood cells and renal medulla continue to utilise glucose while insulin-dependent tissues like muscle stop taking up glucose. This results in release of glycogen stores of the liver to maintain normal blood glucose level. Subsequently, hepatic gluconeogenesis from other sources such as breakdown of proteins takes place.

2. **Proteins** Protein stores and the triglycerides of adipose tissue have enough energy for about 3 months in an individual. *Proteins* breakdown to release amino acids which are used as fuel for hepatic gluconeogenesis so as to maintain glucose needs of the brain. This results in nitrogen imbalance due to excretion of nitrogen compounds as urea.

3. **Fats** After about one week of starvation, protein breakdown is decreased while *triglycerides* of adipose tissue breakdown to form glycerol and fatty acids. The fatty acids are converted into ketone bodies in the liver which are used by most organs including brain in place of glucose. Starvation can then continue till all the body fat stores are exhausted following which death occurs.

PROTEIN-ENERGY MALNUTRITION

The inadequate consumption of protein and energy as a result of primary dietary deficiency or conditioned deficiency may cause loss of body mass and adipose tissue, resulting in protein energy or protein calorie malnutrition (PEM or PCM). The primary deficiency is more frequent due to socioeconomic factors limiting the quantity and quality of dietary intake, particularly prevalent in the developing countries of Africa, Asia and South America. The impact of deficiency is marked in infants and children.

The spectrum of *clinical syndromes* produced as a result of PEM includes the following (Fig. 9.7):
1. *Kwashiorkor* which is related to protein deficiency though calorie intake may be sufficient.
2. *Marasmus* is starvation in infants occurring due to overall lack of calories.

The salient features of the two conditions are contrasted in Table 9.3. However, it must be remembered that mixed forms of kwashiorkor-marasmus syndrome may also occur.

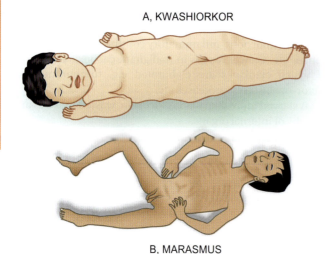

Figure 9.7 ▶ Two forms of PEM.

METALS AND TRACE ELEMENTS

Several minerals in trace amounts are essential for health since they form components of enzymes and cofactors for metabolic functions. Besides *calcium* and *phosphorus* required for vitamin D manufacture, others include: *iron, copper, iodine, zinc, selenium, manganese, nickel, chromium, molybdenum, fluorine*. However, out of these, the dietary deficiency of first five trace elements is associated with deficiency states which are discussed in detail in respective chapters later. These are as under:

i) *Iron:* Microcytic hypochromic anaemia.
ii) *Calcium:* Reduced bone mass, osteoporosis.
iii) *Phosphorus:* Rickets, osteomalacia.
iv) *Copper:* Muscle weakness, neurologic defect, anaemia, growth retardation.
v) *Iodine:* Goitre and hyperthyroidism, cretinism.
vi) *Zinc:* Growth retardation, infertility, alopecia.
vii) *Selenium:* Cardiomyopathy, muscle degeneration.
viii) *Fluoride:* Dental caries.
ix) *Manganese*: Impaired growth and skeletal development.
x) *Molybdenum*: Severe neurological abnormalities.

 GIST BOX 9.4 — Nutritional Disorders

❖ For good health, humans require energy-providing nutrients (proteins, fats and carbohydrates), vitamins, minerals, water and some non-essential nutrients.
❖ The nutritional deficiency may be *primary* due to either the lack or decreased amount of essential nutrients in diet, or *secondary* or conditioned deficiency occurring as a result of the various factors such as interference in ingestion, absorption, excretion, or increased nutritional demand.
❖ Dietary imbalance and overnutrition may lead to obesity. Effects of obesity are hyperinsulinaemia, type 2 diabetes, hypertension, atherosclerosis, non-alcoholic fatty liver disease, cholelithiasis, hyperventilation, and osteoarthritis.
❖ Starvation is a state of overall deprivation of nutrients i.e. glucose, proteins and fats.
❖ The inadequate consumption of protein and energy cause loss of body mass and adipose tissue, resulting in protein energy or protein calorie malnutrition (PEM or PCM). It is of 2 types: *kwashiorkor* which is related to protein deficiency though calorie intake may be sufficient, and *marasmus* which is starvation in infants occurring due to overall lack of calories.

Table 9.3   Contrasting features of kwashiorkor and marasmus.

FEATURE	KWASHIORKOR	MARASMUS
Definition	Protein deficiency with sufficient calorie intake	Starvation in infants with overall lack of calories
Clinical features	Occurs in children between 6 months and 3 years of age	Common in infants under 1 year of age
	Growth failure	Growth failure
	Wasting of muscles but preserved adipose tissues	Wasting of all tissues including muscles and adipose tissues
	Oedema, localised or generalised, present	Oedema absent
	Enlarged fatty liver	No hepatic enlargement
	Serum proteins low	Serum proteins low
	Anaemia present	Anaemia present
	'Flag sign'—alternate bands of light (depigmented) and dark (pigmented) hair	Monkey-like face, protuberant abdomen, thin limbs
Morphology	Enlarged fatty liver	No fatty liver
	Atrophy of different tissues and organs but subcutaneous fat preserved	Atrophy of different tissues and organs including subcutaneous fat

Chapter 9: Environmental, Nutritional and Vitamin Deficiency Disorders

❖ Besides calcium and phosphorus, several trace elements required in diet may produce deficiency states. Most important ones are due to iron, copper, iodine and zinc.

DISORDERS OF VITAMINS

Vitamins are organic substances which cannot be synthesised within the body and are essential for maintenance of normal structure and function of cells. Thus, these substances must be provided in the human diet. Most of the vitamins are of plant or animal origin so that they normally enter the body as constituents of ingested plant food or animal food. They are required in minute amounts in contrast to the relatively large amounts of essential amino acids and fatty acids. Vitamins do not play any part in production of energy.

ETIOLOGY OF VITAMIN DEFICIENCIES In the developing countries, *multiple deficiencies* of vitamins and other nutrients are common due to generalised malnutrition of dietary origin. In the developed countries, *individual vitamin deficiencies* are noted more often, particularly in children, adolescent, pregnant and lactating women, and in some due to poverty. General secondary causes of conditioned nutritional deficiencies listed already (i.e. interference in ingestion, absorption, utilization, excretion) can result in vitamin deficiency in either case. Chronic alcoholism is a common denominator in many of vitamin deficiencies. A few other noteworthy features about vitamins are as under:
1. While vitamin deficiency as well as its excess may occur from another disease, the states of excess and deficiency themselves also cause disease.
2. Vitamins in high dose can be used as drugs.

CLASSIFICATION OF VITAMINS Vitamins are conventionally divided into 2 groups: fat-soluble and water-soluble.

1. Fat-soluble vitamins There are 4 fat-soluble vitamins: A, D, E and K. They are absorbed from intestine in the presence of bile salts and intact pancreatic function. Their deficiencies occur more readily due to conditioning factors (*secondary deficiency*). Beside the deficiency syndromes of these vitamins, a state of *hypervitaminosis* due to excess of vitamin A and D also occurs.

2. Water-soluble vitamins This group conventionally consists of vitamin C and members of B complex group. Besides, choline, biotin and flavonoids are new additions to this group. Water-soluble vitamins are more readily absorbed from small intestine. Deficiency of these vitamins is mainly due to *primary (dietary) factors*. Being water soluble, these vitamins are more easily lost due to cooking or processing of food.

Table 9.4 sums up the various clinical disorders produced by vitamin deficiencies.

FAT-SOLUBLE VITAMINS

Vitamin A (Retinol)

PHYSIOLOGY Vitamin A or retinol is a fat-soluble alcohol. It is available in diet in 2 forms:
◈ *As preformed retinol,* the dietary sources of which are animal-derived foods such as yolk of eggs, butter, whole milk, fish, liver, kidney.
◈ *As provitamin precursor carotenoid,* which is derived from β-carotene-containing foods such as yellow plants and vegetables e.g. carrots, potatoes, pumpkins, mangoes, spinach. β-carotene can be absorbed intact or converted in the intestinal mucosa to form retinaldehyde which is subsequently reduced to retinol.

Retinol is stored in the liver cells and released for transport to peripheral tissues after binding to retinol-binding protein found in blood.

The **physiologic functions** of retinol are as follows:
1. *Maintenance of normal vision in reduced light.* This involves formation of 2 pigments by oxidation of retinol: *rhodopsin*, a light sensitive pigment in reduced light synthesised in the rod cells, and *iodopsins* sensitive in bright light and formed in cone cells of retina. These pigments then transform the radiant energy into nerve impulses.
2. *Maintenance of structure and function of specialised epithelium.* Retinol plays an important role in the synthesis of glycoproteins of the cell membrane of specialised epithelium such as mucus-secreting columnar epithelium in glands and mucosal surfaces, respiratory epithelium and urothelium.
3. *Maintenance of normal cartilaginous and bone growth.*
4. *Increased immunity* against infections in children.
5. *Anti-proliferative effect.* β-carotene has anti-oxidant properties and may cause regression of certain non-tumorous skin diseases, premalignant conditions and certain cancers.

LESIONS IN VITAMIN A DEFICIENCY Nutritional deficiency of vitamin A is common in countries of South-East Asia, Africa, Central and South America whereas malabsorption syndrome may account for conditioned vitamin A deficiency in developed countries.

MORPHOLOGIC FEATURES Consequent to vitamin A deficiency, following pathologic changes are seen (Fig. 9.8):

1. Ocular lesions Lesions in the eyes are most obvious. *Night blindness* is usually the first sign of vitamin A deficiency. As a result of replacement metaplasia of mucus-secreting cells by squamous cells, there is dry and scaly scleral conjunctiva (*xerophthalmia*). The lacrimal duct also shows hyperkeratosis. Corneal ulcers may occur which may get infected and cause *keratomalacia*. *Bitot's spots* may appear which are focal triangular areas of opacities due to accumulation of keratinised epithelium. If these occur on cornea, they impede transmission of light. Ultimately, infection, scarring and opacities lead to *blindness*.

Table 9.4	Vitamin deficiencies.	
	VITAMINS	**DEFICIENCY DISORDERS**
I.	**FAT-SOLUBLE VITAMINS**	
	Vitamin A *(Retinol)*	Ocular lesions (night blindness, xerophthalmia, keratomalacia, Bitot's spots, blindness) Cutaneous lesions (xeroderma) Other lesions (squamous metaplasia of respiratory epithelium, urothelium and pancreatic ductal epithelium, subsequent anaplasia; retarded bone growth)
	Vitamin D *(Calcitriol)*	Rickets in growing children Osteomalacia in adults Hypocalcaemic tetany
	Vitamin E *(α-Tocopherol)*	Degeneration of neurons, retinal pigments, axons of peripheral nerves; denervation of muscles Reduced red cell lifespan Sterility in male and female animals
	Vitamin K	Hypoprothrombinaemia (in haemorrhagic disease of newborn, biliary obstruction, malabsorption, anticoagulant therapy, antibiotic therapy, diffuse liver disease)
II.	**WATER-SOLUBLE VITAMINS**	
	Vitamin C *(Ascorbic acid)*	Scurvy (haemorrhagic diathesis, skeletal lesions, delayed wound healing, anaemia, lesions in teeth and gums)
	Vitamin B Complex	
	(i) Thiamine (Vitamin B_1)	Beriberi ('dry' or peripheral neuritis, 'wet' or cardiac manifestations, 'cerebral' or Wernicke-Korsakoff's syndrome)
	(ii) Riboflavin (Vitamin B_2)	Ariboflavinosis (ocular lesions, cheilosis, glossitis, dermatitis)
	(iii) Niacin/Nicotinic acid (Vitamin B_3)	Pellagra (dermatitis, diarrhoea, dementia)
	(iv) Pyridoxine (Vitamin B_6)	Vague lesions (convulsions in infants, dermatitis, cheilosis, glossitis, sideroblastic anaemia)
	(v) Folate/Folic acid	Megaloblastic anaemia
	(vi) Cyanocobalamin (Vitamin B_{12})	Megaloblastic anaemia Pernicious anaemia
	(vii) Biotin	Mental and neurological symptoms
	Choline	Fatty liver, muscle damage
	Flavonoids	Preventive of neurodegenerative disease, osteoporosis, diabetes

2. Cutaneous lesions The skin develops papular lesions giving toad-like appearance (*xeroderma*). This is due to follicular hyperkeratosis and keratin plugging in the sebaceous glands.

3. Other lesions These are as under:
i) *Squamous metaplasia of respiratory epithelium* of bronchus and trachea may predispose to respiratory infections.
ii) *Squamous metaplasia of pancreatic ductal epithelium* may lead to obstruction and cystic dilatation.
iii) *Squamous metaplasia of urothelium* of the pelvis of kidney may predispose to pyelonephritis and perhaps to renal calculi.
iv) Long-standing metaplasia may cause progression to *anaplasia* under certain circumstances.

v) *Bone growth* in vitamin A deficient animals is retarded.
vi) *Immune dysfunction* may occur due to damaged barrier epithelium and compromised immune defenses.
vii) *Pregnant women* may have increased risk of maternal infection, mortality and impaired embryonic development.

HYPERVITAMINOSIS A Very large doses of vitamin A can produce toxic manifestations in children as well as in adults. These may be *acute or chronic.*

Acute toxicity This results from a single large dose of vitamin A. The effects include neurological manifestations resembling brain tumour e.g. headache, vomiting, stupor, papilloedema.

Chronic toxicity Clinical manifestations of chronic vitamin A excess are as under:

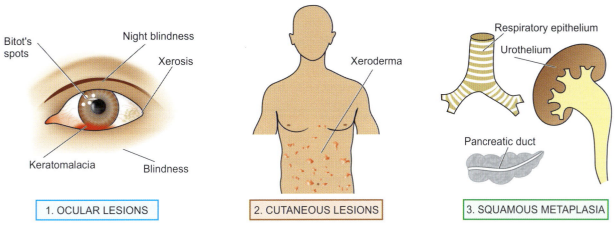

Figure 9.8 ▶ Lesions resulting from vitamin A deficiency.

i) *Neurological* such as severe headache and disordered vision due to increased intracranial pressure.
ii) *Skeletal pains* due to loss of cortical bone by increased osteoclastic activity as well as due to exostosis.
iii) *Cutaneous involvement* may be in the form of pruritus, fissuring, sores at the corners of mouth and coarseness of hair.
iv) *Hepatomegaly* with parenchymal damage and fibrosis.
v) *Hypercarotenaemia* is yellowness of palms and skin due to excessive intake of β-carotene containing foods like carrots or due to inborn error of metabolism.

The effects of toxicity usually disappear on stopping excess of vitamin A intake.

Vitamin D (Calcitriol)

PHYSIOLOGY This fat-soluble vitamin exists in 2 activated *sterol forms:*
- Vitamin D_2 or *calciferol;* and
- Vitamin D_3 or *cholecalciferol.*

The material originally described as vitamin D_1 was subsequently found to be impure mixture of sterols. Since vitamin D_2 and D_3 have similar metabolism and functions, they are therefore referred to as vitamin D.

There are 2 *main sources* of vitamin D:

i) Endogenous synthesis 80% of body's need of vitamin D is met by endogenous synthesis from the action of ultraviolet light on 7-dehydrocholesterol widely distributed in oily secretions of the skin. The vitamin so formed by irradiation enters the body directly through the skin. Pigmentation of the skin reduces the beneficial effects of ultraviolet light.

ii) Exogenous sources The other source of vitamin D is diet such as deep sea fish, fish oil, eggs, butter, milk, some plants and grains.

Irrespective of the source of vitamin D, it must be converted to its *active metabolites* (25-hydroxy vitamin D and 1,25-dihydroxy vitamin D or calcitriol) after its metabolism in the liver and kidney for being functionally active **(Fig. 9.9)**.

1, 25-dihydroxy vitamin D (calcitriol) is 5-10 times more potent biologically than 25-hydroxy vitamin D. The production of calcitriol by the kidney is regulated by:
i) plasma levels of calcitriol (hormonal feedback);
ii) plasma calcium levels (hypocalcaemia stimulates synthesis); and
iii) plasma phosphorus levels (hypophosphataemia stimulates synthesis).

The main storage site of vitamin D is the adipose tissue rather than the liver which is the case with vitamin A.

The main **physiologic functions** of the most active metabolite of vitamin D, calcitriol, are mediated by its binding to nuclear receptor superfamily, vitamin D receptor, expressed on a wide variety of cells. These actions are as under:

1. Maintenance of normal plasma levels of calcium and phosphorus The major essential function of vitamin D is

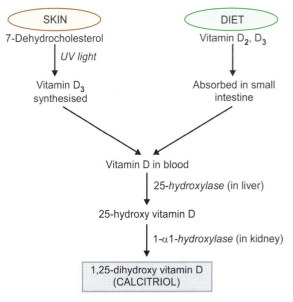

Figure 9.9 ▶ Normal metabolism of vitamin D.

to promote mineralisation of bone. This is achieved by the following actions of vitamin D:

i) *Intestinal absorption* of calcium and phosphorus is stimulated by vitamin D.

ii) *On bones* Vitamin D is normally required for mineralisation of epiphyseal cartilage and osteoid matrix. However, in hypocalcaemia, vitamin D collaborates with parathyroid hormone and causes osteoclastic resorption of calcium and phosphorus from bone so as to maintain the normal blood levels of calcium and phosphorus.

iii) *On kidneys* Vitamin D stimulates reabsorption of calcium at distal renal tubular level, though this function is also parathyroid hormone-dependent.

2. Anti-proliferative effects   Vitamin D receptor is expressed on the parathyroid gland cells by which active form of vitamin D causes anti-proliferative action on parathyroid cells and suppresses the parathormone gene. Besides, vitamin D receptor is also expressed on cells of organs which do not have any role in mineral ion homeostasis and has antiproliferative effects on them e.g. in skin, breast cancer cells, prostate cancer cells.

LESIONS IN VITAMIN D DEFICIENCY   Deficiency of vitamin D may result from:

i) reduced endogenous synthesis due to inadequate exposure to sunlight;

ii) dietary deficiency of vitamin D;

iii) malabsorption of lipids due to lack of bile salts such as in intrahepatic biliary obstruction, pancreatic insufficiency and malabsorption syndrome;

iv) derangements of vitamin D metabolism as occur in kidney disorders (chronic renal failure, nephrotic syndrome, uraemia), liver disorders (diffuse liver disease) and genetic disorders; and

v) resistance of end-organ to respond to vitamin D.

Deficiency of vitamin D from any of the above mechanisms results in 3 types of lesions:

1. rickets in growing children;
2. osteomalacia in adults; and
3. hypocalcaemic tetany due to neuromuscular dysfunction.

RICKETS   The primary defects in rickets are:
- interference with mineralisation of bone; and
- deranged endochondral and intramembranous bone growth.

The pathogenesis of lesions in rickets is better understood by contrasting them with sequence of changes in normal bone growth as outlined in **Table 9.5**.

MORPHOLOGIC FEATURES   Rickets occurs in growing children from 6 months to 2 years of age. The disease has the following lesions and clinical characteristics **(Fig. 9.10)**:

Skeletal changes   These are as under:

i) *Craniotabes* is the earliest bony lesion occurring due to small round unossified areas in the membranous bones of the skull, disappearing within 12 months of birth. The skull looks square and box-like.

ii) *Harrison's sulcus* appears due to indrawing of soft ribs on inspiration.

iii) *Rachitic rosary* is a deformity of chest due to cartilaginous overgrowth at costochondral junction.

iv) *Pigeon-chest deformity* is the anterior protrusion of sternum due to action of respiratory muscles.

v) *Bow legs* occur in ambulatory children due to weak bones of lower legs.

vi) *Knocked knees* may occur due to enlarged ends of the femur, tibia and fibula.

Table 9.5   Contrasting features of rickets with normal bone growth.

	NORMAL BONE GROWTH	RICKETS
I.	ENDOCHONDRAL OSSIFICATION (OCCURRING IN LONG TUBULAR BONES)	
	i. Proliferation of cartilage cells at the epiphyses followed by provisional mineralisation	i. Proliferation of cartilage cells at the epiphyses followed by inadequate provisional mineralisation
	ii. Cartilage resorption and replacement by osteoid matrix	ii. Persistence and overgrowth of epiphyseal cartilage; deposition of osteoid matrix on inadequately mineralised cartilage resulting in enlarged and expanded costochondral junctions
	iii. Mineralisation to form bone	iii. Deformed bones due to lack of structural rigidity
	iv. Normal vascularisation of bone	iv. Irregular overgrowth of small blood vessels in disorganised and weak bone
II.	INTRAMEMBRANOUS OSSIFICATION (OCCURRING IN FLAT BONES)	
	Mesenchymal cells differentiate into osteoblasts which develop osteoid matrix and subsequent mineralisation	Mesenchymal cells differentiate into osteoblasts with laying down of osteoid matrix which fails to get mineralised resulting in soft and weak flat bones

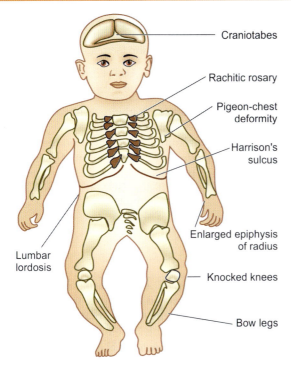

Figure 9.10 ▶ Lesions in rickets.

vii) *Lower epiphyses of radius may be enlarged.*
viii) *Lumbar lordosis* is due to involvement of the spine and pelvis.

Biochemical changes These are as follows:
i) Lowered levels of active metabolites of vitamin D (25-hydroxy vitamin D and 1, 25-dihydroxy vitamin D).
ii) Plasma calcium levels are normal or slightly low.
iii) Plasma phosphate levels are lowered.
iv) Plasma alkaline phosphatase is usually raised due to osteoblastic activity.

Vitamin D-dependent rickets is an autosomal dominant disorder of vitamin D. The disease responds rapidly to administration of 1,25-dihydroxy vitamin D.

OSTEOMALACIA Osteomalacia is the adult counterpart of rickets in which there is failure of mineralisation of the osteoid matrix. It may occur following dietary deficiency, poor endogenous synthesis of vitamin D, or as a result of conditioned deficiency.

MORPHOLOGIC FEATURES Due to deficiency of vitamin D, osteoid matrix laid down fails to get mineralised. In H & E stained microscopic sections, this is identified by widened and thickened osteoid seams (stained pink) and decreased mineralisation at the borders between osteoid and bone (stained basophilic). *von Kossa's stain* for calcium may be employed to mark out the wide seams of unstained osteoid while the calcified bone is stained black. In addition, there may be increased osteoclastic activity and fibrosis of marrow.

Clinical features Osteomalacia is characterised by:
i) muscular weakness;
ii) vague bony pains;
iii) fractures following trivial trauma;
iv) incomplete or greenstick fractures; and
v) looser's zones or pseudofractures at weak places in bones.

Biochemical changes These are:
i) normal or low serum calcium levels;
ii) plasma phosphate levels lowered; and
iii) raised serum alkaline phosphatase due to increased osteoblastic activity.

It may be worthwhile to note here that another chronic disorder of skeleton seen in elderly, *osteoporosis,* is clinically similar but biochemically different disease (Chapter 30).

HYPERVITAMINOSIS D Very large excess of vitamin D may cause increased intestinal absorption of calcium and phosphorus, leading to hypercalcaemia, hyperphosphataemia and increased bone resorption. These changes may result in the following effects:
i) increased urinary excretion of calcium and phosphate;
ii) predisposition to renal calculi;
iii) osteoporosis; and
iv) widespread metastatic calcification, more marked in the renal tubules, arteries, myocardium, lungs and stomach.

Vitamin E (α-Tocopherol)

PHYSIOLOGY Out of many naturally-occurring tocoferols and tocotrienols, α-tocopherol is biologically the most active fat soluble compound for humans. Vitamin E is found in most of the ordinary foods such as vegetables, grains, nuts and oils. It is absorbed from the intestine and transported in blood in the form of chylomicrons. It is stored in fat depots, liver and muscle.

The main **physiologic functions** of vitamin E are as under:

1. *Anti-oxidant activity* Active form of vitamin E acts as an antioxidant and prevents the oxidative degradation of cell membranes containing phospholipids.

2. *Scavenger of free radicals* Vitamin E scavenges free radicals formed by redox reaction in the body (page 34) and thus maintains the integrity of the cell.

3. *Inhibits prostaglandin synthesis.*

4. *Activates protein kinase C and phospholipase A_2.*

LESIONS IN VITAMIN E DEFICIENCY The deficiency of vitamin E is mainly by conditioning disorders affecting its absorption and transport such as abetalipoproteinaemia, intra- and extrahepatic biliary cholestasis, cystic fibrosis of the pancreas and malabsorption syndrome. Low birth weight neonates, due to physiologic immaturity of the liver and bowel, may also develop vitamin E deficiency. Lesions of vitamin E deficiency are as follows:

1. *Neurons* with long axons develop degeneration in the posterior columns of spinal cord.

2. *Peripheral nerves* may also develop myelin degeneration in the axons.
3. *Skeletal muscles* may develop denervation.
4. *Retinal pigmentary degeneration* may occur.
5. *Red blood cells* deficient in vitamin E such as in premature infants have reduced lifespan.
6. In experimental animals, vitamin E deficiency can produce *sterility* in both male and female animals.

Vitamin K

PHYSIOLOGY Vitamin K (*K for Koagulations in Danish*) exists in nature in *2 forms:*

◆ Vitamin K_1 or *phylloquinone,* obtained from exogenous dietary sources such as most green leafy vegetables; and

◆ Vitamin K_2 or *menaquinone,* produced endogenously by normal intestinal flora. Phylloquinone can be converted into menaquinone in some organs.

Like other fat-soluble vitamins, vitamin K is absorbed from the small intestine and requires adequate bile flow and intact pancreatic function.

The main **physiologic function** of vitamin K is in hepatic microsomal carboxylation reaction for vitamin K-dependent coagulation factors (most importantly factor II or prothrombin; others are factors VII, IX and X).

LESIONS IN VITAMIN K DEFICIENCY Since vitamin K is necessary for the manufacture of prothrombin, its deficiency leads of *hypoprothrombinaemia* (page 411). Estimation of plasma prothrombin, thus, affords a simple *in vitro* test for determining whether there is deficiency of vitamin K. Subjects with levels below 70% of normal should receive therapy with vitamin K.

Because most of the green vegetables contain vitamin K and that it can be synthesised endogenously, vitamin K deficiency is frequently a conditioned deficiency. The conditions which may bring about vitamin K deficiency are as follows:

1. Haemorrhagic disease of newborn The newborn infants are deficient in vitamin K because of minimal stores of vitamin K at birth, lack of established intestinal flora for endogenous synthesis and limited dietary intake since breast milk is a poor source of vitamin K. Hence the clinical practice is to routinely administer vitamin K at birth.

2. Biliary obstruction Bile is prevented from entering the bowel due to biliary obstruction which prevents the absorption of this fat-soluble vitamin. Surgery in patients of obstructive jaundice, therefore, leads to marked tendency to bleeding.

3. Due to malabsorption syndrome Patients suffering from malabsorption of fat develop vitamin K deficiency e.g. coeliac disease, sprue, pancreatic disease, hypermotility of bowel etc.

4. Due to anticoagulant therapy Patients on warfarin group of anticoagulants have impaired biosynthesis of vitamin K-dependent coagulation factors.

5. Due to antibiotic therapy Use of broad-spectrum antibiotics and sulfa drugs reduces the normal intestinal flora.

6. Diffuse liver disease Patients with diffuse liver disease (e.g. cirrhosis, amyloidosis of liver, hepatocellular carcinoma, hepatoblastoma) have hypoprothrombinaemia due to impaired synthesis of prothrombin. Administration of vitamin K to such patients is of no avail since liver, where prothrombin synthesis utilising vitamin K takes place, is diseased.

WATER-SOLUBLE VITAMINS

Vitamin C (Ascorbic Acid)

PHYSIOLOGY Vitamin C exists in natural sources as L-ascorbic acid closely related to glucose. The major sources of vitamin C are citrus fruits such as orange, lemon, grape fruit and some fresh vegetables like tomatoes and potatoes. It is present in small amounts in meat and milk. The vitamin is easily destroyed by heating so that boiled or pasteurised milk may lack vitamin C. It is readily absorbed from the small intestine and is stored in many tissues, most abundantly in adrenal cortex.

The **physiologic functions** of vitamin C are due to its ability to carry out *oxidation-reduction reactions:*

$$\text{L-Ascorbic Acid} \rightleftharpoons \text{Dehydro L-Ascorbic acid} + 2H^+ + 2e$$

1. Vitamin C has been found to have *antioxidant* properties and can scavenge free radicals.

2. Ascorbic acid is required for hydroxylation of proline to form hydroxyproline which is an essential component of *collagen.*

3. Besides collagen, it is necessary for the *ground substance* of other mesenchymal structures such as osteoid, chondroitin sulfate, dentin and cement substance of vascular endothelium.

4. Vitamin C being a *reducing substance* has other functions such as:
◆ hydroxylation of dopamine to norepinephrine;
◆ maintenance of folic acid levels by preventing oxidation of tetrahydrofolate; and
◆ role in iron metabolism in its absorption, storage and keeping it in reduced state.

LESIONS IN VITAMIN C DEFICIENCY Vitamin C deficiency in the food or as a conditioned deficiency results in scurvy. The lesions and clinical manifestations of scurvy are seen more commonly at two peak ages: in early childhood and in the very aged. These are as under **(Fig. 9.11):**

Chapter 9: Environmental, Nutritional and Vitamin Deficiency Disorders

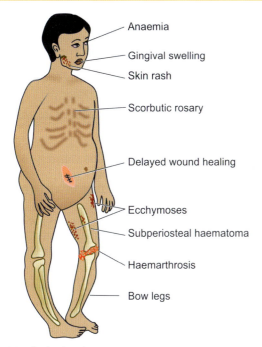

Figure 9.11 ▶ Lesions in scurvy.

1. **Haemorrhagic diathesis** A marked tendency to bleeding is characteristic of scurvy. This may be due to deficiency of intercellular cement which holds together the cells of capillary endothelium. There may be haemorrhages in the skin, mucous membranes, gums, muscles, joints and underneath the periosteum.

2. **Skeletal lesions** These changes are more pronounced in growing children. The most prominent change is the *deranged formation of osteoid matrix and not deranged mineralisation* (c.f. the pathological changes underlying rickets already described). Growing tubular bones as well as flat bones are affected. The epiphyseal ends of growing long bones have cartilage cells in rows which normally undergo provisional mineralisation. However, due to vitamin C deficiency, the next step of laying down of osteoid matrix by osteoblasts is poor and results in failure of resorption of cartilage. Consequently, mineralised cartilage under the widened and irregular epiphyseal plates project as *scorbutic rosary*. The skeletal changes are further worsened due to haemorrhages and haematomas under the periosteum and bleeding into the joint spaces.

3. **Delayed wound healing** There is delayed healing of wounds in scurvy due to following:
  ◆ deranged collagen synthesis;
  ◆ poor preservation and maturation of fibroblasts; and
  ◆ localisation of infections in the wounds.

4. **Anaemia** Anaemia is common in scurvy. It may be the result of haemorrhage, interference with formation of folic acid or deranged iron metabolism. Accordingly, anaemia is most often normocytic normochromic type; occasionally it may be megaloblastic or even iron deficiency type.

5. **Lesions in teeth and gums** Scurvy may interfere with development of dentin. The gums are soft and swollen, may bleed readily and get infected commonly.

6. **Skin rash** Hyperkeratotic and follicular rash may occur in scurvy.

Vitamin B Complex

The term vitamin B was originally coined for a substance capable of curing beriberi (B from beriberi). Now, vitamin B complex is commonly used for *a group of essential compounds which are biochemically unrelated but occur together in certain foods* such as green leafy vegetables, cereals, yeast, liver and milk. Most of the vitamins in this group are involved in metabolism of proteins, carbohydrates and fats.

The principal members of vitamin B complex are thiamine (vitamin B_1), riboflavin (vitamin B_2), niacin or nicotinic acid (vitamin B_3), pantothenic acid (vitamin B_5), pyridoxine (vitamin B_6), folate (folic acid), cyanocobalamin (vitamin B_{12}) and biotin. There is no definite evidence that any clinical disorder results from deficiency of pantothenic acid (vitamin B_5).

Thiamine (Vitamin B_1)

PHYSIOLOGY Thiamine was the first in the family of vitamin B complex group and hence named B_1. Thiamine hydrochloride is available in a variety of items of diet such as peas, beans, pulses, yeast, green vegetable roots, fruits, meat, pork, rice and wheat bran. The vitamin is lost in refined foods such as polished rice, white flour and white sugar. A few substances in the diet (strong tea, coffee) act as *anti-thiamines*. Since the vitamin is soluble in water, considerable amount of the vitamin is lost during cooking of vegetables. The vitamin is absorbed from the intestine either by passive diffusion or by energy-dependent transport. Reserves of vitamin B_1 are stored in the skeletal muscles, heart, liver, kidneys and bones.

The main **physiologic function** of thiamine is in carbohydrate metabolism. Thiamine after absorption is phosphorylated to form thiamine pyrophosphate which is functionally active compound. This compound acts as coenzyme for carboxylase so as to decarboxylate pyruvic acid, synthesises ATP and also participates in the synthesis of fat from carbohydrate. In addition, thiamin plays a role in peripheral nerve conduction by an unknown mechanism.

LESIONS IN THIAMINE DEFICIENCY Thiamine deficiency can occur from primary or conditioned causes, chronic alcoholism being an important cause. The deficiency state leads to failure of complete combustion of carbohydrate and accumulation of pyruvic acid. This results in beriberi which

produces lesions at 3 target tissues (peripheral nerves, heart and brain). Accordingly, beriberi is of 3 types:
- dry beriberi (*peripheral neuritis*);
- wet beriberi (*cardiac manifestations*), and
- cerebral beriberi (*Wernicke-Korsakoff's syndrome*).

It is worth-noting that lesions in beriberi are mainly located in the nervous system and heart. This is because the energy requirement of the brain and nerves is solely derived from oxidation of carbohydrates which is deranged in beriberi, while lesions in the heart appear to arise due to reduced ATP synthesis in beriberi which is required for cardiac functions.

The features of 3 forms of beriberi are as under:

1. Dry beriberi (peripheral neuritis) This is marked by neuromuscular symptoms such as weakness, paraesthesia and sensory loss. The nerves show polyneuritis, myelin degeneration and fragmentation of axons.

2. Wet beriberi (cardiac manifestations) This is characterised by cardiovascular involvement, generalised oedema, serous effusions and chronic passive congestion of viscera. The heart in beriberi is flabby (due to thin and weak myocardium), enlarged and globular in appearance due to 4-chamber dilatation **(Fig. 9.12)**.

Microscopic examination of the heart shows hydropic degeneration of myocardial fibres, loss of striations, interstitial oedema and lymphocytic infiltration.

3. Cerebral beriberi (Wernicke-Korsakoff's syndrome) It consists of the following features:

i) *Wernicke's encephalopathy* occurs more often due to conditioned deficiencies such as in chronic alcoholism. It is characterised by degeneration of ganglia cells, focal demyelination and haemorrhage in the nuclei surrounding the region of ventricles and aqueduct.

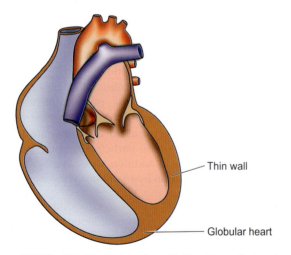

Figure 9.12 ▶ Wet (Cardiac) beriberi. Flabby, thin-walled, enlarged and globular appearance of the heart due to four-chamber dilatation.

Microscopic examination shows degeneration and necrosis of neurons, hypertrophy-hyperplasia of small blood vessels and haemorrhages.

ii) *Korsakoff's psychosis* results from persistence of psychotic features following brain haemorrhage in Wernicke's encephalopathy.

Riboflavin (Vitamin B$_2$)

PHYSIOLOGY Riboflavin used to be called 'yellow respiratory enzyme' (*flavus* = yellow), now known as 'cytochrome oxidase enzyme' which is important in view of its role as cellular respiratory coenzyme. The vitamin is usually distributed in plant and animal foods such as the liver, beef, mutton, pork, eggs, milk and green vegetables. Like other water-soluble vitamins, it is rapidly absorbed from the bowel and stored in tissues like liver.

LESIONS IN RIBOFLAVIN DEFICIENCY Lesions due to primary or conditioned deficiency of riboflavin (*ariboflavinosis*) are as follows:

1. *Ocular lesions* consist of vascularisation of normally avascular cornea due to proliferation of capillaries from limbus. Subsequently, conjunctivitis, interstitial keratitis and corneal ulcers may develop.

2. *Cheilosis* and *angular stomatitis* are characterised by occurrence of fissures and cracks at the angles of mouth.

3. *Glossitis* is development of red, cyanosed and shiny tongue due to atrophy of mucosa of tongue (*'bald tongue'*).

4. *Skin changes* appear in the form of scaly dermatitis resembling seborrheic dermatitis on nasolabial folds on the face, scrotum and vulva.

5. *Anaemia* may develop in some cases.

Niacin or Nicotinic Acid (Vitamin B$_3$)

PHYSIOLOGY As with thiamine and riboflavin, niacin or nicotinic acid or vitamin B$_3$ is also widely distributed in plant and animal foods such as the liver, kidney, meat, green vegetables and whole grain cereals. Niacin includes biologically active derivative *nicotinamide* which is essential for the formation of 2 oxidative coenzymes (*dehydrogenases*):
- NAD (nicotinamide adenine dinucleotide) which is required for dehydrogenation in the metabolism of fat, carbohydrates and proteins.
- NADP (nicotinamide adenine dinucleotide phosphate) which is essential for dehydrogenation in the hexose monophosphate shunt of glucose metabolism.

LESIONS IN NIACIN DEFICIENCY Deficiency of niacin causes pellagra, so named because of the rough skin of such patients (Italian *pelleagra* = rough skin). Pellagra may result from dietary deficiency in those who largely subsist on maize since niacin in maize is present in bound form and is hence not absorbable. Since niacin can be endogenously synthesised from tryptophan, a diet deficient in this amino acid or disorders of tryptophan metabolism such as in carcinoid syndrome or Hartnup syndrome results in niacin deficiency.

Lesions in pellagra are characterised by *3Ds*:
1. *Dermatitis:* The sun-exposed areas of skin develop erythema resembling sunburn. This may progress to chronic type of dermatitis with blister formation.
2. *Diarrhoea:* Lesions similar to those seen in skin may develop in mucous membrane of the alimentary tract resulting in glossitis, lesions in the mouth, oesophagus, stomach and colon and cause diarrhoea, nausea, vomiting and burning sensation.
3. *Dementia:* Degeneration of neurons of the brain and of spinal tract results in neurological symptoms such as dementia, peripheral neuritis, ataxia and visual and auditory disturbances.

TOXICITY OF NIACIN Toxicity due to administration of high doses of niacin as therapy for dyslipidaemia has been observed but not due to dietary excess. It is characterised by flushing of skin and liver derangement.

Pyridoxine (Vitamin B$_6$)

PHYSIOLOGY Pyridoxine or vitamin B$_6$ is widely distributed in all animal and plant foods such as meat, liver, eggs, green vegetables and whole grain cereals. Pyridoxine exists in 3 closely related naturally-occurring substances—*pyridoxine, pyridoxal* and *pyridoxamine*. All of these can be converted into biologically active coenzyme, pyridoxal 5-phosphate.

The major **physiologic functions** of pyridoxine are related to:
i) fat metabolism;
ii) protein metabolism;
iii) amino acid metabolism such as decarboxylation of amino acids, transmethylation of methionine, conversion of tryptophan to niacin;
iv) steroid metabolism;
v) neurotransmitter synthesis; and
vi) haem synthesis.

LESIONS IN PYRIDOXINE DEFICIENCY Vitamin B$_6$ deficiency may result from inadequate dietary intake or may result from secondary deficiency such as increased demand in pregnancy and lactation, chronic alcoholism and intake of certain drugs (e.g. isoniazid in the treatment of tuberculosis, penicillamine, oestrogen in oral contraceptives etc).

The **lesions** of pyridoxine deficiency include the following:
1. Convulsions in infants born to mothers who had been administered large doses of vitamin B$_6$ for hyperemesis gravidarum (pyridoxine dependence)
2. Dermatitis and seborrhoea
3. Cheilosis and angular stomatitis
4. Glossitis (bald tongue)
5. Neuropathy
6. Depression, confusion
7. Sideroblastic anaemia.

Folate (Folic Acid) and Cyanocobalamin (Vitamin B$_{12}$)

Both these vitamins included in the B complex group are required for red cell formation. Their deficiency leads to megaloblastic anaemia which is discussed in Chapter 22.

Biotin

PHYSIOLOGY Biotin is a water-soluble vitamin and a member of vitamin B complex group. It is available in food sources such as organ meat, soya beans, egg yolk; however egg-white has a protein avidin which binds to biotin and blocks its bioavailability.

The major **physiologic functions** of biotin are as under:
1. In gene expression
2. In gluconeogenesis
3. In fatty acid synthesis
4. In catabolism of certain amino acids such as leucine
5. As carrier of CO_2 in carboxylase enzymes.

LESIONS IN BIOTIN DEFICIENCY Biotin deficiency is rare and develops due to inborn errors of metabolism and in patients on parenteral nutrients devoid of biotin. The lesions of biotin deficiency are as under:
1. Mental and neurologic symptoms such as hallucination, depression, paraesthesia
2. Anorexia
3. Nausea
4. Scaly, seborrhoeic dermatitis
5. In infants, hypotonia, alopecia and rash near ears.

In concluding the discussion of vitamin B complex, it must be mentioned that many of the animal and plant foods contain vitamin B complex group of vitamins. Their deficiency, whether primary from poverty, ignorance etc, or secondary from conditioning factors like chronic alcoholism, is more frequently *multiple vitamin deficiency*. Hence, the clinical practice is to administer combination of these members of vitamin B complex.

CHOLINE

PHYSIOLOGY Choline is precursor form of acetylcholine and betaine. Choline is widely distributed as lecithin in foods such as egg yolk, milk, wheat and organ meat. Choline is also synthesised in the liver.

The major **physiologic functions** of choline are as under:
1. In maintenance structural integrity of cell membranes
2. Intramembrane signalling pathways
3. In cholinergic neurotransmission
4. In metabolism of lipids and cholesterol.

LESIONS IN CHOLINE DEFICIENCY Choline deficiency develops in patients on choline-free parenteral nutrients. The lesions of choline deficiency are as under:
1. Fatty liver with deranged liver enzymes
2. Skeletal muscle damage with elevated CPK levels.

FLAVONOIDS

PHYSIOLOGY Flavonoids are a form of polyphenols present in several fruits and vegetables and are the constituents which impart colour, flavour and taste to these edible products. Particular food and vegetables rich in flavonoids are berries, grapes, apples, broccoli, onions, legumes etc.

The major **physiologic functions** of flavonoids are as under:
1. As antioxidants
2. In cell signaling pathways

LESIONS IN FLAVONOID DEFICIENCY Flavonoids have been a recent addition to the family of vitamins. Present data on animal experiments and human clinical studies indicates that they play a role in prevention of neurodegenerative diseases, osteoporosis and diabetes.

GIST BOX 9.5	Disorders of Vitamins

- There are 4 fat-soluble vitamins: A, D, E and K. Water-soluble vitamins consist of vitamin C and members of B complex group; in addition choline, biotin and flavonoids are newer members of this group.
- Vitamin A deficiency causes ocular lesions (night blindness, xerophthalmia, Bitot's spots), xeroderma, and squamous metaplasia of various specialised epithelia (respiratory, pancreatic ductal, urothelium). A state of hypervitaminosis A may produce an acute and chronic toxicity.
- Vitamin D is derived from endogenous (synthesis from UV light) and exogenous (sea fish, eggs, butter) sources. Its deficiency may produce rickets in growing children and osteomalacia in adults. Hypervitaminosis D may lead to hypercalcaemia, hyperphosphataemia and increased bone resorption.
- Vitamin E deficiency may cause degeneration of neurons, peripheral nerves and retinal pigment.
- Vitamin K deficiency causes hypoprothrombinaemia and may produce haemorrhagic disease of newborn.
- Vitamin C deficiency results in scurvy having lesions and clinical manifestations in early childhood and in the very aged. These are haemorrhagic diathesis, skeletal derangements and delayed healing.
- The principal members of vitamin B complex and their deficiency diseases are: thiamine (vitamin B_1) causing beriberi; riboflavin (vitamin B_2) causing lesions on cornea and angle of mouth; niacin or nicotinic acid (vitamin B_3) causing pellagra having 3 Ds (dermatitis, diarrhoea, dementia); pantothenic acid (vitamin B_5) not known to cause any deficiency state; pyridoxine (vitamin B_6) causing dermatitis and seborrhea; cyanocobalamin (vitamin B_{12}) and folate (folic acid) responsible for megaloblastic anaemia; and rare deficiency of biotin may cause mental and neurological symptoms.
- Besides, deficiency of choline may cause fatty liver and flavonoids act as antioxidants.

DIET AND CANCER

Before closing the discussion of nutritional pathology, it is worthwhile to sum up relationship of these factors to carcinogenesis discussed in Chapter 19. There are three possible mechanisms on which the story of this relationship can be built up:

1. Dietary Content of Exogenous Carcinogens

i) The most important example in this mechanism comes from naturally-occurring carcinogen *aflatoxin* which is strongly associated with high incidence of hepatocellular carcinoma in those consuming grain contaminated with mould, *Aspergillus flavus*.

ii) *Artificial sweeteners* (e.g. saccharine cyclomates), food additives and pesticide contamination of food are implicated as carcinogens derived from diet.

2. Endogenous Synthesis of Carcinogens or Promoters

i) In the context of etiology of *gastric carcinoma*, nitrites, nitrates and amines from the digested food are transformed in the body to carcinogens—nitrosamines and nitrosamides.

ii) In the etiology of *colon cancer*, low fibre intake and high animal-derived fats are implicated. High fat diet results in rise in the level of bile acids and their intermediate metabolites produced by intestinal bacteria which act as carcinogens. The low fibre diet, on the other hand, does not provide adequate protection to the mucosa and reduces the stool bulk and thus increases the time the stools remain in the colon.

iii) In the etiology of *breast cancer*, epidemiologic studies have implicated the role of animal proteins, fats and obesity but the evidence is yet unsubstantiated.

3. Inadequate Protective Factors

As already mentioned, some components of diet such as *vitamin C, A, E, selenium,* and *β-carotenes* have protective role against cancer. These substances in normal amounts in the body act as antioxidants and protect the cells against free radical injury but their role of supplementation in diet as prevention against cancer is unproven.

GIST BOX 9.6	Diet and Cancer

- Diet plays an important role in health and disease.
- Mechanisms of components of diet acting in carcinogenesis are due to certain exogenous carcinogenic agents in diet, endogenous synthesis of carcinogens or their promoters, and dietary content poor in protective factors against cancer, mainly antioxidants.

Section II — Inflammation and Healing, Immunity and Hypersensitivity, Infections and Infestations

Chapter 10: Inflammation: Acute
Chapter 11: Inflammation: Chronic and Granulomatous
Chapter 12: Healing of Tissues
Chapter 13: Infectious and Parasitic Diseases
Chapter 14: Diseases of Immunity including AIDS

10 Inflammation: Acute

INFLAMMATION—INTRODUCTION

DEFINITION AND CAUSES Inflammation is defined as the local response of living mammalian tissues to injury from any agent. It is a body defense reaction in order to eliminate or limit the spread of injurious agent, followed by removal of the necrosed cells and tissues.

The injurious agents causing inflammation may be as under:
1. *Infective agents* like bacteria, viruses and their toxins, fungi, parasites.
2. *Immunological agents* like cell-mediated and antigen-antibody reactions.
3. *Physical agents* like heat, cold, radiation, mechanical trauma.
4. *Chemical agents* like organic and inorganic poisons.
5. *Inert materials* such as foreign bodies.

Thus, *inflammation is distinct from infection*—inflammation is a protective response by the body to a variety of etiologic agents (infectious or non-infectious), while infection is invasion into the body by harmful microbes and their resultant ill-effects by toxins. Inflammation involves 2 basic processes with some overlapping, viz. early *inflammatory response* and later followed by *healing*. Though both these processes generally have protective role against injurious agents, inflammation and healing may cause considerable harm to the body as well e.g. anaphylaxis to bites by insects or reptiles, drugs, toxins, atherosclerosis, chronic rheumatoid arthritis, fibrous bands and adhesions in intestinal obstruction.

It may be appreciated that "immunity or immune reaction" and "inflammatory response" by the host are both interlinked protective mechanisms in the body—inflammation is the visible response to an immune reaction, while activation of immune response is almost essential before inflammatory response appears.

SIGNS OF INFLAMMATION The Roman writer Celsus in 1st century A.D. named the famous 4 *cardinal signs of inflammation* as:
i) *rubor* (redness);
ii) *tumor* (swelling);
iii) *calor* (heat); and
iv) *dolor* (pain).

To these, fifth sign *functio laesa* (loss of function) was later added by Virchow. The word inflammation means burning. This nomenclature had its origin in old times but now we know that burning is only one of the features of inflammation.

TYPES OF INFLAMMATION Depending upon the defense capacity of the host and duration of response, inflammation can be classified as acute and chronic.

A. *Acute inflammation* is of short duration (lasting less than 2 weeks) and represents the early body reaction, resolves quickly and is usually followed by healing.

The main features of acute inflammation are:
1. accumulation of fluid and plasma at the affected site;
2. intravascular activation of platelets; and
3. polymorphonuclear neutrophils as inflammatory cells.

Sometimes, the acute inflammatory response may be quite severe and is termed as *fulminant acute inflammation.*

B. *Chronic inflammation* is of longer duration and occurs after delay, either after the causative agent of acute inflammation persists for a long time, or the stimulus is such that it induces chronic inflammation from the beginning. A variant, *chronic active inflammation*, is the type of chronic inflammation in which during the course of disease there are acute exacerbations of activity.

The characteristic feature of chronic inflammation is presence of chronic inflammatory cells such as lymphocytes, plasma cells and macrophages, granulation tissue formation, and in specific situations as granulomatous inflammation.

Section II: Inflammation and Healing, Immunity and Hypersensitivity, Infections and Infestations

In some instances, the term *subacute inflammation* is used for the state of inflammation between acute and chronic.

| GIST BOX 10.1 | Introduction to Inflammation |

- Inflammation is the local response of living mammalian tissues to injury from any agent which could be microbial, immunological, physical or chemical agents.
- Cardinal signs of inflammation are: redness, swelling, heat, pain and loss of function.
- Inflammation is of 2 types: acute when due to early response by the body and is of short duration, and chronic when it is for longer duration and occurs after delay and is characterised by response of chronic inflammatory cells.

ACUTE INFLAMMATORY RESPONSE

Acute inflammatory response by the host to any agent is a continuous process but for the purpose of discussion, it can be divided into following two events:
I. Vascular events
II. Cellular events

Intimately linked to these two processes is the release of mediators of acute inflammation, which is also discussed just afterwards.

I. VASCULAR EVENTS

Alteration in the microvasculature (arterioles, capillaries and venules) is the earliest response to tissue injury. These alterations include: haemodynamic changes and changes in vascular permeability.

Haemodynamic Changes

The earliest features of inflammatory response result from changes in the vascular flow and calibre of small blood vessels in the injured tissue. The sequence of these changes is as under:

1. Irrespective of the type of cell injury, immediate vascular response is of **transient vasoconstriction** of arterioles. With mild form of injury, the blood flow may be re-established in 3-5 seconds while with more severe injury the vasoconstriction may last for about 5 minutes.

2. Next follows **persistent progressive vasodilatation** which involves mainly the arterioles, but to a lesser extent, affects other components of the microcirculation like venules and capillaries. This change is obvious within half an hour of injury. Vasodilatation results in increased blood volume in microvascular bed of the area, which is responsible for redness and warmth at the site of acute inflammation.

3. Progressive vasodilatation, in turn, may elevate the **local hydrostatic pressure** resulting in transudation of fluid into the extracellular space. This is responsible for swelling at the local site of acute inflammation.

4. **Slowing or stasis** of microcirculation follows which causes increased concentration of red cells, and thus, raised blood viscosity.

5. Stasis or slowing is followed by **leucocytic margination** or peripheral orientation of leucocytes (mainly neutrophils) along the vascular endothelium. The leucocytes stick to the vascular endothelium briefly, and then move and migrate through the gaps between the endothelial cells into the extravascular space. This process is known as *emigration* (page 111).

TRIPLE RESPONSE The features of haemodynamic changes in inflammation are best demonstrated by the **Lewis experiment.** Lewis induced the changes in the skin of inner aspect of forearm by firm stroking with a blunt point. The reaction so elicited is known as *triple response* or *red line response* consisting of the following (Fig. 10.1):

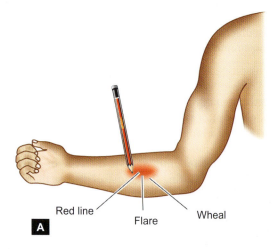
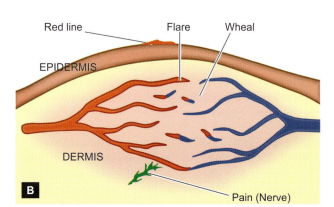

Figure 10.1 ▶ A, 'Triple response' elicited by firm stroking of skin of forearm with a pencil. B, Diagrammatic view of microscopic features of triple response of the skin.

i) Red line appears within a few seconds after stroking and is due to local vasodilatation of capillaries and venules.

ii) Flare is the bright reddish appearance or flush surrounding the red line and results from vasodilatation of the adjacent arterioles.

iii) Wheal is the swelling or oedema of the surrounding skin occurring due to transudation of fluid into the extravascular space.

These features, thus, elicit the classical signs of inflammation—redness, heat and swelling, to which fourth feature, pain, has been added.

Altered Vascular Permeability

PATHOGENESIS In and around the inflamed tissue, there is accumulation of oedema fluid in the interstitial compartment which comes from blood plasma by its escape through the endothelial wall of peripheral vascular bed. In the initial stage, the escape of fluid is due to vasodilatation and consequent elevation in hydrostatic pressure. This is transudate in nature. But subsequently, the characteristic inflammatory oedema, exudate, appears by increased vascular permeability of microcirculation. The differences between transudate and exudate are summarised in **Table 15.1** (*see* page 226).

The appearance of inflammatory oedema due to increased vascular permeability of microvascular bed is explained on the basis of **Starling's hypothesis**. According to this, normally the fluid balance is maintained by two opposing sets of forces:

i) Forces that cause **outward movement** of fluid from microcirculation: These are *intravascular hydrostatic pressure* and *colloid osmotic pressure of interstitial fluid*.

ii) Forces that cause **inward movement** of interstitial fluid into circulation: These are *intravascular colloid osmotic pressure* and *hydrostatic pressure of interstitial fluid*.

Whatever little fluid is left in the interstitial compartment is drained away by lymphatics and, thus, no oedema results normally **(Fig. 10.2, A)**.

However, in inflamed tissues, the endothelial lining of microvasculature becomes more leaky. Consequently, intravascular colloid osmotic pressure decreases and osmotic pressure of the interstitial fluid increases resulting in excessive outward flow of fluid into the interstitial compartment which is exudative inflammatory oedema **(Fig. 10.2, B)**.

PATTERNS OF INCREASED VASCULAR PERMEABILITY Increased vascular permeability in acute inflammation by which normally non-permeable endothelial layer of microvasculature becomes leaky can have following patterns and mechanisms which may be acting singly or more often in combination **(Fig. 10.3)**:

i) Contraction of endothelial cells This is the most common mechanism of increased leakiness that affects venules exclusively while capillaries and arterioles remain unaffected. The endothelial cells develop temporary gaps between them due to their contraction resulting in vascular

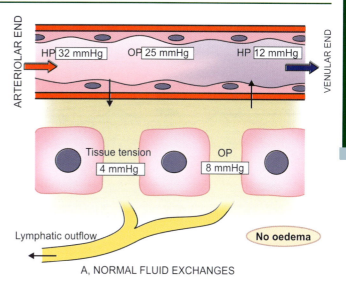

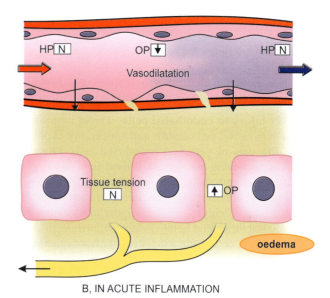

Figure 10.2 ▶ Fluid interchange between blood and extracellular fluid (ECF). (HP = hydrostatic pressure, OP = osmotic pressure).

leakiness. It is mediated by the release of histamine, bradykinin and other chemical mediators. The response begins immediately after injury, is usually reversible, and is for short duration (15-30 minutes).

An example of such *immediate transient response* is mild thermal injury of skin of forearm.

ii) Contraction or mild endothelial damage In this mechanism, there is structural re-organisation of the cytoskeleton of endothelial cells that causes reversible retraction at the intercellular junctions or mild form of endothelial damage. This change affects venules and capillaries and is mediated by cytokines such as interleukin-1 (IL-1) and tumour necrosis factor (TNF)-α. The onset of response occurs

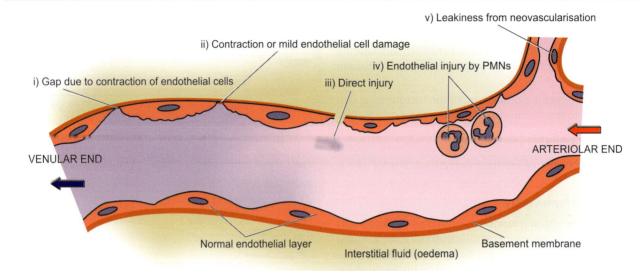

Figure 10.3 ▶ Schematic illustration of pathogenesis of increased vascular permeability in acute inflammation. The serial numbers in the figure correspond to five numbers described in the text.

after delay of 4-6 hours following injury and lasts for several hours to days.

Classic example of *delayed and prolonged leakage* is appearance of sunburns mediated by ultraviolet radiation.

iii) Direct injury to endothelial cells Direct injury to the endothelium causes cell necrosis and appearance of physical gaps at the sites of detached endothelial cells. Process of thrombosis involving platelets and fibrin is initiated at the site of damaged endothelial cells. The change affects all levels of microvasculature (venules, capillaries and arterioles). The increased permeability may either appear immediately after injury and last for several hours or days *(immediate sustained leakage)*, or may occur after a delay of 2-12 hours and last for hours or days *(delayed prolonged leakage)*.

The examples of *immediate sustained leakage* are severe bacterial infections while delayed prolonged leakage may occur following moderate thermal injury and radiation injury.

iv) Leucocyte-mediated endothelial injury Adherence of leucocytes to the endothelium at the site of inflammation may result in activation of leucocytes. The activated leucocytes release proteolytic enzymes and toxic oxygen species which may cause endothelial injury and increased vascular leakiness. This form of increased vascular leakiness affects mostly venules and is a *late response*.

The examples are seen in sites where leucocytes adhere to the vascular endothelium e.g. in pulmonary venules and capillaries.

v) Leakiness in neovascularisation In addition, the newly formed capillaries under the influence of vascular endothelial growth factor (VEGF) during the process of repair and in tumours are excessively leaky.

These mechanisms are summarised in **Table 10.1**.

II. CELLULAR EVENTS

The cellular phase of inflammation consists of 2 processes:
1. exudation of leucocytes; and
2. phagocytosis.

Exudation of Leucocytes

The escape of leucocytes from the lumen of microvasculature to the interstitial tissue is the most important feature of inflammatory response. In acute inflammation, polymorphonuclear neutrophils (PMNs) comprise the first line of body defense, followed later by monocytes and macrophages.

The changes leading to migration of leucocytes are as follows **(Fig. 10.4)**:

1. CHANGES IN THE FORMED ELEMENTS OF BLOOD In the early stage of inflammation, the rate of flow of blood is increased due to vasodilatation. But subsequently, there is slowing or stasis of bloodstream. With stasis, changes in the normal axial flow of blood in the microcirculation take place. The normal axial flow consists of central stream of cells comprised by leucocytes and RBCs and peripheral cell-free layer of plasma close to vessel wall. Due to slowing and stasis, the central stream of cells widens and peripheral plasma zone becomes narrower because of loss of plasma by exudation. This phenomenon is known as *margination*. As a result of this redistribution, neutrophils of the central column come close to the vessel wall; this is known as *pavementing*.

2. ROLLING AND ADHESION Peripherally marginated and pavemented neutrophils slowly roll over the endothelial cells lining the vessel wall *(rolling phase)*. This is followed by transient bond between the leucocytes and endothelial

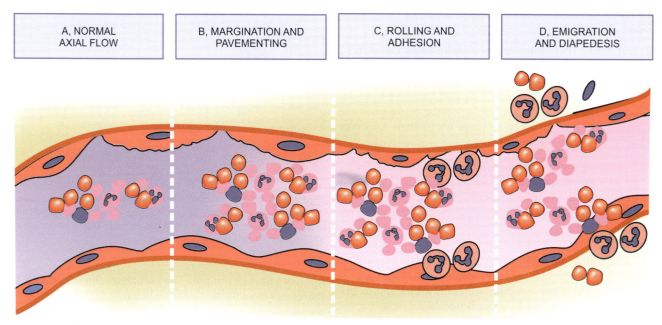

Figure 10.4 ▶ Sequence of changes in the exudation of leucocytes. A, Normal axial flow of blood with central column of cells and peripheral zone of cell-free plasma. B, Margination and pavementing of neutrophils with narrow plasmatic zone. C, Adhesion of neutrophils to endothelial cells with pseudopods in the intercellular junctions. D, Emigration of neutrophils and diapedesis with damaged basement membrane.

cells becoming firmer *(adhesion phase)*. The following cell adhesion molecules (CAMs) bring about rolling and adhesion phases:

i) **Selectins** These are a group of CAMs expressed on the surface of activated endothelial cells and are structurally composed of lectins or lectin-like protein molecules the most important of which is s-Lewis X molecule. Their role is to recognise and bind to glycoproteins and glycolipids on the cell surface of neutrophils. There are 3 types of selectins:

❖ *P-selectin* (*p*reformed and stored in endothelial cells and platelets, also called CD62) is involved in rolling.
❖ *E-selectin* (synthesised by cytokine-activated *e*ndothelial cells, also named ECAM) is associated with both rolling and adhesion.
❖ *L-selectin* (expressed on the surface of *l*ymphocytes and neutrophils, also called LCAM) is responsible for homing

Table 10.1	Mechanisms of increased vascular permeability.			
MECHANISM	MICROVASCULATURE	RESPONSE TYPE	PATHOGENESIS	EXAMPLES
1. Endothelial cell contraction	Venules	Immediate transient (last for 15-30 min)	Histamine, bradykinin, others	Mild thermal injury
2. Contraction or mild endothelial injury	Venules, capillaries	Somewhat delayed (in 4-6 hrs) prolonged (for 24 hrs to days)	IL-1, TNF-α	Sunburns
3. Direct endothelial cell injury	Arterioles, venules, capillaries	Immediate prolonged (hrs to days), or delayed (2-12 hrs) prolonged (hrs to days)	Cell necrosis and detachment	Moderate to severe burns, severe bacterial infection, radiation injury
4. Leucocyte-mediated endothelial injury	Venules, capillaries	Delayed, prolonged	Leucocyte activation	Pulmonary venules and capillaries
5. Neovascularisation	All levels	Any type	Angiogenesis, VEGF	Healing, tumours

of circulating lymphocytes to the endothelial cells in lymph nodes.

ii) **Integrins** These are a family of endothelial cell surface proteins having alpha (or CD11) and beta (CD18) subunits, which are activated during the process of loose and transient adhesions between endothelial cells and leucocytes. At the same time the receptors for integrins on the neutrophils are also stimulated. This process brings about firm adhesion between leucocyte and endothelium.

iii) **Immunoglobulin gene superfamily adhesion molecules** This group consists of a variety of immunoglobulin molecules present on most cells of the body. These partake in cell-to-cell contact through various other CAMs and cytokines. They have a major role in recognition and binding of immunocompetent cells as under:

❖ Intercellular adhesion molecule-1 (ICAM-1, also called CD54) and vascular cell adhesion molecule-1 (VCAM-1, also named CD106) allow a tighter adhesion and stabilise the interaction between leucocytes and endothelial cells.

❖ Platelet-endothelial cell adhesion molecule-1 (PECAM-1) or CD31 is involved in leucocyte migration from the endothelial surface.

3. EMIGRATION After sticking of neutrophils to endothelium, the former move along the endothelial surface till a suitable site between the endothelial cells is found where the neutrophils throw out cytoplasmic pseudopods. Subsequently, the neutrophils lodged between the endothelial cells and basement membrane cross the basement membrane by damaging it locally with secreted collagenases and escape out into the extravascular space; this is known as *emigration*. The damaged basement membrane is repaired almost immediately. As already mentioned, neutrophils are the dominant cells in acute inflammatory exudate in the first 24 hours, and monocyte-macrophages appear in the next 24-48 hours. However, neutrophils are short-lived (24-48 hours) while monocyte-macrophages survive much longer.

Simultaneous to emigration of leucocytes, escape of red cells through gaps between the endothelial cells, *diapedesis*, takes place. It is a passive phenomenon—RBCs being forced out either by raised hydrostatic pressure or may escape through the endothelial defects left after emigration of leucocytes. Diapedesis gives haemorrhagic appearance to the inflammatory exudate.

4. CHEMOTAXIS The transmigration of leucocytes after crossing several barriers (endothelium, basement membrane, perivascular myofibroblasts and matrix) to reach the interstitial tissues is a chemotactic factor-mediated process called chemotaxis. The concept of chemotaxis is well illustrated by *Boyden's chamber experiment*. In this, a

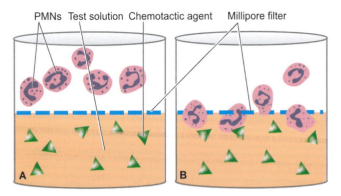

Figure 10.5 ▶ The Boyden's chamber with millipore filter, shown by dotted line. A, Suspension of leucocytes above is separated from test solution below. B, Lower half of chamber shows migration of neutrophils towards chemotactic agent.

millipore filter (3 μm pore size) separates the suspension of leucocytes from the test solution in tissue culture chamber. If the test solution contains chemotactic agent, the leucocytes migrate through the pores of filter towards the chemotactic agent **(Fig. 10.5)**.

The following agents act as potent chemotactic substances for neutrophils:

i) Leukotriene B4 (LT-B4), a product of lipooxygenase pathway of arachidonic acid metabolites

ii) Components of complement system (C5a and C3a in particular)

iii) Cytokines (Interleukins, in particular IL-8)

iv) Soluble bacterial products (such as formylated peptides).

In addition to neutrophils, other inflammatory cells too respond and partake in inflammation having specific chemokines, e.g. monocyte chemoattractant protein (MCP-1), eotaxin chemotactic for eosinophils, NK cells for recognising virally infected cells etc.

Phagocytosis

Phagocytosis is defined as the process of engulfment of solid particulate material by the cells (cell-eating). The cells performing this function are called *phagocytes*. There are 2 main types of phagocytic cells:

i) Polymorphonuclear neutrophils (PMNs) which appear early in acute inflammatory response, sometimes called as *microphages*.

ii) Circulating monocytes and fixed tissue mononuclear phagocytes, commonly called as *macrophages*.

Neutrophils and macrophages on reaching the tissue spaces produce several proteolytic enzymes—lysozyme, protease, collagenase, elastase, lipase, proteinase, gelatinase, and acid hydrolases. These enzymes degrade collagen

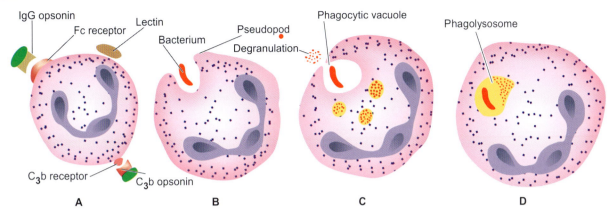

Figure 10.6 ▶ Stages in phagocytosis of a foreign particle. A, Opsonisation of the particle. B, Pseudopod engulfing the opsonised particle. C, Incorporation within the cell (phagocytic vacuole) and degranulation. D, Phagolysosome formation after fusion of lysosome of the cell.

and extracellular matrix. Phagocytosis of the microbe by polymorphs and macrophages involves the following 3 steps (Fig. 10.6):
1. Recognition and attachment
2. Engulfment
3. Killing and degradation

1. RECOGNITION AND ATTACHMENT
Phagocytosis is initiated by the expression of cell surface receptors on macrophages which recognise microorganisms: *mannose receptor* and *scavenger receptor*. The process of phagocytosis is further enhanced when the microorganisms are coated with specific proteins, *opsonins*, from the serum and the process is called opsonisation (meaning preparing for eating). Opsonins establish a bond between bacteria and the cell membrane of phagocytic cell. The main opsonins present in the serum and their corresponding receptors on the surface of phagocytic cells (PMNs or macrophages) are as under:

i) *IgG opsonin* is the Fc fragment of immunoglobulin G; it is the naturally-occurring antibody in the serum that coats the bacteria while the PMNs possess receptors for the same.

ii) *C3b opsonin* is the fragment generated by activation of complement pathway. It is strongly chemotactic for attracting PMNs to bacteria.

iii) *Lectins* are carbohydrate-binding proteins in the plasma which bind to bacterial cell wall.

2. ENGULFMENT
The opsonised particle or microbe bound to the surface of phagocyte is ready to be engulfed. This is accomplished by formation of cytoplasmic pseudopods around the particle due to activation of actin filaments beneath cell wall, enveloping it in a phagocytic vacuole. Eventually, plasma membrane enclosing the particle breaks from the cell surface so that membrane-lined phagocytic vacuole or phagosome becomes internalised in the cell and lies free in the cell cytoplasm. The phagosome fuses with one or more lysosomes of the cell and form bigger vacuole called phagolysosome.

3. KILLING AND DEGRADATION
Next is the stage of killing and degradation of microorganism to dispose it off which is the major function of phagocytes as scavenger cells. The microorganisms after being killed by antibacterial substances are degraded by hydrolytic enzymes. However, this mechanism fails to kill and degrade some bacteria like tubercle bacilli.

In general, following mechanisms are involved in disposal of microorganisms:

A. *Intracellular mechanisms:*
i) Oxidative bactericidal mechanism by oxygen free radicals
   a) MPO-dependent
   b) MPO-independent
ii) Oxidative bactericidal mechanism by lysosomal granules
iii) Non-oxidative bactericidal mechanism

B. *Extracellular mechanisms:*
These mechanisms are discussed below.

A. INTRACELLULAR MECHANISMS Intracellular metabolic pathways are involved in killing microbes, more commonly by oxidative mechanism and less often by non-oxidative pathways.

i) Oxidative bactericidal mechanism by oxygen free radicals An important mechanism of microbicidal killing is by oxidative damage by the production of reactive oxygen metabolites (O'_2, H_2O_2, OH', $HOCl$, HOI, $HOBr$).

A phase of increased oxygen consumption ('respiratory burst') by activated phagocytic leucocytes requires the essential presence of NADPH oxidase.

NADPH-oxidase present in the cell membrane of phagosome reduces oxygen to superoxide ion (O'_2):

Section II: Inflammation and Healing, Immunity and Hypersensitivity, Infections and Infestations

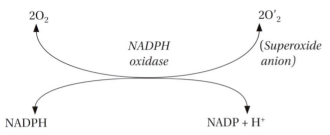

Superoxide is subsequently converted into H_2O_2 which has bactericidal properties:

$$2O'_2 + 2H^+ \longrightarrow H_2O_2$$
(Hydrogen peroxide)

This type of bactericidal activity is carried out either via enzyme myeloperoxidase (MPO) present in the azurophilic granules of neutrophils and monocytes, or independent of enzyme MPO, as under:

a) *MPO-dependent killing.* In this mechanism, the enzyme MPO acts on H_2O_2 in the presence of halides (chloride, iodide or bromide) to form hypohalous acid (HOCl, HOI, HOBr). This is called *H_2O_2-MPO-halide system* and is more potent antibacterial system in polymorphs than H_2O_2 alone:

$$H_2O_2 \xrightarrow[Cl',\ Br',\ I']{MPO} HOCl + H_2O$$
(Hypochlorous acid)

b) *MPO-independent killing.* Mature macrophages lack the enzyme MPO and they carry out bactericidal activity by producing OH^- ions and superoxide singlet oxygen (O') from H_2O_2 in the presence of O'_2 (Haber-Weiss reaction) or in the presence of Fe^{++} (Fenton reaction):

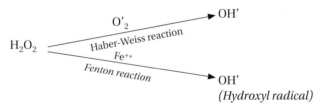

Reactive oxygen metabolites are particularly useful in eliminating microbial organisms that grow within phagocytes e.g. *Mycobacterium tuberculosis, Histoplasma capsulatum.*

ii) Oxidative bactericidal mechanism by lysosomal granules In this mechanism, the preformed granule-stored products of neutrophils and macrophages are discharged or secreted into the phagosome and the extracellular environment. While the role of MPO is already highlighted above, other substances liberated by degranulation of macrophages and neutrophils are protease, trypsinase, phospholipase, and alkaline phosphatase. Progressive degranulation of neutrophils and macrophages along with oxygen free radicals degrades proteins i.e. induces proteolysis.

iii) Non-oxidative bactericidal mechanism Some agents released from the granules of phagocytic cells do not require oxygen for bactericidal activity. These include the following:

a) Granules Some of liberated lysosomal granules do not cause killing by oxidative damage but cause lysis of microbe within phagosome. These are lysosomal hydrolases, permeability increasing factors, cationic proteins (defensins), lipases, proteases, DNAases.

b) Nitric oxide Nitric oxide is a reactive free radicals similar to oxygen free radicals which is formed by nitric oxide synthase. It is produced by endothelial cells as well as by activated macrophages. Nitric oxide is another potent mechanism of microbial killing.

B. EXTRACELLULAR MECHANISMS Following mechanisms explain the bactericidal activity at extracellular level:

i) Granules Degranulation of macrophages and neutrophils explained above continues to exert its effects of proteolysis outside the cells as well.

ii) Immune mechanisms Immune-mediated lysis of microbes takes place outside the cells by mechanisms of cytolysis, antibody-mediated lysis and by cell-mediated cytotoxicity (Chapter 14).

GIST BOX 10.2 — Acute Inflammatory Response

- The sequential haemodynamic changes are: an initial transient vasoconstriction, followed by persistent progressive vasodilatation, raised local hydrostatic pressure and transudation in extracellular space. Next, there is emigration of leucocytes from the capillary wall due to slowing and stasis in microcirculation.
- There is increased vascular permeability and appearance of inflammatory oedema. It has different mechanisms and various patterns: contraction of endothelial cells, mild to severe endothelial damage, direct or leucocyte-mediated injury to endothelial cells and leakiness in neovascularisation.
- Cellular phase of inflammation consists of exudation of leucocytes and phagocytosis.
- Leucocyte exudation begins from change of normal axial blood flow to slowing and stasis. This is followed by margination, pavementing, rolling, adhesion, and finally emigration of leucocytes to the extravascular space.
- Phagocytosis is cellular eating. The process of engulfment of foreign particulate material involves its initial recognition and opsonisation. The mechanisms of phagocytosis are largely intracellular (oxidative and non-oxidative bactericidal) and a few extracellular mechanisms.

MEDIATORS OF INFLAMMATION

These are a large and increasing number of endogenous chemical substances which mediate the process of acute inflammation.

Mediators of inflammation have some common properties as under:

1) These mediators are released either *from the cells or are derived from plasma proteins*:

◆ Cell-derived mediators are released either from their storage in the cell granules or are synthesised in the cells.

◆ The most common site of synthesis of plasma-derived mediators is the liver. After their release from the liver, these mediators require activation.

2) All mediators are *released in response to certain stimuli*. These stimuli may be a variety of injurious agents, dead and damaged tissues, or even one mediator stimulating release of another. The latter are called secondary mediators which may perform the function of the initial mediator or may have opposing action.

3) Mediators *act on different targets*. They may have similar action on different target cells or differ in their action on different target cells. They may act on cells which formed them or on other body cells.

4) *Range of actions* of different mediators are: increased vascular permeability, vasodilatation, chemotaxis, fever, pain and tissue damage.

5) Mediators have *short lifespan* after their release. After release, they are rapidly removed from the body by various mechanisms e.g. by enzymatic inactivation, antioxidants, regulatory proteins or may even decay spontaneously.

Two main groups of substances acting as chemical mediators of inflammation are those released *from the cells and those from the plasma proteins,* (Table 10.2) while their range of actions in acute inflammation are shown in Fig. 10.7.

I. CELL-DERIVED MEDIATORS

1. VASOACTIVE AMINES Two important pharmacologically active amines that have role in the early inflammatory response (first one hour) are histamine and 5-hydroxytryptamine (5-HT) or serotonin; another addition to this group is neuropeptides.

i) Histamine It is stored in the granules of mast cells, basophils and platelets. Histamine is released from these cells by various agents as under:

a) Stimuli or substances inducing acute inflammation e.g. heat, cold, irradiation, trauma, irritant chemicals, immunologic reactions etc.

Table 10.2 Mediators of inflammation.

I. CELL-DERIVED MEDIATORS
1. Vasoactive amines (Histamine, 5-hydroxytryptamine, neuropeptides)
2. Arachidonic acid metabolites (Eicosanoids)
    i. Metabolites via cyclo-oxygenase pathway (prostaglandins, thromboxane A_2, prostacyclin, resolvins)
    ii. Metabolites via lipo-oxygenase pathway (5-HETE, leukotrienes, lipoxins)
3. Lysosomal components (from PMNs, macrophages)
4. Platelet activating factor
5. Cytokines (IL-1, IL-6, IL-8, IL-12, IIL-17, TNF-α, TNF-β, IFN-γ, chemokines)
6. Free radicals (Oxygen metabolites, nitric oxide)

II. PLASMA PROTEIN-DERIVED MEDIATORS (PLASMA PROTEASES) Products of:
1. The kinin system
2. The clotting system
3. The fibrinolytic system
4. The complement system

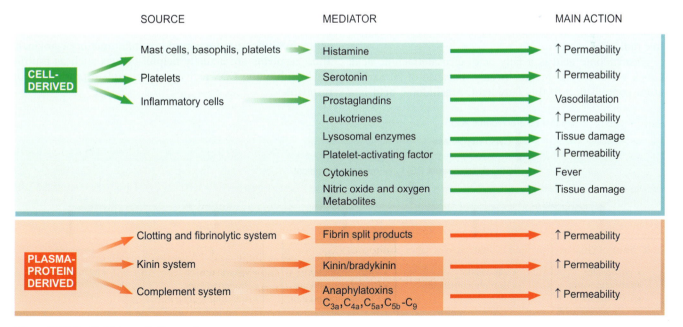

Figure 10.7 ▶ Mediators of inflammation.

b) Anaphylatoxins like fragments of complement C3a, and C5a, which increase vascular permeability and cause oedema in tissues.

c) Histamine-releasing factors from neutrophils, monocytes and platelets.

d) Interleukins.

The main *actions* of histamine are: vasodilatation, increased vascular (venular) permeability, itching and pain. Stimulation of mast cells and basophils also releases products of arachidonic acid metabolism including the release of *slow-reacting substances of anaphylaxis (SRS-As)*. The SRS-As consist of various leukotrienes (LTC_4, LTD_4 and LTE_4) (page 117).

ii) 5-Hydroxytryptamine (5-HT or serotonin) It is present in tissues like chromaffin cells of GIT, spleen, nervous tissue, mast cells and platelets. The actions of 5-HT are similar to histamine but it is a less potent mediator of increased vascular permeability and vasodilatation than histamine. It may be mentioned here that carcinoid tumour is a serotonin-secreting tumour.

iii) Neuropeptides Another class of vasoactive amines is tachykinin neuropeptides such as substance P, neurokinin A, vasoactive intestinal polypeptide (VIP) and somatostatin. These small peptides are produced in the central and peripheral nervous systems.

The major proinflammatory *actions* of these neuropeptides are as follows:
a) Increased vascular permeability.
b) Transmission of pain stimuli.
c) Mast cell degranulation.

2. ARACHIDONIC ACID METABOLITES (EICOSANOIDS)

Arachidonic acid metabolites or eicosanoids are the most potent mediators of inflammation, much more than oxygen free radicals.

Arachidonic acid is a fatty acid, eicosatetraenoic acid; Greek word '*eikosa*' means 'twenty' because of 20 carbon atom composition of this fatty acid. Arachidonic acid is a constituent of the phospholipid cell membrane, besides its presence in some constituents of diet. Arachidonic acid is released from the cell membrane by phospholipases. It is then activated to form arachidonic acid metabolites or eicosanoids by one of the following 2 pathways: via cyclo-oxygenase pathway or via lipo-oxygenase pathway:

i) Metabolites via cyclo-oxygenase pathway: Prostaglandins, thromboxane A_2, prostacyclin The name 'prostaglandin' was first given to a substance found in human seminal fluid but now the same substance has been isolated from a number of other body cells. Prostaglandins and related compounds are also called *autocoids* because these substances are mainly autocrine or paracrine agents. The terminology used for prostaglandins is abbreviation as PG followed by suffix of an alphabet and a serial number e.g. PGG_2, PGE_2 etc.

Cyclo-oxygenase (COX), a fatty acid enzyme present as COX-1 and COX-2, acts on activated arachidonic acid to form prostaglandin endoperoxide (PGG_2). PGG_2 is enzymatically transformed into PGH_2 with generation of free radical of oxygen. PGH_2 is further acted upon by enzymes and results in formation of the following 3 metabolites **(Fig. 10.8)**:

a) *Prostaglandins (PGD_2, PGE_2 and PGF_2-α)*. PGD_2 and PGE_2 act on blood vessels and cause increased venular permeability, vasodilatation and bronchodilatation and inhibit inflammatory cell function. PGF_2-α induces vasodilatation and bronchoconstriction.

b) *Thromboxane A_2 (TXA_2)*. Platelets contain the enzyme thromboxane synthetase and hence the metabolite, thromboxane A_2, formed is active in platelet aggregation, besides its role as a vasoconstrictor and broncho-constrictor.

c) *Prostacyclin (PGI_2)*. PGI_2 induces vasodilatation, bronchodilatation and inhibits platelet aggregation.

d) *Resolvins* are another derivative of COX pathway which act by inhibiting production of pro-inflammatory cytokines. Thus, resolvins are actually helpful—drugs such as aspirin act by inhibiting COX activity and stimulate production of resolvins.

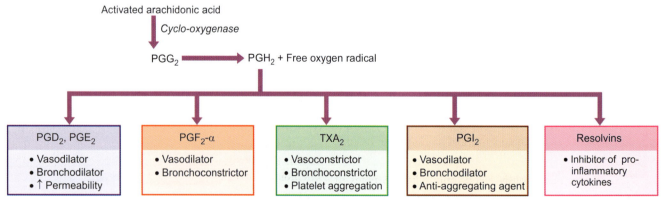

Figure 10.8 ▶ Arachidonic acid metabolites via cyclooxygenase pathway.

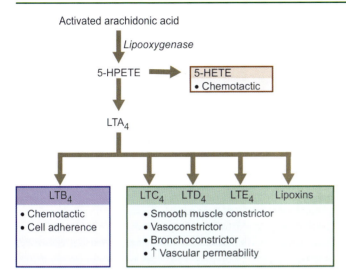

Figure 10.9 ▶ Arachidonic acid metabolites via lipooxygenase pathway.

It may be mentioned here that some of the major anti-inflammatory drugs act by inhibiting activity of the enzyme COX; e.g. non-steroidal anti-inflammatory drugs (NSAIDs), COX-2 inhibitors.

ii) Metabolites via lipo-oxygenase pathway: 5-HETE, leukotrienes, lipoxins The enzyme, lipo-oxygenase, a predominant enzyme in neutrophils, acts on activated arachidonic acid to form hydroperoxy eicosatetraenoic acid (5-HPETE) which on further peroxidation forms following 2 metabolites (Fig. 10.9):

a) *5-HETE* (hydroxy compound), an intermediate product, is a potent chemotactic agent for neutrophils.

b) *Leukotrienes* (LT) are so named as they were first isolated from leucocytes. Firstly, unstable leukotriene A_4 (LTA_4) is formed which is acted upon by enzymes to form LTB_4 (chemotactic for phagocytic cells and stimulates phagocytic cell adherence) while LTC_4, LTD_4 and LTE_4 have common actions by causing smooth muscle contraction and thereby induce vasoconstriction, bronchoconstriction and increased vascular permeability; hence they are also called as slow-reacting substances of anaphylaxis (SRS-As).

c) *Lipoxins* (LX) act to regulate and counterbalance actions of leukotrienes. Lipooxygenase-12 present in platelets acts on LTA_4 derived from neutrophils and forms LXA_4 and LXB_4.

3. LYSOSOMAL COMPONENTS The inflammatory cells—neutrophils and monocytes, contain lysosomal granules which on release elaborate a variety of mediators of inflammation. These are as under:

i) Granules of neutrophils Neutrophils have 3 types of granules: primary or azurophil, secondary or specific, and tertiary.

a) *Primary or azurophil granules* are large azurophil granules which contain functionally active enzymes. These are myeloperoxidase, acid hydrolases, acid phosphatase, lysozyme, defensin (cationic protein), phospholipase, cathepsin G, elastase, and protease.

b) *Secondary or specific granules* contain alkaline phosphatase, lactoferrin, gelatinase, collagenase, lysozyme, vitamin-B_{12} binding proteins, plasminogen activator.

c) *Tertiary granules or C particles* contain gelatinase and acid hydrolases.

Myeloperoxidase causes oxidative lysis by generation of oxygen free radicals, acid hydrolases act within the cell to cause destruction of bacteria in phagolysosome while proteases attack on the extracellular constituents such as basement membrane, collagen, elastin, cartilage etc.

However, degradation of extracellular components like collagen, basement membrane, fibrin and cartilage by proteases results in harmful tissue destruction which is kept in check by presence of antiproteases like α1-antitrypsin and α2-macroglobulin.

ii) Granules of monocytes and tissue macrophages These cells on degranulation also release mediators of inflammation like acid proteases, collagenase, elastase and plasminogen activator. However, they are more active in chronic inflammation than acting as mediators of acute inflammation.

4. PLATELET ACTIVATING FACTOR (PAF) It is released from IgE-sensitised basophils or mast cells, other leucocytes, endothelium and platelets. Apart from its action on platelet aggregation and release reaction, the actions of PAF as mediator of inflammation are:
i) increased vascular permeability;
ii) vasodilatation in low concentration and vasoconstriction otherwise;
iii) bronchoconstriction;
iv) adhesion of leucocytes to endothelium; and
v) chemotaxis.

5. CYTOKINES Cytokines are polypeptide substances produced by activated lymphocytes *(lymphokines)* and activated monocytes *(monokines)*. The term *chemokine* is used for a family of substances which act as chemoattractants for inflammatory cells.

All these agents may act on 'self' cells which produced them or on other cells. Although over 200 cytokines have been described, major cytokines and their role in inflammation are as under (Table 10.3):

a) **Interleukins (IL-1, IL-6, IL-8, IL-12, IL-17)** While IL-1 and IL-6 are active in mediating acute inflammation, IL-12 and IL-17 play a potent role in chronic inflammation. IL-8 is a chemokine for acute inflammatory cells:

IL-1 is elaborated by several body cells-monocytes and macrophages, B lymphocytes, fibroblasts, endothelial and

Section II: Inflammation and Healing, Immunity and Hypersensitivity, Infections and Infestations

Table 10.3 Major cytokines in inflammation.

CYTOKINE	CELL SOURCE	CELL TARGET	MAIN ACTIONS
IL-1	Monocytes/macrophages, B cells, fibroblasts, endothelial cells, some epithelial cells	All cells	• Expression of adhesion molecules • Emigration of neutrophils and macrophages • Role in fever and shock • Hepatic production of acute phase protein
IL-6	Same as for IL-1	T and B cells, Epithelial cells, hepatocytes, Monocytes/macrophages	• Hepatic production of acute phase protein • Differentiation and growth of T and B cells
IL-8	Monocytes/macrophages, T cells, neutrophils, fibroblasts, endothelial cells, epithelial cells	Neutrophils, basophils, T cells, monocytes/macrophages, endothelial cells	• Induces migration of neutrophils, macrophages and T cells • Stimulates release of histamine from basophils • Stimulates angiogenesis
IL-12	Macrophages, dendritic cells, neutrophils	T cells, NK cells	• Induces formation of T helper cells and killer cells • Promotes CTL cytolytic activity • Increases production of IFN-γ • Decreases production of IL-17
IL-17	CD4+T cells	Fibroblasts, endothelial cells, epithelial cells	• Increases secretion of other cytokines • Migration of neutrophils and monocytes
TNF-α	Monocytes/macrophages, mast cells/basophils, eosinophils, B cells, T cells, NK cells	All cells except RBCs	• Hepatic production of acute phase protein • Systemic features (fever, shock, anorexia) • Expression of endothelial adhesion molecules • Enhanced leucocyte cytotoxicity • Induction of pro-inflammatory cytokines
IFN-γ	T cells, NK cells	All cells	• Activation of macrophages and NK cells • Stimulates secretion of Igs by B cells • Differentiation of T helper cells
MCP-1	Fibroblasts, smooth muscle cells, blood mononuclear cells	Monocytes/macrophages, NK cells, T cells	• Chemoattractant for monocytes, T cells and NK cells • Stimulates release of histamine from basophils
Eotaxin	Alveolar cells, myocardium	Eosinophils, basophils	• Chemoattractant for eosinophils and basophils • Induces allergic pulmonary disease
PF-4	Platelets, megakaryocytes	Fibroblasts, endothelial cells	• Chemoattractant for fibroblasts • Inhibitory to haematopoietic precursors and endothelial cell proliferation

IL=interleukin; TNF=tumour necrosis factor; IFN=interferon; MCP=monocyte chemotactic protein; PF=platelet factor.

some epithelial cells. Similarly, it can target all body cells. Its major actions are:
◈ expression of adhesion molecules;
◈ emigration of neutrophils and macrophages;
◈ role in fever and shock; and
◈ hepatic production of acute phase protein.

IL-6 is similar in its sources and target cells of action. Its major role are:
◈ hepatic production of acute phase protein; and
◈ differentiation and growth of T and B cells.

IL-8 is also elaborated by the same cells as for IL-2 and IL-6 except that it is secreted by T cells instead of B lymphocytes. Its target cells are neutrophils, basophils, T cells, monocytes/macrophages, endothelial cells. IL-8 is chemokine and its major actions are:

◈ induces migration of neutrophils, macrophages and T cells;
◈ stimulates release of histamine from basophils; and
◈ stimulates angiogenesis.

IL-12 is synthesised by macrophages, dendritic cells and neutrophils while it targets T cells and NK cells. Its major actions in chronic inflammation are as under:
◈ induces formation of T helper cells and killer cells;
◈ promotes CTL cytolytic activity;
◈ increases production of IFN-γ; and
◈ decreases production of IL-17.

IL-17 is formed by CD4+T cells while it targets fibroblasts, endothelial cells and epithelial cells. Its action in chronic inflammation are:

- increased secretion of other cytokines; and
- migration of neutrophils and monocytes.

b) Tumour necrosis factor (TNF-α and β) TNF-α is a mediator of acute inflammation while TNF-β is involved in cellular cytotoxicity and in development of spleen and lymph nodes. TNF-α is formed by various cells (Monocytes/macrophages, mast cells/basophils, eosinophils, B cells, T cells, NK cells) while TNF-β is formed by B and T lymphocytes only. Both can target all body cells except erythrocytes. Major actions of TNF-α are:
- hepatic production of acute phase proteins;
- systemic features (fever, shock, anorexia);
- expression of endothelial adhesion molecules;
- enhanced leucocyte cytotoxicity; and
- induction of pro-inflammatory cytokines.

c) Interferon (IFN)-γ It is produced by T cells and NK cells and may act on all body cells. It acts as mediator of acute inflammation as under:
- activation of macrophages and NK cells;
- stimulates secretion of immunoglobulins by B cells; and
- role in differentiation of T helper cells.

d) Other chemokines (IL-8, MCP-1, eotaxin, PF-4) Besides IL-8, a few other chemoattractants for various cells are as under:

MCP-1 is elaborated by fibroblasts, smooth muscle cells, and peripheral blood mononuclear cells. Its actions are:
- chemoattractant for monocytes, T cells and NK cells; and
- Stimulates release of histamine from basophils.

Eotaxin is formed by alveolar cells of the lung and in the heart. Its actions are:
- chemoattractant for eosinophils and basophils; and
- induces allergic pulmonary disease.

PF-4 is formed by platelets and megakaryocytes and may act on fibroblasts and endothelial cells. Its actions are:
- chemoattractant for fibroblasts; and
- inhibitory to haematopoietic precursors and angiogenesis.

6. FREE RADICALS: OXYGEN METABOLITES AND NITRIC OXIDE Free radicals act as potent mediator of inflammation:

i) *Oxygen-derived metabolites* are released from activated neutrophils and macrophages and include superoxide oxygen (O'_2), H_2O_2, OH' and toxic NO products. These oxygen-derived free radicals have the following actions in inflammation:
a) Endothelial cell damage and thereby increased vascular permeability.
b) Activation of protease and inactivation of antiprotease causing tissue matrix damage.
c) Damage to other cells.

The actions of free radicals are counteracted by anti-oxidants present in tissues and serum which play a protective role (page 32).

ii) *Nitric oxide (NO)* was originally described as vascular relaxation factor produced by endothelial cells. Now it is known that NO is formed by activated macrophages during the oxidation of arginine by the action of enzyme, NO synthase. NO plays the following roles in mediating inflammation:
a) Vasodilatation
b) Anti-platelet activating agent
c) Possibly microbicidal action.

II. PLASMA PROTEIN-DERIVED MEDIATORS (PLASMA PROTEASES)

These include various products derived from activation and interaction of 4 interlinked systems: kinin, clotting, fibrinolytic and complement. Each of these systems has its inhibitors and accelerators in plasma with negative and positive feedback mechanisms respectively.

Hageman factor (factor XII) of clotting system plays a key role in interactions of the four systems. Activation of factor XII *in vivo* by contact with basement membrane and bacterial endotoxins, and *in vitro* with glass or kaolin, leads to activation of clotting, fibrinolytic and kinin systems. In inflammation, activation of factor XII is brought about by contact of the factor leaking through the endothelial gaps. The end-products of the activated clotting, fibrinolytic and kinin systems activate the complement system that generate permeability factors. These permeability factors, in turn, further activate clotting system.

The inter-relationship among 4 systems is summarised in Fig. 10.10.

1. THE KININ SYSTEM This system on activation by factor XIIa generates bradykinin, so named because of the slow contraction of smooth muscle induced by it. First, kallikrein is formed from plasma prekallikrein by the action of prekallikrein activator which is a fragment of factor XIIa. Kallikrein then acts on high molecular weight kininogen to form bradykinin (Fig. 10.11).

Bradykinin acts in the early stage of inflammation and its effects include:
i) smooth muscle contraction;
ii) vasodilatation;
iii) increased vascular permeability; and
iv) pain.

2. THE CLOTTING SYSTEM Factor XIIa initiates the cascade of the clotting system resulting in formation of fibrinogen which is acted upon by thrombin to form fibrin and fibrinopeptides (Fig. 10.12).

The actions of fibrinopeptides in inflammation are:
i) increased vascular permeability;
ii) chemotaxis for leucocyte; and
iii) anticoagulant activity.

3. THE FIBRINOLYTIC SYSTEM This system is activated by plasminogen activator, the sources of which include kallikrein of the kinin system, endothelial cells and leucocytes. Plasminogen activator acts on plasminogen present as component of plasma proteins to form plasmin. Further breakdown of fibrin by plasmin forms fibrinopeptides or fibrin split products (Fig. 10.13).

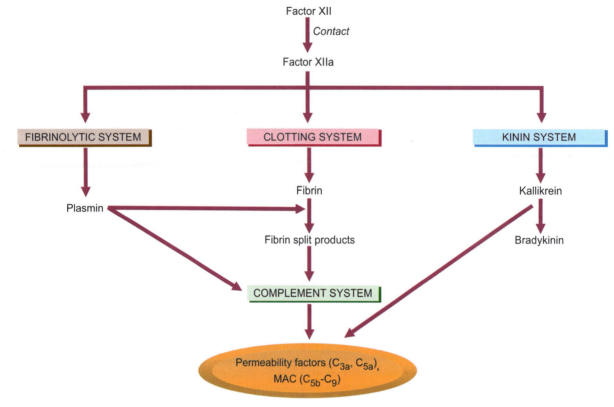

Figure 10.10 ▶ Inter-relationship among clotting, fibrinolytic, kinin and complement systems.

The actions of plasmin in inflammation are as follows:
i) activation of factor XII to form prekallikrein activator that stimulates the kinin system to generate bradykinin;
ii) splits off complement C3 to form C3a which is a permeability factor; and
iii) degrades fibrin to form fibrin split products which increase vascular permeability and are chemotactic to leucocytes.

4. THE COMPLEMENT SYSTEM The activation of complement system can occur either:
i) by *classic pathway* through antigen-antibody complexes; or
ii) by *alternate pathway* via non-immunologic agents such as bacterial toxins, cobra venoms and IgA.

Complement system on activation by either of these two pathways yields activated products which include anaphylatoxins (C3a, C4a and C5a), and membrane attack complex (MAC) i.e. C5b,C6,7,8,9.

The actions of activated complement system in inflammation are as under:
◈ C3a, C5a, C4a (anaphylatoxins) activate mast cells and basophils to release of histamine, cause increased vascular permeability causing oedema in tissues, augments phagocytosis.
◈ C3b is an opsonin.
◈ C5a is chemotactic for leucocytes.
◈ Membrane attack complex (MAC) (C5b-C9) is a lipid dissolving agent and causes holes in the phospholipid membrane of the cell.

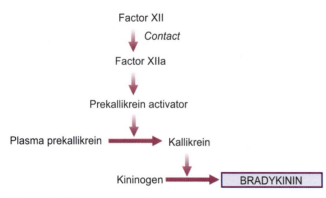

Figure 10.11 ▶ Pathway of kinin system.

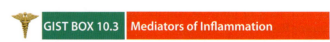

GIST BOX 10.3 — Mediators of Inflammation

❖ These are endogenous chemical substances which mediate the process of acute inflammation.
❖ They have some common properties: i) they are released either from the cells or are derived from plasma proteins, ii) they are released in response to certain stimuli,

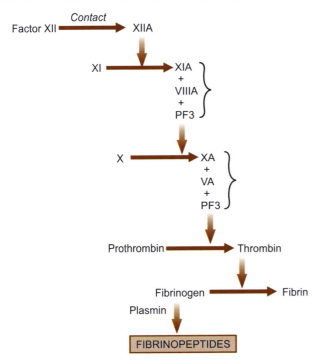

Figure 10.12 ▶ Pathway of the clotting system.

- iii) they act on different targets, iv) they have a short lifespan after their release, v) they have several actions, most important being increased vascular permeability.
- ❖ Cell-derived mediators of inflammation are: vasoactive amines (histamine, 5HT, neuropeptides), arachidonic acid metabolites (prostaglandins, 5-HETE, leukotrienes, lipoxins), lysosomal components, platelet activating factor, cytokines (ILs, TNF, IFN, chemokines) and free radicals (oxygen metabolites and nitric oxide).
- ❖ Plasma protein derived mediators are products of kinin, clotting, fibrinolytic and complement system.

REGULATION OF INFLAMMATION

The onset of inflammatory responses outlined above may have potentially damaging influence on the host tissues as evident in hypersensitivity conditions. Such self-damaging

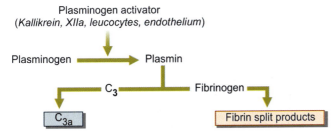

Figure 10.13 ▶ Activation of fibrinolytic system.

effects are kept in check by the host regulatory mechanisms in order to resolve inflammation. These mechanisms are as follows:

i) **Acute phase reactants** A variety of acute phase reactant (APR) proteins are released in plasma in response to tissue trauma and infection. Their major role is to protect the normal cells from harmful effects of toxic molecules generated in inflammation and to clear away the waste material. APRs include the following:

i) *Certain cellular protection factors* (e.g. α1-antitrypsin, α1-chymotrypsin, α2-antiplasmin, plasminogen activator inhibitor): They protect the tissues from cytotoxic and proteolytic damage.

ii) *Some coagulation proteins* (e.g. fibrinogen, plasminogen, von Willebrand factor, factor VIII): They generate factors to replace those consumed in coagulation.

iii) *Transport proteins* (e.g. ceruloplasmin, haptoglobin): They carry generated factors.

iv) *Immune agents* (e.g. serum amyloid A and P component, C-reactive protein or CRP): CRP is an opsonising agent for phagocytosis and its levels are a useful indicator of inflammation in the body.

v) *Stress proteins* (e.g. heat shock proteins—HSP, ubiquitin): They are molecular chaperons who carry the toxic waste within the cell to the lysosomes (page 14).

vi) *Antioxidants* (e.g. ceruloplasmin) are active in elimination of excess of oxygen free radicals.

The APR are synthesised mainly in the liver, and to some extent in macrophages. APR along with systemic features of fever and leucocytosis is termed 'acute phase response'. Deficient synthesis of APR leads to severe form of disease in the form of chronic and repeated inflammatory responses.

ii) **Corticosteroids** The endogenous corticosteroids act as anti-inflammatory agents. Their levels are raised in infection and trauma by self-regulating mechanism.

iii) **Free cytokine receptors** The presence of freely circulating soluble receptors for cytokines in the serum correlates directly with disease activity.

iv) **Anti-inflammatory chemical mediators** As already described, PGE_2 or prostacyclin have both pro-inflammatory as well as anti-inflammatory actions.

GIST BOX 10.4 — Regulators of Inflammation

- ❖ Normally, inflammation is kept in check by the inbuilt regulatory system to resolve its harmful effects.
- ❖ These substances are acute phase reactant proteins, endogenous glucocorticoids, cytokine receptors and certain anti-inflammatory mediators (e.g. prostacyclin).

THE INFLAMMATORY CELLS

The cells participating in acute and chronic inflammation are circulating leucocytes, plasma cells, tissue macrophages and inflammatory giant cells. The structure, function and production of these cells are dealt with in detail in Chapter 24. Here, it is pertinent to describe their role in inflammation. Their morphology, characteristics and functions are summarised in **Table 10.4**.

POLYMORPHONUCLEAR NEUTROPHILS (PMNs)

Commonly called as neutrophils or polymorphs, these cells along with basophils and eosinophils are together known as granulocytes due to the presence of granules in their cytoplasm. These granules contain many substances like proteases, myeloperoxidase, lysozyme, esterase, aryl sulfatase, acid and alkaline phosphatase, and cationic proteins. The diameter of neutrophils ranges from 10 to 15 µm and are

Table 10.4 Morphology and functions of inflammatory cells.

MORPHOLOGY	FEATURES	MEDIATORS
A, POLYMORPH	i. Initial phagocytosis of bacteria and foreign body ii. Acute inflammatory cell	i. Primary granules (MPO, lysozyme, cationic proteins, acid hydrolases, elastase) ii. Secondary granules (lysozyme, alk. phosph, collagenase, lactoferrin) iii. Tertiary granules (gelatinase, cathepsin) iv. Reactive oxygen metabolites
B, MONOCYTE/MACROPHAGE	i. Bacterial phagocytosis ii. Chronic inflammatory cell iii. Regulates lymphocyte response	i. Acid and neutral hydrolases (lysosomal) ii. Cationic protein iii. Phospholipase iv. Prostaglandins, leukotrienes v. IL-1
C, LYMPHOCYTE	i. Humoral and cell-mediated immune responses ii. Chronic inflammatory cell iii. Regulates macrophage response	i. B cells: antibody production ii. T cells: delayed hypersensitivity, cytotoxicity
D, PLASMA CELL	i. Derived from B cells ii. Chronic inflammatory cell	i. Antibody synthesis ii. Antibody secretion
E, EOSINOPHIL	i. Allergic states ii. Parasitic infestations iii. Chronic inflammatory cell	i. Reactive oxygen metabolites ii. Lysosomal (major basic protein, cationic protein, eosinophil peroxidase, neurotoxin) iii. PGE_2 synthesis
F, BASOPHIL/MAST CELL	i. Receptor for IgE molecules ii. Electron-dense granules	i. Histamine ii. Leukotrienes iii. Platelet activating factor

actively motile (Table 10.4, A). These cells comprise 40-75% of circulating leucocytes and their number is increased in blood (neutrophilia) and tissues in acute bacterial infections. These cells arise in the bone marrow from stem cells (page 418).

The functions of neutrophils in inflammation are as follows:

i) Initial phagocytosis of microorganisms as they form the first line of body defense in bacterial infection. The steps involved are adhesion of neutrophils to vascular endothelium, emigration through the vessel wall, chemotaxis, engulfment, degranulation, killing and degradation of the foreign material.

ii) Engulfment of antigen-antibody complexes and non-microbial material.

iii) Harmful effect of neutrophils are by causing basement membrane destruction of the glomeruli and small blood vessels in immunologic cell injury.

EOSINOPHILS

These are slightly larger than neutrophils but are fewer in number, comprising 1 to 6% of total blood leucocytes (Table 10.4, E). Eosinophils share many structural and functional similarities with neutrophils like their production in the bone marrow, locomotion, phagocytosis, lobed nucleus and presence of granules in the cytoplasm containing a variety of enzymes, of which major basic protein and eosinophil cationic protein are the most important which have bactericidal and toxic action against helminthic parasites. However, granules of eosinophils are richer in myeloperoxidase than neutrophils and lack lysozyme. High level of steroid hormones leads to fall in number of eosinophils and even disappearance from blood.

The absolute number of eosinophils is increased in the following conditions and, thus, they partake in inflammatory responses associated with these conditions:
i)   allergic conditions;
ii) parasitic infestations;
iii) skin diseases; and
iv) certain malignant lymphomas.

BASOPHILS AND MAST CELLS

The basophils comprise about 1% of circulating leucocytes and are morphologically and functionally similar to their tissue counterparts, mast cells. These cells contain coarse basophilic granules in the cytoplasm and a polymorphonuclear nucleus (Table 10.4, F). These granules are laden with heparin and histamine. Basophils and mast cells have receptors for IgE and degranulate when cross-linked with antigen.

The role of these cells in inflammation are:
i)   in immediate and delayed type of hypersensitivity reactions; and
ii) release of histamine by IgE-sensitised basophils.

LYMPHOCYTES

Next to neutrophils, these cells are the most numerous of the circulating leucocytes in adults (20-45%). Apart from blood, lymphocytes are present in large numbers in spleen, thymus, lymph nodes and mucosa-associated lymphoid tissue (MALT). They have scanty cytoplasm and consist almost entirely of nucleus (Table 10.4, C).

Their role in antibody formation (B lymphocytes) and in cell-mediated immunity (T lymphocytes) has been discussed in Chapter 14; in addition these cells participate in the following types of inflammatory responses:

i)   *In tissues*, they are dominant cells in chronic inflammation and late stage of acute inflammation.

ii) *In blood*, their number is increased (lymphocytosis) in chronic infections like tuberculosis.

PLASMA CELLS

These cells are larger than lymphocytes with more abundant cytoplasm and an eccentric nucleus which has cart-wheel pattern of chromatin (Table 10.4, D). Plasma cells are normally not seen in peripheral blood. They develop from B lymphocytes and are rich in RNA and γ-globulin in their cytoplasm. There is an interrelationship between plasmacytosis and hyperglobulinaemia. These cells are most active in antibody synthesis.

Their number is increased in the following conditions:
i)   prolonged infection with immunological responses e.g. in syphilis, rheumatoid arthritis, tuberculosis;
ii) hypersensitivity states; and
iii) multiple myeloma.

MONONUCLEAR-PHAGOCYTE SYSTEM (RETICULOENDOTHELIAL SYSTEM)

This cell system includes cells derived from 2 sources with common morphology, function and origin (Table 10.4, B). These are as under:

A. Blood monocytes   These comprise 4-8% of circulating leucocytes.

B. Tissue macrophages   These include the following cells in different tissues:
  i)   Macrophages or phagocytes in inflammation.
  ii) Histiocytes which are macrophages present in connective tissues.
  iii) Epithelioid cells are modified macrophages seen in granulomatous inflammation.
  iv) Kupffer cells are macrophages of the liver.
  v)   Alveolar macrophages (type II pneumocytes) in the lungs.
  vi) Reticulum cells are macrophages/histiocytes of the bone marrow.
  vii) Tingible body macrophages of germinal centres of the lymph nodes.

viii) Littoral cells of the splenic sinusoids.
ix) Osteoclasts in the bones.
x) Microglial cells of the brain.
xi) Langerhans' cells/dendritic histiocytes of the skin.
xii) Hoffbaüer cells of the placenta.
xiii) Mesangial cells of the glomerulus.

The mononuclear phagocytes are the scavenger cells of the body as well as participate in immune system of the body (Chapter 14); their functions in inflammation are as under:

Role of macrophages in inflammation The functions of mononuclear-phagocyte cells are as under:

i) *Phagocytosis* (cell eating) and *pinocytosis* (cell drinking).

ii) *Macrophages on activation* by lymphokines released by T lymphocytes or by non-immunologic stimuli elaborate a variety of biologically active substances as under:
  a) Proteases like collagenase and elastase which degrade collagen and elastic tissue.
  b) Plasminogen activator which activates the fibrinolytic system.
  c) Products of complement.
  d) Some coagulation factors (factor V and thromboplastin) which convert fibrinogen to fibrin.
  e) Chemotactic agents for other leucocytes.
  f) Metabolites of arachidonic acid.
  g) Growth promoting factors for fibroblasts, blood vessels and granulocytes.
  h) Cytokines like interleukin-1 and TNF-$\alpha\alpha$.
  i) Oxygen-derived free radicals.

GIANT CELLS

A few examples of multinucleate giant cells exist in normal tissues (e.g. osteoclasts in the bones, trophoblasts in placenta, megakaryocytes in the bone marrow). However, in chronic inflammation when the macrophages fail to deal with particles to be removed, they fuse together and form multinucleated giant cells. Besides, morphologically distinct giant cells appear in some tumours also. Some of the common types of giant cells are described below (Fig. 10.14):

A. Giant cells in inflammation:

i) *Foreign body giant cells* These contain numerous nuclei (up to 100) which are uniform in size and shape and resemble the nuclei of macrophages. These nuclei are scattered throughout the cytoplasm. These are seen in chronic infective granulomas, leprosy and tuberculosis.

ii) *Langhans' giant cells* These are seen in tuberculosis and sarcoidosis. Their nuclei are like the nuclei of macrophages and epithelioid cells. These nuclei are arranged either around the periphery in the form of horseshoe or ring, or are clustered at the two poles of the giant cell.

iii) *Touton giant cells* These multinucleated cells have vacuolated cytoplasm due to lipid content e.g. in xanthoma.

iv) *Aschoff giant cells* These multinucleate giant cells are derived from cardiac histiocytes and are seen in rheumatic nodule (page 502).

B. Giant cells in tumours:

i) *Anaplastic cancer giant cells* These are larger, have numerous nuclei which are hyperchromatic and vary in size and shape (page 273). These giant cells are not derived from macrophages but are formed from dividing nuclei of the neoplastic cells e.g. carcinoma of the liver, various soft tissue sarcomas etc.

ii) *Reed-Sternberg cells* These are also malignant tumour giant cells which are generally binucleate and are seen in various histologic types of Hodgkin's lymphomas (page 445).

iii) *Osteoclastic giant cells of bone tumour* Giant cell tumour of the bones or osteoclastoma has uniform distribution of osteoclastic giant cells spread in the stroma.

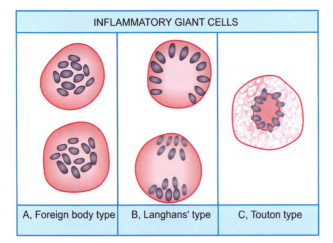
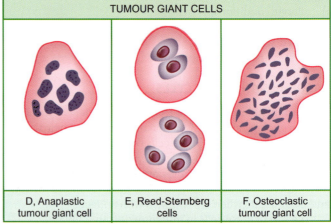

Figure 10.14 ▶ Giant cells of various types. A, Foreign body giant cell with uniform nuclei dispersed throughout the cytoplasm. B, Langhans' giant cells with uniform nuclei arranged peripherally or clustered at the two poles. C, Touton giant cell with circular pattern of nuclei and vacuolated cytoplasm. D, Anaplastic tumour giant cell with nuclei of variable size and shape. E, Reed-Sternberg cell. F, Osteoclastic tumour giant cell.

> **GIST BOX 10.5 The Inflammatory Cells**
>
> - Cells participating in acute and chronic inflammation are circulating leucocytes, plasma cells, tissue macrophages and inflammatory giant cells.
> - Polymorphs or neutrophils are the first line of defense against invading agents and perform initial phagocytosis.
> - Eosinophils participate in allergic conditions, parasitic infestations and certain skin diseases.
> - Basophils and mast cells are involved in immediate and delayed type of hypersensitivity reactions.
> - Lymphocytes are immunocompetent cells—B cells in humoral immunity and T cells in cell-mediated immunity. Besides, lymphocytes are the dominant cells in chronic inflammation.
> - Plasma cells develop from B cells and are immunoglobulin-synthesising cells and are seen in chronic inflammation.
> - Mononuclear phagocyte system is comprised by circulating monocytes and tissue macrophages. These are scavenger cells of the body.
> - Different types of giant cells are seen in different inflammatory conditions. The types of giant cells are foreign body, Langhans' touton and Aschoff giant cells.

ACUTE INFLAMMATION—FACTORS, MORPHOLOGY, EFFECTS, FATE

FACTORS DETERMINING VARIATION IN INFLAMMATORY RESPONSE

Although acute inflammation is typically characterised by vascular and cellular events with emigration of neutrophilic leucocytes, not all examples of acute inflammation show infiltration by neutrophils. On the other hand, some chronic inflammatory conditions are characterised by neutrophilic infiltration. For example, *typhoid fever* is an example of acute inflammatory process but the cellular response in it is lymphocytic; *osteomyelitis* is an example of chronic inflammation but the cellular response in this condition is mainly neutrophilic.

The variation in inflammatory response depends upon a number of factors and processes. These may pertain to the organisms and the host:

Factors Involving the Organisms

i) Types of injury and infection For example, skin reacts to herpes simplex infection by formation of vesicle and to streptococcal infection by formation of boil; lung reacts to pneumococci by occurrence of lobar pneumonia while to tubercle bacilli it reacts by granulomatous inflammation.

ii) Virulence Many species and strains of organisms may have varying virulence e.g. the three strains of *Corynebacterium diphtheriae (gravis, intermedius and mitis)* produce the same diphtherial exotoxin but in different amount.

iii) Dose The concentration of organism in small doses produces usually local lesions while larger dose results in more severe spreading infections.

iv) Portal of entry Some organisms are infective only if administered by particular route e.g. *Vibrio cholerae* is not pathogenic if injected subcutaneously but causes cholera if swallowed.

v) Product of organisms Some organisms produce enzymes that help in spread of infections e.g. hyaluronidase by *Clostridium welchii*, streptokinase by streptococci, staphylokinase and coagulase by staphylococci.

Factors Involving the Host

i) Systemic diseases Certain acquired systemic diseases in the host are associated with impaired inflammatory response e.g. diabetes mellitus, chronic renal failure, cirrhosis of the liver, chronic alcoholism, bone marrow suppression from various causes (drugs, radiation, idiopathic). These conditions render the host more susceptible to infections.

ii) Immune status of host Patients who are immunosuppressed from congenital or acquired immunodeficiency have lowered inflammatory response and spread of infections occurs rapidly e.g. in AIDS, congenital immunodeficiency diseases, diabetes mellitus, protein calorie malnutrition, starvation.

iii) Congenital neutrophil defects Congenital defects in neutrophil structure and functions result in reduced inflammatory response.

iv) Leukopenia Patients with low WBC count with neutropenia or agranulocytosis develop spreading infection.

v) Site or type of tissue involved For example, the lung has loose texture as compared to bone and, thus, both tissues react differently to acute inflammation.

vi) Local host factors For instance, ischaemia, presence of foreign bodies and chemicals cause necrosis and thus cause more harm.

MORPHOLOGY OF ACUTE INFLAMMATION

Inflammation of an organ is usually named by adding the suffix-*itis* to its Latin name e.g. appendicitis, hepatitis, cholecystitis, meningitis etc. A few examples of acute inflammation are described below:

APPENDICITIS

Acute inflammation of the appendix, acute appendicitis, is the most common acute abdominal condition confronting the surgeon. The condition is seen more commonly in older children and young adults, and is uncommon at the extremes of age. The disease is seen more frequently in the West and in affluent societies which may be due to variation in diet—a diet with low bulk or cellulose and high protein intake more often causes appendicitis.

ETIOPATHOGENESIS The most common mechanism is obstruction of the lumen from various etiologic factors that leads to increased intraluminal pressure. This presses upon the blood vessels to produce ischaemic injury which in turn favours the bacterial proliferation and hence acute appendicitis. The common causes of appendicitis are as under:

A. Obstructive:
1. Faecolith
2. Calculi
3. Foreign body
4. Tumour
5. Worms (especially *Enterobius vermicularis*)
6. Diffuse lymphoid hyperplasia, especially in children.

B. Non-obstructive:
1. Haematogenous spread of generalised infection
2. Vascular occlusion
3. Inappropriate diet lacking roughage.

MORPHOLOGIC FEATURES. Grossly, the appearance depends upon the stage at which the acutely-inflamed appendix is examined. In *early acute appendicitis,* the organ is swollen and serosa shows hyperaemia. In well-developed acute inflammation called *acute suppurative appendicitis,* the serosa is coated with fibrinopurulent exudate and engorged vessels on the surface. In further advanced cases called *acute gangrenous appendicitis,* there is necrosis and ulcerations of mucosa which extend through the wall so that the appendix becomes soft and friable and the surface is coated with greenish-black gangrenous necrosis **(Fig. 10.15)**.

Microscopically, the most important diagnostic histological criterion is the *neutrophilic infiltration of the muscularis*. In early stage, the other changes besides acute inflammatory changes, are congestion and oedema of the appendiceal wall. In later stages, the mucosa is sloughed off, the wall becomes necrotic, the blood vessels may get thrombosed and there may be neutrophilic abscesses in the wall. In either case, an impacted foreign body, faecolith, or concretion may be seen in the lumen **(Fig. 10.16)**.

Thus, there is good correlation between macroscopic and microscopic findings in acute appendicitis.

CLINICAL COURSE. The patient presents with features of acute abdomen as under:
1. Colicky pain, initially around umbilicus but later localised to right iliac fossa
2. Nausea and vomiting
3. Pyrexia of mild grade
4. Abdominal tenderness
5. Increased pulse rate
6. Neutrophilic leucocytosis.

An attack of acute appendicitis predisposes the appendix to repeated attacks *(recurrent acute appendicitis)* and thus surgery has to be carried out. If appendicectomy is done at a later stage following acute attack *(interval appendicectomy),* pathological changes of healing by fibrosis of the wall and chronic inflammation are observed.

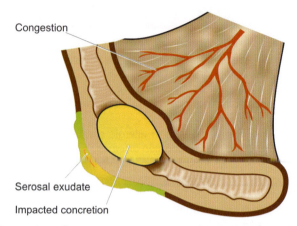

Figure 10.15 ▶ Acute appendicitis. Gross appearance of longitudinally opened appendix showing impacted faecolith in the lumen and exudate on the serosa.

COMPLICATIONS. If the condition is not adequately managed, the following complications may occur:

1. Peritonitis A perforated appendix as occurs in gangrenous appendicitis may cause localised or generalised peritonitis.

2. Appendix abscess This is due to rupture of an appendix giving rise to localised abscess in the right iliac fossa. This abscess may spread to other sites such as between the liver and diaphragm (subphrenic abscess), into the pelvis between the urinary bladder and rectum, and in the females may involve uterus and fallopian tubes.

3. Adhesions Late complications of acute appendicitis are fibrous adhesions to the greater omentum, small intestine and other abdominal structures.

4. Portal pylephlebitis Spread of infection into mesenteric veins may produce septic phlebitis and liver abscess.

5. Mucocele Distension of distal appendix by mucus following recovery from an attack of acute appendicitis is referred to as mucocele. It occurs generally due to proximal obstruction but sometimes may be due to a benign or malignant neoplasm in the appendix. An infected mucocele may result in formation of *empyema* of the appendix.

ULCER

Ulcers are local defects on the surface of an organ produced by inflammation. Common sites for ulcerations are the stomach, duodenum, intestinal ulcers in typhoid fever, intestinal tuberculosis, bacillary and amoebic dysentery, ulcers of legs due to varicose veins etc. In the acute stage, there is infiltration by polymorphs with vasodilatation while long-standing ulcers develop infiltration by lymphocytes, plasma cells and macrophages with associated fibroblastic proliferation and scarring.

Chapter 10: Inflammation: Acute

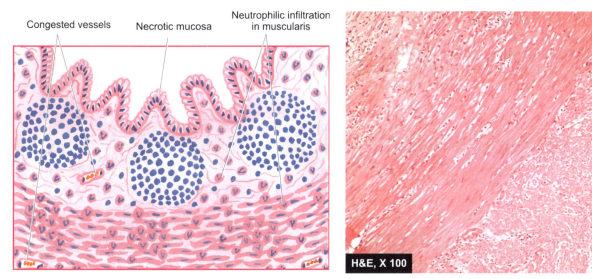

Figure 10.16 ▶ Acute appendicitis. Microscopic appearance showing diagnostic neutrophilic infiltration into the muscularis. Other changes present are necrosis of mucosa and periappendicitis.

SUPPURATION (ABSCESS FORMATION)

When acute bacterial infection is accompanied by intense neutrophilic infiltrate in the inflamed tissue, it results in tissue necrosis. A cavity is formed which is called an abscess and contains purulent exudate or pus and the process of abscess formation is known as suppuration. The bacteria which cause suppuration are called pyogenic.

Microscopically, pus is creamy or opaque in appearance and is composed of numerous dead as well as living neutrophils, some red cells, fragments of tissue debris and fibrin. In old pus, macrophages and cholesterol crystals are also present **(Fig. 10.17).**

An abscess may be discharged to the surface due to increased pressure inside or may require drainage by the surgeon. Due to tissue destruction, resolution does not occur but instead healing by fibrous scarring takes place.

Some of the common examples of abscess formation are as under:
i) *Boil or furuncle* which is an acute inflammation via hair follicles in the dermal tissues.
ii) *Carbuncle* is seen in untreated diabetics and occurs as a loculated abscess in the dermis and soft tissues of the neck.
iii) *Cellulitis*. It is a diffuse inflammation of soft tissues resulting from spreading effects of substances like hyaluronidase released by some bacteria.

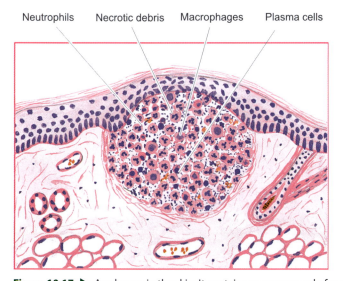
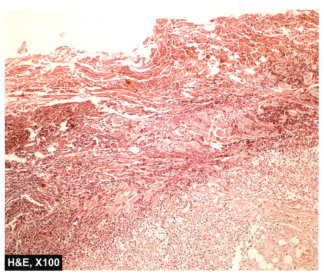

Figure 10.17 ▶ An abscess in the skin. It contains pus composed of necrotic tissue, debris, fibrin, RBCs and dead and living neutrophils. Some macrophages are seen at the periphery.

SYSTEMIC EFFECTS OF ACUTE INFLAMMATION

The account of acute inflammation given so far now above is based on local tissue responses. However, acute inflammation is associated with systemic effects as well. These include fever, leucocytosis, lymphangitis-lymphadenitis and shock.

1. **Fever** occurs due to bacteraemia. It is thought to be mediated through release of factors like prostaglandins, interleukin-1 and TNF-α in response to infection.

2. **Leucocytosis** commonly accompanies the acute inflammatory reactions, usually in the range of 15,000-20,000/μl. When the counts are higher than this with 'shift to left' of myeloid cells, the blood picture is described as leukaemoid reaction. Usually, in bacterial infections there is neutrophilia; in viral infections lymphocytosis; and in parasitic infestations, eosinophilia. Typhoid fever, an example of acute inflammation, however, induces leucopenia with relative lymphocytosis.

3. **Lymphangitis-lymphadenitis** is one of the important manifestations of localised inflammatory injury. The lymphatics and lymph nodes that drain the inflamed tissue show reactive inflammatory changes in the form of lymphangitis and lymphadenitis. This response represents either a nonspecific reaction to mediators released from inflamed tissue or is an immunologic response to a foreign antigen. The affected lymph nodes may show hyperplasia of lymphoid follicles (follicular hyperplasia) and proliferation of mononuclear phagocytic cells in the sinuses of lymph node (sinus histiocytosis) (Chapter 24).

4. **Shock** may occur in severe cases. Massive release of cytokine TNF-α, a mediator of inflammation, in response to severe tissue injury or infection results in profuse systemic vasodilatation, increased vascular permeability and intravascular volume loss. The net effect of these changes is hypotension and shock. Systemic activation of coagulation pathway may occur leading to microthrombi throughout the body and result in disseminated intravascular coagulation (DIC), bleeding and death.

FATE OF ACUTE INFLAMMATION

The acute inflammatory process can culminate in one of the following outcomes (Fig. 10.18):

1. **Resolution** It means complete return to normal tissue following acute inflammation. This occurs when tissue changes are slight and the cellular changes are reversible e.g. resolution in lobar pneumonia.

2. **Healing** When the tissue loss in acute inflammation is superficial, healing takes place by regeneration. However, when the tissue destruction is extensive, then healing occurs by fibrosis.

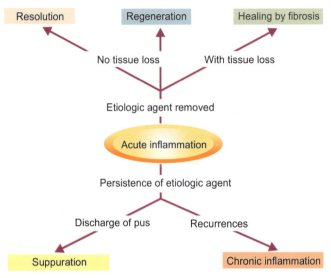

Figure 10.18 ▶ Fate of acute inflammation.

3. **Suppuration** When the pyogenic bacteria causing acute inflammation result in severe tissue necrosis, the process progresses to suppuration. Initially, there is intense neutrophilic infiltration. Subsequently, mixture of neutrophils, bacteria, fragments of necrotic tissue, cell debris and fibrin comprise pus which is contained in a cavity to form an abscess. The abscess, if not drained, may get organised by dense fibrous tissue, and in time, get calcified.

4. **Chronic inflammation** Persisting or recurrent acute inflammation may progress to chronic inflammation in which the processes of inflammation and healing proceed side by side.

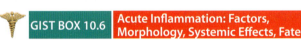

- The variation in inflammatory response depends upon factors pertaining to the organisms (type, virulence, dose, route of entry) or host factors (systemic diseases, immune status, defect in neutrophil function, type of tissue).
- Morphologic patterns of acute inflammation are various forms of exudates, pseudomembranous inflammation, ulcers, abscesses, cellulitis, and bacterial infection through blood (bacteraemia, septicaemia, pyaemia).
- Besides local effects, acute inflammation produces systemic manifestations such as fever, leucocytosis, lymphangitis and shock.
- Acute inflammation may have variety of outcomes: resolution, healing (by regeneration or by fibrosis), suppuration or may end up in chronic inflammation.

11 Inflammation: Chronic and Granulomatous

CHRONIC INFLAMMATION

Chronic inflammation is defined as a prolonged process in which tissue destruction and inflammation occur at the same time.

Chronic inflammation may occur by one of the following 3 ways:

1. Chronic inflammation following acute inflammation When the tissue destruction is extensive, or the bacteria survive and persist in small numbers at the site of acute inflammation e.g. in osteomyelitis, pneumonia terminating in lung abscess.

2. Recurrent attacks of acute inflammation When repeated bouts of acute inflammation culminate in chronicity of the process e.g. in recurrent urinary tract infection leading to chronic pyelonephritis, repeated acute infection of gallbladder leading to chronic cholecystitis.

3. Chronic inflammation starting *de novo* When the infection with organisms of low pathogenicity is chronic from the beginning e.g. infection with *Mycobacterium tuberculosis*.

GENERAL FEATURES OF CHRONIC INFLAMMATION

Though there may be differences in chronic inflammatory response depending upon the tissue involved and causative organisms, there are some basic similarities amongst various types of chronic inflammation. Following general features characterise any chronic inflammation:

1. MONONUCLEAR CELL INFILTRATION Chronic inflammatory lesions are infiltrated by mononuclear inflammatory cells like phagocytes and lymphoid cells. Phagocytes are represented by circulating monocytes, tissue macrophages, epithelioid cells and sometimes, multinucleated giant cells. The macrophages comprise the most important cells in chronic inflammation. These may appear at the site of chronic inflammation from:
  i) chemotactic factors and adhesion molecules for continued infiltration of macrophages;
  ii) local proliferation of macrophages; and
  iii) longer survival of macrophages at the site of inflammation.

The blood monocytes on reaching the extravascular space transform into tissue macrophages. Besides the role of macrophages in phagocytosis, they may get activated in response to stimuli such as cytokines (lymphokines) and bacterial endotoxins. On activation, macrophages release several biologically active substances e.g. acid and neutral proteases, oxygen-derived reactive metabolites and cytokines. These products bring about tissue destruction, neovascularisation and fibrosis.

Other chronic inflammatory cells include lymphocytes, plasma cells, eosinophils and mast cells. In chronic inflammation, lymphocytes and macrophages influence each other and release mediators of inflammation.

2. TISSUE DESTRUCTION OR NECROSIS Tissue destruction and necrosis are central features of most forms of chronic inflammatory lesions. This is brought about by activated macrophages which release a variety of biologically active substances e.g. protease, elastase, collagenase, lipase, reactive oxygen radicals, cytokines (IL-1, IL-8, TNF-α), nitric oxide, angiogenesis growth factor etc.

3. PROLIFERATIVE CHANGES As a result of necrosis, proliferation of small blood vessels and fibroblasts is stimulated resulting in formation of inflammatory granulation tissue. Eventually, healing by fibrosis and collagen laying takes place.

SYSTEMIC EFFECTS OF CHRONIC INFLAMMATION

Chronic inflammation is associated with the following systemic features:

1. Fever Invariably there is mild fever, often with loss of weight and weakness.

2. Anaemia As discussed in Chapter 22, chronic inflammation is accompanied by anaemia of varying degree.

3. Leucocytosis As in acute inflammation, chronic inflammation also has leucocytosis but generally there is relative lymphocytosis in these cases.

4. ESR ESR is elevated in all cases of chronic inflammation.

5. Amyloidosis Long-term cases of chronic suppurative inflammation may develop secondary systemic (AA) amyloidosis.

TYPES OF CHRONIC INFLAMMATION

Conventionally, chronic inflammation is subdivided into 2 types:

1. Chronic non-specific inflammation When the irritant substance produces a non-specific chronic inflammatory reaction with formation of granulation tissue and healing by fibrosis, it is called chronic non-specific inflammation e.g. chronic osteomyelitis, chronic ulcer, lung abscess. A variant of this type of chronic inflammatory response is chronic suppurative inflammation in which infiltration by polymorphs and abscess formation (features seen in acute inflammation) are additional features e.g. actinomycosis.

2. **Chronic granulomatous inflammation** In this, the injurious agent causes a characteristic histologic tissue response by formation of granulomas e.g. tuberculosis, leprosy, syphilis, actinomycosis, sarcoidosis etc.

| GIST BOX 11.1 | Chronic Inflammation—General Aspects |

❖ Chronic inflammation may result either following acute inflammation or after its recurrent attacks, or may start afresh.
❖ A few general features of chronic inflammation are infiltration by mononuclear cells, tissue destruction and proliferation of blood vessels and fibroblasts.
❖ Chronic inflammation may produce systemic features such as fever, anaemia, leucocytosis, raised ESR and development of secondary amyloidosis in longstanding cases.
❖ Chronic inflammation is of 2 main types: non-specific and granulomatous type.

GRANULOMATOUS INFLAMMATION

Granuloma is defined as a circumscribed, tiny lesion, about 1 mm in diameter, composed predominantly of collection of modified macrophages called epithelioid cells, and rimmed at the periphery by lymphoid cells. The word *'granuloma'* is derived from *granule* meaning circumscribed granule-like lesion, and *-oma* which is a suffix commonly used for true tumours but here it indicates a localised inflammatory mass or collection of macrophages.

PATHOGENESIS OF GRANULOMA Formation of granuloma is a type IV granulomatous hypersensitivity reaction (page 215). It is a protective defense reaction by the host but eventually causes tissue destruction because of persistence of the poorly digestible antigen e.g. *Mycobacterium tuberculosis, M. leprae,* suture material, particles of talc etc.

The sequence in evolution of granuloma is schematically shown in **Fig. 11.1** and is briefly outlined below:

1. **Engulfment by macrophages** Macrophages and monocytes engulf the antigen and try to destroy it. But since the antigen is poorly degradable, these cells fail to digest and degrade the antigen, and instead undergo morphologic changes to transform into epithelioid cells.

2. **CD4+ T cells** Macrophages, being antigen-presenting cells, having failed to deal with the antigen, present it to CD4+ T lymphocytes. These lymphocytes get activated and elaborate lymphokines (IL-1, IL-2, interferon-γ, TNF-α).

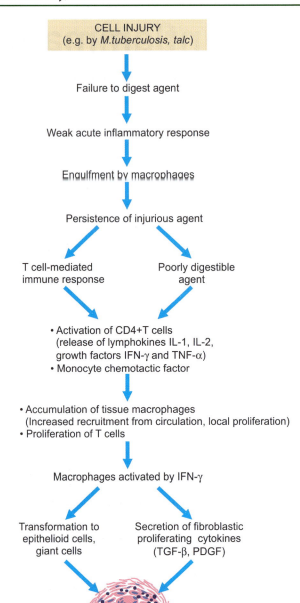

Figure 11.1 ▶ Mechanism of evolution of a granuloma (IL=interleukin; IFN= interferon; TNF = tumour necrosis factor).

3. **Cytokines** Various cytokines formed by activated CD4+ T cells and also by activated macrophages perform the following roles:

i) *IL-1 and IL-2* stimulate proliferation of more T cells.

ii) *Interferon-γ* activates macrophages.

iii) TNF-α promotes fibroblast proliferation and activates endothelium to secrete prostaglandins which have a role in vascular response in inflammation.

iv) Growth factors (transforming growth factor-β, platelet-derived growth factor) elaborated by activated macrophages stimulate fibroblast growth.

Thus, a granuloma is formed having macrophages modified as epithelioid cells in the centre, with some interspersed multinucleate giant cells, surrounded peripherally by lymphocytes (mainly T cells), and healing by fibroblasts or collagen depending upon the age of granuloma.

COMPOSITION OF GRANULOMA In general, a granuloma has the following structural composition:

1. Epithelioid cells These are so called because of their epithelial cell-like appearance. They are modified macrophages/histiocytes which are somewhat elongated cells having slipper-shaped nucleus. The nuclear chromatin of these cells is vesicular and lightly-staining, while the cytoplasm is abundant, pale-staining with hazy outlines so that the cell membrane of adjacent epithelioid cells is closely apposed. Epithelioid cells are weakly phagocytic.

2. Multinucleate giant cells Multinucleate giant cells are formed by fusion of adjacent epithelioid cells and may have 20 or more nuclei. These nuclei may be arranged at the periphery like the horseshoe or as a ring, or may be clustered at the two poles (Langhans' giant cells), or they may be present centrally (foreign body giant cells). The former are commonly seen in tuberculosis while the latter are common in foreign body tissue reactions. Like epithelioid cells, these giant cells are weakly phagocytic but produce secretory products which help in removing the invading agents.

3. Lymphoid cells As a cell-mediated immune reaction to antigen, the host response by lymphocytes is integral to composition of a granuloma. Plasma cells indicative of accelerated humoral immune response are present in some types of granulomas.

4. Necrosis Necrosis may be a feature of some granulomatous conditions e.g. central caseation necrosis in tuberculosis, so called, because of its dry cheese-like appearance.

5. Fibrosis Fibrosis is a feature of healing by proliferating fibroblasts at the periphery of granuloma.

The classical example of granulomatous inflammation is the tissue response to tubercle bacilli which is called *tubercle* seen in tuberculosis (page 132). A fully-developed tubercle is about 1 mm in diameter with central area of caseation necrosis, surrounded by epithelioid cells and one to several multinucleated giant cells (commonly Langhans' type), surrounded at the periphery by lymphocytes and bounded by fibroblasts and fibrous tissue (Fig. 11.2).

Major differences between acute and chronic inflammation are summed up in Table 11.1.

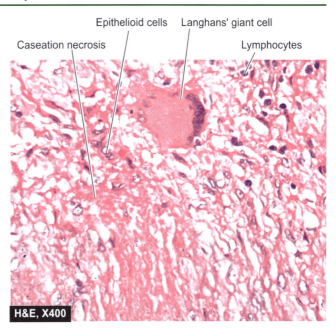

Figure 11.2 ▶ Morphology of a tubercle. There is central caseation necrosis, surrounded by elongated epithelioid cells having characteristic slipper-shaped nuclei, with interspersed Langhans' giant cells. Periphery shows lymphocytes.

GIST BOX 11.2 Chronic Granulomatous Inflammation—General Aspects

❖ A granuloma is a circumscribed collection of epithelioid cells surrounded at the periphery by lymphocytes and may contain a few multinucleate giant cells.
❖ A granuloma is formed as a host inflammatory response to a poorly degradable agent by eliciting delayed type hypersensitivity (type IV reaction).
❖ Formation of a granuloma involves engulfment of the invading agent by the macrophages, failure to degrade the antigen, morphologic change of macrophages to epithelioid cells, and incoming CD4+ T cells which elaborate various cytokines which contribute to proliferation and activation of cells.
❖ A granuloma may have necrosis in the centre and eventually heals by fibrosis.
❖ Granulomatous diseases include infections (bacterial, fungal, parasitic) autoimmune inflammatory, and reaction to foreign bodies.

EXAMPLES OF GRANULOMATOUS INFLAMMATION

Granulomatous inflammation is typical of reaction to poorly digestible agents elicited by tuberculosis, leprosy, fungal infections, schistosomiasis, foreign particles etc. A comprehensive list of important examples of granulomatous conditions, their etiologic agents and salient features, is given

Section II: Inflammation and Healing, Immunity and Hypersensitivity, Infections and Infestations

Table 11.1 Major differences between acute and chronic inflammation.

FEATURE	ACUTE INFLAMMATION	CHRONIC INFLAMMATION
1. Onset and Duration	• Within short time • Lasts for short duration	• After delay • Lasts longer
2. Cardinal Signs	Invariably present	Generally imperceptible
3. Pathogenesis	• Vascular events: haemodynamic changes, increased vascular permeability • Cellular events: exudation of leucocytes, Phagocytosis • Role of chemical mediators and regulators	• Following acute inflammation • Recurrent attacks of acute inflammation • Chronic inflammation from beginning
4. Main Inflammatory Cells	• Neutrophils • Eosinophils • Lymphomononuclear cells (late) • Pus cells	• Lymphocytes • Plasma cells • Monocytes/macrophages (epithelioid cells in granulomas) • Giant cells (foreign body, Langhans')
5. Plasma Exudation	Present	May or may not be present
6. Systemic Effects	• Fever: high grade • Leucocytosis (neutropphilic, eosinophilic) • Lymphadenitis-lymphangiitis • Septic shock (in severe acute infection)	• Fever: mild • Leucocytosis (lymphocytic, monocytic) • Lymphadenitis-lymphangiitis • Raised ESR • Anaemia • Amyloidosis (in long-term cases)
7. Main Morphology	• Abscesses (suppuration) • Ulcers • Through blood (Bacteraemia, septicaemia, pyaemia)	• Chronic non-specific inflammation (infectious, others) • Granulomatous inflammation (tuberculosis, leprosy, sarcoidosis, syphilis, actinomycosis, Crohn's disease etc)
8. Fate	• Resolution • Healing (regeneration, fibrosis) • Chronicity	• Resolution • Healing (regeneration, fibrosis) • Dystrophic calcification
9. Common Examples	Pyogenic abscess, cellulitis, bacterial pneumonia, pyaemia	Granulation tissue, granulomatous inflammation (tuberculosis, leprosy etc), chronic osteomyelitis

in Table 11.2. The principal examples (marked with asterisk in the table) are discussed below while a few others appear in relevant Chapters later.

TUBERCULOSIS

Tissue response in tuberculosis represents classical example of chronic granulomatous inflammation in humans.

INCIDENCE In spite of great advances in chemotherapy and immunology, tuberculosis still continues to be a major public health problem in the entire world, more common in developing countries of Asia, Africa and Latin America. In fact, half the total number of cases in the world are shared by India and China. Other factors contributing to higher incidence of tuberculosis are malnutrition, inadequate medical care, poverty, crowding, chronic debilitating conditions like uncontrolled diabetes, alcoholism and immunocompromised states. In the Western countries, there has been a resurgence of tuberculosis due to HIV-AIDS. Observations in different populations suggest that besides these factors, genetic factors also play a key role in innate resistance to infection with *M. tuberculosis* and in the development of disease, which is responsible for differing degree of susceptibility to tuberculosis. However, the exact incidence of disease cannot be determined as all patients infected with *M. tuberculosis* may not develop the clinical disease and many cases remain reactive to tuberculin without developing symptomatic disease.

HIV-ASSOCIATED TUBERCULOSIS HIV-infected individuals have very high incidence of tuberculosis all over the world. Vice-versa, rate of HIV infection in patients of tuberculosis is very high. Moreover, HIV-infected individual on acquiring infection with tubercle bacilli develops active disease rapidly (within a few weeks) rather than after months or years. Pulmonary tuberculosis in HIV presents in typical manner. However, it is more often sputum smear-negative but often culture-positive. Extra-pulmonary tuberculosis is more common in HIV disease and manifests commonly by involving lymph nodes, pleura, pericardium, and tuberculous meningitis. Infection with *M. avium-intracellulare* (avian or bird strain) is common in patients with HIV/AIDS.

Table 11.2 Principal granulomatous conditions.

	CONDITIONS	ETIOLOGIC AGENT	SPECIAL CHARACTERISTICS
I.	**BACTERIAL**		
1.	Tuberculosis*	Mycobacterium tuberculosis	Tuberculous granulomas with central caseation necrosis; acid-fast bacilli.
2.	Leprosy*	Mycobacterium leprae	Foamy histiocytes with acid-fast bacilli (lepromatous); epithelioid cell granulomas (tuberculoid).
3.	Syphilis*	Treponema pallidum	Gummas composed of histiocytes; plasma cell infiltration; central necrosis.
4.	Granuloma inguinale (Donovanosis)	C. donovani (Donovan body)	Anal and genital lesions; macrophages and neutrophils show Donovan bodies.
5.	Brucellosis (Mediterranean fever)	Brucella abortus	Dairy infection to humans; enlarged reticuloendothelial organs (lymph nodes, spleen, bone marrow); non-specific granulomas.
6.	Cat scratch disease	Bartonella henselae	Lymphadenitis; reticuloendothelial hyperplasia; granulomas with central necrosis and neutrophils.
7.	Tularaemia (Rabbit fever)	Francisella (Pasteurella) tularensis	Necrosis and suppuration (acute); tubercles hard or with minute central necrosis (chronic).
8.	Glanders	Actinobacillus mallei	Infection from horses and mules; subcutaneous lesions and lymphadenitis; infective granulomas.
II.	**FUNGAL**		
1.	Actinomycosis* (bacterial)	Actinomycetes israelii	Cervicofacial, abdominal and thoracic lesions; granulomas and abscesses with draining sinuses; sulphur granules.
2.	Blastomycosis	Blastomyces dermatitidis	Cutaneous, systemic and lung lesions; suppuration; ulceration and granulomas.
3.	Cryptococcosis	Cryptococcus neoformans	Meninges, lungs and systemic distribution; organism yeast-like with clear capsule.
4.	Coccidioidomycosis	Coccidioides immitis	Meninges, lungs and systemic distribution; granulomas and abscesses; organism cyst containing endospores.
III.	**PARASITIC**		
	Schistosomiasis (Bilharziasis)	Schistosoma mansoni, haematobium, japonicum	Eggs and granulomas in gut, liver, lung; schistosome pigment; eosinophils in blood and tissue.
IV.	**MISCELLANEOUS**		
1.	Sarcoidosis*	Unknown	Non-caseating granulomas (hard tubercles); asteroid and Schaumann bodies in giant cells.
2.	Crohn's disease (Regional enteritis)	Unknown ? Bacteria, ?? Viruses	Transmural chronic inflammatory infiltrates; non-caseating sarcoid-like granulomas.
3.	Silicosis	Silica dust	Lung lesions, fibrocollagenous nodules.
4.	Berylliosis	Metallic beryllium	Sarcoid-like granulomas in lungs; fibrosis; inclusions in giant cells (asteroids, Schaumann bodies, crystals).
5.	Foreign body granulomas	Talc, suture, oils, wood splinter etc.	Non-caseating granulomas with foreign body giant cells; demonstration of foreign body.

*Diseases discussed in this chapter.

CAUSATIVE ORGANISM Tubercle bacillus or Koch's bacillus (named after discovery of the organism by Robert Koch in 1882) called *Mycobacterium tuberculosis* causes tuberculosis in the lungs and other tissues of the human body. The organism is a strict aerobe and thrives best in tissues with high oxygen tension such as in the apex of the lung.

Out of various pathogenic strains for human disease included in *Mycobacterium tuberculosis* complex, currently the most common is *M. tuberculosis hominis* (human strain), while *M. tuberculosis bovis* (bovine strain) used to be common pathogen to human beings during the era of consumption of unpasteurised milk but presently constitutes a small number of human cases. Other less common strains included in the complex are *M. africanum* (isolated from patients from parts of Africa), *M. microti*, *M. pinnipedii* and *M. canettii*. A non-pathogenic strain, *M. smegmatis*, is found in the smegma and as contaminant in the urine of both men and women.

M. tuberculosis hominis is a slender rod-like bacillus, 0.5 µm by 3 µm, is neutral on Gram staining, and can be demonstrated by the following methods:

1. *Acid fast (Ziehl-Neelsen) staining* The acid fastness of the tubercle bacilli is due to mycolic acids, cross-linked fatty acids and other lipids in the cell wall of the organism making it impermeable to the usual stains. It takes up stain by heated carbol fuchsin and resists decolourisation by acids and alcohols (acid fast and alcohol fast) and can be decoloured by 20% sulphuric acid (compared to 5% sulphuric acid for decolourisation for *M. leprae* which are less acid fast) **(Fig. 11.3)**. However, false positive AFB staining may occur due to *Nocardia*, *Rhodococcus*, *Legionella*, and some protozoa such as *Isospora* and *Cryptosporidium*.

2. *Fluorescent methods* This method is quite reliable and employs use of fluorescent dyes such as auramine and rhodamine. Mycobacteria also show autofluorescence which is quite an economical method of demonstration of the organism.

3. *Culture* of the organism from sputum or from any other material in Lowenstein-Jensen (L.J.) medium by conventional method has high specficity but takes a long time (8-12 weeks). Currently, rapid methods (e.g. Bactec culture, high pressure liquid chromatography or HPLC of mycolic acids) are also available reducing the bacteriologic confirmation to 2-3 weeks.

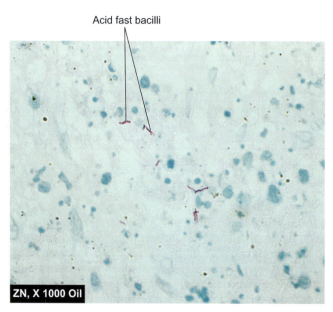

Figure 11.3 ▶ Tuberculosis of the lymph nodes showing presence of acid-fast bacilli in Ziehl-Neelsen staining.

4. *Guinea pig inoculation* method by subcutaneous injection of the organisms is rarely used now.

5. *Molecular methods* such as nucleic acid amplification (e.g. PCR) are the most useful methods for species confirmation and for distinction between *M. tuberculosis* and non-tuberculous mycobacteria because the treatment between the two is quite different.

6. *Immunohistochemical stain* with anti-MBP 64 antibody stain can be used to demonstrate the organism.

ATYPICAL MYCOBACTERIA (NON-TUBERCULOUS MYCOBACTERIA) The term atypical mycobacteria or non-tuberculous mycobacteria (NTM) is used for mycobacterial species other than *M. tuberculosis* complex and *M. leprae*. NTM are widely distributed in the environment and are, therefore, also called as *environmental mycobacteria*. They too are acid fast. Occasionally, human tuberculosis may be caused by NTM which are non-pathogenic to guinea pigs and resistant to usual anti-tubercular drugs.

Conventionally, NTM are classified on the basis of colour of colony produced in culture and the speed of growth in media:

Rapid growers These organisms grow fast on solid media (within 7 days) but are less pathogenic than others. Examples include *M. abscessus*, *M. fortuitum*, *M. chelonae*.

Slow growers These species grow mycobacteria on solid media (in 2-3 weeks). Based on the colour of colony formed, they are further divided into the following:

Photochromogens: These organisms produce yellow pigment in the culture grown in light.

Scotochromogens: Pigment is produced, whether the growth is in light or in dark.

Non-chromogens: No pigment is produced by the bacilli and the organism is closely related to avium bacillus.

The examples of slow growers are *M. avium-intracellulare*, *M. kansasii*, *M. ulcerans* and *M. fortuitum*.

The infection by NTM is acquired directly from the environment, unlike person-to-person transmission of classical tuberculosis. They produce human disease, *atypical mycobacteriosis,* similar to tuberculosis but are much less virulent. The lesions produced may be granulomas, nodular collection of foamy cells, or acute inflammation.

Five patterns of the disease are recognised:
i) Pulmonary disease produced by *M. kansasii* or *M. avium-intracellulare*.
ii) Lymphadenitis caused by *M. avium-intracellulare* or *M. scrofulaceum*.
iii) Ulcerated skin lesions produced by *M. ulcerans* or *M. marinum*.
iv) Abscesses caused by *M.fortuitum* or *M. chelonae*.
v) Bacteraemias by *M. avium-intracellulare* as seen in immunosuppressed patients of AIDS.

MODE OF TRANSMISSION Human beings acquire infection with tubercle bacilli by one of the following routes:

1. *Inhalation* of organisms present in fresh cough droplets or in dried sputum from an open case of pulmonary tuberculosis.

2. *Ingestion* of the organisms leads to development of tonsillar or intestinal tuberculosis. This mode of infection of human tubercle bacilli is from self-swallowing of infected sputum of an open case of pulmonary tuberculosis, or ingestion of bovine tubercle bacilli from milk of diseased cows.

3. *Inoculation* of the organisms into the skin may rarely occur from infected postmortem tissue.

4. *Transplacental route* results in development of congenital tuberculosis in foetus from infected mother and is a rare mode of transmission.

SPREAD OF TUBERCULOSIS The disease spreads in the body by various routes:

1. Local spread This takes place by macrophages carrying the bacilli into the surrounding tissues.

2. Lymphatic spread Tuberculosis is primarily an infection of lymphoid tissues. The bacilli may pass into lymphoid follicles of pharynx, bronchi, intestines or regional lymph nodes resulting in regional tuberculous lymphadenitis which is typical of childhood infections. Primary complex is primary focus with lymphangitis and lymphadenitis.

3. Haematogenous spread This occurs either as a result of tuberculous bacillaemia because of the drainage of lymphatics into the venous system or due to caseous material escaping through ulcerated wall of a vein. This produces millet seed-sized lesions in different organs of the body like lungs, liver, kidneys, bones and other tissues and is known as miliary tuberculosis.

4. By the natural passages Infection may spread from:
i) lung lesions into pleura (tuberculous pleurisy);
ii) transbronchial spread into the adjacent lung segments;
iii) tuberculous salpingitis into peritoneal cavity (tuberculous peritonitis);
iv) infected sputum into larynx (tuberculous laryngitis);
v) swallowing of infected sputum (ileocaecal tuberculosis); and
vi) renal lesions into ureter and down to trigone of bladder.

PATHOGENESIS (HYPERSENSITIVITY AND IMMUNITY)
Hypersensitivity or allergy, and immunity or resistance, play a major role in the development of lesions in tuberculosis. Tubercle bacilli as such do not produce any toxins. Tissue changes seen in tuberculosis are not the result of any exotoxin or endotoxin but are instead the result of host response to the organism which is by way of development of delayed type hypersensitivity (or type IV hypersensitivity) and immunity. Both these host responses develop as a consequence of several lipids present in the microorganism as under:

1. Mycosides such as 'cord factor' which are essential for growth and virulence of the organism in the animals.

2. Glycolipids present in the mycobacterial cell wall like 'Wax-D' which acts as an adjuvant acting along with tuberculoprotein.

Hypersensitivity and immunity are closely related and are initiated through CD4+ T lymphocytes sensitised against specific antigens in tuberculin (i.e. cell-mediated immunity). As a result of this sensitisation, lymphokines are released from T cells which induce increased microbicidal activity of the macrophages.

It has been known since the time of Robert Koch that the tissue reaction to tubercle bacilli is different in healthy animal not previously infected (primary infection) from an animal who is previously infected (secondary infection), the best experiment being on guinea pig because this animal does not possess any natural resistance to tubercle bacilli.

1. In the primary infection, intradermal injection of tubercle bacilli into the skin of a healthy guinea pig evokes no visible reaction for 10-14 days. After this period, a nodule develops at the inoculation site which subsequently ulcerates and heals poorly as the guinea pig, unlike human beings, does not possess any natural resistance. The regional lymph nodes also develop tubercles. This process is a manifestation of delayed type hypersensitivity (type IV reaction) and is comparable to primary tuberculosis in children although healing invariably occurs in children.

2. In the secondary infection, the sequence of changes is different. When the tubercle bacilli are injected into the skin of the guinea pig who has been previously infected with tuberculosis 4-6 weeks earlier, the sequence and duration of development of lesions is different. In 1-2 days, the site of inoculation is indurated and dark, attaining a diameter of about 1 cm. The skin lesion ulcerates which heals quickly and the regional lymph nodes are not affected. This is called *Koch's phenomenon* and is indicative of hypersensitivity and immunity in the host which is guinea pig in this case.

Similar type of changes can be produced if injection of live tubercle bacilli is replaced with old tuberculin (OT) which is used in skin tests in human beings.

Immunisation against tuberculosis Protective immunisation against tuberculosis is induced by injection of attenuated strains of bovine type of tubercle bacilli, *Bacille Calmette-Guérin* (BCG). Cell-mediated immunity with consequent delayed hypersensitivity reaction develops with healing of the lesion, but the cell-mediated immunity persists, rendering the host tuberculin-positive and hence immune. While BCG vaccination is routinely done at birth in countries with high prevalence of tuberculosis, it has never been recommended in US for general use due to lower prevalence of tuberculosis and the impact of the test on interpretation of skin test.

Tuberculin (Mantoux) skin test (TST) This test is done by intradermal injection of 0.1 ml of tuberculoprotein, purified protein derivative (PPD). Delayed type of hypersensitivity develops in individuals who are having or have been previously infected with tuberculous infection which is identified as an indurated area of more than 15 mm in 72 hours; reaction larger than 15 mm is unlikely to be due to previous BCG vaccination. Patients having disseminated tuberculosis may show negative test due to release of large amount of tuberculoproteins from the endogenous lesions masking the hypersensitivity test. A positive test is indicative of cell-mediated hypersensitivity to tubercular antigens but does not distinguish between infection and disease.

The test may be *false positive* in atypical mycobacterial infection and previous BCG vaccination, *false negative* in cutaneous anergy (due to weakened immune system), sarcoidosis, some viral infections, Hodgkin's disease, recent tuberculous (8-10 weeks of exposure) infection and fulminant tuberculosis.

EVOLUTION OF TUBERCLE The sequence of events which takes place when tubercle bacilli are introduced into the tissue culminating in development of a tubercle, are as under (Fig. 11.4):

1. When the tubercle bacilli are injected intravenously into the guinea pig, the bacilli are lodged in pulmonary capillaries where an *initial response of neutrophils* is evoked which are rapidly destroyed by the organisms. However, in general, 2 types of cells are essential for a response to tubercle bacilli: *macrophages and T cells.*

2. After about 12 hours, there is *progressive infiltration by macrophages.* This is due to coating of tubercle bacilli with serum complement factors C2a and C3b which act as opsonins and attract the macrophages. Macrophages dominate the picture throughout the remaining life of the lesions. If the tubercle bacilli are, however, inhaled into the lung alveoli, macrophages predominate the picture from the beginning.

3. The macrophages start *phagocytosing* the tubercle bacilli and either try to kill the bacteria or die away themselves. In the latter case, there is production of nitric oxide radicals having antimycobacterial properties and also cause increased synthesis of cytokines (TNF-α and IL-1) resulting in proliferation of macrophages locally as well as increased recruitment from blood monocytes.

4. As a part of body's immune response, T and B cells are activated. Activated CD4+T cells elaborate cytokines, IFN-γ and IL-2. These cytokines and their regulators determine the host's response by infiltrating macrophages-monocytes and develop the cell-mediated *delayed type hypersensitivity reaction.* Qualitative and quantitative defects of CD4+ cells in HIV explain their poor ability to deal with tubercle bacilli and hence their proneness to disseminated tuberculosis.

5. B cells form antibodies but *humoral immunity* plays little role in body's defense against tubercle bacilli. However, recent evidence suggests the role of LAM (lipoarabinomannan) antibodies in preventing dissemination of tuberculosis in children.

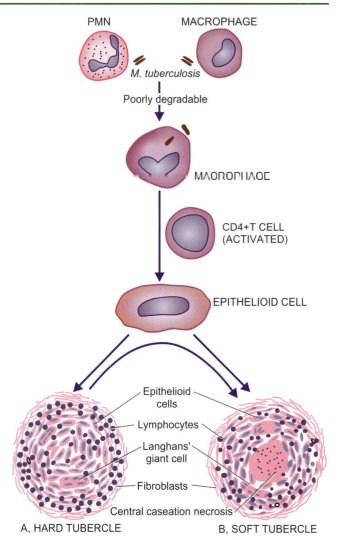

Figure 11.4 ▶ Schematic evolution of tubercle. In fully formed granuloma, the centre is composed of granular caseation necrosis, surrounded by epithelioid cells and Langhans' giant cells and peripheral rim of lymphocytes bounded by fibroblasts.

6. In 2-3 days, the macrophages undergo structural changes as a result of immune mechanisms—the cytoplasm becomes pale and eosinophilic and their nuclei become elongated and vesicular. These modified macrophages resemble epithelial cells and are called *epithelioid cells* (i.e. epithelial like).

7. The epithelioid cells in time aggregate into tight clusters or *granulomas.* Release of cytokines in response to sensitised CD4+T cells and some constituents of mycobacterial cell wall play a role in formation of granuloma.

8. Some macrophages, unable to destroy tubercle bacilli, fuse together and form *multinucleated giant cells.* These giant cells may be Langhans' type having peripherally arranged nuclei in the form of horseshoe or ring, or clustered at the two poles of the giant cell; or they may be foreign body type having centrally placed nuclei.

9. Around the mass or cluster of epithelioid cells and a few giant cells, a zone of lymphocytes and plasma cells is formed which is further surrounded by fibroblasts. The lesion at this stage is called *hard tubercle* due to absence of central necrosis.

10. Within 10-14 days, the centre of the cellular mass begins to undergo caseation necrosis, characterised by cheesy appearance and high lipid content. This stage is called *soft tubercle* which is the hallmark of tuberculous lesions. The development of caseation necrosis is possibly due to interaction of mycobacteria with activated T cells (CD4+ helper T cells via IFN-γ and CD8+ suppressor T cells directly) as well as by direct toxicity of mycobacteria on macrophages. *Microscopically*, caseation necrosis is structureless, eosinophilic and granular material with nuclear debris.

11. The soft tubercle which is a fully-developed granuloma with caseous centre does not favour rapid proliferation of tubercle bacilli. *Acid-fast bacilli* are difficult to find in these lesions and may be demonstrated at the margins of recent necrotic foci and in the walls of the cavities.

The **fate of a granuloma** is variable:

i) The caseous material may undergo liquefaction and extend into surrounding soft tissues, discharging the contents on the surface. This is called *cold abscess* although there are no pus cells in it.

ii) In tuberculosis of tissues like bones, joints, lymph nodes and epididymis, sinuses are formed and the *sinus tracts* are lined by tuberculous granulation tissue.

iii) The adjacent granulomas may *coalesce* together enlarging the lesion which is surrounded by progressive fibrosis.

iv) In the granuloma enclosed by fibrous tissue, calcium salts may get deposited in the caseous material *(dystrophic calcification)* and sometimes the lesion may even get ossified over the years.

TYPES OF TUBERCULOSIS

Lung is the main organ affected in tuberculosis while amongst the extra-pulmonary sites, lymph node involvement is most common. Depending upon the type of tissue response and age, the infection with tubercle bacilli is of 2 main types:

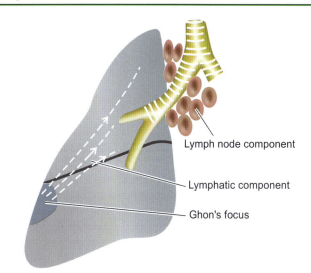

Figure 11.5 ▶ The primary complex is composed of 3 components: Ghon's focus, draining lymphatics, and hilar lymph nodes.

primary and secondary tuberculosis; their salient differences are given in Table 11.3.

A. Primary Tuberculosis

The infection of an individual who has not been previously infected or immunised is called *primary tuberculosis* or *Ghon's complex* or *childhood tuberculosis*.

Primary complex or Ghon's complex is the lesion produced in the tissue of portal of entry with foci in the draining lymphatic vessels and lymph nodes. The most commonly involved tissues for primary complex are lungs and hilar lymph nodes. Other tissues which may show primary complex are tonsils and cervical lymph nodes, and in the case of ingested bacilli the lesions may be found in small intestine and mesenteric lymph nodes.

The incidence of disseminated form of progressive primary tuberculosis is particularly high in immunocompromised host e.g. in patients of AIDS.

Primary complex or Ghon's complex in lungs consists of 3 components (Fig. 11.5):

Table 11.3	Differences between primary and secondary tuberculosis.	
FEATURE	PRIMARY TUBERCULOSIS	SECONDARY TUBERCULOSIS
1. Age	Mostly children	Children and adults
2. Organs	Almost exclusive in lungs	Lungs, lymph nodes, other organs (genitourinary tract, bones, meninges, brain, eye, liver, spleen, intestines, skin etc.
3. Lesions	Ghon's complex (lung lesion as consolidation, lymphatic vessel and hilar lymph nodes lesions)	Tubercles, extensive caseation, miliary lesions, cavitation, fibrocaseous lesions, caseous pneumonia, pleurisy/effusion
4. Fate	Healing by fibrosis, calcification, may get reactivated in weakened immunity	Consolidation, parenchymal nodules, thickened pleura, amyloidosis, reactivation of healed lesion in impaired immunity and AIDS

1. **Pulmonary component** Lesion in the lung is the primary focus or Ghon's focus. It is 1-2 cm solitary area of tuberculous pneumonia located peripherally under a patch of pleurisy, in any part of the lung but more often in subpleural focus in the upper part of lower lobe.

2. **Lymphatic vessel component** The lymphatics draining the lung lesion contain phagocytes containing bacilli and may develop beaded, miliary tubercles along the path of hilar lymph nodes.

3. **Lymph node component** This consists of enlarged hilar and tracheo-bronchial lymph nodes in the area drained. The affected lymph nodes are matted and show caseation necrosis. Nodal lesions are potential source of re-infection later (Fig. 11.6, A).

> *Microscopically,* the lesions of primary tuberculosis have the following features (Fig. 11.6, B):
> i) Tuberculous granulomas with peripheral fibrosis.
> ii) Extensive caseation necrosis in the centers of granulomas.
> iii) Old lesions have fibrosis and calcification.

In the case of primary tuberculosis of the alimentary tract due to ingestion of tubercle bacilli, a small primary focus is seen in the intestine with enlarged mesenteric lymph nodes producing *tabes mesenterica*. The enlarged and caseous mesenteric lymph nodes may rupture into peritoneal cavity and cause tuberculous peritonitis.

FATE OF PRIMARY TUBERCULOSIS Primary complex may have one of the following sequelae (Fig. 11.7):

1. The lesions of primary tuberculosis of the lung commonly do not progress but instead heal by *fibrosis,* and in time undergo *calcification* and even *ossification.*

2. In some cases, the primary focus in the lung continues to grow and the caseous material is disseminated through bronchi to the other parts of the same lung or the opposite lung. This is called *progressive primary tuberculosis.*

3. At times, bacilli may enter the circulation through erosion in a blood vessel and spread by haematogenous route to other tissues and organs. This is called *primary miliary tuberculosis* and the lesions may be seen in organs like the liver, spleen, kidney, brain and bone marrow.

4. In certain circumstances like in lowered resistance and increased hypersensitivity of the host, the healed lesions of primary tuberculosis may get reactivated. The bacilli lying dormant in acellular caseous material or healed lesion are activated and cause *progressive secondary tuberculosis.* It affects children more commonly but immunocompromised adults may also develop this kind of progression.

B. Secondary Tuberculosis

The infection of an individual who has been previously infected or sensitised is called *secondary,* or *post-primary* or *reinfection,* or *chronic tuberculosis.*

The infection may occur from (Fig. 11.8):
◈ *endogenous source* such as reactivation of dormant primary complex; or
◈ *exogenous source* such as fresh dose of reinfection by the tubercle bacilli.

Secondary tuberculosis occurs most commonly in lungs. Other sites and tissues which can be involved are lymph nodes, tonsils, pharynx, larynx, small intestine and skin. Secondary tuberculosis of lungs and intestines is discussed below.

Secondary Pulmonary Tuberculosis

The lesions in secondary pulmonary tuberculosis usually begin as 1-2 cm apical area of consolidation of the lung,

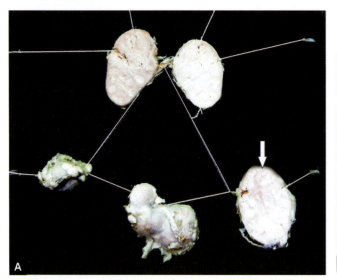
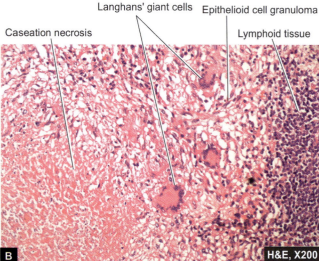

Figure 11.6 ▶ Caseating granulomatous lymphadenitis. A, Cut section of matted mass of lymph nodes shows merging capsules and large areas of caseation necrosis (arrow). B, Caseating epithelioid cell granulomas with a few Langhans' giant cells in the cortex of lymph node.

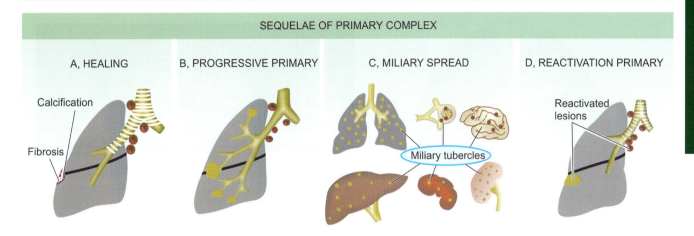

Figure 11.7 ▶ Sequelae of primary complex. A, Healing by fibrosis and calcification. B, Progressive primary tuberculosis spreading to the other areas of the same lung or opposite lung. C, Miliary spread to lungs, liver, spleen, kidneys and brain. D, Progressive secondary pulmonary tuberculosis from reactivation of dormant primary complex.

which, in time, may develop a small area of central caseation necrosis and peripheral fibrosis. It occurs by lympho-haematogenous spread of infection from primary complex to the apex of the affected lung where the oxygen tension is high and favourable for growth of aerobic tubercle bacilli. *Microscopically*, the appearance is typical of tuberculous granulomas with caseation necrosis.

Patients with HIV infection previously exposed to tuberculous infection have particularly high incidence of reactivation of primary tuberculosis. The pattern of lesions in such cases is similar to that of primary tuberculosis i.e. with involvement of hilar lymph nodes rather than cavitary and apical lesions in the lung. In addition, infection with *M. avium-intracellulare* occurs more frequently in cases of AIDS.

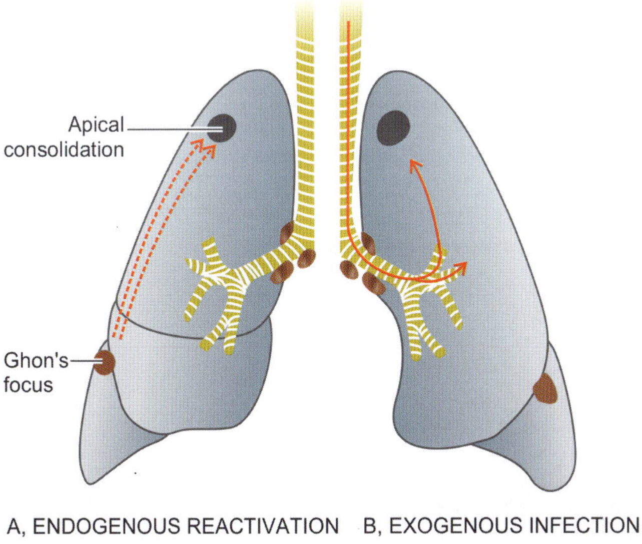

FATE OF SECONDARY PULMONARY TUBERCULOSIS
The subapical lesions in lungs can have the following course:

1. The lesions may *heal* with fibrous scarring and calcification.

2. The lesions may *coalesce* together to form larger area of tuberculous pneumonia and produce progressive secondary pulmonary tuberculosis with the following pulmonary and extrapulmonary involvements:
i) Fibrocaseous tuberculosis
ii) Tuberculous caseous pneumonia
iii) Miliary tuberculosis
iv) Tuberculous empyema

FIBROCASEOUS TUBERCULOSIS The original area of tuberculous pneumonia undergoes peripheral healing and massive central caseation necrosis which may:

❖ either break into a bronchus from a cavity *(cavitary or open fibrocaseous tuberculosis)*; or

❖ remain, as a soft caseous lesion without drainage into a bronchus or bronchiole to produce a non-cavitary lesion *(chronic fibrocaseous tuberculosis)*.

The cavity provides favourable environment for proliferation of tubercle bacilli due to high oxygen tension. The cavity may communicate with bronchial tree and becomes the source of spread of infection *('open tuberculosis')*. The open case of secondary tuberculosis may implant tuberculous lesion on the mucosal lining of air passages producing *endobronchial and endotracheal tuberculosis*. Ingestion of sputum containing tubercle bacilli from endogenous pulmonary lesions may produce *laryngeal and intestinal tuberculosis*.

Figure 11.8 ▶ Progressive secondary tuberculosis. A, Endogenous infection from reactivation of dormant primary complex. B, Exogenous infection from fresh dose of tubercle bacilli.

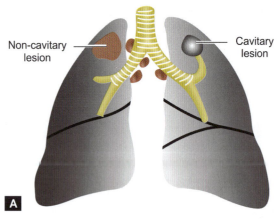 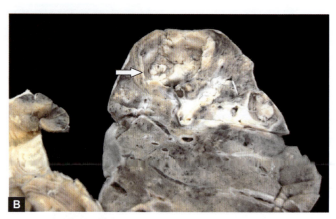

Figure 11.9 ▶ Fibrocaseous tuberculosis. A, Non-cavitary (chronic) fibrocaseous tuberculosis (left) and cavitary/open fibrocaseous tuberculosis (right). B, Chronic fibrocaseous tuberculosis lung. Sectioned surface shows a cavity in the apex of the lung (arrow). There is consolidation of lung parenchyma surrounding the cavity.

Grossly, tuberculous cavity is spherical with thick fibrous wall, lined by yellowish, caseous, necrotic material and the lumen is traversed by thrombosed blood vessels. Around the wall of cavity are seen foci of consolidation. The overlying pleura may also be thickened (Fig. 11.9).

Microscopically, the wall and lumen of cavity shows eosinophilic, granular, caseous material which may show foci of dystrophic calcification. Widespread coalesced tuberculous granulomas composed of epithelioid cells, Langhans' giant cells and peripheral mantle of lymphocytes and having central caseation necrosis are seen. The outer wall of cavity shows fibrosis (Fig. 11.10).

Complications of cavitary secondary tuberculosis are as follows:

a) Aneurysms of patent arteries crossing the cavity producing haemoptysis.
b) Extension to pleura producing bronchopleural fistula.
c) Tuberculous empyema from deposition of caseous material on the pleural surface.
d) Thickened pleura from adhesions of parietal pleura.

TUBERCULOUS CASEOUS PNEUMONIA The caseous material from a case of secondary tuberculosis in an individual with high degree of hypersensitivity may spread to rest of the lung producing caseous pneumonia (Fig. 11.11, A).

Microscopically, the lesions show exudative reaction with oedema, fibrin, polymorphs and monocytes but numerous tubercle bacilli can be demonstrated in the exudates (Fig. 11.11, B).

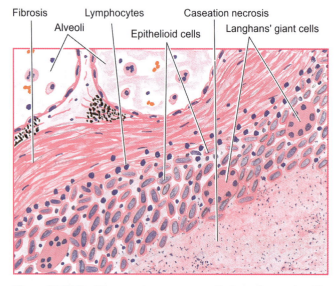 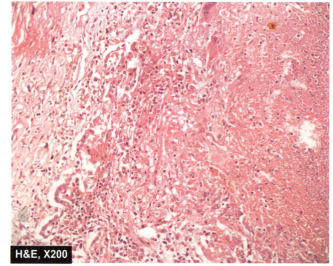

Figure 11.10 ▶ Microscopic appearance of lesions of secondary fibrocaseous tuberculosis of the lung showing wall of the cavity.

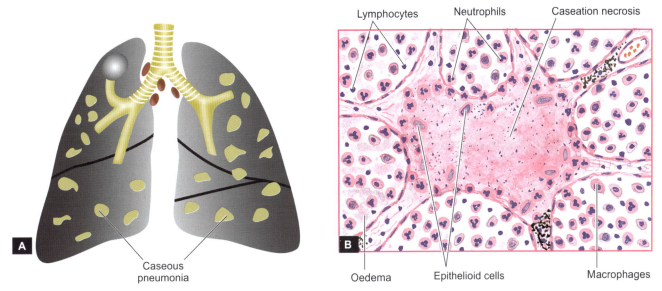

Figure 11.11 ▶ A, Bilateral tuberculous caseous pneumonia. B, Tuberculous caseous pneumonia showing exudative reaction. In AFB staining, these cases have numerous acid-fast bacilli (not shown here).

MILIARY TUBERCULOSIS This is lymphohaematogenous spread of tuberculous infection from primary focus or later stages of tuberculosis. The spread may occur to systemic organs or isolated organ. The spread is either by entry of infection into pulmonary vein producing disseminated or isolated organ lesion in different extra-pulmonary sites (e.g. liver, spleen, kidney, brain, meninges, genitourinary tract and bone marrow) (Fig. 11.12), or into pulmonary artery restricting the development of miliary lesions within the lung (Fig. 11.13).

Grossly, the miliary lesions are millet seed-sized (1 mm diameter), yellowish, firm areas without grossly visible caseation necrosis.

Microscopically, the lesions show the structure of tubercles with minute areas of caseation necrosis (Fig. 11.14).

TUBERCULOUS EMPYEMA The caseating pulmonary lesions of tuberculosis may be associated with pleurisy (pleuritis, pleural effusion) as a reaction and is expressed as

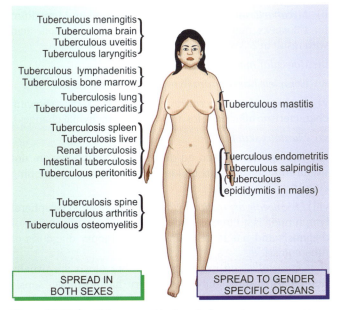

Figure 11.12 ▶ Miliary spread by lymphohaematogenous route.

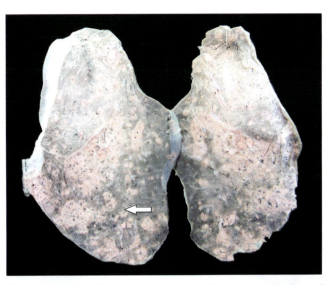

Figure 11.13 ▶ Miliary tuberculosis lung. The sectioned surface of the lung parenchyma shows presence of minute millet-seed sized tubercles.

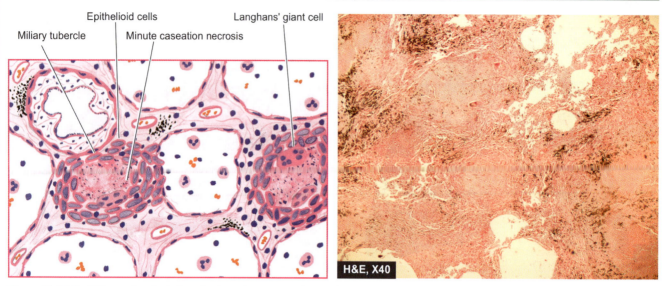

Figure 11.14 ▶ Miliary tubercles in lung having minute areas of central caseation necrosis.

a serous or fibrinous exudates. Pleural effusion may heal by fibrosis and obliterate the pleural space (thickened pleura by chronic pleuritis). Occasionally, pleural cavity may contain caseous material and develop into tuberculous empyema.

Fig. 11.15 depicts various pulmonary and pleural lesions in tuberculosis.

Clinical Features and Diagnosis of Tuberculosis

The clinical manifestations in tuberculosis may be variable depending upon the location, extent and type of lesions. However, in secondary pulmonary tuberculosis which is the common type, the usual clinical features are as under:

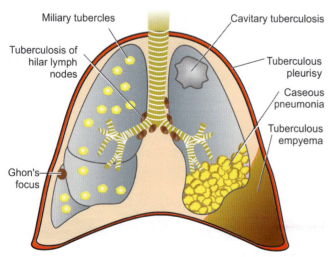

Figure 11.15 ▶ Spectrum of lesions in the lungs and pleura in all types of pulmonary tuberculosis.

1. **Referable to lungs**—such as productive cough (may be with haemoptysis), pleural effusion, dyspnoea, orthopnoea etc. Chest X-ray may show typical apical changes like pleural effusion, nodularity, and miliary or diffuse infiltrates in the lung parenchyma.

2. **Systemic features**—such as fever, night sweats, fatigue, loss of weight and appetite. Long-standing and untreated cases of tuberculosis may develop systemic secondary amyloidosis.

The *diagnosis* is made by the following tests:

i) *AFB microscopy* of diagnostic specimen such as sputum, aspirated material.

ii) *Mycobacterial culture* (traditional method on LJ medium for 4-8 weeks, newer rapid method by HPLC of mycolic acid with result in 2-3 weeks).

iii) *Molecular methods* such as PCR.

iv) *Complete haemogram* (lymphocytosis and raised ESR).

v) *Radiographic procedures* e.g. chest X-ray showing characteristic hilar nodules and other parenchymal changes).

vi) *Mantoux skin test*.

vii) *Serologic tests* based on detection of antibodies are not useful although these are being advocated in some developing countries.

viii) *Fine needle aspiration cytology* of an enlarged peripheral lymph node is quite useful and easy way for confirmation of diagnosis and has largely replaced the biopsy diagnosis of tuberculosis.

Causes of death in pulmonary tuberculosis are usually pulmonary insufficiency, pulmonary haemorrhage, sepsis due to disseminated miliary tuberculosis, cor pulmonale or secondary amyloidosis.

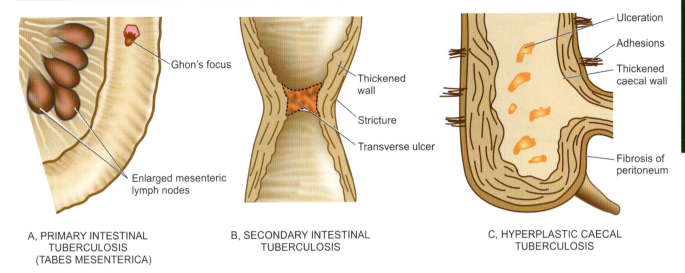

Figure 11.16 ▶ Intestinal tuberculosis, three patterns.

Intestinal Tuberculosis

Intestinal tuberculosis can occur in 3 forms—primary, secondary and hyperplastic caecal tuberculosis.

1. PRIMARY INTESTINAL TUBERCULOSIS Though an uncommon disease in the developed countries of the world, primary tuberculosis of the ileocaecal region is quite common in developing countries including India. In the pre-pasteurisation era, it used to occur by ingestion of unpasteurised cow's milk infected with *Mycobacterium bovis*. But now-a-days due to control of tuberculosis in cattle and pasteurisation of milk, virtually all cases of intestinal tuberculosis are caused by *M. tuberculosis*. The predominant changes are in the mesenteric lymph nodes without any significant intestinal lesion.

Grossly, the affected lymph nodes are enlarged, matted and caseous (tabes mesenterica). Eventually, there is healing by fibrosis and calcification **(Fig. 11.16, A)**.

Microscopically, in the initial stage, there is primary complex or Ghon's focus in the intestinal mucosa as occurs elsewhere in primary tuberculous infection. Subsequently, the mesenteric lymph nodes are affected which show typical tuberculous granulomatous inflammatory reaction with caseation necrosis. Tuberculous peritonitis may occur due to spread of the infection.

2. SECONDARY INTESTINAL TUBERCULOSIS Self-swallowing of sputum in patients with active pulmonary tuberculosis may cause secondary intestinal tuberculosis, most commonly in the terminal ileum and rarely in the colon.

Grossly, the intestinal lesions are more prominent than the lesions in regional lymph nodes as in secondary pulmonary tuberculosis **(Fig. 11.16, B)**. The lesions begin in the Peyer's patches or the lymphoid follicles with formation of small ulcers that spread through the lymphatics to form large ulcers which are *transverse to the long axis of the bowel,* (*c.f.* typhoid ulcers of small intestine, page 168). These ulcers may be coated with caseous material. Serosa may be studded with visible tubercles. In advanced cases, transverse fibrous strictures and intestinal obstruction are seen **(Fig. 11.17, A, B)**.

Histologically, the tuberculous lesions in the intestine are similar to those observed elsewhere i.e. presence of tubercles. Mucosa and submucosa show ulceration and the muscularis may be replaced by variable degree of fibrosis **(Fig. 11.17, C)**. Tuberculous peritonitis may be observed.

3. HYPERPLASTIC ILEOCAECAL TUBERCULOSIS This is a variant of occurring secondary to pulmonary tuberculosis.

Grossly, the terminal ileum, caecum and/or ascending colon are thick-walled with mucosal ulceration. Clinically, the lesion is palpable and may be mistaken for carcinoma **(Fig. 11.16, C)**.

Microscopically, the presence of caseating tubercles distinguishes the condition from Crohn's disease in which granulomas are non-caseating. Besides, bacteriological evidence by culture or animal inoculation and Mantoux test are helpful in differential diagnosis of the two conditions.

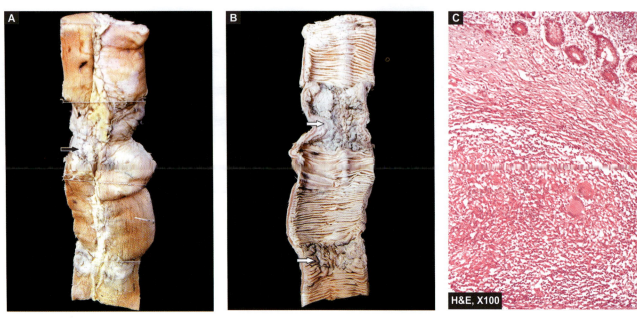

Figure 11.17 ▶ Intestinal tuberculosis. A, The external surface of small intestine shows stricture and a lymph node in section having caseation necrosis (arrow). B, The lumen shows characteristic transverse ulcers and two strictures (arrow). The wall of intestine in the area of narrowed lumen is thickened. C, Microscopy of intestine shows caseating epithelioid cell granulomas in the intestinal wall.

GIST BOX 11.3 — Tuberculosis

- In tuberculosis, tissue response to the causative organism, *Mycobacterium tuberculosis* (a strict aerobe) is a classic example of caseating granulomatous inflammation associated with Langhans' and foreign body giant cells.
- The organism is acid-fast bacillus (AFB) which can be demonstrated by Ziehl-Neelsen staining.
- Tubercle bacilli contain mycoside cord factor essential for growth of the organism and glycolipids in the bacterial cell wall.
- Tuberculosis is worldwide in distribution, more common in developing countries. Other factors include malnutrition, poverty and chronic debilitating diseases and immunocompromised states like AIDS.
- Infection is commonly transmitted by inhalation of cough droplets from an infected individual and self-ingestion of infected sputum. The disease may spread locally, and by lymphohaematogenous route.
- Primary tuberculosis is infection of an individual who has not been previously infected, also called childhood tuberculosis or Ghon's complex. It affects lung most commonly and the tissue response is by formation of a small area of consolidation in the lung, and granulomatous involvement of lymphatic vessel and hilar lymph nodes.
- Secondary pulmonary tuberculosis includes fibrocaseous (cavitary) type, tuberculous caseous pneumonia, military spread to various organs and tuberculous pleurisy.
- Common methods of diagnosis of pulmonary tuberculosis are demonstration of the organism in the sputum, haematologic tests (raised ESR), positive Mantoux skin test, and X-ray chest. Fine needle aspiration of enlarged lymph nodes is a convenient method of confirmation of diagnosis.
- Intestinal tuberculosis can occur as primary, secondary or hyperplastic ileocaecal type. In a classic case, there are multiple transverse ulcers and strictures causing intestinal obstruction.

LEPROSY

Leprosy or Hansen's disease (after discovery of the causative organism by Hansen in 1874), was first described in ancient Indian text going back to 6th Century BC, is a chronic non-fatal infectious disease. It affects mainly the cooler parts of the body such as the skin, mouth, respiratory tract, eyes, peripheral nerves, superficial lymph nodes and testis. The earliest and main involvement in leprosy is of the skin and nerves. However, in bacteraemia from endothelial colonisation or by bacilli filtered from blood by reticuloendothelial system, other organs such as the liver, spleen, bone marrow and regional lymph nodes are also involved. Advanced cases may develop secondary amyloidosis and renal disease, both of which are of immunologic origin.

Causative Organism

The disease is caused by *Mycobacterium leprae* which closely resembles *Mycobacterium tuberculosis* but the organism is less acid-fast. The organisms in tissues appear as compact rounded masses *(globi)* or are arranged in parallel fashion like *cigarettes-in-pack*.

M. leprae can be demonstrated in tissue sections, in split skin smears by splitting the skin, scrapings from cut edges of dermis, and in nasal smears by the following techniques:

1. *Acid-fast (Ziehl-Neelsen or ZN) staining* The staining procedure is similar as for demonstration of *M. tuberculosis* but can be decolourised by lower concentration (5%) of sulphuric acid (less acid-fast).

2. *Fite-Faraco staining* procedure is a modification of Z.N. procedure and is considered better for more adequate staining of tissue sections (Fig. 11.18).

3. *Gomori methenamine silver (GMS)* staining can also be employed.

4. *Molecular methods* e.g. PCR.

5. *IgM antibodies to PGL-1 antigen* seen in 95% cases of lepromatous leprosy but only in 60% cases of tuberculoid leprosy.

The slit smear technique gives a reasonable quantitative measure of *M. leprae* when stained with Z.N. method and examined under 100x oil objective for determining the density of bacteria in the lesion *(bacterial index, BI)*. B.I. is scored from 1+ to 6+ (range from 1 to 10 bacilli per 100 fields to >1000 per field) as *multibacillary* leprosy while B.I. of 0+ is termed *paucibacillary*.

Although lepra bacilli were the first bacteria identified for causing human disease, *M. leprae* remains one of the few bacterial species which is yet to be cultured on artificial media. Nine-banded armadillo, a rodent, acts as an experimental animal model as it develops leprosy which is histopathologically and immunologically similar to human leprosy.

Incidence

The disease is endemic in areas with hot and moist climates and in poor tropical countries. Leprosy is almost exclusively a disease of a few developing countries in Asia, Africa and Latin America. According to the WHO, 8 countries—India, China, Nepal, Brazil, Indonesia, Myanmar (Burma), Madagascar and Nigeria, together constitute about 80% of leprosy cases, of which India accounts for one-third of all the registered leprosy cases globally. In India, the disease is seen more commonly in states of Tamil Nadu, Bihar, Puducherry, Andhra Pradesh, Odisha, West Bengal and Assam. Very few cases are now seen in Europe and the United States.

Mode of Transmission

Leprosy is a slow communicable disease and the incubation period between first exposure and appearance of signs of disease varies from 2 to 20 years (average about 3 years). The infectivity may be from the following sources:

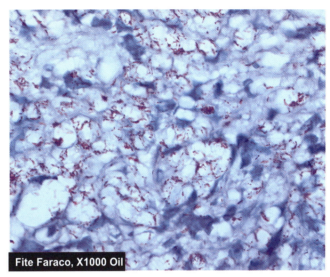

Figure 11.18 ▶ Lepra bacilli in LL are seen as globi and cigarettes-in-a-pack appearance inside the foam macrophages (Fite-Faraco stain).

1. *Direct contact* with untreated leprosy patients who shed numerous bacilli from damaged skin, nasal secretions, mucous membrane of mouth and hair follicles.

2. *Materno-foetal transmission* across the placenta.

3. Transmission from *milk* of leprosy affected mother to infant.

Immunology of Leprosy

Like in tuberculosis, the immune response in leprosy is also T cell-mediated delayed hypersensitivity (type IV reaction) but the two diseases are quite dissimilar as regards immune reactions and lesions. *M. leprae* do not produce any toxins but instead the damage to tissues is immune-mediated. This is due to the following peculiar aspects in immunology of leprosy:

1. **Antigens of leprosy bacilli** Lepra bacilli have several antigens. The bacterial cell wall contains large amount of *M. leprae*-specific phenolic glycolipid (PGL-1) and another surface antigen, lipo-arabinomannan (LAM). These antigens of the bacilli determine the immune reaction of host lymphocytes and macrophages. Another unique feature of leprosy bacilli is invasion in peripheral nerves which is due to binding of trisaccharide of *M. leprae* to basal lamina of Schwann cells.

2. **Genotype of the host** Genetic composition of the host as known by MHC class (or HLA type) determines which antigen of leprosy bacilli shall interact with host immune cells. Accordingly, the host response to the leprosy bacilli in different individuals is variable.

3. **T cell response** There is variation in T cell response in two main forms of leprosy:

i) Unlike tubercle bacilli, there is not only *activation* of CD4+ T cells but also of CD8+ T cells.

ii) CD4+ T cells in lepra bacilli infected persons act not only as helper and promoter cells but also assume the role of *cytotoxicity*.

iii) The two subpopulations of CD4+ T cells (or T helper cells)—T_H 1 cells and T_H 2 cells, elaborate different types of *cytokines* in response to stimuli from the lepra bacilli and macrophages.

iv) In tuberculoid leprosy, the response is largely by CD4+ T cells, while in lepromatous leprosy although there is excess of CD8+ T cells (suppressor T) but the macrophages and suppressor T cells fail to destroy the bacilli due to *CD8+ T cell defect*.

4. **Humoral response** Though the patients of lepromatous leprosy have humoral components such as high levels of immunoglobulins (IgG, IgA, IgM) and antibodies to mycobacterial antigens but these antibodies do not have any protective role against lepra bacilli.

Based on the above unique immunologic features in leprosy, lesions in leprosy are classified into 5 distinct clinicopathologic types and three forms of reactional leprosy (described below), and an intradermal immunologic test, lepromin test.

LEPROMIN TEST It is not a diagnostic test but is used for classifying leprosy on the basis of immune response. Intradermal injection of lepromin, an antigenic extract of *M. leprae,* reveals delayed hypersensitivity reaction in patients of tuberculoid leprosy:

1) An early positive reaction appearing as an indurated area in 24-48 hours is called *Fernandez reaction.*
2) A delayed granulomatous lesion appearing after 3-4 weeks is called *Mitsuda reaction.*

Patients of lepromatous leprosy are negative by the lepromin test.

The test indicates that cell-mediated immunity is greatly suppressed in lepromatous leprosy while patients of tuberculoid leprosy show good immune response. Delayed type of hypersensitivity is conferred by T helper cells. The granulomas of tuberculoid leprosy have sufficient T helper cells and fewer T suppressor cells at the periphery while the cellular infiltrates of lepromatous leprosy lack T helper cells.

Classification

RIDLEY AND JOPLING'S CLASSIFICATION Traditionally, two main forms of leprosy are distinguished:
1. Lepromatous type representing *low resistance*; and
2. Tuberculoid type representing *high resistance.*

Salient differences between these two forms of leprosy are summarised in **Table 11.4**.

Since both these types of leprosy represent two opposite poles of host immune response, these are also called *polar forms* of leprosy. Cases not falling into either of the two poles are classified as *borderline* and *indeterminate types*.

Based on clinical, histologic and immunologic features, modified Ridley and Jopling's classification divides leprosy into 5 groups as under:

TT—Tuberculoid Polar *(High resistance)*
BT—Borderline Tuberculoid
BB—Mid Borderline (Dimorphic)
BL—Borderline Lepromatous
LL—Lepromatous Polar *(Low resistance)*

VARIANTS In addition, not included in Ridley-Jopling's classification are following types:

◆ *Indeterminate leprosy* This is an initial non-specific stage of any type of leprosy.

◆ *Pure neural leprosy* In these cases, skin lesions which are the cardinal feature of leprosy are absent but instead neurologic involvement is the main feature.

◆ *Histoid leprosy* Described by Wade in 1963, this is a variant of LL in which the skin lesions resemble nodules of dermatofibroma and the lesions are highly positive for lepra bacilli.

Table 11.4	Differences between lepromatous and tuberculoid leprosy.	
FEATURE	LEPROMATOUS LEPROSY	TUBERCULOID LEPROSY
1. Skin lesions	Symmetrical, multiple, hypopigmented, erythematous, maculopapular or nodular (leonine facies).	Asymmetrical, single or a few lesions, hypopigmented and erythematous macular.
2. Nerve involvement	Present but sensory disturbance is less severe.	Present with distinct sensory disturbance.
3. Histopathology	Collection of foamy macrophages or lepra cells in the dermis separated from epidermis by a 'clear zone'.	Hard tubercle similar to granulomatous lesion, eroding the basal layer of epidermis; no clear zone.
4. Bacteriology	Lepra cells highly positive for lepra bacilli seen as 'globi' or 'cigarettes-in-pack' appearance (multibacillary type).	Lepra bacilli few, seen in destroyed nerves as granular or beaded forms (paucibacillary type).
5. Immunity	Suppressed (low resistance).	Good immune response (high resistance).
6. Lepromin test	Negative	Positive

REACTIONAL LEPROSY Based on shift in immune status or in patients of leprosy on treatment, two types of reactional leprosy are distinguished: type I (reversal reactions), and type II (erythema nodosum leprosum).

Type I: Reversal reactions The polar forms of leprosy do not undergo any change in clinical and histopathological picture. The borderline groups are unstable and may move across the spectrum in either direction with upgrading or downgrading of patient's immune state. Accordingly, there may be two types of borderline reaction:

◈ *Upgrading reaction* is characterised by increased cell-mediated immunity and occurs in patients of borderline lepromatous (BL) type on treatment who upgrade or shift towards tuberculoid type.

◈ *Downgrading reaction* is characterised by lowering of cellular immunity and is seen in borderline tuberculoid (BT) type who downgrade or shift towards lepromatous type.

Type II: Erythema nodosum leprosum (ENL) ENL occurs in lepromatous patients after treatment. It is characterised by tender cutaneous nodules, fever, iridocyclitis, synovitis and lymph node involvement.

Histopathology of Leprosy

Usually, skin biopsy from the margin of lesions is submitted for diagnosis and for classification of leprosy. The histopathologic diagnosis of multibacillary leprosy like LL and BL offers no problem while the indeterminate leprosy and tuberculoid lesions are paucibacillary and their diagnosis is made together with clinical evidence.

In general, for histopathologic evaluation in all suspected cases of leprosy, the following general *features* should be looked for:
i) Cell type of granuloma
ii) Nerve involvement
iii) Bacterial load
iv) Presence and absence of lymphocytes
v) Relation of granuloma with epidermis and adenexa.

The salient features in major types of leprosy are as follows.

1. **Lepromatous leprosy:**
The following features characterise lepromatous polar leprosy (Fig. 11.19):
i) In the dermis, there is proliferation of macrophages with foamy change, particularly around the blood vessels, nerves and dermal appendages. The foamy macrophages are called *'lepra cells'* or *Virchow cells.*
ii) The lepra cells are heavily laden with acid-fast bacilli demonstrated with AFB staining. The AFB may be seen as compact globular masses *(globi)* or arranged in parallel fashion like *'cigarettes-in-pack'* (see Fig. 11.18).
iii) The dermal infiltrate of lepra cells characteristically does not encroach upon the basal layer of epidermis and is separated from epidermis by a subepidermal uninvolved *clear zone.*
iv) The *epidermis* overlying the lesions is thinned out, flat and may even ulcerate.

2. **Tuberculoid leprosy:**
The polar tuberculoid form presents the following histological features (Fig. 11.20):
i) The dermal lesions show granulomas resembling *hard tubercles* composed of epithelioid cells, Langhans' giant cells and peripheral mantle of lymphocytes.

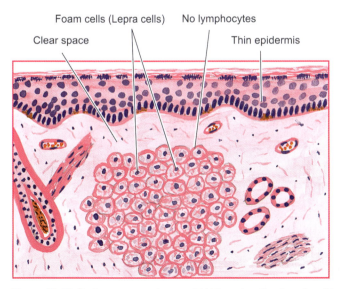
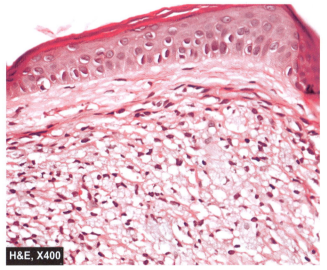

Figure 11.19 ▶ Lepromatous leprosy (LL). There is collection of proliferating foam macrophages (lepra cells) in the dermis, sparse lymphocytes and a clear subepidermal zone.

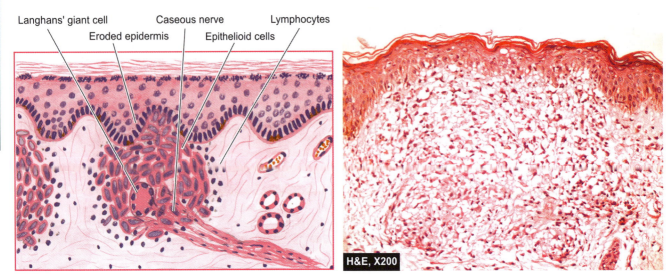

Figure 11.20 ▶ Tuberculoid leprosy (TT). Granuloma eroding the basal layer of the epidermis. The granuloma is composed of epithelioid cells with sparse Langhans' giant cells and many lymphocytes.

ii) Lesions of tuberculoid leprosy have predilection for *dermal nerves* which may be destroyed and infiltrated by epithelioid cells and lymphocytes.
iii) The granulomatous infiltrate erodes the basal layer of epidermis i.e. there is *no clear zone*.
iv) The *lepra bacilli* are few and seen in destroyed nerves.

3. **Borderline leprosy:**
The histopathologic features of the three forms of borderline leprosy are as under:
i) *Borderline tuberculoid (BT)* form shows epithelioid cells and plentiful lymphocytes. There is a narrow clear subepidermal zone. Lepra bacilli are scanty and found in nerves.
ii) *Borderline lepromatous (BL)* form shows predominance of histiocytes, a few epithelioid cells and some irregularly dispersed lymphocytes. Numerous lepra bacilli are seen.
iii) *Mid-borderline (BB)* or dimorphic form shows sheets of epithelioid cells with no giant cells. Some lymphocytes are seen in the peri-neurium. Lepra bacilli are present, mostly in nerves.

4. **Indeterminate leprosy:**
The histopathologic features are non-specific so that the diagnosis of non-specific chronic dermatitis may be made. However, a few features help in suspecting leprosy as under:
i) Lymphocytic or mononuclear cell infiltrate, localised particularly around skin adnexal structures like hair follicles and sweat glands or around blood vessels.
ii) Nerve involvement, if present, is strongly supportive of diagnosis.
iii) Confirmation of diagnosis is made by finding of lepra bacilli.

5. **Pure neural leprosy:**
Histopathologic features described in skin lesion of various forms of leprosy may be seen in the nerve biopsy specimens. Pure neural leprosy may be AFB positive or AFB negative.

6. **Histoid leprosy:**
Following features characterise these lesions:
i) Whorls and fascicles of spindle cells in the upper dermis after a clear subepidermal space.
ii) On close scrutiny, these cells have foamy cytoplasm.
iii) The cytoplasm of these cells is laden with lepra bacilli.

7. **Reactional leprosy:**
Two types of reactional leprosy show the following features:

Type I reaction: Reversal reactions. These may be upgrading or downgrading type of reaction:

Upgrading reaction shows an increase of lymphocytes, oedema of the lesions, necrosis in the centre and reduced B.I.

Downgrading reaction shows dispersal and spread of the granulomas and increased presence of lepra bacilli.

Type II reaction: ENL The lesions in ENL show infiltration by neutrophils and eosinophils and prominence of vasculitis. Inflammation often extends deep into the subcutaneous fat causing panniculitis. Bacillary load is increased. Secondary amyloidosis may follow repeated attacks of ENL in leprosy.

Clinical Features

The two main forms of leprosy show distinctive clinical features:

Chapter 11: Inflammation: Chronic and Granulomatous

1. Lepromatous leprosy:

i) The skin lesions in LL are generally symmetrical, multiple, slightly hypopigmented and erythematous macules, papules, nodules or diffuse infiltrates. The nodular lesions may coalesce to give *leonine facies* appearance.

ii) The lesions are hypoaesthetic or anaesthetic but the sensory disturbance is not as distinct as in TT.

2. Tuberculoid leprosy:

i) The skin lesions in TT occur as either single or as a few asymmetrical lesions which are hypopigmented and erythematous macules.

ii) There is a distinct sensory impairment.

Long-term cases of either type may develop secondary amyloidosis. Anti-leprosy vaccines have been developed but are undergoing human trials yet. Since the incubation period of leprosy is quite long, the efficacy of such vaccines will be known after a number of years.

GIST BOX 11.4 — Leprosy

- Leprosy or Hansen's disease, is a chronic infectious disease that affects mainly the cooler parts of the body such as the skin, mouth, respiratory tract, eyes, peripheral nerves, superficial lymph nodes and testis.
- The disease is caused by *Mycobacterium leprae* which closely resembles *Mycobacterium tuberculosis* but is less acid-fast.
- The disease spreads by close contact for a long duration, often lasting for several years.
- Based on clinical, pathologic and immunologic features, leprosy is classified into polar tuberculoid (high resistance), polar lepromatous (low resistance), and borderline towards either type. A few variants are reactional (type I upgrading and downgrading, type II or ENL) histoid, and pure neural leprosy.
- Lepromatous type has foam cell granulomas (multibacillary on lepra stain) while tuberculoid type has epithelioid cell granulomas (paucibacillary on lepra stain).

SYPHILIS

Syphilis is a venereal (sexually-transmitted) disease caused by spirochaetes, *Treponema pallidum*. Other treponemal diseases are yaws, pinta and bejel. The word 'syphilis' is derived from the name of the mythological handsome boy, Syphilus, who was cursed by Greek God Apollo with the disease.

Causative Organism

T. pallidum is a coiled spiral filament 10 µm long that moves actively in fresh preparations. The organism cannot be stained by the usual methods and can be demonstrated in the exudates and tissues by:

1. *dark ground illumination (DGI)* in fresh preparation;
2. *fluorescent antibody technique*;
3. *silver impregnation techniques*; and
4. *nucleic acid amplification* technique by PCR.

The organism has not been cultivated in any culture media but experimental infection can be produced in rabbits and chimpanzees. The organism is rapidly destroyed by cold, heat, and antiseptics.

Incidence

Since the advent of penicillin therapy in 1943, syphilis has shown a decline in incidence. However, the disease continues to have global presence. Most commonly affected regions in the world are in Sub-Saharan Africa, South America, and South East Asia. Male homosexuals are at greater risk. Some African countries have very high incidence of congenital syphilis and also responsible for high rate of stillbirths.

Immunology

T. pallidum does not produce any endotoxin or exotoxin. The pathogenesis of the lesions appears to be due to host immune response.

There are two types of serological tests for syphilis: treponemal and non-treponemal.

A. Treponemal serological tests These tests measure antibody to *T. pallidum* antigen and are more useful and sensitive for the diagnosis of syphilis:

i) *Fluorescent treponemal antibody-absorbed (FTA-ABS) test*.

ii) *Agglutinin assays* e.g. microhaemagglutination assay for *T. pallidum* (MHA-TP), and Serodia TP-PA; the latter is more sensitive.

iii) *T. pallidum passive haemagglutination (TPHA) test*.

B. Non-treponemal serological tests These tests measure non-specific reaginic antibodies IgM and IgG immunoglobulins directed against cardiolipin-lecithin-cholesterol complex and are more commonly used. These tests are as under:

i) *Reiter protein complement fixation (RPCF) test*: Test of choice for rapid diagnosis.

ii) *Venereal Disease Research Laboratory (VDRL) or Rapid Plasma Reagin (RPR) test*: Wassermann described a complement fixing antibody against antigen of human syphilitic tissue. This antigen is used in the Standard Test for Syphilis (STS) in Wassermann complement fixing test and VDRL test.

Mode of Transmission

Syphilitic infection can be transmitted by the following routes:
1. *Sexual intercourse* is the most common route of infection and results in lesions on glans penis, vulva, vagina and cervix.

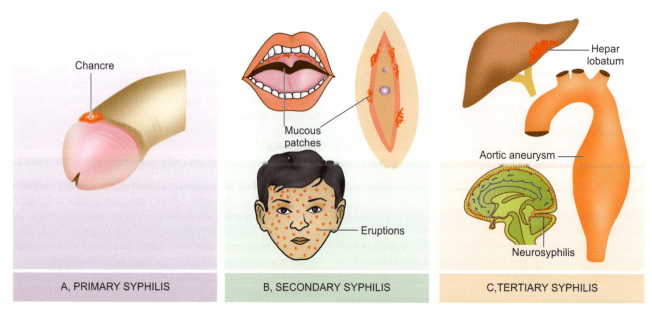

Figure 11.21 ▶ Organ involvement in various stages of acquired syphilis. A, *Primary syphilis*: Primary lesion is 'chancre' on glans penis. B, *Secondary syphilis:* Mucocutaneous lesions—mucous patches on oral and vaginal mucosa and generalised skin eruptions. C, *Tertiary syphilis:* Localised lesion as gumma of liver with scarring (hepar lobatum); diffuse lesions (right) in aorta (aneurysm, narrowing of mouths of coronary ostia and incompetence of aortic valve ring) and nervous system.

2. *Intimate person-to-person contact* with lesions on lips, tongue or fingers.
3. *Transfusion* of infected blood.
4. *Materno-foetal transmission* in congenital syphilis if the mother is infected.

Stages of Acquired Syphilis

Acquired syphilis is divided into 3 stages depending upon the period after which the lesions appear and the type of lesions. These are: primary, secondary and tertiary syphilis.

PRIMARY SYPHILIS Typical lesion of primary syphilis is *chancre* which appears on genitals or at extra-genital sites in 2-4 *weeks* after exposure to infection **(Fig. 11.21,A)**. Initially, the lesion is a painless papule which ulcerates in the centre. The fully-developed chancre is an indurated lesion with central ulceration accompanied by regional lymphadenitis. The chancre heals without scarring, even in the absence of treatment.

Histologically, the chancre has the following features:
i) Dense infiltrate of mainly plasma cells, some lymphocytes and a few macrophages.
ii) Perivascular aggregation of mononuclear cells, particularly plasma cells (periarteritis and endarteritis).
iii) Proliferation of vascular endothelium.

Antibody tests are positive in 1-3 weeks after the appearance of chancre. Spirochaetes can be demonstrated in the exudates by DGI.

SECONDARY SYPHILIS Inadequately treated patients of primary syphilis develop *mucocutaneous lesions* and painless lymphadenopathy in *2-3 months* after the exposure **(Fig. 11.21,B)**. Mucocutaneous lesions may be in the form of the mucous patches on mouth, pharynx and vagina; and generalised skin eruptions and condyloma lata in anogenital region.

Antibody tests are always positive at this stage. Secondary syphilis is *highly infective stage* and spirochaetes can be easily demonstrated in the mucocutaneous lesions.

TERTIARY SYPHILIS After a latent period of appearance of secondary lesions and about *2-3 years* following first exposure, tertiary lesions of syphilis appear. Lesions of tertiary syphilis are much less infective than the other two stages and spirochaetes can be demonstrated with great difficulty. These lesions are of 2 main types **(Fig. 11.21, C)**:

i) Syphilitic gumma It is a solitary, localised, rubbery lesion with central necrosis, seen in organs like liver, testis, bone and brain. In the liver, the gumma is associated with scarring of hepatic parenchyma *(hepar lobatum)*.

Histologically, the structure of gumma shows the following features **(Fig. 11.22)**:
a) Central coagulative necrosis resembling caseation but is less destructive so that outlines of necrosed cells can still be faintly seen.
b) Surrounding zone of palisaded macrophages with many plasma cells, some lymphocytes, giant cells and fibroblasts.

Chapter 11: Inflammation: Chronic and Granulomatous

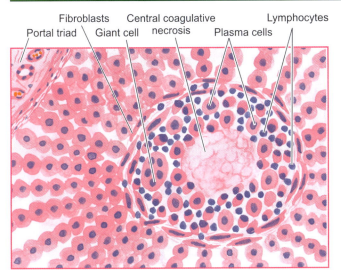

Figure 11.22 ▶ Typical microscopic appearance in the case of syphilitic gumma of the liver. Central coagulative necrosis is surrounded by palisades of macrophages and plasma cells marginated peripherally by fibroblasts.

ii) Diffuse lesions of tertiary syphilis The lesions appear following widespread dissemination of spirochaetes in the body. The diffuse lesions are predominantly seen in cardiovascular and nervous systems. Briefly, these lesions are as under:

a) *Cardiovascular syphilis* mainly involves thoracic aorta. The wall of aorta is weakened and dilated due to syphilitic aortitis and results in aortic aneurysm, incompetence of aortic valve and narrowing of mouths of coronary ostia.

b) *Neurosyphilis* may manifest as:
◆ meningovascular syphilis affecting chiefly the meninges;
◆ tabes dorsalis affecting the spinal cord; and
◆ general paresis affecting the brain.

CONGENITAL SYPHILIS Congenital syphilis may develop in a foetus of more than 16 weeks gestation who is exposed to maternal spirochaetaemia. The major morphologic features are as under:

i) Saddle-shaped nose deformity due to destruction of bridge of the nose.
ii) The characteristic 'Hutchinson's teeth' which are small, widely spaced, peg-shaped permanent teeth.
iii) Mucocutaneous lesions of acquired secondary syphilis.
iv) Bony lesions like epiphysitis and periostitis.
v) Interstitial keratitis with corneal opacity.
vi) Diffuse fibrosis in the liver.
vii) Interstitial fibrosis of lungs.
viii) If the foetus with congenital syphilis is born dead, it is premature, with macerated skin, enlarged spleen and liver, and with syphilitic epiphysitis.

Histologically, the basic morphology of lesions in syphilis is seen in all the affected organs: perivascular plasma cell rich inflammatory infiltrate and endothelial cell proliferation. Many spirochaetes can be demonstrated in involved tissues.

GIST BOX 11.5 — Syphilis

❖ Syphilis is a venereal (sexually-transmitted) disease caused by spirochaetes, *Treponema pallidum*, most often by sexual intercourse.
❖ The organism can be demonstrated directly in tissue fluids by dark ground immunisation, fluorescent method. Supportive laboratory tests are antibody tests such as VDRL, STS, FTA.
❖ Syphilis has 3 clinicopathologic stages: primary, secondary and tertiary. Characteristically, these lesions are plasma cell rich.
❖ Typical lesion of primary syphilis is *chancre* which appears on genitals or at extra-genital sites in 2-4 weeks after exposure to infection. These lesions are positive for spirochaetes.
❖ Secondary syphilis has mucocutaneous lesions and painless lymphadenopathy. Spirochaetes may be seen in the lesions.
❖ Tertiary stage occurs after a latent period lasting 2-3 years and its lesions are in form of gummas (in liver or testis), and as diffuse lesions (cardiovascular and neurosyphilis).
❖ Babies with congenital syphilis have saddle nose deformity and wide short teeth.

ACTINOMYCOSIS

Actinomycosis is a chronic suppurative disease caused by anaerobic bacteria, *Actinomycetes israelii*. The disease is conventionally included in mycology though the causative organism is filamentous bacteria and not true fungus although its name sounds like one. The disease is worldwide in distribution. The organisms are commensals in the oral cavity, alimentary tract and vagina. The infection is always endogenous in origin and not by person-to-person contact. The organisms invade, proliferate and disseminate in favourable conditions like break in mucocutaneous continuity, some underlying disease etc.

MORPHOLOGIC FEATURES Depending upon the anatomic location of lesions, actinomycosis is of 4 types: cervicofacial, thoracic, abdominal, and pelvic **(Fig. 11.23)**.

1. Cervicofacial actinomycosis This is the commonest form (60%) and has the best prognosis. The infection enters from tonsils, carious teeth, periodontal disease or trauma following tooth extraction. Initially, a firm swelling

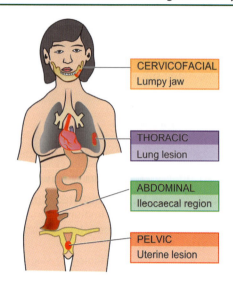

Figure 11.23 ▶ Actinomycosis, sites and routes of infection.

develops in the lower jaw ('lumpy jaw'). In time, the mass breaks down and abscesses and sinuses are formed. The discharging pus contains typical tiny yellow sulphur granules. The infection may extend into adjoining soft tissues and may destroy the bone.

2. **Thoracic actinomycosis** The infection in the lungs is due to aspiration of the organism from oral cavity or extension of infection from abdominal or hepatic lesions. Initially, the disease resembles pneumonia but subsequently the infection spreads to the whole of lung, pleura, ribs and vertebrae.

3. **Abdominal actinomycosis** This type is common in appendix, caecum and liver. The abdominal infection results from swallowing of organisms from oral cavity or extension from thoracic cavity.

4. **Pelvic actinomycosis** Infection in the pelvis occurs as a complication of intrauterine contraceptive devices (IUCDs).

Microscopically, irrespective of the location of actinomycosis, the following features are seen (Fig. 11.24):

i) The inflammatory reaction is a granuloma with central suppuration. There is formation of abscesses in the centre of lesions and at the periphery chronic inflammatory cells, giant cells and fibroblasts are seen.

ii) The centre of each abscess contains the bacterial colony, 'sulphur granule', characterised by radiating filaments (hence previously known as *ray fungus*) with hyaline, eosinophilic, club-like ends representing secreted immunoglobulins, best highlighted in Masson's trichrome stain.

iii) Bacterial stains reveal the organisms as gram-positive filaments, nonacid-fast, which stain positively with Gomori's methenamine silver (GMS) staining.

GIST BOX 11.6 Actinomycosis

- Actinomycosis is a chronic suppurative disease caused by *Actinomycetes israelii*. Though the name of disease sounds like a fungus, it is caused by anaerobic bacteria.
- Depending upon the anatomic location, actinomycosis is of 4 types: cervicofacial (commonest as lumpy jaw), thoracic, abdominal, and pelvic.
- Microscopically, the lesions have an abscess containing the bacterial colony as sulphur granule.

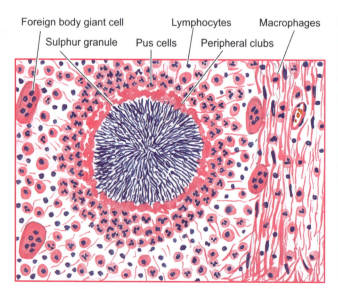
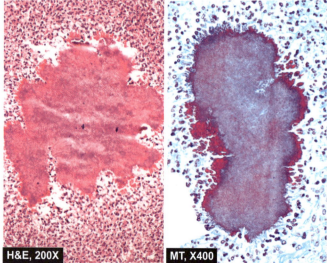

Figure 11.24 ▶ Actinomycosis. Microscopic appearance of sulphur granule lying inside an abscess. The margin of the colony shows hyaline filaments highlighted by Masson's trichrome stain (right photomicrograph).

SARCOIDOSIS (BOECK'S SARCOID)

Sarcoidosis is a multisystem disease of unknown etiology. It is worldwide in distribution and affects adults from 20-40 years of age. The disease may be asymptomatic or may have organ dysfunction such as respiratory complaints or cutaneous or ocular lesions. The disease is characterised by the presence of non-caseating epithelioid cell granulomas ('sarcoid granuloma') in the affected tissues and organs, notably lymph nodes, lungs and skin. Other sites are the uvea of the eyes, spleen, salivary glands, liver and bones of hands and feet.

ETIOLOGY AND PATHOGENESIS The cause of sarcoidosis remains unknown. However, the disease has immune pathogenesis but the antigenic trigger that stimulates the disease process is still unknown. No single etiologic agent or consistent genetic locus has been identified. However, the disease appears to involve 3 interlinked factors:
1. Disturbed immune system
2. Genetic predisposition
3. Exposure to environmental agent

1. **Disturbed immune system** The disease is characterised by granulomatous tissue reaction, indicative of expression of cell-mediated immune mechanism.

◆ Antigen-presenting cells (i.e. macrophages) present an unknown antigen to helper T cells.

◆ These clusters of macrophages and helper T cells on activation release several cytokines—IL-2, IFN-γ, IL-8, IL-10, IL-12, IL-18 and TNF.

◆ These multiple cytokines form the granuloma in which macrophages predominate but T cells have a necessary role in initial inflammatory reaction.

2. **Genetic predisposition** Although no consistent genetic loci have been found, there is increased risk of development of sarcoidosis in certain HLA haplotype, HLA-DRB1, HLA-A1, HLA-B8.

3. **Exposure to environmental agent** The environmental agent acting as antigen which initiates the immunologic response has eluded the workers. Infectious agents have been suspected; these include mycobacteria or their antigenic proteins, *Propionibacter acnes*, rickettsia, and atypical mycobacteria.

KVEIM'S TEST It is a useful intradermal diagnostic test based on immune pathogenesis of disease. The antigen prepared from involved lymph node or spleen is injected intradermally. In a positive test, nodular lesion appears in 3-6 weeks at the inoculation site which on microscopic examination shows presence of non-caseating granulomas.

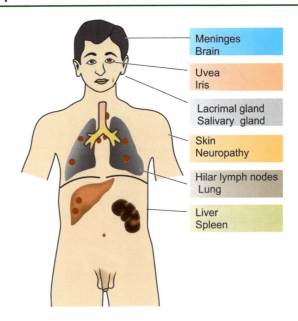

Figure 11.25 ▶ Common locations of lesions in sarcoidosis. The lesions are predominantly seen in lymph nodes and throughout lung parenchyma.

MORPHOLOGIC FEATURES The lesions in sarcoidosis are generalised and may affect various organs and tissues at sometime in the course of disease, but brunt of the disease is borne by the lungs and lymph nodes **(Fig. 11.25)**.

Microscopically, the diagnosis is generally made by exclusion of other causes of granulomatous inflammation. However, following features are seen **(Fig. 11.26)**:
1. The diagnostic feature in sarcoidosis of any organ or tissue is the *non-caseating sarcoid granuloma,* composed of epithelioid cells, Langhans' and foreign body giant cells and surrounded peripherally by fibroblasts. However, at times fibrinoid necrosis may be seen in the centre of granuloma.
2. Typically, granulomas of sarcoidosis are *'naked'* i.e. either devoid of peripheral rim of lymphocytes or there is paucity of lymphocytes.
3. In late stage, the granuloma is either *enclosed by hyalinised fibrous tissue* or is replaced by hyalinised fibrous mass.
4. The giant cells in sarcoid granulomas contain certain *cytoplasmic inclusions* as follows:
i) *Asteroid bodies* which are eosinophilic and stellate-shaped structures.
ii) *Schaumann's bodies or conchoid (conch like) bodies* which are concentric laminations of calcium and of iron salts, complexed with proteins.
iii) *Birefringent cytoplasmic crystals* which are colourless.
Similar types of inclusions are also observed in chronic berylliosis.

Section II: Inflammation and Healing, Immunity and Hypersensitivity, Infections and Infestations

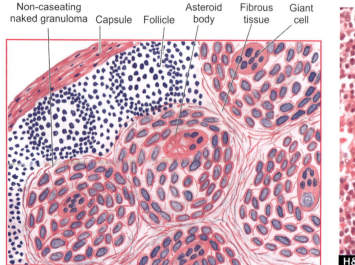 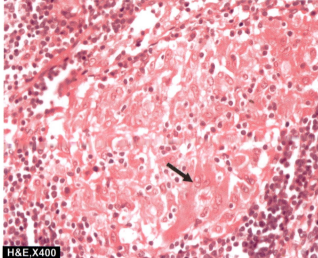

Figure 11.26 ▶ Sarcoidosis in lymph node. Characteristically, there are non-caseating epithelioid cell granulomas which have paucity of lymphocytes. A giant cell with inclusions is also seen in the photomicrograph (arrow).

 GIST BOX 11.7 | **Sarcoidosis**

❖ Sarcoidosis is a multisystem disease of unknown etiology. It is worldwide in distribution and affects adults from 20-40 years of age.
❖ The disease is characterised by the presence of non-caseating epithelioid cell granulomas ('sarcoid granuloma') in the affected tissues and organs, notably lymph nodes, lungs, skin and eyes.
❖ The cause of sarcoidosis remains unknown. However, the disease has immune pathogenesis and involves interplay of 3 factors: disturbed cellular immune function, genetic predisposition and exposure to an unknown environmental agent.

12. Healing of Tissues

Healing is the body's response to injury in an attempt to restore normal structure and function. It involves 2 processes:
- *Regeneration* when healing takes place by proliferation of parenchymal cells and usually results in complete restoration of the original tissues.
- *Repair* when healing takes place by proliferation of connective tissue resulting in fibrosis and scarring.

At times, both these processes take place simultaneously.

REGENERATION AND REPAIR

REGENERATION

Some parenchymal cells are short-lived while others have a longer lifespan. In order to maintain proper structure of tissues, these cells are under the constant regulatory control of their cell cycle. These include growth factors such as: epidermal growth factor, fibroblast growth factor, platelet-derived growth factor, endothelial growth factor, transforming growth factor-β.

Cell cycle is defined as the period between two successive cell divisions and is divided into 4 unequal phases (Fig. 12.1):
- *M (mitosis) phase:* Phase of mitosis.
- *G1 (gap 1) phase:* The daughter cell enters G1 phase after mitosis.
- *S (synthesis) phase:* During this phase, the synthesis of nuclear DNA takes place.
- *G2 (gap 2) phase:* After completion of nuclear DNA duplication, the cell enters G2 phase.
- *G0 (gap 0) phase:* This is the quiescent or resting phase of the cell after an M phase.
- Period between the mitosis is called *interphase*.

Not all cells of the body divide at the same pace. Some mature cells do not divide at all while others complete a cell cycle every 16-24 hours. The main difference between slowly-dividing and rapidly-dividing cells is the duration of G1 phase.

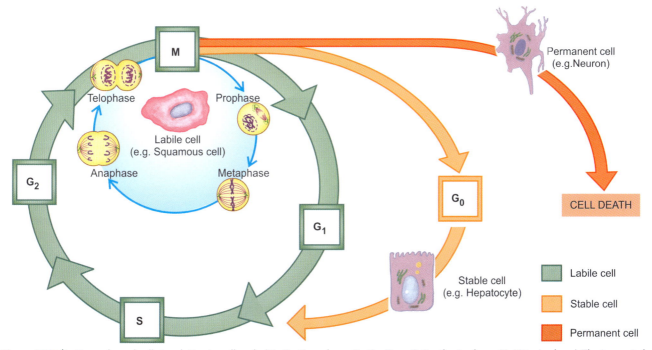

Figure 12.1 ▶ Parenchymal cells in relation to cell cycle (G_0–Resting phase; G_1, G_2–Gaps; S–Synthesis phase; M–Mitosis phase). The inner circle *shown with green line* represents cell cycle for labile cells; circle *shown with yellow-orange line* represents cell cycle for stable cells; and the circle *shown with red line* represents cell cycle for permanent cells. Compare them with traffic signals—green stands for *'go'* applies here to dividing labile cells; yellow-orange signal for *'ready to go'* applies here to stable cells which can be stimulated to enter cell cycle; and red signal for *'stop'* here means non-dividing permanent cells.

Depending upon their capacity to divide, the cells of the body can be divided into 3 groups: labile cells, stable cells, and permanent cells.

1. Labile cells These cells continue to multiply throughout life under normal physiologic conditions. These include: surface epithelial cells of the epidermis, alimentary tract, respiratory tract, urinary tract, vagina, cervix, uterine endometrium, haematopoietic cells of bone marrow and cells of lymph nodes and spleen.

2. Stable cells These cells decrease or lose their ability to proliferate after adolescence but retain the capacity to multiply in response to stimuli throughout adult life. These include: parenchymal cells of organs like liver, pancreas, kidneys, adrenal and thyroid; mesenchymal cells like smooth muscle cells, fibroblasts, vascular endothelium, bone and cartilage cells.

3. Permanent cells These cells lose their ability to proliferate around the time of birth. These include: neurons of nervous system, skeletal muscle and cardiac muscle cells.

RELATIONSHIP OF PARENCHYMAL CELLS WITH CELL CYCLE
If the three types of parenchymal cells described above are correlated with the phase of cell cycle, following inferences can be derived **(Fig. 12.1)**:
1. Labile cells which are continuously dividing cells remain in the cell cycle from one mitosis to the next.
2. Stable cells are in the resting phase (G0) but can be stimulated to enter the cell cycle.
3. Permanent cells are non-dividing cells which have left the cell cycle and die after injury.

Regeneration of any type of parenchymal cells involves the following 2 processes:
i) Proliferation of original cells from the margin of injury with migration so as to cover the gap.
ii) Proliferation of migrated cells with subsequent differentiation and maturation so as to reconstitute the original tissue.

CELL CYCLE SIGNALING PATHWAYS
Mitosis is controlled by genes which encode for release of specific protein molecules that promote or inhibit the process of mitosis at different steps. Mitosis-promoting protein molecules are *cyclins A, B and E*. These cyclins activate *cyclin-dependent kinases (CDKs)* which act in conjunction with cyclins. After the mitosis is complete, cyclins and CDKs are degraded and the residues of used molecules are taken up by cytoplasmic caretaker proteins, *ubiquitin*, to the peroxisome for further degradation.

REPAIR

Repair is the replacement of injured tissue by fibrous tissue. Two processes are involved in repair:
- Granulation tissue formation
- Contraction of wounds

Repair response takes place by participation of mesenchymal cells (consisting of connective tissue stem cells, fibrocytes and histiocytes), endothelial cells, macrophages, platelets, and the parenchymal cells of the injured organ.

Granulation Tissue Formation

The term granulation tissue derives its name from slightly granular and pink appearance of the tissue. Each granule corresponds histologically to proliferation of new small blood vessels which are slightly lifted on the surface by thin covering of fibroblasts and young collagen.

The following 3 phases are observed in the formation of granulation tissue **(Fig. 12.2)**:

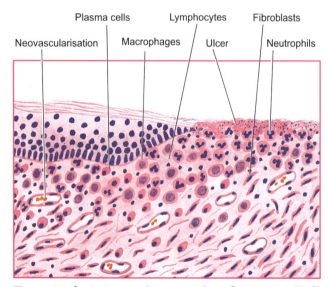
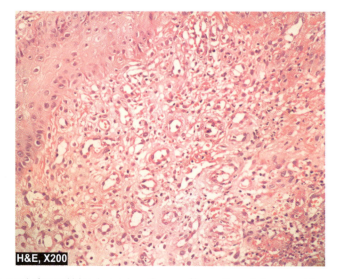

Figure 12.2 ▶ Active granulation tissue has inflammatory cell infiltrate, newly formed blood vessels and young fibrous tissue in loose matrix.

1. **PHASE OF INFLAMMATION** Following trauma, blood clots at the site of injury. There is acute inflammatory response with exudation of plasma, neutrophils and some monocytes within 24 hours.

2. **PHASE OF CLEARANCE** Combination of proteolytic enzymes liberated from neutrophils, autolytic enzymes from dead tissues cells, and phagocytic activity of macrophages clear off the necrotic tissue, debris and red blood cells.

3. **PHASE OF INGROWTH OF GRANULATION TISSUE** This phase consists of 2 main processes: angiogenesis or neovascularisation, and fibrogenesis.

i) **Angiogenesis (neovascularisation)** Formation of new blood vessels at the site of injury takes place by proliferation of endothelial cells from the margins of severed blood vessels. Initially, the proliferated endothelial cells are solid buds but within a few hours develop a lumen and start carrying blood. The newly formed blood vessels are more leaky, accounting for the oedematous appearance of new granulation tissue. Soon, these blood vessels differentiate into muscular arterioles, thin-walled venules and true capillaries.

The process of angiogenesis is stimulated with proteolytic destruction of basement membrane. Angiogenesis takes place under the influence of following factors:

a) Vascular endothelial growth factor (VEGF) elaborated by mesenchymal cells while its receptors are present in endothelial cells only.

b) Platelet-derived growth factor (PDGF), transforming growth factor-β (TGF-β), basic fibroblast growth factor (bFGF) and surface integrins are all associated with cellular proliferation.

ii) **Fibrogenesis** The newly formed blood vessels are present in an amorphous ground substance or matrix. The new fibroblasts have features intermediate between those of fibroblasts and smooth muscle cells (*myofibroblasts*). Collagen fibrils begin to appear by about 6th day. The myofibroblasts have surface receptors for fibronectin molecules which form bridges between collagen fibrils. As maturation proceeds, more and more collagen is formed while the number of active fibroblasts and new blood vessels decreases. This results in formation of inactive looking scar; this process is known as *cicatrisation*.

| GIST BOX 12.1 | Healing: Regeneration and Repair |

❖ Healing is the body's response to injury in an attempt to restore normal structure and function. It involves 2 processes: regeneration and repair.
❖ Regeneration is restoration to original tissue by proliferation of parenchymal cells while repair is healing by proliferation of connective tissue resulting in fibrosis and scarring.
❖ Regeneration depends upon the dividing ability of parenchymal cells. Labile cells continue to divide throughout life (e.g. epidermis, mucosa), stable cells decrease or lose their ability to proliferate (e.g. liver, kidneys) while permanent cells cease to regenerate around the time of birth (e.g. neurons, myocardium).
❖ Repair is healing by formation of granulation tissue. It involves initial inflammatory reaction by the body, followed by clearance by proteolytic enzymes, and phase of angiogenesis and proliferation of fibroblasts.

HEALING OF SKIN WOUNDS

Healing of skin wounds provides a classical example of combination of regeneration and repair described above. Wound healing can be accomplished in one of the following two ways:

◈ Healing by first intention *(primary union)*
◈ Healing by second intention *(secondary union)*.

HEALING BY FIRST INTENTION (PRIMARY UNION)

This is defined as healing of a wound which has the following characteristics:
i) clean and uninfected;
ii) surgically incised;
iii) without much loss of cells and tissue; and
iv) edges of wound are approximated by surgical sutures.

The sequence of events in primary union is illustrated in **Fig. 12.3** and described below:

1. **Initial haemorrhage** Immediately after injury, the space between the approximated surfaces of incised wound is filled with blood which then clots and seals the wound against dehydration and infection.

2. **Acute inflammatory response** This occurs within 24 hours with appearance of polymorphs from the margins of incision. By 3rd day, polymorphs are replaced by macrophages.

3. **Epithelial changes** Basal cells of epidermis from both the cut margins start proliferating and migrating towards incisional space in the form of epithelial spurs. A well-approximated wound is covered by a layer of epithelium in 48 hours. The migrated epidermal cells separate the underlying viable dermis from the overlying necrotic material and clot, forming *scab* which is cast off. The basal cells from the margins continue to divide. By 5th day, a multilayered new epidermis is formed which is differentiated into superficial and deeper layers.

4. **Organisation** By 3rd day, fibroblasts also invade the wound area. By 5th day, new collagen fibrils start forming which dominate till healing is completed. In 4 weeks, the scar tissue with scanty cellular and vascular elements, a few inflammatory cells and epithelialised surface is formed.

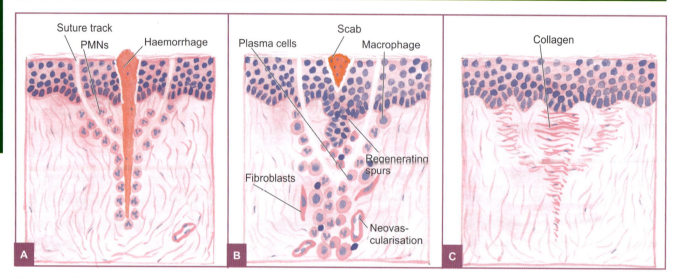

Figure 12.3 ▶ Primary union of skin wounds. A, The incised wound as well as suture track on either side are filled with blood clot and there is inflammatory response from the margins. B, Spurs of epidermal cells migrate along the incised margin on either side as well as around the suture track. Formation of granulation tissue also begins from below. C, Removal of suture at around 7th day results in scar tissue at the sites of incision and suture track.

5. **Suture tracks** Each suture track is a separate wound and incites the same phenomena as in healing of the primary wound i.e. filling the space with haemorrhage, some inflammatory cell reaction, epithelial cell proliferation along the suture track from both margins, fibroblastic proliferation and formation of young collagen. When sutures are removed around 7th day, much of epithelialised suture track is avulsed and the remaining epithelial tissue in the track is absorbed. However, sometimes the suture track gets infected *(stitch abscess)*, or the epithelial cells may persist in the track *(implantation or epidermal cysts)*.

Thus, the scar formed in a sutured wound is neat due to close apposition of the margins of wound; the use of adhesive tapes or metal clips avoids removal of stitches and its complications.

HEALING BY SECOND INTENTION (SECONDARY UNION)

This is defined as healing of a wound having the following characteristics:
i) open with a large tissue defect, at times infected;
ii) having extensive loss of cells and tissues; and
iii) the wound is not approximated by surgical sutures but is left open.

The basic events in secondary union are similar to primary union but differ in having a larger tissue defect which has to be bridged. Hence, healing takes place from the base upward and also from the margins inwards. Healing by second intention is slow and results in a large, at times ugly, scar as compared to rapid healing and neat scar of primary union.

The sequence of events in secondary union is illustrated in **Fig. 12.4** and described below:

1. **Initial haemorrhage** As a result of injury, the wound space is filled with blood and fibrin clot which dries.

2. **Inflammatory phase** There is an initial acute inflammatory response followed by appearance of macrophages which clear off the debris as in primary union.

3. **Epithelial changes** As in primary healing, the epidermal cells from both the margins of wound proliferate and migrate into the wound in the form of epithelial spurs till they meet in the middle and re-epithelialise the gap completely. However, the proliferating epithelial cells do not cover the surface fully until granulation tissue from base has started filling the wound space. In this way, pre-existing viable connective tissue is separated from necrotic material and clot on the surface, forming *scab* which is cast off. In time, the regenerated epidermis becomes stratified and keratinised.

4. **Granulation tissue** Main bulk of secondary healing is by granulations. Granulation tissue is formed by proliferation of fibroblasts and neovascularisation from the adjoining viable elements. The newly-formed granulation tissue is deep red, granular and very fragile. With time, the scar on maturation becomes pale and white due to increase in collagen and decrease in vascularity. Specialised structures of the skin like hair follicles and sweat glands are not replaced unless their viable residues remain which may regenerate.

5. **Wound contraction** Contraction of wound is an important feature of secondary healing, not seen in primary healing. Due to the action of myofibroblasts present in granulation tissue, the wound contracts to one-third to one-fourth of its original size.

6. **Presence of infection** Bacterial contamination of an open wound delays the process of healing due to release

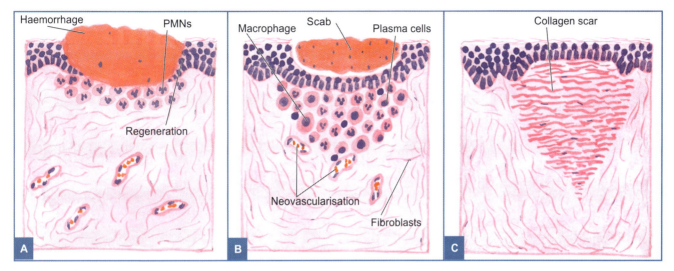

Figure 12.4 ▶ Secondary union of skin wounds. A, The open wound is filled with blood clot and there is inflammatory response at the junction of viable tissue. B, Epithelial spurs from the margins of wound meet in the middle to cover the gap and separate the underlying viable tissue from necrotic tissue at the surface forming scab. C, After contraction of the wound, a scar smaller than the original wound is left.

of bacterial toxins that provoke necrosis, suppuration and thrombosis. Surgical removal of dead and necrosed tissue, *debridement*, helps in preventing the bacterial infection of open wounds.

Differences between primary and secondary union of wounds are given in Table 12.1.

COMPLICATIONS OF WOUND HEALING

During the course of healing, following complications may occur:

1. *Infection* The wound may get infected due to entry of bacteria which delays the healing.
2. *Implantation (epidermal) cyst* Formation of implantation epidermoid cyst may occur due to persistence of epithelial cells in the wound after healing.
3. *Pigmentation* Healed wounds may at times have rust-like colour due to staining with haemosiderin. Some coloured particulate material left in the wound may persist and impart colour to the healed wound.
4. *Deficient scar formation* This may occur due to inadequate formation of granulation tissue.
5. *Incisional hernia* A weak scar, especially after a laparotomy, may be either the site of bursting open of a wound early (wound dehiscence), or later an incisional hernia may occur at this site.
6. *Hypertrophied scars and keloid formation* At times, the scar formed is excessive, ugly and painful. Excessive formation of collagen in healing may result in keloid *(claw-like)* formation, seen more commonly in blacks. Hypertrophied scars differ from keloid in that they are confined to the borders of the initial wound while keloids have tumour-like projection of connective tissue.
7. *Excessive contraction* An exaggeration of wound contraction may result in formation of contractures or cicatrisation e.g. Dupuytren's (palmar) contracture, plantar

Table 12.1	Differences between primary and secondary union of wounds.	
FEATURE	PRIMARY UNION	SECONDARY UNION
1. Cleanliness of wound	Clean	Unclean
2. Infection	Generally uninfected	May be infected
3. Margins	Surgical clean	Irregular
4. Sutures	Used	Not used
5. Healing	Scanty granulation tissue at the incised gap and along suture tracks	Exuberant granulation tissue to fill the gap
6. Outcome	Neat linear scar	Contracted irregular wound
7. Complications	Infrequent, epidermal inclusion cyst formation	Suppuration, may require debridement

contracture and Peyronie's disease (contraction of the cavernous tissues of penis).

8. *Neoplasia* Rarely, scar may be the site for development of carcinoma later e.g. squamous cell carcinoma in Marjolin's ulcer i.e. a scar following burns on the skin.

EXTRACELLULAR MATRIX— WOUND CONTRACTION AND STRENGTH

The wound starts contracting after 2-3 days and the process is completed by the 14th day. During this period, the wound is reduced by approximately 80% of its original size. Contracted wound results in rapid healing since lesser surface area of the injured tissue has to be replaced. The wound is strengthened by proliferation of fibroblasts and myofibroblasts which get structural support from the extracellular matrix (ECM). In addition to providing structural support, ECM can direct cell migration, attachment, differentiation and organisation.

ECM is not a static structure but the matrix proteins comprising it undergo marked remodelling during foetal life which slows down in adult tissues. These matrix proteins are degraded by a family of metalloproteinases which act under regulatory control of inhibitors of metalloproteinases.

ECM has five main components: collagen, adhesive glycoproteins, basement membrane, elastic fibres, and proteoglycans.

1. **COLLAGEN** Collagens are a family of proteins which provide structural support to the multicellular organism. It is the main component of tissues such as fibrous tissue, bone, cartilage, valves of heart, cornea, basement membrane etc.

Collagen is synthesised and secreted by a complex biochemical mechanism on ribosomes. The collagen synthesis is stimulated by various growth factors and is degraded by collagenase. Regulation of collagen synthesis and degradation take place by various local and systemic factors so that the collagen content of normal organs remains constant. On the other hand, defective regulation of collagen synthesis leads to hypertrophied scar, fibrosis, and organ dysfunction.

Depending upon the biochemical composition, 18 types of collagen have been identified called collagen *type I to XVIII,* many of which are unique for specific tissues. Type I collagen is normally present in the skin, bone and tendons and accounts for 90% of collagen in the body:

◆ Type I, III and V are *true fibrillar collagen* which form the main portion of the connective tissue during healing of wounds in scars.

◆ Other types of collagen are *non-fibrillar* and amorphous material seen as component of the basement membranes.

Morphologically, the smallest units of collagen are *collagen fibrils,* which align together in parallel bundles to form *collagen fibres,* and then *collagen bundles.*

2. **ADHESIVE GLYCOPROTEINS** Various adhesive glycoproteins act as glue for the ECM and the cells. These consist of fibronectin, tenascin (cytotactin) and thrombospondin:

i) **Fibronectin** (*nectere* = to bind) is the best characterised glycoprotein in ECM and has binding properties to other cells and ECM. It is of two types—plasma and tissue fibronectin.

◆ *Plasma fibronectin* is synthesised by the liver cells and is trapped in basement membrane such as during filtration through the renal glomerulus.

◆ *Tissue fibronectin* is formed by fibroblasts, endothelial cells and other mesenchymal cells. It is responsible for the primitive matrix such as in the foetus, and in wound healing.

ii) **Tenascin or cytotactin** is the glycoprotein associated with fibroblasts and appears in wound about 48 hours after injury. It disappears from mature scar tissue.

iii) **Thrombospondin** is mainly synthesised by granules of platelets. It functions as adhesive protein for keratinocytes and platelets but is inhibitory to attachment of fibroblasts and endothelial cells.

3. **BASEMENT MEMBRANE** Basement membranes are periodic acid-Schiff (PAS)-positive amorphous structures that lie underneath epithelia of different organs and endothelial cells. They consist of collagen type IV and laminin.

4. **ELASTIC FIBRES** While the tensile strength in tissue comes from collagen, the ability to recoil is provided by elastic fibres. Elastic fibres consist of 2 components—elastin glycoprotein and elastic microfibril. Elastases degrade the elastic tissue e.g. in inflammation, emphysema etc.

5. **PROTEOGLYCANS** These are a group of molecules having 2 components—an essential carbohydrate polymer (called polysaccharide or glycosaminoglycan), and a protein bound to it, and hence the name proteoglycan. Various proteoglycans are distributed in different tissues as under:
i) *Chondroitin sulphate*—abundant in cartilage, dermis
ii) *Heparan sulphate*—in basement membranes
iii) *Dermatan sulphate*—in dermis
iv) *Keratan sulphate*—in cartilage
v) *Hyaluronic acid*—in cartilage, dermis.

In wound healing, the deposition of proteoglycans precedes collagen laying.

The strength of wound also depends upon certain factors such as the site of injury, depth of incision and area of wound. After removal of stitches on around 7th day, the wound strength is approximately 10% which reaches 80% in about 3 months.

FACTORS INFLUENCING HEALING

Two types of factors influence the wound healing: those acting locally, and those acting in general.

A. LOCAL FACTORS:

1. *Infection* is the most important factor acting locally which delays the process of healing.

2. *Poor blood supply* to wound slows healing e.g. injuries to face heal quickly due to rich blood supply while injury to leg with varicose ulcers having poor blood supply heals slowly.

3. *Foreign bodies* including sutures interfere with healing and cause intense inflammatory reaction and infection.

4. *Movement* delays wound healing.

5. Exposure to *ionising radiation* delays granulation tissue formation.

6. Exposure to *ultraviolet light* facilitates healing.

7. *Type, size and location* of injury determines whether healing takes place by resolution or organisation.

B. SYSTEMIC FACTORS:

1. *Age.* Wound healing is rapid in young and somewhat slow in aged and debilitated people due to poor blood supply to the injured area in the latter.

2. *Nutrition.* Deficiency of constituents like protein, vitamin C (scurvy), vitamin A and zinc delays the wound healing.

3. *Systemic infection* delays wound healing.

4. *Administration of glucocorticoids* has anti-inflammatory effect.

5. *Uncontrolled diabetics* are more prone to develop infections and hence delay in healing.

6. *Haematologic abnormalities* like defect of neutrophil functions (chemotaxis and phagocytosis), and neutropenia and bleeding disorders slow the process of wound healing.

> **GIST BOX 12.2 | Healing of Skin Wounds**
>
> ❖ Healing of skin wounds can be accomplished by first intention *(primary union)* and by second intention *(secondary union).*
> ❖ Primary union is healing of a wound which is clean and uninfected, surgically incised, without much loss of cells and tissue. In this, edges of wound are approximated by surgical sutures.
> ❖ Secondary union of a wound is for open with a large tissue defect which are at times infected, having extensive loss of cells and tissues. Here, the wound is not approximated by surgical sutures.
> ❖ The basic events in both primary and secondary union are similar but differ in having a larger tissue defect in secondary union which has to be bridged. Hence, healing takes place from the base upward as well as from the margins inwards.
> ❖ The healing by second intention is slow and results in a large, at times ugly, scar as compared to rapid healing and neat scar of primary union.
> ❖ Complications of wound healing are infection, inclusion cyst formation, pigmentation, incisional hernia, hypertrophied scar and contracture.
> ❖ The wound is strengthened by proliferation of fibroblasts and myofibroblasts which get structural support from the extracellular matrix (ECM).
> ❖ ECM is comprised by collagen, adhesive glycoproteins, basement membrane, elastic tissue and proteoglycans.
> ❖ Various local and systemic factors may influence wound healing.

HEALING IN SPECIALISED TISSUES

Healing of the skin wound provides an example of general process of healing by regeneration and repair. However, in certain specialised tissues, either regeneration or repair may predominate. Some of these examples are described here.

FRACTURE HEALING

Healing of fracture by callus formation depends upon some clinical considerations whether the fracture is:

◈ *traumatic* (in previously normal bone), or *pathological* (in previously diseased bone);

◈ *complete or incomplete* like green-stick fracture; and

◈ *simple* (closed), *comminuted* (splintering of bone), or *compound* (communicating to skin surface).

However, basic events in healing of any type of fracture are similar and resemble healing of skin wound to some extent.

◈ **Primary union of fractures** occurs when the ends of fracture are approximated surgically by application of compression clamps or metal plates. In these cases, bony union takes place with formation of medullary callus without periosteal callus formation. The patient can be made ambulatory early but there is more extensive bone necrosis and slow healing.

◈ **Secondary union** is more common form of fracture healing when the plaster casts are applied for immobilisation of a fracture. Though it is a continuous process, secondary bone union is described under the following 3 headings:
i) Procallus formation
ii) Osseous callus formation
iii) Remodelling

These processes are illustrated in **Fig. 12.5** and described below:

I. PROCALLUS FORMATION Steps involved in the formation of procallus are as follows:

1. Haematoma forms due to bleeding from torn blood vessels, filling the area surrounding the fracture. Loose meshwork is formed by blood and fibrin clot which acts as framework for subsequent granulation tissue formation.

2. Local inflammatory response occurs at the site of injury with exudation of fibrin, polymorphs and macrophages. The macrophages clear away the fibrin, red blood cells, inflammatory exudate and debris. Fragments of necrosed bone are scavenged by macrophages and osteoclasts.

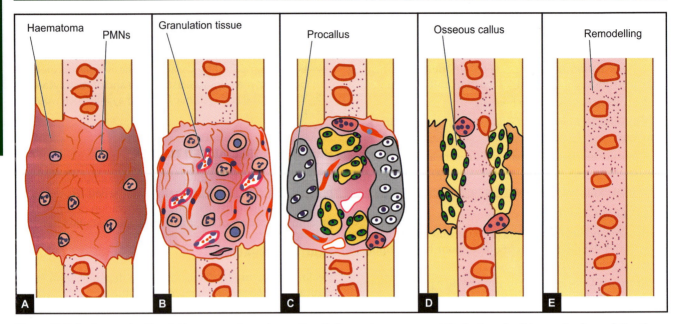

Figure 12.5 ▶ Fracture healing. A, Haematoma formation and local inflammatory response at the fracture site. B, Ingrowth of granulation tissue with formation of soft tissue callus. C, Formation of procallus composed of woven bone and cartilage with its characteristic fusiform appearance and having 3 arbitrary components—external, intermediate and internal callus. D, Formation of osseous callus composed of lamellar bone following clearance of woven bone and cartilage. E, Remodelled bone ends; the external callus cleared away. Intermediate callus converted into lamellar bone and internal callus developing bone marrow cavity.

3. **Ingrowth of granulation tissue** begins with neovascularisation and proliferation of mesenchymal cells from periosteum and endosteum. A soft tissue callus is thus formed which joins the ends of fractured bone without much strength.

4. **Callus composed of woven bone and cartilage** starts within the first few days. The cells of inner layer of the periosteum have osteogenic potential and lay down collagen as well as osteoid matrix in the granulation tissue (Fig. 12.6). The osteoid undergoes calcification and is called *woven bone callus*. A much wider zone over the cortex on either side of fractured ends is covered by the woven bone callus and united to bridge the gap between the ends, giving spindle-shaped or fusiform appearance to the union. In poorly immobilised fractures (e.g. fracture ribs), the subperiosteal osteoblasts may form cartilage at the fracture site. At times, callus is composed of woven bone as well as cartilage, temporarily immobilising the bone ends.

This stage is called provisional callus or procallus formation and is arbitrarily divided into *external, intermediate* and *internal procallus*.

II. OSSEOUS CALLUS FORMATION The procallus acts as scaffolding on which osseous callus composed of lamellar bone is formed. The woven bone is cleared away by incoming osteoclasts and the calcified cartilage disintegrates. In their place, newly-formed blood vessels and osteoblasts invade, laying down osteoid which is calcified and lamellar bone is formed by developing Haversian system concentrically around the blood vessels.

III. REMODELLING During the formation of lamellar bone, osteoblastic laying and osteoclastic removal are taking place remodelling the united bone ends, which after sometime, is

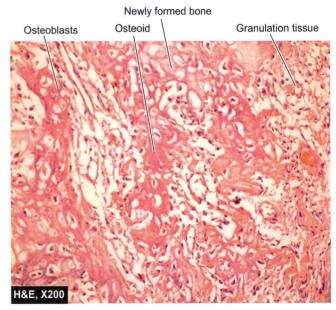

Figure 12.6 ▶ Callus formation in fracture healing.

indistinguishable from normal bone. The external callus is cleared away, compact bone (cortex) is formed in place of intermediate callus and the bone marrow cavity develops in internal callus.

Complications of Fracture Healing

These are as under:

1. **Fibrous union** may result instead of osseous union if the immobilisation of fractured bone is not done. Occasionally, a false joint may develop at the fracture site (pseudo-arthrosis).

2. **Non-union** may result if some soft tissue is interposed between the fractured ends.

3. **Delayed union** may occur from causes of delayed wound healing in general such as infection, inadequate blood supply, poor nutrition, movement and old age.

HEALING OF NERVOUS TISSUE

CENTRAL NERVOUS SYSTEM The nerve cells of the brain, spinal cord and ganglia are permanent cells, and therefore once destroyed are not replaced. Axons of CNS also do not show any significant regeneration. The damaged neuroglial cells, however, may show proliferation of astrocytes called gliosis.

PERIPHERAL NERVOUS SYSTEM In contrast to the cells of CNS, the peripheral nerves show limited regeneration, mainly from proliferation of Schwann cells and fibrils from distal end. The pathologic reactions of the PNS in response to injury may be in the form of one of the types of degenerations causing *peripheral neuropathy* or formation of a *traumatic neuroma*. There are 3 main types of degenerative processes in the PNS—Wallerian degeneration, axonal degeneration and segmental demyelination (Fig. 12.7):

Wallerian degeneration Wallerian degeneration occurs after transection of the axon which may be as a result of knife wounds, compression, traction and ischaemia. Following transection, initially there is accumulation of organelles in the proximal and distal ends of the transection sites. Subsequently, the axon and myelin sheath distal to the transection site undergo disintegration upto the next node of Ranvier, followed by phagocytosis. The process of regeneration occurs by sprouting of axons and proliferation of Schwann cells from the proximal end.

Axonal degeneration In axonal degeneration, degeneration of the axon begins at the peripheral terminal and proceeds backward towards the nerve cell body. The cell body often undergoes chromatolysis. There is Schwann cell proliferation in the region of axonal degeneration. The loss of axonal integrity occurs, probably as a result of some primary metabolic disturbance within the axon itself. Changes similar to those seen in Wallerian degeneration are present but regenerative reaction is limited or absent.

Segmental demyelination Segmental demyelination is similar to demyelination within the brain. Segmental demyelination is loss of myelin of the segment between two consecutive nodes of Ranvier, leaving a denuded axon segment. The axon, however, remains intact. Schwann cell proliferation generally accompanies demyelination. This results in remyelination of the affected axon. Repeated episodes of demyelination and remyelination are associated with concentric proliferation of Schwann cells around axons producing *'onion bulbs'* found in hypertrophic neuropathy.

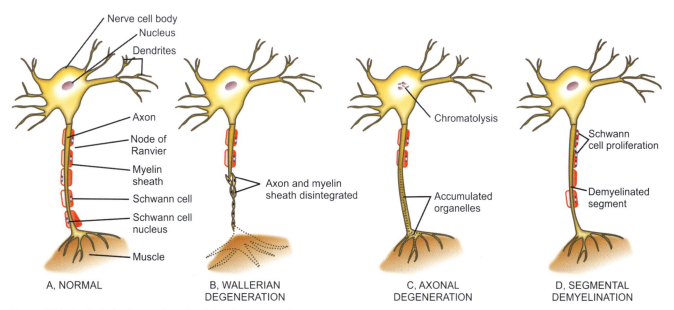

Figure 12.7 ▶ Pathologic reaction of peripheral nerve to injury.

Traumatic neuroma Normally, the injured axon of a peripheral nerve regenerates at the rate of approximately 1 mm per day. However, if the process of regeneration is hampered due to an interposed haematoma or fibrous scar, the axonal sprouts together with Schwann cells and fibroblasts form a peripheral mass called as traumatic or stump neuroma.

HEALING OF MUSCLE

SKELETAL MUSCLE The regeneration of striated muscle is similar to peripheral nerves. On injury, the cut ends of muscle fibres retract but are held together by stromal connective tissue. The injured site is filled with fibrinous material, polymorphs and macrophages. After clearance of damaged fibres by macrophages, one of the following two types of regeneration of muscle fibres can occur:

❖ If the muscle sheath is intact, sarcolemmal tubes containing histiocytes appear along the endomysial tube which, in about 3 months time, restores properly oriented muscle fibres e.g. in Zenker's degeneration of muscle in typhoid fever.

❖ If the muscle sheath is damaged, it forms a disorganised multinucleate mass and scar composed of fibrovascular tissue e.g. in Volkmann's ischaemic contracture.

SMOOTH MUSCLE Non-striated muscle has limited regenerative capacity e.g. appearance of smooth muscle in the arterioles in granulation tissue. However, in large destructive lesions, the smooth muscle is replaced by permanent scar tissue.

CARDIAC MUSCLE Destruction of heart muscle is replaced by fibrous tissue. However, in situations where the endomysium of individual cardiac fibre is intact (e.g. in diphtheria and coxsackie virus infections), regeneration of cardiac fibres may occur in young patients.

HEALING OF MUCOSAL SURFACES

The cells of mucosal surfaces have very good regeneration and are normally being lost and replaced continuously e.g. mucosa of alimentary tract, respiratory tract, urinary tract, uterine endometrium etc. This occurs by proliferation from margins, migration, multilayering and differentiation of epithelial cells in the same way as in the epidermal cells in healing of skin wounds.

HEALING OF SOLID EPITHELIAL ORGANS

Following gross tissue damage to organs like the kidney, liver and thyroid, the replacement is by fibrous scar e.g. in chronic pyelonephritis and cirrhosis of liver. However, in parenchymal cell damage with intact basement membrane or intact supporting stromal tissue, regeneration may occur. For example:

❖ *In tubular necrosis* of the kidney with intact basement membrane, proliferation and slow migration of tubular epithelial cells may occur to form renal tubules again.

❖ *In viral hepatitis,* if part of the liver lobule is damaged with intact stromal network, proliferation of hepatocytes may result in restoration of liver lobule.

| GIST BOX 12.3 | Healing in Specialised Tissues |

❖ Fracture healing may be primary union when the ends of fracture are approximated as is done by application of compression clamps. In these cases, bony union takes place with formation of medullary callus without periosteal callus formation.
❖ Secondary union of fractures is more common and includes procallus and osseous callus formation followed by remodelling of the bone.
❖ While neurons of the brain and spinal cord lose their ability for regeneration and fail to get replaced, healing of peripheral nerves occurs from limited regeneration, mainly from proliferation of Schwann cells and fibrils from distal end. There are 3 main types of degenerative processes in the peripheral nerves—Wallerian degeneration, axonal degeneration and segmental demyelination.
❖ Regeneration of skeletal muscle is similar to peripheral nerves, while damaged myocardium heals by fibrosis. Smooth muscle, however, has limited regenerative capacity.
❖ Healing of mucosal surfaces is by regeneration of the epithelial surface and replaced continuously.
❖ Healing of organs such as kidneys, liver and thyroid is by limited regeneration and some healing by fibrosis.

STEM CELL CONCEPT OF HEALING—REGENERATIVE MEDICINE

Currently, the field of stem cell biology has emerged at the forefront of healing of injured tissue, treatment of diseases and holds promise for tissue transplantation in future.

Stem cells are the primitive cells which have 2 main properties:

i) They have capacity for self renewal.

ii) They can be coaxed into multilineage differentiation (i.e. into any of about 220 types of cells e.g. red cells, myocardial fibres, neurons etc).

Stem cells exist in both embryos and in adult tissues:

❖ In embryos, they function to generate new organs and tissues; their presence for organogenesis has been an established fact.

❖ In adults, they normally function to replace cells during the natural course of cell turnover. For example, stem cells in the bone marrow which spontaneously differentiate into mature haematopoietic cells, has been known for a long time.

However, what is new about stem cells is as follows:

i) Stem cells exist in almost all adult tissues called somatic stem cells and are less numerous.

ii) Other sources of stem cells are embryos and umbilical cord blood; these stem cells are more numerous.

iii) Stem cells can be harvested and grown in the laboratory into a desired cell lineage by transdifferentiation i.e. these cells are pluripotent.

iv) Homing of transfused stem cells is their innate abilty to travel to the desired site in the body and thus they get engrafted there morphologically and functionally.

Some of the major clinical trials on applications of stem cells underway are in the following directions:

1. **Bone marrow stem cells** Haematopoietic stem cells, marrow stromal cells and stem cells sourced from umbilical cord blood have been used for treatment of various forms of blood cancers and other blood disorders for about three decades. However, their use for treatment of other diseases by transdifferentiation is relatively new.

2. **Neuron stem cells** These cells are capable of generating neurons, astrocytes and oligodendroglial cells. It may be possible to use these cells in neurodegenerative diseases such as Parkinsonism and Alzheimer's disease, and in spinal cord injury. Thus, the accepted concept that neurons do not regenerate may not hold true anymore.

3. **Islet cell stem cells** Clinical trials are under way for use of adult mesenchymal stem cells for islet cells in type 1 diabetes.

4. **Cardiac stem cells** It is now known that the heart has cardiac stem cells which have capacity to repair myocardium after infarction.

5. **Skeletal muscle stem cells** Although skeletal muscle cells do not divide when injured, stem cells of muscle have capacity to regenerate.

6. **Adult eye stem cells** The cornea of the eye contains stem cells in the region of limbus. These limbal stem cells have a potential therapeutic use in corneal opacities and damage to the conjunctiva.

7. **Skin stem cells** In the skin, the stem cells are located in the region of hair follicle and sebaceous glands. These stem cells contribute to repair of damaged epidermis. While healing in adults normally takes place with formation of scar and loss of hair, stem cells would elicit a response similar to wound healing in foetal tissue where the healing is by regeneration.

8. **Liver stem cells** In the liver, the stem cells are located in the canal of Hering which connects the bile ductules with hepatocytes. These cells can cause regeneration of fulminant damage to the liver or in chronic hepatitis.

9. **Intestinal stem cells** Crypts of the intestine contain stem cells which form the villi.

10. **Lung tissue stem cells** Clinical trials on the repair of injured lung parenchyma in patients of chronic obstructive pulmonary disease (COPD) is going on.

However, it may be mentioned here that except the bone marrow stem cell therapy and in the cornea, all other clinical trials to test the abilities of different types of stem cells to treat certain diseases and replace injured tissues are in experimental stage, costly and controversial, but are anticipated to have vast usefulness in future.

> **GIST BOX 12.4** **Stem Cell Concept of Healing: Regenerative Medicine**
>
> ❖ Stem cell biology is at the forefront of healing of injured tissue, treatment of diseases and holds promise for tissue transplantation in future.
> ❖ Stem cells are the primitive cells having capacity for self-renewal and that they can be modulated into multilineage differentiation.
> ❖ Stem cells exist in embryos where they are more numerous compared to those in adult tissues where they are fewer.
> ❖ Their presence in the bone marrow has been known for long and they have been used for blood cancers and other blood disorders.
> ❖ However, use of bone marrow stem cells for other diseases and sourcing of adult stem cells from other organs and their use for damaged organ is relatively new.

13 Infectious and Parasitic Diseases

INTRODUCTION

Microorganisms, namely bacteria, viruses, fungi and parasites, are present everywhere—in the soil, water, atmosphere and on the body surfaces, and are responsible for a large number of infectious diseases in human beings. Some microorganisms are distributed throughout the world while others are limited to certain geographic regions only. In general, tropical and developing countries are particularly affected more by infectious diseases than the developed countries.

❖ There are several examples of certain *infectious diseases* which are not so common in the developed world now but they continue to be major health problems in the developing countries e.g. tuberculosis, leprosy, typhoid fever, cholera, measles, pertussis, malaria, amoebiasis, pneumonia etc.

❖ *Vaccines* have, however, been successful in controlling or eliminating some diseases all over the world e.g. smallpox, poliomyelitis, measles, pertussis etc. Similarly, insecticides have helped in controlling malaria to an extent.

❖ However, infections still rank very high *as a cause of death* in the world. Reasons for this trend are not difficult to seek:

i) Development of newer and antibiotic-resistant strains of microorganisms; classic example is that of methicillin-resistant *Staph. aureus* (MRSA).

ii) Administration of immunosuppressive therapy to patients with malignant tumours and transplanted organs making them susceptible to *opportunistic infections*.

iii) Increasing number of patients reporting to hospital for different illnesses but instead many developing hospital-acquired infections.

iv) Lastly, discovery in 1981 of previously unknown deadly disease i.e. acquired immunodeficiency syndrome (AIDS) caused by human immunodeficiency virus (HIV).

While talking of microbial infective diseases, let us not forget the fact that many microorganisms may actually benefit mankind. Following is the range of *host-organism inter-relationship*, which may vary quite widely:

1. *Symbiosis* i.e. cooperative association between two dissimilar organisms beneficial to both.
2. *Commensalism* i.e. two dissimilar organisms living together benefitting one without harming the other.
3. *True parasitism* i.e. two dissimilar organisms living together benefitting the parasite but harming the host.
4. *Saprophytism* i.e. organisms thriving on dead tissues.

Besides microorganisms, a modified infectious host protein present in the mammalian CNS has been identified called *prion protein*. Prions are transmissible agents similar to infectious particles but lack nucleic acid. These agents are implicated in the etiology of spongiform encephalopathy (including kuru), bovine spongiform encephalopathy (or mad cow disease) and Creutzfeldt-Jakob disease or CJD (associated with corneal transplantation). (Dr Prusiner who discovered prion protein was awarded Nobel Prize in medicine in 1997).

Transmission of infectious diseases requires a chain of events and is the consequence of inter-relationship between disease-producing properties of microorganisms and host-defense capability against the invading organisms. Briefly, chain in transmission of infections and factors determining this host-microorganism relationship are given below:

Chain in Transmission of Infectious Diseases

Transmission of infections occurs following a chain of events pertaining to various parameters as under:

i) Reservoir of pathogen Infection occurs from the source of reservoir of pathogen. It may be a human being (e.g. in influenza virus), animal (e.g. dog for rabies), insect (e.g. mosquito for malaria), or soil (e.g. enterobiasis).

ii) Route of infection Infection is transmitted from the reservoir to the human being by different routes, usually from breach in the mucosa or the skin, at the portal of exit from the reservoir as well as the portal of entry in the susceptible host. In general, the organism is transmitted to the site where it would normally flourish e.g. *N. gonorrhoeae* usually inhabits the male and female urethra and, therefore, the route of transmission would be sexual contact.

iii) Mode of transmission The organism may be transmitted directly by physical contact or by faecal contamination (e.g. spread of eggs in hookworm infestation), or indirectly by fomites (e.g. insect bite).

iv) Susceptible host The organism would colonise the host if the host has good immunity but such a host can pass on infection to others. However, if the host is old, debilitated, malnourished, or immunosuppressed due any etiology, he is susceptible to have manifestations of infection.

Key to management of infection lies in breaking or blocking this chain for transmission and spread of infection.

Factors Relating to Infectious Agents

Microbial factors favouring transmission of infections are as under:

1. Mode of entry Microorganisms causing infectious diseases may gain entry into the body by various routes e.g.
i) through ingestion (external route);
ii) inoculation (parenteral method);
iii) inhalation (respiration);
iv) perinatally (vertical transmission);
v) by direct contact (contagious infection); and
vi) by contaminated water, food, soil, environment or from an animal host (zoonotic infections).

2. Spread of infection Microorganisms after entering the body may spread further through the phagocytic cells, blood vessels and lymphatics.

3. Virulence of organisms Many species and strains of organisms may have varying virulence e.g. the three strains of *C. diphtheriae (gravis, intermedius* and *mitis)* produce the same diphtherial exotoxin but in different amounts.

4. Production of toxins Bacteria liberate toxins which have effects on cell metabolism. *Endotoxins* are liberated on lysis of the bacterial cell while *exotoxins* are secreted by bacteria and have effects at distant sites too.

5. Product of organisms Some organisms produce enzymes that help in spread of infections e.g. hyaluronidase by *Cl. welchii*, streptokinase by streptococci, staphylokinase and coagulase by staphylococci.

Factors Relating to Host

Microorganisms invade human body when defenses are not adequate. These factors include the following:

1. Physical barrier A break in the continuity of the skin and mucous membranes allows the microorganisms to enter the body.

2. Chemical barrier Mucus secretions of the oral cavity and the alimentary tract and gastric acidity prevent bacterial colonisation.

3. Effective drainage Natural passages of the hollow organs like respiratory, gastrointestinal, urinary and genital system provide a way to drain the excretions effectively. Similarly, ducts of various glands are the conduits of drainage of secretions. Obstruction in any of these passages promotes infection.

4. Immune defense mechanisms These include the phagocytic leucocytes of blood (polymorphs and monocytes), phagocytes of tissues (mononuclear-phagocyte system) and the immune system as discussed in Chapter 14.

Some of the common diseases produced by pathogenic microorganisms are discussed in this chapter. Each group of microorganisms discussed here is accompanied by a Table listing diseases produced by them. These lists of diseases are in no way complete but include only important and common examples. No attempts will be made to give details of organisms as that would mean repeating what is given in the textbooks of Microbiology. Instead, salient clinico-pathologic aspects of these diseases are highlighted.

Methods of Identification

The organisms causing infections and parasitic diseases may be identified by routine H & E stained sections in many instances **(Table 13.1)**. However, confirmation in most cases requires either application of special staining techniquesor is confirmed by molecular biologic methods **(Fig. 13.1)**. In addition, culture of lesional tissue should be carried out for species identification and drug sensitivity. Generally, the organism is looked for at the advancing edge of the lesion in the tissue section rather than in the necrotic centre.

Table 13.1 Methods of identification of microorganisms.

1. BACTERIA
   i. Gram stain: Most bacteria
   ii. Acid fast stain: Mycobacteria, Nocardia
   iii. Giemsa: Campylobacteria
2. FUNGI
   i. Silver stain: Most fungi
   ii. Periodic acid-Schiff (PAS): Most fungi
   iii. Mucicarmine: Cryptococci
3. PARASITES
   i. Giemsa: Malaria, Leishmania
   ii. Periodic acid-Schiff: Amoebae
   iii. Silver stain: Pneumocystis
4. ALL CLASSES INCLUDING VIRUSES
   i. Culture
   ii. *In situ* hybridisation
   iii. DNA analysis
   iv. Polymerase chain reaction (PCR)

GIST BOX 13.1 Infections and Infestations: Introduction

- Certain infectious diseases continue to be major health problems in the developing countries e.g. tuberculosis, leprosy, typhoid fever, cholera, measles, pertussis, malaria, amoebiasis, pneumonia etc.
- Factors pertaining to the organism and the host determine the outcome of any microbial infection.
- Microbial factors favouring transmission of infections are its mode of entry, spread of infection, virulence, production of toxins, and other products.
- Host factors favouring invasion by microorganisms are breach in physical and chemical barrier, block in drainage, impaired immunity.

Section II: Inflammation and Healing, Immunity and Hypersensitivity, Infections and Infestations

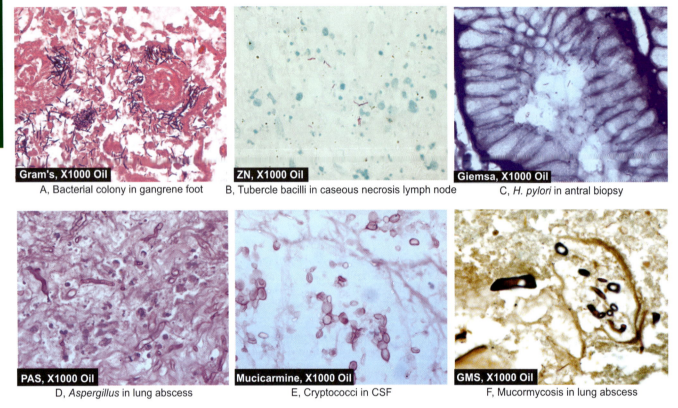

Figure 13.1 ▶ Common stains used for demonstration of microbes. A, Gram's stain. B, Ziehl-Neelsen (ZN) or AFB stain. C, Giemsa stain. D, Periodic acid Schiff (PAS) stain. E, Mucicarmine stain. F, Gomori methenamine silver (GMS) stain.

❖ Identification of organism is done by routine H & E stain, special stains (Gram's, Giemsa, AFB, PAS, GMS), culture and molecular methods.

DISEASES CAUSED BY BACTERIA, SPIROCHAETES AND MYCOBACTERIA

In order to gain an upper hand in human host, bacteria must resist early engulfment by neutrophils. They survive and damage the host in a variety of ways such as by generation of toxins (e.g. gas-forming anaerobes), by forming a slippery capsule that resists attachment to macrophages (e.g. pneumococci), by inhibition of fusion of phagocytic vacuoles with lysosomes (e.g. tubercle bacilli) etc.

Table 13.2 provides an abbreviated classification of bacterial diseases and their etiologic agents. A few common and important examples amongst these are discussed below.

ENTERIC FEVER (TYPHOID FEVER)

The term enteric fever is used to describe acute infection caused by *Salmonella typhi* (typhoid fever) or *Salmonella paratyphi* (paratyphoid fever). Besides these 2 salmonellae, *Salmonella typhimurium* causes food poisoning.

PATHOGENESIS The typhoid bacilli are ingested through contaminated food or water. During the initial asymptomatic incubation period of about 2 weeks, the bacilli invade the lymphoid follicles and Peyer's patches of the small intestine and proliferate. Following this, the bacilli invade the bloodstream causing bacteraemia, and the characteristic clinical features of the disease like continuous rise in temperature and 'rose spots' on the skin are observed. Immunological reactions (Widal's test) begin after about 10 days and peak titres are seen by the end of the third week. Eventually, the bacilli are localised in the intestinal lymphoid tissue (producing typhoid intestinal lesions), in the mesenteric lymph nodes (leading to haemorrhagic lymphadenitis), in the liver (causing foci of parenchymal necrosis), in the gallbladder (producing typhoid cholecystitis), and in the spleen (resulting in splenic reactive hyperplasia).

MORPHOLOGIC FEATURES The lesions are observed in the intestines as well as in other organs.

1. INTESTINAL LESIONS *Grossly,* terminal ileum is affected most often, but lesions may be seen in the jejunum and colon. Peyer's patches show oval typhoid ulcers with their *long axis along the length of the bowel* (*c.f.* tuberculous ulcers of small intestine, page 143). The base of the

Chapter 13: Infectious and Parasitic Diseases

Table 13.2	Diseases caused by bacteria, spirochaetes and mycobacteria.
DISEASE	ETIOLOGIC AGENT
1. Typhoid (enteric) fever*	*Salmonella typhi*
2. Plague	*Yersinia pestis*
3. Anthrax	*Bacillus anthracis*
4. Whooping cough* (pertussis)	*Bordetella pertussis*
5. Chancroid	*Haemophilus ducreyi*
6. Donovanosis (granuloma inguinale)	*Calymmatobacterium donovani*
7. Lymphogranuloma venereum	*Chlamydia trachomatis*
8. Cat-scratch disease*	*Bartonella henselae*
9. Gonorrhoea	*Neisseria gonorrhoeae*
10. Cholera	*Vibrio cholerae*
11. Shigellosis*	*S. dysenteriae, S. flexneri, S. boydii, S. sonnei*
12. Brucellosis	*B. melitensis, B. abortus, B. suis, B. canis*
13. Diphtheria	*Corynebacterium diphtheriae*
14. Lobar pneumonia*	*Streptococcus pneumoniae, Staphylococcus aureus, Haemophilus influenzae, Klebsiella pneumoniae*
15. Bronchopneumonia*	*Staphylococci, Streptococci, K. pneumoniae, H. influenzae*
16. Bacterial meningitis	*Escherichia coli, H. influenzae, Neisseria meningitidis, Streptococcus pneumoniae*
17. Bacterial endocarditis (page 507)	*Staphylococcus aureus, Streptococcus viridans*
18. Other staphylococcal infections*	*S. aureus, S. epidermidis, S. saprophyticus*
19. Streptococcal infections*	*S. pyogenes, S. faecalis, S. pneumoniae. S. viridans*
20. *E. coli* infections (Urinary tract infection)	*Escherichia coli*
21. Clostridial diseases*	
i) Gas gangrene	*C. perfringens*
ii) Tetanus	*C. tetani*
iii) Botulism	*C. botulinum*
iv) Clostridial food poisoning	*C. perfringens*
v) Necrotising enterocolitis	*C. perfringens*
22. Tuberculosis (page 132)	*Mycobacterium tuberculosis*
23. Leprosy (page 144)	*Mycobacterium leprae*
24. Syphilis (page 149)	*Treponema pallidum*
25. Actinomycosis (page 151)	*Actinomyces israelii*
26. Nocardiosis	*Nocardia asteroides*
27. Lyme disease	*Borrelia burgdorferi*

*Diseases discussed in this chapter.

ulcers is black due to sloughed mucosa. The margins of the ulcers are slightly raised due to inflammatory oedema and cellular proliferation. There is never significant fibrosis and hence fibrous stenosis seldom occurs in healed typhoid lesions. The regional lymph nodes are invariably enlarged (Fig. 13.2, A).

Microscopically, there is hyperaemia, oedema and cellular proliferation consisting of phagocytic histiocytes (showing characteristic erythrophagocytosis), lymphocytes and plasma cells. Though enteric fever is an example of acute inflammation, neutrophils are invariably absent from the cellular infiltrate and this is reflected in the leucopenia with neutropenia and relative lymphocytosis in the peripheral blood (Fig. 13.2, B).

The main **complications** of the intestinal lesions of typhoid are perforation of the ulcers and haemorrhage.

2. OTHER LESIONS Besides the intestinal involvement, various other organs and tissues showing pathological changes in enteric fever are as under:

i) *Mesenteric lymph nodes*—haemorrhagic lymphadenitis.
ii) *Liver*—foci of parenchymal necrosis.
iii) *Gallbladder*—typhoid cholecystitis.
iv) *Spleen*—splenomegaly with reactive hyperplasia.
v) *Kidneys*—nephritis.
vi) *Abdominal muscles*—Zenker's degeneration.
vii) *Joints*—arthritis.
viii) *Bones*—osteomyelitis.
ix) *Meninges*—meningitis.
x) *Testis*—orchitis.

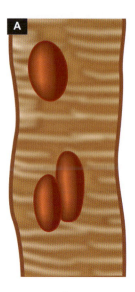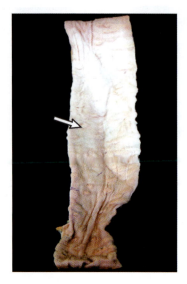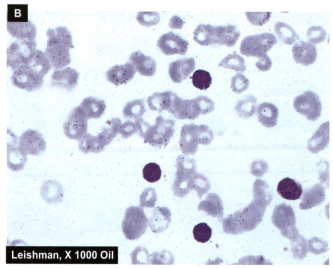

Figure 13.2 ▶ A, Typhoid ulcers in the small intestine appear characteristically oval with their long axis parallel to the long axis of the bowel. B, Blood picture in typhoid fever showing neutropenia and relative lymphocytosis.

Persistence of organism in the gallbladder or urinary tract may result in passage of organisms in the faeces or urine creating a 'carrier state' which is a source of infection to others.

SHIGELLOSIS (BACILLARY DYSETENRY)

Shigellosis or bacillary dysentery is the term used for infection by *Shigella* species: *S. dysenteriae, S. flexneri, S. boydii* and *S. sonnei*. Infection occurs by faeco-oral route and is seen with poor personal hygiene, in densely populated areas, and with contaminated food and water. The common housefly plays a role in spread of infection.

Grossly, the lesions are mainly found in the colon and occasionally in the ileum. Superficial transverse ulcerations of mucosa of the bowel wall occur in the region of lymphoid follicles but perforation is seldom seen. The intervening intact mucosa is hyperaemic and oedematous. Following recovery from the acute attack, complete healing usually takes place.

Microscopically, the mucosa overlying the lymphoid follicles is necrosed. The surrounding mucosa shows congestion, oedema and infiltration by neutrophils and lymphocytes. The mucosa may be covered by greyish-yellow *'pseudomembrane'* composed of fibrinosuppurative exudate.

Complications of bacillary dysentery are haemorrhage, perforation, stenosis, polyarthritis and iridocyclitis.

PNEUMONIAS

Pneumonia is defined as acute inflammation of the lung parenchyma distal to the terminal bronchioles (consisting of the respiratory bronchiole, alveolar ducts, alveolar sacs and alveoli). The terms 'pneumonia' and 'pneumonitis' are often used synonymously for inflammation of the lungs, while 'consolidation' (meaning solidification) is the term used for gross and radiologic appearance of the lungs in pneumonia.

PATHOGENESIS The microorganisms gain entry into the lungs by one of the following four routes:

1. *Inhalation* of the microbes present in the air.
2. *Aspiration* of organisms from the nasopharynx or oropharynx.
3. *Haematogenous spread* from a distant focus of infection.
4. *Direct spread* from an adjoining site of infection.

The normal lung is free of bacteria because of the presence of a number of lung defense mechanisms at different levels such as nasopharyngeal filtering action, mucociliary action of the lower respiratory airways, the presence of phagocytosing alveolar macrophages and immunoglobulins. Failure of these defense mechanisms and presence of certain predisposing factors result in pneumonias. These conditions are as under:

1. Altered consciousness The oropharyngeal contents may be aspirated in states causing unconsciousness e.g. in coma, cranial trauma, seizures, cerebrovascular accidents, drug overdose, alcoholism etc.

2. Depressed cough and glottic reflexes Depression of effective cough may allow aspiration of gastric contents e.g.

in old age, pain from trauma or thoracoabdominal surgery, neuromuscular disease, weakness due to malnutrition, kyphoscoliosis, severe obstructive pulmonary diseases, endotracheal intubation and tracheostomy.

3. **Impaired mucociliary transport** The normal protection offered by mucus-covered ciliated epithelium in the airways from the larynx to the terminal bronchioles is impaired or destroyed in many conditions favouring passage of bacteria into the lung parenchyma. These conditions are cigarette smoking, viral respiratory infections, immotile cilia syndrome, inhalation of hot or corrosive gases and old age.

4. **Impaired alveolar macrophage function** Pneumonias may occur when alveolar macrophage function is impaired e.g. by cigarette smoke, hypoxia, starvation, anaemia, pulmonary oedema and viral respiratory infections.

5. **Endobronchial obstruction** Effective clearance mechanism is interfered in endobronchial obstruction from tumour, foreign body, cystic fibrosis and chronic bronchitis.

6. **Immunocompromised states** Disorders of lymphocytes including congenital and acquired immunodeficiencies (e.g. AIDS, debility, senility, immunosuppressive therapy) and granulocyte abnormalities may predispose to pneumonia.

CLASSIFICATION There are several classification schemes for pneumonias:

I. On the basis of the *anatomic region* of the lung parenchyma involved, pneumonias are traditionally classified into 3 main types:
1. Lobar pneumonia
2. Bronchopneumonia (or Lobular pneumonia)
3. Interstitial pneumonia.

II. Based on the *clinical settings* in which infection occurred, pneumonias are classified as under:
1. Community-acquire pneumonia
2. Health care-associated pneumonia (including hospital-acquired pneumonia)
3. Ventilator-associated pneumonia

III. Based on *etiology and pathogenesis*, pneumonias are classified as under:
A. Bacterial pneumonia
B. Viral pneumonia
C. Pneumonias from other etiologies.

In the present discussion, a combined approach of etiologic and morphologic classification will be followed.

Bacterial Pneumonia

Bacterial infection of the lung parenchyma is the most common cause of pneumonia or consolidation of one or both the lungs. Two types of acute bacterial pneumonias are distinguished—lobar pneumonia and broncho-(lobular-) pneumonia, each with distinct etiologic agent and morphologic changes. Another type distinguished by some workers separately is *confluent pneumonia* which combines the features of both lobar and bronchopneumonia and involves larger (confluent) areas in both the lungs irregularly, while others consider this as a variant of bronchopneumonia.

Lobar Pneumonia

Lobar pneumonia is an acute bacterial infection of a part of a lobe, the entire lobe, or even two lobes of one or both the lungs.

ETIOLOGY Based on the etiologic microbial agent causing lobar pneumonia, following types of lobar pneumonia are described:

1. **Pneumococcal pneumonia** More than 90% of all lobar pneumonias are caused by *Streptococcus pneumoniae*, a lancet-shaped diplococcus. Out of various types, type 3 *S. pneumoniae* causes particularly virulent form of lobar pneumonia. Pneumococcal pneumonia in majority of cases is community-acquired infection.

2. **Staphylococcal pneumonia** *Staphylococcus aureus* causes pneumonia by haematogenous spread of infection from another focus or after viral infections.

3. **Streptococcal pneumonia** β-haemolytic streptococci may rarely cause pneumonia such as in children after measles or influenza, in severely debilitated elderly patients and in diabetics.

4. **Pneumonia by gram-negative aerobic bacteria** Less common causes of lobar pneumonia are gram-negative bacteria like *Haemophilus influenzae, Klebsiella pneumoniae (Friedlander's bacillus), Pseudomonas, Proteus* and *Escherichia coli, H. influenzae* commonly causes pneumonia in children below 3 years of age after a preceding viral infection.

MORPHOLOGIC FEATURES Laennec's original description divides lobar pneumonia into 4 sequential pathologic phases: *stage of congestion* (initial phase), *red hepatisation* (early consolidation), *grey hepatisation* (late consolidation) and *resolution*. However, these classic stages seen in untreated cases are found much less often nowadays due to early institution of antibiotic therapy and improved medical care.

In lobar pneumonia, as the name suggests, part of a lobe, a whole lobe, or two lobes are involved, sometimes bilaterally. The lower lobes are affected most commonly. The sequence of pathologic changes described below represents the inflammatory response of lungs in bacterial infection.

1 STAGE OF CONGESTION: INITIAL PHASE (Fig. 13.3, A) The initial phase represents the early acute inflammatory response to bacterial infection that lasts for 1 to 2 days.

Grossly, the affected lobe is enlarged, heavy, dark red and congested. Cut surface exudes blood-stained frothy fluid.

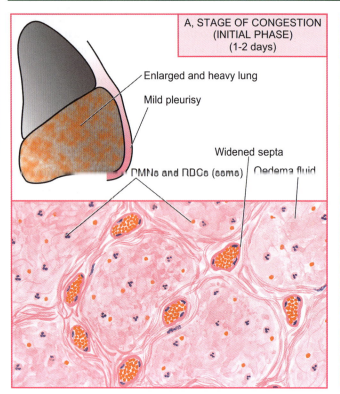
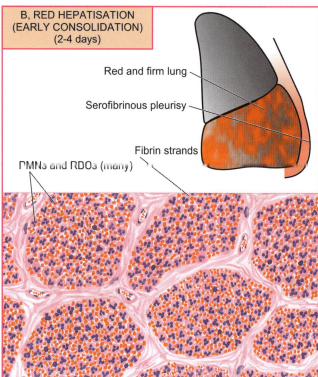
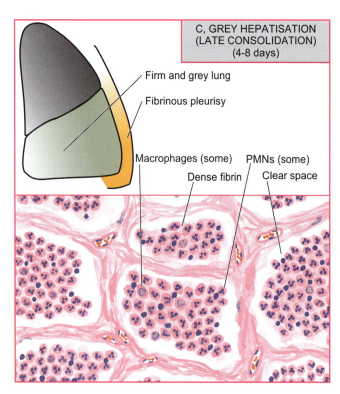
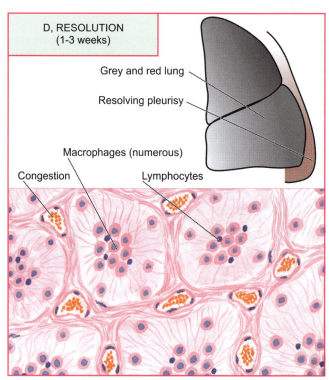

Figure 13.3 ▶ Four stages of lobar pneumonia, showing correlation of gross appearance of the lung with microscopic features in each stage. For details consult the text.

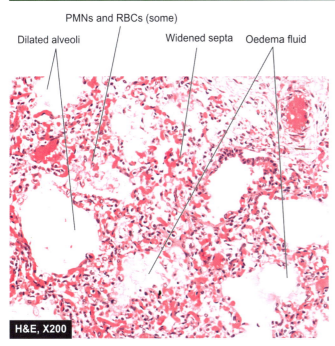

Figure 13.4 ▶ Lobar pneumonia, acute congestion stage. There is congestion of septal walls while the air spaces contain pale oedema fluid and a few red cells.

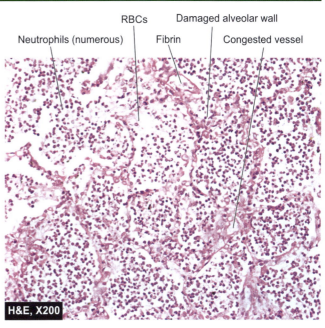

Figure 13.5 ▶ Lobar pneumonia, red hepatisation stage. The alveoli are filled with cellular exudates composed of neutrophils admixed with some red cells.

Histologically, typical features of acute inflammatory response to the organisms are seen. These are as under (Fig. 13.4):
i) Dilatation and congestion of the capillaries in the alveolar walls.
ii) Pale eosinophilic oedema fluid in the air spaces.
iii) A few red cells and neutrophils in the intra-alveolar fluid.
iv) Numerous bacteria demonstrated in the alveolar fluid by Gram's staining.

2. RED HEPATISATION: EARLY CONSOLIDATION (Fig. 13.3, B) This phase lasts for 2 to 4 days. The term hepatisation in pneumonia refers to liver-like consistency of the affected lobe on cut section.

Grossly, the affected lobe is red, firm and consolidated. The cut surface of the involved lobe is airless, red-pink, dry, granular and has liver-like consistency. The stage of red hepatisation is accompanied by serofibrinous pleurisy.

Histologically, the following features are observed (Fig. 13.5):
i) The oedema fluid of the preceding stage is replaced by strands of fibrin.
ii) There is marked cellular exudate of neutrophils and extravasation of red cells.
iii) Many neutrophils show ingested bacteria.
iv) The alveolar septa are less prominent than in the first stage due to cellular exudation.

3. GREY HEPATISATION: LATE CONSOLIDATION (Fig. 13.3, C) This phase lasts for 4 to 8 days.

Grossly, the affected lobe is firm and heavy. The cut surface is dry, granular and grey in appearance with liver-like consistency (Fig. 13.6, A). The change in colour from red to grey begins at the hilum and spreads towards the periphery. Fibrinous pleurisy is prominent.

Histologically, the following changes are present (Fig. 13.6, B):
i) The fibrin strands are dense and more numerous.
ii) The cellular exudate of neutrophils is reduced due to disintegration of many inflammatory cells as evidenced by their pyknotic nuclei. The red cells are also fewer. The macrophages begin to appear in the exudate.
iii) The cellular exudate is often separated from the septal walls by a thin clear space.
iv) The organisms are less numerous and appear as degenerated forms.

4. RESOLUTION (Fig. 13.3, D) This stage begins by 8th to 9th day if no chemotherapy is administered and is completed in 1 to 3 weeks. However, antibiotic therapy induces resolution on about 3rd day. Resolution proceeds in a progressive manner.

Grossly, the previously solid fibrinous constituent is liquefied by enzymatic action, eventually restoring the normal aeration in the affected lobe. The process of softening begins centrally and spreads to the periphery.

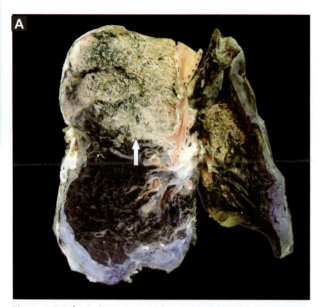
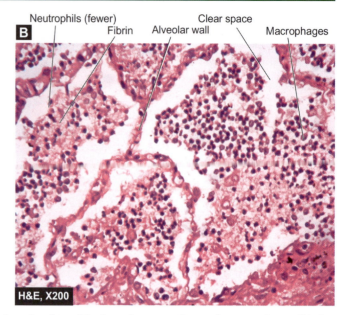

Figure 13.6 ▶ Lobar pneumonia, grey hepatisation stage. A, The sectioned surface of the lung shows grey-brown, firm area of consolidation (liver-like) affecting a lobe (arrow). B, The cellular exudate in the alveolar lumina is lying separated from the septal walls by a clear space. The infiltrate in the lumina is composed of neutrophils and macrophages.

The cut surface is grey-red or dirty brown and frothy, yellow, creamy fluid can be expressed on pressing. The pleural reaction may also show resolution but may undergo organisation leading to fibrous obliteration of pleural cavity.

Histologically, the following features are noted:
i) Macrophages are the predominant cells in the alveolar spaces, while neutrophils diminish in number. Many of the macrophages contain engulfed neutrophils and debris.
ii) Granular and fragmented strands of fibrin in the alveolar spaces are seen due to progressive enzymatic digestion.
iii) Alveolar capillaries are engorged.
iv) There is progressive removal of fluid content as well as cellular exudate from the air spaces, partly by expectoration but mainly by lymphatics, resulting in restoration of normal lung parenchyma with aeration.

COMPLICATIONS Since the advent of antibiotics, serious complications of lobar pneumonia are uncommon. However, they may develop in neglected cases and in patients with impaired immunologic defenses. These are as under:

1. Organisation In about 3% of cases, resolution of the exudate does not occur but instead it undergoes organisation. There is ingrowth of fibroblasts from the alveolar septa resulting in fibrosed, tough, airless leathery lung tissue. This type of post-pneumonic fibrosis is called *carnification.*

2. Pleural effusion About 5% of treated cases of lobar pneumonia develop inflammation of the pleura with effusion. The pleural effusion usually resolves but sometimes may undergo organisation with fibrous adhesions between visceral and parietal pleura.

3. Empyema Less than 1% of treated cases of lobar pneumonia develop encysted pus in the pleural cavity termed empyema.

4. Lung abscess A rare complication of lobar pneumonia is formation of lung abscess, especially when there is secondary infection by other organisms.

5. Metastatic infection Occasionally, infection in the lungs and pleural cavity in lobar pneumonia may extend into the pericardium and the heart causing purulent pericarditis, bacterial endocarditis and myocarditis. Other forms of metastatic infection encountered rarely in lobar pneumonias are otitis media, mastoiditis, meningitis, brain abscess and purulent arthritis.

CLINICAL FEATURES Classically, the onset of lobar pneumonia is sudden. The major symptoms are: shaking chills, fever, malaise with pleuritic chest pain, dyspnoea and cough with expectoration which may be mucoid, purulent or even bloody. The common physical findings are fever, tachycardia, and tachypnoea, and sometimes cyanosis if the patient is severely hypoxaemic. There is generally a marked neutrophilic leucocytosis. Blood cultures are positive in about 30% of cases. Chest radiograph may reveal consolidation. Culture of the organisms in the sputum and antibiotic sensitivity are most significant investigations for institution of specific antibiotics. The response to antibiotics is usually rapid with clinical improvement in 48 to 72 hours after the initiation of antibiotics.

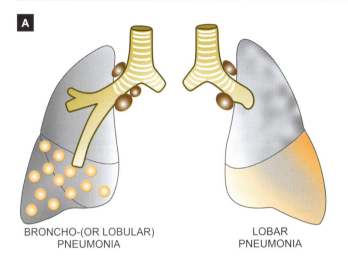
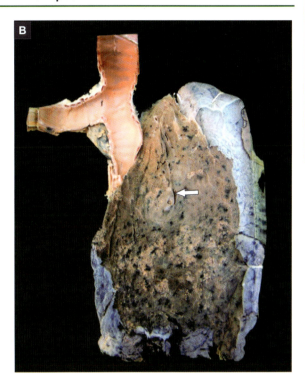

Figure 13.7 ▶ A, Gross appearance of bronchopneumonia contrasted with that of lobar pneumonia. B, The pleural surface of the specimen of the lung shows serofibrinous exudate. The sectioned surface shows multiple, small, grey-brown, firm, patchy areas of consolidation around bronchioles (arrow), while the intervening lung is spongy.

Bronchopneumonia (Lobular Pneumonia)

Bronchopneumonia or lobular pneumonia is infection of the terminal bronchioles that extends into the surrounding alveoli resulting in patchy consolidation of the lung. The condition is particularly frequent at the extremes of life (i.e. in infancy and old age), as a terminal event in chronic debilitating diseases and as a secondary infection following viral respiratory infections such as influenza, measles etc.

ETIOLOGY Common organisms responsible for bronchopneumonia are staphylococci, streptococci, pneumococci, *Klebsiella pneumoniae, Haemophilus influenzae,* and gram-negative bacilli like *Pseudomonas* and coliform bacteria.

MORPHOLOGIC FEATURES Grossly, bronchopneumonia is identified by patchy areas of red or grey consolidation affecting one or more lobes, frequently found bilaterally and more often involving the lower zones of the lungs due to gravitation of the secretions. On cut surface, these patchy consolidated lesions are dry, granular, firm, red or grey in colour, 3 to 4 cm in diameter, slightly elevated over the surface and are often centred around a bronchiole (Fig. 13.7). These patchy areas are best picked up by passing the fingertips on the cut surface.

Histologically, the following features are observed (Fig. 13.8):
i) Acute bronchiolitis.
ii) Suppurative exudate, consisting chiefly of neutrophils, in the peribronchiolar alveoli.
iii) Thickening of the alveolar septa by congested capillaries and leucocytic infiltration.
iv) Less involved alveoli contain oedema fluid.

COMPLICATIONS The complications of lobar pneumonia may occur in bronchopneumonia as well. However, complete resolution of bronchopneumonia is uncommon. There is generally some degree of destruction of the bronchioles resulting in foci of bronchiolar fibrosis that may eventually cause bronchiectasis.

CLINICAL FEATURES The patients of bronchopneumonia are generally infants or elderly individuals. There may be history of preceding bed-ridden illness, chronic debility, aspiration of gastric contents or upper respiratory infection. For initial 2 to 3 days, there are features of acute bronchitis but subsequently signs and symptoms similar to those of lobar pneumonia appear. Blood examination usually shows a neutrophilic leucocytosis. Chest radiograph shows mottled, focal opacities in both the lungs, chiefly in the lower zones.

The salient features of the two main types of bacterial pneumonias are contrasted in Table 13.3.

WHOOPING COUGH (PERTUSSIS)

Whooping cough is a highly communicable acute bacterial disease of childhood caused by *Bordetella pertussis*. The use of DPT vaccine has reduced the prevalence of whooping cough in different populations.

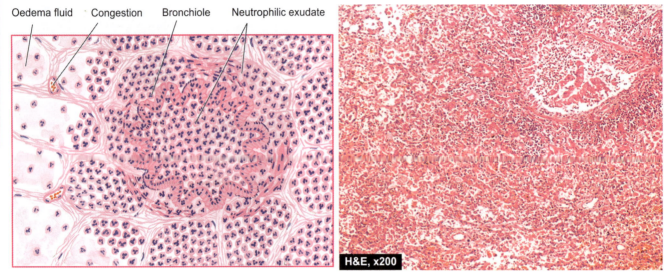

Figure 13.8 ▶ Microscopic appearance of bronchopneumonia. The bronchioles as well as the adjacent alveoli are filled with exudate consisting chiefly of neutrophils. The alveolar septa are thickened due to congested capillaries and neutrophilic infiltrate.

The causative organism, *B. pertussis,* has strong tropism for the brush border of the bronchial epithelium. The organisms proliferate here and stimulate the bronchial epithelium to produce abundant tenacious mucus. Within 7-10 days after exposure, catarrhal stage begins which is the most infectious stage. There is low grade fever, rhinorrhoea, conjunctivitis and excess tear production. Paroxysms of cough occur with characteristic 'whoop'. The condition is self-limiting but may cause death due to asphyxia in infants. *B. pertussis* produces a heat-labile toxin, a heat-stable endotoxin, and a lymphocytosis-producing factor called histamine-sensitising factor.

Microscopically, the lesions in the respiratory tract consist of necrotic bronchial epithelium covered by thick mucopurulent exudate. In severe cases, there is mucosal erosion and hyperaemia. The peripheral blood shows marked lymphocytosis up to 90% **(Fig. 13.9)** and enlargement of lymphoid follicles in the bronchial mucosa and peribronchial lymph nodes.

Table 13.3 Contrasting features of lobar pneumonia and bronchopneumonia.

	FEATURE	LOBAR PNEUMONIA	BRONCHOPNEUMONIA
1.	Definition	Acute bacterial infection of a part of a lobe of one or both lungs, or the entire lobe/s	Acute bacterial infection of the terminal bronchioles extending into adjoining alveoli
2.	Age group	More common in adults	Commoner at extremes of age: infants and old age
3.	Predisposing factors	More often affects healthy individuals	Pre-existing diseases e.g. chronic debility, terminal illness, flu, measles
4.	Common etiologic agents	Pneumococci, *Klebsiella pneumoniae*, staphylococci, streptococci	Staphylococci, streptococci, *Pseudomonas*, *Haemophilus influenzae*
5.	Pathologic features	Typical case passes through stages of congestion (1-2 days), early (2-4 days) and late consolidation (4-8 days), followed by resolution (1-3 weeks)	Patchy consolidation with central granularity, alveolar exudation, thickened septa
6.	Investigations	Neutrophilic leucocytosis, positive blood culture, X-ray shows consolidation	Neutrophilic leucocytosis, positive blood culture, X-ray shows mottled focal opacities
7.	Prognosis	Better response to treatment, resolution common, prognosis good	Response to treatment variable, organisation may occur, prognosis poor
8.	Complications	Less common; pleural effusion, empyema, lung abscess, organisation	Bronchiectasis may occur; other complications same as for lobar pneumonia

Chapter 13: Infectious and Parasitic Diseases

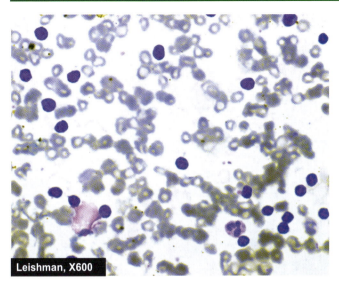

Figure 13.9 ▶ Marked peripheral blood lymphocytosis in whooping cough.

CAT-SCRATCH DISEASE

Another condition related to LGV, cat-scratch disease, is caused by *Bartonella henselae,* an organism linked to rickettsiae but unlike rickettsiae this organism can be grown in culture. The condition occurs more commonly in children (under 18 years of age). There is regional nodal enlargement which appears about 2 weeks after cat-scratch, and sometimes after thorn injury. The lymphadenopathy is self-limited and regresses in 2-4 months.

Microscopically, the changes in lymph node are characteristics:
i) Initially, there is formation of non-caseating sarcoid-like granulomas.
ii) Subsequently, there are neutrophilic abscesses surrounded by pallisaded histiocytes and fibroblasts, an appearance simulating LGV discussed above.
iii) The organism is extracellular and can be identified by silver stains.

STAPHYLOCOCCAL INFECTIONS

Staphylococci are gram-positive cocci which are present everywhere—in the skin, umbilicus, nasal vestibule, stool etc. Three species are pathogenic to human beings: *Staph. aureus, Staph. epidermidis* and *Staph. saprophyticus.* Most staphylococcal infections are caused by *Staph. aureus.* Staphylococcal infections are among the commonest antibiotic-resistant hospital-acquired infection in surgical wounds.

A wide variety of suppurative diseases are caused by *Staph. aureus* which includes the following **(Fig. 13.10):**

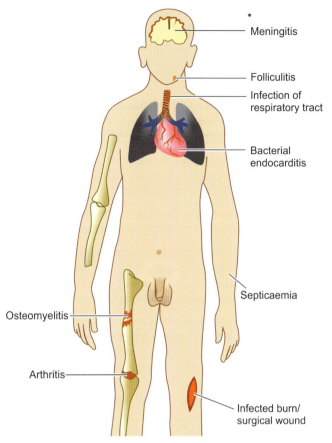

Figure 13.10 ▶ Suppurative diseases caused by *Staphylococcus aureus.*

1. **Infections of skin** Staphylococcal infections of the skin are quite common. The infection begins from lodgement of cocci in the hair root due to poor hygiene and results in obstruction of sweat or sebaceous gland duct. This is termed *folliculitis.* Involvement of adjacent follicles results in larger lesions called *furuncle.* Further spread of infection horizontally under the skin and subcutaneous tissue causes *carbuncle* or *cellulitis. Styes* are staphylococcal infection of the sebaceous glands of Zeis, the glands of Moll and eyelash follicles. *Impetigo* is yet another staphylococcal skin infection common in school children in which there are multiple pustular lesions on face forming honey-yellow crusts. *Breast abscess* may occur following delivery when staphylococci are transmitted from infant having neonatal sepsis or due to stasis of milk.

2. **Infections of burns and surgical wounds** These are quite common due to contamination from the patient's own nasal secretions or from hospital staff. Elderly, malnourished, obese patients and neonates have increased susceptibility.

3. **Infections of the upper and lower respiratory tract** Small children under 2 years of age get staphylococcal

infections of the respiratory tract commonly. These include pharyngitis, bronchopneumonia, staphylococcal pneumonia and its complications.

4. Bacterial arthritis Septic arthritis in the elderly is caused by *Staph. aureus*.

5. Infection of bone (Osteomyelitis) Young boys having history of trauma or infection may develop acute staphylococcal osteomyelitis (page 585).

6. Bacterial endocarditis Acute and subacute bacterial endocarditis are complications of infection with *Staph. aureus* and *Staph. epidermidis* (page 507).

7. Bacterial meningitis Surgical procedures on central nervous system may lead to staphylococcal meningitis.

8. Septicaemia Staphylococcal septicaemia may occur in patients with lowered resistance or in patients having underlying staphylococcal infections. Patients present with features of bacteraemia such as shaking chills and fever.

9. Toxic shock syndrome Toxic shock syndrome is a serious complication of staphylococcal infection characterised by fever, hypotension and exfoliative skin rash. The condition affected young menstruating women who used tampons of some brands which when kept inside the vagina caused absorption of staphylococcal toxins from the vagina.

STREPTOCOCCAL INFECTIONS

Streptococci are also gram-positive cocci but unlike staphylococci, they are more known for their non-suppurative autoimmune complications than suppurative inflammatory responses. Streptococcal infections occur throughout the world but their problems are greater in underprivileged populations where antibiotics are not instituted readily.

The following groups and subtypes of streptococci have been identified and implicated in different streptococcal diseases (Fig. 13.11):

1. *Group A or Streptococcus pyogenes,* also called β-haemolytic streptococci, are involved in causing upper respiratory tract infection and cutaneous infections (erysipelas). In addition, β-haemolytic streptococci are involved in autoimmune reactions in the form of rheumatic heart disease (RHD) (page 500).

2. *Group B or Streptococcus agalactiae* produces infections in the newborn and is involved in non-suppurative post-streptococcal complications such as RHD and acute glomerulonephritis.

3. *Group C and G streptococci* are responsible for respiratory infections.

4. *Group D or Streptococcus faecalis,* also called enterococci are important in causation of urinary tract infection, bacterial endocarditis, septicaemia etc.

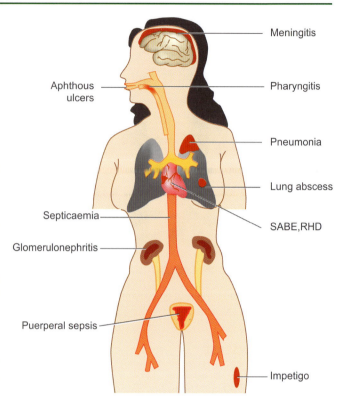

Figure 13.11 ▶ Diseases caused by streptococci.

5. *Untypable α-haemolytic streptococci* such as *Streptococcus viridans* constitute the normal flora of the mouth and may cause bacterial endocarditis.

6. *Pneumococci or Streptococcus pneumoniae* are etiologic agents for bacterial pneumonias, meningitis and septicaemia.

CLOSTRIDIAL DISEASES

Clostridia are gram-positive spore-forming anaerobic microorganisms found in the gastrointestinal tract of herbivorous animals and man. These organisms may undergo vegetative division under anaerobic conditions, and sporulation under aerobic conditions. These spores are passed in faeces and can survive in unfavourable conditions. On degeneration of these microorganisms, the plasmids are liberated which produce many toxins responsible for the following clostridial diseases depending upon the species (Fig. 13.12):

1. Gas gangrene by *C. perfringens*
2. Tetanus by *C. tetani*
3. Botulism by *C. botulinum*
4. Clostridial food poisoning by *C. perfringens*
5. Necrotising enterocolitis by *C. perfringens*.

GAS GANGRENE Gas gangrene is a rapidly progressive and fatal illness in which there is myonecrosis of previously healthy skeletal muscle due to elaboration of myotoxins by

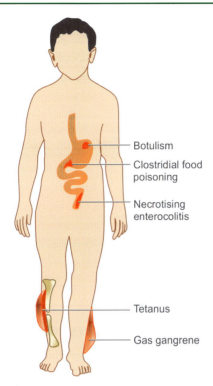

Figure 13.12 ▶ Diseases caused by clostridia.

some species of clostridia. In majority of cases (80-90%), the source of myotoxins is *C. perfringens* Type A; others are *C. novyi* and *C. septicum*. Generally, traumatic wounds and surgical procedures are followed by contamination with clostridia and become the site of myonecrosis. The incubation period is 2 to 4 days. The most common myotoxin produced by *C. perfringens* Type A is the alpha toxin which is a lecithinase. The prevention of gas gangrene lies in debridement of damaged tissue in which the clostridia thrive. The lesion has serosanguineous discharge with odour and contains gas bubbles. There is very scanty inflammatory reaction at the site of gas gangrene.

TETANUS Tetanus or 'lock jaw' is a severe acute neurologic syndrome caused by tetanus toxin, tetanospasmin, which is a neurotoxic exotoxin elaborated by *C. tetani*. The spores of the microorganism present in the soil enter the body through a penetrating wound. In underdeveloped countries, tetanus in neonates is seen due to application of soil or dung on the umbilical stump. The degenerated microorganisms liberate the tetanus neurotoxin which causes neuronal stimulation and spasm of muscles. The incubation period of the disease is 1-3 weeks. The earliest manifestation is lock-jaw or trismus. Rigidity of muscles of the back causes backward arching or opisthotonos. Death occurs due to spasm of respiratory and laryngeal muscles.

BOTULISM Botulism is characterised by symmetric paralysis of cranial nerves, limbs and trunk. The condition occurs following ingestion of food contaminated with neurotoxins of *C. botulinum* and less often by contamination of a penetrating wound. The spores of *C. botulinum* are capable of surviving in unfavourable conditions and contaminate vegetables and other foods, especially if improperly stored or canned. The symptoms of botulism begin to appear within 12 to 36 hours of ingestion of food containing the neurotoxins (type A to type G). The toxins resist gastric digestion and are absorbed from the upper portion of small intestine and enter the blood. On reaching the cholinergic nerve endings, the toxin binds to membrane receptors and inhibits release of acetylcholine resulting in paralysis and respiratory failure.

CLOSTRIDIAL FOOD POISONING Clostridial food poisoning is caused by enterotoxin elaborated by *C. perfringens*. Out of five serotypes of *C. perfringens*, type A and C produce alpha-enterotoxin that causes food poisoning. These serotypes of organism are omnipresent in the environment and thus clostridial poisoning occurs throughout the world. Food poisoning from *C. perfringens* is mostly from ingestion of meat and its products which have been allowed to dry resulting in dehydration and anaerobic conditions suitable for growth of *C. perfringens*. The contaminated meat contains vegetative form of the organism and no preformed enterotoxin (unlike botulism where preformed neurotoxin of *C. botulinum* is ingested). On ingestion of the contaminated meat, α-enterotoxin is produced in the intestine. Symptoms of the food poisoning appear within 12 hours of ingestion of contaminated meat and recovery occurs within 2 days.

NECROTISING ENTEROCOLITIS Necrotising enterocolitis or 'pig bel' is caused by beta-enterotoxin produced by *C. perfringens* Type C. The condition occurs especially in undernourished children who suddenly indulge in overeating such as was first reported participation in pig feasts by poor children in New Guinea and hence the name 'pig bel'. Adults do not develop the condition due to good antibody response.

Ingestion of contaminated pork by malnourished children who normally take protein-deficient vegetarian diet causes elaboration of β-enterotoxin. The symptoms appear within 48 hours after ingestion of contaminated meat. These include: severe abdominal pain, distension, vomiting and passage of bloody stools. Milder form of disease runs a course similar to other forms of gastroenteritis while fulminant 'pig bel' may result in death of the child.

Grossly, the disease affects small intestine segmentally. The affected segment of bowel shows green, necrotic pseudomembrane covering the necrotic mucosa and there is associated peritonitis. Advanced cases may show perforation of the bowel wall.

Microscopically, there is transmural infiltration by acute inflammatory cell infiltrate with changes of mucosal infarction, oedema and haemorrhage. The pseudomembrane consists of necrotic epithelium with entangled bacilli.

GIST BOX 13.2 — Diseases caused by Bacteria

- Enteric fever is acute infection caused by *Salmonella* (typhoid fever). There are oval ulcers along the long axis of the small intestine and may be complicated by perforation.
- Bacterial food poisoning may be caused by staphylococci, *Clostridia*, and *Salmonella*.
- Dysentery is diarrhoea with abdominal cramps, tenesmus and passage of mucus in the stools, and may be bacillary and amoebic.
- Pneumonia or consolidation is acute inflammation of the lung parenchyma distal to the terminal bronchioles. These occur in settings of altered consciousness, impaired immunity, endobronchial obstruction etc. Pneumonias are classified on location in the part of lung, clinical settings and etiology. Bacterial pneumonias may be located in a lobe (lobar) or terminal bronchiole (bronchopneumonia).
- Lobar pneumonia is caused by pneumococci, staphylococci, streptococci and gram-negative organisms. It passes through stages of congestion, red and grey hepatisation, and resolution.
- Bronchopneumonia is patchy areas of consolidation around terminal bronchioles.
- Whooping cough is a highly communicable acute bacterial disease of childhood caused by Bordetella-pertussis and is characterised by respiratory mucosal erosions and lymphocytosis.
- Cat-scratch disease is caused by Bartonella henselae, an organism linked to rickettsiae.
- Staphylococci cause wide variety of suppurative infections such as skin, burn wounds, upper and lower respirtory tract, joints, bones and meninges.
- Streptococci are known for their non-suppurative autoimmune complications such as in rheumatic heart disease and acute glomerulonephritis.
- Clostridia are spore forming Gram-positive anaerobic bacteria and cause gas gangrene, tetanus, botulism and food poisoning.

DISEASES CAUSED BY FUNGI

Of the large number of known fungi, only a few are infective to human beings. Many of the human fungal infections are opportunistic i.e. they occur in conditions with impaired host immune mechanisms. Such conditions include defective neutrophil function, administration of corticosteroids, immunosuppressive therapy and immunodeficiency states (congenital and acquired). A list of common fungal infections of human beings is given in **Table 13.4**. A few important representative examples are discussed below.

Table 13.4 Diseases caused by fungi.

DISEASE	ETIOLOGIC AGENT
1. Pneumocystis pneumonia*	*Pneumocystis jirovecii*
2. Mycetoma*	*Madurella mycetomatis*
3. Aspergillosis*	*Aspergillus fumigatus, A. flavus, A. niger*
4. Blastomycosis	*Blastomyces dermatitidis*
5. Candidiasis*	*Candida albicans*
6. Coccidioidomycosis	*Coccidioides immitis*
7. Cryptococcosis	*Cryptococcus neoformans*
8. Histoplasmosis	*Histoplasma capsulatum*
9. Rhinosporidiosis*	*Rhinosporidium seeberi*
10. Superficial mycosis*	*Microsporum, Trichophyton, Epidermophyton*

*Conditions discussed in this chapter.

FUNGAL INFECTIONS OF LUNG (FUNGAL PNEUMONIAS)

Fungal infections of the lung are more common than tuberculosis in the US. These infections in healthy individuals are rarely serious but in immunosuppressed individuals may prove fatal. Some common examples of fungal infections of the lung are briefly given below:

Pneumocystis Pneumonia

Pneumocystis is an opportunistic fungal infection of the lungs. The original species *P. carinii* infects rats while *P. jirovecii* causes pneumonia by inhalation of the organisms in neonates and immunosuppressed people. Almost 100% cases of HIV/AIDS develop opportunistic infection during the course of disease, most commonly *Pneumocystis* pneumonia. Other immunosuppressed groups are patients on chemotherapy for organ transplant and tumours, malnutrition, agammaglobulinaemia etc.

MORPHOLOGIC FEATURES *Grossly,* the affected parts of the lung are consolidated, dry and grey.

Microscopically, the features are as under:
i) Interstitial pneumonitis with thickening and mononuclear infiltration of the alveolar walls.
ii) Alveolar lumina contain pink frothy fluid having the organisms **(Fig. 13.13)**.
iii) By Grocott's methenamine-silver (GMS) stain, the characteristic oval or crescentic cysts, about 5 µm in diameter and surrounded by numerous tiny black dot-like organism *P. Jirovecii* are demonstrable in the frothy fluid.
iv) No significant inflammatory exudate is seen in the air spaces.

Chapter 13: Infectious and Parasitic Diseases

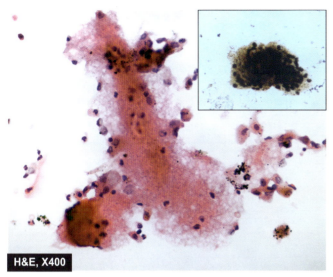

Figure 13.13 ▶ *Pneumocystis* pneumonia. Smears from the sputum show frothy vacuolated exudate containing the organisms. Inbox shows Grocott's silver methenamine stain positivity for the organisms.

CLINICAL FEATURES There is rapid onset of dyspnoea, tachycardia, cyanosis and non-productive cough. If untreated, it causes death in one or two weeks. Chest radiograph shows diffuse alveolar and interstitial infiltrate.

Other Fungal Infections of Lung

1. **Aspergillosis** Aspergillosis is the most common fungal infection of the lung caused by *Aspergillus fumigatus* that grows best in cool, wet climate. The infection may result in *allergic bronchopulmonary aspergillosis, aspergilloma* and *necrotising bronchitis*. Immunocompromised persons develop more serious manifestations of aspergillus infection, especially in leukaemic patients on cytotoxic drug therapy and HIV/AIDS. Extensive haematogenous spread of aspergillus infection may result in widespread changes in lung tissue due to arterial occlusion, thrombosis and infarction.

Grossly, pulmonary aspergillosis may occur within pre-existing pulmonary cavities or in bronchiectasis as fungal ball.

Microscopically, the fungus may appear as a tangled mass within the cavity. The organisms are identified by their characteristic morphology—thin septate hyphae with dichotomous branching at acute angles which stain positive for fungal stains such as PAS and silver impregnation technique (Fig. 13.14). The wall of the cavity shows chronic inflammatory cells.

2. **Mucormycosis** Mucormycosis or phycomycosis is caused by *Mucor* and *Rhizopus*. The infection in the lung occurs in a similar way as in aspergillosis. The pulmonary lesions are especially common in patients of *diabetic ketoacidosis*. Mucor is distinguished by its broad, non-parallel, nonseptate hyphae which branch at an obtuse angle. Mucormycosis is more often angioinvasive, and disseminates; hence it is more destructive than aspergillosis (see **Fig. 13.1, F).**

3. **Candidiasis** Candidiasis or moniliasis caused by *Candida albicans* is a normal commensal in oral cavity, gut and

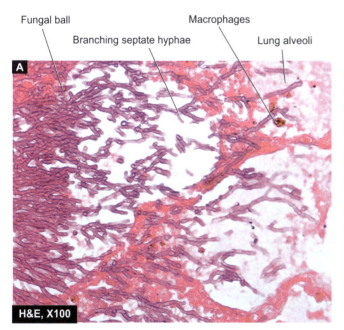
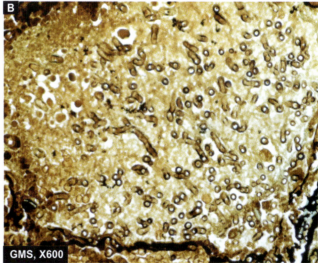

Figure 13.14 ▶ Aspergillosis lung. A, Acute angled septate hyphae lying in necrotic debris and acute inflammatory exudates in lung abscess. B, Organisms, *Apergillus flavus*, are best identified with a special stain for fungi, Gomory's methenamine silver (GMS).

vagina but attains pathologic form in immunocompromised host. Angioinvasive growth of the organism may occur in the airways.

4. **Histoplasmosis** It is caused by oval organism, *Histoplasma capsulatum,* by inhalation of infected dust or bird droppings. The condition may remain asymptomatic or may produce lesions similar to the Ghon's complex.

5. **Cryptococcosis** It is caused by *Cryptococcus neoformans* which is round yeast having a halo around it due to shrinkage in tissue sections. The infection occurs from infection by inhalation of pigeon droppings. The lesions in the body may range from a small parenchymal granuloma in the lung to cryptococcal meningitis.

6. **Coccidioidomycosis** Coccidioidomycosis is caused by *Coccidioidesimmitis* which are spherical spores. The infection in human beings is acquired by close contact with infected dogs. The lesions consist of peripheral parenchymal granuloma in the lung.

7. **Blastomycosis** It is an uncommon condition caused by *Blastomyces dermatitidis.* The lesions result from inhalation of spores in the ground. Pathological features may present as Ghon's complex-like lesion, as a pneumonic consolidation, and as multiple skin nodules.

MYCETOMA

Mycetoma is a chronic suppurative infection involving a limb, shoulder or other tissues and is characterised by draining sinuses. The material discharged from the sinuses is in the form of grains consisting of colonies of fungi or bacteria. Mycetomas are of 2 main types:

◆ *Mycetoma* caused by actinomyces (higher bacteria) also called actinomycetoma comprises about 60% of cases (page 151).

◆ *Eumycetoma* caused by true fungi, *Madurella mycetomatis* or *Madurella grisea,* comprises the remaining 40% of the cases.

Eumycetomas are particularly common in Northern and tropical Africa, Southern Asia and tropical America. The organisms are inoculated directly from soil into barefeet, from carrying of contaminated sacks on the shoulders, and into the hands from infected vegetation.

MORPHOLOGIC FEATURES After several months of infection, the affected site, most commonly foot, is swollen and hence the name 'madura foot'. The lesions extend deeply into the subcutaneous tissues, along the fascia and eventually invade the bones. They drain through sinus tracts which discharge purulent material and black grains. The surrounding tissue shows granulomatous reaction (Fig. 13.15).

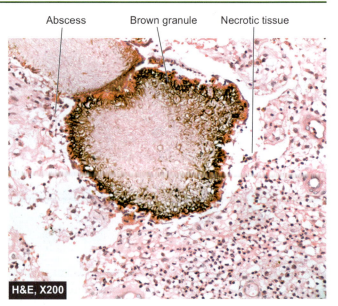

Figure 13.15 ▶ Madura foot. Brown granule lying in necrotic tissue in the discharging sinus.

CANDIDIASIS

Candidiasis is an opportunistic fungal infection caused most commonly by *Candida albicans* and occasionally by *Candida tropicalis.* In human beings, Candida species are present as normal flora of the skin and mucocutaneous areas, intestines and vagina. The organism becomes pathogenic when the balance between the host and the organism is disturbed. Various predisposing factors are: impaired immunity, prolonged use of oral contraceptives, long-term antibiotic therapy, corticosteroid therapy, diabetes mellitus, obesity, pregnancy etc.

MORPHOLOGIC FEATURES Candida produces superficial infections of the skin and mucous membranes, or may invade deeper tissues as described under:

1. Oral thrush This is the commonest form of mucocutaneous candidiasis seen especially in early life. Full-fledged lesions consist of creamy white pseudomembrane composed of fungi covering the tongue, soft palate, and buccal mucosa. In severe cases, ulceration may be seen.

2. Candidal vaginitis Vaginal candidiasis or monilial vaginitis is characterised clinically by thick, yellow, curdy discharge. The lesions form pseudomembrane of fungi on the vaginal mucosa. They are quite pruritic and may extend to involve the vulva (vulvovaginitis) and the perineum.

3. Cutaneous candidiasis Candidal involvement of nail folds producing change in the shape of nail plate (paronychia) and colonisation in the intertriginous areas of the skin, axilla, groin, infra- and inter-mammary, inter-gluteal folds and interdigital spaces are some of the common forms of cutaneous lesions caused by *Candida albicans* (Fig. 13.16).

Chapter 13: Infectious and Parasitic Diseases

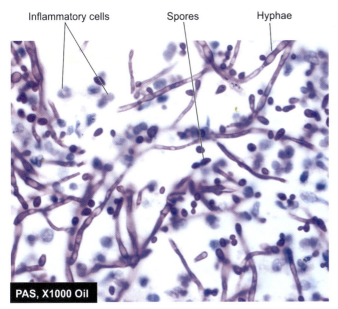

Figure 13.16 ▶ Candidiasis of the ulcer in the skin.

4. Systemic candidiasis Invasive candidiasis is rare and is usually a terminal event of an underlying disorder associated with impaired immune system. The organisms gain entry into the body through an ulcerative lesion on the skin and mucosa or may be introduced by iatrogenic means such as via intravenous infusion, peritoneal dialysis or urinary catheterisation. The lesions of systemic candidiasis are most commonly encountered in kidneys as ascending pyelonephritis and in heart as candidal endocarditis.

RHINOSPORIDIOSIS NOSE

Rhinosporidiosis is caused by a fungus, *Rhinosporidium seeberi*. Typically it occurs in a nasal polyp but may be found in other locations like nasopharynx, larynx and conjunctiva. The disease is common in India and Sri Lanka and sporadic in other parts of the world.

Microscopically, besides the structure of inflammatory or allergic polyp, large number of organisms of the size of erythrocytes with chitinous wall are seen in the thick-walled *sporangia*. Each sporangium may contain a few thousand spores. On rupture of a sporangium, the spores are discharged into the submucosa or on to the surface of the mucosa. The intervening tissue consists of inflammatory granulation tissue (plasma cells, lymphocytes, histiocytes, neutrophils) while the overlying epithelium shows hyperplasia, focal thinning and occasional ulceration (Fig. 13.17).

CUTANEOUS SUPERFICIAL MYCOSIS

Dermatophytes cause superficial mycosis of the skin, the important examples being *Microsporum, Trichophyton* and *Epidermophyton*. These superficial fungi are spread by direct contact or by fomites and infect tissues such as the skin, hair and nails. Examples of diseases pertaining to these tissues are as under:
◈ *Tinea capitis* characterised by patchy alopecia affecting the scalp and eyebrows.
◈ *Tinea barbae* is acute folliculitis of the beard.
◈ *Tinea corporis* is dermatitis with formation of erythematous papules.

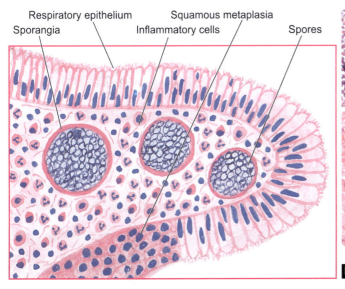
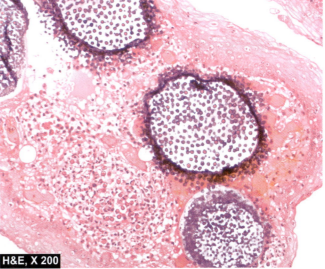

Figure 13.17 ▶ Rhinosporidiosis in a nasal polyp. The spores are present in sporangia as well as are intermingled in the inflammatory cell infiltrate.

The diagnosis of dermatophytosis is made by light microscopic examination of skin scrapings after addition of sodium or potassium hydroxide solution. Other methods include fungal culture and demonstration of fungus in tissue sections.

> **GIST BOX 13.3 Diseases caused by Fungi**
>
> ❖ Opportunistic fungi occur in conditions with impaired host immunity.
> ❖ Almost 100% cases of HIV/AIDS develop opportunistic infection during the course of disease, most commonly *Pneumocystis* pneumonia. Other immunosuppressed groups are patients on chemotherapy for organ transplant and tumours, malnutrition, agammaglobulinaemia. Other common fungal infections of lung are aspergillosis, mucormycosis, candidiasis etc.
> ❖ *Mycetoma* is a chronic suppurative infection caused by either actinomyces (higher bacteria) also called actinomycetoma, or *eumycetomas* caused by true fungi (madura foot).
> ❖ Candidiasis is an opportunistic fungal infection caused commonly by *Candida albicans* and produces superficial infections of the skin and mucous membranes e.g. oral thrush, candidal vaginitis, cutaneous candidiasis.
> ❖ Rhinosporidiosis presents as nasal polyp and has sporangia of fungus.
> ❖ Superficial mycosis of the skin are caused by dermatophytes and produce tinea of various tissues.

Table 13.5 Diseases caused by viruses.

	DISEASE	ETIOLOGIC AGENT
1.	Viral haemorrhagic fevers*	Arthropod-borne (arbo) viruses
2.	Influenza [Bird flu, H5N1, Swine flu (H1N1)]*	Influenza virus type A
3.	Viral encephalitis	Arthropod-borne (arbo) viruses
4.	Rabies*	Rabies virus (arboviruses)
5.	Poliomyelitis	Poliovirus
6.	Smallpox (Variola)	Variola virus
7.	Chickenpox (varicella)*	Varicella-zoster virus
8.	Herpes simplex and herpes genitalis*	Herpes simplex virus (HSV-I and HSV-II)
9.	Herpes zoster*	Varicella-zoster virus
10.	Viral hepatitis (page 537)	Hepatotropic viruses
11.	Cytomegalovirus inclusion disease	Cytomegalovirus (CMV)
12.	Infectious mononucleosis (page 424)	Epstein-Barr virus (EBV)
13.	Measles (Rubeola)	Measles virus
14.	German measles (Rubella)	Rubella virus
15.	Mumps (page 526)	Mumps virus
16.	Viral respiratory infections	Adenovirus, echovirus, rhinovirus, coxsackie virus, influenza A, B and C, etc.
17.	Viral gastroenteritis	Rotaviruses, Norwalk-like viruses

*Diseases discussed in this chapter.

DISEASES CAUSED BY VIRUSES

Viral diseases are the most common cause of human illness. However, many of the viral infections remain asymptomatic while others produce viral disease. Another peculiar feature of viral infection is that a single etiologic agent may produce different diseases in the same host depending upon host immune response and age at infection e.g. varicella-zoster virus is causative for chickenpox as well as herpes zoster. Viruses are essentially intracellular parasites. Depending upon their nucleic acid genomic composition, they may be single-stranded or double-stranded, RNA or DNA viruses. A list of common viruses and diseases caused by them is given in Table 13.5. Oncogenic viruses and their role in neoplasms are discussed on page 303. A few common and important viral diseases are described below.

VIRAL HAEMORRHAGIC FEVERS

Viral haemorrhagic fevers are a group of acute viral infections which have common features of causing haemorrhages, shock and sometimes death. Viruses causing haemorrhagic fevers were earlier called *arthropod-borne (or arbo) viruses* since their transmission to humans was considered to be from arthropods. However, now it is known that all such viruses are not transmitted by arthropod vectors alone and hence now such haemorrhagic fevers are classified according to the routes of transmission and other epidemiologic features into 4 groups:

1. Mosquito-borne (e.g. yellow fever, dengue fever, chikungunya, Rift Valley fever)

2. Tick-borne (e.g. Crimean haemorrhagic fever, Kyasanur Forest disease)

3. Zoonotic (e.g. Korean haemorrhagic fever, Lassa fever)

4. Marburg virus disease and Ebola virus disease by unknown route.

Of these, mosquito-borne viral haemorrhagic fevers in which *Aedes aegypti* mosquitoes are vectors, are the most common problem the world over, especially in developing countries. Two important examples of Aedes mosquito-borne viral haemorrhagic fevers are yellow fever and dengue fever, which are discussed here.

Yellow Fever

Yellow fever is the oldest known viral haemorrhagic fever restricted to some regions of Africa and South America. Monkeys carry the virus without suffering from illness and the virus is transmitted from them to humans by *Aedes aegypti* as vector.

Yellow fever is characterised by the following clinical features: Sudden onset of high fever, chills, myalgia, headache, jaundice, hepatic failure, renal failure, bleeding disorders and hypotension.

MORPHOLOGIC FEATURES Major pathologic changes are seen in the liver and kidneys.

Liver The characteristic changes include:
i) midzonal necrosis;
ii) Councilman bodies; and
iii) microvesicular fat.

Kidneys The kidneys show the following changes:
i) coagulative necrosis of proximal tubules;
ii) accumulation of fat in the tubular epithelium; and
iii) haemorrhages.

Patients tend to recover without sequelae; death rate is less than 5%, death resulting from hepatic or renal failure, and petechial haemorrhages in the brain.

Dengue Haemorrhagic Fever (DHF)

The word dengue is derived from African word *'denga'* meaning fever with haemorrhages. Dengue is caused by virus transmitted by bites of mosquito *Aedes aegypti*; the transmission being highest during and after rainy season when mosquitos are numerous. DHF was first described in 1953 when it struck Philippines. Since then, DHF has been regularly reported from tropics and subtropics—South East Asia, Latin America and Pacific Islands. Since 1996, cases are seen every year in North India in the post-monsoon rain period.

Dengue occurs in two forms:

1. *Dengue fever or break-bone fever* in an uncomplicated way is a self-limited febrile illness affecting muscles and joints with severe back pain due to myalgia (and hence the name 'break-bone' fever).

2. *Dengue haemorrhagic fever (DHF)*, on the other hand, is a severe and potentially fatal form of acute febrile illness characterised by cutaneous and intestinal haemorrhages due to thrombocytopenia, haemoconcentration, hypovolaemic shock and neurologic disturbances. DHF is most common in children under 15 years of age.

There are 4 types of dengue viruses and all of them produce similar clinical syndrome. These viruses infect blood monocytes, lymphocytes and endothelial cells. This initiates complement activation and consumptive coagulopathy including thrombocytopenia. The entire process takes place rapidly and may evolve over a period of a few hours. If patient is treated appropriately at this stage, there is rapid and dramatic recovery. But in untreated cases, *dengue shock syndrome* develops and death occurs.

MORPHOLOGIC FEATURES Predominant *organ changes in DHF* are due to following:
i) Focal haemorrhages and congestion
ii) Increased vascular permeability resulting in oedema in different organs
iii) Coagulopathy with thrombocytopenia
iv) Haemoconcentration.

Diagnosis of DHF is confirmed by the following tests:
1. Serologic testing for detection of antibodies
2. Detection of virus by immunofluorescence method and monoclonal antibodies
3. Rapid methods such as reverse transcriptase-PCR and fluorogenic-ELISA.

The main abnormalities in **investigations in DHF** are as under:
i) Leucopenia with relative lymphocytosis, sometimes with atypical lymphocytes
ii) Thrombocytopenia
iii) Elevated haematocrit due to haemoconcentration
iv) X-ray chest showing bilateral pleural effusion
v) Deranged liver function tests (elevated transaminases, hypoalbuminaemia and reversed A:G ratio)
vi) Prolonged coagulation tests (prothrombin time, activated partial thromboplastin time and thrombin time)

At autopsy, the predominant organ changes observed are as follows:
i) *Brain:* Intracranial haemorrhages, cerebral oedema, dengue encephalitis.
ii) *Liver:* Enlarged; necrosis of hepatocytes and Kupffer cells, Reye's syndrome in children.
iii) *Kidneys:* Petechial haemorrhages and features of renal failure.
iv) *Muscles and joints:* Perivascular mononuclear cell infiltrate.

Chikungunya Virus Infection

The word chikungunya means "that which bends up" and is derived from the language in Africa where this viral disease was first found in human beings. Chikungunya virus infection is primarily a disease in nonhuman primates but the infection is transmitted to humans by *A. aegypti* mosquito. The disease is endemic in parts of Africa and Asia and occurs sporadically elsewhere.

◆ *Clinically,* the disease is characterised by abrupt onset of fever, severe arthralgia (producing bending posture of patient due to pain and hence the name), migratory polyarthritis affecting small joints, chills, headache, anorexia, nausea, abdominal pain, rash, petechiae and ocular symptoms such as photophobia.

- *Major laboratory findings* include leucopenia, mild thrombocytopenia, elevated transaminases and raised CRP.

INFLUENZA VIRUS INFECTIONS

Influenza virus infection is an important and common form of communicable disease, especially prevalent as a seasonal infection in the developed countries. Its general clinical features range from a mild afebrile illness similar to common cold by appearance of sudden fever, headache, myalgia, malaise, chills and respiratory tract manifestations such as cough, soar throat to a more severe form of acute respiratory illness and lymphadenopathy. Various forms of influenza virus infections have occurred as an outbreak at different times, sometimes with alarming morbidity and mortality in the world. Seasonal flu vaccine is administered to population at high risk in developed countries.

ETIOLOGIC AGENT Influenza virus is a single-stranded RNA virus belonging to coronaviruses. Depending upon its antigenic characteristics of the nucleoprotein and matrix, 3 distinct types are known: A, B and C. Out of these, influenza type A is responsible for most serious and severe forms of outbreaks in human beings while types B and C cause a milder form of illness. Type A influenza virus is further subtyped based on its 2 viral surface features:

Haemagglutinin (H) H antigen elicits host immune response by antibodies and determines the future protection against influenza A viruses. There are 16 distinct H subtypes of type A influenza viruses.

Neuraminidase (N) Antibody response against N antigen limits the spread of viral infection and is responsible for reduction of infection. N antigen of influenza A exists in 9 subtypes.

Thus, the subtypes of influenza A viruses are designated by denoting serial subtype numbers of H and N antigens as H1N1, H2N2 etc.

Influenza A viruses infect human beings, birds, pigs and horses. In view of a high antigenic variation in H and N components, influenza A viruses are responsible for many known epidemics and pandemics in history and in present times. Major antigenic variation in H or N antigens is called *antigenic shift* while minor variation is termed *antigenic drift*. In general, population at high risk are immunosuppressed patients, elderly individuals and infants.

Two of the known subtypes of influenza A viruses which have affected the human beings in recent times are as under:
- Avian influenza virus A/H5N1 commonly called "bird flu".
- Swine influenza virus A/H1N1 commonly called "swine flu".

These two entities are briefly discussed below.

Bird Flu ((Influenza A/H5N1)

H5N1 subtype of the influenza type A virus infection causes severe acute respiratory syndrome (SARS) which is the human form of bird flu or avian influenza with having similar symptomatology. Every year, there have been outbreaks in poultry birds in different parts of the world resulting in slaughtering of millions of infected chickens every year. Human outbreak of the disease called SARS re-emerged in December 2003 in southern China, Hong Kong and Vietnam and then spread to other countries in Asia, Europe and America. Since then, every year there have been seasonal outbreaks in the human form of the disease in high winter and has so far affected 15 countries and taken a toll of over 250 lives. Its rapidly downhill and fatal clinical course and an apprehension of pandemic has sent alarm bells all over world for quarantine.

PATHOGENESIS SARS is caused by influenza type A/H5N1 respiratory virus, also called SARS-associated coronaviruses (SARS-CoV). Though it is not fatal for wild birds, it can kill poultry birds and people. Humans acquire infection through contaminated nasal, respiratory and faecal material from infected birds. An individual who has human flu and also gets infected with bird flu, then the hybrid virus so produced is highly contagious and causes lethal disease. No person-to-person transmission has been reported so far but epidemiologists fear that if it did occur it will be a global epidemic. Humans do not have immune protection against avian viruses.

LABORATORY DIAGNOSIS Following abnormalities in laboratory tests are noted:
1. Almost normal-to-low TLC with lymphopaenia in about half the cases, mostly due to fall in CD4+ T cells.
2. Thrombocytopenia.
3. Elevated liver enzymes: aminotransferases, creatine kinase and LDH.
4. Virus isolation by reverse transcriptase-PCR on respiratory sample, plasma, urine or stool.
5. Tissue culture.
6. Detection of serum antibodies by ELISA or immunofluorescence.

CLINICOPATHOLOGICAL FEATURES Typically, the disease begins with influenza-like features such as fever, cough, dyspnoea, sore throat, muscle aches and eye infection. Soon, the patient develops viral pneumonia evident on X-ray chest and acute respiratory distress (hence the term SARS), and terminally kidney failure.

There is apprehension of an epidemic of SARS, if the avian virus mutates and gains the ability to cause person-to-person infection. Since currently vaccine is yet being developed, the available measures are directed at prevention of infection such as by culling (killing of the infected poultry birds) and isolation of infected case.

Swine Flu (Influenza A/H1N1)

H1N1 influenza type A flu which appeared last in 1977-78 as a mild form of pandemic reappeared in April 2009 as an outbreak in Mexico but soon spread elsewhere. Presently, the disease spread to 39 countries including US. In view of rising number of cases, with about 10,000 confirmed cases and about 100 deaths attributed to swine flu from all over the world, the WHO sounded worldwide alert of a pandemic.

PATHOGENESIS H1N1 influenza type A virus is primarily an infection in pigs with low mortality in them. Human beings acquire infection by direct contact with infected pigs. However, further transmission of H1N1 flu occurs by person-to-person contact such as by coughing, sneezing etc but it is not known to occur from eating pork.

CLINICAL FEATURES The disease has the usual flu-like clinical features, but additionally one-third of cases have been found to have diarrhoea and vomiting.

Since human beings do not have immune protection by antibody response against H1N1 influenza type A and the usual seasonal flu vaccine does not provide protection against H1N1, personal hygiene and prophylaxis remain the mainstay of further spread of disease.

VARICELLA ZOSTER VIRUS INFECTION

Varicella zoster virus is a member of herpes virus family and causes chickenpox (varicella) in non-immune individuals and herpes zoster (shingles) in those who had chickenpox in the past.

Varicella or chickenpox It is an acute vesicular exanthem occurring in non-immune persons, especially children. The condition begins as an infection of the nasopharynx. On entering the blood stream, viraemia is accompanied by onset of fever, malaise and anorexia. Maculopapular skin rash, usually on the upper trunk and face, develops in a day or two. This is followed by formation of vesicles which rupture and heal with formation of scabs. A few cases may develop complications which include pneumonia, hepatitis, encephalitis, carditis, orchitis, arthritis, and haemorrhages.

Herpes zoster or shingles It is a recurrent, painful, vesicular eruption caused by reactivation of dormant varicella zoster virus in an individual who had chickenpox in the earlier years. The condition is infectious and spreads to children. The virus during the latent period resides in the dorsal root spinal ganglia or in the cranial nerve ganglia. On reactivation, the virus spreads from the ganglia to the sensory nerves and to peripheral nerves. Unlike chickenpox, the vesicles in shingles are seen in one or more of the sensory dermatomes and along the peripheral nerves. The lesions are particularly painful as compared with painless eruptions in chickenpox.

HERPES SIMPLEX VIRUS INFECTION

Two of the herpes simplex viruses (HSV)—type 1 and 2, cause 'fever blisters' and herpes genitalis respectively.

HSV-1 causes vesicular lesions on the skin, lips and mucous membranes. The infection spreads by close contact. The condition is particularly severe in immunodeficient patients and neonates while milder attacks of infection cause fever-blisters on lips, oral mucosa and skin. Severe cases may develop complications such as meningoencephalitis and keratoconjunctivitis. Various stimuli such as fever, stress and respiratory infection reactivate latent virus lying in the ganglia and result in recurrent attacks of blisters.

HSV-2 causes herpes genitalis characterised by vesicular and necrotising lesions on the cervix, vagina and vulva. Like HSV-1 infection, lesions caused by HSV-2 are also recurrent and develop in non-immune individuals. Latency of HSV-2 infection is similar to HSV-1 and the organisms are reactivated by stimuli such as menstruation and sexual intercourse.

RABIES

Rabies is a fatal form of encephalitis in humans caused by rabies virus. The virus is transmitted into the human body by the bite of infected carnivores e.g. dog, wolf, fox and bats. The virus spreads from the contaminated saliva of these animals. The organism enters a peripheral nerve and then travels to the spinal cord and brain. A latent period of 10 days to 3 months may elapse between the bite and onset of symptoms. Since the virus localises at the brainstem, it produces classical symptoms of difficulty in swallowing and painful spasm of the throat termed hydrophobia. Other clinical features such as irritability, seizure and delirium point towards viral encephalopathy. Death occurs within a period of a few weeks.

> *Microscopically,* neurons of the brainstem show characteristic Negri bodies which are intracytoplasmic, deeply eosinophilic inclusions.

GIST BOX 13.4 | Diseases caused by Viruses

- Mosquito-borne viral haemorrhagic fevers in which Aedes aegypti mosquitoes are vectors, are the most common problem the world over, especially in developing countries, and include yellow fever, dengue fever, chikungunya.
- Chikungunya is primarily a disease in nonhuman primates but the infection is transmitted to humans by *A. aegypti* mosquito.
- Influenza virus infection is an important and common form of communicable disease, especially prevalent as a seasonal infection in the developed countries.
- Two of the known subtypes of influenza A viruses which have affected the mankind in recent times are avian influenza virus A/H5N1 commonly called "bird flu" and swine influenza virus A/H1N1 commonly called "swine flu".
- Varicella zoster virus is a member of herpes virus family and causes chickenpox (varicella) in non-immune individuals and herpes zoster (shingles) in those who had chickenpox in the past.

❖ Two of the herpes simplex viruses (HSV)—type 1 and 2, cause 'fever blisters' and herpes genitalis.
❖ Rabies is a fatal form of encephalitis in humans caused by rabies virus.

DISEASES CAUSED BY PARASITES

Diseases caused by parasites (protozoa and helminths) are quite common and comprise a very large group of infestations and infections in human beings. Parasites may cause disease due to their presence in the lumen of the intestine, due to infiltration into the blood stream, or due to their presence inside the cells. A brief list of parasitic diseases is given in Table 13.6. These diseases form a distinct subject of study called Parasitology; only a few conditions causing tissue changes are briefly considered below.

AMOEBIASIS

Amoebiasis is caused by *Entamoeba histolytica,* named for its lytic action on tissues. It is the most important intestinal infection of man. The condition is particularly more common in tropical and subtropical areas with poor sanitation.

The parasite occurs in 2 forms:

◈ a *trophozoite form* which is active adult form seen in the tissues and diarrhoeal stools; and

◈ a *cystic form* seen in formed stools but not in the tissues.

The trophozoite form can be stained positively with PAS stain in tissue sections while amoebic cysts having four nuclei can be identified in stools. The cysts are the infective stage of the parasite and are found in contaminated water or food. The trophozoites are formed from the cyst stage in the intestine and colonise in the caecum and large bowel. The trophozoites as well as cysts are passed in stools but the trophozoites fail to survive outside or are destroyed by gastric secretions.

MORPHOLOGIC FEATURES The lesions of amoebiasis include amoebic dysentery, amoebic colitis, amoeboma, amoebic liver abscess and spread of lesions to other sites (Fig. 13.18).

Table 13.6	Diseases caused by parasites.
DISEASE	ETIOLOGIC AGENT
A. PROTOZOAL DISEASES	
1. Chagas' disease (Trypanosomiasis)	*Trypanosoma cruzi*
2. Leishmaniasis (Kala-azar)	*L. tropica, L. braziliensis, L. donovani*
3. Malaria*	*Plasmodium vivax, P. falciparum, P. ovale, P. malariae*
4. Toxoplasmosis	*Toxoplasma gondii*
5. Amoebiasis*	*Entamoeba histolytica*
6. Giardiasis	*Giardia lamblia*
7. Babesiosis	*Babesia microti* and *B divergens*
B. HELMINTHIC DISEASES	
1. Ascariasis	*Ascaris lumbricoides*
2. Enterobiasis (oxyuriasis)	*Enterobius vermicularis*
3. Hookworm disease	*Ancylostoma duodenale*
4. Trichinosis	*Trichinella spiralis*
5. Filariasis*	*Wuchereria bancrofti*
6. Visceral larva migrans	*Toxocara canis*
7. Cutaneous larva migrans	*Strongyloides stercoralis*
8. Schistosomiasis (Bilharziasis)	*Schistosoma haematobium*
9. Clonorchiasis	*Clonorchis sinensis*
10. Fascioliasis	*Fasciola hepatica*
11. Echinococcosis (Hydatid disease)*	*Echinococcus granulosus*
12. Cysticercosis*	*Taenia solium*

*Diseases discussed in this chapter

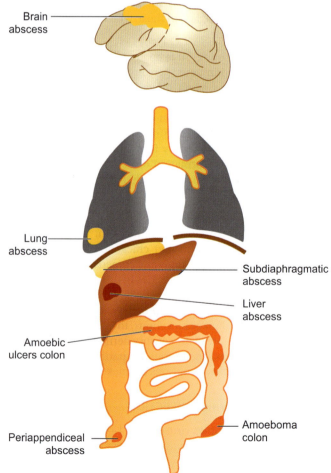

Figure 13.18 ▶ Lesions of amoebiasis.

Amoebic dysentery This is due to infection by *Entamoeba histolytica*. It is more prevalent in the tropical countries and primarily affects the large intestine. Infection occurs from ingestion of cyst form of the parasite. The cyst wall is dissolved in the small intestine from where the liberated amoebae pass into the large intestine. Early intestinal lesions appear as small areas of elevation on the mucosal surface.

Amoebic colitis, the most common type of amoebic infection begins as a small area of necrosis of mucosa which may ulcerate. In advanced cases, typical flask-shaped ulcers having narrow neck and broad base are seen. They are more conspicuous in the caecum, rectum and in the flexures. These ulcerative lesions may enlarge, develop undermining of margins of the ulcer due to lytic action of the trophozoite and have necrotic bed. Such chronic amoebic ulcers are described as flask-shaped ulcers due to their shape **(Fig. 13.19, A)**. *Microscopically,* the ulcerated area shows chronic inflammatory reaction consisting of lymphocytes, plasma cells, macrophages and eosinophils. The trophozoites of *Entamoeba* are seen in the inflammatory exudate and are concentrated at the advancing margin of the lesion. Intestinal amoebae characteristically have ingested red cells in their cytoplasm. Oedema and vascular congestion are present in the area surrounding the ulcers **(Fig. 13.19, B)**.

Complications of intestinal amoebic ulcers are: amoebic liver abscess or amoebic hepatitis, perforation, haemorrhage and formation of amoeboma which is a tumour-like mass.

Amoeboma is the inflammatory thickening of the wall of large bowel resembling carcinoma of the colon. *Microscopically*, the lesion consists of inflammatory granulation tissue, fibrosis and clusters of trophozoites at the margin of necrotic with viable tissue.

Amoebic liver abscess may be formed by invasion of the radicle of the portal vein by trophozoites. Amoebic liver abscess may be single or multiple. The amoebic abscess contains yellowish-grey amorphous liquid material in which trophozoites are identified at the junction of the viable and necrotic tissue.

Other sites where spread of amoebic infection may occur are peritonitis by perforation of amoebic ulcer of colon, extension to the lungs and pleura by rupture of amoebic liver abscess, haematogenous spread to cause amoebic carditis and cerebral lesions, cutaneous amoebiasis via spread of rectal amoebiasis or from anal intercourse.

MALARIA

Malaria is a protozoal disease caused by any one or combination of four species of plasmodia: *Plasmodium vivax, Plasmodium falciparum, Plasmodium ovale* and *Plasmodium malariae*. While *Plasmodium falciparum* causes malignant malaria, the other three species produce benign form of illness. These parasites are transmitted by bite of female *Anopheles* mosquito. The disease is endemic in several parts of the world, especially in tropical Africa, parts of South and Central America, India and South-East Asia.

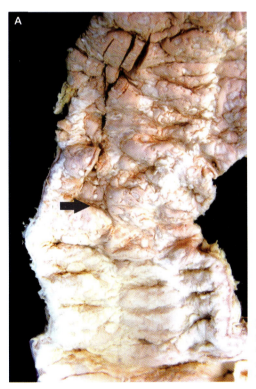

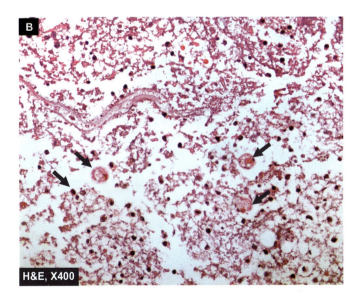

Figure 13.19 ▶ Amoebic ulcers large intestine. A, The luminal surface shows multiple ulcers some of which are deep and are flask-shaped with narrow neck and broad base (arrow) containing necrotic tissue and undermined margins. B, Trophozoites of *Entamoeba histolytica* are seen at the margin of ulcer (arrow).

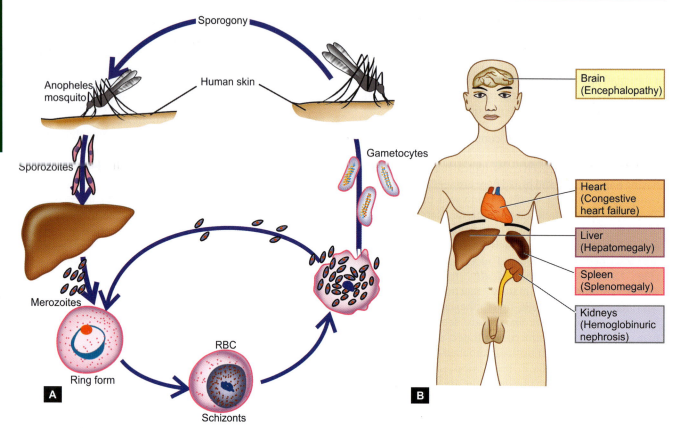

Figure 13.20 ▶ Life cycle of malaria (A) and major pathological changes in organs (B).

The life cycle of plasmodia is complex and is diagrammatically depicted in Fig. 13.20, A. *P. falciparum* differs from other forms of plasmodial species in 4 respects:
i) It does not have exo-erythrocytic stage.
ii) Erythrocytes of any age are parasitised while other plasmodia parasitise juvenile red cells.
iii) One red cell may contain more than one parasite.
iv) The parasitised red cells are sticky causing obstruction of small blood vessels by thrombi, a feature which is responsible for extraordinary virulence of *P. falciparum*.

The main clinical features of malaria are cyclic peaks of high fever accompanied by chills, anaemia and splenomegaly.

MORPHOLOGIC FEATURES Parasitisation and destruction of erythrocytes are responsible for major pathologic changes as under (Fig. 13.20, B):
1. Malarial pigment liberated by destroyed red cells accumulates in the phagocytic cells of the reticuloendothelial system resulting in enlargement of the spleen and liver *(hepatosplenomegaly)*.
2. In falciparum malaria, there is massive absorption of haemoglobin by the renal tubules producing *blackwater fever (haemoglobinuric nephrosis)*.
3. At autopsy, *cerebral malaria* is characterised by congestion and petechiae on the white matter.
4. Parasitised erythrocytes in falciparum malaria are sticky and get attached to endothelial cells resulting in obstruction of capillaries of deep organs such as of the brain leading to hypoxia and death. If the patient lives, *microhaemorrhages* and *microinfarcts* may be seen in the brain.

The diagnosis of malaria is made by demonstration of malarial parasite in thin or thick blood films or sometimes in histologic sections (Fig. 13.21). Differential diagnosis has to be made from babesiosis which is caused by malaria-like protozoa, *Babesia microti* and *B. divergens* and transmitted by deer-tick that also causes the Lyme disease.

Major complications occur in severe falciparum malaria which may have manifestations of cerebral malaria (coma), hypoglycaemia, renal impairment, severe anaemia, haemoglobinuria, jaundice, pulmonary oedema, and acidosis followed by congestive heart failure and hypotensive shock.

FILARIASIS

Wuchereria bancrofti and *Brugia malayi* are responsible for causing Bancroftian and Malayan filariasis in different geographic regions. The lymphatic vessels inhabit the adult worm, especially in the lymph nodes, testis and epididymis.

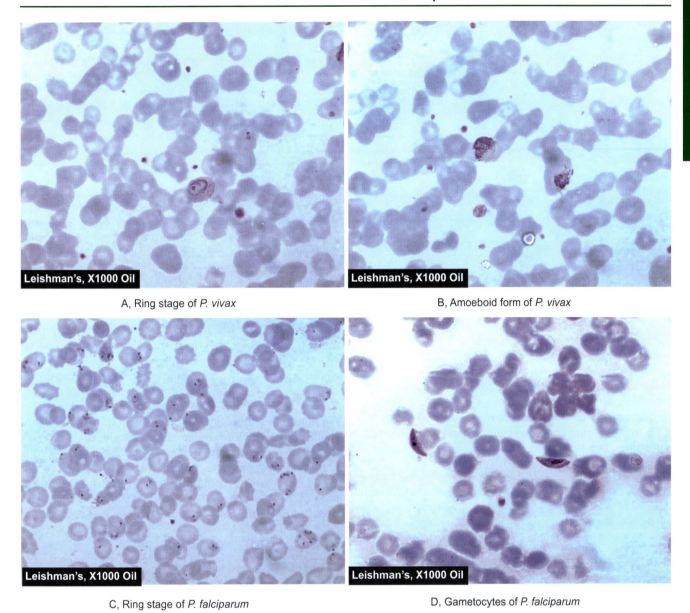

Figure 13.21 ▶ Malarial parasite in blood film—various stages of two main species, *P. vivax* and *P. falciparum*.

Microfilariae seen in the circulation are produced by the female worm **(Fig. 13.22)**. Majority of infected patients remain asymptomatic. Symptomatic cases may have two forms of disease—an acute form and a chronic form.

◈ *Acute form* of filariasis presents with fever, lymphangitis, lymphadenitis, epididymo-orchitis, urticaria, eosinophilia and microfilariaemia.

◈ *Chronic form* of filariasis is characterised by lymphadenopathy, lymphoedema, hydrocele and elephantiasis.

MORPHOLOGIC FEATURES The most significant histologic changes are due to the presence of adult worms in the lymphatic vessels causing lymphatic obstruction and lymphoedema. The regional lymph nodes are enlarged and their sinuses are distended with lymph. The tissues surrounding the blocked lymphatics are infiltrated by chronic inflammatory cell infiltrate consisting of lymphocytes, histiocytes, plasma cells and eosinophils. Chronicity of the process causes enormous thickening and induration of the skin of legs and scrotum resembling the hide of an elephant and hence the name *elephantiasis*. *Chylous ascites* and *chyluria* may occur due to rupture of the abdominal lymphatics.

CYSTICERCOSIS

Cysticercosis is an infection by the larval stage of *Taenia solium*, the pork tapeworm. The adult tapeworm resides in

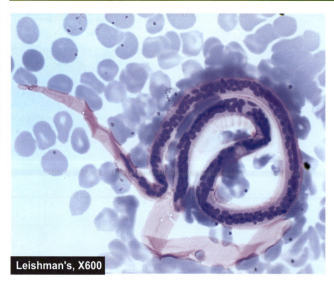

Figure 13.22 ▶ Microfilariae in blood film.

sites are the brain, skeletal muscle and skin (Fig. 13.23). Cysticercus consists of a round to oval white cyst, about 1 cm in diameter, contains milky fluid and invaginated scolex with birefringent hooklets. The cysticercus may remain viable for a long time and incite no inflammation. But when the embryo dies, it produces granulomatous reaction with eosinophils. Later, the lesion may become scarred and calcified (Fig. 13.24).

HYDATID DISEASE (ECHINOCOCCOSIS)

Hydatid disease occurs as a result of infection by the larval cyst stage of the tapeworm, *Echinococcus granulosus*. The dog is the common definite host, while man, sheep and cattle are the intermediate hosts. The dog is infected by eating the viscera of sheep containing hydatid cysts. The infected faeces of the dog contaminate grass and farmland from where the ova are ingested by sheep, pigs and man. Thus, man can acquire infection by handling dogs as well as by eating contaminated vegetables. The ova ingested by man are liberated from the chitinous wall by gastric juice and pass through the intestinal mucosa from where they are carried to the liver by portal venous system. These are trapped in the hepatic sinusoids where they eventually develop into hydatid cyst. About 70% of hydatid cysts develop in the liver which acts as the first filter for ova. However, ova which pass through the liver enter the right side of the heart and are caught in the pulmonary capillary bed and form pulmonary hydatid cysts. Some ova which enter the systemic circulation give rise to hydatid cysts in the brain, spleen, bone and muscles.

The disease is common in sheep-raising countries such as Australia, New Zealand and South America. The *uncomplicated hydatid cyst* of the liver may be silent or may

the human intestines. The eggs are passed in human faeces which are ingested by pigs or they infect vegetables. These eggs then develop into larval stages in the host, spread by blood to any site in the body and form cystic larvae termed *cysticercus cellulosae*. Human beings may acquire infection by the larval stage by eating undercooked pork ('measly pork'), by ingesting uncooked contaminated vegetables, and sometimes, by autoinfection.

MORPHOLOGIC FEATURES The cysticercus may be single or there may be multiple cysticerci in the different tissues of the body. The cysts may occur virtually anywhere in body and accordingly produce symptoms; most common

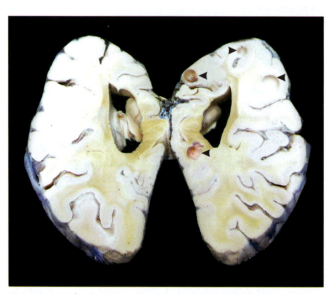

Figure 13.23 ▶ Numerous cysticerci in the base of the brain.

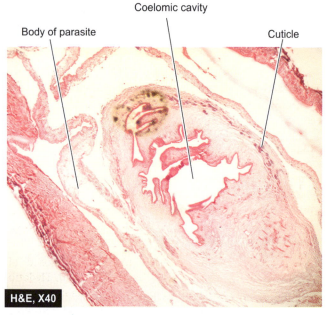

Figure 13.24 ▶ Cysticercus in skeletal muscle. The worm is seen in the cyst while the cyst wall shows palisade layer of histiocytes.

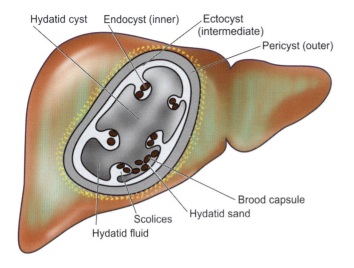
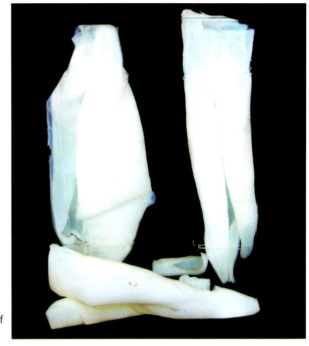

Figure 13.25 ▶ Hydatid cyst in the liver. The cyst wall is composed of whitish membrane resembling the membrane of a hard boiled egg.

produce dull ache in the liver area and some abdominal distension.

Complications of hydatid cyst include its rupture (e.g. into the peritoneal cavity, bile ducts and lungs), secondary infection and hydatid allergy due to sensitisation of the host with cyst fluid. The diagnosis is made by peripheral blood eosinophilia, radiologic examination and serologic tests such as indirect haemagglutination test and Casoni skin test.

MORPHOLOGIC FEATURES Hydatid cyst grows slowly and may eventually attain a size over 10 cm in diameter in about 5 years. *E. granulosus* generally causes unilocular hydatid cyst while *E. multilocularis* results in multilocular or alveolar hydatid disease in the liver.

The cyst wall is composed of 3 distinguishable zones—outer *pericyst,* intermediate characteristic *ectocyst* and inner *endocyst* (Fig. 13.25):

1. Pericyst is the outer host inflammatory reaction consisting of fibroblastic proliferation, mononuclear cells, eosinophils and giant cells, eventually developing into dense fibrous capsule which may even calcify.

2. Ectocyst is the intermediate layer composed of characteristic acellular, chitinous, laminated hyaline material (Fig. 13.26).

3. Endocyst is the inner germinal layer bearing daughter cysts (brood-capsules) and scolices projecting into the lumen.

Hydatid sand is the grain-like material composed of numerous scolices present in the hydatid fluid. Hydatid fluid, in addition, contains antigenic proteins so that its liberation into circulation gives rise to pronounced eosinophilia or may cause anaphylaxis.

TORCH COMPLEX

Acronym 'TORCH' complex refers to development of common complex of symptoms in infants due to infection with different microorganisms that include: *T*oxoplasma, *O*thers, *R*ubella, *C*ytomegalovirus, and *H*erpes simplex virus; category of 'Others' refers to infections such as hepatitis B, coxsackievirus B, mumps and poliovirus. The infection may be acquired by the foetus during intrauterine life, or perinatally and damage the foetus or infant. Since the symptoms produced by TORCH group of organisms are indistinguishable from each other, it is a common practice to test for all the four main TORCH agents in a suspected pregnant mother or infant.

It has been estimated that TORCH complex infections have an overall incidence of 1-5% of all live born children. All the microorganisms in the TORCH complex are transmitted transplacentally and, therefore, infect the foetus from the mother.

◈ Herpes and cytomegalovirus infections are common intrapartum infections acquired venereally.

◈ Toxoplasmosis is a protozoal infection acquired by contact with cat's faeces or by ingestion of raw uncooked meat.

◈ Rubella or German measles is teratogenic in pregnant mothers.

◈ Cytomegalovirus and herpesvirus infections are generally transmitted to foetus by chronic carrier mothers.

An infectious mononucleosis-like disease is present in about 10% of mothers whose infants have *Toxoplasma* infection. Genital herpes infection is present in 20% of mothers whose newborn babies suffer from herpes infection. Rubella infection during acute stage in the first 10 weeks of pregnancy is more harmful to the foetus than at later stage of

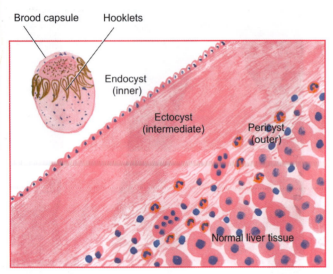
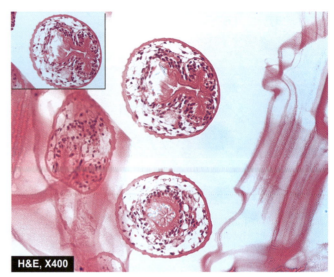

Figure 13.26 ▶ Microscopy shows three layers in the wall of hydatid cyst. Inbox in the right photomicrograph shows a scolex with a row of hooklets.

gestation. Symptoms of cytomegalovirus infection are present in less than 1% of mothers who display antibodies to it.

The classic features of syndrome produced by TORCH complex are seen in congenital rubella. The features include: ocular defects, cardiac defects, CNS manifestations, sensori-neural deafness, thrombocytopenia and hepatosplenomegaly **(Fig. 13.27)**.

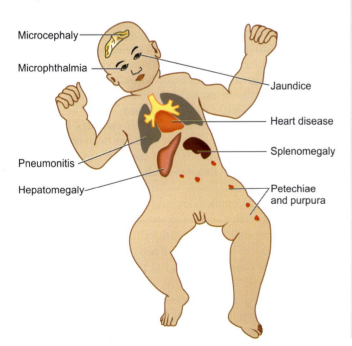

Figure 13.27 ▶ Lesions produced by TORCH complex infection in foetus *in utero*.

The foetal damage caused by TORCH complex infection is irreparable and, therefore, prevention and immunisation are the best modes of therapy.

 GIST BOX 13.5 — **Diseases caused by Parasites and TORCH Complex**

❖ Amoebiasis is caused by *Entamoeba histolytica* and the lesions produced are amoebic dysentery, amoebic colitis, amoeboma, amoebic liver abscess.
❖ Malaria is a protozoal disease caused by any one or combination of four species of plasmodia: *Plasmodium vivax, Plasmodium falciparum, Plasmodium ovale* and *Plasmodium malariae*.
❖ *Wuchereria bancrofti* and *Brugia malayi* cause Bancroftian and Malayan filariasis. The lymphatic vessels inhabit the adult worm, especially in the lymph nodes, testis and epididymis, while microfilariae are seen in the circulation.
❖ Cysticercosis is infection by the larval stage of *Taenia solium*, the pork tapeworm, and produces cystic larvae in different tissues called cysticercosis cellulosae.
❖ Hydatid cyst has endocyst, ectocyst and pericyst and it occurs as a result of infection by the tapeworm larvae, *Echinococcus granulosus*.
❖ TORCH complex refers to development of symptoms in infants due to infection with *T*oxoplasma, *O*thers, *R*ubella, *C*ytomegalovirus, and *H*erpes simplex virus; category of 'Others' refers to infections such as hepatitis B, coxsackievirus B, mumps and poliovirus.

14 Diseases of Immunity including AIDS

THE IMMUNE SYSTEM

Immunity and immunopathology are proverbial two edges of 'double-edged sword' i.e. it is a defense mechanism but it can be injurious to the human body in a variety of ways.

Broadly speaking, immunity or body defense mechanism is divided into 2 types, natural (innate) and specific (adaptive), which are interlinked to each other in their functions:

Natural or innate immunity is *non-specific* and is considered as the first line of defense without antigenic specificity. It has 2 major components:
a) *Humoral:* comprised by complement.
b) *Cellular:* consists of neutrophils, macrophages, and natural killer (NK) cells.

Specific or adaptive immunity is *specific* and is characterised by antigenic specificity. It too has 2 main components:
a) *Humoral:* consisting of antibodies formed by B cells.
b) *Cellular:* mediated by T cells.

The **major functions of immune system** are as under:
i) Recognition of self from non-self
ii) Mounting a specific response against non-self
iii) Memory of what was earlier recognised as non-self
iv) Antibody formation
v) Cell-mediated reactions

While normal function of immunity is for body defense, its failure or derangement in any way results in diseases of the immune system which are broadly classified into the following 4 groups (Fig. 14.1):

1. **Immunodeficiency disorders** are characterised by deficient or absent cellular and/or humoral immune functions. This group is comprised by a list of *primary and secondary immunodeficiency diseases* including the dreaded *acquired immunodeficiency syndrome (AIDS)*.

2. **Hypersensitivity reactions** are characterised by hyperfunction or inappropriate response of the immune system and cover the various mechanisms of *immunologic tissue injury*.

3. **Autoimmune diseases** occur when the immune system fails to recognise 'self' from 'non-self'. A growing number of *autoimmune and collagen diseases* are included in this group.

4. **Possible immune disorders** in which the immunologic mechanisms are suspected in their etiopathogenesis. Classical example of this group is *amyloidosis* (Chapter 7).

Before discussing these diseases, it is important to briefly review the normal structure and function of the immune system (immunophysiology) discussed below.

In any discussion of immunity, a few terms and definitions are commonly used as follows:

◆ An **antigen (Ag)** is defined as a substance, usually protein in nature, which when introduced into the tissues stimulates antibody production.

◆ **Hapten** is a non-protein substance which has no antigenic properties, but on combining with a protein can form a new antigen capable of forming antibodies.

◆ An **antibody (Ab)** is a protein substance produced as a result of antigenic stimulation. Circulating antibodies are immunoglobulins (Igs) of which there are 5 classes: IgG, IgA, IgM, IgE and IgD.

◆ An antigen may induce **specifically sensitised cells** having the capacity to recognise, react and neutralise the injurious agent or organisms.

◆ Antigen may combine with antibody to form **antigen-antibody complex**. The reaction of Ag with Ab *in vitro* may be *primary* or *secondary phenomena*; the secondary reaction induces a number of processes such as agglutination, precipitation, immobilisation, neutralisation, lysis and complement fixation. *In vivo*, the Ag-Ab reaction may cause tissue damage.

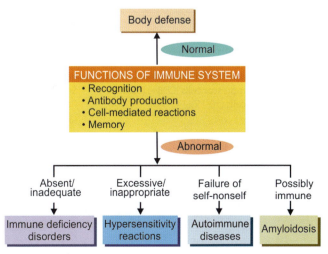

Figure 14.1 ▶ Pathophysiology of diseases of immune system.

ORGANS AND CELLS OF IMMUNE SYSTEM

Although functioning as a system, the organs of immune system are distributed at different places in the body. These are as under:

a) Primary lymphoid organs:
i) Thymus
ii) Bone marrow

b) Secondary lymphoid organs:
i) Lymph nodes
ii) Spleen
iii) MALT (Mucosa-Associated Lymphoid Tissue located in the respiratory tract and GIT).

These organs have been described in the related chapters in the book.

CELLS OF IMMUNE SYSTEM

The cells comprising immune system are as follows:
i) Lymphocytes
ii) Monocytes and macrophages
iii) Mast cells and basophils
iv) Neutrophils
v) Eosinophils

While morphologic aspects of these cells are covered elsewhere in the book, their immune functions are briefly considered below and summarised in **Table 14.1**.

Lymphocytes

Lymphocyte is the master of human immune system. Morphologically, lymphocytes appear as a homogeneous group but functionally two major lymphocyte populations, *T and B lymphocytes*, are identified; while a third type, *NK (natural killer) cells*, comprises a small percentage of circulating lymphocytes having the distinct appearance of *large granular lymphocytes*.

Just as other haematopoietic cells, all three subtypes of lymphocytes are formed from lymphoid precursor cells in the bone marrow. However, unlike other haematopoietic cells, lymphocytes undergo maturation and differentiation in the bone marrow (B cells) and thymus (T cells) and acquire certain genetic and immune surface characters which determine their type and function; this is based on *cluster of differentiation* (CD) molecule on their surface. CD surface protein molecules belong to immunoglobulin superfamily of cell adhesion molecules (CAMs). About 350 different surface CD molecules have been identified so far, which can be identified by 'CD markers' by specific monoclonal antibody stain employing immunohistochemistry or by flow cytometry. B and T lymphocytes proliferate into '*memory cells*' imparting long lasting immunity against specific antigens. While B cells differentiate into plasma cells which form specific antibodies, T cells get functionally activated on coming in contact with appropriate antigen.

Upon coming in contact with antigen, the macrophage (i.e. specialised antigen-presenting cell such as dendritic cell) and the major histocompatibility complex (MHC) in the macrophage, determine whether the invading antigen is to be presented to B cells or T cells. Some strong antigens that cannot be dealt by antibody response from B cells such as certain microorganisms (e.g. viruses, mycobacteria *M. tuberculosis* and *M. leprae*), cancer cells, tissue transplantation antigen etc, are presented to T cells.

Features and functions of subtypes of lymphocytes are summed up below and illustrated diagrammatically in **Fig. 14.2**.

Table 14.1	Cells of the immune system and their functions.
CELLS	**FUNCTIONS**
1. Lymphocytes (20-50%)	Master of immune system
i) B-cells (10-15%)	Antibody-based humoral reactions, transform to plasma cells
Plasma cells	Secrete immunoglobulins
ii) T-cells (75-80%)	Cell-mediated immune reactions
a) T-helper cells (CD4+) (60%)	Promote and enhance immune reaction by elaboration of cytokines
b) T-suppressor cells (CD8+) (30%)	Suppress immune reactions but are directly cytotoxic to antigen
c) NK-cells (10-15%)	Part of natural or innate immunity; cause antibody-dependent cell-mediated cytotoxicity (ADCC)
2. Monocytes-macrophages (~5%)	Antigen recognition Phagocytosis Secretory function Antigen presentation
3. Mast cells and basophils (0-1%)	Allergic reactions Wound healing
4. Neutrophils (40-75%)	First line of defense against microorganisms and other small antigens
5. Eosinophils (1-6%)	Allergic reactions Helminthiasis

The figures in brackets denote percentage of cells in circulation.

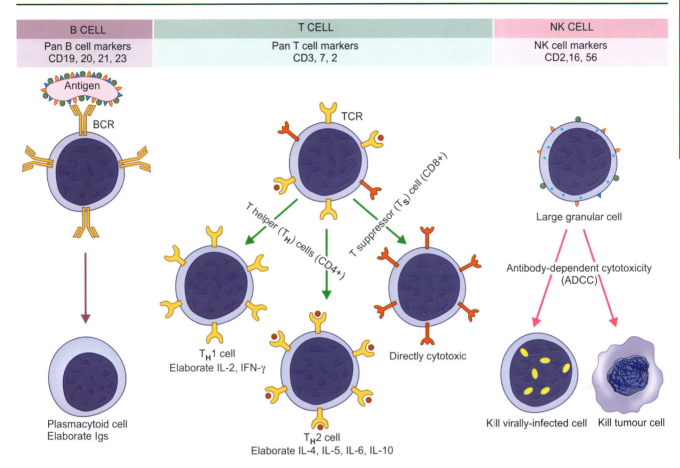

Figure 14.2 ▶ Schematic representation of functions of B and T lymphocytes and NK cells. (BCR = B cell receptor, TCR = T cell receptor).

B CELLS These cells are involved in humoral immunity by inciting antibody response. B cells in circulation comprise about 10-15% of lymphocytes. On coming in contact with antigen (e.g. invading microorganisms), B cells are activated to proliferate and transform into plasmacytoid lymphocytes and then into plasma cells. Depending upon the maturation stage of B cells, specific CD molecules appear on the cell surface which can be identified by CD markers. Common B cell markers are: CD 19, 20, 21, 23. These cells also possess B cell receptors (BCR) for surface immunoglobulins (IgM and IgG) and Fc receptor for attaching to antibody molecule. T cell help is provided to B cells by a subset of T helper cells, $T_H 2$, by elaborated interleukins (IL-4, IL-5, IL-10, IL-13).

T CELLS These cells are implicated in inciting cell-mediated immunity and delayed type of hypersensitivity. T cells in circulation comprise 75-80% of lymphocytes. Pan T cell markers are CD3, CD7 and CD2. Besides, T cells also carry receptor (TCR) for recognition of MHC molecules. Depending upon functional activity, T cells have two major subtypes: *T helper (or CD4+) cells* and *T suppressor (or CD8+) cells*.

T helper cells Abbreviated as T_H cells, these cells promote and enhance the immune reaction and are also termed as *T-regulatory cells*. They carry CD4 molecule on their surface and hence are also called *CD4+ cells*. CD4+ cells in circulation are about twice the number of CD8+ cells (CD4+/CD8 ratio 2:1). These cells act by elaboration of variety of cytokines. Depending upon the type of cytokines elaborated, these T_H cells are further of two subclasses: $T_H 1$ and $T_H 2$.

◈ *$T_H 1$ cells* elaborate IL-2 and interferon (IFN)-γ.

◈ *$T_H 2$ cells* elaborate IL-4, IL-5, IL-6, and IL-10.

CD4+ cells are predominantly involved in cell-mediated reactions to viral infections (e.g. in HIV), tissue transplant reactions and tumour lysis.

T suppressor cells Abbreviated as T_S cells, they suppress immune reactions but are cytotoxic and actually destroy the invading antigen; hence are also termed as *cytotoxic T lymphocytes (CTL)*. These cells carry CD8 molecule on their surface and hence are also called *CD8+ cells*. CD8+ cells in circulation are about half the number of CD4+ cells. Compared

Table 14.2	Differences between T and B lymphocytes.	
FEATURE	T CELLS	B CELLS
1. Origin	Bone marrow → Thymus	Bone marrow → Bursa (in fowl); mucosa-associated lymphoid tissue (MALT)
2. Lifespan	Small T cells: months to years T cell blasts: several days	Small B cells: less than 1 month B cell blasts: several days
3. Location		
(i) Lymph nodes	Perifollicular (paracortical)	Germinal centres, medullary cords
(ii) Spleen	Periarteriolar	Germinal centres, red pulp
(iii) Peyer's patches	Perifollicular	Central follicles
4. Presence in circulation	75-80%	10-15%
5. Surface markers		
(i) Ag receptors	Present	Absent
(ii) Surface Ig	Absent	Present
(iii) Fc receptor	Absent	Present
(iv) Complement receptor	Absent	Present
(v) CD markers	T_H cells CD4, 3, 7, 2 T_S cells CD8, 3, 7, 2	CD19, 20, 21, 23
6. Functions	(i) CMI via cytotoxic T cells positive for CD3 and CD4 (ii) Delayed hypersensitivity via CD4+ T cells (iii) Immunoregulation of other T cells, B cells and stem cells via T helper (CD4+) or T suppressor (CD8+) cells	(i) Role in humoral immunity by synthesis of specific antibodies (Igs) (ii) Precursors of plasma cells

to CD4+ cells which act by elaboration of cytokines, CD8+ cells are directly cytotoxic to the antigen.

CD8+ cells are particularly involved in destroying cells infected with viruses, foreign cells and tumour cells.

Contrasting features of B and T cells are given in Table 14.2.

NATURAL KILLER (NK) CELLS NK cells comprise about 10-15% of circulating lymphocytes. These lymphocytes do not have B or T cell markers, nor are these cells dependent upon thymus for development unlike CD4+ and CD8+ T cells. NK cells carry surface molecules of CD2, CD16 and CD56, but negative for T cell marker CD3. NK cells are morphologically distinct from B and T cells in being *large granular lymphocytes*.

NK cells are part of the natural or innate immunity. These cells recognise antibody-coated target cells and bring about killing of the target directly; this process is termed as *antibody-dependent cell-mediated cytotoxicity (ADCC)*. This mechanism is particularly operative against viruses and tumour cells.

Monocytes and Macrophages

The role of macrophages in inflammation consisting of circulating monocytes, organ-specific macrophages and histiocytes has been described in Chapter 10. Circulating monocytes are immature macrophages and constitute about 5% of peripheral leucocytes. They remain in circulation for about 3 days before they enter tissues to become macrophages. The macrophage subpopulations such as the dendritic cells (in the lymphoid tissue) and Langerhans' cells (in the epidermis) are characterised by the presence of dendritic cytoplasmic processes and are active in the immune system.

Salient features and important immune functions of macrophages are as follows:

1. Antigen recognition They possess cell surface receptors to several extracellular molecules—receptor for cytokines, component of complement (C3b), selectins, integrins and Fc (constant fragment) of antibody. These receptors recognise the organisms and initiate intracellular mechanism in macrophages. Antigen to become recognisable can also get coated by antibodies or complement, the process being termed as *opsonisation*. Macrophages have capacity to distinguish self from non-self by presence of human leucocyte antigens (HLA) or major histocompatibility complex (MHC) discussed below.

2. Phagocytosis Antigen that has been recognised by the macrophages due to availability of above-mentioned surface receptors, or the opsonised antigen, is ready to be engulfed by the process of cell-eating by macrophages explained on page 112.

3. Secretory function Macrophages secrete important substances as follows:

i) *Cytokines* (IL-1, IL-2, IL-6, IL-8, IL-10, IL-12, tumour necrosis factor-α) and *prostaglandins* (PGE, thromboxane-A, leukotrienes) which are chemical mediators of inflammation and activate other leucocytes.

ii) *Secretion of proteins involved in wound healing* e.g. collagenase, elastase, fibroblast growth factor, angiogenesis factor.

iii) *Acute phase reactants* e.g. fibronectin, microglobulin, complement components.

4. Antigen presentation When macrophages are unable to lyse an antigen or an organism, the next best course adopted by them is to act as antigen-presenting cells for presenting to immunocompetent T cells (subtype CD4+ or CD8+ cells), or to B cells. Accordingly, the lymphoid cell would then deal with such antigen.

Basophils and Mast Cells

Basophils are a type of circulating granulocytes (0-1%) while mast cells are their counterparts seen in tissues, especially in connective tissue around blood vessels and in submucosal location. Basophils and mast cells have IgE surface receptor; thus on coming in contact with antigen binding to IgE (e.g. allergic reaction to parasites), these cells get activated and release granules i.e. they degranulate. These granules contain active substances such as histamine, platelet activating factor, heparin and certain chemical mediators (e.g. prostaglandins, leukotrienes).

Mast cells and basophils are thus involved in mediating inflammation in allergic reactions and have a role in wound healing.

Neutrophils

Polymorphonuclear neutrophils (PMNs) are normally the most numerous of the circulating leucocytes (40-75%). The cytoplasm of PMNs contains lysosomal granules of three types: primary (azurophilic), secondary, and tertiary.

PMNs have similar function to those of macrophages and are therefore appropriately referred to as '*microphages*' owing to their role as first line of defense against an invading foreign organism in the body. However, these cells have limitation of size and type of organisms to be engulfed e.g. while they are capable of acting against bacteria and small foreign particulate material but not against viruses and large particles.

Eosinophils

Eosinophils are also circulating granulocytes (1-6%). These cells play a role in allergic reactions and in intestinal helminthiasis. The granules of eosinophils contain lysosomal enzymes, peroxidases, and chemical mediators of inflammation (e.g. prostaglandins, leukotrienes). On coming in contact with IgE opsonised antigen (e.g. helminths), eosinophils degranulate and release the chemicals stored in granules and incite inflammation.

CYTOKINES

Cytokines are immunomodulating agents composed of soluble proteins, peptides and glycoproteins secreted by haematopoietic and non-haematopoietic cells in response to various stimuli. Their main role is in molecular interaction between various cells of the immune system described above and are critical in innate as well as in adaptive immune responses. Cytokines are named according to their presumed targets or possible functions e.g. monokines, colony stimulating factor etc. Presently, about 200 cytokines have been identified. Many of these cytokines have further subtypes as alpha, beta, or are identified by numbers.

CLASSIFICATION Based on structural similarity, cytokines are grouped in following 3 main categories:

i) *Haematopoietin family*: G-CSF, GM-CSF, erythropoietin, thrombopoietin, Various interleukins (IL) such as IL-2, IL-3, IL-4, IL-5, IL-6, IL-7, IL-9.

ii) *IL-1α and IL-1 β, tumour necrosis factor (TNF, cachectin), platelet-derived growth factor (PDGF), transforming growth factor (TGF)-β family.*

iii) *Chemokine family:* These regulate movement of cells and act through G-protein-derived receptors e.g. IL-8, monocyte chemokine protein (MCP), eotaxin, platelet factor (PF) 4.

CYTOKINE RECEPTORS There are 5 members of family of cytokine receptors:

i) *Immunoglobulin (Ig) superfamily* is the largest group composed of cell surface receptors and extracellular secreted proteins e.g. IL-1 receptors type 1, type 2 etc.

ii) *Haematopoietic growth factor type 1 receptor family* includes receptors or their subunits shared with several interleukins (IL-3, IL-5, IL-11, IL-12, leukaemia inhibitory factor, granulocyte-monocyte colony stimulating factor receptor).

iii) *IFN type II receptor family* includes receptors for IFN-γ, IFN-β.

iv) *TNF receptor family* members are TNF-R1 and TNF-R2, CD40 (B cell marker), CD27 and CD30 (found on activated T and B cells).

v) *Trans-membrane helix receptor family* is linked to GTP-binding proteins and includes two important chemokines, chemokine receptor type 4 (CXCR4) and β-chemokine receptor type 5 (CCR5), implicated in binding and entry of HIV into CD4+ host cells.

MODE OF ACTION OF CYTOKINES Cytokines may act in one of the following 3 ways:

1) *Autocrine* when a cytokine acts on the cell which produced it.

2) *Paracrine* when it acts on another target cell in the vicinity.

3) *Endocrine* when the cytokine secreted in circulation acts on a distant target.

Inflammasomes are the cytoplasmic protein complexes found in macrophages and neutrophils; they activate caspases and thereby convert interleukins from their inactive form to active form, and thus play a role in producing inflammation in innate immunity.

Cytokines are involved in following actions:

1. Regulation of growth Actions of cytokines in signaling pathways have been studied in detail. They act via haematopoietins and their receptors, which activate Janus family of protein tyrosine kinases (JAK). There is binding of 4 JAK kinases: JAK1, JAK2, JAK3, and tyk2, to receptors causing phosphorylation of target molecules. This promotes mitogen-activated protein kinase pathway. Besides, a substrate of JAKs, signal tranducer and activator of transcription (abbreviated as STAT) family of transcription factors, act on the DNA of the nucleus and thus regulate gene expression.

2. Inflammatory mediators Some cytokines are potent mediators of inflammation e.g. lymphokines, monokines, IL-1, IL-8, TNF-α and β, IFN-γ. This aspect is discussed on page 114.

3. Activation of immune system The immune system is activated by binding of cytokine to specific cell-surface receptors after the cell has interacted with the antigen.

4. Cytokine storm Overstimulation of cytokines can trigger cytokine storm which is a potentially fatal condition.

| GIST BOX 14.1 | The Immune System |

- Body immunity is divided into 2 types, natural (innate) and specific (adaptive), both of which are interlinked and inter-dependent. Each of these has humoral and cellular components.
- The organs of immune system are the thymus, bone marrow, lymph nodes, spleen, and MALT.
- The cells of immune system include lymphocytes, monocytes and macrophages, basophils and mast cells, neutrophils and eosinophils.
- Lymphocytes are the master of immune system. Their functional types are B (10-15%), T (75-80%) and NK (10-15%) cells. T cells have further subpopulations: T helper (type 1 and 2) (CD4+) and T suppressor (CD8+) cells.
- B cells incite antibody response, T cells mediate cellular immunity (CD8+ in cytotoxicity, CD4+ by elaboration of various cytokines) and NK cells are part of innate immunity.
- Monocytes-macrophages are involved in antigen recognition, presentation, phagocytosis and elaboration of certain cytokines.
- Cytokines are immunomodulating proteins or peptides secreted by various cells of the body in response to stimuli. These include haematopoietins, interleukins, interferon, colony stimulating factor, tumour necrosis factor, growth factors, chemokines, and their receptors.
- Inflammasomes have a role in producing inflammation in innate immunity by activation of caspases and thereby activate interleukins.
- Cytokines are involved in growth regulation by cell signaling pathways, inflammation and in activation of immune system.

HLA SYSTEM AND MAJOR HISTOCOMPATIBILITY COMPLEX

Though not a component of immune system, HLA system is described here as it is considered important in the regulation of the immune system and is part of immunoglobulin superfamily of cell adhesion molecules (CAMs). HLA stands for *Human Leucocyte Antigens* because these are antigens or genetic proteins in the body that determine one's own tissue from non-self (histocompatibility) and were first discovered on the surface of leucocytes. Subsequently, it was found that HLA are actually gene complexes of proteins on the surface of all nucleated cells of the body and platelets. Since these complexes are of immense importance in matching donor and recipient for organ transplant, they are called *major histocompatibility complex (MHC) or HLA complex.*

Out of various genes for histocompatibility, most of the transplantation antigens or MHC are located on short arm (p) of *chromosome 6*; these genes occupy four regions or loci—A, B, C and D, and exhibit marked variation in allelic genes at each locus. Therefore, the product of HLA antigens is highly polymorphic. The letter w in some of the genes (e.g. Dw3, Cw4, Bw15 etc) refers to the numbers allocated to them at international workshops.

Depending upon the characteristics of MHC, they have been divided into 3 classes **(Fig. 14.3)**:

◆ **Class I MHC antigens** have loci as HLA-A, HLA-B and HLA-C. CD8+ (i.e. T suppressor) lymphocytes carry receptors for class I MHC; these cells are used to identify class I antigen on them.

◆ **Class II MHC antigens** have single locus as HLA-D. These antigens have further 3 loci: DR, DQ and DP. Class II MHC is identified by B cells and CD4+ (i.e. T helper) cells.

◆ **Class III MHC antigens** are some components of the complement system (C2 and C4) coded on HLA complex but are not associated with HLA expression and are not used in antigen identification.

In view of high polymorphism of class I and class II genes, they have a number of alleles on loci numbered serially like HLA-A 1, HLA-A 2, HLA-A 3 etc.

MHC antigens present on the cell surface help the macrophage in its function of recognition of bacterial antigen i.e. they help to identify self from foreign, and accordingly present the foreign antigen to T cells (CD4+ or CD8+) or to B cells.

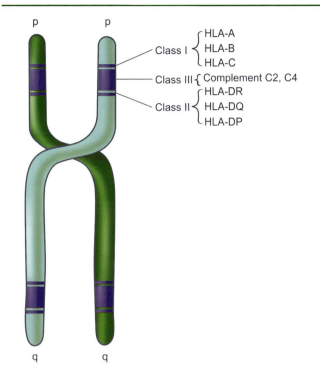

Figure 14.3 ▶ HLA system and loci on short arm of chromosome 6.

ROLE OF HLA COMPLEX The HLA complex is significant in a number of ways:

1. **Organ transplantation** Historically, the major importance of HLA system is in matching donor and recipient for tissue transplantation. The recipient's immune system can recognise the histocompatibility antigens on the donor organ and accordingly accept it or reject it. Both humoral as well as cell-mediated immune responses are involved in case of genetically non-identical transplants.

2. **Regulation of the immune system** Class I and II histocompatibility antigens play a role in regulating both cellular and humoral immunity:
◈ *Class I MHC antigens* regulate the function of cytotoxic T cells (CD8+ subpopulation) e.g. in virus infections.
◈ *Class II MHC antigens* regulate the function of helper T cells (CD4+ subpopulation).

3. **Association of diseases with HLA*** An increasing number of diseases have been found to have association with some specific histocompatibility antigens. These disorders include the following:
◈ *Autoimmune disorders* e.g. rheumatoid arthritis, coeliac disease, Sjogren's syndrome, SLE, chronic active hepatitis.
◈ *Spondyloarthropathies* e.g. ankylosing spondylitis, Reiter's syndrome.
◈ *Endocrinopathies* e.g. type 1 diabetes mellitus.
◈ *Neurologic* e.g. myasthenia gravis

The mechanism of HLA association with diseases is complex and heterogeneous involving multiple steps causing activation of T cells.

GIST BOX 14.2 — HLA System and Major Histocompatibility Complex

❖ HLA system or MHC is composed of antigenic proteins present on all nucleate cells of the body and platelets.
❖ MHC or transplantation antigens are located on short arm of chromosome 6, and has 4 regions or loci: A, B, C and D.
❖ There are 3 classes of antigens. Class I antigens are located on CD8+ cells and have loci as HLA-A, HLA-B and HLA-C. Class II antigens have a single locus, HLA-D and is identified on B cells and CD4+ cells. Class III MHC antigens are components of complement, C2 and C4, but are not used for antigen identification.
❖ Main roles of HLA complex are in organ transplantation, regulation of immune system and its association with certain diseases.

TRANSPLANT REJECTION

According to the genetic relationship between donor and recipient, transplantation of tissues is classified into 4 groups:

1. *Autografts* are grafts in which the donor and recipient is the same individual.

2. *Isografts* are grafts between the donor and recipient of the same genotype.

3. *Allografts* are those in which the donor is of the same species but of a different genotype.

4. *Xenografts* are those in which the donor is of a different species from that of the recipient.

All types of grafts have been performed in human beings but xenografts have been found to be rejected invariably due to genetic disparity. Presently, surgical skills exist for skin grafts and for organ transplants such as kidney, heart, lungs, liver, pancreas, cornea and bone marrow. But most commonly practised are skin grafting, and kidney and bone marrow transplantation. For any successful tissue transplant without immunological rejection, matched major histocompatibility locus antigens (HLA) between the donor and recipient are of paramount importance as discussed already. Greater the genetic disparity between donor and recipient in HLA system, stronger and more rapid will be the rejection reaction.

---

*HLA association with common autoimmune diseases (in chronologic order) are: HLA-DR2=**M**ultiple sclerosis; HLA-DR3=**D**iabetes mellitus type 2; HLA-DR4=**A**rthritis, rheumatoid; HLA-DR5=**A**naemia pernicious and **H**ashimoto's thyroiditis. These can be remembered by the mnemonic as: doctor (**DR**) will turn into **MD** one day, and the thought fills you with a feeling of **MD AAH**! (as HLA-DR association with serial number 2 to 5 and corresponding first letter of each of these diseases as MD AAH).

Besides the rejection reaction, a peculiar problem occurring especially in bone marrow transplantation is *graft-versus-host (GVH) reaction*. In humans, GVH reaction results when immunocompetent cells are transplanted to an immunodeficient recipient e.g. treating severe combined immunodeficiency by bone marrow transplantation. The clinical features of GVH reaction include: fever, weight loss, anaemia, dermatitis, diarrhoea, intestinal malabsorption, pneumonia and hepatosplenomegaly. The intensity of GVH reaction depends upon the extent of genetic disparity between the donor and recipient.

MECHANISMS OF GRAFT REJECTION

Except for autografts and isografts, an immune response against allografts is inevitable. The development of immuno-suppressive drugs has made the survival of allografts in recipients possible. Rejection of allografts involves both cell-mediated and humoral immunity.

1. CELL-MEDIATED IMMUNE REACTIONS These are mainly responsible for graft rejection and are mediated by T cells. The lymphocytes of the recipient on coming in contact with HLA antigens of the donor are sensitised in case of incompatibility. Sensitised T cells in the form of cytotoxic T cells (CD8+) as well as by hypersensitivity reactions initiated by T helper cells (CD4+) attack the graft and destroy it.

2. HUMORAL IMMUNE REACTIONS In addition to the cell-mediated immune reactions, a role for humoral antibodies in certain rejection reactions has been suggested. These include: *preformed circulating antibodies* due to *pre-sensitisation* of the recipient before transplantation e.g. by blood transfusions and previous pregnancies, or in *non-sensitised individuals* by complement dependent cytotoxicity, antibody-dependent cell-mediated cytotoxicity (ADCC) and antigen-antibody complexes.

TYPES OF REJECTION REACTIONS

Based on the underlying mechanism and time period, rejection reactions are classified into 3 types: hyperacute, acute and chronic.

1. HYPERACUTE REJECTION Hyperacute rejection appears within minutes to hours of placing the transplant and destroys it. It is mediated by preformed humoral antibody against donor-antigen. Cross-matching of the donor's lymphocytes with those of the recipient before transplantation has diminished the frequency of hyperacute rejection.

Grossly, hyperacute rejection is recognised by the surgeon soon after the vascular anastomosis of the graft is performed to the recipient's vessels. The organ becomes swollen, oedematous, haemorrhagic, purple and cyanotic rather than gaining pink colour.

Histologically, the characteristics of Arthus reaction are present. There are numerous neutrophils around dilated and obstructed capillaries which are blocked by fibrin and platelet thrombi. Small segments of blood vessel wall may become necrotic and there is necrosis of much of the transplanted organ. Small haemorrhages are common.

2. ACUTE REJECTION This usually becomes evident within a few days to a few months of transplantation. Acute graft rejection may be mediated by cellular or humoral mechanisms. Acute cellular rejection is more common than acute humoral rejection.

Microscopically, the features of the two forms are as under:

i) Acute cellular rejection is characterised by extensive infiltration in the interstitium of the transplant by lymphocytes (mainly T cells), a few plasma cells, monocytes and a few polymorphs. There is damage to the blood vessels and there are foci of necrosis in the transplanted tissue.

ii) Acute humoral rejection appears due to poor response to immunosuppressive therapy. It is characterised by acute rejection vasculitis and foci of necrosis in small vessels. The mononuclear cell infiltrate is less marked as compared to acute cellular rejection and consists mostly of B lymphocytes.

3. CHRONIC REJECTION Chronic rejection may follow repeated attacks of acute rejection or may develop slowly over a period of months to a year or so. The underlying mechanisms of chronic rejection may be immunologic or ischaemic. Patients with chronic rejection of renal transplant show progressive deterioration in renal function as seen by rising serum creatinine levels.

Microscopically, in chronic rejection of transplanted kidney, the changes are intimal fibrosis, interstitial fibrosis and tubular atrophy. Renal allografts may develop glomerulonephritis by transmission from the host, or rarely may develop *de novo* glomerulonephritis.

GIST BOX 14.3 | Transplant Rejection

- Tissue transplants are most often allografts and are done for skin, bone marrow and various solid organs. HLA matching between donor and recipient is always done before tissue transplantation.
- Graft versus host (GVH) reaction occurs when bone marrow cells are transplanted from an immunocompetent donor to an immunodeficient host.
- Graft rejection of other solid organs is mediated mainly by cell-mediated immune reactions via T cells (cytotoxic CD8+ cells and by hypersensitivity reaction initiated by CD4+ cells) and to some extent via humoral immune responses.

> ❖ Rejection reactions may be *hyperacute* appearing within minutes to hours, *acute* becoming evident within a few days to a few months, and *chronic rejection* occurring after repeated attacks of acute rejection or developing slowly.

DISEASES OF IMMUNITY

As already illustrated in Fig. 14.1, diseases of immunity may be classified into following main groups:
1. Immunodeficiency diseases
2. Hypersensitivity diseases
3. Autoimmune diseases.

IMMUNODEFICIENCY DISEASES

Failure or deficiency of immune system, which normally plays a protective role against infections, manifests by occurrence of repeated infections in an individual having immunodeficiency diseases.

Traditionally, immunodeficiency diseases are classified into 2 types:

A. *Primary immunodeficiencies* are usually the result of genetic or developmental abnormality of the immune system.

B. *Secondary immunodeficiencies* arise from acquired suppression of the immune system, the most important example being acquired immunodeficiency syndrome (AIDS).

Since the first description of a primary immunodeficiency disease was made by Bruton in 1952, more and more primary and secondary immunodeficiency syndromes have been added over the years.

A list of most immunodeficiency diseases with the possible defect in the immune system is given in **Table 14.3**, while an account of AIDS is given here.

Table 14.3 Immunodeficiency diseases.

DISEASE	DEFECT
A. PRIMARY IMMUNODEFICIENCY DISEASES	
1. *Severe combined immunodeficiency diseases (Combined deficiency of T cells, B cells and Igs):*	
(i) Reticular dysgenesis	Failure to develop primitive marrow reticular cells
(ii) Thymic alymphoplasia	No lymphoid stem cells
(iii) Agammaglobulinaemia (Swiss type)	No lymphoid stem cells
(iv) Wiscott-Aldrich syndrome	Cell membrane defect of haematopoietic stem cells; associated features are thrombocytopenia and eczema
(v) Ataxia telangiectasia	Defective T cell maturation
2. *T cell defect:* DiGeorge's syndrome (thymic hypoplasia)	Epithelial component of thymus fails to develop
3. *B cell defects (antibody deficiency diseases):*	
(i) Bruton's X-linked agammaglobulinaemia	Defective differentiation from pre-B to B cells
(ii) Autosomal recessive agammaglobulinaemia	Defective differentiation from pre-B to B cells
(iii) IgA deficiency	Defective maturation of IgA synthesising B cells
(iv) Selective deficiency of other Ig types	Defective differentiation from B cells to specific Ig-synthesising plasma cells
(v) Immune deficiency with thymoma	Defective pre-B cell maturation
4. *Common variable immunodeficiencies (characterised by decreased Igs and serum antibodies and variable CMI):*	
(i) With predominant B cell defect	Defective differentiation of pre-B to mature B cells
(ii) With predominant T cell defect	
(a) Deficient T helper cells	Defective differentiation of thymocytes to T helper cells
(b) Presence of activated T suppressor cells	T cell disorder of unknown origin
(iii) With autoantibodies to B and T cells	Unknown differentiation defect
B. SECONDARY IMMUNODEFICIENCY DISEASES	
1. Infections	AIDS (HIV virus); other viral, bacterial and protozoal infections
2. Cancer	Chemotherapy by antimetabolites; irradiation
3. Lymphoid neoplasms (lymphomas, lymphoid leukaemias)	Deficient T and B cell functions
4. Malnutrition	Protein deficiency
5. Sarcoidosis	Impaired T cell function
6. Autoimmune diseases	Administration of high dose of steroids toxic to lymphocytes
7. Transplant cases	Immunosuppressive therapy

Acquired Immunodeficiency Syndrome (AIDS)

Since the initial recognition of AIDS in the United States in 1981, tremendous advances have taken place in the understanding of this dreaded disease as regards its epidemiology, etiology, immunology, pathogenesis, clinical features and morphologic changes in various tissues and organs of the body. Although antiretroviral therapy is being widely used all over the world for such patients, efforts at finding a HIV vaccine have not succeeded so far.

EPIDEMIOLOGY AIDS is pandemic in distribution and is seen in all continents. As per UNAIDS Global Report 2014, an estimated 37 million people are living with AIDS globally (70% in Sub-Saharan Africa), out of which 50% are women and 3.3 million children under 15 years of age. About 1.2 million people are dying from AIDS every year and 2 million cases are being added every year (about 6000 new cases added per day). Regionwise, besides Sub-Saharan Africa, other countries in order of decreasing incidence of AIDS are South and South-East Asia, Latin America, Eastern Europe, Central Asia, North America, while Oceania region has the lowest incidence. It has been seen that new HIV infection has declined by about 35% decline since 2000 and also marginal fall in the number of deaths from HIV. The burden of AIDS in India is estimated at 2.4 million cases; epicentre of the epidemic lies in the states of Maharashtra, Tamil Nadu and Andhra Pradesh which together comprise about 50% of all HIV positive cases (mostly contracted heterosexually), while North-East state of Manipur accounts for 8% of all cases (more often among intravenous drug abusers).

ETIOLOGIC AGENT AIDS is caused by an RNA (retrovirus) virus called human immunodeficiency virus (HIV). There are 4 members of human retroviruses in 2 groups:

◆ *Transforming viruses*: These are human T cell leukaemia-lymphoma virus (HTLV) I and II and are implicated in leukaemia and lymphoma (page 309).

◆ *Cytopathic viruses*: This group includes HIV-1 and HIV-2, causing two forms of AIDS. Most common cause of AIDS in the world including US is HIV-1, while HIV-2 is etiologic agent for AIDS in cases from West Africa and parts of India. Both HIV-1 and HIV-2 are zoonotic infections and their origin can be traced to a species of chimpanzees who are natural reservoir of HIV and most likely source of original infection.

HIV-I virion or virus particle is spherical in shape and 100-140 nm in size **(Fig. 14.4)**:

◆ It contains a *core* having *core proteins*, chiefly p24 and p18, two strands of genomic RNA and the enzyme, reverse transcriptase.

◆ The core is covered by a *double layer of lipid membrane* derived from the outer membrane of the infected host cell during budding process of virus. The membrane is studded with *2 envelope glycoproteins, gp120 and gp41*, in the positions shown.

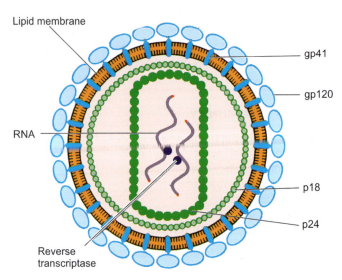

Figure 14.4 ▶ Schematic representation of HIV virion or virus particle. The particle has core containing proteins, p24 and p18, two strands of viral RNA, and enzyme reverse transcriptase. Bilayer lipid membrane is studded with 2 viral glycoproteins, gp120 and gp 41, in the positions shown.

Besides other genes, **three important genes** code for the respective components of virion:
i) *gag (group antigen)* for core proteins,
ii) *pol (polymerase)* for reverse transcriptase, and
iii) *env (envelope)* for the envelope proteins.

These genes and viral components act as markers for the laboratory diagnosis of HIV infection. Besides, there is *tat (transcription activator)* gene for viral functions such as amplification of viral genes, viral budding and replication.

ROUTES OF TRANSMISSION Transmission of HIV infection occurs by one of following three routes and it varies in different populations:

1. Sexual transmission Sexual contact is the main mode of spread and constitutes 75% of all cases of HIV transmission. Most cases of AIDS in the industrialised world such as in the US occur in *homosexual* or *bisexual males* while *heterosexual promiscuity* seems to be the dominant mode of HIV infection in Africa and Asia. Other sexually transmitted diseases (STDs) may act as cofactors for spread of HIV, in particular gonorrhoeal and chlamydial infection. Transmission from male-to-male and male-to-female is more potent route than that from female-to-male.

2. Transmission via blood and blood products This mode of transmission is the next largest group (25%) and occurs in 3 types of high-risk populations:
i) *Intravenous drug abusers* by sharing needles, syringes etc comprise a large group in the US.
ii) *Haemophiliacs* who have received large amounts of clotting factor concentrates from pooled blood components from multiple donors.

iii) *Recipients of HIV-infected blood and blood products* who have received multiple transfusions of whole blood or components like platelets and plasma.

3. **Perinatal transmission** HIV infection occurs from infected mother to the newborn during pregnancy *transplacentally*, or in immediate post-partum period *through contamination* with maternal blood, infected amniotic fluid or breast milk.

4. **Occupational transmission** There have been a small number of health care workers (HCW), laboratory workers and those engaged in disposal of waste of sharps who have developed HIV infection by occupational exposure to HIV-infected material, most often by needle-stick injury. It is imperative that these workers follow the CDC guidelines for *universal precautions* which include disinfecting and sterilising all reusable devices and use of bleaching solution for disinfecting all blood spillage.

5. **Transmission by other body fluids** Although besides blood, HIV has been isolated and identified from a number of body fluids such as saliva, tears, sweat, urine, semen, vaginal secretions, cervical secretions, breast milk, CSF, synovial, pleural, peritoneal and pericardial fluid, there is no definite evidence that HIV transmission can occur by any of these fluids; isolated cases of such infection reported are in likelihood due to concomitant contamination with HIV-infected blood.

It may, however, be understood regarding spread of HIV infection that *AIDS cannot be transmitted by* casual non-sexual contact like shaking hands, hugging, sharing household facilities like beds, toilets, utensils etc.

It should also be appreciated that HIV contaminated waste products can be *sterilised and disinfected* by most of the chemical germicides used in laboratories at a much lower concentration. These are: sodium hypochlorite (liquid chlorine bleach) (1-10% depending upon amount of contamination with organic material such as blood, mucus), formaldehyde (5%), ethanol (70%), glutaraldehyde (2%), β-propionolactone. HIV is also heat-sensitive and can be inactivated at 56°C for 30 min.

PATHOGENESIS The pathogenesis of HIV infection is largely related to the *depletion of CD4+ T cells (helper T cells) resulting in profound immunosuppression.*

Various aspects in the sequence of events is shown schematically in **Fig. 14.5** and is outlined below:

1. **Selective tropism for CD4 molecule receptor** gp120 envelope glycoprotein of HIV has selective tropism for cells containing CD4 molecule receptor on their surface. These cells most importantly are CD4+ T cells (T helper cells); other such cells include monocyte-macrophages, microglial cells, epithelial cells of the cervix, Langerhans cells of the skin and follicular dendritic cells. Initially, HIV on entering the body via any route described above has tropism for macrophages

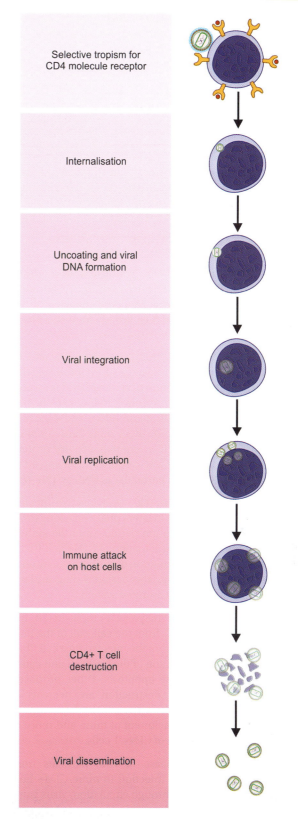

Figure 14.5 ▶ Sequence of events in the pathogenesis of HIV infection.

(M-tropic) while later it becomes either dual tropic or T-tropic only and thus affects mainly CD4+ T cells which are the main target of attack by HIV.

2. Internalisation gp120 of the virion combines with CD4 receptor, but for fusion of virion with the host cell membrane, a chemokine coreceptor (CCR) is necessary. Once HIV has combined with CD4 receptor and CCR, gp41 glycoprotein of envelope is internalised in the CD4+ T cell membrane.

3. Uncoating and viral DNA formation Once the virion has entered the T cell cytoplasm, reverse transcriptase of the viral RNA forms a single-stranded DNA. Using the single-stranded DNA as a template, DNA polymerase copies it to make it double-stranded DNA, while destroying the original RNA strands. Viral DNA so formed has frequent mutations making the HIV quite resistant to anti-retroviral therapy.

4. Viral integration The viral DNA so formed may initially remain *unintegrated* in the affected cell but later viral integrase protein inserts the viral DNA into nucleus of the host T cell and *integrates* in the host cell DNA. At this stage, viral particle is termed as *HIV provirus*.

5. Viral replication HIV provirus having become part of host cell DNA, host cell DNA transcripts for viral RNA with presence of *tat* gene. Multiplication of viral particles is further facilitated by release of cytokines from T helper cells (CD4+ T cells): $T_H 1$ *cells* elaborating IL-2 and IFN-γ, and $T_H 2$ *cells* elaborating IL-4, IL-5, IL6, IL-10. RNA viral particles thus fill the cytoplasm of host T cell where they acquire protein coating. Released cytokines are also responsible for spread of infection to other body sites, in particular to CNS by TNF-α.

6. Latent period and immune attack In an inactive infected T cell, the infection may remain in latent phase for a long time, accounting for the long incubation period. Immune system does act against the virus by participation of CD4+ and CD8+ T cells, macrophages and by formation of antibodies to mount attack against the virus. However, this period is short and the virus soon overpowers the host immune system.

7. CD4+ T cell destruction Viral particles replicated in the CD4+ T cells start forming *buds* from the cell wall of the host cell. As these particles detach from the infected host cell, they damage part of the cell membrane of the host cell and cause death of host CD4+ T cells by apoptosis. Other proposed mechanisms of CD4+ T cell destruction are necrosis of precursors of CD4+ cells by the virus and by formation of syncytial giant cells due to attachment of more and more of gp120 molecules to the surface of CD4+ T cells.

8. Viral dissemination Release of viral particles from infected host cell spreads the infection to more CD4+ host cells and produces viraemia. Through circulation, virus gains entry to the lymphoid tissues (lymph nodes, spleen) where it multiplies further; thus these tissues become the dominant site of virus reservoir rather than circulation.

9. Impact of HIV infection on other immune cells HIV infects other cells of the host immune system and also affects non-infected lymphoid cells.

i) *Other cells of the immune system:* These cells are circulating monocytes, macrophage in tissues and dendritic follicular cells of lymph nodes. HIV-infected monocytes-macrophages do not get destroyed but instead become a reservoir of HIV infection. Infected dendritic follicular cells of the lymph nodes causes massive enlargement of follicle centres and account for persistent generalised lymphadenopathy in AIDS.

ii) *Non-infected lymphoid cells:* These cells include B cells, NK cells and CD8+ T cells. B cells do not have receptors for HIV but the number of B cells slowly declines, their function of immunoglobulin synthesis is impaired due to lack of their activation by depleting CD4+ T cells, and there may be non-specific hypergammaglobulinaemia. NK cells are also reduced due to lack of cytokines from depleted CD4+ T cells. CD8+ cells show lymphocytosis but the cells having intact function of ADCC are reduced, possibly due to quantitative loss of CD4+ T cell and their qualitative dysfunction (reversal of CD4+ T cells: CD8+ T cell ratio).

The net result of immunological changes in the host due to HIV infection lead to profound immunosuppression rendering the host susceptible to opportunistic infections and tumours, to which the patient ultimately succumbs.

10. HIV infection of nervous system Out of non-lymphoid organ involvement, HIV infection of nervous system is the most serious and 75-90% of AIDS patients may demonstrate some form of neurological involvement at autopsy. It infects microglial cells, astrocytes and oligodendrocytes as under:

i) *Infection carried to the microglia* of the nervous system by *HIV infected CD4+ monocyte-macrophage subpopulation or endothelial cells.*

ii) *Direct infection* of astrocytes and oligodendrocytes.

iii) Neurons are not invaded by HIV but are affected due to attachment of gp120 and by release of *cytokines* by HIV-infected macrophages.

A summary of major abnormalities in the immune system in AIDS is given in Table 14.4.

NATURAL HISTORY HIV infection progresses from an early acute syndrome to a prolonged asymptomatic state to advanced disease. Thus, there are different clinical manifestations at different stages. Generally, in an immunocompetent host, the biologic course passes through following 3 phases **(Table 14.5):**

1. Acute HIV syndrome Entry of HIV into the body is heralded by the following sequence of events:

i) High levels of plasma *viraemia* due to replication of the virus.

ii) Virus-specific immune response by formation of anti-HIV antibodies (*seroconversion*) after 3-6 weeks of initial exposure to HIV.

Chapter 14: Diseases of Immunity including AIDS

Table 14.4	Major abnormalities in immune system in AIDS.
1.	**T CELL ABNORMALITIES**
	i) Lymphopenia
	ii) CD4+ T cell depletion
	iii) CD8+ T cell lymphocytosis
	iv) Reversal of CD4: CD8 cell ratio
	v) Decreased production of cytokines by CD4+ T cells
	vi) Decreased antibody-dependent cellular cytotoxicity (ADCC) by CD8+ T cells
2.	**B CELL ABNORMALITIES**
	i) No direct viral damage
	ii) Decreased Ig production
	iii) Polyclonal activation
	iv) Hypergammaglobulinaemia
	v) Circulating immune complexes
3.	**NK CELL ABNORMALITIES**
	i) No direct viral damage
	ii) Depressed number
	iii) Decreased cytotoxicity
4.	**MONOCYTE-MACROPHAGE CELL ABNORMALITIES**
	i) No destruction
	ii) Decreased chemotaxis
	iii) Decreased cytotoxicity

iii) Initially, sudden marked reduction in *CD4+ T cells* (helper T cells) followed by return to normal levels.

iv) Rise in *CD8+ T cells* (cytotoxic T cells).

v) Appearance of self-limited non-specific *acute viral illness* (flu-like or infectious mononucleosis-like) in 50-70% of adults within 3-6 weeks of initial infection. Manifestations include: sore throat, fever, myalgia, skin rash, and sometimes, aseptic meningitis. These symptoms resolve spontaneously in 2-3 weeks.

2. Middle chronic phase Initial acute seroconversion illness is followed by a phase of competition between HIV and the host immune response as under:

i) *Viraemia* due to viral replication in the lymphoid tissue continues which is initially not as high but with passage of time viral load increases due to crumbling host defenses.

ii) Chronic stage, depending upon host immune system, may continue as long as *10 years*.

iii) Although *CD 4+ T cells* continue to proliferate but net result is moderate fall in CD4+ T cell counts.

iv) Cytotoxic CD8+ T cell count remains high.

v) Clinically, it may be a stage of *latency* and the patient may remain asymptomatic, or may develop mild constitutional symptoms and persistent generalised lymphadenopathy.

3. Final crisis phase This phase is characterised by profound immunosuppression and onset of full-blown AIDS and has the following features:

i) Marked increase in *viraemia*.

ii) The time period from HIV infection through chronic phase into full-blown AIDS may last *7-10 years and culminate in death*.

iii) *CD 4+ T cells* are markedly reduced (below 200 per µl).

The average survival after the onset of full-blown AIDS is about 2 years.

Children often have a rapidly progressive disease and full-blown AIDS occurring at 4 to 8 years of age.

REVISED CDC HIV CLASSIFICATION SYSTEM The Centers for Disease Control and Prevention (CDC), US in 1993 revised the classification system for HIV infection in adults and children based on 2 parameters: clinical manifestations and CD4+ T cell counts.

According to this system, irrespective of presence of symptoms, any HIV-infected individual having CD4+ T cell count of <200/µl is labelled as AIDS.

CDC defining criteria divide AIDS into 3 categories: A, B and C, each of which is further subdivided, based on CD4+ T cell count, into three subtypes: A1, B1, C1 (CD4+ T cell count ≥500/µl), A2, B2, C2 (CD4+ T cell count 200-499/µl), and A3, B3, C3 (CD4+ T cell count <200/µl) **(Table 14.5)**:

Clinical category A Includes a variety of conditions: asymptomatic case, persistent generalised lymphadenopathy (PGL), and acute HIV syndrome.

Table 14.5	Natural history and revised CDC HIV/AIDS classification.		
PHASE	**EARLY, ACUTE**	**MIDDLE, CHRONIC**	**FINAL, CRISIS**
Period after infection	3-6 weeks	10-12 years	Any period up to death
CDC clinical category	Category A: Asymptomatic infection Acute HIV syndrome PGL	Category B: Symptomatic disease (neither A nor C) Condition secondary to impaired CMI	Category C: AIDS indicator defining conditions
CD4 + T cell categories			
≥ 500/µl	A1	B1	C1
200-499/µl	A2	B2	C2
< 200/µl	A3	B3	C3
(CDC = Centers for Disease Control, Atlanta, USA; PGL = Persistent generalised lymphadenopathy; CME= cell mediated immunity).			

Clinical category B Includes symptomatic cases and includes conditions secondary to impaired cell-mediated immunity e.g. bacillary dysentery, mucosal candidiasis, fever, oral hairy leukoplakia, ITP, pelvic inflammatory disease, peripheral neuropathy, cervical dysplasia and carcinoma in situ cervix etc.

Clinical category C This category includes conditions listed for AIDS surveillance case definition. These are mucosal candidiasis, bacterial infections (e.g. tuberculosis), fungal infections (e.g. histoplasmosis), parasitic infections (e.g. *Pneumocystis* pneumonia), malnutrition, cancer uterine cervix and wasting of muscles etc.

Similarly, there are revised parameters for *paediatric HIV classification* in which age-adjusted CD4+ T cell counts are given that are relatively higher in each corresponding category.

PATHOLOGICAL LESIONS AND CLINICAL MANIFESTATIONS OF HIV/AIDS HIV/AIDS affects all body organs and systems. In general, clinical manifestations and pathological lesions in different organs and systems are owing to progressive deterioration of body's immune system. Disease progression occurs in all untreated patients, even if the disease is apparently latent. Antiretroviral treatment blocks and slows the progression of the disease.

Pathological lesions and clinical manifestations in HIV disease can be explained by 4 mechanisms:

i) Due to viral infection directly: The major targets are immune system, central nervous system and lymph nodes (persistent generalised lymphadenopathy).

ii) Due to opportunistic infections: Deteriorating immune system provides the body an opportunity to harbour microorganisms. A list of common opportunistic infectious agents affecting HIV/AIDS is given in **Fig. 14.6**.

iii) Due to secondary tumours: End-stage of HIV/AIDS is characterised by development of certain secondary malignant tumours **(Fig 14.6)**

iv) Due to drug treatment: Drugs used in the treatment produce toxic effects. These include antiretroviral treatment, aggressive treatment of opportunistic infections and tumours.

Based on above mechanisms, salient clinical features and pathological lesions in different organs and systems are briefly outlined below and illustrated in **Fig. 14.6**. However, it may be mentioned here that many of the pathological lesions given below may not become clinically apparent during life and may be noted at autopsy alone.

1. Wasting syndrome Most important systemic manifestation corresponding to body's declining immune function is wasting syndrome defined as 'involuntary loss of body weight by more than 10%'. It occurs due to multiple factors such as malnutrition, increased metabolic rate, malabsorption, anorexia, and ill-effects of multiple opportunistic infections.

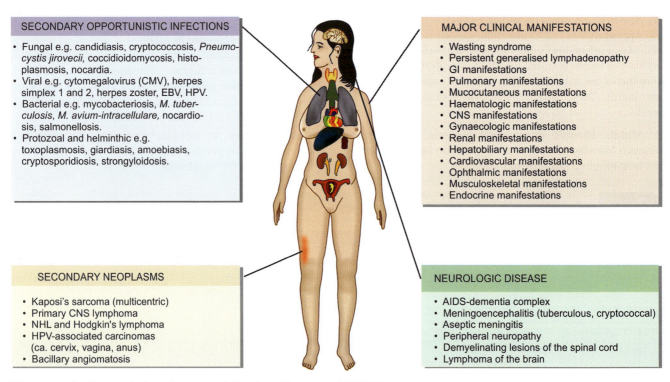

Figure 14.6 ▶ Major pathological lesions and clinical manifestations of HIV/AIDS.

2. Persistent generalised lymphadenopathy In early asymptomatic stage during the course of disease, some patients may develop persistent generalised lymphadenopathy (PGL). PGL is defined as presence of enlarged lymph nodes >1 cm at two or more extrainguinal sites for >3 months without an obvious cause. There is marked cortical follicular hyperplasia, due to proliferation of CD8+ T cells, B cells and dendritic follicular histiocytes. HIV infected CD4+ T cells are seen in the mantle zone. In advanced cases of AIDS, lymph nodes show progressive depletion of lymphoid cells, or there may be occurrence of opportunistic infection (e.g. *M. avium intracellulare, Histoplasma, Toxoplasma*) or appearance of secondary tumours in the lymphoid tissue (e.g. Kaposi's sarcoma, lymphoma).

3. GI lesions and manifestations Almost all patients with HIV infection develop gastrointestinal manifestations. These include: chronic watery or bloody diarrhoea, oral, oropharyngeal and oesophageal candidiasis, anorexia, nausea, vomiting, mucosal ulcers, abdominal pain. These features are due to opportunistic infections (e.g. *Candida, Clostridium, Shigella, Salmonella, Giardia, Entamoeba histolytica, Cryptosporidium,* CMV). Advanced cases may develop secondary tumours in GIT (e.g. Kaposi's sarcoma, lymphoma).

4. Pulmonary lesions and manifestations Symptoms pertaining to lungs develop in about 50-75% of cases and are a major cause of death in HIV/AIDS. These features are largely due to opportunistic infections causing pneumonia e.g. with *Pneumocystis jirovecii, M. tuberculosis,* CMV, *Histoplasma,* and *Staphylococci.* Lung abscess too may develop. Other pulmonary manifestations include adult respiratory distress syndrome and secondary tumours (e.g. Kaposi's sarcoma, lymphoma).

5. Mucocutaneous lesions and manifestations Symptoms due to mucocutaneous involvement occur in about 50 to 75% cases. Mucocutaneous viral exanthem in the form of erythematous rash is seen at the onset of primary infection itself. Other mucocutaneous manifestations are allergic (e.g. drug reaction, seborrhoeic dermatitis), infectious (viral infections such as herpes, varicella zoster, EB virus, HPV; bacterial infections such as *M. avium, Staph. aureus*; fungal infections such as *Candida, Cryptococcus, Histoplasma*) and neoplastic (e.g. Kaposi's sarcoma, squamous cell carcinoma, basal cell carcinoma, cutaneous lymphoma).

6. Haematologic lesions and manifestations Involvement of haematopoietic system is common during the course of HIV/AIDS. These include: anaemia, leucopenia, and thrombocytopenia. These changes are due to bone marrow suppression from several mechanisms: infections such as by HIV, mycobacteria, fungi, and parvoviruses, or by lymphomatous involvement.

7. CNS lesions and manifestations Neurological manifestations occur in almost all cases during the course of disease and are an important cause of mortality and morbidity. These may be inflammatory, demyelinating and degenerative conditions. HIV encephalopathy or AIDS-associated dementia complex, is an AIDS defining condition and manifests clinically with deteriorating cognitive symptoms. Other pathological lesions in HIV/AIDS are meningitis (tuberculous, cryptococcal) demyelinating lesions of the spinal cord, and peripheral neuropathy and lymphoma of the brain.

8. Gynaecologic lesions and manifestations Gynaecologic symptoms are due to monilial (candidal) vaginitis, cervical dysplasia, carcinoma cervix, and pelvic inflammatory disease.

9. Renal lesions and manifestations Features of renal impairment may appear due to HIV-associated nephropathy and genitourinary tract infections including pyelonephritis.

10. Hepatobiliary lesions and manifestations Manifestations of hepatobiliary tract are due to development of coinfection with hepatitis B or C, due to occurrence of other infections and due to drug-induced hepatic injury. The lesions include steatosis, granulomatous hepatitis and opportunistic infections (*M. tuberculosis, Mycobacterium avium intracellulare, Histoplasma*).

11. Cardiovascular lesions and manifestations Diseases affecting the heart are common autopsy findings and include a form of dilated cardiomyopathy called HIV-associated cardiomyopathy, pericardial effusion in advanced disease as a reaction to opportunistic infection, lymphoma and Kaposi's sarcoma.

12. Ophthalmic lesions HIV associated ocular manifestations occur from opportunistic infections (e.g. CMV retinitis), HIV retinopathy, and secondary tumours.

13. Musculoskeletal lesions These include osteoporosis, osteopaenia, septic arthritis, osteomyelitis and polymyositis.

14. Endocrine lesions Several metabolic derangements may occur during the course of disease. Syndrome of lipodystrophy (buffalo hump) due to dyslipidaemia, hyperinsulinaemia and hyperglycaemia may occur. Besides, abnormality of thyroid function, hypogonadism and inappropriate release of ADH may be associated.

LESIONS AND MANIFESTATIONS IN PAEDIATRIC AIDS
Children develop clinical manifestations of AIDS more rapidly than adults. Besides development of opportunistic infections and tumours, neurologic impairment in children cause slowing of development and growth.

DIAGNOSIS OF HIV/AIDS The investigations of a suspected case of HIV/AIDS are categorised into 3 groups: tests for establishing HIV infection, tests for defects in immunity, and tests for detection of opportunistic infections

Table 14.6	Tests for diagnosis of HIV/AIDS.

1. TESTS FOR ESTABLISHING HIV INFECTION

　i) Antibody tests:
　　a) ELISA
　　b) Western blot
　ii) Direct detection of HIV
　　a) p24 antigen capture assay
　　b) HIV RNA assay
　　c) NA-PCR
　　d) Culture of HIV

2. TESTS FOR DEFECTS IN IMMUNITY

　i) CD4+ T cell count: Fall
　ii) CD8+ cell count: Increased
　iii) Ratio of CD4+ T cell/CD8+ T cell count: Reversed
　iv) Lymphopenia
　v) Hypergammaglobulinaemia
　vi) Increased β-2 microglobulin level
　vii) Platelet count: Thrombocytopenia

3. TESTS FOR DETECTION OF OPPORTUNISTIC INFECTION AND SECONDARY TUMOURS

　i) FNAC/exfoliative cytology
　ii) Biopsy

and secondary tumours. However, usually initial testing for antibodies is done against HIV by ELISA and confirmation by Western blot or immunofluorescence test. These tests are as under **(Table 14.6)**:

1. Tests for establishing HIV infection These include antibody tests and direct detection of HIV.

i) Antibody tests These tests are as under:

a) *ELISA* Initial screening is done by serologic test for antibodies by enzyme-linked immunosorbent assay (ELISA) against *gag* and *env* proteins. The term *window period* is used for the initial 2 to 4 weeks period when the patient is infectious but the screening test is negative, while *seroconversion* is the term used for appearance of antibodies. Besides, ELISA may be false positive in autoantibodies, liver disease, recent vaccination against flu, and other viral infections.

b) *Western blot* If ELISA is positive, confirmation is done by Western blot for presence of specific antibodies against all three HIV antigens: *gag, pol and env*.

ii) Direct detection of HIV These tests are as follows:

a) *p24* antigen capture assay.

b) *HIV RNA* assay methods by reverse transcriptase (RT) PCR, branched DNA, nucleic acid sequence-based amplification (NucliSens).

c) *DNA-PCR* by amplification of proviral DNA.

d) *Culture* of HIV from blood monocytes and CD4+ T cells.

2. Tests for defects in immunity These tests are used for diagnosis as well as for monitoring treatment of cases.

i) *CD4+ T cell counts.* Progressive fall in number of CD4+ T cells is of paramount importance in diagnosis and staging as CDC categories as described above.

ii) Rise in CD8+ T cells.

iii) Reversal of CD4+ to CD8+ T cell ratio.

iv) Lymphopenia.

v) Polyclonal hypergammaglobulinaemia.

vi) Increased β-2 microglobulin levels.

vii) Platelet count revealing thrombocytopenia.

3. Tests for detection of opportunistic infections and secondary tumours Diagnosis of organs involved in opportunistic infection and specific tumours secondary to HIV/AIDS is made by aspiration or biopsy methods as for the corresponding primary disease.

GIST BOX 14.4　Immunodeficiency Diseases and HIV-AIDS

❖ Immunodeficiency diseases may be *primary* (usually the result of genetic or developmental abnormality of the immune system) or *secondary* (from acquired suppression of the immune system), the most important example being acquired immunodeficiency syndrome (AIDS).

❖ AIDS has pandemic distribution and is seen in all continents. As per current estimates, 35 million people are living with AIDS globally, Sub-Saharan Africa having the largest number of cases.

❖ It is caused by *retrovirus*, HIV-1 or HIV-2, the former being much more common etiologic agent in most parts of the world.

❖ The routes of spread of infection are: sexual (both homo- and heterosexual), via blood route and by use of contaminated blood products, perinatal transmission to the newborn from infected mothers, needle stick injuries, and rarely from other body fluids.

❖ Mechanism of acquiring disease is by selective tropism of HIV for CD4 molecule located on CD4+ helper T cells and other such cells. The virus internalises in the target cell, uncoats and forms double stranded viral DNA, which then integrates into the host cell DNA, forming HIV provirus. Virus replicates inside the cytoplasm and ultimately destroys the host CD4+T cells. The viral particles then disseminate to the other lymphoid tissues, creating a reservoir of organism in the host.

❖ As per CDC, HIV is defined by clinical features and by CD4+ T cell count <200/μl. Its categories are: A=asymptomatic case, acute HIV syndrome or with PGL; B=symptomatic case due to impaired CMI; and C=having AIDS indicator conditions.

❖ AIDS involves multiple systems and affects almost all organs. The main pathologic lesions in full-blown case are due to opportunistic infections, secondary tumours and CNS manifestations.

❖ Diagnosis of AIDS is made by tests to establish infection (antibody testing by ELISA, confirmation by Western blot), and to detect defect in immunity (low CD4 cell counts and reversal of CD4+:CD8+ cells).

HYPERSENSITIVITY REACTIONS (IMMUNOLOGIC TISSUE INJURY)

Hypersensitivity is defined as an exaggerated or inappropriate state of normal immune response with onset of adverse effects on the body. The lesions of hypersensitivity are a form of antigen-antibody reaction. These lesions are termed as hypersensitivity reactions or immunologic tissue injury, of which 4 types are described: type I, II, III and IV. Depending upon the *rapidity, duration and type* of the immune response, these 4 types of hypersensitivity reactions are grouped into either immediate or delayed type:

1. **Immediate type** in which on administration of antigen, the reaction occurs immediately (within seconds to minutes). Immune response in this type is mediated largely by *humoral antibodies* (B cell mediated). Immediate type of hypersensitivity reactions include *type I, II and III*.

2. **Delayed type** in which the reaction is slower in onset and develops within 24-48 hours and the effect is prolonged. It is mediated by *cellular response* (T cell mediated) and it includes *Type IV reaction*.

The etiopathogenesis and examples of immunologic tissue injury by the 4 types of hypersensitivity reactions are discussed below and are summarised in Table 14.7.

Type I: Anaphylactic (Atopic) Reaction

Type I hypersensitivity is defined as a state of rapidly developing or anaphylactic type of immune response to an antigen (i.e. allergen) to which the individual is previously sensitised (anaphylaxis is the opposite of prophylaxis). The reaction appears within 15-30 minutes of exposure to antigen.

ETIOLOGY Type I reaction is mediated by *humoral antibodies of IgE type or reagin antibodies* in response to antigen. Following hypotheses have been proposed:

1. **Genetic basis** There is evidence that ability to respond to antigen and produce IgE are both linked to genetic basis. For example, there is a 50% chance that a child born to both parents allergic to an antigen, may have similar allergy. Further support to this hypothesis comes from observations of high levels of IgE in hypersensitive individuals and low level of suppressor T cells that control the immune response are observed in persons with certain HLA types (in particular HLA-B8).

2. **Environmental pollutants** Another proposed hypothesis is that environmental pollutants increase mucosal permeability and thus may allow increased entry of allergen into the body, which in turn leads to raised IgE level.

Table 14.7	Comparative features of 4 types of hypersensitivity reactions.			
FEATURE	TYPE I (ANAPHYLACTIC, ATOPIC)	TYPE II (ANTIBODY-MEDIATED, CYTOTOXIC)	TYPE III (IMMUNE-COMPLEX, ARTHUS REACTION)	TYPE IV (DELAYED, T CELL-MEDIATED)
1. Definition	Rapidly developing immune response in a previously sensitised person	Reaction of humoral antibodies that attack cell surface antigens and cause cell lysis	Results from deposition of antigen-antibody complexes on tissues	Cell-mediated slow and prolonged response
2. Peak action time	15-30 minutes	15-30 minutes	Within 6 hours	After 24 hours
3. Mediated by	IgE antibodies	IgG or IgM antibodies	IgG, IgM antibodies	Cell-mediated
4. Etiology	Genetic basis, pollutants, viral infections	HLA-linked, exposure to foreign tissues/cells	Persistence of low grade infection, environmental antigens, autoimmune process	CD8+ T cells, cutaneous antigens
5. Examples	i. Systemic anaphylaxis (administration of antisera and drugs, stings) ii. Local anaphylaxis (hay fever, bronchial asthma, food allergy, cutaneous, angioedema)	i. Cytotoxic antibodies to blood cells (autoimmune haemolytic anaemia, transfusion reactions, erythroblastosis foetalis, ITP, leucopenia, drug-induced) ii. Cytotoxic antibodies to tissue components (Graves' disease, myasthenia gravis, male sterility, type I DM, hyperacute reaction against organ transplant)	i. Immune complex glomerulonephritis ii. Goodpasture's syndrome iii. Collagen diseases (SLE, rheumatoid arthritis) iv. PAN v. Drug-induced vasculitis	i. Reaction against mycobacterial antigen (tuberculin reaction, tuberculosis, tuberculoid leprosy) ii. Reaction against virus-infected cells iii. Reaction against tumour cells

3. Concomitant factors An alternate hypothesis is that allergic response in type I reaction may be linked to simultaneous occurrence of certain viral infections of upper respiratory tract in a susceptible individual.

PATHOGENESIS Type I reaction includes participation by B lymphocytes and plasma cells, mast cells and basophils, neutrophils and eosinophils. The underlying mechanism is as follows **(Fig. 14.7, A)**:

i) During *first contact* of the host with the antigen, *sensitisation takes place*. In response to initial contact with antigen, circulating B lymphocytes get activated and differentiate to form IgE-secreting plasma cells. IgE antibodies so formed bind to the Fc receptors present in plenty on the surface of mast cells and basophils, which are the main effector cells of type I reaction. Thus, these cells are now fully sensitised for the next event.

ii) During the *second contact* with the same antigen, IgE antibodies on the surface of mast cells-basophils are so firmly bound to Fc receptors that it sets in cell damage—membrane lysis, influx of sodium and water and *degranulation* of mast cells-basophils.

iii) The released granules contain important chemicals and enzymes with *proinflammatory* properties— histamine, serotonin, vasoactive intestinal peptide (VIP), chemotactic factors of anaphylaxis for neutrophils and eosinophils, leukotrienes B4 and D4, prostaglandins (thromboxane A2, prostaglandin D2 and E2) and platelet activating factor. The effects of these agents are:
i) increased vascular permeability;
ii) smooth muscle contraction;
iii) early vasoconstriction followed by vasodilatation;
iv) shock;
v) increased gastric secretion;
vi) increased nasal and lacrimal secretions; and
vii) increased migration of eosinophils and neutrophils at the site of local injury as well as their rise in blood (eosinophilia and neutrophilia).

EXAMPLES OF TYPE I REACTION The manifestations of type I reaction may be variable in severity and intensity. It may manifest as a local irritant (skin, nose, throat, lungs etc), or sometimes may be severe and life-threatening anaphylaxis. Common allergens which may incite local or systemic type I reaction are as under:

Systemic anaphylaxis:
i) Administration of antisera e.g. anti-tetanus serum (ATS).
ii) Administration of drugs e.g. penicillin.
iii) Sting by wasp or bee.

The clinical features of systemic anaphylaxis include itching, erythema, contraction of respiratory bronchioles, diarrhoea, pulmonary oedema, pulmonary haemorrhage, shock and death.

Local anaphylaxis:
i) Hay fever (seasonal allergic rhinitis) due to pollen sensitisation of conjunctiva and nasal passages.
ii) Bronchial asthma due to allergy to inhaled allergens like house dust.
iii) Food allergy to ingested allergens like fish, cow's milk, eggs etc.
iv) Cutaneous anaphylaxis due to contact of antigen with skin characterised by urticaria, wheal and flare.
v) Angioedema, an autosomal dominant inherited disorder characterised by laryngeal oedema, oedema of eyelids, lips, tongue and trunk.

Type II: Antibody-mediated (Cytotoxic) Reaction

Type II or cytotoxic reaction is defined as reaction by humoral antibodies that attack cell surface antigens on the specific cells and tissues and cause lysis of target cells. Type II reaction too appears generally within 15-30 minutes after exposure to antigen but in myasthenia gravis and thyroiditis it may appear after longer duration.

ETIOLOGY AND PATHOGENESIS In general, type II reactions have participation by complement system, tissue macrophages, platelets, natural killer cells, neutrophils and eosinophils while main antibodies are IgG and IgM class. Type II hypersensitivity is tissue-specific and reaction occurs after antibodies bind to tissue specific antigens, most often on blood cells. The mechanism involved is as under **(Fig. 3.7, B)**:

i) The antigen on the surface of target cell (foreign cell) attracts and binds Fab portion of the antibody (IgG or IgM) forming antigen-antibody complex.
ii) The unattached Fc fragment of antibodies (IgG or IgM) forms a link between the antigen and complement.
iii) The antigen-antibody binding with Fc forming a link causes activation of classical pathway of serum complement which generates activated complement component, C3b, by splitting C4 and C2 by C1.
iv) Activated C3b bound to the target cell acts as an opsonin and attracts phagocytes to the site of cell injury and initiates phagocytosis.
v) Antigen-antibody complex also activates complement system and exposes membrane attack complex (MAC i.e. C5b-C9) that attacks and destroys the target cell.

EXAMPLES OF TYPE II REACTION Examples of type II reaction are mainly on blood cells and some other body cells and tissues.

1. Cytotoxic antibodies to blood cells These are more common. Some examples are as under:

i) *Autoimmune haemolytic anaemia* in which the red cell injury is brought about by autoantibodies reacting with antigens present on red cell membrane. Antiglobulin test (direct Coombs' test) is employed to detect the antibody on red cell surface (page 387).

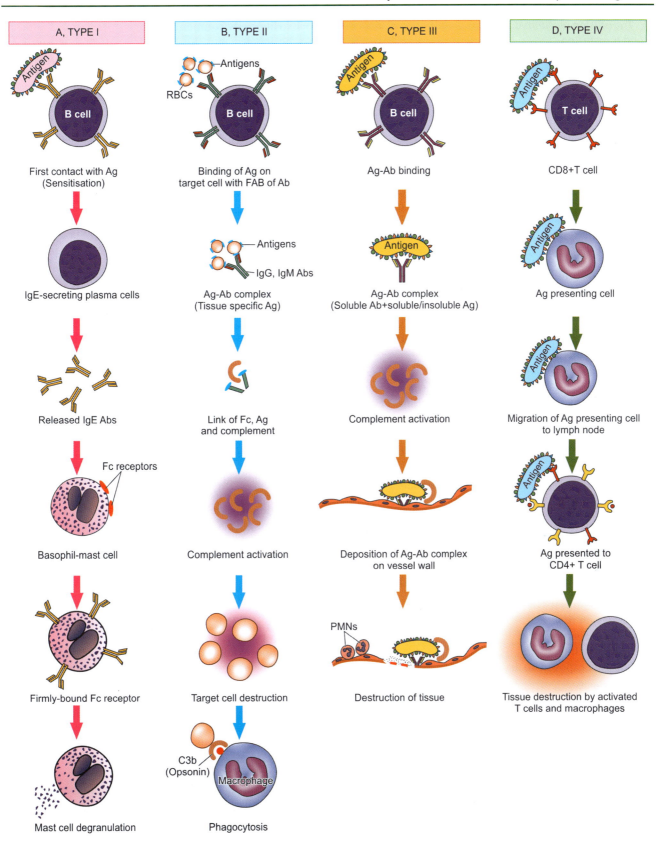

Figure 14.7 ▶ Schematic representation of pathogenesis of 4 types of immunological tissue injury.

ii) *Transfusion reactions* due to incompatible or mismatched blood transfusion.

iii) Haemolytic disease of the newborn (*erythroblastosis foetalis*) in which the foetal red cells are destroyed by maternal isoantibodies crossing the placenta.

iv) *Immune thrombocytopenic purpura* (ITP) is the immunologic destruction of platelets by autoantibodies reacting with surface components of normal plaletets.

v) *Leucopenia with agranulocytosis* may be caused by autoantibodies to leucocytes causing their destruction.

vi) *Drug-induced cytotoxic antibodies* are formed in response to administration of certain drugs like penicillin, methyl dopa, rifampicin etc. The drugs or their metabolites act as haptens binding to the surface of blood cells to which the antibodies combine, bringing about destruction of cells.

2. Cytotoxic antibodies to tissue components Cellular injury may be brought about by autoantibodies reacting with some components of tissue cells in certain diseases.

i) In *Graves' disease* (primary hyperthyroidism), thyroid autoantibody is formed which reacts with the TSH receptor to cause hyperfunction and proliferation.

ii) In *myasthenia gravis*, antibody to acetylcholine receptors of skeletal muscle is formed which blocks the neuromuscular transmission at the motor end-plate, resulting in muscle weakness.

iii) In *male sterility*, antisperm antibody is formed which reacts with spermatozoa and causes impaired motility as well as cellular injury.

iv) In *type 1 diabetes mellitus*, islet cell autoantibodies are formed which react against islet cell tissue.

v) In *hyperacute rejection reaction*, antibodies are formed against donor antigen.

vi) *Goodpasture syndrome* having GBM as antigen.

Type III: Immune Complex Mediated (Arthus) Reaction

Type III reactions result from deposition of antigen-antibody complexes on tissues, which is followed by activation of the complement system and inflammatory reaction, resulting in cell injury. The onset of type III reaction takes place about 6 hours after exposure to the antigen.

ETIOLOGY Type III reaction is not tissue specific and occurs when antigen-antibody complexes fail to get removed by the body's immune system. There are 3 types of possible etiologic factors precipitating type III reaction:

1. Persistence of low-grade microbial infection A low-grade infection with bacteria or viruses stimulates a somewhat weak antibody response. Persistence of infection (antigen) and corresponding weak antibody response leads to chronic antigen-antibody complex formation. Since these complexes fail to get eliminated from body fluids, they are instead deposited in tissues e.g. in blood vessel wall, glomeruli, joint tissue etc.

2. Extrinsic environmental antigen Exogenous antigens may be inhaled into the lungs e.g. antigens derived from moulds, plants or animals. The inhaled antigen combines with antibody in the alveolar fluid and forms antigen-antibody complex which is deposited in the alveolar walls.

3. Autoimmune process Another sequence in type III reaction can be formation of autoantibodies against own tissue (self antigen) forming autoantibody-self antigen complex. Such self antigens can be circulating (e.g. IgA) or tissue derived (e.g. DNA). Immune complexes containing both components from body's own system can thus be deposited in tissues.

PATHOGENESIS It may be mentioned here that both type II and type III reactions have antigen-antibody complex formation but the two can be distinguished—antigen in type II is tissue specific while in type III it is not so. Moreover the mechanism of cell injury in type II is direct but in type III it is by deposition of antigen-antibody complex on tissues and subsequent sequence of cell injury takes place.

Type III reaction has participation by IgG and IgM antibodies, neutrophils, mast cells and complement. The sequence of underlying mechanism is as under **(Fig. 14.7, C)**:

i) Immune complexes are formed by interaction of soluble antibody and soluble or insoluble antigen.

ii) Immune complexes which fail to get removed from body fluid get deposited into tissues. Generally, small and intermediate sized antibodies and antigens precipitate out of the body fluid and get deposited in tissues.

iii) Fc component of antibody links with complement and activates classical pathway of complement resulting in formation of C3a, C5a and membrane attack complex.

iv) C3a stimulates release of histamine from mast cells and its resultant effects of increased vascular permeability and oedema.

v) C5a releases proinflammatory mediators and chemotactic agents for neutrophils.

vi) Accumulated neutrophils and macrophages in the tissue release cytokines and result in tissue destruction.

EXAMPLES OF TYPE III REACTION Common examples of cell injury by type III injury are as under:

i) Immune complex glomerulonephritis in which the antigen may be glomerular basement membrane (GBM) or exogenous agents (e.g. Streptococcal antigen).

ii) SLE in which there is nuclear antigen (DNA, RNA) and there is formation of anti-nuclear and anti-DNA autoantibodies.

iii) Rheumatoid arthritis in which there is nuclear antigen.

iv) Farmer's lung in which actinomycetes-contaminated hay acts as antigen.

v) Polyarteritis nodosa and Wegener's granulomatosis with antineutrophil cytoplasmic antigen.

vi) Henoch-Schönleinpurpura in which respiratory viruses act as antigen.

vii) Drug-induced vasculitis in which the drug acts as antigen.

Type IV: Delayed Hypersensitivity (T Cell-Mediated) Reaction

Type IV or delayed hypersensitivity reaction is tissue injury by T cell-mediated immune response without formation of antibodies (contrary to type I, II and III) but is instead a slow and prolonged response. The reaction occurs about 24 hours after exposure to antigen and the effect is prolonged which may last up to 14 days.

ETIOLOGY AND PATHOGENESIS Type IV reaction involves role of mast cells and basophils, macrophages and CD8+ T cells. Briefly, the mechanism of type IV reaction is as under (Fig. 14.7, D):

i) The antigen is recognised by CD8+ T cells (cytotoxic T cells) and is processed by antigen presenting cells.

ii) Antigen-presenting cells migrate to lymph node where antigen is presented to helper T cells (CD4+ T cells).

iii) Helper T cells release cytokines that stimulate T cell proliferation and activate macrophages.

iv) Activated T cells and macrophages release proinflammatory mediators and cause cell destruction.

EXAMPLES OF TYPE IV REACTION Type IV reaction can explain tissue injury in following common examples:
1. Reaction against mycobacterial infection e.g. tuberculin reaction, granulomatous reaction in tuberculosis, leprosy.
2. Reaction against virally infected cells.
3. Reaction against malignant cells in the body.
4. Reaction against organ transplantation e.g. transplant rejection, graft versus host reaction.

GIST BOX 14.5 — Hypersensitivity Reactions (Immunologic Tissue Injury)

- Depending upon the *rapidity, duration and type* of the immune response, there are 4 types of hypersensitivity reactions grouped into two categories: immediate (type I, II, and III) and delayed type (type IV).
- *Type I (or anaphylactic) hypersensitivity* is a state of rapidly developing or anaphylactic type of immune response to an antigen (i.e. allergen) to which the individual is previously sensitised. The reaction appears within 15-30 minutes of exposure to antigen. It is mediated by humoral antibodies of IgE type for which mast cells and basophils play a key role.
- *Type II or cytotoxic reaction* is a reaction by humoral antibodies that attack cell surface antigens on the specific cells and tissues and cause lysis of target cells. Type II reaction is tissue-specific and occurs after antibodies (IgG or IgM) bind to tissue specific antigens, most often on blood cells.
- *Type III reactions* result from deposition of antigen-antibody complexes on tissues, which is followed by activation of the complement system and inflammatory reaction and tissue injury. Antigen in type II reaction is not tissue specific.
- *Type IV or delayed hypersensitivity* is tissue injury by T cell-mediated immune response without formation of antibodies. The reaction occurs about 24 hours (delayed) after exposure to antigen and the response is prolonged.

AUTOIMMUNE DISEASES

Autoimmunity is a state in which the body's immune system fails to distinguish between 'self' and 'non-self' and reacts by formation of autoantibodies against one's own tissue antigens. In other words, there is loss of tolerance to one's own tissues; *autoimmunity is the opposite of immune tolerance.*

Immune tolerance is a normal phenomenon present since foetal life and is defined as the ability of an individual to recognise self tissues and antigens. Normally, the immune system of the body is able to distinguish self from non-self antigens by the following mechanisms:

1. *Clonal elimination* According to this theory, during embryonic development, T cells maturing in the thymus acquire the ability to distinguish self from non-self. These T cells are then eliminated by apoptosis for the tolerant individual.

2. *Concept of clonal anergy* According to this mechanism, T lymphocytes which have acquired the ability to distinguish self from non-self are not eliminated but instead become non-responsive and inactive.

3. *Suppressor T cells* According to this mechanism, the tolerance is achieved by a population of specific suppressor T cells which do not allow the antigen-responsive cells to proliferate and differentiate.

Pathogenesis (Theories) of Autoimmunity

Normally, the body's response to self antigens (autoimmunity) is prevented by three major processes:

1. *Sequestration* of autoantigens and thus their unavailability for autoimmune response.

2. *Generation and maintenance* of tolerance or anergy by T and B lymphocytes in the body.

3. *Regulatory mechanisms* limiting response by the immune system.

The mechanisms by which the immune tolerance of the body is broken causes autoimmunity. These mechanisms or theories of autoimmunity may be exogenous or endogenous, and include immunological, genetic, and microbial factors, which may be interacting:

1. Immunological factors Failure of immunological mechanisms of tolerance initiates autoimmunity as follows:

i) *Polyclonal activation of B cells* B cells may be directly activated by stimuli such as infection with microorganisms and their products leading to bypassing of T cell tolerance.

ii) *Generation of self-reacting B cell clones* may also lead to bypassing of T cell tolerance.

iii) *Decreased T suppressor and increased T helper cell activity.* Loss of T suppressor cell and increase in T helper cell activities may lead to high levels of autoantibody production by B cells contributing to autoimmunity.

iv) *Fluctuation of anti-idiotype network control* may cause failure of mechanisms of immune tolerance.

v) *Sequestered antigen released from tissues* 'Self-antigen' which is completely sequestered may act as 'foreign-antigen' if introduced into the circulation later. For example, in trauma to the testis, there is formation of anti-sperm antibodies against spermatozoa; similar is the formation of autoantibodies against lens crystallin.

2. **Genetic factors** There is evidence in support of genetic factors in the pathogenesis of autoimmunity as under:

i) There is increased expression of *Class II HLA antigens* on tissues involved in autoimmunity. The presence of HLA-B27 is associated with several autoimmune diseases.

ii) There is increased *familial incidence* of some forms of the autoimmune disorders.

iii) There is higher incidence of autoimmune diseases in *twins* favouring genetic basis.

3. **Microbial factors** Infection with microorganisms, particularly viruses (e.g. EBV infection), and less often bacteria (e.g. streptococci, *Klebsiella*) and mycoplasma, has been implicated in triggering the pathogenesis of autoimmune diseases. However, a definite evidence in support is lacking.

Types and Examples of Autoimmune Diseases

Autoimmune diseases are a growing number of such diseases in which autoimmunity is either mediated by formation of immune complexes or they are mediated by T cells. In order to classify a disease as autoimmune, it is necessary to demonstrate that immune response in the body is elicited by self antigen and has caused the specific pathologic change. In general, presumptive evidence of autoimmune disease is made based on a few criteria, both laboratory and clinical, listed in Table 14.8.

Table 14.8	Criteria for diagnosis of autoimmune diseases.

LABORATORY EVIDENCE
1. Presence and documentation of relevant autoantibodies in the serum
2. Demonstration of T cell reactivity to self antigen
3. Lymphocytic infiltrate in the pathologic lesion
4. Production of cytokines by helper T cells e.g. interferon γ, interleukin 4
5. Evidence to support production of pathologic lesions in the tissues by transplacental transmission
6. Transfer of an autoimmune disease to an experimental animal by administration of autoantibodies

CLINICAL EVIDENCE
1. Association of other autoimmune disease
2. Improved therapeutic response to immunosuppressive agents
3. Family history of autoimmune disease

Depending upon the type of autoantibody formation, the autoimmune diseases are broadly classified into 2 groups:

1. **Organ specific (Localised) diseases** In these, the autoantibodies formed react specifically against an organ or target tissue component and cause its chronic inflammatory destruction. The tissues affected are endocrine glands (e.g. thyroid, pancreatic islets of Langerhans, adrenal cortex), alimentary tract, blood cells and various other tissues and organs.

2. **Organ non-specific (Systemic) diseases** These are diseases in which a number of autoantibodies are formed which react with antigens in many tissues and thus cause systemic lesions. The examples of this group are various systemic collagen diseases.

However, a few autoimmune diseases overlap between these two main categories.

Based on these 2 main groups, a list of common autoimmune (or immune-mediated inflammatory) diseases is presented in Table 14.9 and illustrated in Fig. 14.8. Some of

Table 14.9	Autoimmune diseases.

ORGAN NON-SPECIFIC (SYSTEMIC)
1. Systemic lupus erythematosus*
2. Rheumatoid arthritis
3. Scleroderma (Systemic sclerosis)*
4. Inflammatory myopathies (polymyositis, dermatomyositis, inclusion body myositis)*
5. Polyarteritis nodosa (PAN)
6. Sjögren's syndrome*
7. Wegener's granulomatosis

ORGAN SPECIFIC (LOCALISED)
1. *ENDOCRINE GLANDS*
    i) Hashimoto's (autoimmune) thyroiditis
    ii) Graves' disease
    iii) Type 1 diabetes mellitus
    iv) Idiopathic Addison's disease
2. *ALIMENTARY TRACT*
    i) Autoimmune atrophic gastritis in pernicious anaemia
    ii) Ulcerative colitis
    iii) Crohn's disease
3. *BLOOD CELLS*
    i) Autoimmune haemolytic anaemia
    ii) Autoimmune thrombocytopenia
    iii) Pernicious anaemia
4. *OTHERS*
    i) Myasthenia gravis
    ii) Autoimmune orchitis
    iii) Autoimmune encephalomyelitis
    iv) Goodpasture's syndrome
    v) Primary biliary cirrhosis
    vi) Lupoid hepatitis
    vii) Membranous glomerulonephritis
    viii) Autoimmune skin diseases

*Diseases discussed in this chapter.

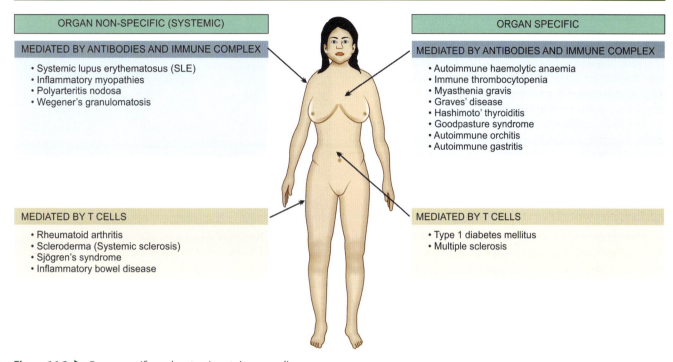

Figure 14.8 ▶ Organ specific and systemic autoimmune diseases.

the systemic autoimmune diseases *(marked with asterisk)* are discussed in this chapter while others from both the groups are described later in the relevant chapters.

Systemic Lupus Erythematosus (SLE)

SLE is the classical example of systemic autoimmune or collagen diseases. The disease derives its name *'lupus'* from the Latin word meaning 'wolf' since initially this disease was believed to affect skin only and eat away skin like a wolf. However, now 2 forms of lupus erythematosus are described:

1. **Systemic or disseminated form** is characterised by acute and chronic inflammatory lesions widely scattered in the body and there is presence of various nuclear and cytoplasmic autoantibodies in the plasma.

2. **Discoid form** is characterised by chronic and localised skin lesions involving the bridge of nose and adjacent cheeks without any systemic manifestations. Rarely, discoid form may develop into disseminated form.

ETIOLOGY The exact etiology of SLE is not known. However, there is role of heredity and certain environmental factors:

1. *Genetic factors* Genetic predisposition to develop autoantibodies to nuclear and cytoplasmic antigens in SLE is due to the immunoregulatory function of class II HLA genes implicated in the pathogenesis of SLE.

2. *Environmental factors* Various other factors express the genetic susceptibility of an individual to develop clinical disease. These factors are:

i) certain drugs e.g. penicillamine D;
ii) certain viral infections e.g. EBV infection; and
iii) certain hormones e.g. oestrogen.

PATHOGENESIS Interaction between susceptibility genes and environmental factors results in abnormal immune responses by formation of various autoantibodies. Autoantibodies against nuclear and cytoplasmic components of the cells are demonstrable in plasma by immunofluorescence tests in almost all cases of SLE. Some of the important *antinuclear antibodies (ANAs)* or antinuclear factors (ANFs) against different nuclear antigens are as under:

i) Antinuclear antibodies (ANA) These are the antibodies against common nuclear antigen that includes DNA as well as RNA. These are demonstrable in about 98% cases and are used as screening test.

ii) Antibodies to double-stranded (anti-dsDNA) This is the most specific for SLE, especially in high titres, and is present in 70% cases.

iii) Anti-Smith antibodies (anti-Sm) These antibodies appear against Smith antigen which is part of ribonucleoproteins. It is also specific for SLE but is seen in about 25% cases.

iv) Other non-specific antibodies Besides above, there are several other antibody tests which lack specificity for SLE. These are as follows:

a) Anti-ribonucleoproteins (anti-RNP) seen in 40% cases of SLE but seen more often in Sjögren's syndrome.

b) Anti-histone antibody, which is antibody against histone associated with DNA in chromatin, is seen particularly in cases of drug-induced lupus than in SLE.
c) Antiphospholipid antibodies (APLA) or lupus anticoagulant are tests for thrombotic complications in cases of SLE.
d) Anti-ribosomal P antibody is antibody against protein in ribosomes and is seen in CNS lupus.

The source of these autoantibodies as well as hypergammaglobulinaemia seen in SLE is the **polyclonal activation of B cells** brought about by following immunologic derangements:
i) an inherited defect in B cells;
ii) stimulation of B cells by micro-organisms;
iii) T helper cell hyperactivity; and
iv) T suppressor cell defect.

Two types of immunologic tissue injury can occur in SLE:

1. *Type II hypersensitivity* is characterised by formation of autoantibodies against blood cells (red blood cells, platelets, leucocytes) and results in haematologic derangement in SLE.

2. *Type III hypersensitivity* is characterised by antigen-antibody complex (commonly DNA-anti-DNA antibody; sometimes Ig-anti-Ig antibody complex) which is deposited at sites such as renal glomeruli, walls of small blood vessels etc.

LE CELL PHENOMENON This was the first diagnostic laboratory test described for SLE. The test is based on the principle that ANAs cannot penetrate the intact cells and thus cell nuclei should be exposed to bind them with the ANAs. The binding of exposed nucleus with ANAs results in homogeneous mass of nuclear chromatin material which is called *LE body or haematoxylin body*.

LE cell is a phagocytic leucocyte, commonly polymorphonuclear neutrophil, and sometimes a monocyte, which engulfs the homogeneous nuclear material of the injured cell. For demonstration of LE cell phenomenon *in vitro*, the blood sample is traumatised to expose the nuclei of blood leucocytes to ANAs. This results in binding of denatured and damaged nucleus with ANAs. The ANA-coated denatured nucleus is chemotactic for phagocytic cells.
◆ If this mass is engulfed by a neutrophil, displacing the nucleus of neutrophil to the rim of the cell, it is called *LE cell* (Fig. 14.9).
◆ If the mass, more often an intact lymphocyte, is phagocytosed by a monocyte, it is called *Tart cell*.

LE cell test is positive in 70% cases of SLE while newer and more sensitive immunofluorescence tests for autoantibodies listed above are positive in almost all cases of SLE. A few other conditions may also show positive LE test e.g. rheumatoid arthritis, lupoid hepatitis, penicillin sensitivity etc.

MORPHOLOGIC FEATURES The manifestations of SLE are widespread in different visceral organs and as erythematous cutaneous eruptions. The principal lesions are renal, vascular, cutaneous and cardiac; other organs and tissues involved are serosal linings (pleuritis, pericarditis), joints (synovitis), spleen (vasculitis), liver (portal triaditis), lungs (interstitial pneumonitis, fibrosing alveolitis), CNS (vasculitis) and in blood (autoimmune haemolytic anaemia, thrombocytopaenia).

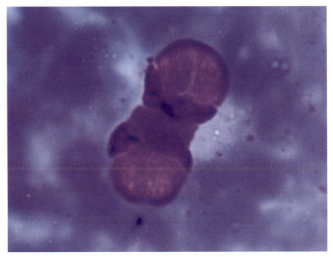

Figure 14.9 ▶ Typical LE cell. There are two LE cells having rounded masses of amorphous nuclear material (LE body) which has displaced the lobes of neutrophil to the rim of the cell.

Histologically, the characteristic lesion in SLE is *fibrinoid necrosis* which may be seen in the connective tissue, beneath the endothelium in small blood vessels, under the mesothelial lining of pleura and pericardium, under the endothelium in endocardium, or under the synovial lining cells of joints.

Table 14.10 summarises the morphology of lesions in different organs and tissues in SLE.

CLINICAL FEATURES SLE, like most other autoimmune diseases, is more common in women in their 2nd to 3rd decades of life. As obvious from Table 14.10, SLE is a multi-system disease and thus a wide variety of clinical features may be present. The severity of disease varies from mild to intermittent to severe and fulminant. Usually targeted organs are musculoskeletal system, skin, kidneys, nervous system, lungs, heart and blood vessels, GI system, and haematopoietic system. Fatigue and myalgia are present in most cases throughout the course of disease. Severe form of illness occurs with fever, weight loss, anaemia and organ related manifestations.

The disease usually runs a long course of flare-ups and remissions; renal failure is the most frequent cause of death.

Scleroderma (Systemic Sclerosis)

Just like SLE, scleroderma was initially described as a skin disease characterised by progressive fibrosis. But now, 2 main types are recognised:

Chapter 14: Diseases of Immunity including AIDS

Table 14.10 Morphology of major lesions in SLE.

1. **RENAL LESIONS (LUPUS NEPHRITIS)**
   EM-shows large deposits in mesangium, subepithelium or subendothelium.
   IM-shows granular deposits of immune complex (IgG and C3) on capillaries, mesangium and tubular basement membranes.
   Six WHO classes of lupus nephritis based on patterns:
   Class I: Minimal disease lupus nephritis: Seen in <5% cases.
   LM shows no change.
   IF shows mesangial deposits.
   Class II: Mesangial proliferative lupus nephritis: Seen in 10-25% cases.
   LM shows mesangial expansion; pure mesangial hypercellularity.
   IF shows subepithelial or subendothelial deposits.
   Class III: Focal lupus nephritis: Seen in 20-35% cases.
   LM shows focal or segmental endothelial and mesangial cell proliferation in <50% glomeruli.
   IF shows focal subendothelial deposits.
   Three subclasses:
   - *Class IIIA*: Active lesions (focal proliferative).
   - *Class IIIA/C*: Active on chronic lesions (focal proliferative and sclerosing).
   - *Class IIIC*: Chronic inactive lesions with scars (focal sclerosing).

   Class IV: Diffuse lupus nephritis: Seen in 35-60% cases.
   LM shows diffuse, segmental or global involvement of ≥50% glomeruli; proliferation of endothelial, mesangial and epithelial cells; epithelial crescents.
   IF shows diffuse subendothelial deposits.
   Two subclasses:
   - *Class IV-S*: 50% of involved glomeruli have segmental lesions.
   - *Class IV-G*: 50% of involved glomeruli have global lesions.

   Each of these subclasses (IV-S and IV-G) has active, active on chronic, and chronic lesions.
   Class V: Membranous lupus nephritis: Seen in 10-15% cases.
   LM shows diffuse basement membrane thickening.
   IF shows global or segmental subepithelial deposits.
   May be seen in combination with class III or IV.
   Class VI: Advanced sclerotic lupus nephritis: Seen as end-stage disease.
   LM shows global sclerosis of ≥ 90% of glomeruli.

2. **LESIONS OF SMALL BLOOD VESSELS (ACUTE NECROTISING VASCULITIS)**
   Affects all tissues; commonly skin and muscles involved.
   LM shows fibrinoid deposits in the vessel wall; perivascular infiltrate of mononuclear cells.

3. **CUTANEOUS LESIONS (ERYTHEMATOUS ERUPTIONS)**
   Butterfly area on nose and cheek.
   LM shows liquefactive degeneration of basal layer of epidermis, oedema at dermoepidermal junction; acute necrotising vasculitis in dermis.
   IF shows immune complex deposits (IgG and C3) at dermoepidermal junction.

4. **CARDIAC LESIONS (LIBMAN-SACKS ENDOCARDITIS)**
   Vegetations on mitral and tricuspid valves, may extend to mural endocardium, chordae tendineae.
   LM of vegetations shows fibrinoid material, necrotic debris, inflammatory cells, haematoxylin bodies may be present; connective tissue of endocardium and myocardium may show focal inflammwation and necrotising vasculitis.

(LM = Light microscopy; IF = Immunofluorescence microscopy).

1. *Diffuse scleroderma* in which the skin shows widespread involvement and may progress to involve visceral structures.

2. *CREST syndrome* characterised by *C*alcinosis (C), *R*aynaud's phenomenon (R), *E*sophageal hypomotility (E), *S*clerodactyly (S) and *T*elangiectasia (T).

ETIOPATHOGENESIS There is role of following 2 factors in its etiology:

1. *Susceptibility genes* as seen in occurrence of disease in families and in twins.

2. *Certain environmental factors* e.g. CMV infection, and role of common shared environmental exposure of certain agents as seen by prevalence of disease in some geographic location.

Antinuclear antibodies are detected in majority of cases of systemic sclerosis. Thus, immunologic mechanisms have been implicated in the pathogenesis of lesions in systemic sclerosis which finally cause activation of fibroblasts. The *immune mechanisms* leading to stimulation of fibroblasts act in the following ways:

i) *Elaboration of cytokines* such as by fibroblast growth factor and chemotactic factors by activated T cells and macrophages.

ii) *Endothelial cell injury* due to cytotoxic damage to endothelium from autoantibodies or antigen-antibody complexes. This results in aggregation and activation of platelets which increases vascular permeability and stimulates fibroblastic proliferation.

MORPHOLOGIC FEATURES Disseminated visceral involvement as well as cutaneous lesions are seen in systemic sclerosis.

1. Skin changes Skin is involved diffusely, beginning distally from fingers and extending proximally to arms, shoulders, neck and face. In advanced stage, the fingers become claw-like and face mask-like.

Microscopically, changes are progressive from early to late stage.

◈ *Early stage* shows oedema and degeneration of collagen. The small-sized blood vessels are occluded and there is perivascular infiltrate of mononuclear cells.

◈ *Late stage* reveals thin and flat epidermis. Dermis is largely replaced by compact collagen and there is hyaline thickening of walls of dermal blood vessels. In advanced cases subcutaneous calcification may occur.

2. Kidney changes Involvement of kidneys is seen in majority of cases of systemic sclerosis. The lesions are prominent in the walls of interlobular arteries which develop changes resembling malignant hypertension. There is thickening of tunica intima due to concentric proliferation of intimal cells and fibrinoid necrosis of vessel wall.

3. Smooth muscle of GIT Muscularis of the alimentary tract, particularly oesophagus, is progressively atrophied and replaced by fibrous tissue.

4. Skeletal muscle The interstitium of skeletal muscle shows progressive fibrosis and degeneration of muscle fibres with associated inflammatory changes.

5. Cardiac muscle Involvement of interstitium of the heart may result in heart failure.

6. Lungs Diffuse fibrosis may lead to contraction of the lung substance. There may be epithelium-lined honey-combed cysts of bronchioles.

7. Small arteries The lesions in small arteries show endarteritis due to intimal proliferation and may be the cause for Raynaud's phenomenon.

CLINICAL FEATURES Systemic sclerosis is more common in middle-aged women. The clinical manifestations include:
i) claw-like flexion deformity of hands;
ii) Raynaud's phenomenon;
iii) oesophageal fibrosis causing dysphagia and hypomotility;
iv) malabsorption syndrome;
v) respiratory distress;
vi) malignant hypertension;
vii) pulmonary hypertension; and
viii) biliary cirrhosis.

Inflammatory Myopathies

This group includes three conditions having common clinical feature of progressive skeletal muscle weakness: polymyositis, dermatomyositis and inclusion body myositis.

ETIOPATHOGENESIS All the three forms of inflammatory myositis appear to have an autoimmune etiology. This is supported by following:
1. Association with other autoimmune (collagen) diseases.
2. Presence of various autoantibodies against nuclear and cytoplasmic antigens in 20% cases.
3. Presence of humoral immune mechanism in dermatomyositis as observed by B cell infiltration in the lesions.
4. In polymyositis and inclusion body myositis, T cell mediated cytotoxicity is implicated as seen by CD8+ T cells along with macrophages in the lesions.
5. Some non-immune factors such as viral infection with coxsackie B, influenza, Epstein-Barr, CMV etc in triggering autoimmune mechanism has been suggested.

MORPHOLOGIC FEATURES There is symmetric involvement of skeletal muscles such as those of pelvis, shoulders, neck, chest and diaphragm.
Histologically, vacuolisation and fragmentation of muscle fibres and numerous inflammatory cells are present. In late stage, muscle fibres are replaced by fat and fibrous tissue.

CLINICAL FEATURES It is a multi-system disease characterised by:
i) progressive muscle weakness, mainly proximal;
ii) skin rash, typically with heliotropic erythema and periorbital oedema;
iii) dysphagia due to involvement of pharyngeal muscles;
iv) respiratory dysfunction; and
v) association with deep-seated malignancies.

Sjögren's Syndrome

Sjögren's syndrome is characterised by the *triad* of dry eyes *(keratoconjunctivitis sicca),* dry mouth *(xerostomia),* and *rheumatoid arthritis.* The combination of the former two symptoms is called *sicca syndrome.*

ETIOPATHOGENESIS Both humoral and cellular immune mechanisms have been implicated in the etiopathogenesis of lesions in Sjögren's syndrome:
i) There is B lymphocyte hyperactivity as seen by rise of monoclonal immunoglobulins in 25% cases.
ii) Presence of antinuclear antibodies in about 90% of cases.
iii) Positive rheumatoid factor in 25% of cases.
iv) Infiltration by T lymphocytes in exocrine glands.
v) Association of disease with certain HLA class II genes.
vi) Association with other autoimmune diseases.

MORPHOLOGIC FEATURES *In early stage,* the lacrimal and salivary glands show periductal infiltration by lymphocytes and plasma cells, which at times may form lymphoid follicles (pseudolymphoma). *In late stage,* glandular parenchyma is replaced by fat and fibrous tissue. The ducts are also fibrosed and hyalinised.

CLINICAL FEATURES The disease is common in women in 4th to 6th decades of life. It is clinically characterised by the following:
i) Symptoms *referable to eyes* such as blurred vision, burning and itching.
ii) Symptoms *referable to xerostomia* such as fissured oral mucosa, dryness, and difficulty in swallowing.
iii) Symptoms due to *glandular involvement* such as enlarged and inflamed lacrimal gland (Mikulicz's syndrome is involvement of parotid along with lacrimal gland).
iv) Symptoms due to *systemic involvement* referable to lungs, CNS and skin.

Reiter Syndrome

This syndrome is characterised by a triad of features: arthritis, conjunctivitis and urethritis. There may be mucocutaneous lesions, on palms, soles, oral mucosa and genitalia. Antinuclear antibodies and RA factor are usually negative. About 75% cases of Reiter syndrome are positive for genetic marker, HLA-B27.

GIST BOX 14.6 — Autoimmune Diseases

- Depending upon the type of autoantibody formation, the autoimmune diseases are broadly classified into 2 groups: organ specific (localised) and organ non-specific (or systemic).
- SLE is the classical example of systemic autoimmune or collagen diseases. Autoantibodies against nuclear (ANAs) and cytoplasmic components of the cells are demonstrable in plasma by immunofluorescence tests in almost all cases of SLE e.g. ANA, anti-ds-DNA, antiSm etc. LE cell test is positive in 70% cases. SLE is a multisystem disease and affects chiefly kidneys (lupus nephritis), skin, small blood vessels, and heart.
- Scleroderma or systemic sclerosis may occur as diffuse form or as CREST syndrome. The disease involves skin, kidneys, GIT, skeletal muscle, heart and lungs.
- Inflammatory myopathies are a group of 3 diseases having common clinical feature of progressive skeletal muscle weakness: polymyositis, dermatomyositis and inclusion body myositis.
- Sjögren's syndrome is characterised by the *triad* of dry eyes (keratoconjunctivitis sicca), dry mouth (xerostomia), and rheumatoid arthritis.

Section III ▶ Fluid and Haemodynamic Disorders

▶ **SECTION CONTENTS**

Chapter 15: Derangements of Body Fluids
Chapter 16: Blood Flow Volume Disorders
Chapter 17: Obstructive Haemodynamic Derangements

15 Derangements of Body Fluids

HOMEOSTASIS

Many workers have pointed out that life on the earth probably arose in the sea, and that the body water which is the environment of the cells, consisting of "salt water" is similar to the ancient ocean. The sea within us flows through blood and lymph vessels, bathes the cells as well as lies within the cells. However, water within the body contains several salts that include sodium, chloride, potassium, calcium, magnesium, phosphate, and other electrolytes. Although it appears quite tempting to draw comparison between environment of the cell and the ancient oceans, it would be rather an oversimplification in considering the cellular environment to be wholly fluid ignoring the presence of cells, fibres and ground substance.

Claude Bernarde (1949) first coined the term *internal environment or milieu interieur* for the state in the body in which the interstitial fluid that bathes the cells and the plasma, together maintain the normal morphology and function of the cells and tissues of the body. The mechanism by which the constancy of the internal environment is maintained and ensured is called the *homeostasis*. For this purpose, living membranes with varying permeabilities such as vascular endothelium and the cell wall play important role in exchange of fluids, electrolytes, nutrients and metabolites across the compartments of body fluids.

The normal composition of internal environment consists of the following components (Fig. 15.1):

1. WATER Water is the principal and essential constituent of the body. The total body water in a normal adult male comprises 50-70% (average 60%) of the body weight and about 10% less in a normal adult female (average 50%). Thus, the body of a normal male weighing 65 kg contains approximately 40 litres of water. The total body water (assuming average of 60%) is distributed into 2 main compartments of body fluids separated from each other by membranes freely permeable to water. These are as under (Fig. 15.2):

i) Intracellular fluid compartment This comprises about 33% of the body weight, the bulk of which is contained in the muscles.

ii) Extracellular fluid compartment This constitutes the remaining 27% of body weight containing water. Included in this are the following 4 subdivisions of extracellular fluid (ECF):

a) Interstitial fluid including lymph fluid constitutes the major proportion of ECF (12% of body weight).

b) Intravascular fluid or blood plasma comprises about 5% of the body weight. Plasma content is about 3 litres of fluid out of 5 litres of total blood volume.

c) Mesenchymal tissues such as dense connective tissue, cartilage and bone contain body water that comprises about 9% of the body weight.

d) Transcellular fluid constitutes 1% of body weight. This is the fluid contained in the secretions of secretory cells of the body e.g. skin, salivary glands, mucous membranes of alimentary and respiratory tracts, pancreas, liver and biliary tract, kidneys, gonads, thyroid, lacrimal gland and CSF.

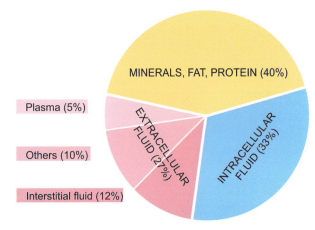

Figure 15.1 ▶ Distribution of body fluid compartments.

Chapter 15: Derangements of Body Fluids

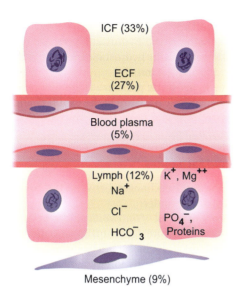

Figure 15.2 ▶ Body fluid compartments (ICF = intracellular fluid compartment; ECF = extracellular fluid compartment).

2. **ELECTROLYTES** The concentration of cations (positively charged) and anions (negatively charged) is different in intracellular and extracellular fluids:

◆ *In the intracellular fluid,* the main cations are potassium and magnesium and the main anions are phosphates and proteins. It has low concentration of sodium and chloride.

◆ *In the extracellular fluid,* the predominant cation is sodium and the principal anions are chloride and bicarbonate. Besides these, a small proportion of non-diffusible proteins and some diffusible nutrients and metabolites such as glucose and urea are present in the ECF.

The essential difference between the two main subdivisions of ECF is the higher protein content in the plasma than in the interstitial fluid which plays an important role in maintaining fluid balance.

The **major functions** of electrolytes are as follows:
i) Electrolytes are the main solutes in the body fluids for maintenance of acid-base equilibrium.
ii) Electrolytes maintain the proper osmolality and volume of body fluids (*Osmolality* is the solute concentration per kg water, compared from *osmolarity* which is the solute concentration per litre solution).
iii) The concentration of certain electrolytes determines their specific physiologic functions e.g. the effect of calcium ions on neuromuscular excitability. The concentration of the major electrolytes is expressed in milliequivalent (mEq) per litre so as to compare the values directly with each other. In order to convert mg per dl into mEq per litre, the following formula is used:

$$\text{mEq/L} = \frac{\text{mg/dl}}{\text{Eq weight of element}} \times 10$$

NORMAL WATER AND ELECTROLYTE BALANCE (GIBBS-DONNAN EQUILIBRIUM)

Normally, a state of balance exists between the amount of water absorbed into the body and the amount eliminated from the body. The water and electrolytes are distributed nearly constantly in different body fluid compartments:
1. Water is normally *absorbed* into the body from the bowel or is introduced parenterally; average intake being 2800 ml per day.
2. Water is *eliminated* from the body via:
i) kidneys in the urine (average 1500 ml per day);
ii) via the skin as insensible loss in perspiration or as sweat (average 800 ml per day), though there is wide variation in loss via sweat depending upon weather, temperature, fever and exercise;
iii) via the lungs in exhaled air (average 400 ml per day); and
iv) minor losses via the faeces (average 100 ml per day) and lacrimal, nasal, oral, sexual and mammary (milk) secretions.

The cell wall as well as capillary endothelium are entirely permeable to water but they differ in their permeability to electrolytes. Capillary wall is completely permeable to electrolytes while the cell membrane is somewhat impermeable. As mentioned earlier, concentration of potassium and phosphate are high in the intracellular fluid whereas concentration of sodium and chloride are high in the ECF. The osmotic equilibrium between the two major body fluid compartments is maintained by the passage of water from or into the intracellular compartment. The 2 main subdivisions of ECF—blood plasma and interstitial fluid, are separated from each other by capillary wall which is freely permeable to water but does not allow free passage of macro-molecules of plasma proteins resulting in higher protein content in the plasma.

ACID-BASE BALANCE

Besides changes in the volume of fluids in the compartments, changes in ionic equilibrium affecting the acid-base balance of fluids occur. In terms of body fluids,
◆ an *acid* is a molecule or ion which is capable of giving off a hydrogen ion (H^+ ion donor); and
◆ a base is a molecule or ion which is capable of taking up hydrogen ion (H^+ ion acceptor).

A number of acids such as carbonic, phosphoric, sulfuric, lactic, hydrochloric and ketoacids are formed during normal metabolic activity. However, carbonic acid is produced in largest amount as it is the end-product of aerobic tissue activity. In spite of these acids, the pH of the blood is kept constant at 7.4 ± 0.05 in health.

The pH of blood and acid-base balance are regulated in the body as follows:

1. **BUFFER SYSTEM** Buffers are substances which have weak acids and strong bases and limit the change in H^+ ion concentration to the normal range. They are the first line

of defense for maintaining acid-base balance and do so by taking up H⁺ ions when the pH rises. The most important buffer which regulates the pH of blood is *bicarbonate-carbonic acid system* followed by *intracellular buffering action of haemoglobin* and *carbonic anhydrase* in the red cells.

2. **PULMONARY MECHANISM** During respiration, CO_2 is removed by the lungs depending upon the partial pressure of CO_2 in the arterial blood. With ingestion of high quantity of acid-forming salts, ventilation is increased as seen in acidosis in diabetic ketosis and uraemia.

3. **RENAL MECHANISM** The other route by which H⁺ ions can be excreted from the body is in the urine. Here, H⁺ ions secreted by the renal tubular cells are buffered in the glomerular filtrate by:

i) combining with phosphates to form phosphoric acid;

ii) combining with ammonia to form ammonium ions; and

iii) combining with filtered bicarbonate ions to form carbonic acid.

However, carbonic acid formed is dissociated to form CO_2 which diffuses back into the blood to reform bicarbonate ions.

PRESSURE GRADIENTS AND FLUID EXCHANGES

Besides water and electrolytes (or crystalloids), both of which are freely interchanged between the interstitial fluid and plasma, the ECF contains colloids (i.e. proteins) which minimally cross the capillary wall. These substances exert pressures responsible for exchange between the interstitial fluid and plasma.

Normal Fluid Pressures

1. **OSMOTIC PRESSURE** This is the pressure exerted by the chemical constituents of the body fluids. Accordingly, osmotic pressure may be of the following types **(Fig. 15.3, A)**:

◆ **Crystalloid osmotic pressure** exerted by electrolytes present in the ECF and comprises the major portion of the total osmotic pressure.

◆ **Colloid osmotic pressure (Oncotic pressure)** exerted by proteins present in the ECF and constitutes a small part of the total osmotic pressure but is more significant physiologically. Since the protein content of the plasma is higher than that of interstitial fluid, oncotic pressure of plasma is higher (average 25 mmHg) than that of interstitial fluid (average 8 mmHg).

◆ **Effective oncotic pressure** is the difference between the higher oncotic pressure of plasma and the lower oncotic pressure of interstitial fluid and is *the force that tends to draw fluid into the vessels.*

2. **HYDROSTATIC PRESSURE** This is the pressure of fluid in capillary and interstitial fluid.

◆ **Capillary pressure** There is considerable *pressure gradient* at the two ends of capillary loop—being higher at the arteriolar end (average 32 mmHg) than at the venular end (average 12 mmHg).

◆ **Tissue tension** is the hydrostatic pressure of interstitial fluid and is lower than the hydrostatic pressure in the capillary at either end (average 4 mmHg).

◆ **Effective hydrostatic pressure** is the difference between the higher hydrostatic pressure in the capillary and the lower tissue tension; it is *the force that drives fluid through the capillary wall into the interstitial space.*

Normal Fluid Exchanges

Normally, the fluid exchanges between the body compartments take place as under:

◆ *At the arteriolar end of the capillary*, the balance between the hydrostatic pressure (32 mmHg) and plasma oncotic pressure (25 mmHg) is the hydrostatic pressure of 7 mmHg which is the outward-driving force so that a small quantity of fluid and solutes leave the vessel to enter the interstitial space.

◆ *At the venular end of the capillary*, the balance between the hydrostatic pressure (12 mmHg) and plasma oncotic pressure (25 mmHg) is the oncotic pressure of 13 mmHg which is the inward-driving force so that the fluid and solutes re-enter the plasma.

◆ *Tissue fluid* left after exchanges across the capillary wall escapes into the lymphatics from where it is finally drained into venous circulation.

◆ *Tissue factors* (i.e. oncotic pressure of interstitial fluid and tissue tension) are normally small and insignificant forces opposing the plasma oncotic pressure and capillary hydrostatic pressure, respectively.

GIST BOX 15.1 | Homeostasis

❖ The mechanism by which constancy of the internal environment is maintained and ensured is called the homeostasis. Living membranes such as cell wall and vascular endothelium play important role in exchanges of fluid, electrolytes, nutrients and metabolites.

❖ Total body water is about 60% of the body weight and is divided into intracellular (33%) and extracellular compartments (27%). Intracellular fluid has low concentration of sodium and chloride while extracellular compartment has high sodium, chloride and bicarbonate; plasma has high protein content compared from interstitial fluid.

❖ Effective oncotic pressure is the difference between the higher oncotic pressure of plasma and the lower oncotic pressure of interstitial fluid and *is the force that tends to draw fluid into the vessels.*

❖ Effective hydrostatic pressure is the difference between the higher hydrostatic pressure in the capillary and the lower tissue tension; it *is the force that drives fluid through the capillary wall into the interstitial space.*

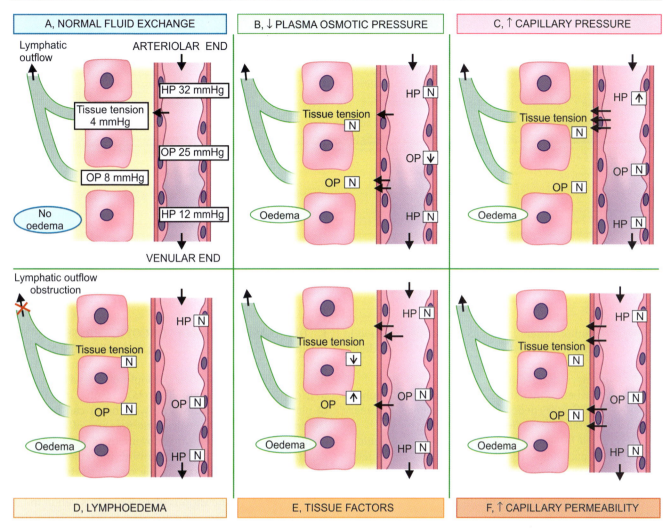

Figure 15.3 ▶ Diagrammatic representation of pathogenesis of oedema (OP = oncotic pressure; HP = hydrostatic pressure). A, Normal pressure gradients and fluid exchanges between plasma, interstitial space and lymphatics. B, Mechanism of oedema by decreased plasma oncotic pressure and hypoproteinaemia. C, Mechanism of oedema by increased hydrostatic pressure in the capillary. D, Mechanism of lymphoedema. E, Mechanism by tissue factors (increased oncotic pressure of interstitial fluid and lowered tissue tension). F, Mechanism of oedema by increased capillary permeability.

DISTURBANCES OF BODY WATER

The common derangements of body water are as follows:
1. Oedema
2. Dehydration
3. Overhydration
   These are discussed below.

OEDEMA

Definition and Types

The Greek word *oidema* means swelling. *Oedema is defined as abnormal and excessive accumulation of "free fluid" in the interstitial tissue spaces and serous cavities*. The presence of abnormal collection of fluid within the cell is sometimes called intracellular oedema but should more appropriately be called hydropic degeneration (page 36).

◈ *Free fluid in body cavities:* Commonly called as effusion, it is named according to the body cavity in which the fluid accumulates. For example, ascites (if in the peritoneal cavity), hydrothorax or pleural effusion (if in the pleural cavity), and hydropericardium or pericardial effusion (if in the pericardial cavity).

◈ *Free fluid in interstitial space:* Commonly termed as oedema, the fluid lies free in the interstitial space between the cells and can be displaced from one place to another. In the case of oedema in the subcutaneous tissues, momentary pressure of finger produces a depression known as *pitting*

Section III: Fluid and Haemodynamic Disorders

Table 15.1 Differences between transudate and exudate.

	FEATURE	TRANSUDATE	EXUDATE
1.	Definition	Filtrate of blood plasma without changes in endothelial permeability	Oedema of inflamed tissue associated with increased vascular permeability
2.	Character	Non-inflammatory oedema	Inflammatory oedema
3.	Protein content	Low (less than 1 gm/dl); mainly albumin, low fibrinogen; hence no tendency to coagulate	High (2.5-3.5 gm/dl), readily coagulates due to high content of fibrinogen and other coagulation factors
4.	Glucose content	Same as in plasma	Low (less than 60 mg/dl)
5.	Specific gravity	Low (less than 1.015)	High (more than 1.018)
6.	pH	> 7.3	<7.3
7.	LDH	Low	High
8.	Effusion LDH/ Serum LDH ratio	< 0.6	>0.6
9.	Cells	Few cells, mainly mesothelial cells and cellular debris	Many cells, inflammatory as well as parenchymal
10.	Examples	Oedema in congestive cardiac failure	Purulent exudate such as pus

oedema. The other variety is *non-pitting* or *solid oedema* in which no pitting is produced on pressure e.g. in myxoedema, elephantiasis.

Oedema may be of 2 main types:
1. *Localised* when limited to an organ or limb e.g. lymphatic oedema, inflammatory oedema, allergic oedema, pulmonary oedema, cerebral oedema etc.
2. *Generalised (anasarca or dropsy)* when it is systemic in distribution, particularly noticeable in the subcutaneous tissues e.g. renal oedema, cardiac oedema, nutritional oedema.

Depending upon fluid composition, oedema fluid may be:
◆ *transudate* which is more often the case, such as in oedema of cardiac and renal disease; or
◆ *exudate* such as in inflammatory oedema.

The differences between transudate and exudate are tabulated in Table 15.1.

Pathogenesis of Oedema

Oedema is caused by mechanisms that interfere with normal fluid balance of plasma, interstitial fluid and lymph flow. The following mechanisms may be operating singly or in combination to produce oedema:
1. Decreased plasma oncotic pressure
2. Increased capillary hydrostatic pressure
3. Lymphatic obstruction
4. Tissue factors (increased oncotic pressure of interstitial fluid, and decreased tissue tension)
5. Increased capillary permeability
6. Sodium and water retention.

These mechanisms are discussed below and illustrated in Fig. 15.3:

1. DECREASED PLASMA ONCOTIC PRESSURE The plasma oncotic pressure exerted by the total amount of plasma proteins tends to draw fluid into the vessels normally. A fall in the total plasma protein level (hypoproteinaemia of less than 5 g/dl, mainly hypoalbuminaemia), results in lowering of plasma oncotic pressure in a way that it can no longer counteract the effect of hydrostatic pressure of blood. This results in increased outward movement of fluid from the capillary wall and decreased inward movement of fluid from the interstitial space causing oedema **(Fig. 15.3, B)**. Hypoproteinaemia usually produces generalised oedema (anasarca). Out of the various plasma proteins, albumin has four times higher plasma oncotic pressure than globulin; thus it is mainly hypoalbuminaemia (albumin below 2.5 g/dl) that generally results in oedema.

The **examples** of oedema by this mechanism are seen in the following conditions:
i) *Oedema of renal disease* e.g. in nephrotic and nephritic syndrome.
ii) *Ascites* of liver disease e.g. in cirrhosis of the liver.
iii) *Oedema due to other causes* of hypoproteinaemia e.g. in protein-losing enteropathy.

2. INCREASED CAPILLARY HYDROSTATIC PRESSURE
The hydrostatic pressure of the capillary is the force that normally tends to drive fluid through the capillary wall into the interstitial space by counteracting the force of plasma oncotic pressure. A rise in the hydrostatic pressure at the venular end of the capillary which is normally low (average 12 mmHg) to a level more than the plasma oncotic pressure results in minimal or no reabsorption of fluid at the venular end, consequently leading to oedema **(Fig. 15.3,C)**.

The **examples** of oedema by this mechanism are seen in the following disorders:

i) *Oedema of cardiac disease* e.g. in congestive cardiac failure, constrictive pericarditis.
ii) *Ascites of liver disease* e.g. in cirrhosis of the liver.
iii) *Passive congestion* e.g. in mechanical obstruction due to thrombosis of veins of the lower legs, varicosities, pressure by pregnant uterus, tumours etc.
iv) *Postural oedema* e.g. transient oedema of feet and ankles due to increased venous pressure seen in individuals whose job involves standing for long hours such as traffic constables and nurses.

3. LYMPHATIC OBSTRUCTION Normally, the interstitial fluid in the tissue spaces escapes by way of lymphatics. Obstruction to outflow of these channels causes localised oedema, known as lymphoedema **(Fig. 15.3,D)**.

The **examples** of lymphoedema include the following:
i) *Removal of axillary lymph nodes* in radical mastectomy for carcinoma of the breast causing lymphoedema of the affected arm.
ii) *Pressure from outside* on the main abdominal or thoracic duct such as due to tumours, effusions in serous cavities etc may produce lymphoedema. At times, the main lymphatic channel may rupture and discharge chyle into the pleural cavity (chylothorax) or into peritoneal cavity (chylous ascites).
iii) *Inflammation of the lymphatics* as seen in filariasis (infection with *Wuchereria bancrofti*) results in chronic lymphoedema of scrotum and legs known as elephantiasis, a form of non-pitting oedema.
iv) *Occlusion of lymphatic channels* by malignant cells may result in lymphoedema.
v) *Milroy's disease or hereditary lymphoedema* is due to abnormal development of lymphatic channels. It is seen in families and the oedema is mainly confined to one or both the lower limbs.

4. TISSUE FACTORS The two forces acting in the interstitial space—oncotic pressure of the interstitial space and tissue tension, are normally quite small and insignificant to counteract the effects of plasma oncotic pressure and capillary hydrostatic pressure respectively. However, in some situations, the tissue factors in combination with other mechanisms play a role in causation of oedema **(Fig. 15.3, E)**. These are as under:
i) *Elevation of oncotic pressure of interstitial fluid* as occurs due to increased vascular permeability and inadequate removal of proteins by lymphatics.
ii) *Lowered tissue tension* as seen in *loose subcutaneous tissues* of eyelids and external genitalia.

5. INCREASED CAPILLARY PERMEABILITY An intact capillary endothelium is a semipermeable membrane which permits the free flow of water and crystalloids but allows minimal passage of plasma proteins normally. However, when the capillary endothelium is injured by various 'capillary poisons' such as toxins and their products (e.g. histamine, anoxia, venoms, certain drugs and chemicals), the capillary permeability to plasma proteins is enhanced due to development of gaps between the endothelial cells, causing leakage of plasma proteins into interstitial fluid. This, in turn, causes reduced plasma oncotic pressure and elevated oncotic pressure of interstitial fluid, consequently producing oedema **(Fig. 15.3, F)**.

The **examples** of oedema due to increased vascular permeability are seen in the following conditions:
i) *Generalised oedema* occurring in systemic infections, poisonings, certain drugs and chemicals, anaphylactic reactions and anoxia.
ii) *Localised oedema* A few examples are as under:
◈ *Inflammatory oedema* as seen in infections, allergic reactions, insect-bite, irritant drugs and chemicals. It is generally exudate in nature.
◈ *Angioneurotic oedema* is an acute attack of localised oedema occurring on the skin of face and trunk and may involve lips, larynx, pharynx and lungs. It is possibly neurogenic or allergic in origin.

6. SODIUM AND WATER RETENTION The mechanism of oedema by sodium and water retention in extravascular compartment is best described in relation to derangement in normal regulatory mechanism of sodium and water balance.

Natrium (Na) is the Latin term for sodium. Normally, about 80% of sodium is reabsorbed by the proximal convoluted tubule under the influence of either intrinsic renal mechanism or extra-renal mechanism while retention of water is affected by release of antidiuretic hormone **(Fig. 15.4)**:

◈ **Intrinsic renal mechanism** is activated in response to sudden reduction in the effective arterial blood volume (hypovolaemia) e.g. in severe haemorrhage. Hypovolaemia stimulates the arterial baroreceptors present in the carotid sinus and aortic arch which, in turn, send the sympathetic outflow via the vasomotor centre in the brain. As a result of this, renal ischaemia occurs which causes reduction in the glomerular filtration rate, decreased excretion of sodium in the urine and consequent retention of sodium.

◈ **Extra-renal mechanism** involves the secretion of aldosterone, a sodium-retaining hormone, by the *renin-angiotensin-aldosterone system*. Renin is an enzyme secreted by the granular cells in the juxta-glomerular apparatus. Its release is stimulated in response to low concentration of sodium in the tubules. Its main action is stimulation of the angiotensinogen which is α_2-globulin or renin substrate present in the plasma. On stimulation, angiotensin I, a decapeptide, is formed in the plasma which is subsequently converted into angiotensin II, an octapeptide, in the lungs and kidneys by angiotensin converting enzyme (ACE). Angiotensin II stimulates the adrenal cortex to secrete aldosterone hormone. Aldosterone increases sodium reabsorption in the renal tubules and sometimes causes a rise in the blood pressure.

◈ **ADH mechanism** Retention of sodium leads to retention of water secondarily under the influence of anti-diuretic

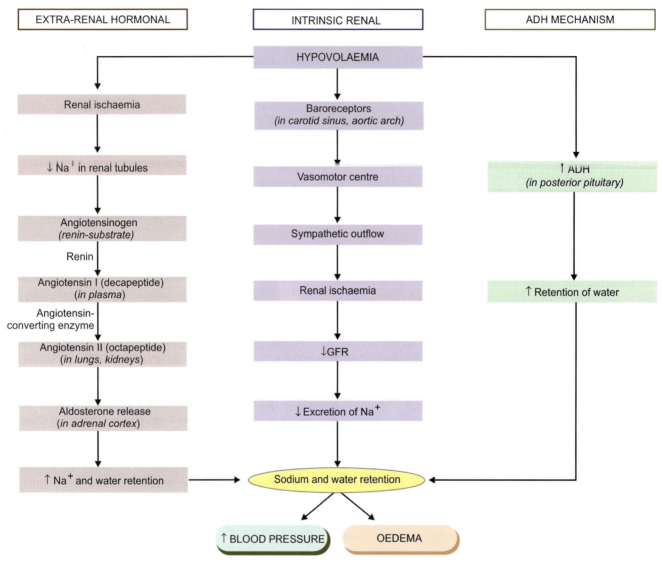

Figure 15.4 ▶ Mechanisms involved in oedema by sodium and water retention.

hormone (ADH) or vasopressin. This hormone is secreted by the cells of the supraoptic and paraventricular nuclei in the hypothalamus and is stored in the neurohypophysis (posterior pituitary). The release of ADH is stimulated by increased concentration of sodium in the plasma and hypovolaemia. Large amounts of ADH produce highly concentrated urine.

Thus, the possible factors responsible for causing oedema by excessive retention of sodium and water in the extravascular compartment via stimulation of intrinsic renal and extra-renal mechanisms as well as via release of ADH are as under:

i) Reduced glomerular filtration rate in response to hypovolaemia.
ii) Enhanced tubular reabsorption of sodium and consequently its decreased renal excretion.
iii) Increased filtration factor i.e. increased filtration of plasma from the glomerulus.
iv) Decreased capillary hydrostatic pressure associated with increased renal vascular resistance.

The **examples** of oedema by these mechanisms are as under:
i) *Oedema of cardiac disease* e.g. in congestive cardiac failure.
ii) *Ascites* of liver disease e.g. in cirrhosis of liver.
iii) *Oedema of renal disease* e.g. in nephrotic and nephritic syndrome.

Important Types of Oedema

As observed from the pathogenesis of oedema just described, more than one mechanism may be involved in many

Table 15.2	Contrasting features of nephrotic and acute nephritic syndromes.		
	FEATURE	NEPHROTIC SYNDROME	ACUTE NEPHRITIC SYNDROME
1.	Proteinuria	Heavy (>3 gm per 24 hrs)	Mild (<3 gm per 24 hrs)
2.	Hypoalbuminaemia	Present	Uncommons
3.	Oedema	Marked, generalised peripheral	Mild, in loose tissues
4.	Mechanism of oedema	↓ plasma osmotic pressure, Na$^+$ and water retention	Na$^+$ and water retention
5.	Haematuria	Absent	Present, microscopic
6.	Hypertension	Present in advanced disease	Present
7.	Hyperlipidaemia	Present	Absent
8.	Lipiduria	Present	Absenta
9.	Oliguria	Present in advanced disease	Present
10.	Hypercoagulability	Present	Absenta

examples of localised and generalised oedema. Some of the important examples are described below.

Renal Oedema

Generalised oedema occurs in certain diseases of renal origin such as in nephrotic syndrome, nephritic syndrome, and in renal failure due to acute tubular injury. Differences between nephritic and nephritic syndrome are summed up in Table 15.2.

1. Oedema in nephrotic syndrome Since there is persistent and heavy proteinuria (albuminuria) in nephrotic syndrome, there is hypoalbuminaemia causing decreased plasma oncotic pressure resulting in severe generalised oedema *(nephrotic oedema)*. The hypoalbuminaemia also causes fall in the plasma volume activating renin-angiotensin-aldosterone mechanism which results in retention of sodium and water, thus setting in a vicious cycle which persists till the albuminuria continues. Similar type of mechanism operates in the pathogenesis of oedema in protein-losing enteropathy, adding further support to the role of protein loss in the causation of oedema.

The *nephrotic oedema* is classically more severe, generalised and marked and is present in the subcutaneous tissues as well as in the visceral organs.

Grossly, the affected organ is enlarged and heavy with tense capsule.

Microscopically, the oedema fluid separates the connective tissue fibres of subcutaneous tissues. Depending upon the protein content, the oedema fluid may appear homogeneous, pale, eosinophilic, or may be deeply eosinophilic and granular.

2. Oedema in nephritic syndrome Oedema occuring in conditions with diffuse glomerular disease such as in acute diffuse glomerulonephritis and rapidly progressive glomerulonephritis is termed *nephritic oedema*. In contrast to nephrotic oedema, nephritic oedema is primarily not due to hypoproteinaemia because of low albuminuria but is largely due to excessive reabsorption of sodium and water in the renal tubules via renin-angiotensin-aldosterone mechanism. The protein content of oedema fluid in glomerulonephritis is quite low (less than 0.5 g/dl).

The *nephritic oedema* is usually mild as compared to nephrotic oedema and begins in the loose tissues such as on the face around eyes, ankles and genitalia. Oedema in these conditions is usually not affected by gravity (unlike cardiac oedema).

The salient differences between the nephrotic and nephritic oedema are outlined in Table 15.3.

3. Oedema in acute tubular injury Acute tubular injury following shock or toxic chemicals results in gross oedema of the body. The damaged tubules lose their capacity for selective reabsorption and concentration of the glomerular filtrate, resulting in excessive retention of water and electrolytes, and consequent oliguria. Besides, there is rise in blood urea.

Table 15.3	Differences between nephrotic and nephritic oedema.		
	FEATURE	NEPHROTIC OEDEMA	NEPHRITIC OEDEMA
1.	Cause	Nephrotic syndrome	Glomerulonephritis (acute, rapidly progressive)
2.	Proteinuria	Heavy	Moderate
3.	Protein content	High (>1 g/dl)	Low (<0.5 g/dl)
4.	Mechanism	↓ Plasma oncotic pressure, Na$^+$ and water retention	Na$^+$ and water retention
5.	Degree of oedema	Severe, generalised	Mild
6.	Distribution	Subcutaneous tissues as well as visceral organs	Loose tissues mainly (face, eyes, ankles, genitalia)

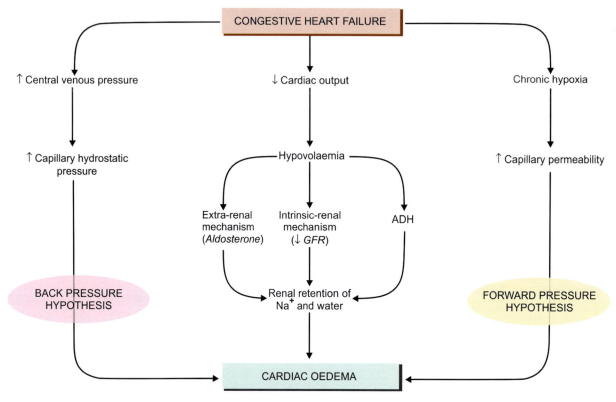

Figure 15.5 ▶ Mechanisms involved in the pathogenesis of cardiac oedema.

Cardiac Oedema

Generalised oedema develops in right-sided and congestive cardiac failure. Pathogenesis of cardiac oedema is explained on the basis of the following mechanisms (Fig. 15.5):
1. Reduced cardiac output causes hypovolaemia which stimulates intrinsic-renal and extra-renal hormonal (renin-angiotensin-aldosterone) mechanisms as well as ADH secretion resulting in *sodium and water retention* (as discussed above) and consequent oedema.
2. Due to heart failure, there is elevated central venous pressure which is transmitted backward to the venous end of the capillaries, raising the capillary hydrostatic pressure and consequent transudation; this is known as *back pressure hypothesis*.
3. Chronic hypoxia may injure the capillary endothelium causing increased capillary permeability and result in oedema; this is called *forward pressure hypothesis*. However, this theory lacks support since the oedema by this mechanism is exudate whereas the cardiac oedema is typically transudate.

In left heart failure, the changes are, however, different. There is venous congestion, particularly in the lungs, causing pulmonary oedema rather than generalised oedema.

Cardiac oedema is influenced by gravity and is thus characteristically *dependent oedema* i.e. in an ambulatory patient it is on the lower extremities, while in a bed-ridden patient oedema appears on the sacral and genital areas. The accumulation of fluid may also occur in serous cavities.

Pulmonary Oedema

Acute pulmonary oedema is the most important form of local oedema as it causes serious functional impairment. However, it has special features and differs from oedema elsewhere in that the fluid accumulation is not only in the tissue space but also in the pulmonary alveoli.

ETIOPATHOGENESIS The hydrostatic pressure in the pulmonary capillaries is much lower (average 10 mmHg). Normally the plasma oncotic pressure is adequate to prevent the escape of fluid into the interstitial space and hence lungs are normally free of oedema. Pulmonary oedema can result from either the elevation of pulmonary hydrostatic pressure or the increased capillary permeability (Fig. 15.6).

1. **Elevation in pulmonary hydrostatic pressure (Haemodynamic oedema)** In heart failure, there is increase in the pressure in pulmonary veins which is transmitted to pulmonary capillary bed. This results in imbalance between pulmonary hydrostatic pressure and the plasma oncotic pressure so that excessive fluid moves out of pulmonary capillaries into the

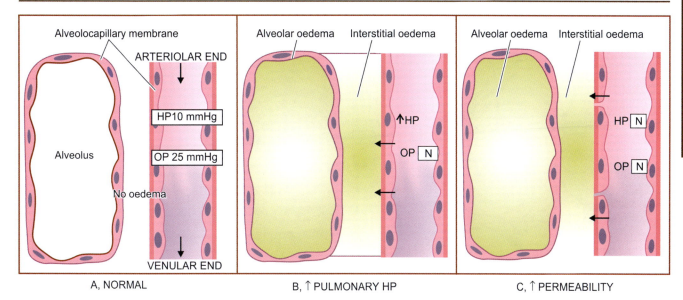

Figure 15.6 ▶ Mechanisms involved in the pathogenesis of pulmonary oedema. A, Normal fluid exchange at the alveolocapillary membrane (capillary endothelium and alveolar epithelium). B, Pulmonary oedema via elevated pulmonary hydrostatic pressure. C, Pulmonary oedema via increased vascular permeability.

interstitium of the lungs. Simultaneously, the endothelium of the pulmonary capillaries develops fenestrations permitting passage of plasma proteins and fluid into the interstitium. The interstitial fluid so collected is cleared by the lymphatics present around the bronchioles, small muscular arteries and veins. As the capacity of the lymphatics to drain the fluid is exceeded (about ten-fold increase in fluid), the excess fluid starts accumulating in the interstitium *(interstitial oedema)* i.e. in the loose tissues around bronchioles, arteries and in the lobular septa. This causes thickening of the alveolar walls. Up to this stage, no significant impairment of gaseous exchange occurs. However, prolonged elevation of hydrostatic pressure and due to high pressure of interstitial oedema, the alveolar lining cells break and the alveolar air spaces are flooded with fluid *(alveolar oedema)* driving the air out of alveoli, thus seriously hampering the lung function.

Examples of pulmonary oedema by this mechanism are seen in left heart failure, mitral stenosis, pulmonary vein obstruction, thyrotoxicosis, cardiac surgery, nephrotic syndrome and obstruction to the lymphatic outflow by tumour or inflammation.

2. Increased vascular permeability (Irritant oedema) The vascular endothelium as well as the alveolar epithelial cells (alveolo-capillary membrane) may be damaged causing increased vascular permeability so that excessive fluid and plasma proteins leak out, initially into the interstitium and subsequently into the alveoli.

This mechanism explains pulmonary oedema in conditions such as in fulminant pulmonary and extra-pulmonary infections, inhalation of toxic substances, aspiration, shock, radiation injury, hypersensitivity to drugs or antisera, uraemia and adult respiratory distress syndrome (ARDS).

3. Acute high altitude oedema Individuals climbing to high altitude suddenly without halts and without waiting for acclimatisation to set in, suffer from serious circulatory and respiratory ill-effects. The deleterious effects begin to appear often after an altitude of 2500 metres is reached. These changes include appearance of oedema fluid in the lungs, congestion and widespread minute haemorrhages. These changes can cause death within a few days. The underlying mechanism is due to anoxic damage to the pulmonary vessels. However, if acclimatisation to high altitude is allowed to take place, the individual develops polycythaemia, raised pulmonary arterial pressure, increased pulmonary ventilation and a rise in heart rate and increased cardiac output, and thus the ill-effects do not appear.

MORPHOLOGIC FEATURES Irrespective of the underlying mechanism in the pathogenesis of pulmonary oedema, the fluid accumulates more in the basal regions of lungs. The thickened interlobular septa along with their dilated lymphatics may be seen in chest X-ray as linear lines perpendicular to the pleura and are known as *Kerley's lines*.

Grossly, the lungs in pulmonary oedema are heavy, moist and subcrepitant. Cut surface exudes frothy fluid (mixture of air and fluid).

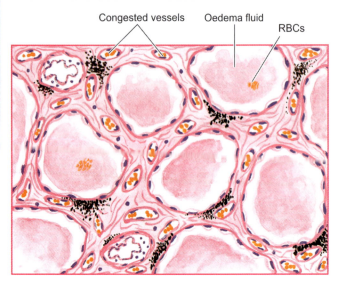
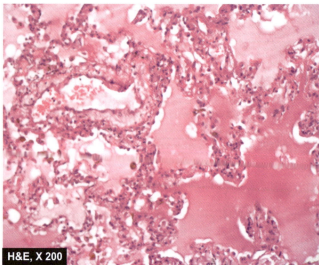

Figure 15.7 ▶ Pulmonary oedema. The alveolar capillaries are congested. The alveolar spaces as well as interstitium contain eosinophilic, granular, homogeneous and pink proteinaceous oedema fluid alongwith some RBCs and inflammatory cells.

Microscopically, the alveolar capillaries are congested. Initially, the excess fluid collects in the interstitial lung spaces in the septal walls (interstitial oedema). Later, the fluid fills the alveolar spaces (alveolar oedema). Oedema fluid in the interstitium as well as the alveolar spaces, appears as eosinophilic, granular and pink proteinaceous material, often admixed with some RBCs and alveolar macrophages, also called heart failure cells **(Fig. 15.7)**. Organisation of alveolar oedema may be seen as brightly eosinophilic pink lines along the alveolar margin called *hyaline membrane.*

Long-standing pulmonary oedema is prone to get infected by bacteria producing hypostatic pneumonia which may be fatal.

Cerebral Oedema

Cerebral oedema or swelling of the brain is the most life-threatening example of oedema. The mechanism of fluid exchange in the brain differs from elsewhere in the body since there are no draining lymphatics in the brain but instead, the function of fluid-electrolyte exchange is performed by the blood-brain barrier located at the endothelial cells of the capillaries.

Cerebral oedema can be of 3 types: vasogenic, cytotoxic and interstitial.

1. **VASOGENIC OEDEMA** This is the most common type and its mechanism is similar to oedema in other body sites from increased filtration pressure or increased capillary permeability. Vasogenic oedema is prominent around cerebral contusions, infarcts, brain abscess and some tumours.

Grossly, the white matter is swollen, soft, with flattened gyri and narrowed sulci. Sectioned surface is soft and gelatinous.

Microscopically, there is separation of tissue elements by the oedema fluid and swelling of astrocytes. The perivascular (Virchow-Robin) space is widened and clear halos are seen around the small blood vessels.

2. **CYTOTOXIC OEDEMA** In this type, the blood-brain barrier is intact and the fluid accumulation is intracellular. The underlying mechanism is disturbance in the cellular osmoregulation as occurs in some metabolic derangements, acute hypoxia and with some toxic chemicals.

Microscopically, the cells are swollen and vacuolated. In some situations, both vasogenic and cytotoxic cerebral oedema result e.g. in purulent meningitis.

3. **INTERSTITIAL OEDEMA** This type of cerebral oedema occurs when the excessive fluid crosses the ependymal lining of the ventricles and accumulates in the periventricular white matter. This mechanism is responsible for oedema in non-communicating hydrocephalus.

Hepatic Oedema

Briefly, the mechanisms involved in causation of oedema of the legs and ascites in cirrhosis of the liver is as under (page 557):

i) There is *hypoproteinaemia* due to impaired synthesis of proteins by the diseased liver.
ii) Due to portal hypertension, there is increased venous pressure in the abdomen, and hence *raised hydrostatic pressure*.
iii) Failure of inactivation of aldosterone in the diseased liver and hence *hyperaldosteronism*.
iv) Secondary stimulation of renin-angiotensin mechanism promoting *sodium and water retention*.

Nutritional Oedema

Oedema due to nutritional deficiency of proteins (kwashiorkor, prolonged starvation, famine, fasting), vitamins (beri-beri due to vitamin B_1 deficiency) and chronic alcoholism occurs on legs but sometimes may be more generalised. The main contributing factors are hypoproteinaemia and sodium-water retention related to metabolic abnormalities. In kwashiorkor occurring in children in economically deprived communities in Africa and Asia, oedema is associated with characteristic mucocutaneous ulceration and depigmentation of the hair, all of which revert back to normal on adequate nutrition.

Myxoedema

Myxoedema from hypothyroidism is a form of non-pitting oedema occurring on skin of face and other parts of the body as also in the internal organs due to excessive deposition of glycosaminoglycans in the interstitium. Microscopically, it appears as basophilic mucopolysaccharides.

DEHYDRATION

Dehydration is a state of pure deprivation of water leading to sodium retention and hence a state of hypernatraemia. In other words, there is only loss of water without loss of sodium. Clinically, the patients present with intense thirst, mental confusion, fever, and oliguria.

ETIOLOGY Pure water deficiency is less common than salt depletion but can occur in the following conditions:

1. **GI excretion:**
i) Severe vomitings
ii) Diarrhoea
iii) Cholera

2. **Renal excretion:**
i) Acute renal failure in diuretic phase
ii) Extensive use of diuretics
iii) Endocrine diseases e.g. diabetes insipidus, Addison's disease

3. **Loss of blood and plasma:**
i) Severe injuries, severe burns
ii) During childbirth

4. **Loss through skin:**
i) Excessive perspiration
ii) Hyperthermia

5. **Accumulation in body cavities:**
i) Sudden development of ascites
ii) Acute intestinal obstruction with accumulation of fluid in the bowel.

MORPHOLOGICAL FEATURES There are no particular pathological changes in organs, except in advanced cases when the organs are dark and shrunken. However, there are haematological and biochemical changes.

❖ There is haemoconcentration as seen by increased PCV and raised haemoglobin.

❖ In late stage, there is rise in blood urea and serum sodium.

❖ Renal shutdown and a state of shock may develop.

OVERHYDRATION

Overhydration is increased extracellular fluid volume due to pure water excess or water intoxication. Clinically, the patients present with disordered cerebral function e.g. nausea, vomiting, headache, confusion and in severe cases convulsions, coma, and even death.

ETIOLOGY Overhydration is generally an induced condition and is encountered in the following situations:

1. **Excessive unmonitored intravascular infusion:**
i) Normal saline (0.9% sodium chloride)
ii) Ringer lactate

2. **Renal retention of sodium and water:**
i) Congestive heart failure
ii) Acute glomerulonephritis
iii) Cirrhosis
iv) Cushing's syndrome
v) Chronic renal failure

MORPHOLOGICAL FEATURES Sudden weight gain is a significant parameter of excess of fluid accumulation. Haematological and biochemical changes include the following:

❖ Reduced PCV.

❖ Reduced plasma electrolytes and lowered plasma proteins.

Besides disturbances of body water discussed above, derangements of electrolytes (most commonly hypo- and hypernatraemia, hypo- and hyperkalaemia), altered pH of blood and acid-base imbalance (e.g. metabolc acidosis and alkalosis, respiratory acidosis and alkalosis) are other clinically significant abnormalities.

GIST BOX 15.2 — Disturbances of Body Water

- Oedema is abnormal and excessive accumulation of "free fluid" in the interstitial tissue spaces and serous cavities.
- Oedema may be localised when limited to an organ or limb, and generalised (anasarca or dropsy) when it is systemic in distribution, particularly noticeable in the subcutaneous tissues.
- Depending upon fluid composition, oedema fluid may be transudate which is more often the case, such as in oedema of cardiac and renal disease; or exudate such as in inflammatory oedema.
- Various mechanisms operating singly or in combination to produce oedema are: decreased plasma oncotic pressure, increased capillary hydrostatic pressure, lymphatic obstruction, tissue factors (increased oncotic pressure of interstitial fluid, and decreased tissue tension), increased capillary permeability, and sodium and water retention.
- Generalised oedema of renal origin occurs in nephrotic syndrome, nephritic syndrome, and in renal failure due to acute tubular injury.
- Cardiac oedema is generalised and dependent type and develops in right-sided and congestive cardiac failure.
- Acute pulmonary oedema results from either the elevation of pulmonary hydrostatic pressure or the increased capillary permeability from various causes.
- In cerebral oedema, fluid-electrolyte exchange occurs at the blood-brain barrier because there are no lymphatics. Cerebral oedema can be vasogenic, cytotoxic and interstitial.
- Dehydration is pure deprivation of water leading to sodium retention and a state of hypernatraemia.
- Overhydration is increased extracellular fluid volume due to pure water excess or water intoxication.

16 Blood Flow Volume Disorders

The principles of blood flow are called haemodynamics. Normal circulatory function requires uninterrupted flow of blood from the left ventricle to the farthest capillaries in the body; return of the blood from systemic capillary network into the right ventricle; and from the right ventricle to the farthest pulmonary capillaries and back to the left atrium (Fig. 16.1). There are three essential requirements to maintain normal blood flow and perfusion of tissues: normal anatomic features, normal physiologic controls for blood flow, and normal biochemical composition of the blood.

Derangements of blood flow or haemodynamic disturbances are considered under 2 broad headings:

I. *Disturbances in the volume of the circulating blood* These include: hyperaemia and congestion, haemorrhage and shock. These are discussed in this chapter.

II. *Circulatory disturbances of obstructive nature* These are: thrombosis, embolism, ischaemia and infarction. These are discussed in Chapter 17.

HYPERAEMIA AND CONGESTION

Hyperaemia and congestion are the terms used for localised increase in the volume of blood within dilated vessels of an organ or tissue.

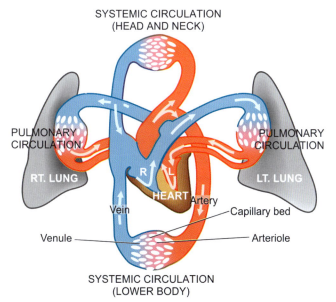

Figure 16.1 ▶ Normal haemodynamic flow of blood in the body.

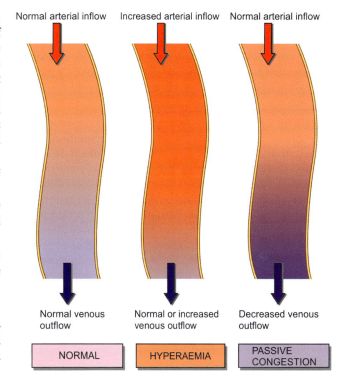

Figure 16.2 ▶ Schematic representation of abnormal accumulation of blood in the arteriovenous capillary bed causing hyperaemia and passive congestion.

❖ Increased volume of blood from arterial and arteriolar dilatation (i.e. increased inflow) is referred to as *hyperaemia or active hyperaemia*.

❖ Impaired venous drainage (i.e. diminished outflow) is called *venous congestion or passive hyperaemia* (Fig. 16.2).

If the condition develops rapidly it is called *acute*, while more prolonged and gradual response is known as *chronic*.

ACTIVE HYPERAEMIA

The dilatation of arteries, arterioles and capillaries is effected either through sympathetic neurogenic mechanism or via the release of vasoactive substances. The affected tissue or organ is pink or red in appearance (erythema).

The *examples* of active hyperaemia are seen in the following conditions:

i) Inflammation e.g. congested vessels in the walls of alveoli in pneumonia

ii) Blushing i.e. flushing of the skin of face in response to emotions
iii) Menopausal flush
iv) Muscular exercise
v) High-grade fever
vi) Goitre
vii) Arteriovenous malformations

Clinically, hyperaemia is characterised by redness and raised temperature in the affected part.

PASSIVE HYPERAEMIA (VENOUS CONGESTION)

The dilatation of veins and capillaries due to impaired venous drainage results in passive hyperaemia or venous congestion, commonly referred to as *passive congestion*. Congestion may be acute or chronic, the latter being more common and is called *chronic venous congestion* (CVC). The affected tissue or organ is bluish in colour due to accumulation of venous blood (cyanosis). Obstruction to the venous outflow may be local or systemic. Accordingly, venous congestion is of 2 types:

◆ *Local venous congestion* results from obstruction to the venous outflow from an organ or part of the body e.g. portal venous obstruction in cirrhosis of the liver, outside pressure on the vessel wall as occurs in tight bandage, plasters, tumours, pregnancy, hernia etc, or intraluminal occlusion by thrombosis.

◆ *Systemic (General) venous congestion* is engorgement of veins e.g. in left-sided and right-sided heart failure and diseases of the lungs which interfere with pulmonary blood flow like pulmonary fibrosis, emphysema etc. Usually the fluid accumulates upstream to the specific chamber of the heart which is initially affected (page 470). For example, in *left-sided heart failure* (such as due to mechanical overload in aortic stenosis, or due to weakened left ventricular wall as in myocardial infarction) pulmonary congestion (or CVC lungs) results, whereas in *right-sided heart failure* (such as due to pulmonary stenosis or pulmonary hypertension) systemic venous congestion (i.e. CVC of systemic organs) results. **Fig. 16.3** illustrates the mechanisms involved in passive or venous congestion of different organs.

Morphology of CVC of Organs

CVC Lung

Chronic venous congestion of the lung occurs in left heart failure (e.g. in rheumatic mitral stenosis) resulting in rise in pulmonary venous pressure.

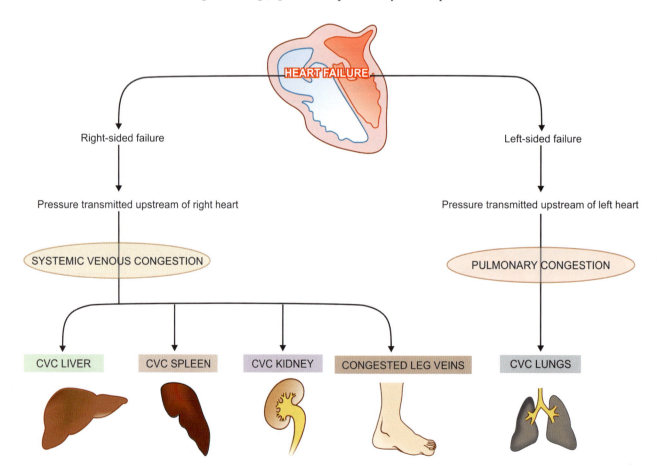

Figure 16.3 ▶ Schematic representation of mechanisms involved in chronic venous congestion (CVC) of different organs.

Chapter 16: Blood Flow Volume Disorders

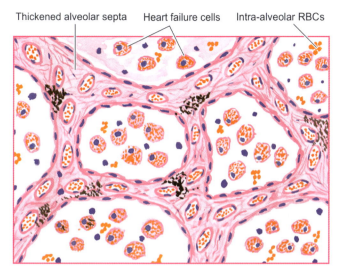
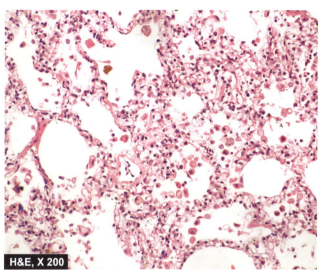

Figure 16.4 ▶ CVC lung. The alveolar septa are widened and thickened due to congestion, oedema and mild fibrosis. The alveolar lumina contain heart failure cells (alveolar macrophages containing haemosiderin pigment).

Grossly, the lungs are heavy and firm in consistency. The sectioned surface is dark and rusty brown in colour, referred to as *brown induration* of the lungs.

Histologically, the features are as under:

i) The alveolar septa are widened due to presence of interstitial oedema and dilated and congested capillaries in the septal wall. There is also slight increase in fibrous connective tissue in the alveolar septa.

ii) Rupture of dilated and congested capillaries may result in minute intra-alveolar haemorrhages. The breakdown of erythrocytes liberates haemosiderin pigment which is taken up by alveolar macrophages, called as *heart failure cells,* seen in the alveolar lumina. The brown induration observed on the cut surface of the lungs is due to the pigmentation and fibrosis (Fig. 16.4).

CVC Liver

Chronic venous congestion of the liver occurs in right heart failure and sometimes due to occlusion of inferior vena cava and hepatic vein.

Grossly, the liver is enlarged and tender and the capsule is tense. Cut surface shows characteristic *nutmeg** appearance due to red and yellow mottled appearance, corresponding to congested centre of lobules and fatty peripheral zone respectively (Fig. 16.5).

Microscopically, the changes of passive congestion are more marked in the centrilobular zone (zone 3) which is farthest from blood supply (periportal zone, zone 1) and thus bears the brunt of hypoxia the most.

i) The central veins as well as the adjacent sinusoids are distended and filled with blood. The centrilobular hepatocytes undergo degenerative changes, and eventually *centrilobular haemorrhagic necrosis* occurs.

ii) Long-standing cases may show fine centrilobular fibrosis and regeneration of hepatocytes, resulting in cardiac cirrhosis (Chapter 19).

iii) The peripheral zone of the lobule is less severely affected by chronic hypoxia and shows some *fatty change* in the hepatocytes (Fig. 16.6).

CVC Spleen

Chronic venous congestion of the spleen occurs in right heart failure and in portal hypertension from cirrhosis of liver.

Grossly, the spleen in early stage is slightly to moderately enlarged (up to 250 g as compared to normal 150 g), while in long-standing cases there is progressive enlargement and may weigh up to 500 to 1000 g. The organ is deeply congested, tense and cyanotic. Sectioned surface is grey-tan (Fig. 16.7).

Microscopically, the features are as under (Fig. 16.8):

i) *Red pulp* is enlarged due to congestion and marked sinusoidal dilatation and there are areas of recent and old haemorrhages. Sinusoids may get converted into capillaries (capillarisation of sinusoids).

ii) There is *hyperplasia* of *reticuloendothelial cells* in the red pulp of the spleen (splenic macrophages).

---

*Nutmeg (vernacular name *jaiphal*) is the seed of a spice tree that grows in India, and is used in cooking as spice for giving flavours.

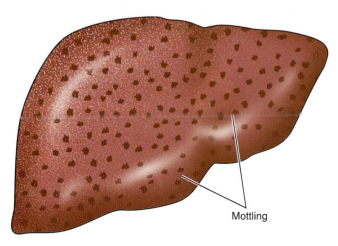
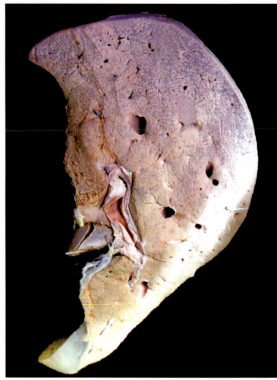

Figure 16.5 ▶ Nutmeg liver. The cut surface shows mottled appearance—alternate pattern of dark congestion and pale fatty change.

iii) There is *fibrous thickening* of the capsule and of the trabeculae.
iv) Some of haemorrhages overlying fibrous tissue get deposits of haemosiderin pigment and calcium salts; these organised structures are termed as *Gamna-Gandy bodies* or siderofibrotic nodules.

v) Firmness of the spleen in advanced stage is seen more commonly in hepatic cirrhosis (*congestive splenomegaly*) and is the commonest cause of hypersplenism (Chapter 24).

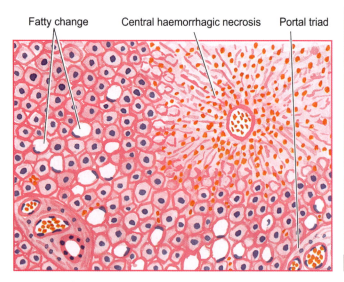
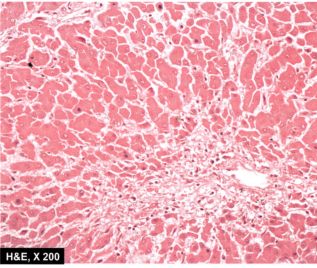

Figure 16.6 ▶ CVC liver. The centrilobular zone shows marked degeneration and necrosis of hepatocytes accompanied by haemorrhage while the peripheral zone shows mild fatty change of liver cells.

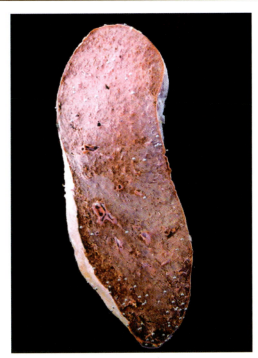

Figure 16.7 ▶ CVC spleen (Congestive splenomegaly). Sectioned surface shows that the spleen is heavy and enlarged in size. The colour of sectioned surface is grey-tan.

CVC Kidney

Grossly, the kidneys are slightly enlarged and the medulla is congested.

Microscopically, the changes are rather mild. The tubules may show degenerative changes like cloudy swelling and fatty change. The glomeruli may show mesangial proliferation.

HAEMORRHAGE

Haemorrhage is the escape of blood from a blood vessel. The bleeding may occur *externally, or internally* into the serous cavities (e.g. haemothorax, haemoperitoneum, haemopericardium), or into a hollow viscus. Extravasation of blood into the tissues with resultant swelling is known as *haematoma*. Large extravasations of blood into the skin and mucous membranes are called *ecchymoses. Purpuras* are small areas of haemorrhages (up to 1 cm) into the skin and mucous membrane, whereas *petechiae* are minute pinhead-sized haemorrhages. Microscopic escape of erythrocytes into loose tissues may occur following marked congestion and is known as *diapedesis*.

ETIOLOGY The blood loss may be large and sudden *(acute),* or small repeated bleeds may occur over a period of time *(chronic).* The various causes of haemorrhage are as under:

1. *Trauma* to the vessel wall e.g. penetrating wound in the heart or great vessels, during labour etc.

2. *Spontaneous haemorrhage* e.g. rupture of an aneurysm, septicaemia, bleeding diathesis (such as purpura), acute leukaemias, pernicious anaemia, scurvy.

3. *Inflammatory lesions of the vessel wall* e.g. bleeding from chronic peptic ulcer, typhoid ulcers, blood vessels traversing a tuberculous cavity in the lung, syphilitic involvement of the aorta, polyarteritis nodosa.

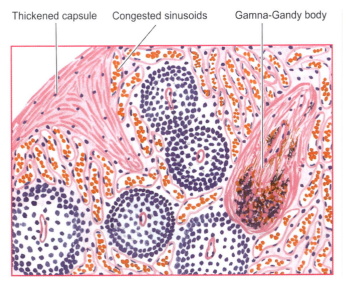
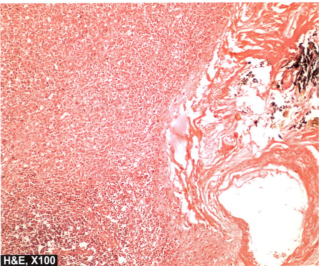

Figure 16.8 ▶ CVC spleen. The sinuses are dilated and congested. There is increased fibrosis in the red pulp, capsule and the trabeculae. A Gamna-Gandy body is also seen.

4. *Neoplastic invasion* e.g. haemorrhage following vascular invasion in carcinoma of the tongue.
5. *Vascular diseases* e.g. atherosclerosis.
6. *Elevated pressure within the vessels* e.g. cerebral and retinal haemorrhage in systemic hypertension, severe haemorrhage from varicose veins due to high pressure in the veins of legs or oesophagus.

EFFECTS The effects of blood loss depend upon 3 main factors:
i) amount of blood loss;
ii) speed of blood loss; and
iii) site of haemorrhage.

The loss up to 20% of blood volume suddenly or slowly generally has little clinical effects because of compensatory mechanisms. A sudden loss of 33% of blood volume may cause death, while loss of up to 50% of blood volume gradually over a period of 24 hours may not be necessarily fatal. However, chronic blood loss generally produces iron deficiency anaemia, whereas acute haemorrhage may lead to serious immediate consequences such as hypovolaemic shock.

GIST BOX 16.1 — Hyperaemia, Congestion and Haemorrhage

- Increased volume of blood from arterial and arteriolar dilatation (i.e. increased inflow) is referred to as hyperaemia or active hyperaemia, while impaired venous drainage (i.e. diminished outflow) is called venous congestion or passive hyperaemia.
- Congestion may be acute or chronic, the latter being more common and is called chronic venous congestion (CVC).
- Systemic venous congestion is engorgement of veins e.g. in left-sided heart failure (CVC lungs), right-sided heart failure (CVC liver, spleen, kidneys, other sites).
- Haemorrhage is the escape of blood from a blood vessel. The bleeding may occur externally, or internally into the serous cavities, into a hollow viscus, or in to skin and mucous membranes.
- Rapid loss of above 33% of blood volume is more serious than gradual blood loss of 50% in 24 hours.

SHOCK

DEFINITION

Shock is a life-threatening clinical syndrome of cardiovascular collapse characterised by:
◆ an acute reduction of effective circulating blood volume (hypotension); and
◆ an inadequate perfusion of cells and tissues (hypoperfusion).

If uncompensated, these mechanisms may lead to impaired cellular metabolism and death.

Thus, by definition *"true (or secondary) shock"* is a circulatory imbalance between oxygen supply and oxygen requirements at the cellular level, and is also called as circulatory shock and is the type which is commonly referred to as 'shock' if not specified.

The term *"initial (or primary) shock"* is used for transient and usually a benign vasovagal attack resulting from sudden reduction of venous return to the heart caused by neurogenic vasodilatation and consequent peripheral pooling of blood e.g. immediately following trauma, severe pain or emotional overreaction such as due to fear, sorrow or surprise. Clinically, patients of primary shock suffer from the attack lasting for a few seconds or minutes and develop brief unconsciousness, weakness, sinking sensation, pale and clammy limbs, weak and rapid pulse, and low blood pressure. Another type of shock which is not due to circulatory derangement is *anaphylactic shock* from type 1 immunologic (amaphylactic) reaction (page 211).

CLASSIFICATION AND ETIOLOGY

Although in a given clinical case, two or more factors may be involved in causation of true shock, a simple etiologic classification of shock syndrome divides it into following 3 major types and a few other variants (Table 16.1):

1. Hypovolaemic shock This form of shock results from inadequate circulatory blood volume by various etiologic factors that may be *either* from the loss of red cell mass and plasma due to haemorrhage, *or* from the loss of plasma volume alone.

2. Cardiogenic shock Acute circulatory failure with sudden fall in cardiac output from acute diseases of the heart without actual reduction of blood volume (normovolaemia) results in cardiogenic shock.

3. Septic (Toxaemic) shock Severe bacterial infections or septicaemia induce septic shock. It may be the result of Gram-negative septicaemia (endotoxic shock) which is more common, or less often from Gram-positive septicaemia (exotoxic shock).

4. Other types These include the following types:

i) Traumatic shock Shock resulting from trauma is initially due to hypovolaemia, but even after haemorrhage has been controlled, these patients continue to suffer loss of plasma volume into the interstitium of injured tissue and hence is considered separately in some descriptions.

ii) Neurogenic shock Neurogenic shock results from causes of interruption of sympathetic vasomotor supply.

iii) Hypoadrenal shock Hypoadrenal shock occurs from unknown adrenal insufficiency in which the patient fails to respond normally to the stress of trauma, surgery or illness.

PATHOGENESIS

In general, all forms of shock involve following 3 derangements:

Chapter 16: Blood Flow Volume Disorders

Table 16.1	Classification and etiology of shock.

1. HYPOVOLAEMIC SHOCK
    i) Acute haemorrhage
    ii) Dehydration from vomitings, diarrhoea
    iii) Burns
    iv) Excessive use of diuretics
    v) Acute pancreatitis
2. CARDIOGENIC SHOCK
    i) *Deficient emptying e.g.*
        a) Myocardial infarction
        b) Cardiomyopathies
        c) Rupture of the heart, ventricle or papillary muscle
        d) Cardiac arrhythmias
    ii) *Deficient filling e.g.*
        a) Cardiac tamponade from haemopericardium
    iii) *Obstruction to the outflow e.g.*
        a) Pulmonary embolism
        b) Ball valve thrombus
        c) Tension pneumothorax
        d) Dissecting aortic aneurysm
3. SEPTIC SHOCK
    i) *Gram-negative septicaemia (endotoxic shock) e.g.* Infection with *E. coli, Proteus, Klebsiella, Pseudomonas* and *Bacteroides*
    ii) *Gram-positive septicaemia (exotoxic shock) e.g.* Infection with streptococci, pneumococci
4. OTHER TYPES
    i) *Traumatic shock*
        a) Severe injuries
        b) Surgery with marked blood loss
        c) Obstetrical trauma
    ii) *Neurogenic shock*
        a) High cervical spinal cord injury
        b) Accidental high spinal anaesthesia
        c) Severe head injury
    iii) *Hypoadrenal shock*
        a) Administration of high doses of glucocorticoids
        b) Secondary adrenal insufficiency (e.g. in tuberculosis, metastatic disease, bilateral adrenal haemorrhage, idiopathic adrenal atrophy)

i) Reduced effective circulating blood volume.
ii) Reduced supply of oxygen to the cells and tissues with resultant anoxia.
iii) Inflammatory mediators and toxins released from shock-induced cellular injury.

These derangements initially set in compensatory mechanisms (discussed below) but eventually a vicious cycle of cell injury and severe cellular dysfunction lead to breakdown of organ function (Fig. 16.9).

1. Reduced effective circulating blood volume It may result by either of the following mechanisms:
i) by actual loss of blood volume as occurs in hypovolaemic shock; or
ii) by decreased cardiac output without actual loss of blood (normovolaemia) as occurs in cardiogenic shock and septic shock.

2. Impaired tissue oxygenation Following reduction in the effective circulating blood volume from either of the above two mechanisms and from any of the etiologic agents, there is decreased venous return to the heart resulting in decreased cardiac output. This consequently causes reduced supply of oxygen to the organs and tissues and hence tissue anoxia occurs, which sets in cellular injury.

3. Release of inflammatory mediators In response to cellular injury, innate immunity of the body gets activated as a body defense mechanism and causes release of inflammatory mediators but eventually these agents themselves become the cause of cell injury. Endotoxins in bacterial wall in septic shock stimulate massive release of pro-inflammatory mediators (cytokines) but a similar process of release of these agents takes place in late stages of shock from other causes. Several pro-inflammatory mediators are released from monocytes-macrophages, other leucocytes and other body cells, the most important being the tumour necrosis factor-(TNF)-α and interleukin-1 (IL-1) cytokines (Fig. 16.10).

After these general comments on mechanisms in shock, features specific to pathogenesis of three major forms of shock are given below:

PATHOGENESIS OF HYPOVOLAEMIC SHOCK Hypovolaemic shock occurs from inadequate circulating blood volume due to various causes, most often from loss of red cell mass due to haemorrhage and, therefore, also called as haemorrhagic shock. The major effects in this are due to decreased cardiac output and low intracardiac pressure. The severity of clinical features depends upon degree of blood volume lost; accordingly haemorrhagic shock is divided into four types:
i) $\leq$1000 ml: Compensated
ii) 1000-1500 ml: Mild
iii) 1500-2000 ml: Moderate
iv) >2000 ml: Severe

Major clinical features are increased heart rate (tachycardia), low blood pressure (hypotension), low urinary output (oliguria to anuria) and alteration in mental state (agitated to confused to lethargic).

PATHOGENESIS OF CARDIOGENIC SHOCK Cardiogenic shock results from a severe left ventricular dysfunction from various causes such as acute myocardial infarction. The resultant decreased cardiac output has its effects in the form of decreased tissue perfusion and movement of fluid from pulmonary vascular bed into pulmonary interstitial space initially (*interstitial pulmonary oedema*) and later into alveolar spaces (*alveolar pulmonary oedema*).

PATHOGENESIS OF SEPTIC SHOCK Septic shock results most often from Gram-negative bacteria entering the body from genitourinary tract, alimentary tract, respiratory tract

Section III: Fluid and Haemodynamic Disorders

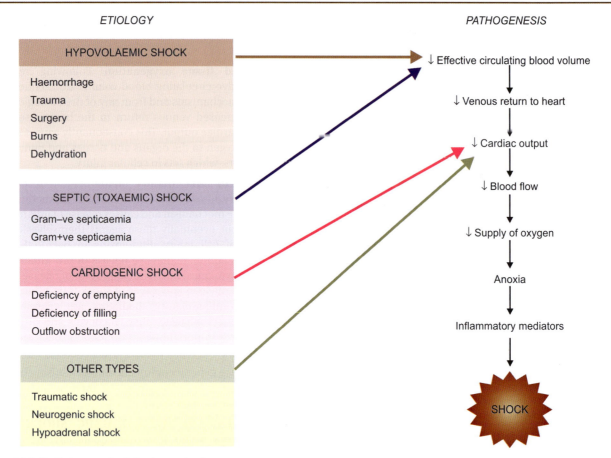

Figure 16.9 ▶ Pathogenesis of circulatory shock.

or skin, and less often from Gram-positive bacteria. In septic shock, there is immune system activation and severe systemic inflammatory response to infection as follows:

i) Activation of macrophage-monocytes Lysis of Gram-negative bacteria releases endotoxin, a lipopolysaccharide (LPS), into circulation where it binds to lipopolysaccharide-binding protein (LBP). The complex of LPS-LBP binds to CD14 molecule on the surface of the monocyte/macrophages which are stimulated to elaborate proinflammatory cytokines, the most important ones being TNF-α and IL-1. The effects of these cytokines are as under:

a) *By altering endothelial cell adhesiveness*: This results in recruitment of more neutrophils which liberate free radicals that cause vascular injury.
b) *Promoting nitric oxide synthase*: This stimulates increased synthesis of nitric oxide which is responsible for vasodilatation and hypotension.

ii) Activation of other inflammatory responses Microbial infection activates other inflammatory cascades which have profound effects in triggering septic shock. These are as under:

a) *Activation of complement pathway*: End-products C5a and C3a induce microemboli and endothelial damage.

b) *Activation of mast cells*: Histamine is released which increases capillary permeability.
c) *Activation of coagulation system*: Enhances development of thrombi.
d) *Activation of kinin system:* Released bradykinin causes vasodilatation and increased capillary permeability.

The net result of above mechanisms is vasodilatation and increased vascular permeability in septic shock. Profound peripheral vasodilatation and pooling of blood causes hyperdynamic circulation in septic shock, in contrast to hypovolaemic and cardiogenic shock. Increased vascular permeability causes development of inflammatory oedema. Disseminated intravascular coagulation (DIC) is prone to develop in septic shock due to endothelial cell injury by toxins. Reduced blood flow produces hypotension, inadequate perfusion of cells and tissues, finally leading to organ dysfunction.

PATHOPHYSIOLOGY (STAGES OF SHOCK)

Although deterioration of the circulation in shock is a progressive and continuous phenomenon and compensatory mechanisms become progressively less effective, historically shock has been divided arbitrarily into 3 stages (Fig. 16.11):

Chapter 16: Blood Flow Volume Disorders

1. Compensated (non-progressive, initial, reversible) shock
2. Progressive decompensated shock
3. Irreversible decompensated shock

COMPENSATED (NON-PROGRESSIVE, INITIAL, REVERSIBLE) SHOCK In the early stage of shock, an attempt is made to maintain adequate cerebral and coronary blood supply by redistribution of blood so that the vital organs (brain and heart) are adequately perfused and oxygenated. This is achieved by activation of various neurohormonal mechanisms causing *widespread vasoconstriction* and by *fluid conservation by the kidney*. If the condition that caused the shock is adequately treated, the compensatory mechanism may be able to bring about recovery and re-establish the normal circulation; this is called compensated or reversible shock. These compensatory mechanisms are as under:

i) Widespread vasoconstriction In response to reduced blood flow (hypotension) and tissue anoxia, the neural and humoral factors (e.g. baroreceptors, chemoreceptors, catecholamines, renin, and angiotensin-II) are activated. All these bring about vasoconstriction, particularly in the vessels of the skin and abdominal viscera. Widespread vasoconstriction is a protective mechanism as it causes increased peripheral resistance, increased heart rate (tachycardia) and increased blood pressure. However, in septic shock, there is initial vasodilatation followed by vasoconstriction. Besides, in severe septic shock there is elevated level of thromboxane A2 which is a potent vasoconstrictor and may augment the cardiac output along with other sympathetic mechanisms. Clinically, cutaneous vasoconstriction is responsible for cool and pale skin in initial stage of shock.

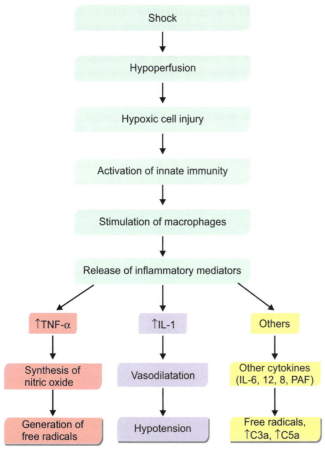

Figure 16.10 ▶ Response of inflammatory mediators in shock.

STAGE	PATHOGENESIS	EFFECTS
COMPENSATED (INITIAL) SHOCK	i) Widespread vasoconstriction ii) Fluid conservation by kidney iii) Stimulation of adrenal medulla	• Tachycardia • Cool clammy skin
PROGRESSIVE DECOMPENSATED SHOCK	i) Pulmonary hypoperfusion ii) Tissue ischaemia	• ↓ Cardiac output • Mental confusion • ↓ Urinary output • Tachypnoea
IRREVERSIBLE DECOMPENSATED SHOCK	i) Progressive vasodilatation ii) ↑ Vascular permeability iii) Myocardial depressant factor (MDF) iv) Pulmonary hypoperfusion v) Anoxic damage vi) Hypercoagulability	• Brain: Hypoxic encephalopathy • Heart: Focal myocardial necrosis • Lungs: ARDS • Kidney: ATN • Adrenals: Necrosis • GI: Haemorrhagic gastroenteropathy • Liver: Necrosis • Blood: DIC

Figure 16.11 ▶ Mechanisms and effects of three stages of shock.

ii) Fluid conservation by the kidney In order to compensate the actual loss of blood volume in hypovolaemic shock, the following factors may assist in restoring the blood volume and improve venous return to the heart:
a) Release of aldosterone from hypoxic kidney by activation of renin-angiotensin-aldosterone mechanism.
b) Release of ADH due to decreased effective circulating blood volume.
c) Reduced glomerular filtration rate (GFR) due to arteriolar constriction.
d) Shifting of tissue fluids into the plasma due to lowered capillary hydrostatic pressure (hypotension).

iii) Stimulation of adrenal medulla In response to low cardiac output, adrenal medulla is stimulated to release excess of catecholamines (epinephrine and non-epinephrine) which increase heart rate and try to increase cardiac output.

PROGRESSIVE DECOMPENSATED SHOCK This is a stage when the patient suffers from some other stress or risk factors (e.g. pre-existing cardiovascular and lung disease) besides persistence of the shock condition; this causes progressive deterioration. The effects of resultant tissue hypoperfusion in progressive decompensated shock are as under:

i) Pulmonary hypoperfusion Decompensated shock worsens pulmonary perfusion and increases vascular permeability resulting in tachypnoea and adult respiratory distress syndrome (ARDS).

ii) Tissue ischaemia Impaired tissue perfusion causes switch from aerobic to anaerobic glycolysis resulting in *metabolic lactic acidosis*. Lactic acidosis lowers the tissue pH which, in turn, makes the vasomotor response ineffective. This results in vasodilatation and peripheral pooling of blood.

Clinically, at this stage the patient develops confusion and worsening of renal function.

IRREVERSIBLE DECOMPENSATED SHOCK When the shock is so severe that in spite of compensatory mechanisms and despite therapy and control of etiologic agent which caused the shock, no recovery takes place, it is called decompensated or irreversible shock. Its effects due to widespread cell injury are as follows:

i) Progressive vasodilatation During later stages of shock, anoxia damages the capillary and venular wall while arterioles become unresponsive to vasoconstrictors listed above and begin to dilate. Vasodilatation results in peripheral pooling of blood which further deteriorates the effective circulating blood volume.

ii) Increased vascular permeability Anoxic damage to tissues releases proinflammatory mediators which cause increased vascular permeability. This results in escape of fluid from circulation into the interstitial tissues thus deteriorating effective circulating blood volume.

iii) Myocardial depressant factor (MDF) Progressive fall in the blood pressure and persistently reduced blood flow to myocardium causes coronary insufficiency and myocardial ischaemia due to release of myocardial depressant factor (MDF). This results in further depression of cardiac function, reduced cardiac output and decreased blood flow.

iv) Worsening pulmonary hypoperfusion Further pulmonary hypoperfusion causes respiratory distress due to pulmonary oedema, tachypnoea and adult respiratory distress syndrome (ARDS).

v) Anoxic damage to heart, kidney and brain Progressive tissue anoxia causes severe metabolic acidosis due to anaerobic glycolysis. There is release of proinflammatory cytokines and other inflammatory mediators and generation of free radicals. Since highly specialised cells of the myocardium, proximal tubular cells of the kidney, and neurons of the CNS are dependent solely on aerobic respiration for ATP generation, there is ischaemic cell death in these tissues.

vi) Hypercoagulability of blood Tissue damage in shock activates coagulation cascade with release of clot promoting factor, thromboplastin and release of platelet aggregator, ADP, which contributes to slowing of blood-stream and vascular thrombosis. In this way, hypercoagulability of blood with consequent microthrombi impair the blood flow and cause further tissue necrosis.

Clinically, at this stage the patient has features of coma, worsened heart function and progressive renal failure due to acute tubular necrosis.

MORPHOLOGIC FEATURES

Eventually, shock is characterised by multisystem failure. The morphologic changes in shock are due to hypoxia resulting in degeneration and necrosis in various organs. The major organs affected are the brain, heart, lungs and kidneys. Morphologic changes are also noted in the adrenals, gastrointestinal tract, liver and other organs. The predominant morphologic changes and their incidence are shown in Fig. 16.12 and described below.

1. HYPOXIC ENCEPHALOPATHY Cerebral ischaemia in compensated shock may produce altered state of consciousness. However, if the blood pressure falls below 50 mmHg as occurs in systemic hypotension in prolonged shock and cardiac arrest, brain suffers from serious ischaemic damage with loss of cortical functions, coma, and a vegetative state.

Grossly, the area supplied by the most distal branches of the cerebral arteries suffers from severe ischaemic necrosis which is usually the border zone between the anterior and middle cerebral arteries.

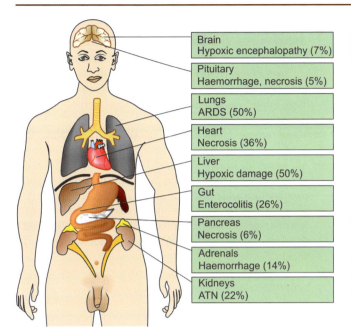

Figure 16.12 ▶ Morphologic features of shock.

Microscopically, the changes are noticeable if ischaemia is prolonged for 12 to 24 hours. Neurons, particularly Purkinje cells, are more prone to develop the effects of ischaemia. The cytoplasm of the affected neurons is intensely eosinophilic and the nucleus is small pyknotic. Dead and dying nerve cells are replaced by gliosis.

2. HEART IN SHOCK The heart is more vulnerable to the effects of hypoxia than any other organ. Heart is affected in cardiogenic as well as in other forms of shock. There are 2 types of morphologic changes in heart in all types of shock:

i) *Haemorrhages and necrosis* There may be small or large ischaemic areas or infarcts, particularly located in the subepicardial and subendocardial region.
ii) *Zonal lesions* These are opaque transverse contraction bands in the myocytes near the intercalated disc.

3. SHOCK LUNG Lungs due to dual blood supply are generally not affected by hypovolaemic shock but in septic shock the morphologic changes in lungs are quite prominent termed 'shock lung'.

Grossly, the lungs are heavy and wet.

Microscopically, changes of adult respiratory distress syndrome (ARDS) are seen. Briefly, the changes include congestion, interstitial and alveolar oedema, interstitial lymphocytic infiltrate, alveolar hyaline membranes, thickening and fibrosis of alveolar septa, and fibrin and platelet thrombi in the pulmonary microvasculature.

4. SHOCK KIDNEY One of the important complications of shock is irreversible renal injury, first noted in persons who sustained crush injuries in building collapses in air raids in World War II. Renal ischaemia following systemic hypotension is considered responsible for renal changes in shock. The end-result is generally anuria and death.

Grossly, the kidneys are soft and swollen. Sectioned surface shows blurred architectural markings.

Microscopically, tubular lesions are seen at all levels of nephron and are referred to as acute tubular necrosis (ATN) which can occur following other causes besides shock. If extensive muscle injury or intravascular haemolysis is also associated, peculiar brown tubular casts are seen.

5. ADRENALS IN SHOCK The adrenals show stress response in shock. This includes release of aldosterone in response to hypoxic kidney, release of glucocorticoids from adrenal cortex and catecholamines like adrenaline from adrenal medulla. In severe shock, acute adrenal haemorrhagic necrosis may occur.

6. HAEMORRHAGIC GASTROENTEROPATHY The hypoperfusion of the alimentary tract in conditions such as shock and cardiac failure may result in mucosal and mural infarction called haemorrhagic gastroenteropathy. This type of non-occlusive ischaemic injury of bowel must be distinguished from full-fledged infarction in which deeper layers of the gut (muscularis and serosa) are also damaged. In shock due to burns, acute stress ulcers of the stomach or duodenum may occur and are known as Curling's ulcers.

Grossly, the lesions are multifocal and widely distributed throughout the bowel. The lesions are superficial ulcers, reddish purple in colour. The adjoining bowel mucosa is oedematous and haemorrhagic.

Microscopically, the involved surface of the bowel shows dilated and congested vessels and haemorrhagic necrosis of the mucosa and sometimes submucosa. Secondary infection may supervene and condition may progress into pseudomembranous enterocolitis.

7. LIVER IN SHOCK *Grossly,* faint nutmeg appearance is seen.

Microscopically, depending upon the time gap between injury and cell death, ischaemic shrinkage, hydropic change, focal necrosis, or fatty change may be seen. Liver function may be impaired.

8. OTHER ORGANS Other organs such as lymph nodes, spleen and pancreas may also show foci of necrosis in shock. In addition, patients who survive acute phase of shock succumb to overwhelming infections due to altered immune status and impaired host defense mechanism.

CLINICAL FEATURES AND COMPLICATIONS

The classical features of decompensated shock are characterised by *depression of 4 vital processes:*
i) Very low blood pressure
ii) Subnormal temperature
iii) Feeble and irregular pulse
iv) Shallow and sighing respiration

In addition, the patients in shock have pale face, sunken eyes, weakness, cold and clammy skin.

Life-threatening complications in shock are due to hypoxic cell injury resulting in immuno-inflammatory responses and activation of various cascades (clotting, complement, kinin). These include the following*:
1. Acute respiratory distress syndrome (ARDS)
2. Disseminated intravascular coagulation (DIC)
3. Acute renal failure (ARF)
4. Multiple organ dysfunction syndrome (MODS)

With progression of the condition, the patient may develop stupor, coma and death.

GIST BOX 16.2 | Shock

- Shock is a clinical syndrome of cardiovascular collapse characterised by an acute reduction of effective circulating blood volume (hypotension) and an inadequate perfusion of cells and tissues (hypoperfusion).
- There are 3 major forms of shock: hypovolaemic, cardiogenic and septic.
- All forms of shock involve 3 mechanisms: reduced effective circulating blood volume, impaired tissue oxygenation and release of proinflammatory mediators.
- Shock is divided into 3 stages: initial reversible stage (compensated shock), progressive decompensated shock and finally the stage of irreversible decompensated shock.
- Shock causes morphologic changes in different organ systems, notably in the brain (hypoxic encephalopathy), heart (haemorrhage and necrosis), lungs (ARDS), kidneys (tubular necrosis), adrenals (haemorrhage and necrosis), liver (focal necrosis), gut (haemorrhagic gastroenteropathy) and other organs.
- Clinically, shock is characterised by low blood pressure, low body temperature, feeble pulse, shallow respiration, pale face and cold clammy skin.

---

*Major complications of shock can be remembered from acronym ADAM: A = ARDS; D = DIC; A = ARF; M = MODS.

17 Obstructive Haemodynamic Derangements

As outlined in previous chapter, derangements of blood flow or haemodynamic disturbances can be broadly grouped under 2 headings:

I. *Disturbances in the volume of the circulating blood* These include: hyperaemia and congestion, haemorrhage and shock; these have been discussed in Chapter 16.

II. *Circulatory disturbances of obstructive nature* These are: thrombosis, embolism, ischaemia and infarction. These are discussed here.

THRMOBOSIS

DEFINITION AND EFFECTS

Thrombosis is the process of formation of solid mass in circulation from the constituents of flowing blood; the mass itself is called a *thrombus*. A term commonly used erroneously synonymous with thrombosis is blood clotting. While *thrombosis* is characterised by events that essentially involve activation of platelets, the process of *clotting* involves only conversion of soluble fibrinogen to insoluble polymerised fibrin. Besides, clotting is also used to denote coagulation of blood *in vitro* e.g. in a test tube. *Haematoma* is the extravascular accumulation of blood e.g. into the tissues. *Haemostatic plugs* are the blood clots formed in healthy individuals at the site of bleeding e.g. in injury to the blood vessel. In other words, haemostatic plug at the cut end of a blood vessel may be considered the simplest form of thrombosis. Haemostatic plugs are useful as they stop escape of blood and plasma, whereas thrombi developing in the unruptured cardiovascular system may be life-threatening by causing one of the following harmful effects:

1. *Ischaemic injury* Thrombi may decrease or stop the blood supply to part of an organ or tissue and cause ischaemia which may subsequently result in infarction.

2. *Thromboembolism* Thrombus or its part may get dislodged and be carried along in the blood stream as embolus to lodge in a distant vessel.

PATHOPHYSIOLOGY

Since the protective haemostatic plug formed as a result of normal haemostasis is an example of thrombosis, it is essential to describe *thrombogenesis* in relation to the normal haemostatic mechanism.

Human beings possess inbuilt system by which the blood remains in fluid state normally and guards against the hazards of thrombosis and haemorrhage. However, injury to the blood vessel initiates haemostatic repair mechanism or thrombogenesis.

Virchow described three primary events which predispose to thrombus formation *(Virchow's triad):* endothelial injury, altered blood flow, and hypercoagulability of blood. To this are added the activation processes that follow these primary events: activation of platelets and of clotting system (Fig. 17.1). These events are discussed below:

1. ENDOTHELIAL INJURY The integrity of blood vessel wall is important for maintaining normal blood flow. An intact endothelium has the following functions:

i) It *protects* the flowing blood from thrombogenic influence of subendothelium.

ii) It elaborates a few *anti-thrombotic* factors (thrombosis inhibitory factors) as follows:

a) Heparin-like substance which accelerates the action of antithrombin III and inactivates some other clotting factors.

b) Thrombomodulin which converts thrombin into activator of protein C, an anticoagulant.

c) Inhibitors of platelet aggregation such as ADPase, PGI_2 (or prostacyclin).

d) Tissue plasminogen activator which accelerates fibrinolytic activity.

iii) It releases a few *prothrombotic factors* which have procoagulant properties (thrombosis favouring factors) as under:

a) Thromboplastin or tissue factor released from endothelial cells.

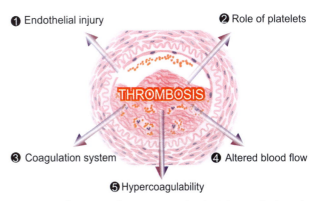

Figure 17.1 ▶ Major factors in pathophysiology of thrombus formation.

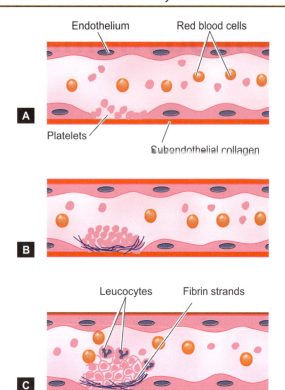

Figure 17.2 ▶ Role of endothelial injury and platelet activation in thrombosis. A, Endothelial injury exposes subendothelial matrix to circulating blood. B, This triggers three platelet steps involving platelet activation: adhesion, release and aggregation. Platelet release is associated with release of granules (alpha granules and dense bodies). C, Concurrent activation of coagulation cascade generates fibrin strands and thrombin, forming a tight meshwork called thrombus.

b) von Willebrand factor that causes adherence of platelets to the subendothelium.
c) Platelet activating factor which is activator and aggregator of platelets.
d) Inhibitor of plasminogen activator that suppresses fibrinolysis.

Vascular injury exposes the subendothelial extracellular matrix or ECM (e.g. collagen, elastin, fibronectin, laminin and glycosaminoglycans) which is thrombogenic and thus plays an important role in initiating haemostasis as well as thrombosis (Fig. 17.2). Injury to vessel wall also causes vasoconstriction of small blood vessels briefly so as to reduce the blood loss. Endothelial injury is of major significance in the formation of arterial thrombi and thrombi of the heart, especially of the left ventricle. A number of factors and conditions may cause vascular injury and predispose to the formation of thrombi. These are as under:
i) Endocardial injury in myocardial infarction, myocarditis, cardiac surgery, prosthetic valves.
ii) Ulcerated plaques in advanced atherosclerosis.
iii) Haemodynamic stress in hypertension.
iv) Arterial diseases.
v) Diabetes mellitus.
vi) Endogenous chemical agents such as hypercholesterolaemia, endotoxins.
vii) Exogenous chemical agents such as cigarette smoke.

2. ROLE OF PLATELETS Following endothelial cell injury, platelets come to play a central role in normal haemostasis as well as in thrombosis. The sequence of events is as under (Fig. 17.2):

i) Platelet adhesion Glycoprotein Ib (GpIb) receptor on the platelets recognises the site of endothelial injury and the circulating platelets adhere to exposed subendothelial ECM *(primary aggregation)*. von Willebrand's factor (vWF), synthesised by the endothelial cells binds to GpIb and forms a firm adhesion of platelets with ECM. Thus, deficiency of vWF (as happens in von Willebrand's disease) or absence of GpIb (as is seen in Bernard-Soulier disease) would result in defective platelet adhesion and cause abnormal bleeding.

ii) Platelet release reaction Activated platelets then undergo release reaction by which the platelet granules are released to the exterior. Two main types of platelet granules are released:

a) Dense bodies Their release liberates ADP (adenosine diphosphate), ionic calcium, 5-HT (serotonin), histamine and epinephrine. Release of contents of dense bodies are more important since ADP is further an activator of platelets, and calcium is required in the coagulation cascade.

b) Alpha granules Their release produces fibrinogen, fibronectin, platelet-derived growth factor (PDGF), platelet factor 4 (an antiheparin) and thrombospondin.

As a sequel to platelet activation and release reaction, the phospholipid complex-platelet factor 3 gets activated which plays important role in the intrinsic pathway of coagulation.

iii) Platelet aggregation Following release of ADP, a potent platelet aggregating agent, aggregation of additional platelets takes place *(secondary aggregation)*. This results in formation of temporary haemostatic plug. However, stable haemostatic plug is formed by the action of fibrin, thrombin and thromboxane A_2.

3. ROLE OF COAGULATION SYSTEM Coagulation mechanism is the conversion of the plasma fibrinogen into solid mass of fibrin. The coagulation system is involved in both haemostatic process and thrombus formation. Fig. 17.3 shows schematic representation of the cascade of intrinsic (blood) pathway, the extrinsic (tissue) pathway, and the common pathway leading to formation of fibrin polymers.

i) In the intrinsic pathway, contact with abnormal surface (e.g. ECM in the subendothelium) leads to activation of factor XII and the sequential interactions of factors XI, IX, VIII

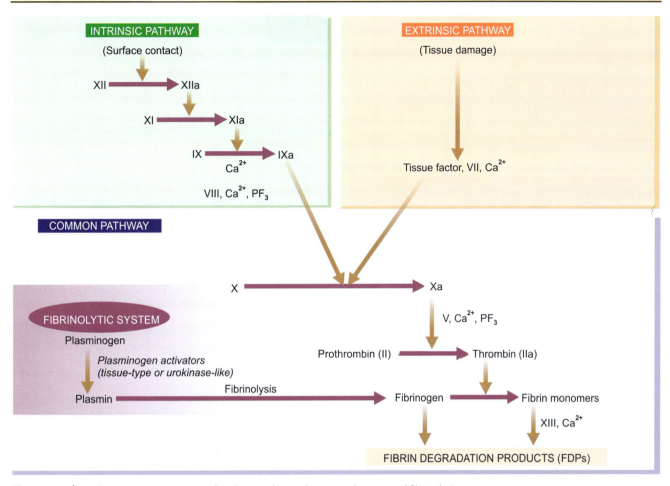

Figure 17.3 ▶ Schematic representation of pathways of coagulation mechanism and fibrinolytic system.

and finally factor X, along with calcium ions (factor IV) and platelet factor 3.

ii) In the extrinsic pathway, tissue damage results in release of tissue factor or thromboplastin. Tissue factor on interaction with factor VII activates factor X.

iii) The common pathway begins where both intrinsic and extrinsic pathways converge to activate factor X which forms a complex with factor Va and platelet factor 3, in the presence of calcium ions. This complex activates prothrombin (factor II) to thrombin (factor IIa) which, in turn, converts fibrinogen to fibrin. Initial monomeric fibrin is polymerised to form insoluble fibrin by activation of factor XIII.

Regulation of coagulation system Normally, the blood is kept in fluid state and the coagulation system is kept in check by controlling mechanisms. These are as under:

i) *Protease inhibitors* These act on coagulation factors so as to oppose the formation of thrombin e.g. antithrombin III, protein C, C1 inactivator, α1-antitrypsin, α2-macroglobulin.

ii) *Fibrinolytic system* Plasmin, a potent fibrinolytic enzyme, is formed by the action of plasminogen activator on plasminogen present in the normal plasma. Two types of plasminogen activators (PA) are identified:

a) *Tissue-type PA* derived from endothelial cells and leucocytes.

b) *Urokinase-like PA* present in the plasma.

Plasmin so formed acts on fibrin to destroy the clot and produces fibrin split products (FSP).

4. ALTERATION OF BLOOD FLOW *Turbulence* means unequal flow while *stasis* means slowing.

i) Normally, there is axial flow of blood in which the most rapidly-moving central stream consists of leucocytes and red cells. The platelets are present in the slow-moving laminar stream adjacent to the central stream while the peripheral stream consists of most slow-moving cell-free plasma close to endothelial layer (Fig. 17.4,A).

ii) Turbulence and stasis occur in thrombosis in which the normal axial flow of blood is disturbed. When blood slows

Section III: Fluid and Haemodynamic Disorders

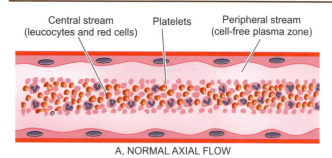

Figure 17.4 ▶ Alterations in flow of blood.

Table 17.1	Causes of thrombophilia (hypercoagulable states).

INHERITED (PRIMARY) FACTORS
 i) Deficiency of antithrombin III
 ii) Deficiency of protein C
 iii) Deficiency of protein S
 iv) Mutation in factor V Leiden
 v) Defects in fibrinolysis (dysfibrinogenaemia, plasminogen disorders)
 vi) Increased levels of coagulations factors (II and VIII)

ACQUIRED (SECONDARY) FACTORS
 a) *Risk factors:*
   i) Advancing age, ii) Prolonged bed-rest, iii) Prolonged immobilisation (e.g. in plaster cast, long distance travel), iv) Cigarette smoking, v) Obesity
 b) *Predisposing clinical conditions:*
   i) Heart diseases (e.g. myocardial infarction, CHF, rheumatic mitral stenosis, cardiomyopathy)
   ii) Vascular diseases (e.g. atherosclerosis, aneurysms of the aorta and other vessels, varicosities of leg veins)
   iii) Hypercoagulable conditions (e.g. polycythaemia, myeloproliferative disorders, dehydration, nephrotic syndrome, disseminated cancers)
   iv) Shock
   v) Tissue damage e.g. trauma, fractures, burns, major surgery on bones, abdomen or brain.
   vi) Late pregnancy and puerperium
   vii) Certain drugs (e.g. anaesthetic agents, oral contraceptives, hormonal replacement therapy).
 c) *Antiphospholipid antibody (APLA) syndrome:*
   i) Lupus anticoagulant antibody
   ii) Anti-cardiolipin antibody

down, the blood cells including platelets marginate to the periphery and form a kind of pavement close to endothelium (margination and pavementing) **(Fig. 17.4,B)**. While stasis allows a higher release of oxygen from the blood, turbulence may actually injure the endothelium resulting in deposition of platelets and fibrin. Formation of arterial and cardiac thrombi is facilitated by *turbulence* in the blood flow, while *stasis* initiates the venous thrombi even without evidence of endothelial injury.

5. HYPERCOAGULABLE STATES (THROMBOPHILIA)

Thrombophilia or hypercoagulable states are a group of conditions having increased risk or predisposition to develop venous thrombosis. These conditions may be hereditary (or primary) or acquired (or secondary) causes **(Table 17.1)**. However, in a given case of thrombosis, several factors are generally present simultaneously.

Hereditary (Primary) factors These include deficiency or mutation of some factors as under:

i) *Deficiency of antithrombin III* It is inherited as autosomal dominant disorder having less than 50% antithrombin III. The condition is associated with recurrent episodes of venous thrombosis.

ii) *Deficiency of protein C and S* Both these are autosomal dominant disorders having either reduced amount of protein C or S, or both, or their functional defect. Clinically, both the conditions are associated with lifelong risk of thrombosis of deep leg veins.

iii) *Mutation in factor V Leiden* This is also an autosomal dominant disorder in which the mutation lies in replacement of arginine by glycine at position 506. It is the most common cause of thrombophilia.

iv) *Defects in fibrinolysis* These include a few rare inherited disorders such as dysfibrinogenaemia and plasminomgen disorders.

v) *Increased levels of coagulations factors (II and VIII).* Elevated level of prothrombin and factor VIII due to genetic mutation may predispose to thrombosis.

Secondary (acquired) factors As listed in **Table 17.1**, thrombosis is favoured by certain risk factors, some predisposing clinical conditions and antiphospholipid antibody (APLA) syndrome. There are 2 types of APLA: lupus anticoagulant antibody and anti-cardiolipin antibody. Presence of either of the two APLA predisposes an individual to recurrent thrombosis: venous in the former and arterial in the latter type. Other features include spontaneous abortions, transient ischaemic attacks, thrombocytopenia, elevation of activated partial thromboplastin time and multi-organ involvement. Patients of SLE may often coexpress lupus anticoagulant.

ORIGIN OF THROMBI AT DIFFERENT SITES

Thrombi may arise from the heart, arteries, veins or in microcirculation by different mechanisms.

CARDIAC THROMBI Thrombi may form in any of the chambers of the heart and on the valve cusps. They are more common in the atrial appendages, especially of the right atrium, and on mitral and aortic valves such as vegetations seen in infective endocarditis and non-bacterial thrombotic endocarditis (page 507). Cardiac thrombi are mural (non-occlusive) as are the mural thrombi encountered in large vessels such as the aorta in atherosclerosis and in aneurysmal dilatations. Rarely, large round thrombus may form and obstruct the mitral valve and is called *ball-valve thrombus*. *Agonal thrombi* are formed shortly before death and may occur in either or both the ventricles. They are composed mainly of fibrin.

ARTERIAL THROMBI The examples of major forms of thrombi formed in the arteries are as under:
i) Aorta: aneurysms, arteritis.
ii) Coronary arteries: atherosclerosis.
iii) Mesenteric artery: atherosclerosis, arteritis.
iv) Arteries of limbs: atherosclerosis, diabetes mellitus, Buerger's disease, Raynaud's disease.
v) Renal artery: atherosclerosis, arteritis.
vi) Cerebral artery: atherosclerosis, vasculitis.

VENOUS THROMBI A few common examples of these are as under:
i) Veins of lower limbs: deep veins of legs, varicose veins.
ii) Popliteal, femoral and iliac veins: postoperative stage, postpartum.
iii) Pulmonary veins: CHF, pulmonary hypertension.
iv) Hepatic and portal vein: portal hypertension.
v) Superior vena cava: infections in head and neck.
vi) Inferior vena cava: extension of thrombus from hepatic vein.
vii) Mesenteric veins: volvulus, intestinal obstruction.
viii) Renal vein: renal amyloidosis.

Distinguishing features between thrombi formed in rapidly-flowing arterial circulation and slow-moving venous blood are given in **Table 17.2**.

CAPILLARY THROMBI Minute thrombi composed mainly of packed red cells are formed in the capillaries in acute inflammatory lesions, vasculitis and in disseminated intravascular coagulation (DIC).

MORPHOLOGIC FEATURES

The general morphologic features of thrombi formed in various locations are as under:

Grossly, thrombi may be of various shapes, sizes and composition depending upon the site of origin. Arterial thrombi tend to be white and mural while the venous thrombi are red and occlusive. Mixed or laminated thrombi are also common and consist of alternate white and red layers called lines of Zahn. Red thrombi are soft, red and gelatinous whereas white thrombi are firm and pale.

Microscopically, the composition of thrombus is determined by the rate of flow of blood i.e. whether it is formed in the rapid arterial and cardiac circulation, or in the slow moving flow in veins. The lines of Zahn are formed by alternate layers of light-staining aggregated platelets admixed with fibrin meshwork and dark-staining layer of red cells. Red (venous) thrombi have more abundant red cells, leucocytes and platelets entrapped in fibrin meshwork. Thus, red thrombi closely resemble blood clots *in vitro* **(Fig. 17.5)**.

Red thrombi (antemortem) have to be distinguished from postmortem clots **(Table 17.3)**.

FATE OF THROMBUS

The outcome of thrombi can be as under **(Fig. 17.6)**:

	FEATURE	ARTERIAL THROMBI	VENOUS THROMBI
1.	Blood flow	Formed in rapidly-flowing blood of arteries and heart	Formed in slow-moving blood in veins
2.	Sites	Common in aorta, coronary, cerebral, iliac, femoral, renal and mesenteric arteries	Common in superficial varicose veins, deep leg veins, popliteal, femoral and iliac veins
3.	Thrombo-genesis	Formed following endothelial cell injury e.g. in atherosclerosis	Formed following venous stasis e.g. in abdominal operations, child-birth
4.	Development	Usually mural, not occluding the lumen completely, may propagate	Usually occlusive, take the cast of the vessel in which formed, may propagate in both directions
5.	Macroscopy	Grey-white, friable with lines of Zahn on surface	Red-blue with fibrin strands and lines of Zahn
6.	Microscopy	Distinct lines of Zahn composed of platelets, fibrin with entangled red and white blood cells	Lines of Zahn with more abundant red cells
7.	Effects	Ischaemia leading to infarcts e.g. in the heart, brain etc	Thromboembolism, oedema, skin ulcers, poor wound healing

Table 17.2 Distinguishing features of arterial and venous thrombi.

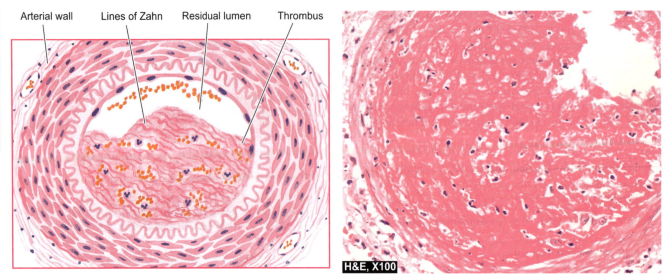

Figure 17.5 ▶ Thrombus in an artery. The thrombus is adherent to the arterial wall and is seen occluding most of the lumen. It shows lines of Zahn composed of granular-looking platelets and fibrin meshwork with entangled red cells and leucocytes.

1. RESOLUTION Thrombus activates the fibrinolytic system with consequent release of plasmin which may dissolve the thrombus completely resulting in resolution. Usually, lysis is complete in small venous thrombi while large thrombi may not be dissolved. Fibrinolytic activity can be accentuated by administration of thrombolytic substances (e.g. urokinase, streptokinase), especially in the early stage when fibrin is in monomeric form e.g. thromobytic therapy in early stage acute myocardial infarction.

2. ORGANISATION If the thrombus is not removed, it starts getting organised. Phagocytic cells (neutrophils and macrophages) appear and begin to phagocytose fibrin and cell debris. The proteolytic enzymes liberated by leucocytes and endothelial cells start digesting coagulum. Capillaries grow into the thrombus from the site of its attachment and fibroblasts start invading the thrombus. Thus, fibrovascular granulation tissue is formed which subsequently becomes dense and less vascular and is covered over by endothelial cells. The thrombus in this way is excluded from the vascular lumen and becomes part of vessel wall. The new vascular channels in it may be able to re-establish the blood flow, called recanalisation. The fibrosed thrombus may undergo hyalinisation and calcification e.g. phleboliths in the pelvic veins.

3. PROPAGATION The thrombus may enlarge in size due to more and more deposition from the constituents of flowing blood. In this way, it may ultimately cause obstruction of some important vessel.

4. THROMBOEMBOLISM The thrombi in early stage and infected thrombi are quite friable and may get detached from the vessel wall. These are released in part or completely in blood-stream as emboli which produce ill-effects at the site of their lodgement.

CLINICAL EFFECTS

Besides differences in mechanism of thrombosis at different sites, clinical effects depend upon not only the site but also on rapidity of formation and nature of thrombi.

1. Cardiac thrombi Large thrombi in the heart may cause sudden death by mechanical obstruction of blood flow or through thromboembolism to vital organs.

2. Arterial thrombi These cause ischaemic necrosis of the deprived part (infarct) which may lead to gangrene. Sudden death may occur following thrombosis of coronary artery.

3. Venous thrombi (Phlebothrombosis) These may cause following effects:
i) Thromboembolism

	FEATURE	ANTEMORTEM THROMBI	POSTMORTEM CLOTS
1.	Gross	Dry, granular, firm and friable	Gelatinous, soft and rubbery
2.	Relation to vessel wall	Adherent to the vessel wall	Weakly attached to the vessel wall
3.	Shape	May or may not fit their vascular contours	Take the shape of vessel or its bifurcation
4.	Microscopy	The surface contains apparent lines of Zahn	The surface is 'chicken fat' yellow covering the underlying red 'currant jelly'

Table 17.3 Distinguishing features of antemortem thrombi and postmortem clots.

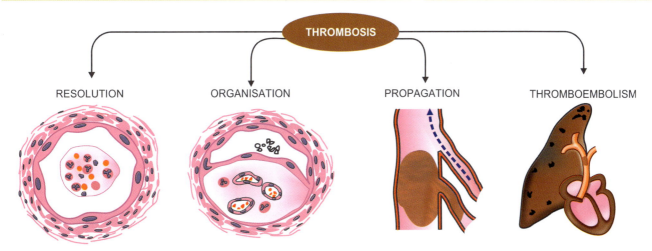

Figure 17.6 ▶ Fate of thrombus.

ii) Oedema of area drained
iii) Poor wound healing
iv) Skin ulcer
v) Painful thrombosed veins (thrombophlebitis)
vi) Painful white leg (phlegmasia alba dolens) due to ileofemoral venous thrombosis in postpartum cases
vii) Thrombophlebitis migrans in cancer.

4. **Capillary thrombi** Microthrombi in microcirculation may give rise to disseminated intravascular coagulation (DIC).

> **GIST BOX 17.1** | **Thrombosis**
>
> ❖ Thrombosis is the process of formation of solid mass in circulation from the constituents of flowing blood; the mass itself is called a thrombus.
> ❖ Thrombogenesis involves interplay of 5 events: endothelial injury, platelets and their release reaction, coagulation system, alterations in the flow of blood and role of certain predisposing conditions and factors causing hypercoagulable states (or thrombophilia).
> ❖ Thrombi may originate in the chambers of the heart, lumina of arteries, veins and microcirculation.
> ❖ The effects of thrombi depend upon their anatomic location, rapidity of formation and nature of thrombi. In general, thrombi produce life-threatening harmful effects by ischaemia and by thromboembolism.
> ❖ Grossly, thrombi are of various shapes, size, consistency and colour. Microscopically, all types of thrombi show lines of Zahn formed by alternate layers of light-staining aggregated platelets and dark-staining red cells.
> ❖ The possible fates of thrombi are resolution, organisation, propagation and thromboembolism.

EMBOLISM

DEFINITION AND TYPES

Embolism is the process of partial or complete obstruction of some part of the cardiovascular system by any mass carried in the circulation; the transported intravascular mass detached from its site of origin is called an *embolus*. Most usual forms of emboli (90%) are thromboemboli i.e. originating from thrombi or their parts detached from the vessel wall.

Emboli may be of various types:

A. Depending upon the matter in the emboli:
i) *Solid* e.g. detached thrombi (thromboemboli), atheromatous material, tumour cell clumps, tissue fragments, parasites, bacterial clumps, foreign bodies.
ii) *Liquid* e.g. fat globules, amniotic fluid, bone marrow.
iii) *Gaseous* e.g. air, other gases.

B. Depending upon whether infected or not:
i) *Bland*, when sterile.
ii) *Septic*, when infected.

C. Depending upon the source of the emboli:
i) *Cardiac emboli* from left side of the heart e.g. emboli originating in the atrium and atrial appendages, infarct in the left ventricle, vegetations of endocarditis.
ii) *Arterial emboli* e.g. in systemic arteries in the brain, spleen, kidney, intestine.
iii) *Venous emboli* e.g. in pulmonary arteries.
iv) *Lymphatic emboli* can also sometimes occur.

D. Depending upon the flow of blood, two special types of emboli are mentioned:
i) *Paradoxical embolus* An embolus which is carried from the venous side of circulation to the arterial side or vice

Section III: Fluid and Haemodynamic Disorders

	Table 17.4	Important types of embolism.
	TYPE	COMMON ORIGIN
1.	Pulmonary embolism	Veins of lower legs
2.	Systemic embolism	Left ventricle (arterial)
3.	Fat embolism	Trauma to bones/soft tissues
4.	Air embolism	Venous: head and neck operations, obstetrical trauma Arterial: cardiothoracic surgery, angiography
5.	Decompression sickness	Descent: divers Ascent: unpressurised flight
6.	Amniotic fluid embolism	Components of amniotic fluid
7.	Atheroembolism	Atheromatous plaques
8.	Tumour embolism	Tumour fragments

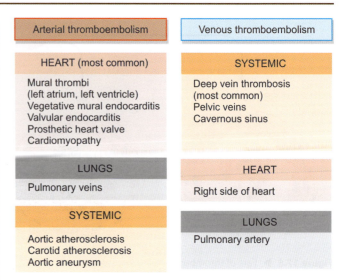

Figure 17.7 ▶ Sources of arterial and venous emboli.

versa, is called *paradoxical or crossed embolus* e.g. through arteriovenous communication such as in patent foramen ovale, septal defect of the heart, and arteriovenous shunts in the lungs.

ii) Retrograde embolus An embolus which travels against the flow of blood is called retrograde embolus. For example, metastatic deposits in the spine from carcinoma prostate in which case the spread occurs by retrograde embolism through intraspinal veins (which normally do not carry the blood from the prostate) which carry tumour emboli from large thoracic and abdominal veins because of increased pressure in body cavities such as during coughing or straining.

Some of the important types of embolism are listed in **Table 17.4** and are described below:

THROMBOEMBOLISM

A detached thrombus or part of a thrombus constitutes the most common type of embolism. These may arise in the arterial or venous circulation **(Fig. 17.7)**:

Arterial (systemic) thromboembolism Arterial emboli may be derived from the following sources:
A. *Causes within the heart* (80-85%): These are mural thrombi in the left atrium or left ventricle, vegetations on the mitral or aortic valves, prosthetic heart valves and cardiomyopathy.
B. *Causes within the arteries:* These include emboli developing in relation to atherosclerotic plaques, aortic aneurysms, pulmonary veins and paradoxical arterial emboli from the systemic venous circulation.

The *effects* of arterial emboli depend upon their size, site of lodgement, and adequacy of collateral circulation. If the vascular occlusion occurs, the following ill-effects may result:
i) *Infarction* of the organ or its affected part e.g. ischaemic necrosis in the lower limbs (70-75%), spleen, kidneys, brain, intestine.

ii) *Gangrene* following infarction in the lower limbs if the collateral circulation is inadequate.
iii) *Arteritis and mycotic aneurysm* formation from bacterial endocarditis.
iv) *Myocardial infarction* may occur following coronary embolism.
v) *Sudden death* may result from coronary embolism or embolism in the middle cerebral artery.

Venous thromboembolism Venous emboli may arise from the following sources:
i) Deep vein thrombosis (DVT) of the lower legs, the most common cause of venous thrombi.
ii) Thrombi in the pelvic veins.
iii) Thrombi in the veins of the upper limbs.
iv) Thrombosis in cavernous sinus of the brain.
v) Thrombi in the right side of heart.

The most significant *effect* of venous embolism is obstruction of pulmonary arterial circulation leading to pulmonary embolism described below.

Pulmonary Thromboembolism

DEFINITION Pulmonary embolism is the most common and fatal form of venous thromboembolism in which there is occlusion of pulmonary arterial tree by thromboemboli. In contrast, pulmonary thrombosis is uncommon and may occur in pulmonary atherosclerosis and pulmonary hypertension. Differentiation of pulmonary thrombosis from pulmonary thromboembolism is tabulated in **Table 17.5**.

ETIOLOGY Pulmonary emboli are more common in hospitalised or bed-ridden patients, though they can occur in ambulatory patients as well. The causes are as follows:
i) Thrombi originating from large veins of lower legs (such as popliteal, femoral and iliac) are the cause in 95% of pulmonary emboli.

Table 17.5	Contrasting features of pulmonary thrombosis and pulmonary thromboembolism.	
FEATURE	PULMONARY THROMBOSIS	PULMONARY THROMBOEMBOLISM
1. Pathogenesis	Locally formed	Travelled from distance
2. Location	In small arteries and branches	In major arteries and branches
3. Attachment to vessel wall	Firmly adherent	Loosely attached or lying free
4. Gross appearance	Head pale, tail red	No distinction in head and tail; smooth-surfaced dry dull surface
5. Microscopy	Platelets and fibrin in layers Lines of Zahn seen	Mixed with blood clot Lines of Zahn rare

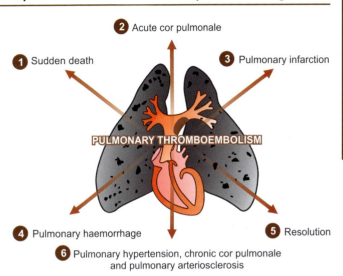

Figure 17.8 ▶ Major consequences of pulmonary embolism.

ii) Less common sources include thrombi in varicosities of superficial veins of the legs, and pelvic veins such as periprostatic, periovarian, uterine and broad ligament veins.

PATHOGENESIS Risk factors for pulmonary thromboembolism are stasis of venous blood and hypercoagulable states. Detachment of thrombi from any of the above-mentioned sites produces a thrombo-embolus that flows through venous drainage into the larger veins draining into right side of the heart.

◆ If the thrombus is large, it is impacted at the bifurcation of the main pulmonary artery *(saddle embolus)*, or may be found in the right ventricle or its outflow tract.

◆ More commonly, there are *multiple emboli*, or a large embolus may be fragmented into many smaller emboli which are then impacted in a number of vessels, particularly affecting the lower lobes of lungs.

◆ Rarely, *paradoxical embolism* may occur by passage of an embolus from right heart into the left heart through atrial or ventricular septal defect. In this way, pulmonary emboli may reach systemic circulation.

CONSEQUENCES OF PULMONARY EMBOLISM Pulmonary embolism occurs more commonly as a complication in patients of acute or chronic debilitating diseases who are immobilised for a long duration. Women in their reproductive period are at higher risk such as in late pregnancy, following delivery and with use of contraceptive pills. The effects of pulmonary embolism depend mainly on the size of the occluded vessel, the number of emboli, and on the cardiovascular status of the patient. Natural history of pulmonary embolism may have following consequences (Fig. 17.8):

i) Sudden death Massive pulmonary embolism results in instantaneous death, without occurrence of chest pain or dyspnoea. However, if the death is somewhat delayed, the clinical features resemble myocardial infarction i.e. severe chest pain, dyspnoea and shock.

ii) Acute cor pulmonale Numerous small emboli may obstruct most of the pulmonary circulation resulting in acute right heart failure. Another mechanism is by release of vasoconstrictor substances from platelets or by reflex vasoconstriction of pulmonary vessels.

iii) Pulmonary infarction Obstruction of relatively small-sized pulmonary arterial branches may result in pulmonary infarction (page 262). The clinical features include chest pain due to fibrinous pleuritis, haemoptysis and dyspnoea due to reduced functioning pulmonary parenchyma.

iv) Pulmonary haemorrhage Obstruction of terminal branches (endarteries) leads to central pulmonary haemorrhage. The clinical features are haemoptysis, dyspnoea, and less commonly, chest pain due to central location of pulmonary haemorrhage. Sometimes, there may be concomitant pulmonary infarction.

v) Resolution Vast majority of small pulmonary emboli (60-80%) are resolved by fibrinolytic activity. These patients are clinically silent owing to bronchial circulation so that lung parenchyma is adequately perfused.

vi) Pulmonary hypertension, chronic cor pulmonale and pulmonary arteriosclerosis These are the sequelae of multiple small thromboemboli undergoing organisation rather than resolution.

SYSTEMIC EMBOLISM

This is the type of arterial embolism that originates commonly from thrombi in the diseased heart, especially in the left ventricle. These heart diseases include myocardial infarction, cardiomyopathy, RHD, congenital heart disease, infective endocarditis, and prosthetic cardiac valves. The emboli are arterial and invariably cause infarction at the sites of lodgement. These sites, in descending order of frequency, are:

lower extremity, brain, and internal visceral organs (spleen, kidneys, intestines). *Thus, the effects and sites of arterial emboli are in striking contrast to venous emboli* which are often lodged in the lungs.

FAT EMBOLISM

Obstruction of arterioles and capillaries by fat globules constitutes fat embolism. If the obstruction in the circulation is by fragments of adipose tissue, it is called fat-tissue embolism.

ETIOLOGY Causes of fat embolism may be traumatic and non-traumatic:

Traumatic causes:

i) Trauma to bones is the most common cause of fat embolism e.g. in fractures of long bones leading to passage of fatty marrow in circulation, concussions of bones, after orthopaedic surgical procedures etc.

ii) Trauma to soft tissue e.g. laceration of adipose tissue and in puerperium due to injury to pelvic fatty tissue.

Non-traumatic causes:

i) Extensive burns

ii) Diabetes mellitus

iii) Fatty liver

iv) Pancreatitis

v) Sickle cell anaemia

vi) Decompression sickness

vii) Inflammation of bones and soft tissues

viii) Extrinsic fat or oils introduced into the body

ix) Hyperlipidaemia

x) Cardiopulmonary bypass surgery

PATHOGENESIS Pathogenesis of fat embolism is explained by following mechanisms which may be acting singly or in combination:

i) Mechanical theory Mobilisation of fluid fat may occur following trauma to the bone or soft tissues. Fat globules released from the injured area may enter venous circulation and finally most of the fat is arrested in the small vessels in the lungs. Some of the fat globules may further pass through lungs and enter into the systemic circulation to lodge in other organs.

ii) Emulsion instability theory This theory explains the pathogenesis of fat embolism in non-traumatic cases. According to this theory, fat emboli are formed by aggregation of plasma lipids (chylomicrons and fatty acids) due to disturbance in natural emulsification of fat.

iii) Intravascular coagulation theory In stress, release of some factor activates disseminated intravascular coagulation (DIC) and aggregation of fat emboli.

iv) Toxic injury theory According to this theory, the small blood vessels of lungs are chemically injured by high plasma levels of free fatty acid, resulting in increased vascular permeability and consequent pulmonary oedema.

CONSEQUENCES OF FAT EMBOLISM Effects of fat embolism depend upon the size and quantity of fat globules, and whether or not the emboli pass through the lungs into the systemic circulation.

i) Pulmonary fat embolism In patients dying after fractures of bones, presence of numerous fat emboli in the capillaries of the lung is a frequent autopsy finding because the small fat globules are not likely to appreciably obstruct the vast pulmonary vascular bed. However, widespread obstruction of pulmonary circulation due to extensive pulmonary embolism can occur and result in sudden death.

Microscopically, the lungs show hyperaemia, oedema, petechial haemorrhages and changes of adult respiratory distress syndrome (ARDS). Pulmonary infarction is usually not a feature of fat embolism because of the small size of globules. In routine stains, the fat globules in the pulmonary arteries, capillaries and alveolar spaces appear as vacuoles. Frozen section is essential for confirmation of globules by fat stains such as Sudan dyes (Sudan black, Sudan III and IV), oil red O and osmic acid.

ii) Systemic fat embolism Some of the fat globules may pass through the pulmonary circulation such as via patent foramen ovale, arteriovenous shunts in the lungs and vertebral venous plexuses, and get lodged in the capillaries of organs like the brain, kidney, skin etc.

◆ **Brain** The pathologic findings in the brain are petechial haemorrhages on the leptomeninges and minute haemorrhages in the parenchyma.

Microscopically, microinfarcts of brain, oedema and haemorrhages are seen. The CNS manifestations include delirium, convulsions, stupor, coma and sudden death.

◆ **Kidney** Renal fat embolism present in the glomerular capillaries, may cause decreased glomerular filtration. Other effects include tubular damage and renal insufficiency.

◆ **Other organs** Besides the brain and kidneys, other findings in systemic fat embolism are petechiae in the skin, conjunctivae, serosal surfaces, fat globules in the urine and sputum.

GAS EMBOLISM

Air, nitrogen and other gases can produce bubbles within the circulation and obstruct the blood vessels causing damage to tissue. Two main forms of gas embolism—air embolism and decompression sickness are described below.

Air Embolism

Air embolism occurs when air is introduced into venous or arterial circulation.

VENOUS AIR EMBOLISM Air may be sucked into systemic veins under the following circumstances:

i) Operations on the head and neck, and trauma The accidental opening of a major vein of the neck like jugular, or neck wounds involving the major neck veins, may allow air to be drawn into venous circulation.

ii) Obstetrical operations and trauma During childbirth by normal vaginal delivery, caesarean section, abortions and other procedures, fatal air embolism may result from the entrance of air into the opened-up uterine venous sinuses and endometrial veins.

iii) Intravenous infusion of blood and fluid Air embolism may occur during intravenous blood or fluid infusions if only positive pressure is employed.

iv) Angiography During venous angiographic procedures, air may be entrapped into a large vein causing air embolism.

The *effects* of venous air embolism depend upon the following factors:

i) Amount of air introduced into the circulation. The volume of air necessary to cause death is variable but usually 100-150 ml of air entry is considered fatal.

ii) Rapidity of entry of a smaller volume of air is important determinant of a fatal outcome.

iii) Position of the patient during or soon after entry of air is another factor. The air bubbles may ascend into the superior vena cava if the position of head is higher than the trunk (e.g. in upright position) and reach the brain.

iv) General condition of the patient e.g. in severely ill patients, as little as 40 ml of air may have serious results.

The mechanism of death is by entrapment of air emboli in the pulmonary arterial trunk in the right heart. If bubbles of air in the form of froth pass further out into pulmonary arterioles, they cause widespread vascular occlusions. If death from pulmonary air embolism is suspected, the heart and pulmonary artery should be opened *in situ* under water so that escaping froth or foam formed by mixture of air and blood can be detected.

ARTERIAL AIR EMBOLISM Entry of air into pulmonary vein or its tributaries may occur in the following conditions:

i) Cardiothoracic surgery and trauma Arterial air embolism may occur following thoracic operations, thoracocentesis, rupture of the lung, penetrating wounds of the lung, artificial pneumothorax etc.

ii) Paradoxical air embolism This may occur due to passage of venous air emboli to the arterial side of circulation through a patent foramen ovale or via pulmonary arteriovenous shunts.

iii) Arteriography During arteriographic procedures, air embolism may occur.

The *effects* of arterial air embolism are in the form of certain characteristic features:

i) Marble skin due to blockage of cutaneous vessels.
ii) Air bubbles in the retinal vessels seen ophthalmoscopically.
iii) Pallor of the tongue due to occlusion of a branch of lingual artery.
iv) Coronary or cerebral arterial air embolism may cause sudden death by much smaller amounts of air than in the venous air embolism.

Decompression Sickness

This is a specialised form of gas embolism known by various names such as caissons disease, divers' palsy or aeroembolism.

PATHOGENESIS Decompression sickness is produced when the individual decompresses suddenly, either from high atmospheric pressure to normal level, or from normal pressure to low atmospheric pressure.

❖ In divers, workers in caissons (diving-bells), offshore drilling and tunnels, who *descend* to high atmospheric pressure, increased amount of atmospheric gases (mainly nitrogen; others are O_2, CO_2) are dissolved in blood and tissue fluids. When such an individual ascends too rapidly i.e. comes to normal level suddenly from high atmospheric pressure, the gases come out of the solution as minute bubbles, particularly in fatty tissues which have affinity for nitrogen. These bubbles may coalesce together to form large emboli.

❖ In aeroembolism, seen in those who *ascend* to high altitudes or air flight in unpressurised cabins, the individuals are exposed to sudden decompression from low atmospheric pressure to normal levels. This results in similar effects as in divers and workers in caissons.

EFFECTS The effects of decompression sickness depend upon the following:
i) Depth or altitude reached
ii) Duration of exposure to altered pressure
iii) Rate of ascent or descent
iv) General condition of the individual

Pathologic changes are more pronounced in sudden decompression from high pressure to normal levels than in those who decompress from low pressure to normal levels. The changes are more serious in obese persons as nitrogen gas is more soluble in fat than in body fluids.

Clinical effects of decompression sickness are of 2 types— acute and chronic.

❖ **Acute form** occurs due to acute obstruction of small blood vessels in the vicinity of joints and skeletal muscles. The condition is clinically characterised by the following:

i) 'The bends', as the patient doubles up in bed due to acute pain in joints, ligaments and tendons.

ii) *'The chokes'* occur due to accumulation of bubbles in the lungs, resulting in acute respiratory distress.
iii) *Cerebral effects* may manifest in the form of vertigo, coma, and sometimes death.

◆ **Chronic form** is due to foci of ischaemic necrosis throughout body, especially the skeletal system. Ischaemic necrosis may be due to embolism *per se,* but other factors such as platelet activation, intravascular coagulation and hypoxia might contribute. The features of chronic form are as under:
i) *Avascular necrosis of bones* e.g. head of femur, tibia, humerus.
ii) *Neurological symptoms* may occur due to ischaemic necrosis in the central nervous system. These include paraesthesia and paraplegia.
iii) *Lung involvement* in the form of haemorrhage, oedema, emphysema and atelactasis may be seen. These result in dyspnoea, nonproductive cough and chest pain.
iv) *Skin manifestations* include itching, patchy erythema, cyanosis and oedema.
v) *Other organs* like parenchymal cells of the liver and pancreas may show lipid vacuoles.

AMNIOTIC FLUID EMBOLISM

This is the most serious, unpredictable and unpreventable cause of maternal mortality. During labour and in the immediate postpartum period, the contents of amniotic fluid may enter the uterine veins and reach right side of the heart resulting in fatal complications. The amniotic fluid components which may be found in uterine veins, pulmonary artery and vessels of other organs are: epithelial squames, vernixcaseosa, lanugo hair, bile from meconium, and mucus. The mechanism by which these amniotic fluid contents enter the maternal circulation is not clear. Possibly, they gain entry either through tears in the myometrium and endocervix, or the amniotic fluid is forced into uterine sinusoids by vigorous uterine contractions.

> ***MORPHOLOGIC FEATURES*** Notable changes are seen in the lungs such as haemorrhages, congestion, oedema and changes of ARDS, and dilatation of right side of the heart. These changes are associated with identifiable amniotic fluid contents within the pulmonary microcirculation.

The *clinical syndrome* of amniotic fluid embolism is characterised by the following features:
i) Sudden respiratory distress and dyspnoea
ii) Deep cyanosis
iii) Cardiovascular shock
iv) Convulsions
v) Coma
vi) Unexpected death

The *cause of death* may not be obvious but can occur as a result of the following mechanisms:
i) Mechanical blockage of the pulmonary circulation in extensive embolism.
ii) Anaphylactoid reaction to amniotic fluid components.
iii) Disseminated intravascular coagulation (DIC) due to liberation of thromboplastin by amniotic fluid.
iv) Haemorrhagic manifestations due to thrombocytopenia and afibrinogenaemia.

ATHEROEMBOLISM

Atheromatous plaques, especially from aorta, may get eroded to form atherosclerotic emboli which are then lodged in medium-sized and small arteries. These emboli consist of cholesterol crystals, hyaline debris and calcified material, and may evoke foreign body reaction at the site of lodgement.

> ***MORPHOLOGIC FEATURES*** Pathologic changes and their effects in atheroembolism are as under:
> i) Ischaemia, atrophy and necrosis of tissue distal to the occluded vessel.
> ii) Infarcts in the organs affected such as the kidneys, spleen, brain and heart.
> iii) Gangrene in the lower limbs.
> iv) Hypertension, if widespread renal vascular lesions are present.

TUMOUR EMBOLISM

Malignant tumour cells invade the local blood vessels and may form tumour emboli to be lodged elsewhere, producing metastatic tumour deposits. Notable examples are clear cell carcinoma of kidney, carcinoma of the lung, malignant melanoma etc (page 275).

MISCELLANEOUS EMBOLI

Various other endogenous and exogenous substances may act as emboli. These may include the following:
i) Fragments of tissue
ii) Placental fragments
iii) Red cell aggregates (sludging)
iv) Bacteria
v) Parasites
vi) Barium emboli following enema
vii) Foreign bodies e.g. needles, talc, sutures, bullets, catheters etc.

 GIST BOX 17.2 | **Embolism**

❖ Embolism is the process of partial or complete obstruction of some part of the cardiovascular system by any mass carried in the circulation.

- ❖ Most common forms of emboli (90%) are thromboemboli originating from thrombi or their detached parts within the heart, arteries or veins.
- ❖ Pulmonary thromboembolism is common and fatal form of venous thromboembolism, most often originating from deep vein thrombosis of the lower legs.
- ❖ Most common form of arterial embolism arises in the thrombi from the left ventricle due to heart diseases.
- ❖ Fat embolism may be traumatic (most often from surgical or accidental trauma to the bones) or from several non-traumatic causes.
- ❖ Gas embolism may be air embolism (arterial or venous) or decompression sickness (in divers or in high altitude).
- ❖ Amniotic fluid embolism is the most serious, unpredictable and unpreventable cause of maternal mortality occurring during labour and in the immediate postpartum period.
- ❖ Other forms of embolism include atheroembolism, tumour embolism etc.

ISCHAEMIA

DEFINITION

Ischaemia is defined as deficient blood supply to part of a tissue relative to its metabolic needs. The cessation of blood supply may be *complete* (complete ischaemia) or *partial* (partial ischaemia). The adverse effects of ischaemia may result from 3 ways:

1. Hypoxia due to deprivation of oxygen to tissues relative to its needs; this is the most important and common cause. It may be of 4 types:

i) *Hypoxic hypoxia*: due to low oxygen in arterial blood.
ii) *Anaemic hypoxia*: due to low level of haemoglobin in blood.
iii) *Stagnant hypoxia*: due to inadequate blood supply.
iv) *Histotoxic hypoxia*: low oxygen uptake due to cellular toxicity.

2. Malnourishment of cells due to inadequate supply of nutrients to the tissue (i.e. glucose, amino acids); this is less important.

3. Inadequate clearance of metabolites which results in accumulation of metabolic waste-products in the affected tissue; this is relevant in some conditions such as muscleache after ischaemia from heavy exercise.

ETIOLOGY

A number of causes may produce ischaemia. These causes are discussed below with regard to different levels of blood vessels:

1. Causes in the heart Inadequate cardiac output resulting from heart block, ventricular arrest and fibrillation from various causes may cause variable degree of hypoxic injury to the brain as under:

i) If the arrest continues for 15 seconds, consciousness is lost.

ii) If the condition lasts for more than 4 minutes, irreversible ischaemic damage to the brain occurs.

iii) If it is prolonged for more than 8 minutes, death is inevitable.

2. Causes in the arteries The commonest and most important causes of ischaemia are due to obstruction in arterial blood supply as under:

i) *Luminal occlusion of artery (intraluminal)*:
   a) Thrombosis
   b) Embolism
ii) *Causes in the arterial walls (intramural)*:
   a) Vasospasm (e.g. in Raynaud's disease)
   b) Hypothermia, ergotism
   c) Arteriosclerosis
   d) Polyarteritis nodosa
   e) Thromboangiitis obliterans (Buerger's disease)
   f) Severed vessel wall
iii) *Outside pressure on an artery (extramural)*:
   a) Ligature
   b) Tourniquet
   c) Tight plaster, bandages
   d) Torsion.

3. Causes in the veins Blockage of venous drainage may lead to engorgement and obstruction to arterial blood supply resulting in ischaemia. The examples include the following:

i) *Luminal occlusion of vein (intraluminal)*:
   a) Thrombosis of mesenteric veins
   b) Cavernous sinus thrombosis
ii) *Causes in the vessel wall of vein (intramural)*:
   a) Varicose veins of the legs
iii) *Outside pressure on vein (extramural)*:
   a) Strangulated hernia
   b) Intussusception
   c) Volvulus

4. Causes in the microcirculation Ischaemia may result from occlusion of arterioles, capillaries and venules. The causes are as under:

i) *Luminal occlusion in microvasculature (intraluminal)*:
a) By red cells e.g. in sickle cell anaemia, red cells parasitised by malaria, acquired haemolytic anaemia, sludging of the blood.
b) By white cells e.g. in chronic myeloid leukaemia
c) By fibrin e.g. defibrination syndrome
d) By precipitated cryoglobulins
e) By fat embolism
f) In decompression sickness.

ii) *Causes in the microvasculature wall (intramural)*:
a) Vasculitis e.g. in polyarteritis nodosa, Henoch-Schönlein purpura, Arthus reaction, septicaemia.
b) Frost-bite injuring the wall of small blood vessels.

iii) *Outside pressure on microvasculature (extramural)*:
a) Bedsores.

FACTORS DETERMINING SEVERITY OF ISCHAEMIC INJURY

The extent of damage produced by ischaemia due to occlusion of arterial or venous blood vessels depends upon a number of factors as under:

1. Anatomic pattern The extent of injury by ischaemia depends upon the anatomic pattern of arterial blood supply of the organ or tissue affected. There are 4 different patterns of arterial blood supply:

i) Single arterial supply without anastomosis Some organs receive blood supply from arteries which do not have significant anastomosis and are thus functional end-arteries. Occlusion of such vessels invariably results in ischaemic necrosis. For example:
a) Central artery of the retina
b) Interlobular arteries of the kidneys.

ii) Single arterial supply with rich anastomosis Arterial supply to some organs has rich interarterial anastomoses so that blockage of one vessel can re-establish blood supply bypassing the blocked arterial branch, and hence infarction is less common in such circumstances. For example:
a) Superior mesenteric artery supplying blood to the small intestine.
b) Inferior mesenteric artery supplying blood to distal colon.
c) Arterial supply to the stomach by 3 separate vessels derived from coeliac axis.
d) Interarterial anastomoses in the 3 main trunks of the coronary arterial system.

iii) Parallel arterial supply Blood supply to some organs and tissues is such that vitality of the tissue is maintained by alternative blood supply in case of occlusion of one. For example:
a) Blood supply to the brain in the region of circle of Willis.
b) Arterial supply to forearm by radial and ulnar arteries.

iv) Double blood supply The effect of occlusion of one set of vessels is modified if an organ has dual blood supply. For example:
a) Lungs are perfused by bronchial circulation as well as by pulmonary arterial branches.
b) Liver is supplied by both portal circulation and hepatic arterial flow.

However, collateral circulation is of little value if the vessels are severely affected with spasm, atheroma or any other such condition.

2. General and cardiovascular status The general status of an individual as regards cardiovascular function is an important determinant to assess the effect of ischaemia. Some of the factors which render the tissues more vulnerable to the effects of ischaemia are as under:
i) Anaemias (sickle cell anaemia, in particular)
ii) Lowered oxygenation of blood (hypoxaemia)
iii) Senility with marked coronary atherosclerosis
iv) Cardiac failure
v) Blood loss
vi) Shock.

3. Type of tissue affected Vulnerability of the tissue of the body to the effect of ischaemia is variable. Mesenchymal tissues are quite resistant to the effect of ischaemia as compared to parenchymal cells of the organs. The following tissues are more vulnerable to ischaemia:
i) Brain (cerebral cortical neurons, in particular).
ii) Heart (myocardial cells).
iii) Kidney (especially epithelial cells of proximal convoluted tubules).

4. Rapidity of development Sudden vascular obstruction results in more severe effects of ischaemia than if it is gradual since there is less time for collaterals to develop.

5. Degree of vascular occlusion Complete vascular obstruction results in more severe ischaemic injury than the partial occlusion.

EFFECTS

The effects of ischaemia are variable and range from 'no change' to 'sudden death'.

1. No effects on the tissues If the collateral channels develop adequately, the effect of ischaemia fails to occur.

2. Functional disturbances These result when collateral channels are able to supply blood during normal activity but the supply is not adequate to withstand the effect of exertion. The examples are angina pectoris and intermittent claudication.

3. Cellular changes Partial and gradual ischaemia may produce cellular changes such as cloudy swelling, fatty change, ischaemic atrophy and replacement fibrosis. Infarction results when the deprivation of blood supply is complete so as to cause necrosis of tissue affected.

4. Sudden death Cause of sudden death from ischaemia is usually myocardial and cerebral infarction.

The most important and common outcome of ischaemia is infarction discussed below. **Fig. 17.9** shows the organs most commonly affected by infarction.

INFARCTION

Infarction is the process of tissue necrosis, usually coagulative type, resulting from ischaemia; the localised area of necrosis so developed is called an *infarct*.

ETIOLOGY

All the causes of ischaemia discussed above can cause infarction. However, there are a few other noteworthy features in infarction:

i) Most commonly, infarcts are caused by interruption in arterial blood supply, called *ischaemic necrosis*.

ii) Less commonly, venous obstruction can produce infarcts termed *stagnant hypoxia*.

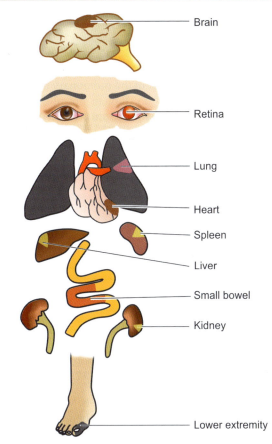

Figure 17.9 ▶ Common locations of systemic infarcts following arterial embolism.

iii) Generally, *sudden, complete, and continuous occlusion* (e.g. thrombosis or embolism) produces infarcts.

iv) Infarcts may be produced by *nonocclusive circulatory insufficiency* as well e.g. incomplete atherosclerotic narrowing of coronary arteries may produce myocardial infarction due to acute coronary insufficiency.

TYPES OF INFARCTS

Infarcts are classified depending upon different features:

1. **According to their colour:**
   i) *Pale or anaemic,* due to arterial occlusion and are seen in compact organs e.g. in the kidneys, heart, spleen.
   ii) *Red or haemorrhagic,* seen in soft loose tissues and are caused either by pulmonary arterial obstruction (e.g. in the lungs) or by arterial or venous occlusion (e.g. in the intestines).

2. **According to their age:**
   i) *Recent or fresh*
   ii) *Old or healed*

3. **According to presence or absence of infection:**
   i) *Bland,* when free of bacterial contamination
   ii) *Septic,* when infected.

PATHOGENESIS

The process of infarction takes place as follows:
i) *Localised hyperaemia* due to local anoxaemia occurs immediately after obstruction of the blood supply.
ii) Within a few hours, the affected part becomes swollen due to *oedema and haemorrhage*. The amount of haemorrhage is variable, being more marked in the lungs and spleen, and less extensive in the kidneys and heart.
iii) *Cellular changes* such as cloudy swelling and degeneration appear early (reversible cell injury), while cell death (irreversible cell injury or necrosis) occurs in 12-48 hours.
iv) There is progressive *proteolysis* of the necrotic tissue and there is lysis of the red cells.
v) *An acute inflammatory reaction and hyperaemia* appear at the same time in the surrounding tissues in response to products of proteolysis.
vi) *Blood pigments*, haematoidin and haemosiderin, liberated by lysis of RBCs are deposited in the infarct. At this stage, most infarcts become pale-grey due to loss of red cells.
vii) Following this, there is progressive *ingrowth of granulation tissue* from the margin of the infarct so that eventually the infarct is replaced by a fibrous scar. Dystrophic calcification may occur sometimes.

MORPHOLOGIC FEATURES

Some general morphological features of infarcts characterise infarcts of all organ sites.

Grossly, general features are as follows:

i) Infarcts of solid organs are usually wedge-shaped, the apex pointing towards the occluded artery and the wide base on the surface of the organ.

ii) Infarcts due to arterial occlusion are generally pale while those due to venous obstruction are haemorrhagic.

iii) Most infarcts become pale later as the red cells are lysed but pulmonary infarcts never become pale due to extensive amount of blood.

iv) Cerebral infarcts are poorly defined with central softening (encephalomalacia).

v) Recent infarcts are generally slightly elevated over the surface while the old infarcts are shrunken and depressed under the surface of the organ.

Microscopically, the general features are as under:

i) Pathognomonic cytologic change in all infarcts is coagulative (ischaemic) necrosis of the affected area of tissue or organ. In cerebral infarcts, however, there is characteristic liquefactive necrosis.

ii) Some amount of haemorrhage is generally present in any infarct.

iii) At the periphery of an infarct, inflammatory reaction is noted. Initially, neutrophils predominate but subsequently macrophages and fibroblasts appear.

Section III: Fluid and Haemodynamic Disorders

Table 17.6 Infarcts of most commonly affected organs.

	LOCATION	GROSS APPEARANCE	OUTCOME
1.	Myocardial infarction	Pale	Frequently lethal
2.	Pulmonary infarction	Haemorrhagic	Less commonly fatal
3.	Cerebral infarction	Haemorrhagic or pale	Fatal if massive
4.	Intestinal infarction	Haemorrhagic	Frequently lethal
5.	Renal infarction	Pale	Not lethal unless massive and bilateral
6.	Infarct spleen	Pale	Not lethal
7.	Infarct liver	Pale	Not lethal
8.	Infarcts lower extremity	Pale	Not lethal

iv) Eventually, the necrotic area is replaced by fibrous scar tissue, which at times may show dystrophic calcification.

v) In cerebral infarcts, the liquefactive necrosis is followed by gliosis i.e. replacement by microglial cells distended by fatty material (gitter cells).

INFARCTS OF DIFFERENT ORGANS

A few representative examples of infarction of some organs (lungs, kidney, liver and spleen) are discussed below. Myocardial infarction (page 491), cerebral infarction (page 40) and infarction of the small intestines (page 46) have been described already.

Table 17.6 sums up the gross appearance and the usual outcome of the common types of infarction.

INFARCT LUNG Embolism of the pulmonary arteries may produce pulmonary infarction, though not always. This is because lungs receive blood supply from bronchial arteries as well, and thus occlusion of pulmonary artery ordinarily does not produce infarcts. However, it may occur in patients who have inadequate circulation such as in chronic lung diseases and congestive heart failure.

Grossly, pulmonary infarcts are classically wedge-shaped with base on the pleura, haemorrhagic, variable in size, and most often in the lower lobes (Fig. 17.10). Fibrinous pleuritis usually covers the area of infarct. Cut surface is dark purple and may show the blocked vessel near the apex of the infarcted area. Old organised and healed pulmonary infarcts appear as retracted fibrous scars.

Microscopically, the characteristic histologic feature is coagulative necrosis of the alveolar walls. Initially, there is infiltration by neutrophils and intense alveolar capillary congestion, but later their place is taken by haemosiderin, phagocytes and granulation tissue (Fig. 17.11).

INFARCT KIDNEY Renal infarction is common, found in up to 5% of autopsies. Majority of them are caused by thromboemboli, most commonly originating from the heart such as in mural thrombi in the left atrium, myocardial infarction, vegetative endocarditis and from aortic aneurysm. Less commonly, renal infarcts may occur due to advanced renal artery atherosclerosis, arteritis and sickle cell anaemia.

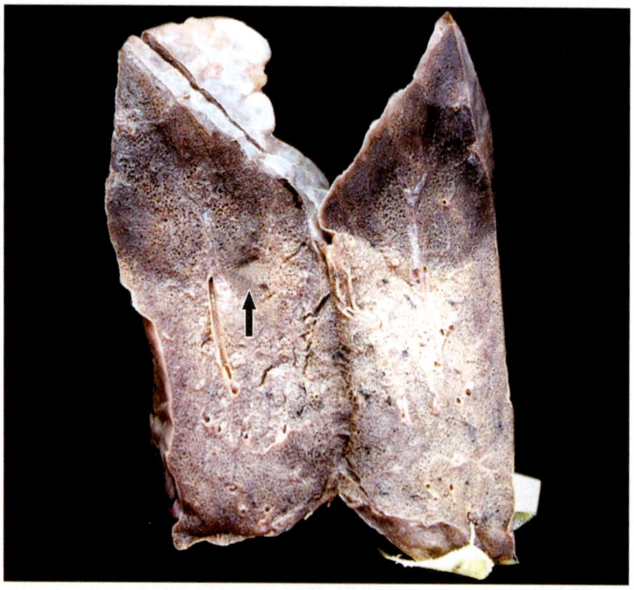

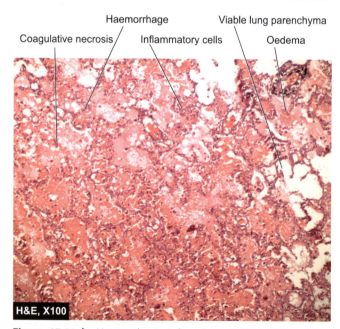

Figure 17.10 ▶ Haemorrhagic infarct lung. The sectioned surface shows dark tan firm areas (arrow) with base on the pleura.

Figure 17.11 ▶ Haemorrhagic infarct lung. Infarcted area shows ghost alveoli filled with blood.

Chapter 17: Obstructive Haemodynamic Derangements

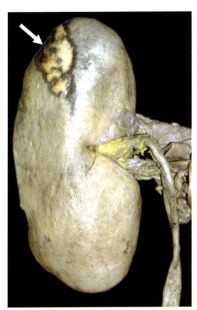

Figure 17.12 ▶ Infarct kidney. The wedge-shaped infarct is slightly depressed on the surface. The apex lies internally and wide base is on the surface. The central area is pale while the margin is haemorrhagic.

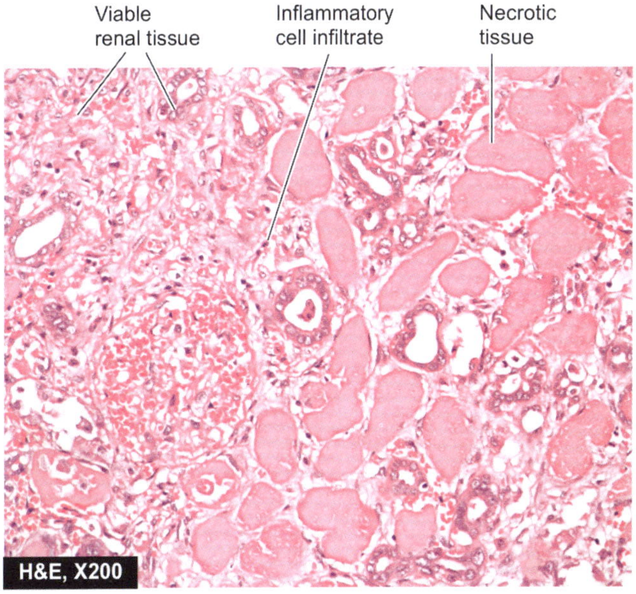

Figure 17.13 ▶ Renal infarct. Renal tubules and glomeruli show typical coagulative necrosis i.e. intact outlines of necrosed cells. There is acute inflammatory infiltrate at the periphery of the infarct.

Grossly, renal infarcts are often multiple and may be bilateral. Characteristically, they are pale or anaemic and wedge-shaped with base resting under the capsule and apex pointing towards the medulla. Generally, a narrow rim of preserved renal tissue under the capsule is spared because it draws its blood supply from the capsular vessels. Cut surface of renal infarct in the first 2 to 3 days is red and congested but by 4th day the centre becomes pale yellow. At the end of one week, the infarct is typically anaemic and depressed below the surface of the kidney (Fig. 17.12).

Microscopically, the affected area shows characteristic coagulative necrosis of renal parenchyma i.e. there are ghosts of renal tubules and glomeruli without intact nuclei and cytoplasmic content. The margin of the infarct shows inflammatory reaction—initially acute but later macrophages and fibrous tissue predominate (Fig. 17.13).

INFARCT SPLEEN Spleen is one of the common sites for infarction. Splenic infarction results from occlusion of the splenic artery or its branches. Occlusion is caused most commonly by thromboemboli arising in the heart (e.g. in mural thrombi in the left atrium, vegetative endocarditis, myocardial infarction), and less frequently by obstruction of microcirculation (e.g. in myeloproliferative diseases, sickle cell anaemia, arteritis, Hodgkin's disease, bacterial infections).

Grossly, splenic infarcts are often multiple. They are characteristically pale or anaemic and wedge-shaped with their base at the periphery and apex pointing towards hilum (Fig.17.14).

Microscopically, the features are similar to those found in anaemic infarcts in kidney. Coagulative necrosis and inflammatory reaction are seen. Later, the necrotic tissue is replaced by shrunken fibrous scar (Fig. 17.15).

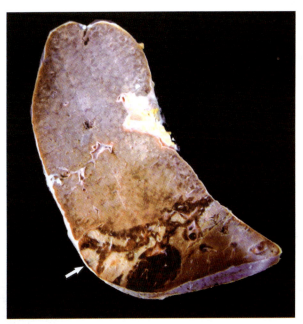

Figure 17.14 ▶ Pale infarct spleen. A wedge-shaped shrunken area of pale colour is seen with base resting under the capsule, while the margin is congested.

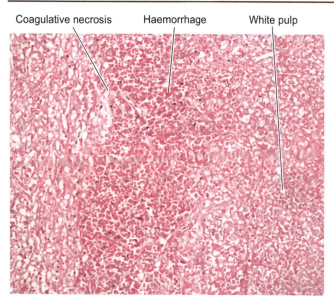

Figure 17.15 ▶ Pale infarct spleen. The affected area shows outlines of cells only due to coagulative necrosis while the margin of infarcted area shows haemorrhage.

INFARCT LIVER Just as in lungs, infarcts in the liver are uncommon due to dual blood supply—from portal vein and from hepatic artery.

◈ Obstruction of the portal vein is usually secondary to other diseases such as hepatic cirrhosis, intravenous invasion of primary carcinoma of the liver, carcinoma of the pancreas and pylephlebitis. Occlusion of portal vein or its branches generally does not produce ischaemic infarction but instead reduced blood supply to hepatic parenchyma causes non-ischaemic infarct called *infarct of Zahn*.

◈ Obstruction of the hepatic artery or its branches, on the other hand, caused by arteritis, arteriosclerosis, bland or septic emboli, results in ischaemic infarcts of the liver.

Grossly, ischaemic infarcts of the liver are usually anaemic but sometimes may be haemorrhagic due to stuffing of the site by blood from the portal vein. Infarcts of Zahn (non-ischaemic infarcts) produce sharply defined red-blue area in liver parenchyma.

Microscopically, ischaemic infarcts show characteristics of pale or anaemic infarcts as in kidney or spleen. Infarcts of Zahn occurring due to reduced portal blood flow over a long duration result in chronic atrophy of hepatocytes and dilatation of sinusoids.

GIST BOX 17.3 | Ischaemia and Infarction

- Ischaemia is defined as deficient blood supply to part of a tissue relative to its metabolic needs.
- Causes of ischaemia may lie in the heart, arteries, veins and microcirculation.
- Adverse effects of ischaemia may result in 3 ways: hypoxia, malnourishment of cells and inadequate clearance of metabolites.
- Severity of ischaemic injury depends upon anatomic pattern of blood supply, general and cardiovascular status, type of tissue affected, and speed of development of ischaemia.
- Most common effect of ischaemia is infarction, generally from coagulative necrosis in most organs, but in the brain it is liquefactive necrosis.
- Some of the common locations of infarcts are: brain, heart, kidneys, spleen, small intestines, and lower extremities. Infarction of lungs and liver is less frequent due to dual blood supply to both these organs.

Section IV ▶ Neoplasia

▶ SECTION CONTENTS

Chapter 18: General Aspects of Neoplasia
Chapter 19: Etiology and Pathogenesis of Neoplasia
Chapter 20: Host-Tumour Relationship and Diagnosis of Neoplasms
Chapter 21: Common Specific Tumours

18 General Aspects of Neoplasia

DEFINITION, NOMENCLATURE AND CLASSIFICATION

INTRODUCTION The term 'neoplasia' means new growth; the new growth produced is called 'neoplasm' or 'tumour'. However, all 'new growths' are not neoplasms since examples of new growth of tissues and cells also exist in the processes of embryogenesis, regeneration and repair, hyperplasia and hormonal stimulation. The proliferation and maturation of cells in normal adults is controlled. Thus, normally some cells proliferate throughout life (labile cells), some have limited proliferation (stable cells), while others do not replicate (permanent cells). On the other hand, neoplastic cells lose control and regulation of replication and form an abnormal mass of tissue.

Therefore, satisfactory definition of a neoplasm or tumour is *'a mass of tissue formed as a result of abnormal, excessive, uncoordinated, autonomous and purposeless proliferation of cells even after cessation of stimulus for growth which caused it.'* The branch of science dealing with the study of neoplasms or tumours is called oncology (*oncos*=tumour, *logos*=study). Neoplasms may be 'benign' when they are slow-growing and localised without causing much difficulty to the host, or 'malignant' when they proliferate rapidly, spread throughout the body and may eventually cause death of the host. The common term used for all malignant tumours is cancer. Hippocrates (460-370 BC) coined the term *karkinos* for cancer of the breast. The word 'cancer' means crab, thus reflecting the true character of cancer since 'it sticks to the part stubbornly like a crab'.

All tumours, benign as well as malignant, have 2 basic components:

◆ *'Parenchyma'* comprised by proliferating tumour cells; parenchyma determines the nature and evolution of the tumour.
◆ *'Supportive stroma'* composed of fibrous connective tissue and blood vessels; it provides the framework on which the parenchymal tumour cells grow.

The tumours derive their nomenclature on the basis of the parenchymal component comprising them. The suffix '*-oma*' is added to denote benign tumours. Malignant tumours of epithelial origin are called *carcinomas*, while malignant mesenchymal tumours are named *sarcomas* (*sarcos* = fleshy) **(Fig. 18.1)**. However, some cancers are composed of highly undifferentiated cells and are referred to as *undifferentiated malignant tumours.*

Although, this broad generalisation regarding nomenclature of tumours usually holds true in majority of instances, some examples contrary to this concept are: *melanoma* for carcinoma of the melanocytes, *hepatoma* for carcinoma of the hepatocytes, *lymphoma* for malignant tumour of the lymphoid tissue, and *seminoma* for malignant tumour of the testis. *Leukaemia* is the term used for cancer of blood forming cells.

SPECIAL CATEGORIES OF TUMOURS Following categories of tumours are examples which defy the generalisation in nomenclature given above:

1. Mixed tumours When two types of tumours are combined in the same tumour, it is called a mixed tumour. For example:

i) Adenosquamous carcinoma is the combination of adenocarcinoma and squamous cell carcinoma in the endometrium.
ii) Adenoacanthoma is the mixture of adenocarcinoma and benign squamous elements in the endometrium.
iii) Carcinosarcoma is the rare combination of malignant tumour of the epithelium (carcinoma) and of mesenchymal tissue (sarcoma) such as in breast and thyroid.
iv) Collision tumour is the term used for morphologically two different cancers in the same organ which do not mix with each other.
v) Mixed tumour of the salivary gland (or pleomorphic adenoma) is the term used for benign tumour having combination of both epithelial and mesenchymal tissue elements.

2. Teratomas These tumours are made up of a mixture of various tissue types arising from totipotent cells derived

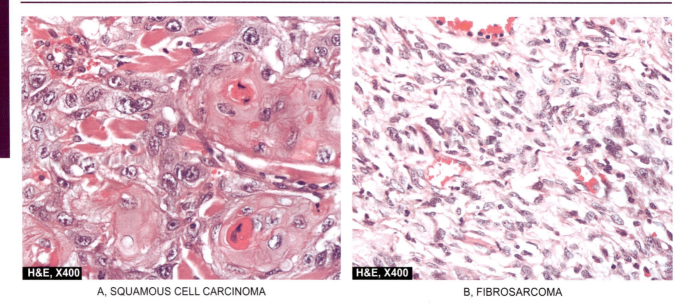

A, SQUAMOUS CELL CARCINOMA   B, FIBROSARCOMA

Figure 18.1 ▶ Examples of carcinoma (epithelial malignant tumour) (A) and sarcoma (mesenchymal malignant tumour) (B).

from the three germ cell layers—ectoderm, mesoderm and endoderm. Most common sites for teratomas are ovaries and testis (*gonadal teratomas*). But they occur at *extra-gonadal sites* as well, mainly in the midline of the body such as in the head and neck region, mediastinum, retroperitoneum, sacrococcygeal region etc. Teratomas may be *benign or mature* (most of the ovarian teratomas) or *malignant or immature* (most of the testicular teratomas).

3. Blastomas (Embryomas) Blastomas or embryomas are a group of malignant tumours which arise from embryonal or partially differentiated cells which would normally form blastema of the organs and tissue during embryogenesis. These tumours occur more frequently in infants and children (under 5 years of age). Some examples of such tumours in this age group are: neuroblastoma, nephroblastoma (Wilms' tumour), hepatoblastoma, retinoblastoma, medulloblastoma, pulmonary blastoma.

4. Hamartoma Hamartoma is benign tumour which is made of mature but disorganised cells of tissues indigenous to the particular organ e.g. hamartoma of the lung consists of mature cartilage, mature smooth muscle and epithelium. Thus, all mature differentiated tissue elements which comprise the bronchus are present in it but are jumbled up as a mass.

5. Choristoma Choristoma is the name given to the ectopic islands of normal tissue. Thus, choristoma is heterotopia but is not a true tumour, though it sounds like one.

CLASSIFICATION Currently, classification of tumours is based on the histogenesis (i.e. cell of origin) and on the anticipated behaviour **(Table 18.1)**. However, it must be mentioned here that the classification described here is only a summary. Detailed classifications of benign and malignant tumours pertaining to different tissues and body systems along with morphologic features of specific tumours appear in the specific chapters of Systemic Pathology later.

 GIST BOX 18.1   **Definition, Nomenclature and Classification of Tumours**

- A neoplasm or tumour is a mass of tissue formed as a result of abnormal, excessive, uncoordinated, autonomous and purposeless proliferation of cells even after removal of stimulus for growth which caused it.
- Neoplasms may be 'benign' when they are slow-growing and localised without causing much difficulty to the host, or 'malignant' when they proliferate rapidly, spread throughout the body and may eventually cause death of the host.
- All tumours have 2 basic components: parenchyma comprised by proliferating tumour cells, and supportive stroma composed of fibrous connective tissue and blood vessels.
- The tumours are named with suffix '-oma' to denote benign tumours. Malignant tumours of epithelial origin are called *carcinomas*, while malignant mesenchymal tumours are named *sarcomas*.
- A few examples of combination of tumours are mixed tumours, teratoma, blastoma, hamartoma, and choristoma.

Table 18.1: Classification of tumours.

TISSUE OF ORIGIN	BENIGN	MALIGNANT
I. TUMOURS OF ONE PARENCHYMAL CELL TYPE		
A. Epithelial Tumours		
1. Squamous epithelium	Squamous cell papilloma	Squamous cell (Epidermoid) carcinoma
2. Transitional epithelium	Transitional cell papilloma	Transitional cell carcinoma
3. Glandular epithelium	Adenoma	Adenocarcinoma
4. Basal cell layer skin	—	Basal cell carcinoma
5. Neuroectoderm	Naevus	Melanoma (Melanocarcinoma)
6. Hepatocytes	Liver cell adenoma	Hepatoma (Hepatocellular carcinoma)
7. Placenta (Chorionic epithelium)	Hydatidiform mole	Choriocarcinoma
B. Non-epithelial (Mesenchymal) Tumours		
1. Adipose tissue	Lipoma	Liposarcoma
2. Adult fibrous tissue	Fibroma	Fibrosarcoma
3. Embryonic fibrous tissue	Myxoma	Myxosarcoma
4. Cartilage	Chondroma	Chondrosarcoma
5. Bone	Osteoma	Osteosarcoma
6. Synovium	Benign synovioma	Synovial sarcoma
7. Smooth muscle	Leiomyoma	Leiomyosarcoma
8. Skeletal muscle	Rhabdomyoma	Rhabdomyosarcoma
9. Mesothelium	—	Mesothelioma
10. Blood vessels	Haemangioma	Angiosarcoma
11. Lymph vessels	Lymphangioma	Lymphangiosarcoma
12. Glomus	Glomus tumour	—
13. Meninges	Meningioma	Invasive meningioma
14. Haematopoietic cells	—	Leukaemias
15. Lymphoid tissue	Pseudolymphoma	Malignant lymphomas
16. Nerve sheath	Neurilemmoma, Neurofibroma	Neurogenic sarcoma
17. Nerve cells	Ganglioneuroma	Neuroblastoma
II. MIXED TUMOURS		
Salivary glands	Pleomorphic adenoma (mixed salivary tumour)	Malignant mixed salivary tumour
III. TUMOURS OF MORE THAN ONE GERM CELL LAYER		
Totipotent cells in gonads or in embryonal rests	Mature teratoma	Immature teratoma

CHARACTERISTICS OF TUMOURS

Majority of neoplasms can be categorised into benign and malignant on the basis of certain clinical features, biologic behaviour and morphological characteristics. However, there are exceptions—a small proportion of tumours have some features suggesting innocent growth while other features point towards a more ominous behaviour. Therefore, it must be borne in mind that based on characteristics of neoplasms, there is a wide variation in the degree of deviation from the normal in all the tumours.

The characteristics of tumours are described under the following headings:
I. Rate of growth
II. Cancer phenotype and stem cells
III. Clinical and gross features
IV. Microscopic features
V. Spread of tumours
 a. Local invasion or direct spread
 b. Metastasis or distant spread

Based on these characteristics, contrasting features of benign and malignant tumours are summarised in Table 18.2 and illustrated in Fig. 18.2. These aspects are discussed below.

RATE OF GROWTH

The tumour cells generally proliferate more rapidly than the normal cells. In general, benign tumours grow slowly and malignant tumours rapidly. However, there are exceptions

Section IV: Neoplasia

Table 18.2 Contrasting features of benign and malignant tumours.

	FEATURE	BENIGN	MALIGNANT
I.	**CLINICAL AND GROSS FEATURES**		
1.	Boundaries	Encapsulated or well-circumscribed	Poorly-circumscribed and irregular
2.	Surrounding tissue	Often compressed	Usually invaded
3.	Size	Usually small	Often larger
4.	Secondary changes	Occur less often	Occur more often
II.	**MICROSCOPIC FEATURES**		
1.	Pattern	Usually resembles the tissue of origin closely	Often poor resemblance to tissue of origin
2.	Basal polarity	Retained	Often lost
3.	Pleomorphism	Usually not present	Often present
4.	Nucleo-cytoplasmic ratio	Normal	Increased
5.	Anisonucleosis	Absent	Generally present
6.	Hyperchromatism	Absent	Often present
7.	Mitoses	May be present but are always typical mitoses	Mitotic figures increased and are generally atypical and abnormal
8.	Tumour giant cells	May be present but without nuclear atypia	Present with nuclear atypia
9.	Chromosomal abnormalities	Infrequent	Invariably present
10.	Function	Usually well maintained	May be retained, lost or become abnormal
III.	**GROWTH RATE**	Usually slow	Usually rapid
IV.	**LOCAL INVASION**	Often compresses the surrounding tissues without invading or infiltrating them	Usually infiltrates and invades the adjacent tissues
V.	**METASTASIS**	Absent	Frequently present
VI.	**PROGNOSIS**	Local complications	Death by local and metastatic complications

to this generalisation. The rate at which the tumour enlarges depends upon 2 main factors:
1. Rate of cell production, growth fraction and rate of cell loss
2. Degree of differentiation of the tumour.

1. Rate of cell production, growth fraction and rate of cell loss Rate of growth of a tumour depends upon 3 important parameters:
i) doubling time of tumour cells,
ii) number of cells remaining in proliferative pool (growth fraction), and
iii) rate of loss of tumour cells by cell shedding.

In general, malignant tumour cells have increased mitotic rate (doubling time) and slower death rate i.e. the cancer cells do not follow normal controls in cell cycle and are immortal. If the rate of cell division is high, it is likely that tumour cells in the centre of the tumour do not receive adequate nourishment and undergo ischaemic necrosis. At a stage when malignant tumours grow relentlessly, they do so because a larger proportion of tumour cells remain in replicative pool but due to lack of availability of adequate nourishment, these tumour cells are either lost by shedding or leave the cell cycle to enter into G_0 (resting phase) or G_1 phase. While dead tumour cells appear as 'apoptotic figures' (page 42), the dividing cells of tumours are seen as normal and abnormal 'mitotic figures' (page 272). Ultimately, malignant tumours grow in size because the cell production exceeds the cell loss.

2. Degree of differentiation Secondly, the rate of growth of malignant tumour is directly proportionate to the degree of dedifferentiation. Poorly differentiated tumours show aggressive growth pattern as compared to better differentiated tumours. Some tumours, after a period of slow growth, may suddenly show spurt in their growth due to development of an aggressive clone of malignant cells. On the other hand, some tumours may cease to grow after sometime. Rarely, a malignant tumour may disappear spontaneously from the primary site, possibly due to necrosis caused by good host immune attack, only to reappear as secondaries elsewhere in the body e.g. choriocarcinoma, malignant melanoma.

The regulation of tumour growth is under the control of growth factors secreted by the tumour cells. Out of various growth factors, important ones modulating tumour biology are listed below and discussed later:
i) Epidermal growth factor (EGF)
ii) Fibroblast growth factor (FGF)
iii) Platelet-derived growth factor (PDGF)

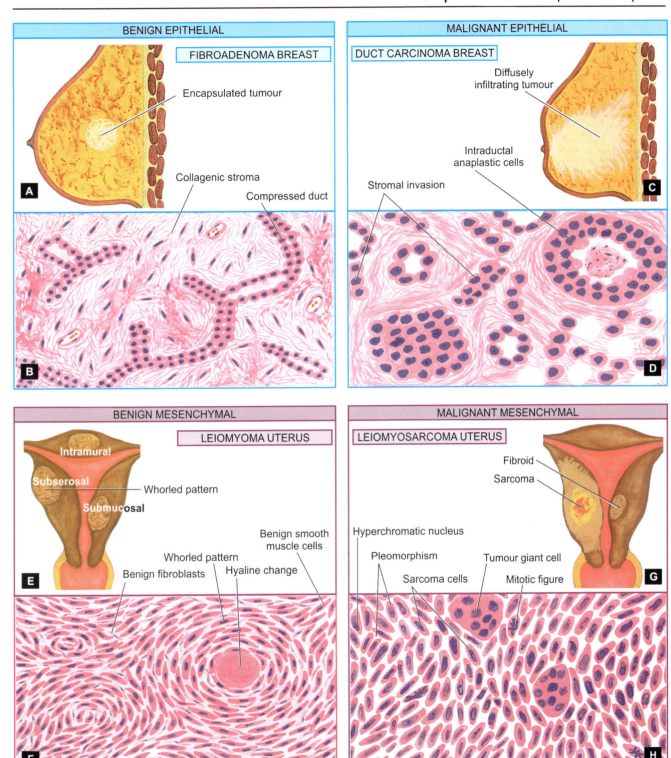

Figure 18.2 ▶ Salient gross and microscopic features of prototypes of benign *(left)* and malignant *(right)* tumours.

iv) Colony stimulating factor (CSF)
v) Transforming growth factors-β (TGF-β)
vi) Interleukins 1 and 6 (IL-1, IL-6)
vii) Vascular endothelial growth factor (VEGF)
viii) Hepatocyte growth factor (HGF)

CANCER PHENOTYPE AND STEM CELLS

Normally growing cells in an organ are related to the neighbouring cells—they grow under normal growth controls, perform their assigned function and there is a balance between the rate of cell proliferation and the rate of cell death including cell suicide (i.e. apoptosis). Thus, normal cells are socially desirable. However, cancer cells exhibit anti-social behaviour as under:
i) Cancer cells disobey the growth controlling signals in the body and thus *proliferate rapidly*.
ii) Cancer cells escape death signals and achieve *immortality*.
iii) Imbalance between cell proliferation and cell death in cancer causes *excessive growth*.
iv) Cancer cells lose properties of differentiation and thus perform *little or no function*.
v) Due to loss of growth controls, cancer cells are genetically unstable and develop *newer mutations*.
vi) Cancer cells over-run their neighbouring tissue and *invade locally*.
vii) Cancer cells have the ability to travel from the site of origin to other sites in the body where they colonise and establish *distant metastasis*.

Cancer cells originate by clonal proliferation of a single progeny of a cell (monoclonality). There is evidence to suggest that cancer cells arise from stem cells normally present in the tissues in small number and are not readily identifiable. These stem cells have the properties of prolonged self-renewal, asymmetric replication and transdifferentiation (i.e. plasticity). These cancer stem cells are called tumour-initiating cells. Their definite existence in acute leukaemias has been known for a few decades and have now been found to be present in some other malignant tumours.

CLINICAL AND GROSS FEATURES

Clinically, benign tumours are generally slow growing, and depending upon the location, may remain asymptomatic (e.g. subcutaneous lipoma), or may produce serious symptoms (e.g. meningioma in the nervous system). On the other hand, malignant tumours grow rapidly, may ulcerate on the surface, invade locally into deeper tissues, may spread to distant sites (metastasis), and also produce systemic features such as weight loss, anorexia and anaemia. In fact, three cardinal clinical features of malignant tumours are: *anaplasia, invasiveness and metastasis* (discussed later).

Gross appearance of benign and malignant tumours may be quite variable and the features may not be diagnostic on the basis of gross appearance alone. However, certain distinctive features characterise almost all tumours compared to neighbouring normal tissue of origin—they have a different colour, texture and consistency. Gross terms such as papillary, fungating, infiltrating, haemorrhagic, ulcerative and cystic are used to describe the macroscopic appearance of the tumours. General gross features of benign and malignant tumours are as under (Figs. 18.2 and 18.3):

◆ *Benign tumours* are generally spherical or ovoid in shape. They are encapsulated or well-circumscribed, freely movable, more often firm and uniform, unless secondary changes like haemorrhage or infarction supervene (Fig. 18.2, A, E).

◆ *Malignant tumours,* on the other hand, are usually irregular in shape, poorly-circumscribed and extend into the adjacent tissues. Secondary changes like haemorrhage, infarction and ulceration are seen more often. Sarcomas typically have fish-flesh like consistency while carcinomas are generally firm (Fig. 18.2, C, G).

MICROSCOPIC FEATURES

For recognising and classifying the tumours, the microscopic characteristics of tumour cells are of greatest importance. These features appreciated in histologic sections are as under:
1. Microscopic pattern
2. Histomorphology of neoplastic cells (differentiation and anaplasia)
3. Tumour angiogenesis and stroma
4. Inflammatory reaction.

1. Microscopic Pattern

The patterns or arrangements of tumour cells are best appreciated under *low power* microscopic examination of the tissue section. Some of the common patterns in tumours are as under:

i) The *epithelial tumours* generally consist of acini, sheets, columns or cords of epithelial tumour cells that may be arranged in solid or papillary pattern (Fig. 18.2, B, D).

ii) The *mesenchymal tumours* have mesenchymal tumour cells arranged as interlacing bundles, fascicles or whorls, lying separated from each other usually by the intercellular matrix substance such as hyaline material in leiomyoma (Fig. 18.2, E), cartilaginous matrix in chondroma, osteoid in osteosarcoma, reticulin network in soft tissue sarcomas etc (Fig. 18.2, H).

iii) Certain tumours have *mixed patterns* e.g. teratoma arising from totipotent cells, pleomorphic adenoma of salivary gland (mixed salivary tumour), fibroadenoma of the breast, carcinosarcoma of the uterus and various other combinations of tumour types.

iv) *Haematopoietic tumours* such as leukaemias and lymphomas often have none or little stromal support.

v) Generally, most benign tumours and low grade malignant tumours *reduplicate* the normal structure of origin more closely so that there is little difficulty in identifying and

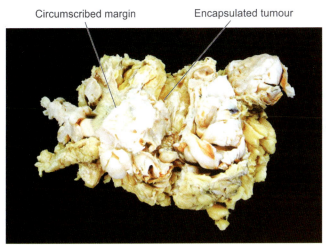
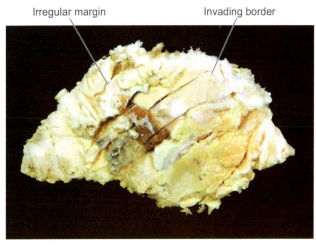

A, FIBROADENOMA BREAST   B, INFILTRATING CARCINOMA BREAST

Figure 18.3 ▶ Gross appearance of a prototype of benign and malignant tumour.

classifying such tumours (Fig. 18.2, B, F). However, anaplastic tumours differ greatly from the arrangement in normal tissue of origin of the tumour and may occasionally pose problems in classifying the tumour.

2. Cytomorphology of Neoplastic Cells (Differentiation and Anaplasia)

The neoplastic cell is characterised by morphologic and functional alterations, the most significant of which are 'differentiation' and 'anaplasia'.

◈ **Differentiation** is defined as the extent of morphological and functional resemblance of parenchymal tumour cells to corresponding normal cells. If the deviation of neoplastic cell in structure and function is minimal as compared to normal cell, the tumour is described as 'well-differentiated' such as most benign and low-grade malignant tumours. 'Poorly differentiated', 'undifferentiated' or 'dedifferentiated' are synonymous terms for poor structural and functional resemblance to corresponding normal cell.

◈ **Anaplasia** is lack of differentiation and is a characteristic feature of most malignant tumours. Depending upon the degree of differentiation, the extent of anaplasia is also variable i.e. poorly differentiated malignant tumours have high degree of anaplasia.

As a result of anaplasia, noticeable morphological and functional alterations in the neoplastic cells are observed which are best appreciated under *higher magnification* of the microscope. These features are as follows and are diagrammatically depicted in Fig. 18.4:

i) Loss of polarity Normally, the nuclei of epithelial cells are oriented along the basement membrane which is termed as basal polarity. This property is based on cell adhesion molecules, particularly selectins. Early in malignancy, tumour cells lose their basal polarity so that the nuclei tend to lie away from the basement membrane (Fig. 18.5).

ii) Pleomorphism The term pleomorphism means variation in size and shape of the tumour cells. The extent of cellular pleomorphism generally correlates with the degree of anaplasia. Tumour cells are often bigger than normal but in some tumours they can be of normal size or smaller than normal (Fig. 18.6).

iii) N:C ratio Generally, the nuclei of malignant tumour cells show more conspicuous changes. Nuclei are enlarged disproportionate to the cell size so that the nucleocytoplasmic ratio is increased from normal 1:5 to 1:1 (Fig. 18.6).

iv) Anisonucleosis Just like cellular pleomorphism, the nuclei too, show variation in size and shape in malignant tumour cells (Fig. 18.6).

v) Hyperchromatism Characteristically, the nuclear chromatin of malignant cell is increased and coarsely clumped. This is due to increase in the amount of nucleoprotein resulting in dark-staining nuclei, referred to as hyperchromatism (Fig. 18.6). Nuclear shape may vary, nuclear membrane may be irregular and nuclear chromatin is clumped along the nuclear membrane.

vi) Nucleolar changes Malignant cells frequently have a prominent nucleolus or nucleoli in the nucleus reflecting increased nucleoprotein synthesis (Fig. 18.6). This may be demonstrated as Nucleolar Organiser Region (NOR) by silver (Ag) staining called AgNOR material.

vii) Mitotic figures The parenchymal cells of poorly-differentiated tumours often show large number of mitoses as compared with benign tumours and well-differentiated

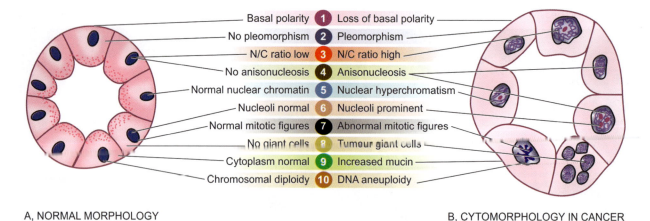

Figure 18.4 ▶ Diagrammatic representation of cytomorphologic features of neoplastic cells. Characteristics of cancer (B) are contrasted with the normal appearance of an acinus (A).

malignant tumours. As stated above, these appear as either normal or abnormal mitotic figures (Fig. 18.7):

◆ *Normal mitotic figures* may be seen in some non-neoplastic proliferating cells (e.g. haematopoietic cells of the bone marrow, intestinal epithelium, hepatocytes etc), in certain benign tumours and some low grade malignant tumours; in sections they are seen as a dark band of dividing chromatin at two poles of the nuclear spindle.

◆ *Abnormal or atypical mitotic figures* are more important in malignant tumours and are identified as tripolar, quadripolar and multipolar spindles in malignant tumour cells.

viii) *Tumour giant cells* Multinucleate tumour giant cells or giant cells containing a single large and bizarre nucleus, possessing nuclear characters of the adjacent tumour cells, are another important feature of anaplasia in malignant tumours (Fig. 18.8).

ix) *Functional (Cytoplasmic) changes* Structural anaplasia in tumours is accompanied with functional anaplasia as appreciated from the cytoplasmic constituents of the tumour cells. The functional abnormality in neoplasms may be quantitative, qualitative, or both.

◆ Generally, benign tumours and better-differentiated malignant tumours continue to function well qualitatively, though there may be *quantitative* abnormality in the product e.g. large or small amount of collagen produced by benign tumours of fibrous tissue, keratin formation in well-

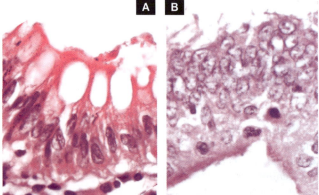

Figure 18.5 ▶ Microscopic appearance of loss of nuclear polarity (B) contrasted with normal basal polarity in columnar epithelium (A). The basement membrane is intact in both.

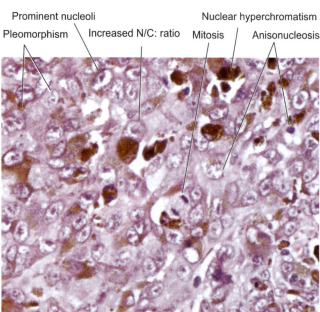

Figure 18.6 ▶ Nuclear features of malignant cells in malignant melanoma—pleomorphism, anisonucleosis, increased N/C: ratio, nuclear hyperchromatism and prominent nucleoli.

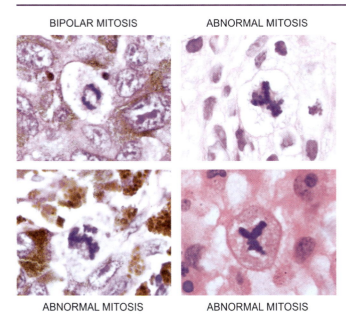

Figure 18.7 ▶ Normal and abnormal (atypical) mitotic figures.

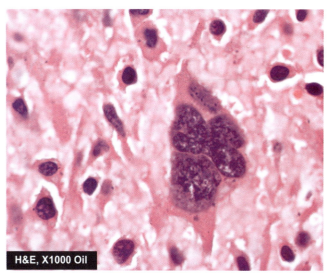

Figure 18.8 ▶ A multinucleate tumour giant cell in osteosarcoma.

differentiated squamous cell carcinoma. In more anaplastic tumours, there is usually quantitative fall in the product made by the tumour cells e.g. absence of keratin in anaplastic squamous cell carcinoma.

◆ There may be both *qualitative and quantitative* abnormality of the cellular function in some anaplastic tumours e.g. multiple myeloma producing abnormal immunoglobulin in large quantities.

◆ Endocrine tumours may cause excessive hormone production leading to characteristic clinical syndromes. Besides the production of hormones by endocrine tumours, hormones or hormone-like substances may be produced by certain tumours quite unrelated to the endocrine glands. This property of tumours is called *ectopic hormone production* e.g. oat cell carcinoma of the lung can secrete ACTH and ADH; less often it may produce gonadotropin, thyrotropin, parathormone, calcitonin and growth hormone. Ectopic erythropoietin may be produced by carcinoma of kidneys, hepatocellular carcinoma and cerebellar haemangioblastoma.

x) *Chromosomal abnormalities* All tumour cells have abnormal genetic composition and on division they transmit the genetic abnormality to their progeny. The chromosomal abnormalities are more marked in more malignant tumours which include deviations in both morphology and number of chromosomes. Most malignant tumours show *DNA aneuploidy*, often in the form of an increase in the number of chromosomes, reflected morphologically by the increase in the size of nuclei.

One of the most important examples of a consistent chromosomal abnormality in human malignancy is the presence of Philadelphia chromosome (named after the city in which it was first described) in 95% cases of chronic myeloid leukaemia. In this, part of the long arm of chromosome 9 is translocated to part of the long arm of chromosome 22 (t 9; 22). Other examples of neoplasms showing chromosomal abnormalities are Burkitt's lymphoma, acute lymphoid leukaemia, multiple myeloma, retinoblastoma, oat cell carcinoma, Wilms' tumour etc.

3. Tumour Angiogenesis and Stroma

The connective tissue along with its vascular network forms the supportive framework on which the parenchymal tumour cells grow and receive nourishment. In addition to variable amount of connective tissue and vascularity, the stroma may have nerves and metaplastic bone or cartilage but no lymphatics.

TUMOUR ANGIOGENESIS In order to provide nourishment to growing tumour, new blood vessels are formed from pre-existing ones (angiogenesis). Its mechanism and the role of angiogenic factors elaborated by tumour cells (e.g. vascular endothelium growth factor or VEGF) is discussed later under molecular pathogenesis of cancer. However, related morphologic features are as under:

i) *Microvascular density* The new capillaries add to the vascular density of the tumour which has been used as a marker to assess the rate of growth of tumours and hence grade the tumours. This is done by counting microvascular density in the section of the tumour.

ii) *Central necrosis* However, if the tumour outgrows its blood supply as occurs in rapidly growing tumours or tumour angiogenesis fails, its core undergoes ischaemic necrosis.

TUMOUR STROMA The collagenous tissue in the stroma may be scanty or excessive. If the stroma is scanty, the tumour

Section IV: Neoplasia

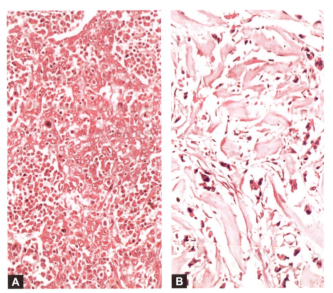

Figure 18.9 ▶ Tumour stroma. A, Medullary carcinoma of breast is rich in parenchymal cells. B, Scirrhous carcinoma of breast having abundant collagenised (desmoplastic) stroma.

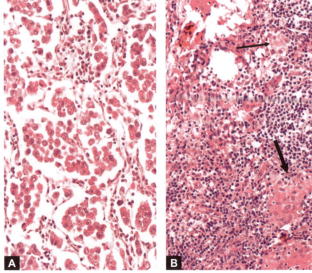

Figure 18.10 ▶ Inflammatory reaction in the stroma of the tumour. A, Lymphocytic reaction in seminoma testis. B, Granulomatous reaction (thick arrow) in Hodgkin's lymphoma (thin arrow for RS cell).

is soft and fleshy (e.g. in sarcomas, lymphomas), while if it is excessive the tumour is hard and gritty (e.g. infiltrating duct carcinoma breast). Growth of fibrous tissue in tumour is stimulated by basic fibroblast growth factor (bFGF) elaborated by tumour cells.

❖ If the epithelial tumour is almost entirely composed of parenchymal cells, it is called *medullary* e.g. medullary carcinoma of the breast **(Fig. 18.9, A)**, medullary carcinoma of the thyroid.

❖ If there is excessive connective tissue stroma in the epithelial tumour, it is referred to as *desmoplasia* and the tumour is hard or *scirrhous* e.g. infiltrating duct carcinoma breast **(Fig. 18.9, B)**, linitis plastica of the stomach.

4. Inflammatory Reaction

At times, prominent inflammatory reaction is present in and around the tumours. It could be the result of ulceration in the cancer when there is secondary infection. The inflammatory reaction in such instances may be acute or chronic. However, some tumours show chronic inflammatory reaction, chiefly of lymphocytes, plasma cells and macrophages, and in some instances granulomatous reaction, as a part of the morphologic features of the tumour, in the absence of ulceration. This is due to cell-mediated immunologic response by the host in an attempt to destroy the tumour. In some cases, such an immune response improves the prognosis.

The *examples* of such reaction are: seminoma testis **(Fig. 18.10)**, malignant melanoma of the skin, lympho-epithelioma of the throat, medullary carcinoma of the breast, choriocarcinoma, Warthin's tumour of salivary glands etc.

GIST BOX 18.2 | Characteristics of Tumours

❖ Neoplasms are categorised into benign and malignant on the basis of certain clinical and morphologic features.

❖ The tumour cells generally proliferate more rapidly than the normal cells; benign tumours grow slowly and malignant tumours rapidly. Tumour enlargement depends upon rate of cell production, growth fraction and rate of cell loss and degree of differentiation of the tumour.

❖ Evidence suggests that cancer cells originate by clonal proliferation of a single progeny of stem cells (monoclonality).

❖ Clinically, benign tumours are generally slow growing and may remain asymptomatic while malignant tumours grow rapidly and may spread locally or to distant sites.

❖ Grossly, benign tumours are generally encapsulated or well-circumscribed, while malignant tumours are usually irregular in shape, poorly-circumscribed and extend into the adjacent tissues.

❖ Microscopic features of tumours are more important for recognising and classifying the tumours. These include microscopic pattern of tumour cells, histomorphology of neoplastic cells, tumour angiogenesis, and stromal reaction.

❖ The neoplastic cells are characterised by morphologic and functional alterations, the most significant of which are 'differentiation' and 'anaplasia'. *Differentiation* is defined as the extent of morphological and functional resemblance of parenchymal tumour cells

to corresponding normal cells. *Anaplasia* is lack of differentiation and is a characteristic feature of most malignant tumours.
* Important features of anaplasia are: loss of polarity, pleomorphism, increased N:C ratio, hyperchromatism, prominent nucleoli, abnormal mitotic figures, qualitative or quantitative cytoplasmic changes, and chromosomal abnormalities.
* Stromal features of significance in tumours are angiogenesis, collagenous stroma (desmoplasia) and inflammatory stromal reaction by the host.

SPREAD OF TUMOURS

One of the cardinal features of malignant tumours is its ability to invade and destroy adjoining tissues (local invasion or direct spread) and disseminate to distant sites (metastasis or distant spread).

LOCAL INVASION (DIRECT SPREAD)

BENIGN TUMOURS Most benign tumours form encapsulated or circumscribed masses that *expand and push aside* the surrounding normal tissues without actually invading, infiltrating or metastasising.

MALIGNANT TUMOURS Malignant tumours also enlarge by expansion and some well-differentiated tumours may be partially encapsulated as well e.g. follicular carcinoma thyroid. But characteristically, they are distinguished from benign tumours by *invasion, infiltration and destruction* of the surrounding tissue, besides spread to distant sites or metastasis (described below). In general, tumours invade via the route of least resistance, though eventually most cancers recognise no anatomic boundaries. Often, cancers extend through tissue spaces, permeate lymphatics, blood vessels, perineural spaces and may penetrate a bone by growing through nutrient foramina. More commonly, the tumours invade thin-walled capillaries and veins than thick-walled arteries. Dense compact collagen, elastic tissue and cartilage are some of the tissues which are sufficiently resistant to invasion by tumours.

Mechanism of direct invasion of malignant tumours is discussed together with that of metastasis below.

METASTASIS (DISTANT SPREAD)

Metastasis (*meta* = transformation, *stasis* = residence) is defined as spread of tumour by invasion in such a way that discontinuous secondary tumour mass/masses are formed at the site of lodgement. *Besides anaplasia, invasiveness and metastasis are the two other most important features to distinguish malignant from benign tumours.* Benign tumours do not metastasise while all the malignant tumours can metastasise, barring a few exceptions like gliomas of the central nervous system and basal cell carcinoma of the skin. Generally, larger, more aggressive and rapidly-growing tumours are more likely to metastasise but there are some exceptions. About one-third of malignant tumours at presentation have evident metastatic deposits while another 20% have occult metastasis.

Routes of Metastasis

Cancers may spread to distant sites by following pathways:
1. Lymphatic spread
2. Haematogenous spread
3. Spread along body cavities and natural passages (Transcoelomic spread, along epithelium-lined surfaces, spread via cerebrospinal fluid, implantation).

1. LYMPHATIC SPREAD *In general, carcinomas metastasise by lymphatic route while sarcomas favour haematogenous route.* However, some sarcomas may also spread by lymphatic pathway. The involvement of lymph nodes by malignant cells may be of two forms:

i) Lymphatic permeation The walls of lymphatics are readily invaded by cancer cells and may form a continuous growth in the lymphatic channels called lymphatic permeation.

ii) Lymphatic emboli Alternatively, the malignant cells may detach to form tumour emboli so as to be carried along the lymph to the next draining lymph node. The tumour emboli enter the lymph node at its convex surface and are lodged in the subcapsular sinus where they start growing **(Fig. 18.11)**. Later, of course, the whole lymph node may be replaced and enlarged by the metastatic tumour **(Fig. 18.12)**. A few characteristics of lymphatic spread of malignant tumors are as follows:

◆ Generally, regional lymph nodes draining the tumour are invariably involved producing *regional nodal metastasis* e.g. from carcinoma breast to axillary lymph nodes, from cancer of the thyroid to lateral cervical lymph nodes, bronchogenic carcinoma to hilar and para-tracheal lymph nodes etc.

◆ However, all regional nodal enlargements are not due to nodal metastasis because necrotic products of tumour and antigens may also incite regional lymphadenitis of *sinus histiocytosis.*

◆ Sometimes lymphatic metastases do not develop first in the lymph node nearest to the tumour because of venouslymphatic anastomoses or due to obliteration of lymphatics by inflammation or radiation, so called *skip metastasis.*

◆ Other times, due to obstruction of the lymphatics by tumour cells, the lymph flow is disturbed and tumour cells spread against the flow of lymph causing *retrograde metastases* at unusual sites e.g. metastasis of carcinoma prostate to the supraclavicular lymph nodes, metastatic deposits from bronchogenic carcinoma to the axillary lymph nodes.

◆ *Virchow's lymph node* is nodal metastasis preferentially to supraclavicular lymph node from cancers of abdominal organs e.g. cancer stomach, colon, and gallbladder.

Section IV: Neoplasia

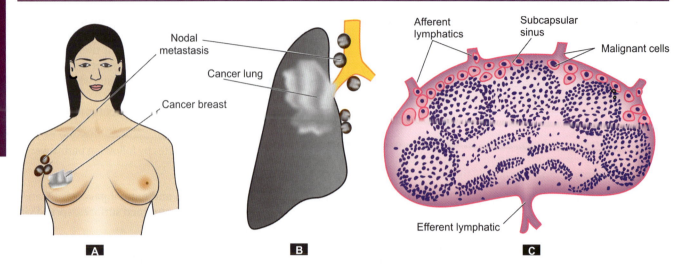

Figure 18.11 ▶ Regional nodal metastasis. A, Axillary nodes involved by carcinoma breast. B, Hilar and para-tracheal lymph nodes involved by bronchogenic carcinoma. C, Lymphatic spread begins by lodgement of tumour cells in subcapsular sinus via afferent lymphatics entering at the convex surface of the lymph node.

It is believed that lymph nodes in the vicinity of tumour perform multiple roles—as initial barrier filter, and in destruction of tumour cells, while later provide fertile soil for growth of tumour cells.

Mechanism of lymphatic route of metastasis is discussed later under biology of invasion and metastasis.

2. HAEMATOGENOUS SPREAD *Blood-borne metastasis is the common route for sarcomas but certain carcinomas also frequently metastasise by this mode,* especially those of the lung, breast, thyroid, kidney, liver, prostate and ovary. The sites where blood-borne metastasis commonly occurs are: the liver, lungs, brain, bones, kidney and adrenals, all of which provide 'good soil' for the growth of 'good seeds', i.e. *seed-soil theory* postulated by Ewing and Paget a century ago. However, a few organs such as the spleen, heart, and skeletal muscle generally do not allow tumour metastasis to grow. Spleen is unfavourable site due to open sinusoidal pattern which does

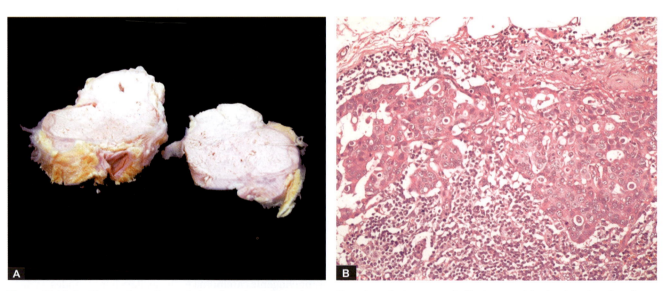

Figure 18.12 ▶ Metastatic carcinoma in lymph nodes. A, Matted mass of lymph nodes is surrounded by increased fat. Sectioned surface shows merging capsules of lymph nodes and replacement of grey brown tissue of nodes by large grey white areas of tumour. B, Masses of malignant cells are seen in the subcapsular sinus and extending into the underlying nodal tissue.

not permit tumour cells to stay there long enough to produce metastasis. In general, only a proportion of cancer cells are capable of clonal proliferation in the proper environment; others die without establishing a metastasis. A few features of haemogenous metastasis are as under:

i) *Systemic veins* drain blood into vena cavae from limbs, head and neck and pelvis. Therefore, cancers of these sites more often metastasise to the lungs.

ii) *Portal veins* drain blood from the bowel, spleen and pancreas into the liver. Thus, tumours of these organs frequently have secondaries in the liver.

iii) *Pulmonary veins* provide another route of spread of not only primary lung cancer but also metastatic growths in the lungs. Blood in the pulmonary veins carrying cancer cells from the lungs reaches left side of the heart and then into systemic circulation and thus may form secondary masses elsewhere in the body.

iv) *Arterial spread* of tumours is less likely because they are thick-walled and contain elastic tissue which is resistant to invasion. Nevertheless, arterial spread may occur when tumour cells pass through pulmonary capillary bed or through pulmonary arterial branches which have thin walls. However, cancers of the kidneys, adrenals, bones, limbs and uterus, which are drained by systemic veins, spread to the lungs via pulmonary artery.

v) *Retrograde spread* by blood route may occur at unusual sites due to retrograde spread after venous obstruction, just as with lymphatic metastases. Important examples are vertebral metastases in cancers of the thyroid and prostate.

Grossly, blood-borne metastases in an organ appear as multiple, rounded nodules of varying size, scattered throughout the organ (Fig. 18.13). Sometimes, the metastasis may grow bigger than the primary tumour. At times, metastatic deposits may come to attention first without an evident primary tumour. In such cases search for primary tumour may be rewarding, but rarely the primary tumour may remain undetected or occult. Metastatic deposits just like primary tumour may cause further dissemination via lymphatics and blood vessels (Fig. 18.14, A).

Microscopically, the secondary deposits generally reproduce the structure of primary tumour (Fig. 18.14, B). However, the same primary tumour on metastasis at different sites may show varying grades of differentiation, apparently due to the influence of local environment surrounding the tumour for its growth.

3. SPREAD ALONG BODY CAVITIES AND NATURAL PASSAGES
Uncommon routes of spread of some cancers are by *seeding* across body cavities and *natural passages* as under:

i) **Transcoelomic spread** Certain cancers invade through the serosal wall of the coelomic cavity so that tumour fragments or clusters of tumour cells break off to be carried in the coelomic fluid and are implanted elsewhere in the body cavity. Peritoneal cavity is involved most often, but occasionally pleural and pericardial cavities are also affected. A few examples of transcoelomic spread are as follows:

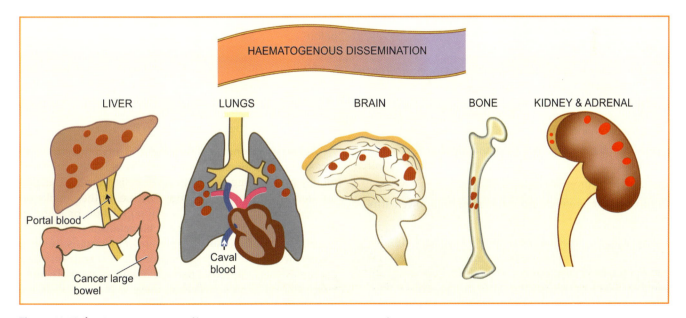

Figure 18.13 ▶ Gross appearance of haematogenous metastases at common sites.

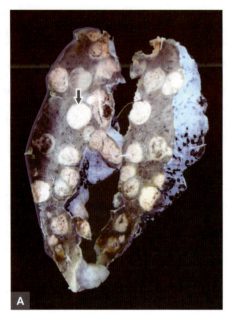 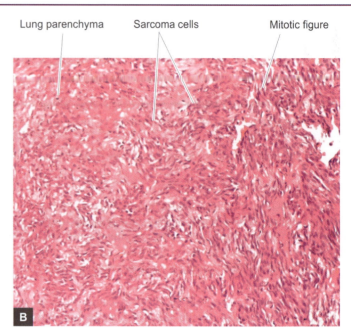

Figure 18.14 ▶ Metastatic sarcoma lung. A, Sectioned surface of the lung shows replacement of slaty-grey spongy parenchyma with multiple, firm, grey-white nodular masses, some having areas of haemorrhages and necrosis. B, Microscopic appearance of pulmonary metastatic deposits from sarcoma.

a) *Carcinoma of the stomach* seeding to both ovaries (Krukenberg tumour).

b) *Carcinoma of the ovary* spreading to the entire peritoneal cavity without infiltrating the underlying organs.

c) *Pseudomyxoma peritonei* is the gelatinous coating of the peritoneum from mucin-secreting carcinoma of the ovary or appendix.

d) *Carcinoma of the bronchus and breast* seeding to the pleura and pericardium.

ii) Spread along epithelium-lined surfaces It is unusual for a malignant tumour to spread along the epithelium-lined surfaces because intact epithelium and mucus coat are quite resistant to penetration by tumour cells. However, exceptionally a malignant tumour may spread through:

a) the fallopian tube from the endometrium to the ovaries or *vice-versa;*

b) through the bronchus into alveoli; and

c) through the ureters from the kidneys into lower urinary tract.

iii) Spread via cerebrospinal fluid Malignant tumour of the ependyma and leptomeninges may spread by release of tumour fragments and tumour cells into the CSF and produce metastases at other sites in the central nervous system.

iv) Implantation There are isolated and rare case reports of spread of some cancers by implantation by surgeon's scalpel, needles, sutures, and direct prolonged contact of cancer of the lower lip causing its implantation to the apposing upper lip.

MECHANISM AND BIOLOGY OF INVASION AND METASTASIS

The process of local invasion and distant spread by lymphatic and haematogenous routes (together called lymphovascular spread) discussed above involves passage through barriers before gaining access to the vascular lumen. This includes making the passage by the cancer cells by dissolution of extracellular matrix (ECM) at three levels—at the basement membrane of tumour itself, at the level of interstitial connective tissue, and at the basement membrane of microvasculature. The following sequential steps are involved which are schematically illustrated in Fig. 18.15.

1. Aggressive clonal proliferation and angiogenesis The first step in the spread of cancer cells is the development of rapidly proliferating clone of cancer cells. This is explained on the basis of *tumour heterogeneity*, i.e. in the population of monoclonal tumour cells, a subpopulation or clone of tumour cells has the right biologic characteristics to complete the steps involved in the development of metastasis. Tumour angiogenesis plays a very significant role in metastasis since the new vessels formed as part of growing tumour are more vulnerable to invasion because these evolving vessels are directly in contact with cancer cells.

2. Tumour cell loosening Normal cells remain glued to each other due to presence of cell adhesion molecules

Chapter 18: General Aspects of Neoplasia

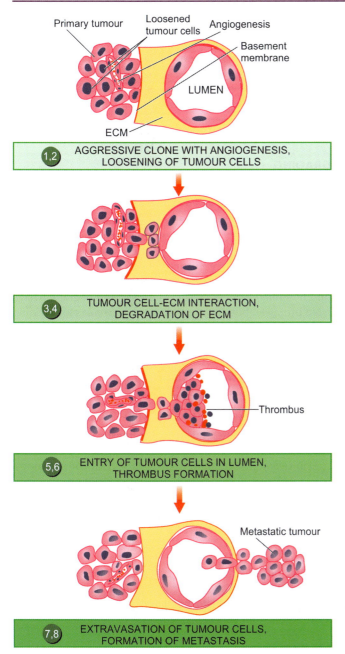

Figure 18.15 ▶ Mechanism and biology of local invasion and metastasis. The serial numbers in the figure correspond to their description in the text.

(CAMs) i.e. E (epithelial)-cadherin. In epithelial cancers, there is either loss or inactivation of E-cadherin and also other CAMs of immunoglobulin superfamily, all of which results in loosening of cancer cells.

3. Tumour cell-ECM interaction Loosened cancer cells are now attached to ECM proteins, mainly *laminin* and *fibronectin*. This attachment is facilitated due to profoundness of receptors on the cancer cells for both these proteins. There is also loss of *integrins*, the transmembrane receptors, further favouring invasion.

4. Degradation of ECM Tumour cells overexpress *proteases* and matrix-degrading enzymes, *metalloproteinases* (e.g. collagenases and gelatinase), while the inhibitors of metalloproteinases are decreased. Another protease, cathepsin D, is also increased in certain cancers. These enzymes bring about dissolution of ECM—firstly basement membrane of tumour itself, then make way for tumour cells through the interstitial matrix, and finally dissolve the basement membrane of the vessel wall.

5. Entry of tumour cells into capillary lumen The tumour cells after degrading the basement membrane are ready to migrate into lumen of capillaries or venules for which the following mechanisms play a role:
i) *Autocrine motility factor (AMF)*, a cytokine derived from tumour cells which stimulates receptor-mediated motility of tumour cells.
ii) *Cleavage products of matrix components* which are formed following degradation of ECM have properties of tumour cell chemotaxis, growth promotion and angiogenesis in the cancer.

After the malignant cells have migrated through the breached basement membrane, these cells enter the lumen of lymphatic and capillary channels.

6. Thrombus formation The tumour cells protruding in the lumen of the capillary are now covered with constituents of the circulating blood and form the thrombus. Thrombus provides nourishment to the tumour cells and also protects them from the immune attack by the circulating host cells. In fact, normally a large number of tumour cells are released into circulation but they are attacked by the host immune cells. Actually a very small proportion of malignant cells (less than 0.1%) in the blood stream survive to develop into metastasis.

7. Extravasation of tumour cells Tumour cells in the circulation (capillaries, venules, lymphatics) may mechanically block these vascular channels and attach to vascular endothelium and then extravasate to the extravascular space. In this way, the sequence similar to local invasion is repeated and the basement membrane is exposed.

8. Survival and growth of metastatic deposit The extravasated malignant cells on lodgement in the right environment grow further under the influence of growth factors produced by host tissues, tumour cells and by cleavage products of matrix components. Some of the growth promoting factors are: PDGF, FGF, TGF-β and VEGF. The metastatic deposits grow further if the host immune defense mechanism fails to eliminate it. Metastatic deposits may further metastasise to the same organ or to other sites by forming emboli.

PROGNOSTIC INDICATORS

Metastasis is a common event in malignant tumours which greatly reduces the survival of the patient. In the biology of tumour, metastasis is a form of unusual cell differentiation in which the tumour cells form disorderly masses at ectopic sites and start growing there. This random phenomenon takes place in a stepwise manner involving only a subpopulation of tumour cells selectively. The process is governed by *inappropriate expression of genes which normally partake in physiologic processes* i.e. it is a genetically programmed phenomenon.

Recent evidence has shown that in metastatic tumours, survival of host is correlated with some clinical and molecular features of tumours which act as *prognostic markers*. These are as under:

i) Clinical prognostic markers: Size, histologic grade, nodal involvement and vascular invasion by the tumour.

ii) Molecular prognostic markers: Molecular markers indicative of poor prognosis in certain specific tumours are as follows:
a) expression of an oncogene by tumour cells *(C-met)*
b) CD 44 molecule
c) Oestrogen receptors
d) Epidermal growth factor receptor
e) Angiogenesis factors and degree of neovascularisation
f) Expression of *metastasis associated gene for nucleic acid* (MAGNA) in the DNA fragment in metastasising tumour.

> **GIST BOX 18.3 Spread and Prognosis of Cancer**
>
> ❖ Malignant tumours invade and destroy adjoining tissues (local invasion or direct spread) and disseminate to distant sites (metastasis or distant spread).
> ❖ Cancers spread to distant sites commonly by lymphatic or haematogenous route, and less commonly along body cavities (transcoelomic spread) and via natural passages (e.g. along bronchus, fallopian tubes, ureters, CSF etc).
> ❖ Carcinomas metastasise more commonly by lymphatic route while sarcomas favour haematogenous route.
> ❖ Common sites of lymphatic metastasis are the regional nodes, while blood-borne metastases are common in the liver, lungs, bones, brain, kidneys and adrenals.
> ❖ Mechanism of direct invasion and metastasis involves passage of cancer cells through the extracellular matrix in the interstitial tissue, basement membranes of the tumour and of the vessel wall.
> ❖ Prognosis of tumours can be assessed by certain general clinical parameters and some molecular tests pertaining to specific tumours.

GRADING AND STAGING OF CANCER

'Grading' and 'staging' are the two systems to predict tumour behaviour and guide therapy after a malignant tumour is detected. *Grading is defined as the gross appearance and microscopic degree of differentiation of the tumour, while staging means extent of spread of the tumour within the patient.* Thus, grading is done on pathologic basis while staging is on clinical grounds.

GRADING

Cancers may be graded grossly and microscopically. Gross features like exophytic or fungating appearance are indicative of less malignant growth than diffusely infiltrating tumours. However, grading is largely based on 2 important histologic features: *the degree of anaplasia, and the rate of growth.* Based on these features, cancers are categorised from grade I as the most differentiated, to grade III or IV as the most undifferentiated or anaplastic. Many systems of grading have been proposed but the one described by *Broders* for dividing squamous cell carcinoma into 4 grades depending upon the degree of differentiation is followed for other malignant tumours as well. *Broders' grading* is as under:

Grade I: Well-differentiated (less than 25% anaplastic cells)

Grade II: Moderately-differentiated (25-50% anaplastic cells)

Grade III: Moderately-differentiated (50-75% anaplastic cells)

Grade IV: Poorly-differentiated or anaplastic (more than 75% anaplastic cells)

However, grading of tumours has several shortcomings. It is subjective and the degree of differentiation may vary from one area of tumour to the other. Therefore, it is common practice with pathologists to grade cancers in descriptive terms (e.g. well-differentiated, undifferentiated, keratinising, non-keratinising etc) rather than giving the tumours grade numbers.

More objective criteria for histologic grading include use of flow cytometry for mitotic cell counts, cell proliferation markers by immunohistochemistry, and by applying image morphometry for cancer cell and nuclear parameters.

STAGING

The extent of spread of cancers can be assessed by 3 ways— by clinical examination, by investigations, and by pathologic examination of the tissue removed. Two important staging systems currently followed are: TNM staging and AJC staging.

TNM staging TNM staging (T for primary *t*umour, N for regional *n*odal involvement, and M for distant *m*etastases) was developed by the UICC (Union InternationaleContre Cancer, Geneva). For each of the 3 components namely T, N and M, numbers are added to indicate the extent of involvement, as under:

T0 to T4: In situ lesion to largest and most extensive primary tumour.

N0 to N3: No nodal involvement to widespread lymph node involvement.

M0 to M2: No metastasis to disseminated haematogenous metastases.

AJC staging American Joint Committee staging divides all cancers into stage 0 to IV, and takes into account all the 3 components of the preceding system (primary tumour, nodal involvement and distant metastases) in each stage.

TNM and AJC staging systems can be applied for staging of most malignant tumours.

Currently, clinical staging of tumours does not rest on routine radiography (X-ray, ultrasound) and exploratory surgery but more modern techniques are available by which it is possible to 'stage' a malignant tumour by these non-invasive techniques. These include use of modern imaging techniques such as *computed tomography (CT)* and *magnetic resonance imaging (MRI)* scan based on tissue density for locating the local extent of tumour and its spread to other organs. Availability of *positron emission tomography (PET)* scan has further overcome the limitation of CT and MRI scan because PET scan facilitates distinction of benign and malignant tumour on the basis of biochemical and molecular processes in tumours. *Radioactive tracer studies in vivo* such as use of iodine isotope 125 bound to specific tumour antibodies is another method by which small number of tumour cells in the body can be detected by imaging of tracer substance bound to specific tumour antigen.

| GIST BOX 18.4 | Grading and Staging of Cancer |

- Grading of tumours is done on pathologic examination and includes the gross appearance and microscopic degree of differentiation of the tumour (e.g. well differentiated, poorly-differentiated).
- Staging of the cancer is clinical and it means the extent of spread of tumour within the patient (e.g. TNM staging, AJC staging).

19 Etiology and Pathogenesis of Neoplasia

EPIDEMIOLOGY OF CANCER

CANCER INCIDENCE

The overall incidence of cancer in a population or a country is known by registration of all cancer cases (cancer registry) and by rate of death from cancer. Worldwide, it is estimated that about 20% of all deaths are cancer-related; in US, cancer is the second most common cause of deaths, next to heart disease. There have been changing patterns in incidence of cancers in both the sexes and in different geographic locations as outlined here. Table 19.1 shows worldwide incidence (in descending order) of 5 most common cancers in men, women, and children. Due to varying etiologic factors, cancers of the cervix and oral cavity are more common in India while cancers of the breast and lung are commoner in the Western populations.

In general, most common cancers in the developed and developing countries are as under:
◆ *Developed countries:* lung, breast, prostate and colorectal.
◆ *Developing countries:* liver, cervix, oral cavity and oesophagus.

About one-third of all cancers worldwide are attributed to 9 *modifiable life-style factors*: tobacco use, alcohol consumption, obesity, physical inactivity, low fiber diet, unprotected sex, polluted air, indoor household smoke, and contaminated injections. Overall, there has been a declining trend in incidence of some of the cancers due to cancer screening programmes e.g. for cancers of the cervix, breast, colorectal region and prostate.

EPIDEMIOLOGIC FACTORS

A lot of clinical and experimental research and epidemiological studies have been carried out in the field of oncology so as to know the possible causes of cancer and mechanisms involved in transformation of a normal cell into a neoplastic cell. It is widely known that no single factor is responsible for development of tumours. The role of some factors in causation of neoplasia is established while that of others is epidemiological and many others are still unknown.

Besides the etiologic role of some agents discussed later, the pattern and incidence of cancer depends upon the following:
A) *Predisposing epidemiologic factors or cofactors* which include a number of endogenous host factors and exogenous environmental factors
B) *Chronic non-neoplastic (pre-malignant) conditions*
C) *Role of hormones in cancer*

The role of these aspects in cancer epidemiology is briefly discussed below.

A. Predisposing Factors

1. FAMILIAL AND GENETIC FACTORS It has long been suspected that familial predisposition and heredity play a role in the development of cancers. In general, the risk of developing cancer in relatives of a known cancer patient is almost three times higher as compared to control subjects. Some of the cancers with familial occurrence are colon, breast, ovary, brain and melanoma. Familial cancers occur at a relatively early age, appear at multiple sites and occur in 2 or more first-degree blood relatives. The overall estimates suggest that genetic cancers comprise about 5% of all cancers. Some of the common examples are as under:

i) Retinoblastoma About 40% of retinoblastomas are familial and show an autosomal dominant inheritance. Carriers of such genetic composition have 10,000 times higher risk of developing retinoblastoma which is often bilateral. Such patients are further predisposed to develop another primary malignant tumour, notably osteogenic sarcoma.

Familial form of retinoblastoma is due to missing of a portion of chromosome 13 where *RB* gene is normally located. In fact, genetic absence of *RB* gene was the first ever tumour suppressor gene identified. Absence of a single copy of *RB* gene predisposes an individual to retinoblastoma and the tumour develops when other copy of *RB* gene from the second parent is also defective.

ii) Adenomatous polyposis coli (APC) This condition has autosomal dominant inheritance. The polypoid adenomas may be seen at birth or in early age. By the age of 50 years,

Table 19.1	Five most common primary cancers in the world.	
	MEN	WOMEN	CHILDREN (UNDER 20)
1.	Prostate (oral cavity in India)	Breast (cervix in India)	Acute leukaemia
2.	Lung	Lung	Gliomas
3.	Colorectal	Colorectal	Bone sarcoma
4.	Urinary bladder	Endometrial	Endocrine
5.	Lymphoma	Lymphoma	Soft tissue sarcoma

almost 100% cases of familial polyposis coli develop cancer of the colon.

iii) Multiple endocrine neoplasia (MEN) A combination of adenomas of pituitary, parathyroid and pancreatic islets (MEN-I) or syndrome of medullary carcinoma thyroid, pheochromocytoma and parathyroid tumour (MEN-II) are encountered in families.

iv) Neurofibromatosis (von Recklinghausen's disease) This condition is characterised by multiple neurofibromas and pigmented skin spots (*cafe aü lait spots*). These patients have family history consistent with autosomal dominant inheritance in 50% of patients.

v) Cancer of the breast Female relatives of breast cancer patients have 2 to 6 times higher risk of developing breast cancer. Inherited breast cancer comprises about 5-10% of all breast cancers. As discussed later, there are two breast cancer susceptibility genes, *BRCA-1* and *BRCA-2*. Mutations in these genes appear in about 3% cases and these patients have about 85% risk of development of breast cancer.

vi) Congenital chromosomal syndromes For example,

a) Down's syndrome or mongolism has trisomy 21; these cases have increased risk of development of acute leukaemia.

b) Klinefelter syndrome associated with an extra X chromosome (47, XXY) has high risk of developing cancer of male breast and extra-gonadal germ cell tumours.

vii) DNA-chromosomal instability syndromes These are a group of pre-neoplastic conditions having defect in DNA repair mechanism. A classical example is xeroderma pigmentosum, an autosomal recessive disorder, characterised by extreme sensitivity to ultraviolet radiation. The patients may develop various types of skin cancers such as basal cell carcinoma, squamous cell carcinoma and malignant melanoma.

2. RACIAL AND GEOGRAPHIC FACTORS Differences in racial incidence of some cancers may be partly attributed to the role of genetic composition but are largely due to influence of the environment and geographic differences affecting the whole population such as climate, soil, water, diet, habits, customs etc. Some of the examples of racial and geographic variations in various cancers are as under:

i) White Europeans and Americans develop most commonly malignancies of the prostate, lung, breast, skin and colorectal region. Liver cancer is uncommon in these races.

ii) Black Africans, on the other hand, have more commonly cancers of the penis, cervix and liver.

iii) Japanese have five times higher incidence of carcinoma of the stomach than the Americans. Breast cancer is uncommon in Japanese women than American women.

iv) South-East Asians, especially of Chinese origin, develop nasopharyngeal cancer more commonly.

v) Indians of both sexes have higher incidence of carcinoma of the oral cavity and upper aerodigestive tract, while in females carcinoma of uterine cervix and of the breast run parallel in incidence. Etiologic factor responsible for liver cancer in India is more often viral hepatitis (HBV and HCV) and subsequent cirrhosis, while in western populations it is more often due to alcoholic cirrhosis.

3. ENVIRONMENTAL AND CULTURAL FACTORS It may seem rather surprising that through out our life we are surrounded by an environment of carcinogens which we eat, drink, inhale and touch. Some of the examples are given below:

i) Cigarette smoking (as well as passive inhalation) is the single most important environmental factor implicated in the etiology of cancer of the lung, oral cavity, pharynx, larynx, nasal cavity and paranasal sinuses, oesophagus, stomach, pancreas, liver, kidney, urinary bladder, uterine cervix and myeloid leukaemia.

ii) Alcohol abuse predisposes to the development of cancer of oropharynx, larynx, oesophagus and liver.

iii) Synergistic interaction of alcohol and tobacco further accentuates the risk of developing cancer of the upper aerodigestive tract and lung.

iv) Cancer of the cervix is linked to a number of factors such as age at first coitus, frequency of coitus, multiplicity of partners, parity etc. Sexual partners of circumcised males have lower incidence of cervical cancer than the partners of uncircumcised males.

v) Penile cancer is rare in the Jews and Muslims as they are customarily circumcised. Carcinogenic component of smegma appears to play a role in the etiology of penile cancer.

vi) Betel nut cancer of the cheek and tongue is quite common in some parts of India due to habitual practice of keeping the bolus of *paan* in a particular place in mouth for a long time.

vii) A large number of **industrial and environmental substances** are carcinogenic and are occupational hazard for some populations. These include exposure to substances like arsenic, asbestos, benzene, vinyl chloride, naphthylamine etc.

viii) Certain constituents of diet have also been implicated in the causation of cancer. Overweight individuals, deficiency of vitamin A and people consuming diet rich in animal fats and low in fibre content are more at risk of developing certain cancers such as colonic cancer. Diet rich in vitamin E, on the other hand, possibly has some protective influence by its antioxidant action.

4. AGE The most significant risk factor for cancer is age. Generally, cancers occur in older individuals past 5th decade of life (two-third of all cancers occur above 65 years of age), though there are variations in age incidence in different forms of cancers. Higher incidence of cancer in advanced age could be due to alteration in the cells of the host, longer exposure to the effect of carcinogen, or decreased ability of the host immune response. Some tumours have two peaks of incidence e.g. acute leukaemias occur in children and in older age group. The biologic behaviour of tumours in children does not always correlate with histologic features. Besides acute leukaemias, *other tumours in infancy and childhood* are: neuroblastoma, nephroblastoma (Wilms' tumour), retinoblastoma, hepatoblastoma, rhabdomyosarcoma, Ewing's sarcoma, teratoma and CNS tumours.

5. SEX Apart from the malignant tumours of organs peculiar to each sex, most tumours are generally more common in men than in women except cancer of the breast, gallbladder, thyroid and hypopharynx. Although there are geographic and racial variations, *cancer of the breast* is the commonest cancer in *women* throughout the world while *lung cancer* is the commonest cancer in *men*. The differences in incidence of certain cancers in the two sexes may be related to the presence of specific sex hormones.

B. Chronic Pre-malignant and Non-neoplastic Conditions

Premalignant lesions are a group of conditions which predispose to the subsequent development of cancer. Such conditions are important to recognise so as to prevent the subsequent occurrence of an invasive cancer. Many of these conditions are characterised by morphologic changes in the cells such as increased nuclear-cytoplasmic ratio, pleomorphism of cells and nuclei, increased mitotic activity, poor differentiation, and sometimes accompanied by chronic inflammatory cells.

Some examples of premalignant lesions are given below:

1. Dysplasia and carcinoma *in situ* (intraepithelial neoplasia) As discussed in Chapter 3, dyspalsia is abnormality in cellular features and may be of varying severity (mild, moderate and marked). Most marked cytological atypia confined to epithelial layers above the basement membrane without invading the basement membrane is called as carcinoma *in situ* or intraepithelial neoplasia (CIN). The common sites are as under:
i)   Uterine cervix at the junction of ecto- and endocervix (Fig. 19.1)
ii) Bronchus
iii) Bowen's disease of the skin
iv) Actinic or solar keratosis
v)   Oral leukoplakia
vi) Barrett's oesophagus developing metaplasia and dysplasia
vii) Intralobular and intraductal carcinoma of the breast.

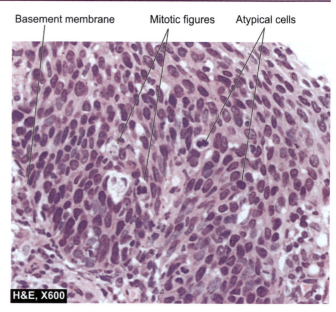

Figure 19.1 ▶ Carcinoma *in situ* of uterine cervix. The atypical dysplastic squamous cells are confined to all the layers of the mucosa but the basement membrane on which these layers rest is intact.

The area involved in carcinoma *in situ* may be single and small, or multifocal. As regards the behaviour of CIN, it may regress and return to normal or may develop into invasive cancer. In some instances such as in cervical cancer, there is a sequential transformation from squamous metaplasia, to epithelial dysplasia, to carcinoma *in situ,* and eventually to invasive cancer.

2. Some benign tumours Commonly, benign tumours do not become malignant. However, there are some exceptions e.g.
i) Multiple adenomas of the large intestine (adenomatous polyposis coli) have high incidence of developing adenocarcinoma.
ii) Neurofibromatosis (von Recklinghausen's disease) may develop into sarcoma.
iii) Pleomorphic adenoma (mixed salivary tumour) may sometimes develop carcinoma (carcinoma e*x*pleomophic adenoma).

3. Miscellaneous conditions Certain inflammatory (both infectious and non-infectious) and hyperplastic conditions are prone to development of cancer, e.g.
i) HPV-induced chronic cervicitis has high risk of developing cervical cancer.
ii) Patients of long-standing ulcerative colitis are predisposed to develop colorectal cancer.
iii) Cirrhosis of the liver has predisposition to develop hepatocellular carcinoma.
iv) *H. pylori* gastritits developing gastric cancer and lymphoma.

v) Chronic bronchitis in heavy cigarette smokers may develop cancer of the bronchus.
vi) Chronic irritation from jagged tooth or ill-fitting denture may lead to cancer of the oral cavity.
vii) Squamous cell carcinoma developing in an old burn scar (Marjolin's ulcer).

C. Hormones and Cancer

Cancer is more likely to develop in organs and tissues which undergo proliferation under the influence of excessive hormonal stimulation. On cessation of hormonal stimulation, such tissues become atrophic. Hormone-sensitive tissues developing tumours are the breast, endometrium, myometrium, vagina, thyroid, liver, prostate and testis. Some examples of hormones influencing carcinogenesis in experimental animals and humans are given below:

1. **OESTROGEN** Examples of oestrogen-induced cancers are as under:

i) In experimental animals Induction of breast cancer in mice by administration of high-dose of oestrogen and reduction of the tumour development following oophorectomy is the most important example. It has been known that associated infection with mouse mammary tumour virus (MMTV or *Bittner milk factor*) has an added influence on the development of breast cancer in mice. Other cancers which can be experimentally induced in mice by oestrogens are squamous cell carcinoma of the cervix, connective tissue tumour of the myometrium, Leydig cell tumour of the testis in male mice, tumour of the kidney in hamsters, and benign as well as malignant tumours of the liver in rats.

ii) In humans Women receiving oestrogen therapy and women with oestrogen-secreting granulosa cell tumour of the ovary have increased risk of developing endometrial carcinoma. Adenocarcinoma of the vagina is seen with increased frequency in adolescent daughters of mothers who had received oestrogen therapy during pregnancy.

2. **CONTRACEPTIVE HORMONES** The sequential types of oral contraceptives increase the risk of developing breast cancer. Other tumours showing a slightly increased frequency in women receiving contraceptive pills for long durations are benign tumours of the liver, and a few patients have been reported to have developed hepatocellular carcinoma.

3. **ANABOLIC STEROIDS** Consumption of anabolic steroids by athletes to increase the muscle mass is not only unethical athletic practice but also increases the risk of developing benign and malignant tumours of the liver.

4. **HORMONE-DEPENDENT TUMOURS** It has been shown in experimental animals that induction of hyperfunction of adenohypophysis is associated with increased risk of developing neoplasia of the target organs following preceding functional hyperplasia. There is tumour regression on removal of the stimulus for excessive hormonal secretion. A few examples of such phenomena are seen in humans:

i) *Prostatic cancer* usually responds to the administration of oestrogens.
ii) *Breast cancer* may regress with oophorectomy, hypophysectomy or on administration of male hormones.
iii) *Thyroid cancer* may slow down in growth with administration of thyroxine that suppresses the secretion of TSH by the pituitary.

GIST BOX 19.1 Epidemiology and Predisposition to Neoplasia

- In general, most common cancers in the developed countries are lung, breast, prostate and colorectal, and in developing countries are liver, cervix, oral cavity and oesophagus.
- Several factors predispose to occurrence of cancers. These are: familial and genetic factors, racial and geographic factors, environmental and cultural factors, age and sex.
- Carcinoma in situ of some sites such as uterine cervix, bronchus, skin, oral cavity etc may progress to cancer and are thus premalignant conditions.
- A few benign conditions may predispose to cancer e.g. colorectal adenomas, neurofibromatosis.
- Some long-standing inflammatory and hyperplastic conditions may develop to cancers e.g. ulcerative colitis, cirrhosis, old burn scar etc.
- High levels of some hormones have a role in predisposition to cancer e.g. hyperoestrogenism associated with higher risk of endometrial cancer, oral contraceptives in breast cancer, testosterone in prostate cancer etc.

MOLECULAR PATHOGENESIS OF CANCER

The mechanism as to how a normal cell is transformed to a cancer cell is complex. At different times, attempts have been made to unravel this mystery by various mechanisms. Currently, a lot of literature continues to accumulate on the pathogenesis of cancer at molecular level.

Before discussing the detailed mechanisms, a general basic concept of cancer at molecular level is briefly outlined below and diagrammatically shown in *Fig. 19.2*.

1. **Monoclonality of tumours** There is strong evidence to support that most human cancers arise from a single clone of cells by genetic transformation or mutation. For example:
i) In a case of multiple myeloma (a malignant disorder of plasma cells), there is production of a single type of immunoglobulin or its chain as seen by monoclonal spike in serum electrophoresis.
ii) Due to inactivation of one of the two X-chromosomes in females (paternal or maternal derived), normal myometrial

Section IV: Neoplasia

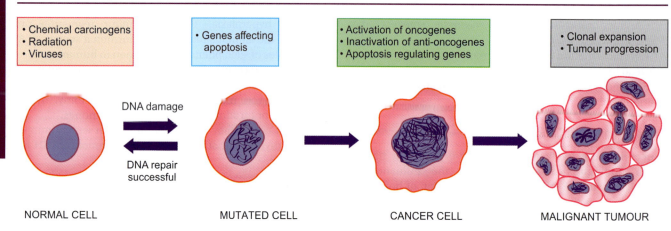

Figure 19.2 ▶ Schematic illustration to show molecular basis of cancer.

cells in the uterus are mosaics with two types of cell populations for glucose-6-phosphatase dehydrogenase (G6PD) isoenzyme A and B. It is observed that all the tumour cells in benign uterine tumours (leiomyoma) contain either A or B genotype of G6PD (i.e. the tumour cells are derived from a single progenitor clone of cell), while the normal myometrial cells are mosaic of both types of cells derived from A as well as B isoenzyme **(Fig. 19.3)**.

2. Field theory of cancer In an organ developing cancer, in the backdrop of normal cells, limited number of cells only grow in to cancer after undergoing sequence of changes under the influence of etiologic agents. This is termed as 'field effect' and the concept called as field theory of cancer.

3. Multi-step process of cancer growth and progression Carcinogenesis is a gradual multi-step process involving many generations of cells. The various etiologic agents may act on the cell one after another (*multi-hit process*). The same process is also involved in further progression of the tumour. Ultimately, the cells so formed are genetically and phenotypically transformed cells having phenotypic features of malignancy—excessive growth, invasiveness and distant metastasis.

4. Genetic theory of cancer Cell growth of normal as well as abnormal types is under genetic control. In cancer, there are either genetic abnormalities in the cell, or there are normal genes with abnormal expression. Thus, the abnormalities in genetic composition may be from inherited or induced mutations (induced by etiologic carcinogenic agents namely: chemicals, viruses, radiation). Eventually, the mutated cells transmit their characters to the next progeny of cells and result in cancer.

5. Genetic regulators of normal and abnormal mitosis In normal cell growth, regulatory genes control mitosis as well as cell ageing, terminating in cell death by apoptosis.

◈ **In normal cell growth,** there are 4 regulatory genes:
i) Proto-oncogenes are growth-promoting genes i.e. they encode for cell proliferation pathway.

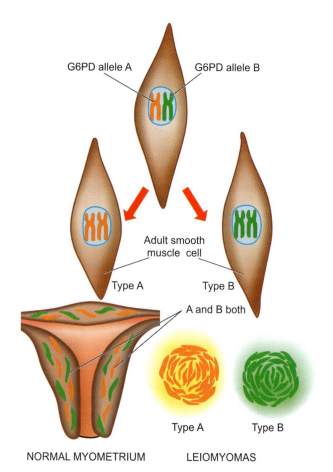

Figure 19.3 ▶ The monoclonal origin of tumour cells in uterine leiomyoma.

ii) Anti-oncogenes are growth-inhibiting or growth suppressor genes.
iii) Apoptosis regulatory genes control the programmed cell death.
iv) DNA repair genes are those normal genes which regulate the repair of DNA damage that has occurred during mitosis and also control the damage to proto-oncogenes and anti-oncogenes.

◈ **In cancer,** the transformed cells are produced by abnormal cell growth due to genetic damage to these normal controlling genes. Thus, corresponding abnormalities in these 4 cell regulatory genes are as under:
i) Activation of growth-promoting oncogenes causing transformation of cell (mutant form of normal proto-oncogene in cancer is termed *oncogene*). Many of these cancer associated genes, oncogenes, were first discovered in viruses, and hence named as *v-onc*. Gene products of oncogenes are called *oncoproteins*. Oncogenes are considered *dominant* since they appear in spite of presence of normal proto-oncogenes.
ii) Inactivation of cancer-suppressor genes (i.e. inactivation of anti-oncogenes) permitting the cellular proliferation of transformed cells. Anti-oncogenes are active in *recessive* form i.e. they are active only if both alleles are damaged.
iii) Abnormal apoptosis regulatory genes which may act as oncogenes or anti-oncogenes. Accordingly, these genes may be active in dominant or recessive form.
iv) Failure of DNA repair genes and thus inability to repair the DNA damage resulting in mutations.

CANCER-RELATED GENES AND CELL GROWTH (HALLMARKS OF CANCER)

It is apparent from the above discussion that genes control the normal cellular growth, while in cancer these controlling genes are altered, typically by mutations. A large number of such cancer-associated genes have been described, each with a specific function in cell growth. Some of these genes are common in many tumours (e.g. *p53* or *TP53*), while others are specific to particular tumours. Therefore, following discussion correlates the role of cancer-related genes with regard to their functions in normal cellular growth.

Genetic basis of cancer includes following *major genetic properties,* also termed as *molecular hallmarks of cancer*:
1. Excessive and autonomous growth: Growth-promoting oncogenes.
2. Refractoriness to growth inhibition: Growth suppressing anti-oncogenes.
3. Escaping cell death by apoptosis: Genes regulating apoptosis and cancer.
4. Avoiding cellular ageing: Telomeres and telomerase in cancer.
5. Continued perfusion of cancer: Cancer angiogenesis.
6. Invasion and distant metastasis: Cancer dissemination.
7. DNA damage and repair system: Mutator genes and cancer.
8. Cancer progression and tumour heterogeneity: Clonal aggressiveness.
9. Cancer a sequential multistep molecular phenomenon: Multistep theory.
10. MicroRNAs in cancer: OncomiRs.

These properties of cancer cells are schematically shown in **Fig. 19.4** and discussed below.

1. Excessive and Autonomous Growth: Growth Promoting Oncogenes

Mutated form of normal protooncogenes in cancer is called oncogenes. In general, overactivity of oncogenes enhances cell proliferation and promotes development of human cancer. About 100 different oncogenes have been described in various cancers. Transformation of proto-oncogene (i.e. normal cell proliferation gene) to oncogenes (i.e. cancer cell proliferation gene) may occur by three mechanisms:

i) Point mutations i.e. an alteration of a single base in the DNA chain. The most important example is *RAS* oncogene carried in many human tumours such as bladder cancer, pancreatic adenocarcinoma, cholangiocarcinoma.

ii) Chromosomal translocations i.e. transfer of a portion of one chromosome carrying protooncogene to another chromosome and making it independent of growth controls. This is implicated in the pathogenesis of leukaemias and lymphomas e.g.
◈ Philadelphia chromosome seen in 95% cases of chronic myelogenous leukaemia in which *c-ABL* protooncogene on chromosome 9 is translocated to BCR of chromosome 22.
◈ In 75% cases of Burkitt's lymphoma, translocation of *c-MYC* proto-oncogene from its site on chromosome 8 to a portion on chromosome 14.

iii) Gene amplification i.e. increasing the number of copies of DNA sequence in protooncogene leading to increased mRNA and thus increased or overexpressed gene product (i.e. oncoproteins). Examples of gene amplification are found in some solid human tumours e.g.
◈ Neuroblastoma having *n-MYC HSR* region.
◈ *ERB-B2* in breast and ovarian cancer.

Most of the oncogenes encode for components of cell signaling system for promoting cell proliferation. Accordingly, these are discussed below under following 5 groups pertaining to different components of cell proliferation signaling systems **(Table 19.2)** and are schematically shown in **Fig. 19.5**:
i) Growth factors
ii) Receptors of growth factors
iii) Cytoplasmic signal transduction proteins
iv) Nuclear transduction factors
v) Cell regulatory proteins

i) Growth factors (GFs) GFs were the first protooncogenes to be discovered which encode for cell proliferation cascade.

Section IV: Neoplasia

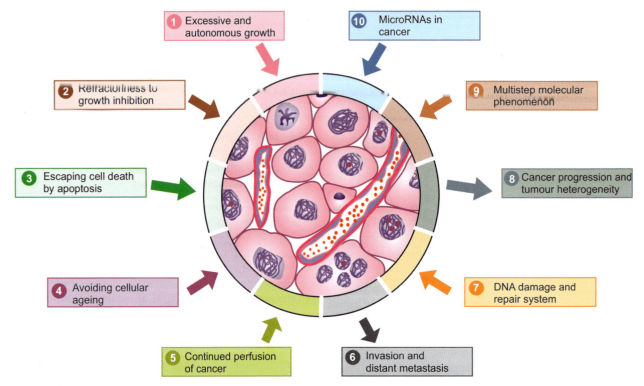

Figure 19.4 ▶ Schematic representation of major properties of cancer in terms of molecular carcinogenesis.

They act by binding to cell surface receptors to activate cell proliferation cascade within the cell. GFs are small polypeptides elaborated by many cells and they normally act on another cell than the one which synthesised it to stimulate its proliferation i.e. *paracrine action*. However, a cancer cell may synthesise a GF and respond to it as well; this way cancer cells acquire growth self-sufficiency.

Most often, growth factor genes in cancer act by overexpression which stimulates large secretion of GFs that stimulate cell proliferation. The examples of such GFs are as under:

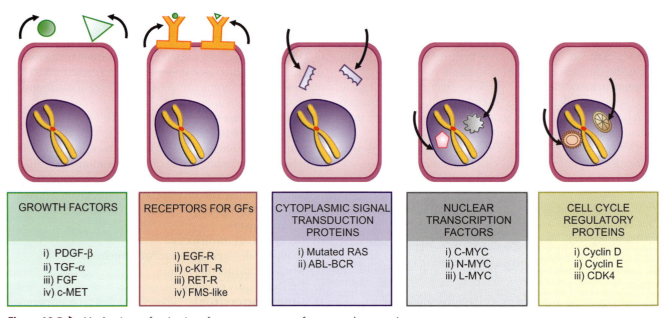

Figure 19.5 ▶ Mechanisms of activation of protooncogenes to form growth promoting oncogenes.

Chapter 19: Etiology and Pathogenesis of Neoplasia

Table 19.2 Important oncogenes, their mechanism of activation and associated human tumours.

	TYPE	PROTO-ONCOGENE	MECHANISM	ASSOCIATED HUMAN TUMOURS
1.	**GROWTH FACTORS**			
	i) PDGF-β	SIS	Overexpression	Gliomas, sarcoma
	ii) TGF-α	RAS	Overexpression	Carcinomas, astrocytoma
	iii) FGF	HST-1	Overexpression	Bowel cancers
		INT-2	Amplification	Breast cancer
	iv) c-MET	HGF	Overexpression	Follicular carcinoma thyroid
2.	**RECEPTORS FOR GROWTH FACTORS**			
	i) EGF receptors	ERB B1 (HER 1)	Overexpression	Squamous cell carcinoma lung, glioblastoma
		ERB B2 (HER 2/neu)	Amplification	Ca breast, ovary, stomach, lungs
	ii) c-KIT receptor (Steel factor)	c-KIT	Point mutation	GIST
	iii) RET receptor	RET	Point mutation	MEN type 2A and type 2B, medullary Ca thyroid
	iv) FMS-like tyrosine kinase receptor	FLT-3 gene	Point mutation	Acute myeloid leukaemia
3.	**CYTOPLASMIC SIGNAL TRANSDUCTION PROTEINS**			
	GTP-bound	RAS	Point mutation	Common in 1/3rd human tumours, Ca lung, colon, pancreas
	Non-GF receptor tyrosine kinase	ABL-BCR	Translocation	CML, acute leukaemias
4.	**NUCLEAR TRANSCRIPTION FACTORS**			
	C-MYC	MYC	Translocation	Burkitt's lymphoma
	N-MYC	MYC	Amplification	Neuroblastoma, small cell Ca lung
	L-MYC	MYC	Amplification	Small cell Ca lung
5.	**CELL CYCLE REGULATORY PROTEINS**			
	Cyclins	Cyclin D	Translocation	Ca breast, liver, mantle cell lymphoma
		Cyclin E	Overexpression	Ca breast
	CDKs	CDK4	Amplification	Glioblastoma, melanoma, sarcomas

a) Platelet-derived growth factor-β (PDGF-β): Overexpression of *SIS* protooncogene that encodes for *PDGF-β* and thus there is increased secretion of *PDGF-β* e.g. in gliomas and sarcomas.

b) Transforming growth factor-α (TGF-α): Overexpression of *TGF-β* gene occurs by stimulation of *RAS* protooncogene and induces cell proliferation by binding to epidermal growth factor *(EGF)* receptor e.g. in carcinoma and astrocytoma.

c) Fibroblast growth factor (FGF): Overexpression of *HST-1* protooncogene and amplification of *INT-2* protoonogene causes excess secretion of *FGF* e.g. in cancer of the bowel and breast.

d) Hepatocyte growth factor (HGF): Overexpression by binding to its receptor *c-MET* e.g. follicular carcinoma thyroid.

ii) Receptors for GFs Growth factors cannot penetrate the cell directly and require to be transported intracellularly by GF-specific cell surface receptors. These receptors are transmembrane proteins and thus have two surfaces: the outer surface of the membrane has an area for binding growth factor, and the inner surface of the membrane has enzyme-activating area which eventually activates cell proliferation pathway.

Most often, mutated form of growth factor receptors stimulate cell proliferation even without binding to growth factors i.e. with little or no growth factor bound to them. Oncogenes encoding for GF receptors include various mechanisms: overexpression, mutation and gene rearrangement. Examples of tumours by mutated receptors for growth factors are as under:

a) EGF receptors: Normal EGF receptor gene is *ERB B1*, and hence this receptor is termed as *EGFR or HER1* (i.e. human epidermal growth factor receptor type 1). *EGFR* (or *HER1*) acts by overexpression of normal GF receptor e.g. in 80% of squamous cell carcinoma of lung and 50% cases of glioblastomas.

Another *EGF* receptor gene called *ERB B2* (or *HER2/neu* or *CD340*) acts by gene amplification e.g. in breast cancer (25% cases), carcinoma of lungs, ovary, stomach.

b) c-KIT receptor: The gene coding for receptor for stem cell factor (or steel factor) is *c-KIT*, that activates tyrosine kinase pathway in cell proliferation. Mutated form of *c-KIT* by point mutation activates receptor for tyrosine kinase e.g. in gastrointestinal stromal tumour (GIST).

c) RET receptor: RET (abbreviation of '*re*arranged during *t*ransfection') protooncogene is a receptor for tyrosine kinase normally expressed in neuroendocrine cells of different tissues. Mutated form by point mutation is seen in MEN type 2A and 2B and in medullary carcinoma thyroid.

d) FMS-like tyrosine kinase receptor: Point mutation of *FLT-3* gene (CD 135) that encodes for *FMS*-like tyrosine kinase receptor has been seen in acute myeloid leukaemia.

iii) Cytoplasmic signal transduction proteins The normal signal transduction proteins in the cytoplasm transduce signal from the GF receptors present on the cell surface, to the nucleus of the cell, to activate intracellular growth signaling pathways.

There are examples of oncogenes having mutated forms of cytoplasmic signaling pathways located in the inner surface of cell membrane in some cancers. These are as under:

a) Mutated RAS gene This is the most common form of oncogene in human tumours, the abnormality being induced by point mutation in *RAS* gene. About a third of all human tumours carry mutated *RAS* gene (*RAS* for *Ra*t *S*arcoma gene where it was first described), seen in examples such as carcinoma colon, lung and pancreas. Normally, the inactive form of *RAS* protein is GDP (guanosinediphosphate)-bound while the activated form is bound to guanosine triphosphate (GTP). GDP/GTP are homologous to G proteins and take part in signal transduction in a similar way just as G proteins act as 'on-off switch' for signal transduction. Normally, active *RAS* protein is inactivated by GTPase activity, while mutated form of *RAS* gene remains unaffected by GTPase, and therefore, continues to signal the cell proliferation.

b) ABL-BCR hybrid gene ABL gene is a non-GF receptor protooncogene having tyrosine kinase activity. *ABL* gene from its normal location on chromosome 9 is translocated to chromosome 22 where it fuses with *BCR* (breakpoint cluster region) gene and forms an *ABL-BCR* hybrid gene which is more potent in signal transduction pathway. *ABL-BCR* hybrid gene is seen in chronic myeloid leukaemia and some acute leukaemias **(Fig. 19.6)**.

iv) Nuclear transcription factors The signal transduction pathway that started with GFs ultimately reaches the nucleus where it regulates DNA transcription and induces the cell to enter into S phase. Out of various nuclear regulatory transcription proteins described, the most important is *MYC* gene located on long arm of chromosome 8. Normally *MYC* protein binds to the DNA and regulates the cell cycle by transcriptional activation and its levels fall immediately after cell enters the cell cycle.

MYC oncogene (originally isolated from myelocytomatosis virus and accordingly abbreviated) is seen most commonly in human tumours. It is associated with persistence of or

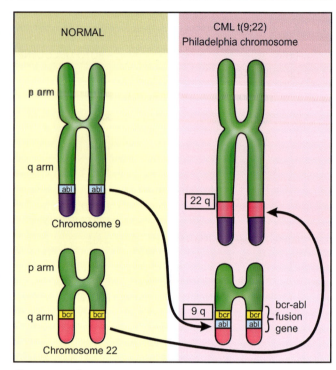

Figure 19.6 ▶ ABL-BCR gene translocation in chronic myeloid leukaemia.

overexpression of *MYC* oncoproteins which, in turn, causes autonomous cell proliferation. The examples of tumours carrying *MYC* oncogene are as under:

a) C-MYC oncogene: Mutated *MYC* gene due to *translocation* t(8;14) seen in Burkitt's lymphoma.

b) N-MYC oncogene: Mutated *MYC* gene due to *amplification* seen in neuroblastoma, small cell carcinoma lung.

c) L-MYC oncogene: Mutated *MYC* gene due to *amplification* seen in small cell carcinoma lung.

v) Cell cycle regulatory proteins Normally, the cell cycle is under regulatory control of cyclins and cyclin-dependent kinases (CDKs) A, B, E and D. Cyclins are so named since they are cyclically synthesised during different phases of the cell cycle and their degradation is also cyclic. Cyclins activate as well as work together with CDKs, while many inhibitors of CDKs (CDKIs) are also known.

Although all steps in the cell cycle are under regulatory controls, G1 → S phase is the most important checkpoint for regulation by oncogenes as well as anti-oncogenes (discussed below). Mutations in cyclins (in particular cyclin D) and CDKs (in particular CDK4) are most important growth promoting signals in cancers. The examples of tumours having such oncogenes are as under:

a) Mutated form of cyclin D protooncogene by translocation seen in mantle cell lymphoma.

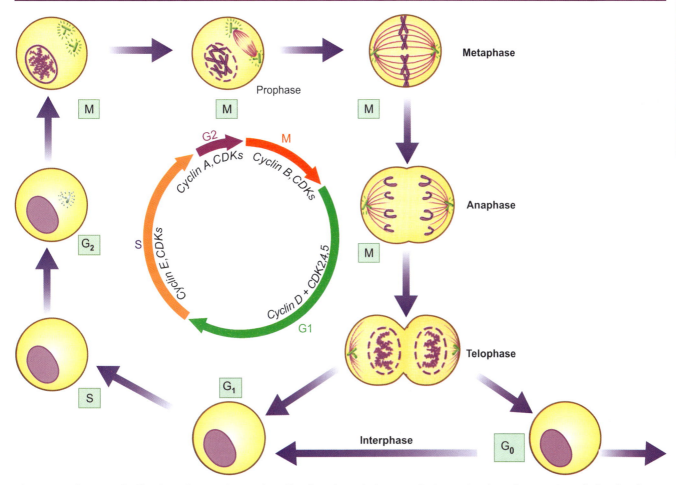

Figure 19.7 ▶ Normal cell cycle and its regulators. The cell cycle is driven by kinases which act when bound to proteins called cyclins, hence known as cyclin-dependent kinases (CDKs).

b) *Mutated form of cyclin E* by overexpression seen in breast cancer.
c) *Mutated form of CDK4* by gene amplification seen in malignant melanoma, glioblastoma and sarcomas.

2. Refractoriness to Growth Inhibition: Growth Suppressing Anti-Oncogenes

The mutation of normal growth suppressor anti-oncogenes results in removal of the brakes for growth; thus the inhibitory effect to cell growth is removed and the abnormal growth continues unchecked. In other words, mutated anti-oncogenes behave like growth-promoting oncogenes.

As compared to the signals and signal transduction pathways for oncogenes described above, the steps in mechanisms of action by growth suppressors are not so well understood. In general, the point of action by anti-oncogenes is also G1 → S phase transition. Normally, anti-oncogenes act by either inducing the dividing cell from the cell cycle to enter into G0 (resting) phase, or by acting in a way that the cell lies in the post-mitotic pool losing its dividing capability **(Fig. 19.7)**. Just as with activation of protooncogenes to become oncogenes, the mechanisms of loss of tumour suppressor actions of genes are due to chromosomal deletions, point mutations and loss of portions of chromosomes.

Major anti-oncogenes implicated in human cancers are as under **(Table 19.3)**:

i) RB gene RB gene is located on long arm (q) of chromosome 13. This is the first ever tumour suppressor gene identified and thus has been amply studied. *RB* gene codes for a nuclear transcription protein called pRB. *RB* gene is termed as master 'brake' in the cell cycle and is virtually present in every human cell. It can exist in both an *active* and an *inactive* form:

◈ *Active form* of RB gene: It blocks cell division by binding to transcription factor, E2F, and thus inhibits the cell from transcription of cell cycle-related genes, thereby *inhibiting* the cell cycle at G1 → S phase i.e. cell cycle is arrested at G1 phase.

Table 19.3: Important tumour-suppressor anti-oncogenes and associated human tumours.

	GENE	LOCATION	ASSOCIATED HUMAN TUMOURS
1.	RB	Nucleus (13q)	Retinoblastoma, osteosarcoma
2.	p53 (TP53)	Nucleus (17p)	Most human cancers, common in Ca lung, head and neck, colon, breast
3.	TGF–β and its receptor	Extracellular	Ca pancreas, colon, stomach
4.	APC and β-catenin proteins	Nucleus, cytosol	Ca colon
5.	Others		
	i) BRCA 1 and 2	Nucleus (*BRCA1* 17q21, *BRCA2* 13q12-13)	Ca breast, ovary
	ii) VHL	Nucleus (3p)	Renal cell carcinoma
	iii) WT 1 and 2	Nucleus (11p)	Wilms' tumour
	iv) NF 1 and 2	Plasma membrane	Neurofibromatosis type 1 and 2

◆ *Inactive form* of *RB* gene: This takes place when RB gene is hyperphosphorylated by cyclin dependent kinases (CDKs) and growth factors bind to their receptors. This removes pRB function from the cell (i.e. the 'brake' on cell division is removed). Resultantly, cell proliferation pathway is stimulated by *permitting* the cell to cross G1 → S phase. Activity of CDKs is inhibited by activation of inhibitory signal, transforming growth factor-β (TGF-β), on cell through activation of inhibitory protein p16.

The mutant form of *RB* gene (i.e. inactivating mutation of *RB* gene) is involved in several human tumours, most commonly in retinoblastoma, the most common intraocular tumour in young children. The tumour occurs in two forms: sporadic and inherited/familial (Fig. 19.8):

◆ *Sporadic retinoblastoma* constitutes about half the cases and affects one eye. These cases have acquired both the somatic mutations in the two alleles in retinal cells after birth.

◆ *Inherited/Familial retinoblastoma* comprises 40% of cases and may be bilateral. In these cases, all somatic cells (retinal as well as non-retinal cells) inherit one mutant *RB* gene from a carrier parent (i.e. germline mutation). Later during life, the other mutational event of second allele affecting the somatic cells occurs. This forms the basis of *two-hit hypothesis* given by Knudson in 1971. Besides retinoblastoma, children inheriting mutant *RB* gene have 200 times greater risk of development of other cancers in early adult life, most notably osteosarcoma; others are cancers of breast, colon and lungs.

ii) *p53* gene (*TP53*) Located on the short arm (p) of chromosome 17, *p53* gene (also termed *TP53* because of molecular weight of 53 kd for the protein) like *pRB* is inhibitory to cell cycle. However, *p53* is normally present in very small amounts and accumulates only after DNA damage.

The two major functions of *p53* in the normal cell cycle are as under:

a) In blocking mitotic activity: p53 inhibits the cyclins and CDKs and prevents the cell to enter G1 phase transiently. This breathing time in the cell cycle is utilised by the cell to repair the DNA damage.

b) In promoting apoptosis: Normally, *p53* acts together with another anti-oncogene, *RB* gene, and identifies the genes that have damaged DNA which cannot be repaired by inbuilt system. *p53* directs such cells to apoptosis by activating apoptosis-inducing *BAX* gene, and thus bringing the defective cells to an end by apoptosis. This process operates in the cell cycle at G1 and G2 phases before the cell enters the S or M phase.

Because of these significant roles in cell cycle, *p53* is called as 'protector of the genome'.

In its mutated form, *p53* ceases to act as protector or as growth suppressor but instead acts like a growth promoter or oncogene. Homozygous loss of *p53* gene allows genetically damaged and unrepaired cells to survive and proliferate resulting in malignant transformation. More than 70% of human cancers have homozygous loss of *p53* by acquired mutations in somatic cells; some common examples are cancers of the lung, head and neck, colon and breast. Besides, mutated *p53* is also seen in the sequential development stages of cancer from hyperplasia to carcinoma *in situ* and into invasive carcinoma.

Less commonly, both alleles of *p53* gene become defective by another way: one allele of p53 mutated by inheritance in germ cell lines rendering the individual to another hit of somatic mutation on the second allele. Just as in *RB* gene, this defect predisposes the individual to develop cancers of multiple organs (breast, bone, brain, sarcomas etc), termed *Li-Fraumeni syndrome.*

iii) Transforming growth factor-β (TGF-β) and its receptor Normally, *TGF-β* is significant inhibitor of cell proliferation, especially in epithelial, endothelial and haematopoietic cells. It acts by binding to *TGF-β* receptor and then the complex so formed acts in G1 phase of cell cycle at two levels:

a) It activates CDK inhibitors (CDKIs) with growth inhibitory effect.

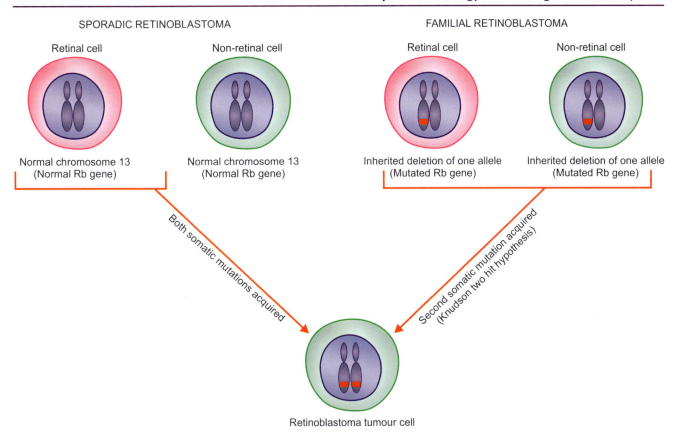

Figure 19.8 ▶ Schematic representation of role of *RB* gene in sporadic and familial retinoblastoma. A, In sporadic form, at birth there is no abnormality of either of two alleles of *RB* gene of retinal and non-retinal cells. Here, two mutations occur after birth involving both alleles of *RB* gene. B, In familial/inherited retinoblastoma, both retinal as well as non-retinal cells have one germline mutation at birth from one of the parents in one allele that encodes for *RB* protein gene. Second mutational event in these cases in the other allele occurs early during life to form homozygous mutation (two hit hypothesis of Hudson).

b) It suppresses the growth promoter genes such as *MYC*, *CDKs* and cyclins.

Mutant form of *TGF-β* gene or its receptor impairs the growth inhibiting effect and thus permits cell proliferation. Examples of mutated form of *TGF-β* are seen in cancers of pancreas, colon, stomach and endometrium.

iv) Adenomatous polyposis coli (APC) gene and β-catenin protein The *APC* gene is normally inhibitory to mitosis, which takes place by a cytoplasmic protein, β-catenin. β-catenin normally has dual functions:
◆ Firstly, it binds to cytoplasmic E-cadherin that is involved in intercellular interactions.
◆ Secondly, it can activate cell proliferation signaling pathway.

In colon cancer cells, *APC* gene is lost and thus β-catenin fails to get degraded, allowing the cancer cells to undergo mitosis without the inhibitory influence of β-catenin.

Patients born with one mutant *APC* gene allele develop large number of polyps in the colon early in life, while after the age of 20 years these cases start developing loss of second *APC* gene allele. It is then that almost all these patients invariably develop malignant transformation of one or more polyps.

v) Other antioncogenes A few other tumour-suppressor genes having mutated germline in various tumours are as under:

a) *BRCA1* and *BRCA2* genes: These are two breast *(BR)* cancer *(CA)* susceptibility genes: *BRCA1* located on chromosome 17q21 and *BRCA2* on chromosome 13q12-13. Women with inherited defect in *BRCA1* gene have very high risk (85%) of developing breast cancer and ovarian cancer (40%). Inherited breast cancer constitutes about 5-10% cases, it tends to occur at a relatively younger age and more often tends to be bilateral.

b) *VHL* gene: von-Hippel-Lindau (VHL) disease is a rare autosomal dominant disease characterised by benign and malignant tumours of multiple tissues. The disease is inherited as a mutation in *VHL* tumour suppressor gene located on chromosome 3p. This results in activation of genes that promote angiogenesis, survival and proliferation; *VHL* gene is found inactivated in 60% cases of renal cell carcinoma.

Table 19.4	Oncogenes versus antioncogenes.		
	FEATURE	ONCOGENE	ANTIONCOGENE
1.	Derived from	Mutated form of normal protooncogenes	Mutated form of normal growth suppressor genes
2.	Genetic abnormality	Mutations (point, translocation, amplification, overexpression) retroviral insertion, DNA damage	Loss of genes by deletion, point mutation and loss of portion of chromosome
3.	Major action	Allows cell proliferation by increased growth promotion pathways	Allows cell proliferation by removal of cell growth suppressor pathway
4.	Level of action in cell	At different levels (cell surface, cytoplasm, mutations)	At different levels (cell surface, cytoplasm, nucleus)
5.	Major types	i) GFs (PDGF-β, TGF-α, FGF, HGF)	i) RB
		ii) GF receptors (EGFR, cKIT, RET)	ii) p53
		iii) Cytoplasmic signal proteins (RAS, BCR-ABL)	iii) TGF-β and its receptor
		iv) Nuclear transcription proteins (MYC)	iv) APC and β-catenin
		v) Cell cycle regular proteins (CDKs, cyclins)	v) Others (BRCA 1 and 2, VHL, WT 1 and 2, NF 1 and 2)

c) **Wilms' tumour (WT) gene:** *WT1* and *WT2* genes are both located on chromosome 11 and normally prevent neoplastic proliferation of cells in embryonic kidney. Mutant form of *WT-1* and *2* are seen in hereditary Wilms' tumour.

d) **Neurofibroma (NF) gene:** *NF* genes normally prevent proliferation of Schwann cells. Two mutant forms are described: *NF1* and *NF2* seen in neurofibromatosis type 1 and type 2.

The contrasting features of growth-promoting oncogenes and growth-suppressing anti-oncogenes are summarised in **Table 19.4**.

3. Escaping Cell Death by Apoptosis: Genes Regulating Apoptosis and Cancer

Besides the role of mutant forms of growth-promoting oncogenes and growth-suppressing anti-oncogenes, another mechanism of tumour growth is by escaping cell death by apoptosis. Apoptosis in normal cell is guided by cell death receptor, *CD95*, resulting in DNA damage. Besides, there is role of some other pro-apoptotic factors (*BAD, BAX, BID* and *p53*) and apoptosis-inhibitors (*BCL2, BCL-X*).

In cancer cells, the function of apoptosis is interfered due to mutations in the above genes which regulate apoptosis in the normal cell. The examples of tumours by this mechanism are as under:

a) ***BCL2* gene** is seen in normal lymphocytes, but its mutant form with characteristic translocation (t14;18) (q32;q21) was first described in B-cell lymphoma and hence the name BCL. It is also seen in many other human cancers such as that of breast, thyroid and prostate. Mutation in *BCL2* gene removes the apoptosis-inhibitory control on cancer cells, thus more live cells undergoing mitosis contributing to tumour growth. Besides, *MYC* oncogene and *p53* tumour suppressor gene are also connected to apoptosis. While *MYC* allows cell growth *BCL2* inhibits cell death; thus *MYC* and *BCL2* together allow cell proliferation. Normally, p53 activates proapoptotic gene *BAX* but mutated *p53* (i.e. absence of *p53*) reduces apoptotic activity and thus allows cell proliferation.

b) ***CD95*** receptors are depleted in hepatocellular carcinoma and hence the tumour cells escape apoptosis.

4. Avoiding Cellular Ageing: Telomeres and Telomerase in Cancer

As discussed in pathology of ageing in Chapter 2, after each mitosis (cell doubling) there is progressive shortening of telomeres which are the terminal tips of chromosomes. Telomerase is the RNA enzyme that helps in repair of such damage to DNA and maintains normal telomere length in successive cell divisions. However, it has been seen that after repetitive mitosis for a maximum of 60 to 70 times, telomeres are lost in normal cells and the cells cease to undergo mitosis. Telomerase is active in normal stem cells but not in normal somatic cells.

Cancer cells in most malignancies have markedly upregulated telomerase enzyme, and hence telomere length is maintained. Thus, cancer cells avoid ageing, mitosis does not slow down or cease, thereby immortalising the cancer cells.

5. Continued Perfusion of Cancer: Tumour Angiogenesis

Cancers can only survive and thrive if the cancer cells are adequately nourished and perfused, as otherwise they cannot grow further. Neovascularisation in the cancers not only supplies the tumour with oxygen and nutrients, but the newly formed endothelial cells also elaborate a few growth factors for progression of primary as well as metastatic cancer. The stimulus for angiogenesis is provided by the release of various factors:

i) Promoters of tumour angiogenesis include the most important *vascular endothelial growth factor (VEGF)* (released from genes in the parenchymal tumour cells) and *basic fibroblast growth factor (bFGF)*.

ii) Anti-angiogenesis factors inhibiting angiogenesis include *thrombospondin-1* (also produced by tumour cells themselves), *angiostatin, endostatin and vasculostatin*. Mutated form of *p53* gene in both alleles in various cancers results in removal of anti-angiogenic role of thrombospondin-1, thus favouring continued angiogenesis.

6. Invasion and Distant Metastasis: Cancer Dissemination

One of the most important characteristic of cancers is invasiveness and metastasis. The mechanisms involved in the biology of invasion and metastasis are discussed already along with spread of tumours (page 278).

7. DNA Damage and Repair System: Mutator Genes and Cancer

Normal cells during complex mitosis suffer from minor damage to the DNA which is detected and repaired before mitosis is completed so that integrity of the genome is maintained. Similarly, small mutational damage to the dividing cell by exogenous factors (e.g. by radiation, chemical carcinogens etc) is also repaired. *p53* gene is held responsible for detection and repair of DNA damage. However, if this system of DNA repair is defective as happens in some inherited mutations (mutator genes), the defect in unrepaired DNA is passed to the next progeny of cells and cancer results.

The examples of mutator genes exist in the following inherited disorders associated with increased propensity to cancer:

i) Hereditary non-polyposis colon cancer (HNPCC or Lynch syndrome) is characterised by hereditary predisposition to develop colorectal cancer. It is due to defect in genes involved in DNA mismatch repair which results in accumulation of errors in the form of mutations in many genes.

ii) Ataxia telangiectasia (AT) has *ATM* (*M* for mutated) gene. These patients have multiple cancers besides other features such as cerebellar degeneration, immunologic derangements and oculo-cutaneous manifestations.

iii) Xeroderma pigmentosum is an inherited disorder in which there is defect in DNA repair mechanism. Upon exposure to sunlight, the UV radiation damage to DNA cannot be repaired. Thus, such patients are more prone to various forms of skin cancers.

iv) Bloom syndrome is an example of damage by ionising radiation which cannot be repaired due to inherited defect and the patients have increased risk to develop cancers, particularly leukaemia.

v) Hereditary breast cancer patients having mutated *BRCA1* and *BRCA2* genes carry inherited defect in DNA repair mechanism. These patients are not only predisposed to develop breast cancer but also cancers of various other organs.

8. Cancer Progression and Heterogeneity: Clonal Aggressiveness

Another feature of note in biology of cancers is that with passage of time cancers become more aggressive; this property is termed *tumour progression*. Clinical parameters of cancer progression are: increasing size of the tumour, higher histologic grade (as seen by poorer differentiation and greater anaplasia), areas of tumour necrosis (i.e. tumour outgrows its blood supply), invasiveness and distant metastasis.

In terms of molecular biology, this attribute of cancer is due to the fact that with passage of time cancer cells acquire more and more *heterogeneity*. This means that though cancer cells remain monoclonal in origin, they acquire more and more mutations which, in turn, produce multiple-mutated subpopulations of more aggressive clones of cancer cells (i.e. heterogeneous cells) in the growth which have tendency to invade, metastasise and be refractory to hormonal influences. Some of these mutations in fact may kill the tumour cells as well.

9. Cancer—A Sequential Multistep Molecular Phenomenon: Multistep Theory

It needs to be appreciated that cancer occurs following several sequential steps of abnormalities in the target cell e.g. initiation, promotion and progression in proper sequence. Similarly, multiple steps are involved at genetic level by which cell proliferation of cancer cells is activated: by activation of growth promoters, loss of growth suppressors, inactivation of intrinsic apoptotic mechanisms and escaping cellular ageing. A classic example of this sequential genetic abnormalities in cancer is seen in adenoma-carcinoma sequence in development of colorectal carcinoma. Recent studies on human genome in cancers of breast and colon have revealed that there is a multistep phenomenon of carcinogenesis at molecular level; on an average a malignant tumour has large number of genetic mutations in cancers.

10. Micro-RNAs in Cancer: Oncomirs

Unlike protein-coding molecules of the cell, microRNAs (or miRNAs) are short non-coding single-stranded RNA transcripts with a length of 20-24 nucleotides only. About 1400 microRNAs of fundamental importance in various biological processes have been identified and the list is increasing.

❖ Normally, microRNAs function as the post-translational gene regulators of cell proliferation, differentiation and survival.

❖ In cancer, microRNAs have an oncogenic role in initiation and progression and are termed as oncogenic microRNAs, abbreviated as *oncomiRs*. These oncogenic microRNAs influence various cellular processes in cancer such as control

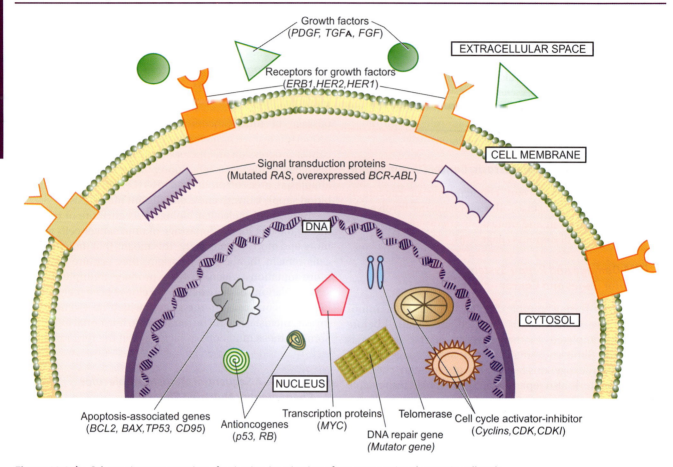

Figure 19.9 ▶ Schematic representation of activation-inactivation of cancer-associated genes in cell cycle.

of proliferation, cell cycle regulation, apoptosis, differentiation, metastasis and metabolism.

The above properties of cancer cells are schematically illustrated in **Fig. 19.9**.

> **GIST BOX 19.2** | **Molecular Basis of Cancer**
>
> ❖ A few properties of cancer render support for its origin at molecular level. For example, most human cancers have a single clone of cellular origin, limited number of cells develop into cancer in a field, cellular growth of cancer is under genetic control with genetic regulators of normal and abnormal mitosis.
> ❖ Normal regulatory genes of cellular growth undergo mutation in cancer. These mutations may occur by alteration in structure of single base in DNA chain by point mutation, by chromosomal translocations, or by increasing number of copies of DNA sequence causing overexpression of gene product.
> ❖ Various cancer-related genes or molecular hallmarks of cancer which undergo such mutational events are: growth promoting oncogenes causing autonomous and excessive growth, removal of brakes on cellular growth by mutation in growth-suppressing antioncogenes, removal of proapoptotic genes making cancer cells immortal, avoiding cellular ageing by mutated telomerase, by continued cancer angiogenesis, by clonal aggressiveness due to cancer heterogeneity, and by short noncoding microRNAs in cancer.

CARCINOGENS AND CARCINOGENESIS

Carcinogenesis or oncogenesis or tumorigenesis means mechanism of induction of tumours (*pathogenesis of cancer*); agents which can induce tumours are called *carcinogens* (*etiology of cancer*). Since the time first ever carcinogen was identified, there has been ever-increasing list of agents implicated in etiology of cancer. There has been still greater accumulation in volumes of knowledge on pathogenesis of cancer, especially due to tremendous strides made in the field of molecular biology and genetics in recent times as discussed already.

Based on implicated causative agents, etiology and pathogenesis of cancer can be discussed under following 3 headings:
A. Chemical carcinogens and chemical carcinogenesis
B. Physical carcinogens and radiation carcinogenesis
C. Biologic carcinogens and viral oncogenesis.

A. CHEMICAL CARCINOGENESIS

The first ever evidence of any cause for neoplasia came from the observation of Sir Percival Pott in 1775 that there was higher incidence of cancer of the scrotal skin in boys engaged in sweeping industrial chimneys in London than in the general population. This inspired the law-makers in London to pass a ruling that these workers should bathe daily and this simple public health measure lowered the cancer incidence of scrotum in these workers. Similar other observations in occupational workers who have skin soaked in industrial oils and reporting higher incidence of cancer of the skin invoked wide interest in soot and coal tar and its constituents as possible carcinogenic agents. The first successful experimental induction of cancer was produced by two Japanese workers (Yamagiwa and Ichikawa) in 1914 in the rabbit's skin by repeatedly painting with coal tar. Since then the list of chemical carcinogens which can experimentally induce cancer in animals and have epidemiological evidence in causing human neoplasia, is ever increasing.

Stages in Chemical Carcinogenesis

The induction of cancer by chemical carcinogens occurs after a delay—weeks to months in the case of experimental animals, and often several years in humans. Other factors that influence the induction of cancer are the dose and mode of administration of carcinogenic chemical, individual susceptibility and various predisposing factors.

Chemical carcinogenesis occurs by induction of mutation in the proto-oncogenes and anti-oncogenes. The phenomena of cellular transformation by chemical carcinogens (as also other carcinogens) is a progressive process involving 3 sequential stages **(Fig. 19.10)**:
◆ Initiation
◆ Promotion
◆ Progression

Initiation of Carcinogenesis

Initiation is the first stage in carcinogenesis induced by initiator chemical carcinogens. The change can be produced

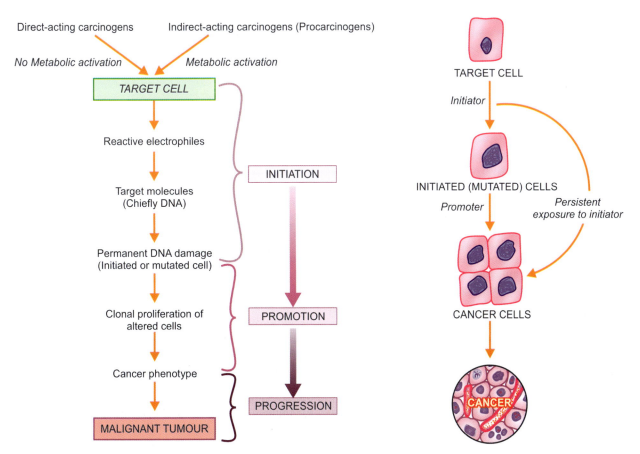

Figure 19.10 ▶ Sequential stages in chemical carcinogenesis (*left*) in evolution of cancer (*right*).

Section IV: Neoplasia

Table 19.5: Important chemical carcinogens.

CARCINOGEN	TUMOUR
I. DIRECT-ACTING CARCINOGENS	
i) Alkylating agents	
a) Anti-cancer drugs (e.g. cyclophosphamide, chlorambucil, busulfan, melphalan, nitrosourea etc)	• Lymphomas
b) β-propiolactone	• AML
c) Epoxides	• Bladder cancer
ii) Acylating agents	
a) Acetyl imidazole	
b) Dimethyl carbamyl chloride	
II. INDIRECT-ACTING CARCINOGENS (PROCARCINOGENS)	
i) Polycyclic, aromatic hydrocarbons (in tobacco, smoke, fossil fuel, soot, tar, minerals oil, smoked animal foods, industrial and atmospheric pollutants)	
a) Anthracenes (benza-, dibenza-, dimethyl benza-)	• Lung cancer
b) Benzapyrene	• Skin cancer
c) Methylcholanthrene	• Cancer of upper aerodigestive tract
ii) Aromatic amines and azo-dyes	
a) β-naphthylamine	• Bladder cancer
b) Benzidine	
c) Azo-dyes (e.g. butter yellow, scarlet red etc)	• Hepatocellular carcinoma
iii) Naturally-occurring products	
a) Aflatoxin Bl	
b) Actinomycin D	
c) Mitomycin C	• Hepatocellular carcinoma
d) Safrole	
e) Betel nuts	
iv) Miscellaneous	
a) Nitrosamines and nitrosamides	• Gastric carcinoma
b) Vinyl chloride monomer	• Angiosarcoma of liver
c) Asbestos	• Bronchogenic carcinoma, mesothelioma
d) Arsenical compounds	• Cancer, skin, lung
e) Metals (e.g. nickel, lead, cobalt, chromium etc)	• Lung cancer
f) Insecticides, fungicides (e.g. aldrin, dieldrin, chlordane etc)	• Cancer in experimental animals
g) Saccharin and cyclomates	

by a single dose of the initiating agent for a short time, though larger dose for longer duration is more effective. The change so induced is sudden, irreversible and permanent. Chemical carcinogens acting as initiators of carcinogenesis can be grouped into 2 categories (Table 19.5):

I. Direct-acting carcinogens These are a few chemical substances (e.g. alkylating agents, acylating agents) which can induce cellular transformation without undergoing any prior metabolic activation.

II. Indirect-acting carcinogens or procarcinogens These require metabolic conversion within the body so as to become 'ultimate' carcinogens having carcinogenicity e.g. polycyclic aromatic hydrocarbons, aromatic amines, azo dyes, naturally-occurring products and others.

In either case, the following steps are involved in transforming 'the target cell' into 'the initiated cell':

1. Metabolic activation Vast majority of chemical carcinogens are indirect-acting or procarcinogens requiring metabolic activation, while direct-acting carcinogens do not require this activation. The indirect-acting carcinogens are activated in the liver by the mono-oxygenases of the cytochrome P-450 system in the endoplasmic reticulum. In some circumstances, the procarcinogen may be detoxified and rendered inactive metabolically.

In fact, following 2 requirements determine the carcinogenic potency of a chemical:
i) Balance between activation and inactivation reaction of the carcinogenic chemical.
ii) Genes that code for cytochrome P-450-dependent enzymes involved in metabolic activation e.g a genotype carrying susceptibility gene *CYP1A1* for the enzyme system has far higher incidence of lung cancer in light smokers as compared to those not having this permissive gene.

Besides these two, additional factors such as age, sex and nutritional status of the host also play some role in determining response of the individual to chemical carcinogen.

2. **Reactive electrophiles** While direct-acting carcinogens are intrinsically electrophilic, indirect-acting substances become electron-deficient after metabolic activation i.e. they become reactive electrophiles. Following this step, both types of chemical carcinogens behave alike and their reactive electrophiles bind to electron-rich portions of other molecules of the cell such as DNA, RNA and other proteins.

3. **Target molecules** The primary target of electrophiles is DNA, producing mutagenesis. The change in DNA may lead to 'the initiated cell' or some form of cellular enzymes may be able to repair the damage in DNA. The classic example of such a situation occurs in xeroderma pigmentosum, a precancerous condition, in which there is hereditary defect in DNA repair mechanism of the cell and thus such patients are prone to develop skin cancer. The carcinogenic potential of a chemical can be tested *in vitro* by Ames' test for mutagenesis (described later).

Any gene may be the target molecule in the DNA for the chemical carcinogen. However, on the basis of chemically induced cancers in experimental animals and epidemiologic studies in human beings, it has been observed that most frequently affected growth promoter oncogene is *RAS* gene mutation and anti-oncogene (tumour suppressor) is *p53* gene mutation.

4. **The initiated cell** The unrepaired damage produced in the DNA of the cell becomes permanent and fixed only if the altered cell undergoes at least one cycle of proliferation. This results in transferring the change to the next progeny of cells so that the DNA damage becomes *permanent* and *irreversible*, which are the characteristics of the initiated cell, vulnerable to the action of promoters of carcinogenesis.

The stimulus for proliferation may come from regeneration of surviving cells, dietary factors, hormone-induced hyperplasia, viruses etc. A few examples are the occurrence of hepatocellular carcinoma in cases of viral hepatitis, association of endometrial hyperplasia with endometrial carcinoma, effect of oestrogen in breast cancer.

Promotion of Carcinogenesis

Promotion is the next sequential stage in the chemical carcinogenesis. Promoters of carcinogenesis are substances such as phorbol esters, phenols, hormones, artificial sweeteners and drugs like phenobarbital. They differ from initiators in the following respects:
i) They do not produce sudden change.
ii) They require application or administration, as the case may be, *following* initiator exposure, for sufficient time and in sufficient dose.
iii) The change induced may be reversible.
iv) They do not damage the DNA *per se* and are thus not mutagenic but instead enhance the effect of direct-acting carcinogens or procarcinogens.
v) Tumour promoters act by further clonal proliferation and expansion of initiated (mutated) cells, and have reduced requirement of growth factor, especially after *RAS* gene mutation.

It may be mentioned here that persistent and sustained application/exposure of the cell to initiator alone unassociated with subsequent application of promoter may also result in cancer. But the *vice versa* does not hold true since neither application of promoter alone, nor its application prior to exposure to initiator carcinogen, would result in transformation of target cell.

Progression of Carcinogenesis

Progression of cancer is the stage when mutated proliferated cell shows phenotypic features of malignancy. These features pertain to morphology, biochemical composition and molecular features of malignancy. Such phenotypic features appear only when the initiated cell starts to proliferate rapidly and in the process acquires more and more mutations. The new progeny of cells that develops after such repetitive proliferation inherits genetic and biochemical characteristics of malignancy.

Carcinogenic Chemicals in Humans

The list of diverse chemical compounds which can produce cancer in experimental animals is a long one but only some of them have sufficient epidemiological evidence in human neoplasia.

Depending upon the mode of action of carcinogenic chemicals, they are divided into 2 broad groups: initiators and promoters (Table 19.5).

Initiator Carcinogens

Chemical carcinogens which can initiate the process of neoplastic transformation are further categorised into 2 subgroups—direct-acting and indirect-acting carcinogens or procarcinogens.

1. **DIRECT-ACTING CARCINOGENS** These chemical carcinogens do not require metabolic activation and fall into 2 classes:

i) **Alkylating agents** This group includes mainly various anti-cancer drugs (e.g. cyclophosphamide, chlorambucil, busulfan, melphalan, nitrosourea etc), β-propiolactone and epoxides. They are weakly carcinogenic and are implicated in the etiology of the lymphomas and leukaemias in human beings.

ii) **Acylating agents** The examples are acetyl imidazole and dimethyl carbamyl chloride.

2. INDIRECT-ACTING CARCINOGENS (PROCARCINOGENS) These are chemical substances which require prior metabolic activation before becoming potent 'ultimate' carcinogens. This group includes vast majority of carcinogenic chemicals. It includes the following 4 categories:

i) Polycyclic aromatic hydrocarbons They comprise the largest group of common procarcinogens which, after metabolic activation, can induce neoplasia in many tissues in experimental animals and are also implicated in a number of human neoplasms. They cause different effects by various modes of administration e.g. by topical application may induce skin cancer, by subcutaneous injection may cause sarcomas, inhalation produces lung cancer, when introduced in different organs by parenteral/metabolising routes may cause cancer of that organ.

Main sources of polycyclic aromatic hydrocarbons are: combustion and chewing of tobacco, smoke, fossil fuel (e.g. coal), soot, tar, mineral oil, smoked animal foods, industrial and atmospheric pollutants. Important chemical compounds included in this group are: anthracenes (benza-, dibenza-, dimethylbenza-), benzapyrene and methylcholanthrene. The following examples have evidence to support the etiologic role of these substances:

a) *Smoking and lung cancer:* There is 20 times higher incidence of lung cancer in smokers of 2 packs (40 cigarettes) per day for 20 years.

b) *Skin cancer:* Direct contact of polycyclic aromatic hydrocarbon compounds with skin is associated with higher incidence of skin cancer. For example, the natives of Kashmir carry an earthen pot containing embers, the *kangri*, under their clothes close to abdomen to keep themselves warm, and skin cancer of the abdominal wall termed *kangri cancer* is common among them.

c) *Tobacco and betel nut chewing and cancer oral cavity:* Cancer of the oral cavity is more common in people chewing tobacco and betel nuts. The *chutta* is a cigar that is smoked in South India (in Andhra Pradesh) with the lighted end in the mouth (i.e. reversed smoking) and such individuals have higher incidence of cancer of the mouth.

ii) Aromatic amines and azo-dyes This category includes the following substances implicated in chemical carcinogenesis:

a) β-*naphthylamine* in the causation of bladder cancer, especially in aniline dye and rubber industry workers.

b) *Benzidine* in the induction of bladder cancer.

c) *Azo-dyes* used for colouring foods (e.g. butter and margarine to give them yellow colour, scarlet red for colouring cherries etc) in the causation of hepatocellular carcinoma.

iii) Naturally-occurring products Some of the important chemical carcinogens derived from plant and microbial sources are aflatoxin B1, actinomycin D, mitomycin C, safrole and betel nuts. Out of these, aflatoxin B1 implicated in causing human hepatocellular carcinoma is the most important, especially when concomitant viral hepatitis B is present. It is derived from the fungus, *Aspergillus flavus,* that grows in stored grains and plants.

iv) Miscellaneous A variety of other chemical carcinogens having a role in the etiology of human cancer are as under:

a) *Nitrosamines and nitrosamides* are involved in gastric carcinoma. These compounds are actually made in the stomach by nitrosylation of food preservatives.

b) *Vinyl chloride monomer* derived from polyvinyl chloride (PVC) polymer in the causation of haemangiosarcoma of the liver.

c) *Asbestos* in bronchogenic carcinoma and mesothelioma, especially in smokers.

d) *Arsenical compounds* in causing epidermal hyperplasia and basal cell carcinoma.

e) *Metals* like nickel, lead, cobalt, chromium etc in industrial workers causing lung cancer.

f) *Insecticides and fungicides* (e.g. aldrin, dieldrin, chlordane) in carcinogenesis in experimental animals.

g) *Saccharin and cyclamates* in cancer in experimental animals.

Promoter Carcinogens

Promoters are chemical substances which lack the intrinsic carcinogenic potential but their application subsequent to initiator exposure helps the initiated cell to proliferate further. These substances include phorbol esters, phenols, certain hormones and drugs.

i) Phorbol esters The best known promoter in experimental animals is *TPA* (tetradecanoylphorbol acetate) which acts by signal induction protein activation pathway.

ii) Hormones Endogenous or exogenous oestrogen excess in promotion of cancers of endometrium and breast, prolonged administration of diethylstilbestrol in the etiology of postmenopausal endometrial carcinoma and in vaginal cancer in adolescent girls born to mothers exposed to this hormone during their pregnancy.

iii) Miscellaneous e.g. dietary fat in cancer of colon, cigarette smoke and viral infections etc.

The feature of initiators and promoters are contrasted in **Table 19.6**.

Tests for Chemical Carcinogenicity

There are 2 main methods of testing chemical compound for its carcinogenicity:

1. EXPERIMENTAL INDUCTION The traditional method is to administer the chemical compound under test to a batch of experimental animals like mice or other rodents

	FEATURE	INITIATOR CARCINOGENS	PROMOTER CARCINOGENS
1.	Mechanism	Induction of mutation	Not mutagenic
2.	Dose	Single for a short time	Repeated dose exposure, for a long time
3.	Response	Sudden response	Slow response
4.	Change	Permanent, irreversible	Change may be reversible
5.	Sequence	Applied first, then followed by promoter	Applied after prior exposure to initiator
6.	Effectivity	Effective alone if exposed in large dose	Not effective alone
7.	Molecular changes	Most common mutation of *RAS* oncogene, *p53* anti-oncogene	Clonal expansion of mutated cells
8.	Examples	Most chemical carcinogens, radiation	Hormones, phorbol esters

Table 19.6 Contrasting features of initiator and promoter carcinogens.

by an appropriate route e.g. painting on the skin, giving orally or parenterally, or by inhalation. The chemical is administered repeatedly, the dose varied, and promoting agents are administered subsequently. After many months, the animal is autopsied and results obtained. However, all positive or negative tests cannot be applied to humans since there is sufficient species variation in susceptibility to particular carcinogen. Besides, the test is rather prolonged and expensive.

2. TESTS FOR MUTAGENICITY (AMES' TEST) A mutagen is a substance that can permanently alter the genetic composition of a cell. Ames' test evaluates the ability of a chemical to induce mutation in the mutant strain of *Salmonella typhimurium* that cannot synthesise histidine. Such strains are incubated with the potential carcinogen to which liver homogenate is added to supply enzymes required to convert procarcinogen to ultimate carcinogen. If the chemical under test is mutagenic, it will induce mutation in the mutant strains of *S. typhimurium* in the form of functional histidine gene, which will be reflected by the number of bacterial colonies growing on histidine-free culture medium (Fig. 19.11). Most of the carcinogenic chemicals tested positive in Ames' test are carcinogenic *in vivo*.

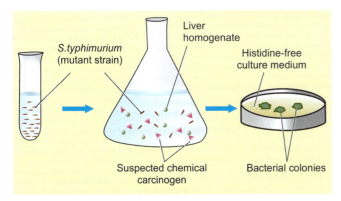

Figure 19.11 ▶ Schematic representation of the Ames' test.

B. PHYSICAL CARCINOGENESIS

Physical agents in carcinogenesis are divided into 2 groups:
1. *Radiation*, both ultraviolet light and ionising radiation, is the most important physical agent. The role of radiation as carcinogenic agent is discussed below while its non-neoplastic complications are described in Chapter 4 (page 34).
2. *Non-radiation* physical agents are the various forms of injury and are less important.

Radiation Carcinogenesis

Ultraviolet (UV) light and ionising radiation are the two main forms of radiation carcinogens which can induce cancer in experimental animals and are implicated in causation of some forms of human cancers. A property common between the two forms of radiation carcinogens is the appearance of mutations followed by a long period of latency after initial exposure, often 10-20 years or even later. Also, radiation carcinogens may act to enhance the effect of another carcinogen (co-carcinogens) and, like chemical carcinogens, may have sequential stages of initiation, promotion and progression in their evolution. Ultraviolet light and ionising radiation differ in their mode of action as described below:

1. ULTRAVIOLET LIGHT The main source of UV radiation is the sunlight; others are UV lamps and welder's arcs. UV light penetrates the skin for a few millimetres only so that its effect is limited to epidermis. The efficiency of UV light as carcinogen depends upon the extent of light-absorbing protective melanin pigmentation of the skin. In humans, excessive exposure to UV rays can cause various forms of skin cancers—squamous cell carcinoma, basal cell carcinoma and malignant melanoma. In support of this is the epidemiological evidence of high incidence of these skin cancers in while race, albinos who do not tan readily, inhabitants of Australia and New Zealand living close to the equator who receive more sunlight, and in farmers and outdoor workers due to the effect of actinic light radiation.

Mechanism UV radiation may have various effects on the cells. The most important is induction of mutation; others are inhibition of cell division, inactivation of enzymes and sometimes causing cell death. The most important biochemical effect of UV radiation is the formation of pyrimidine dimers in DNA. Such UV-induced DNA damage in normal individuals is repaired, while in the predisposed persons who are excessively exposed to sunlight such damage remain unrepaired. The proof in favour of mutagenic effect of UV radiation comes from following recessive hereditary diseases characterised by a defect in DNA repair mechanism and associated with high incidence of cancers:

i) Xeroderma pigmentosum is predisposed to skin cancers at younger age (under 20 years of age).
ii) Ataxia telangiectasia is predisposed to leukaemia.
iii) Bloom's syndrome is predisposed to all types of cancers.
iv) Fanconi's anaemia with increased risk to develop cancer.

Besides, like with other carcinogens, UV radiation also induces mutated forms of oncogenes (in particular *RAS* gene) and anti-oncogenes (*p53* gene).

2. IONISING RADIATION Ionising radiation of all kinds like X-rays, α-, β- and γ-rays, radioactive isotopes, protons and neutrons can cause cancer in animals and in man. Most frequently, radiation-induced cancers are all forms of leukaemias (except chronic lymphocytic leukaemia); others are cancers of the thyroid (most commonly papillary carcinoma), skin, breast, ovary, uterus, lung, myeloma, and salivary glands **(Fig. 19.12)**. The risk is increased by higher dose and with high LET (linear energy transfer) such as in neutrons and α-rays than with low LET as in X-rays and γ-rays. The evidence in support of carcinogenic role of ionising radiation is cited in the following examples:

i) Higher incidence of radiation dermatitis and subsequent malignant tumours of the skin was noted in X-ray workers and radiotherapists who did initial pioneering work in these fields before the advent of safety measures.
ii) High incidence of osteosarcoma was observed in young American watch-working girls engaged in painting the dials with luminous radium who unknowingly ingested radium while using lips to point their brushes.
iii) Miners in radioactive elements have higher incidence of cancers.
iv) Japanese atom bomb survivors of the twin cities of Hiroshima and Nagasaki after World War II have increased frequency of malignant tumours, notably acute and chronic myeloid leukaemias, and various solid tumours of breast, colon, thyroid and lung.
v) Accidental leakage at nuclear power plant in 1985 in Chernobyl (in former USSR, now in Ukraine) has caused long-term hazardous effects of radioactive material to the population living in the vicinity.
vi) It has been observed that therapeutic irradiation results in increased frequency of cancers, e.g. in patients of ankylosing spondylitis, in children with enlarged thymus, and in children exposed to radiation *in utero* during investigations on the mother.
vii) Thorotrast, a thorium-containing contrast medium, used to be employed in radioimaging of abscess cavities in 1940s. These patients were found to have about twice higher incidence of malignant tumours and thus its use was discontinued.
viii) In recent times, there has been debate on the role of electromagnetic radiations emitted by overhead power cables, cellphones and their transmission towers and domestic microwaves in causing cancer. While there is no conclusive link with cancer so far, WHO review report in 2011 has cautioned on *probable* risk of developing brain tumours (glioma and acoustic neuroma) in long-term cellphone users. However, there is no evidence of any health risk by low electromagnetic energy around us from various other sources.

Mechanism Radiation damages the DNA of the cell by one of the 2 possible mechanisms:
i) It may directly alter the cellular DNA.
ii) It may dislodge ions from water and other molecules of the cell and result in formation of highly reactive free radicals that may bring about the damage.

Damage to the DNA resulting in mutagenesis is the most important action of ionising radiation. It may cause chromosomal breakage, translocation, or point mutation.

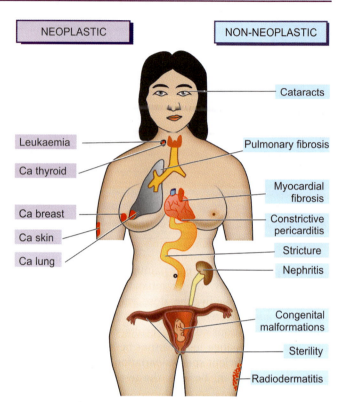

Figure 19.12 ▶ Neoplastic (left) and non-neoplastic complications (right) of ionising radiation.

The effect depends upon a number of factors such as type of radiation, dose, dose-rate, frequency and various host factors such as age, individual susceptibility, immune competence, hormonal influences and type of cells irradiated.

Non-radiation Physical Carcinogenesis

Mechanical injury to the tissues or prolonged contact with certain physical agents has been observed to have higher incidence of certain cancers but without proven basis. A few rare examples of these uncommon associations are as under:
i) Stones in the gallbladder and in the urinary tract having higher incidence of cancers of these organs.
ii) Healed scars following burns or trauma for increased risk of carcinoma of affected skin.
iii) Occupational exposure to asbestos (asbestosis) associated with asbestos-associated tumours of the lung and malignant mesothelioma of the pleura.
iv) Workers engaged in hardwood cutting or engraving having high incidence of adenocarcioma of paranasal sinuses.
v) Surgical implants of inert materials such as plastic, glass etc in prostheses.
vi) Foreign bodies embedded in the body for prolonged duration.

C. BIOLOGIC CARCINOGENESIS

The epidemiological studies on different types of cancers indicate the involvement of transmissible biologic agents in their development, chiefly *viruses*. Other microbial agents implicated in carcinogenesis are as follows:

◆ **Parasites** *Schistosoma haematobium* infection of the urinary bladder is associated with high incidence of squamous cell carcinoma of the urinary bladder in some parts of the world such as in Egypt. *Clonorchis sinensis*, the liver fluke, lives in the hepatic duct and is implicated in causation of cholangiocarcinoma.

◆ **Fungus** *Aspergillus flavus* grows in stored grains and liberates aflatoxin; its human consumption, especially by those with HBV infection, is associated with development of hepatocellular carcinoma.

◆ **Bacteria** *Helicobacter pylori*, a gram-positive spiral-shaped micro-organism, colonises the gastric mucosa and has been found in cases of chronic gastritis and peptic ulcer; its prolonged infection may lead to gastric lymphoma and gastric carcinoma.

However, the role of viruses in the causation of cancer is more significant. Therefore, biologic carcinogenesis is largely *viral carcinogenesis*, described below.

Viral Carcinogenesis

It has been estimated that about 20% of all cancers worldwide are due to persistent virus infection. The association of oncogenic viruses with neoplasia was first observed by an Italian physician Sanarelli in 1889 who noted association between myxomatosis of rabbits with poxvirus. The contagious nature of the common human wart was first established in 1907. Since then, a number of viruses capable of inducing tumours (oncogenic viruses) in experimental animals, and some implicated in humans, have been identified.

Most of the common viral infections (including oncogenic viruses) can be transmitted by one of the 3 routes:

i) *Horizontal transmission* Commonly, viral infection passes from one to another by direct contact, by ingestion of contaminated water or food, or by inhalation as occurs in most contagious diseases. Most of these infections begin on the epithelial surfaces, spread into deeper tissues, and then through haematogenous or lymphatic or neural route disseminate to other sites in the body.

ii) *By parenteral route* such as by inoculation as happens in some viruses by inter-human spread and from animals and insects to humans.

iii) *Vertical transmission*, when the infection is genetically transmitted from infected parents to offsprings.

Based on their nucleic acid content, oncogenic viruses fall into 2 broad groups:
1. Those containing deoxyribonucleic acid are called *DNA oncogenic viruses*.
2. Those containing ribonucleic acid are termed *RNA oncogenic viruses or retroviruses*.

Both types of oncogenic viruses usually have 3 genes and are abbreviated according to the coding pattern by each gene:
i) *gag* gene: codes for group antigen.
ii) *pol* gene: codes for polymerase enzyme.
iii) *env* gene: codes for envelope protein.

Natural history of viral infection can be categorised into primary and persistent:

◆ *Primary viral infections* are majority of the common viral infections in which the infection lasts for a few days to a few weeks and produces clinical manifestations. Primary viral infections are generally cleared by body's innate immunity and specific immune responses. Subsequently, an immunocompetent host is generally immune to the disease or reinfection by the same virus. However, body's immune system is not effective against surface colonization or deep infection or persistence of viral infection.

◆ *Persistence of viral infection or latent infection* in some viruses may occur by acquiring mutations in viruses which resist immune attack by the host, or virus *per se* induces immunosuppression in the host such as HIV.

Viral Oncogenesis: General Aspects

Support to the etiologic role of oncogenic viruses in causation of human cancers is based on the following:
1. Epidemiologic data.
2. Presence of viral DNA in the genome of host target cell.
3. Demonstration of virally induced transformation of human target cells in culture.

4. *In vivo* demonstration of expressed specific transforming viral genes in premalignant and malignant cells.
5. *In vitro* assay of specific viral gene products which produce effects on cell proliferation and survival.

In general, persistence of DNA or RNA viruses may induce mutation in the target host cell, although persistence of viral infection alone is not sufficient for oncogenesis but is one step in the multistep process of cancer development. Generally, RNA viruses have very high mutation rate (e.g. HIV, HCV) than DNA viruses. Mechanisms as to how specific DNA and RNA viruses cause mutation in the host cell are varied, but in general continued presence of DNA or RNA virus in the cell causes activation of growth-promoting pathways or inhibition of tumour-suppressor products in the infected cells. Thus, such virus-infected host cells after having undergone genetic changes enter cell cycle and produce next progeny of transformed cells which have characteristics of autonomous growth and survival completing their role as oncogenic viruses.

General mode of oncogenesis by each group of DNA and RNA oncogenic viruses is briefly considered below:

1. **Mode of DNA viral oncogenesis** Host cells infected by DNA oncogenic viruses may have one of the following 2 results (Fig. 19.13):
i) *Replication* The virus may replicate in the host cell with consequent lysis of the infected cell and release of virions.
ii) *Integration* The viral DNA may integrate into the host cell DNA.

The latter event (integration) results in inducing mutation and thus neoplastic transformation of the host cell, while the former (replication) brings about cell death but no neoplastic transformation. A feature essential for host cell transformation is the expression of virus-specific T-(transforming protein) antigens immediately after infection of the host cell by DNA oncogenic virus (discussed later).

2. **Mode of RNA viral oncogenesis** RNA viruses or retroviruses contain two identical strands of RNA and the enzyme, reverse transcriptase (Fig. 19.14):
i) Reverse transcriptase is RNA-dependent DNA synthetase that acts as a template to synthesise *a single strand of matching viral* DNA i.e. reverse of the normal in which DNA is transcribed into messenger RNA.
ii) The single strand of viral DNA is then copied by DNA-dependent DNA synthetase to form another strand of complementary DNA resulting in *double-stranded viral* DNA or provirus.
iii) The provirus is then integrated into the DNA of the host cell genome and may induce mutation and thus transform the cell into *neoplastic cell*.
iv) Retroviruses are *replication-competent*. The host cells which allow replication of integrated retrovirus are called permissive cells. Non-permissible cells do not permit replication of the integrated retrovirus.

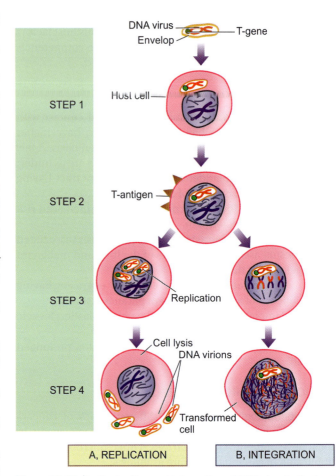

Figure 19.13 ▶ Replication and integration of DNA virus in the host cell.
A, Replication: *Step 1.* The DNA virus invades the host cell. *Step 2.* Viral DNA is incorporated into the host nucleus and T-antigen is expressed immediately after infection. *Step 3.* Replication of viral DNA occurs and other components of virion are formed. The new virions are assembled in the cell nucleus. *Step 4.* The new virions are released, accompanied by host cell lysis. B, Integration: *Steps 1 and 2* are similar as in replication. *Step 3.* Integration of viral genome into the host cell genome occurs which requires essential presence of functional T-antigen. *Step 4.* A 'transformed (neoplastic) cell' is formed.

v) Viral replication begins after integration of the provirus into host cell genome. Integration results in transcription of proviral genes or progenes into messenger RNA which then forms *components of the virus particle*—virion core protein from *gag* gene, reverse transcriptase from *pol* gene, and envelope glycoprotein from *env* gene. The three components of virus particle are then assembled at the plasma membrane of the host cell and the virus particles released by budding off from the plasma membrane, thus completing the process of replication.

With these general comments, we now turn to specific DNA and RNA oncogenic viruses and their specific oncogenic role.

Chapter 19: Etiology and Pathogenesis of Neoplasia

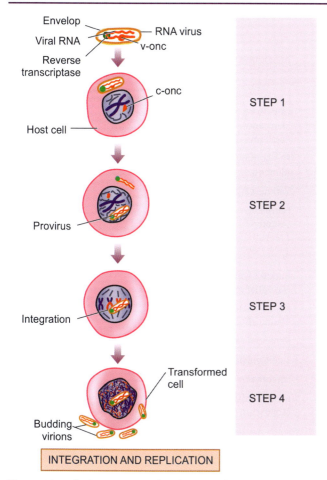

Figure 19.14 ▶ Integration and replication of RNA virus (retrovirus) in the host cell.
Step 1. The RNA virus invades the host cell. The viral envelope fuses with the plasma membrane of the host cell; viral RNA genome as well as reverse transcriptase are released into the cytosol. *Step 2.* Reverse transcriptase acts as template to synthesise single strand of matching viral DNA which is then copied to form complementary DNA resulting in double-stranded viral DNA (provirus). *Step 3.* The provirus is integrated into the host cell genome producing 'transformed host cell.' *Step 4.* Integration of the provirus brings about replication of viral components which are then assembled and released by budding.

DNA Oncogenic Viruses

DNA oncogenic viruses have direct access to the host cell nucleus and are incorporated into the genome of the host cell. DNA viruses are classified into 5 subgroups, each of which is capable of producing neoplasms in different hosts **(Table 19.7)**. These are: Papovaviruses, Herpesviruses, Adenoviruses, Poxviruses and Hepadna viruses.

1. PAPOVAVIRUSES This group consists of the papilloma virus including the human papilloma virus (HPV), polyoma virus and SV-40 (simian vacuolating) virus. These viruses have an etiologic role in following benign and malignant neoplasms in animals and in humans:

i) Papilloma viruses These viruses were the first to be implicated in the etiology of any human neoplasia. These viruses appear to replicate in the layers of stratified squamous epithelium. More than 100 HPV types have been identified; the individual types are associated with different lesions. The following examples of benign and malignant tumours are cited to demonstrate their role in oncogenesis:

In humans—
◈ HPV was first detected as etiologic agent in common *skin warts* or verruca vulgaris (squamous cell papillomas) by Shope in 1933; the condition is infectious. Current evidence supports implication of low-risk HPV types 1, 2, 4 and 7 in common viral warts.
◈ Low-risk HPV types 6 and 11 are involved in the etiology of genital warts (*condyloma acuminata*).
◈ Viral DNA of high-risk HPV types 16, 18, 31, 33 and 45 has been seen in 75-100% cases of *invasive cervical cancer* and its precursor lesions (carcinoma *in situ* and dysplasia) and is strongly implicated.
◈ High-risk HPVs are also involved in causation of *other squamous cell carcinomas* and dysplasias such as of anus, perianal region, vagina, vulva, penis and oral cavity.
◈ HPV types 5 and 8 are responsible for causing an uncommon condition, *epidermodysplasia verruciformis*. The condition is characterised by multiple skin warts and a genetic defect in the cell-mediated immunity. About one-third of cases develop squamous cell carcinoma in the sun-exposed warts.
◈ Some strains of HPV are responsible for causing multiple *juvenile papillomas* of the larynx.

In animals—
◈ Benign warty lesions similar to those seen in humans are produced by different members of the papilloma virus family in susceptible animals such as in rabbits by cottontail rabbit papilloma virus, and in cattle by bovine papilloma virus (BPV).
◈ There is evidence to suggest the association of BPV and cancer of the alimentary tract in cattle.

HPV ONCOGENESIS IN HUMAN CANCER—

Persistent infection with high-risk HPV types in target epithelial cells drives the molecular hallmarks of cancer discussed earlier and directly affect cell growth by following mechanisms:

i) HPV integrates into the host cell DNA which results in overexpression of viral proteins E6 and E7 from high-risk HPV types. E6 and E7 from high-risk HPVs have high affinity for target host cells than these viral oncoproteins from low-risk HPVs.

Table 19.7	DNA oncogenic viruses.		
	VIRUS	HOST	ASSOCIATED TUMOUR
1.	PAPOVAVIRUSES		
	Human papilloma virus	**Humans**	Cervical cancer and its precursor lesions, squamous cell carcinoma at other sites
			Skin cancer in epidermodysplasia verruciformis
			Papillomas (warts) on skin, larynx, genitals (genital warts)
	Papilloma viruses	Cotton-tail rabbits	Papillomas (warts)
		Bovine	Alimentary tract cancer
	Polyoma virus	Mice	Various carcinomas, sarcomas
	SV-40 virus	Monkeys	Harmless
		Hamsters	Sarcoma
		Humans	? Mesothelioma
2.	HERPESVIRUSES		
	Epstein-Barr virus	**Humans**	Burkitt's lymphoma
			Nasopharyngeal carcinoma
	Human herpesvirus 8 (Kaposi's sarcoma herpesvirus)	**Humans**	Kaposi's sarcoma
			Pleural effusion lymphoma
	Lucke' frog virus	Frog	Renal cell carcinoma
	Marek's disease virus	Chickens	T-cell leukaemia-lymphoma
3.	ADENOVIRUSES	Hamsters	Sarcomas
4.	POXVIRUSES	Rabbits	Myxomatosis
		Humans	Molluscum contagiosum, papilloma
5.	HEPADNAVIRUSES		
	Hepatitis B virus	**Humans**	Hepatocellular carcinoma

ii) E6 and E7 viral proteins cause loss of *p53* and *pRB*, the two cell proteins with tumour-suppressor properties. Thus the brakes in cell proliferation are removed, permitting the uncontrolled proliferation.

iii) These viral proteins activate cyclin A and E, and inactivate CDKIs, thus permitting further cell proliferation.

iv) These viral proteins mediate and degrade *BAX*, a proapoptotic gene, thus inhibiting apoptosis.

v) These viral proteins activate telomerase, immortalising the transformed host target cells.

ii) Polyoma virus Polyoma virus occurs as a natural infection in mice.

❖ *In animals*—Polyoma virus infection is responsible for various kinds of carcinomas and sarcomas in immunodeficient (nude) mice and other rodents. In view of its involvement in causation of several unrelated tumours in animals, it was named polyoma.

❖ *In humans*—Polyoma virus infection is not known to produce any human tumour. But it is involved in causation of polyomavirus nephropathy in renal allograft recipients and is also implicated in the etiology of progressive demyelinating leucoencephalopathy, a fatal demyelinating disease.

iii) SV-40 virus Simian vacuolating (SV) virus exists in monkeys without causing any harm but was found in cell cultures being prepared for human polio vaccine in 1960. It was subsequently found that SV-40 could induce sarcoma in hamsters but in humans there is some evidence of involvement of SV-40 infection in mesothelioma of the pleura.

2. HERPESVIRUSES Primary infection of all the herpesviruses in man persists probably for life in a latent stage which can get reactivated later. Important members of herpesvirus family are Epstein-Barr virus, herpes simplex virus type 2 (HSV-2) and human herpesvirus 8 (HHV8), cytomegalovirus (CMV), Lucke's frog virus and Marek's disease virus. Out of these, Lucke's frog virus and Marek's disease virus are implicated in animal tumours only (renal cell carcinoma and T-cell leukaemia-lymphoma respectively). There is no oncogenic role of HSV-2 and CMV in human tumours. The other two—EBV and HHV are implicated in human tumours as under.

EPSTEIN-BARR VIRUS (EBV) EBV infects human B-lymphocytes and epithelial cells and long-term infection stimulates them to proliferate and development of malignancies. EBV is implicated in the following human tumours—Burkitt's lymphoma, anaplastic nasopharyngeal carcinoma, post-transplant lymphoproliferative disease, primary CNS lymphoma in AIDS patients, and Hodgkin's lymphoma. It is also shown to be causative for infectious mononucleosis, a self-limiting disease in humans. The role of EBV in the first two human tumours is given below while others have been discussed elsewhere in relevant chapters.

Burkitt's lymphoma Burkitt's lymphoma was initially noticed in African children by Burkitt in 1958 but is now known to occur in 2 forms—*African endemic form,* and *sporadic form* seen elsewhere in the world. The morphological aspects of the tumour are explained on page 455, while oncogenesis is described here.

There is strong evidence linking Burkitt's lymphoma, a B-lymphocyte neoplasm, with EBV as observed from the following features:

a) Over 90% of Burkitt's lymphomas are EBV-positive in which the tumour cells carry the viral DNA.
b) 100% cases of Burkitt's lymphoma show elevated levels of antibody titers to various EBV antigens.
c) EBV has strong tropism for B lymphocytes. EBV-infected B cells grown in cultures are immortalised i.e. they continue to develop further along B cell-line to propagate their progeny in the altered form.
d) Though EBV infection is almost worldwide in all adults and is also known to cause self-limiting infectious mononucleosis, but the fraction of EBV-infected circulating B cells in such individuals is extremely small.
e) Linkage between Burkitt's lymphoma and EBV infection is very high in African endemic form of the disease and probably in cases of AIDS than in sporadic form of the disease.

However, a few observations, especially regarding sporadic cases of Burkitt's lymphoma, suggest that certain other supportive factors may be contributing. *Immunosuppression* appears to be one such most significant factor. The evidence in favour is as follows:

◆ Normal individuals harbouring EBV-infection as well as cases developing infectious mononucleosis are able to mount good immune response so that they do not develop Burkitt's lymphoma.

◆ In immunosuppressed patients such as in HIV infection and organ transplant recipients, there is marked reduction in body's T-cell immune response and higher incidence of this neoplasm.

◆ It is observed that malaria, which confers immuno-suppressive effect on the host, is prevalent in endemic proportions in regions where endemic form of Burkitt's lymphoma is frequent. This supports the linkage of EBV infection and immunosuppression in the etiology of Burkitt's lymphoma.

Anaplastic nasopharyngeal carcinoma This is the other tumour having close association with EBV infection. The tumour is prevalent in South-East Asia, especially in the Chinese, and in Eskimos. The evidence linking EBV infection with this tumour is as follows:

a) 100% cases of nasopharyngeal carcinoma carry DNA of EBV in nuclei of tumour cells.
b) Individuals with this tumour have high titers of antibodies to various EBV antigens.

However, like in case of Burkitt's lymphoma, there may be some *co-factors* such as genetic susceptibility that account for the unusual geographic distribution.

EBV ONCOGENESIS IN HUMAN CANCER—

Persistent EBV infection is implicated in the causation of malignancies of B lymphocytes and epithelial cells. The mechanism of oncogenesis is as under:

i) Latently infected epithelial cells or B lymphocytes express viral oncogene *LMP1* (latent membrane protein) which is most crucial step in evolution of EBV-associated malignancies. Immunosuppressed individuals are unable to mount attack against EBV infection and thus are more affected.

ii) *LMP1* viral protein dysregulates normal cell proliferation and survival of infected cells and acts like CD40 receptor molecule on B cell surface. Thus, it stimulates B-cell proliferation by activating growth signaling pathways via nuclear factor κB (NF-κB) and *JAK/STAT* pathway.

iii) *LMP-1* viral oncoprotein also activates *BCL2* and thereby prevents apoptosis.

iv) Persistent EBV infection elaborates another viral protein *EBNA-2* (EB virus nuclear antigen) which activates cyclin D in the host cells and thus promotes cell proliferation.

v) In immunocompetent individuals, *LMP1* is kept under control by the body's immune system and in these persons, therefore, lymphoma cells appear only after another characteristic mutation t(8;14) activates growth promoting *MYC* oncogene.

HUMAN HERPESVIRUS 8 (HHV-8) It has been shown that infection with HHV-8 or Kaposi's sarcoma-associated herpesvirus (KSHV) is associated with Kaposi's sarcoma, a vascular neoplasm common in patients of AIDS (page 351). Compared to sporadic Kaposi's sarcoma, the AIDS-associated tumour is multicentric and more aggressive. HHV-8 has lymphotropism and is also implicated in causation of pleural effusion lymphoma and multicentric variant of Castleman's disease.

HHV-8 (KSHV) ONCOGENESIS IN HUMAN CANCER—

i) Viral DNA is seen in nuclei of all tumour cells in Kaposi's sarcoma.

ii) There is overexpression of several KSHV oncoproteins by latently infected cells: v-cyclin, v-interferon regulatory factor (v-IRF) and *LANA* (latency-associated nuclear antigen).

iii) These viral proteins cause increased proliferation and survival of host cells and thus induce malignancy.

3. **ADENOVIRUSES** The human adenoviruses cause upper respiratory infections and pharyngitis.
◆ *In humans,* they are not known to be involved in any tumour.
◆ *In hamsters,* they may induce sarcomas.

4. **POXVIRUSES** This group of oncogenic viruses is involved in the etiology of following lesions:
◆ *In rabbits*—poxviruses cause myxomatosis.
◆ *In humans*—poxviruses cause molluscum contagiosum and may induce squamous cell papilloma.

5. **HEPADNAVIRUSES** *Hepatitis B virus (HBV)* is a member of hepadnavirus (*hepa-* from hepatitis, *-dna* from DNA) family. HBV infection in man causes an acute hepatitis and is responsible for a carrier state, which can result in some cases to chronic hepatitis progressing to hepatic cirrhosis, and onto hepatocellular carcinoma. These lesions and the structure of HBV are described in detail in Chapter 27. Suffice this to say here that there is strong epidemiological evidence linking HBV infection to development of hepatocellular carcinoma as evidenced by the following:
a) The geographic differences in the incidence of hepatocellular carcinoma closely match the variation in prevalence of HBV infection e.g. high incidence in Far-East and Africa.
b) Epidemiological studies in high incidence regions indicate about 200 times higher risk of developing hepatocellular carcinoma in HBV-infected cases as compared to uninfected population in the same area.

Possible mechanism of hepatocellular carcinoma occurring in those harbouring long-standing infection with HBV is chronic destruction of HBV-infected hepatocytes followed by continued hepatocyte proliferation. This process renders the hepatocytes vulnerable to the action of other risk factors such as to aflatoxin causing mutation and neoplastic proliferation.

Evidence has linked an oncogenic role to another hepatotropic virus, hepatitis C virus (HCV) as well which is an RNA virus, while HBV is a DNA virus. HCV is implicated in about half the cases of hepatocellular carcinoma in much the same way as HBV.

HEPATITIS VIRUS ONCOGENESIS IN HUMAN CANCER—
Epidemiologic data firmly support that two hepatotropic viruses, HBV—a DNA virus, and HCV—an RNA virus, are currently involved in causation of 70-80% cases of hepatocellular carcinoma worldwide. Although HBV DNA has been found integrated in the genome of human hepatocytes in many cases of liver cancer which causes mutational changes but a definite pattern is lacking. Thus, exact molecular mechanism as to how HBV and HCV cause hepatocellular carcinoma is yet not quite clear. Probably, multiple factors are involved:
i) Chronic and persistent viral infection with HBV or HCV incites repetitive cycles of inflammation, immune response, cell degeneration/cell death, and regeneration of the hepatocytes which leads to DNA damage of host liver cells.
ii) It is possible that immune response by the host to persistent unresolved infection with these hepatitis viruses becomes defective which promotes tumour development.
iii) On regeneration, proliferation of hepatocytes is stimulated by several growth factors and cytokines elaborated by activated immune cells which contribute to tumour development e.g. factors for angiogenesis, cell survival etc.
iv) Activated immune cells produce nuclear factor κB (NF-κB) that inhibits apoptosis, thus allowing cell survival and growth.
v) HBV genome contains a gene HBx which activates growth signaling pathway.
vi) HBV and HCV do not encode for any specific viral oncoproteins.

RNA Oncogenic Viruses

RNA oncogenic viruses are retroviruses i.e. they contain the enzyme reverse transcriptase (RT), though all retroviruses are not oncogenic **(Table 19.8)**. The enzyme, reverse transcriptase, is required for reverse transcription of viral RNA to synthesise viral DNA strands i.e. reverse of normal—rather than DNA encoding for RNA synthesis, viral RNA transcripts for the DNA by the enzyme RT present in the RNA viruses. RT is a DNA polymerase and helps to form complementary DNA (cDNA) that moves into host cell nucleus and gets incorporated into it.

Based on their activity to transform target cells into neoplastic cells, RNA viruses are divided into 3 subgroups—acute transforming viruses, slow transforming viruses, and human T-cell lymphotropic viruses (HTLV). The former two are implicated in inducing a variety of tumours in animals only while HTLV is causative for human T-cell leukaemia and lymphoma.

1. **ACUTE TRANSFORMING VIRUSES** This group includes retroviruses which transform all the cells infected by them into malignant cells rapidly ('acute'). All the viruses in this group possess one or more viral oncogenes (*v-oncs*). All the members of acute transforming viruses discovered so far are defective viruses in which the particular *v-onc* has substituted other essential genetic material such as *gag, pol* and *env*. These defective viruses cannot replicate by themselves unless the host cell is infected by another 'helper virus'. Acute oncogenic viruses have been identified in tumours in different animals only e.g.
a) Rous sarcoma virus in chickens.
b) Leukaemia-sarcoma viruses of various types such as avian, feline, bovine and primate.

2. **SLOW TRANSFORMING VIRUSES** These oncogenic retroviruses cause development of leukaemias and lymphomas in different species of animals (e.g. in mice, cats and bovine) and include the mouse mammary tumour virus (MMTV) that causes breast cancer in the daughter-mice

Table 19.8: RNA oncogenic viruses.

	VIRUS	HOST	ASSOCIATED TUMOUR
1.	**ACUTE TRANSFORMING VIRUSES**		
	Rous sarcoma virus	Chickens	Sarcoma
	Leukaemia-sarcoma virus	Avian, feline, bovine, primate	Leukaemias, sarcomas
2.	**SLOW TRANSFORMING VIRUSES**		
		Mice, cats, bovine	Leukaemias, lymphomas
	Mouse mammary tumour virus (Bittner milk factor)	Daughter mice	Breast cancer
3.	**HUMAN T-CELL LYMPHOTROPIC VIRUS (HTLV)**		
	HTLV-I	**Human**	Adult T-cell leukaemia lymphoma (ATLL)
	HTLV-II	**Human**	T-cell variant of hairy cell leukaemia
4.	**HEPATITIS C VIRUS**		
	HCV	**Human**	Hepatocellular carcinoma

suckled by the MMTV-infected mother via the causal agent in the mother's milk (*Bittner milk factor*). These viruses have long incubation period between infection and development of neoplastic transformation ('slow'). Slow transforming viruses cause neoplastic transformation by *insertional mutagenesis* i.e. viral DNA synthesised by viral RNA via reverse transcriptase is *inserted* or integrated near the protooncogenes of the host cell resulting in damage to host cell genome (*mutagenesis*) leading to neoplastic transformation.

3. HUMAN T-CELL LYMPHOTROPIC VIRUSES (HTLV)
HTLV is a form of slow transforming virus but is described separately because of 2 reasons:
i) This is the only retrovirus implicated in human cancer.
ii) The mechanism of neoplastic transformation is different from slow transforming as well as from acute transforming viruses.

Four types of HTLVs are recognised—HTLV-1, HTLV-2, HTLV-3 and HTLV-4. It may be mentioned in passing here that the etiologic agent for AIDS, HIV, is also an HTLV (HTLV-3) as described in Chapter 14.

A link between HTLV-1 infection and cutaneous adult T-cell leukaemia-lymphoma (ATLL) has been identified while HTLV-2 is implicated in causation of T-cell variant of hairy cell leukaemia. HTLV-1 is transmitted through sexual contact, by blood, or to infants during breastfeeding. The highlights of this association and mode of neoplastic transformation are as under:
i) Epidemiological studies by tests for antibodies have shown that HTLV-1 infection is endemic in parts of Japan and West Indies where the incidence of ATLL is high. The latent period after HTLV-1 infection is, however, very long (20-30 years).
ii) The initiation of neoplastic process is similar to that for Burkitt's lymphoma except that HTLV-1 has tropism for CD4+T lymphocytes as in HIV infection, while EBV of Burkitt's lymphoma has tropism for B lymphocytes.
iii) As in Burkitt's lymphoma, immunosuppression plays a supportive role in the neoplastic transformation by HTLV-1 infection.

HTLV ONCOGENESIS IN HUMAN CANCER—

The molecular mechanism of ATLL leukaemogenesis by HTLV infection of CD4+ T lymphocytes is not clear. Neoplastic transformation by HTLV-I infection differs from acute transforming viruses because it does not contain *v-onc*, and from other slow transforming viruses because it does not have fixed site of insertion for insertional mutagenesis. Probably, the process is multifactorial:

i) HTLV-1 genome has unique region called pX distinct from other retroviruses, which encodes for two essential viral oncoproteins— *TAX* and *REX*. *TAX* protein up-regulates the expression of cellular genes controlling T-cell replication, while *REX* gene product regulates viral protein production by affecting mRNA expression.

ii) *TAX* viral protein interacts with transcription factor, NF-κB, which stimulates genes for cytokines (interleukins) and their receptors in infected T cells which activates proliferation of T cells by autocrine pathway.

iii) The inappropriate gene expression activates pathway of the cell proliferation by activation of cyclins and inactivation of tumour suppressor genes *CDKN2A/p16* and *p53*, stimulating cell cycle.

iv) Initially, proliferation of infected T cells is polyclonal but subsequently several mutations appear due to *TAX*-based genomic changes in the host cell and monoclonal proliferation of leukaemia occurs.

Viruses and Human Cancer: A Summary

In humans, epidemiological as well as circumstantial evidence has been accumulating since the discovery of

Section IV: Neoplasia

contagious nature of common human wart (papilloma) in 1907 that cancer may have viral etiology. Presently, about 20% of all human cancers worldwide are virally induced. Aside from experimental evidence, the etiologic role of DNA and RNA viruses in a variety of human neoplasms has already been explained above. Here, a summary of different viruses implicated in human tumours is presented (Fig. 19.15):

Benign tumours Following 2 benign conditions which are actually doubtful as tumours have a definite viral etiology:
i) Human wart (papilloma) caused by human papilloma virus
ii) Molluscum contagiosum caused by poxvirus

Malignant tumours The following 8 human cancers have enough epidemiological, serological, and in some cases genomic evidence, that viruses are implicated in their etiology:
i) *Burkitt's lymphoma* by Epstein-Barr virus.
ii) *Nasopharyngeal carcinoma* by Epstein-Barr virus.
iii) *Primary hepatocellular carcinoma* by hepatitis B virus and hepatitis C virus.
iv) *Cervical cancer* by high risk human papilloma virus types (HPV 16 and 18).
v) *Kaposi's sarcoma* by human herpes virus type 8 (HHV-8).
vi) *Pleural effusion B cell lymphoma* by HHV8.
vii) *Adult T-cell leukaemia and lymphoma* by HTLV-1.
viii) *T-cell variant of hairy cell leukaemia* by HTLV-2

Current knowledge and understanding of viral carcinogenesis has provided an opportunity to invent specific vaccines and suggest appropriate specific therapy. For example, hepatitis B vaccines is being widely used to control hepatitis B and is expected to lower incidence of HBV-related hepatocellular carcinoma in high risk populations. HPV vaccine is being used in some countries in young women and is expected to protect them against HPV-associated precancerous lesions of the cervix.

GIST BOX 19.3 — Carcinogens and Carcinogenesis

❖ Important groups of carcinogenic agents having role in carcinogenesis are chemical, physical and biologic agents.
❖ Chemical carcinogenesis occurs by induction of mutation in the proto-oncogenes and anti-oncogenes and goes through sequential stages of initiation, promotion and progression.
❖ Carcinogenic chemicals are of 2 types: direct-acting and indirect-acting.
❖ Direct-acting carcinogens (e.g. alkylating agents, acylating agents) can induce cellular transformation without undergoing any prior metabolic activation.
❖ More common are indirect-acting carcinogens (e.g. polycyclic aromatic hydrocarbons, aromatic amines, azo dyes, naturally-occurring products etc) which require metabolic conversion within the body so as to become 'ultimate' carcinogens.
❖ Physical agents in carcinogenesis are radiation (ultraviolet light and ionising radiation) which is more important, and some non-radiation physical agents.
❖ Excessive exposure to UV rays in humans can cause various forms of skin cancers while ionising radiation is implicated in several human cancers e.g. leukaemias, cancers of the thyroid, skin, breast, ovary, uterus, lung, myeloma, and salivary glands.
❖ Out of biologic agents (viruses, bacteria, parasites, fungi), persistence of DNA or RNA viral infection is of major significance and may induce mutation in the target host cell which is one step in the multistep process of cancer development.
❖ DNA oncogenic viruses with evidence in human cancers are Epstein-Barr virus (Burkitt's lymphoma and nasopharyngeal carcinoma), hepatitis B virus (hepatocellular carcinoma), human papilloma virus types HPV 16 and 18 (carcinoma cervix) and human herpes virus type 8 (Kaposi's sarcoma and pleural effusion B cell lymphoma).
❖ RNA viruses having oncongeic role are HTLV-1 (adult T-cell leukaemia and lymphoma), HTLV-2 (T-cell variant of hairy cell leukaemia) and hepatitis C virus (hepatocellular carcinoma).

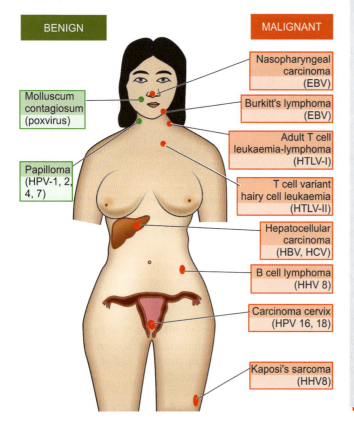

Figure 19.15 ▶ Viruses (in brackets) in human tumours.

20 Host-Tumour Relationship and Diagnosis of Neoplasms

Natural biology of tumours relates to host-tumour inter-relationship that includes response of host against tumour and the effect of tumour on host. Another clinically significant aspect discussed here is the final diagnosis of tumours.

HOST RESPONSE AGAINST TUMOUR (TUMOUR IMMUNOLOGY)

It has long been known that body's immune system can recognise tumour cells as 'non-self' and they attempt to destroy them and limit the spread of cancer. The following observations provide basis for this concept:

1. Certain cancers evoke significant *lymphocytic infiltrate* composed of immunocompetent cells and such tumours have somewhat better prognosis e.g. medullary carcinoma breast (as compared with infiltrating ductal carcinoma), seminoma testis (as compared with other germ cell tumours of testis).

2. Rarely, a cancer may *spontaneously regress* partially or completely, probably under the influence of host defense mechanism. For example, rare spontaneous disappearance of malignant melanoma temporarily from the primary site which may then reappear as metastasis.

3. It is highly unusual to have primary and *secondary tumours in the spleen* due to its ability to destroy the growth and proliferation of tumour cells.

4. Existence of immune surveillance is substantiated by increased frequency of *cancers in immunodeficient host* e.g. in AIDS patients, or development of post-transplant lymphoproliferative disease.

In an attempt to support the above observations and to understand the underlying host defense mechanisms, experimental animal studies involving tumour transplants were carried out. The findings of animal experiments coupled with research on human cancers has led to the concept of immunology of cancer which is discussed under the following headings:
1. Tumour antigens
2. Antitumour immune responses
3. Immunotherapy.

1. TUMOUR ANTIGENS

Tumour cells express surface antigens which have been seen in animals and in some human tumours. Older classification of tumour antigens was based on their surface sharing characteristics on normal versus tumour cells and on their recognition by cytotoxic T lymphocytes CTL (CD8+T cells) on the basis of class I MHC molecules. Accordingly, tumour antigens were categorised into following two types:

i) *Tumour-specific antigens (TSAs)* located on tumour cells and are unique or specific antigens for particular tumour and not shared by normal cells.

ii) *Tumour associated antigens (TAAs)* are present on tumour cells as well as on some normal cells from where the tumour originated.

However, it is now known that TSAs and TAAs can both be present on normal cells and categorisation into TSA and TAA does not hold true. Thus, presently distinction of tumour antigens is based on their recognition by the host immune cells, i.e. CD8+ T cells (CTL), and by the molecular structure of the tumour antigens. Currently, various groups of tumour antigens are as follows:

i) Oncoproteins from mutated oncogenes Protein products derived from mutated oncogenes result in expression of cell surface antigens on tumour cells. The examples include products of *RAS*, *BCR/ABL* and CDK4.

ii) Protein products of tumour suppressor genes In some tumours, protein products of mutated tumour suppressor genes cause expression of tumour antigens on the cell surface. The examples are mutated proteins *p53* and β-catenin.

iii) Overexpressed cellular proteins Some tumours are associated with a normal cellular protein but is excessively expressed in tumour cells and incite host immune response. For example, in melanoma the tumour antigen is structurally normal melanocyte specific protein, tyrosinase, which is overexpressed compared with normal cells. Similarly, *HER2/neu* protein is overexpressed in many cases of breast cancer.

iv) Abnormally expressed cellular proteins Sometimes, a cellular protein is present in some normal cells but is abnormally expressed on the surface of tumour cells of some cancers. The classic example is presence of *MAGE* gene silent in normal adult tissues except in male germ line but *MAGE* genes are expressed on surface of many tumours such as melanoma (abbreviation *MAGE* from 'melanoma antigen' in which it was first found), cancers of liver, lung, stomach and oesophagus. Other examples of similar aberrantly expressed gene products in cancers are *GAGE* (G antigen), *BAGE* (B melanoma antigen) and *RAGE* (renal tumour antigen).

v) Tumour antigens from viral oncoproteins As already discussed above, many oncogenic viruses express viral oncoproteins which result in expression of antigens on tumour cells e.g. viral oncoproteins of HPV (E6, E7) in cervical cancer and EBNA proteins of EBV in Burkitt's lymphoma.

vi) Tumour antigens from randomly mutated genes Various other carcinogens such as chemicals and radiation induce random mutations in the target cells. These mutated cells elaborate protein products targeted by the CTL of the immune system causing expression of tumour antigens.

vii) Cell specific differentiation antigens Normally differentiated cells have cellular antigens which forms the basis of diagnostic immunohistochemistry. Cancers have varying degree of loss of differentiation but particular lineage of the tumour cells can be identified by tumour antigens. For example, various CD markers for various subtypes of lymphomas, prostate specific antigen (PSA) in carcinoma of prostate.

viii) Oncofoetal antigens Oncofoetal antigens such as α-foetoprotein (AFP) and carcinoembryonic antigen (CEA) are normally expressed in embryonic life. But these antigens appear in certain cancers—AFP in liver cancer and CEA in colon cancer which can be detected in serum as cancer markers.

ix) Abnormal cell surface molecules The normal cell expresses surface molecules of glycolipids, glycoproteins, mucins and blood group antigens. In some cancers, there is abnormally changed expression of these molecules. For example, there may be changed blood group antigen, or abnormal expression of mucin in ovarian cancer (CA-125) and in breast cancer (MUC-1).

2. ANTI-TUMOUR IMMUNE RESPONSES

Although both cell-mediated and humoral immunity is mounted by the host against the tumour, significant anti-tumour effector mechanism is mainly cell-mediated. However, despite the existence of immune mechanisms, most of the cancers outsmart these host defenses and gain an upper hand in their battle against the host due to failed immune regulatory mechanisms.

i) Cell-mediated mechanism This is the main mechanism of destruction of tumour cells by the host. The following cellular responses can destroy the tumour cells and induce tumour immunity in humans:
a) *Specifically sensitised cytotoxic T lymphocytes (CTL)* i.e. CD8+ T cells are directly cytotoxic to the target cell and require contact between them and tumour cells. CTL have been found to be effective against virally-induced cancers e.g. in Burkitt's lymphoma (EBV-induced), invasive squamous cell carcinoma of cervix (HPV-induced).
b) *Natural killer (NK) cells* are lymphocytes which after activation by IL-2, destroy tumour cells without sensitisation, either directly or by antibody-dependent cellular cytotoxicity (ADCC). NK cells together with T lymphocytes are the first line of defense against tumour cells and can lyse tumour cells.
c) *Macrophages* are activated by interferon-γ secreted by T-cells and NK-cells, and therefore there is close collaboration of these two subpopulation of lymphocytes and macrophages. Activated macrophages mediate cytotoxicity by production of oxygen free radicals or by tumour necrosis factor.

ii) Humoral mechanism As such there are no anti-tumour humoral antibodies which are effective against cancer cells *in vivo*. However, *in vitro* humoral antibodies may kill tumour cells by complement activation or by antibody-dependent cytotoxicity. Based on this, monoclonal antibody treatment is offered to cases of some types of non-Hodgkin's lymphoma.

iii) Immune regulatory mechanisms Most cancers grow relentlessly in spite of host immunity. This is explained due to deranged controlling mechanisms of immunity as under:
a) During progression of the cancer, immunogenic cells may disappear.
b) Cytotoxic T-cells and NK-cells may play a self-regulatory role.
c) Immunosuppression mediated by various acquired carcinogenic agents (viruses, chemicals, radiation).
d) Immunosuppressive role of factors secreted by tumour cells e.g. transforming growth factor-β.
e) The tumour cells arise from own cells and hence the immune system fails to recognise them as "foreign" which creates a phenomenon of tumour tolerance.

The mechanisms of these immune responses are schematically illustrated in **Fig. 20.1**.

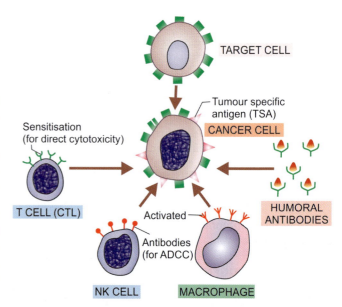

Figure 20.1 ▶ Schematic illustration of immune responses in cancer. For details see the text (CTL = cytotoxic T-lymphocyte; NK cell = natural killer cell; ADCC = antibody-dependent cellular cytotoxicity).

3. CANCER IMMUNOTHERAPY

It is a generally-accepted hypothesis that the best defense against human diseases is our own immune system. As outlined above, in cancer the immune system starts failing and requires to be boosted to become more effective in fighting against cancer. While there is no magic bullet against cancer, immunotherapy has been used as treatment against cancer in combination with other therapies (surgery, radiation, chemotherapy).

i) Non-specific stimulation of the host immune response was initially attempted with BCG, *Corynebacterium parvum* and levamisole, but except slight effect in acute lymphoid leukaemia, it failed to have any significant influence in any other tumour.

ii) Specific stimulation of the immune system was attempted next by immunising the host with irradiated tumour cells but failed to yield desired results because if the patient's tumour within the body failed to stimulate effective immunity, the implanted cells of the same tumour are unlikely to do so.

iii) Current status of immunotherapy is focussed on following three main approaches:

a) *Cellular immunotherapy* consists of infusion of tumour-specific cytotoxic T cells which will increase the population of tumour-infiltrating lymphocytes (TIL). The patient's peripheral blood lymphocytes are cultured with interleukin-2 which generates lymphokine-activated killer cells having potent anti-tumour effect.

b) *Cytokine therapy* is used to build up specific and non-specific host defenses. These include: interleukin-2, interferon-α and -γ, tumour necrosis factor-α, and granulocyte-monocyte colony stimulating factor (GM-CSF).

c) *Monoclonal antibody therapy* is undergoing trial against CD20 molecule of B cells in certain B cell leukaemias and lymphomas.

EFFECT OF TUMOUR ON HOST

Malignant tumours produce more ill-effects than the benign tumours. The effects may be local, or generalised and more widespread.

A. LOCAL EFFECTS

Both benign and malignant tumours cause local effects on the host due to their size or location. Malignant tumours due to rapid and invasive growth potential have more serious effects. Some of the local effects of tumours are as under:

i) Compression Many benign tumours pose only a cosmetic problem. Some benign tumours, however, due to their critical location, have more serious consequences e.g. pituitary adenoma may lead to serious endocrinopathy; a small benign tumour in ampulla of Vater may lead to biliary obstruction.

ii) Mechanical obstruction Benign and malignant tumours in the gut may produce intestinal obstruction.

iii) Tissue destruction Malignant tumours, both primary and metastatic, infiltrate and destroy the vital structures.

iv) Infarction, ulceration, haemorrhage Cancers have a greater tendency to undergo infarction, surface ulceration and haemorrhage than the benign tumours. Secondary bacterial infection may supervene. Large tumours in mobile organs (e.g. an ovarian tumour) may undergo torsion and produce infarction and haemorrhage.

B. SYSTEMIC MANIFESTATIONS

Generalised effects of cancer include cancer cachexia, fever, tumour lysis syndrome and paraneoplastic syndromes.

1. CANCER CACHEXIA Patients with advanced and disseminated cancers terminally have asthenia (emaciation), and anorexia, together referred to as cancer cachexia (meaning wasting). Exact mechanism of cachexia is not clear but it does not occur due to increased nutritional demands of the tumour. Certain cytokines such as tumour necrosis factor α (TNF-α), interleukin-1 and interferon-γ play a contributory role in cachexia. Various other causes of cancer cachexia include necrosis, ulceration, haemorrhage, infection, malabsorption, anxiety, pain, insomnia, hypermetabolism and pyrexia.

2. FEVER Fever of unexplained origin may be presenting feature in some malignancies such as in Hodgkin's disease, adenocarcinoma kidney, osteogenic sarcoma and many other tumours. The exact mechanism of tumour-associated fever is not known but probably the tumour cells themselves elaborate pyrogens.

3. TUMOUR LYSIS SYNDROME This is a condition caused by extensive destruction of a large number of rapidly proliferating tumour cells. The condition is seen more often in cases of lymphomas and leukaemias than solid tumours and may be due to large tumour burden (e.g. in Burkitt's lymphoma), chemotherapy, administration of glucocorticoids or certain hormonal agents (e.g. tamoxifen). It is characterised by hyperuricaemia, hyperkalaemia, hyperphosphataemia and hypocalcaemia, all of which may result in acidosis and renal failure.

4. PARANEOPLASTIC SYNDROMES Paraneoplastic syndromes (PNS) are a group of conditions developing in patients with advanced cancer which are neither explained by direct and distant spread of the tumour, nor by the usual hormone elaboration by the tissue of origin of the tumour. About 10 to 15% of the patients with advanced cancer develop one or more of the syndromes included in the PNS. Rarely, PNS may be the earliest manifestation of a latent cancer.

The various clinical syndromes included in the PNS are as summarised in Table 20.1 and are briefly outlined here:

i) Endocrine syndrome Elaboration of hormones or hormone-like substances by cancer cells of non-endocrine

Table 20.1 Summary of paraneoplastic syndromes.

	CLINICAL SYNDROME	UNDERLYING CANCER	MECHANISM
1.	**ENDOCRINE SYNDROME**		
	i. Hypercalcaemia	Lung (sq. cell Ca), kidney, breast, Adult T-cell leukaemia lymphoma	Parathormone-like protein Vitamin D
	ii. Cushing's syndrome	Lung (small cell carcinoma), pancreas, neural tumours	ACTH or ACTH-like substance
	iii. Inappropriate anti-diuresis	Lung (small cell Ca), prostate, intracranial tumour	ADH or atrial natriuretic factor
	iv. Hypoglycaemia	Pancreas (islet cell tumour), mesothelioma, fibrosarcoma	Insulin or insulin-like substance
	v. Carcinoid syndrome	Bronchial carcinoid tumour, carcinoma pancreas, stomach	Serotonin, bradykinin
	vi. Polycythaemia	Kidney, liver, cerebellar haemangioma	Erythropoietin
2.	**NEUROMUSCULAR SYNDROMES**		
	i. Myasthenia gravis	Thymoma	Immunologic
	ii. Neuromuscular disorders	Lung (small cell Ca), breast	Immunologic
3.	**OSSEOUS, JOINT AND SOFT TISSUE**		
	i. Hypertrophic osteoarthropathy	Lung	Not known
	ii. Clubbing of fingers	Lung	Not known
4.	**HAEMATOLOGIC SYNDROMES**		
	i. Thrombophlebitis (Trousseau's phenomenon)	Pancreas, lung, GIT	Hypercoagulability
	ii. Non-bacterial thrombotic endocarditis	Advanced cancers	Hypercoagulability
	iii. Disseminated intravascular coagulation (DIC)	AML, adenocarcinoma	Chronic thrombotic phenomena
	iv. Anaemia	Thymoma	Unknown
5.	**GASTROINTESTINAL SYNDROMES**		
	i. Malabsorption	Lymphoma of small bowel	Hypoalbuminaemia
6.	**RENAL SYNDROMES**		
	i. Nephrotic syndrome	Advanced cancers	Renal vein thrombosis, systemic amyloidosis
7.	**CUTANEOUS SYNDROMES**		
	i. Acanthosis nigricans	Stomach, large bowel	Immunologic
	ii. Seborrheic dermatitis	Bowel	Immunologic
	iii. Exfoliative dermatitis	Lymphoma	Immunologic
8.	**AMYLOIDOSIS**		
	i. Primary	Multiple myeloma	Immunologic (AL protein)
	ii. Secondary	Kidney, lymphoma, solid tumours	AA protein

origin is called as ectopic hormone production. Some examples are given below:

a) *Hypercalcaemia* Symptomatic hypercalcaemia unrelated to hyperparathyroidism is the most common syndrome in PNS. It occurs from elaboration of parathormone-like substance by tumours such as squamous cell carcinoma of the lung, carcinoma kidney, breast and adult T cell leukaemia lymphoma.

b) *Cushing's syndrome* About 10% patients of small cell carcinoma of the lung elaborate ACTH or ACTH-like substance producing Cushing's syndrome. In addition, cases with pancreatic carcinoma and neurogenic tumours may be associated with Cushing's syndrome.

c) *Polycythaemia* Secretion of erythropoietin by certain tumours such as renal cell carcinoma, hepatocellular carcinoma and cerebellar haemangioma may cause polycythaemia.

d) *Hypoglycaemia* Elaboration of insulin-like substance by fibrosarcomas, islet cell tumours of pancreas and mesothelioma may cause hypoglycaemia.

ii) Neuromyopathic syndromes About 5% of cancers are associated with progressive destruction of neurons throughout the nervous system without evidence of metastasis in the brain and spinal cord. This is probably mediated by immunologic mechanisms. The changes in the neurons may affect the muscles as well. The changes are: peripheral neuropathy, cortical cerebellar degeneration, myasthenia gravis syndrome, polymyositis.

iii) Effects on osseous, joints and soft tissue e.g. hypertrophic pulmonary osteoarthropathy and clubbing of fingers in cases of bronchogenic carcinoma, by unknown mechanism but is probably due to increased blood flow to the limb.

iv) Haematologic and vascular syndrome e.g. venous thrombosis (Trousseau's phenomenon), non-bacterial thrombotic endocarditis, disseminated intravascular coagulation (DIC), leukemoid reaction and normocytic normochromic anaemia occurring in advanced cancers. Autoimmune haemolytic anaemia may be associated with B-cell malignancies.

v) Gastrointestinal syndromes Malabsorption of various dietary components as well as hypoalbuminaemia may be associated with a variety of cancers which do not directly involve small bowel.

vi) Renal syndromes Renal vein thrombosis or systemic amyloidosis may produce nephrotic syndrome in patients with cancer.

vii) Cutaneous syndromes Acanthosis nigricans characterised by the appearance of black warty lesions in the axillae and the groins may appear in the course of adenocarcinoma of gastrointestinal tract. Other cutaneous lesions in PNS include seborrheic dermatitis in advanced malignant tumours and exfoliative dermatitis in lymphomas and Hodgkin's disease.

viii) Amyloidosis Primary amyloid deposits may occur in multiple myeloma whereas renal cell carcinoma and other solid tumours may be associated with secondary systemic amyloidosis.

GIST BOX 20.1 Tumour-Host Interrelationship

❖ The natural history of a neoplasm depends upon host response against tumour (or cancer immunology) and effect of tumour on host.
❖ The existence of host immune defense is supported by the observation of lymphocytic infiltrate in certain tumours with good prognosis, spontaeneous regression of some tumours due to host immune attack and increased incidence of tumours in immunodeficient host.
❖ Tumour cells express a variety of antigens which include: protein products from mutated oncogenes and antioncogenes, overexpression and abnormal expression of normal cellular proteins, virally derived oncoproteins, cell surface differentiation antigens, oncofoetal antigens and abnormal cell surface molecules.
❖ Significant immune response by the host is by cell-mediated immunity exerted by specifically sensitised cytotoxic T cells, natural killer cells and activated macrophages, and to a lesser extent by anti-tumour humoral antibodies.
❖ Malignant tumours produce more ill-effects on the host than the benign tumours and these may be local, or generalised and more widespread.
❖ Local effects of the tumour depend upon the site. These effects are due to mechanical compression, obstruction, tissue destruction and infarction, ulceration and haemorrhage.
❖ Systemic effects are in the form of cancer cachexia, fever, tumour lysis syndrome, and paraneoplastic syndrome.
❖ Paraneoplastic syndrome has several presentations with widespread manifestations. Some of the important features are due to ectopic hormone elaboration, and neuromuscular, osseous, haematologic, gastrointestinal cutaneous and renal manifestations.

PATHOLOGIC DIAGNOSIS OF CANCER

When the diagnosis of cancer is suspected on clinical examination and on other investigations, it must be confirmed. The most certain and reliable method which has stood the test of time is the histological examination of biopsy, though recently many other methods to arrive at the correct diagnosis or confirm the histological diagnosis are available.

1. HISTOLOGICAL METHODS

These methods are most valuable in arriving at the accurate diagnosis and are based on microscopic examination of excised tumour mass or open/needle biopsy from the mass supported with complete clinical and investigative data. The tissue must be fixed in 10% formalin for light microscopic examination and in glutaraldehyde for electron microscopic studies, while quick-frozen section and hormonal analysis are carried out on fresh unfixed tissues. These methods are as under:

i) Paraffin-embedding technique In this, 10% formalin-fixed tissue is used. The representative tissue piece from larger tumour mass or biopsy is processed through a tissue processor having an overnight cycle, embedded in molten paraffin wax for making tissue blocks. These blocks are trimmed followed by fine-sectioning into 3-4 µm sections using rotary microtome for which either fixed knife or disposable blades are used for cutting. These sections are then stained with haematoxylin and eosin (H & E) and examined microscopically.

ii) Frozen section In this technique, unfixed tissue is used and the procedure is generally carried out when the patient is undergoing surgery and is still under anaesthesia. Here, instead of tissue processor and paraffin-embedding, cryostat machine is employed and fresh unfixed tissue is used. The tissue biopsy is quickly frozen to ice at about −25°C that acts as embedding medium and then sectioned. Sections are then ready for rapid H & E or toluidine blue staining. Frozen section is a rapid intraoperative diagnostic procedure for tissues before proceeding to a major radical surgery or may be used to know the extent of presence of cancer at the surgical margin.

The histological diagnosis by either of these methods is made on the basis that morphological features of *benign tumours* resemble those of normal tissue and that they are unable to invade and metastasise, while *malignant tumours* are identified by lack of differentiation in cancer cells termed 'anaplasia' or 'cellular atypia' and may invade as well as metastasise. The light microscopic and ultrastructural characteristics of neoplastic cell have been described earlier on page 267.

2. CYTOLOGICAL METHODS

Cytological methods for diagnosis consist of 2 types of methods: study of cells shed off into body cavities (exfoliative cytology) and study of cells by putting a fine needle introduced under vacuum into the lesion (fine needle aspiration cytology, FNAC).

i) Exfoliative cytology Cytologic smear (Papanicolaou or Pap smear) method was initially employed for detecting dysplasia, carcinoma *in situ* and invasive carcinoma of the uterine cervix. However, its use has now been widely extended to include examination of sputum and bronchial washings; pleural, peritoneal and pericardial effusions; urine, gastric secretions, and CSF. The method is based on microscopic identification of the characteristics of malignant cells which are non-cohesive and loose and are thus shed off or 'exfoliated' into the lumen. However, a 'negative diagnosis' does not altogether rule out malignancy due to possibility of sampling error.

ii) Fine needle aspiration cytology (FNAC) Currently, cytopathology includes not only study of exfoliated cells but also materials obtained from superficial and deep-seated lesions in the body which do not shed off cells freely. The latter method consists of study of cells obtained by a fine needle introduced under vacuum into the lesion, so called *fine needle aspiration cytology (FNAC)*. The superficial masses can be aspirated under direct vision while deep-seated masses such as intra-abdominal, pelvic organs and retroperitoneum are frequently investigated by ultrasound (US)-or computed tomography (CT) guided fine needle aspirations. The smears are fixed in 95% ethanol by wet fixation, or may be air-dried unfixed. While Papanicolaou method of staining is routinely employed in most laboratories for *wet fixed smears,* others prefer H and E due to similarity in staining characteristics in the sections obtained by paraffin-embedding. *Air-dried smears* are stained by May-Grünwald-Giemsa or Leishman stain. FNAC has a diagnostic reliability between 80-97% but it must not be substituted for clinical judgement or compete with an indicated histopathologic biopsy.

3. HISTOCHEMISTRY AND CYTOCHEMISTRY

Histochemistry and cytochemistry are additional diagnostic tools which help the pathologist in identifying the chemical composition of cells, their constituents and their products by special staining methods.

Though immunohistochemical techniques are more useful for tumour diagnosis (see below), many histochemical and cytochemical stains (also called as special stains) are still employed for this purpose. Some of the common examples are summarised in **Table 20.2**.

Table 20.2 Common histochemical/cytochemical stains in tumour diagnosis.

	SUBSTANCE	STAIN
1.	Basement membrane/ collagen	Periodic acid-Schiff (PAS) Reticulin Van Gieson Masson's trichrome
2.	Glycogen	PAS with diastase loss
3.	Glycoproteins, glycolipids, glycomucins *(epithelial origin)*	PAS with diastase persistence
4.	Acid mucin *(mesenchymal origin)*	Alcian blue
5.	Mucin (in general)	Combined Alcian blue-PAS
6.	Argyrophilic/ argentaffin granules	Silver stains
7.	Cross striations	PTAH stain
8.	Enzymes	Myeloperoxidase Acid phosphatase Alkaline phosphatase
9.	Nucleolar organiser regions (NORs)	Colloidal silver stain

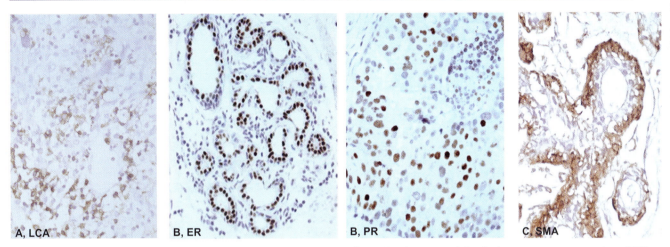

Figure 20.2 ▶ Examples of IHC staining at different sites in the tumour cells. A, Membranous staining for leucocyte common antigen (LCA) or CD45 in lymphomas. B, Cytoplasmic staining for smooth muscle actin (SMA) in myoepithelium on breast acinus. C, Nuclear staining for breast ER-PR receptor studies in breast cancer.

4. IMMUNOHISTOCHEMISTRY

With current technology, it is possible to use routinely processed paraffin-embedded tissue blocks for immunohistochemistry (IHC), thus making profound impact on diagnostic surgical pathology. Earlier, diagnostic surgical pathology used to be considered a subjective science with inter-observer variation, particularly in borderline lesions and lesions of undetermined origin, but use of IHC has added *objectivity, specificity* and *reproducibility* to the surgical pathologist's diagnosis.

IHC is an immunological method of recognising a cell by one or more of its specific components in the cell membrane, cytoplasm or nucleus and are accordingly interpreted (Fig. 20.2). These cell components (called antigens) combine with specific antibodies on the formalin-fixed paraffin sections or cytological smears. The complex of antigen-antibody on slide is made visible for light microscopic identification by either fluorescent dyes ('fluorochromes') or by enzyme system ('chromogens'). The specific antibody against a particular cellular antigen is obtained by hybridoma technique for monoclonal antibody production. These monoclonal antibodies, besides being *specific* against antigen, are highly sensitive in detection of antigenic component, and, therefore, impart objectivity to the subjective tumour diagnosis made by the surgical pathologist.

Various applications of IHC in tumour diagnosis are as under:

i) Tumours of uncertain histogenesis IHC has brought about a revolution in approach to diagnosis of tumours of uncertain origin, primary as well as metastatic from an unknown primary tumour. A panel of antibodies is chosen to resolve such diagnostic problem cases; the selection of antibodies being made is based on clinical history, morphologic features, and results of other relevant investigations. Towards this, IHC stains for *intermediate filaments* (keratin, vimentin, desmin, neurofilaments, and glial fibillary acidic proteins) expressed by the tumour cells are of immense value besides other common IHC stains listed in Table 20.3.

ii) Prognostic markers in cancer The second important application of IHC is to predict the prognosis of tumours by detection of micrometastasis, occult metastasis, and by identification of certain features acquired, or products elaborated, or genes overexpressed, by the malignant cells to predict the biologic behaviour of the tumour. A few examples are: proto-oncogenes (e.g. HER-2/neu overexpression in carcinoma breast), tumour suppressor genes or anti-oncogenes (e.g. *Rb* gene, *p53*), growth factor receptors (e.g. epidermal growth factor receptor or *EGFR*), and tumour cell proliferation markers (e.g. *Ki67*, proliferation cell nuclear antigen *PCNA*).

iii) Prediction of response to therapy IHC is widely used to predict therapeutic response in two important tumours—carcinoma of the breast and prostate. Both these tumours are under the growth regulation of hormones—oestrogen and androgen, respectively. The specific receptors for these growth regulating hormones are located on respective tumour cells. Tumours expressing high level of receptor positivity would respond favourably to removal of the endogenous source of such hormones (oophorectomy in oestrogen-positive breast cancer and orchiectomy in androgen-positive prostatic carcinoma). Alternatively, hormonal therapy is administered to lower their levels: oestrogen therapy in prostatic cancer and androgen therapy in breast cancer. The results of oestrogen-receptors and progesterone-receptors in breast cancer have significant prognostic correlation, though the results of

Table 20.3: Common panel of immunohistochemical stains for tumours of uncertain origin.

	TUMOUR	IMMUNOSTAIN
1.	Epithelial tumours (Carcinomas)	i) Pankeratin (fractions: high and low molecular weight keratins, HMW-K, LMW-K) ii) Epithelial membrane antigen (EMA) iii) Carcinoembryonic antigen (CEA) iv) Neuron-specific enolase (NSE)
2.	Mesenchymal tumours (Sarcomas)	i) Vimentin (general mesenchymal) ii) Desmin (for general myogenic) iii) Muscle specific actin (for general myogenic) iv) Myoglobin (for skeletal myogenic) v) α-1-anti-chymotrypsin (for malignant fibrous histiocytoma) vi) Factor VIII (for vascular tumours) vii) CD34 (endothelial marker)
3.	Special groups	
	a) Melanoma	i) HMB-45 (most specific) ii) Vimentin iii) S-100
	b) Lymphoma	i) Leucocyte common antigen (LCA/CD45) ii) Pan-B (Immunoglobulins, CD20) iii) Pan-T (CD3) iv) CD15, CD30 (RS cell marker for Hodgkin's)
	c) Neural and neuro-endocrine tumours	i) Neurofilaments (NF) ii) NSE iii) GFAP (for glial tumours) iv) Chromogranin (for neuroendocrine)

androgen-receptor studies in prostatic cancer have limited prognostic value.

iv) Infections IHC stains can be applied to confirm infectious agent in tissues by use of specific antibodies against microbial DNA or RNA e.g. detection of viruses (HBV, CMV, HPV, herpesviruses), bacteria (e.g. *Helicobacter pylori*), and parasites (*Pneumocystis jerovecii*) etc.

5. ELECTRON MICROSCOPY

Ultrastructural examination of tumour cells offers selective role in diagnostic pathology. EM examination may be helpful in confirming or substantiating a tumour diagnosis arrived at by light microscopy and immunohistochemistry. A few general features of malignant tumour cells by EM examination can be appreciated:
i) Cell junctions, their presence and type.
ii) Cell surface, e.g. presence of microvilli.
iii) Cell shape and cytoplasmic extensions.
iv) Shape of the nucleus and features of nuclear membrane.
v) Nucleoli, their size and density.
vi) Cytoplasmic organelles—their number is generally reduced.
vii) Dense bodies in the cytoplasm.
viii) Any other secretory product in the cytoplasm e.g. melanosomes in melanoma and membrane-bound granules in endocrine tumours.

6. TUMOUR MARKERS (BIOCHEMICAL ASSAYS)

In order to distinguish from the preceding techniques of tumour diagnosis in which 'stains' are imparted on the tumour cells in section or smear, tumour markers are biochemical assays of products elaborated by the tumour cells in blood or other body fluids. It is, therefore, pertinent to keep in mind that many of these products are produced by normal body cells too, and thus the biochemical estimation of the product in blood or other fluid reflects the total substance and not by the tumour cells alone. These methods, therefore, lack sensitivity as well as specificity and can only be employed for the following:

◆ *Firstly,* as an adjunct to the pathologic diagnosis arrived at by other methods and not for primary diagnosis of cancer.
◆ *Secondly,* it can be used for prognostic and therapeutic purposes.

Tumour markers include: cell surface antigens (or oncofoetal antigens), cytoplasmic proteins, enzymes, hormones and cancer antigens; these are listed in Table 20.4. However, two of the best known examples of oncofoetal antigens secreted by foetal tissues as well as by tumours are alpha-foetoproteins (AFP) and carcinoembryonic antigens (CEA):

i) Alpha-foetoprotein (AFP) This is a glycoprotein synthesised normally by foetal liver cells. Their serum levels are elevated in hepatocellular carcinoma and non-

Table 20.4 Important tumour markers.

	MARKER	CANCER
1.	**ONCOFOETAL ANTIGENS**	
	i. Alpha-foetoprotein (AFP)	Hepatocellular carcinoma, non-seminomatous germ cell tumours of testis
	ii. Carcinoembryonic antigen (CEA)	Cancer of bowel, pancreas, breast
2.	**Enzymes**	
	i. Prostate acid phosphatase (PAP)	Prostatic carcinoma
	ii. Neuron-specific enolase (NSE)	Neuroblastoma, oat cell carcinoma lung
	iii. Lactic dehydrogenase (LDH)	Lymphoma, Ewing's sarcoma
3.	**HORMONES**	
	i. Human chorionic gonadotropin (hCG)	Trophoblastic tumours, non-seminomatous germ cell tumours of testis
	ii. Calcitonin	Medullary carcinoma thyroid
	iii. Catecholamines and vanillylmandelic acid (VMA)	Neuroblastoma, pheochromocytoma
	iv. Ectopic hormone production	Paraneoplastic syndromes
4.	**CANCER ASSOCIATED PROTEINS**	
	i. CA-125	Ovary
	ii. CA 15-3	Breast
	iii. CA 19-9	Colon, pancreas, breast
	iv. CD30	Hodgkin's disease, anaplastic large cell lymphoma (ALCL)
	v. CD25	Hairy cell leukaemia (HCL), adult T cell leukaemia lymphoma (ATLL)
	vi. Monoclonal immunoglobulins	Multiple myeloma, other gammopathies
	vii. Prostate specific antigen (PSA)	Prostate carcinoma

seminomatous germ cell tumours of the testis. Certain non-neoplastic conditions also have increased serum levels of AFP e.g. in hepatitis, cirrhosis, toxic liver injury and pregnancy.

ii) Carcino-embryonic antigen (CEA) CEA is also a glycoprotein normally synthesised in embryonic tissue of the gut, pancreas and liver. Their serum levels are high in cancers of the gastrointestinal tract, pancreas and breast. As in AFP, CEA levels are also elevated in certain non-neoplastic conditions e.g. in ulcerative colitis, Crohn's disease, hepatitis and chronic bronchitis.

7. OTHER MODERN AIDS IN PATHOLOGIC DIAGNOSIS OF TUMOURS

In addition to the methods described above, some other modern diagnostic techniques have emerged for tumour diagnostic pathology but their availability as well as applicability are limited. Briefly, their role in tumour diagnosis is outlined below.

i) Flow cytometry This is a computerised technique by which the detailed characteristics of individual tumour cells are recognised and quantified and the data can be stored for subsequent comparison too. Since for flow cytometry, single cell suspensions are required to 'flow' through the 'cytometer', it can be employed on blood cells and their precursors in bone marrow aspirates and body fluids, and sometimes on fresh-frozen unfixed tissue. The method employs either identification of cell surface antigen (e.g. in classification of leukaemias and lymphomas), or by the DNA content analysis (e.g. aneuploidy in various cancers).

ii) *In situ* hybridisation This is a molecular technique by which nucleic acid sequences (cellular/viral DNA and RNA) can be localised by specifically-labelled nucleic acid probe directly in the intact cell (*in situ*) rather than by DNA extraction (see below). A modification of *in situ* hybridisation technique is fluorescence *in situ* hybridisation (FISH) in which fluorescence dyes applied and is used to detect microdeletions, subtelomere deletions and to look for alterations in chromosomal numbers. *In situ* hybridisation may be used for analysis of certain human tumours by the study of oncogenes aside from its use in diagnosis of viral infection.

iii) Cell proliferation analysis Besides flow cytometry, the degree of proliferation of cells in tumours can be determined by various other methods as under:

a) Mitotic count This is the oldest but still widely used method in routine diagnostic pathology work. The number of cells in mitosis are counted per high power field e.g. in categorising various types of smooth muscle tumours.

b) Radioautography In this method, the proliferating cells are labelled *in vitro* with thymidine and then the tissue processed for paraffin-embedding. Thymidine-labelled cells (corresponding to S-phase) are then counted per 2000 tumour cell nuclei and expressed as thymidine-labelling index. The method is employed as prognostic marker in breast carcinoma.

c) Microspectrophotometric analysis The section is stained with Feulgen reaction which imparts staining to DNA content of the cell and then DNA content is measured by microspectrophotometer. The method is tedious and has limited use.

d) IHC proliferation markers The nuclear antigen specific for cell growth and division is stained by immunohistochemical method and then positive cells are counted under the microscope or by an image analyzer e.g. *Ki-67, MIB-1, PCNA,* cyclins.

e) Nucleolar organiser region (NOR) Nucleolus contains ribosomal components which are formed at chromosomal regions containing DNA called NORs. NORs have affinity for silver. This property is made use in staining the section with silver (AgNOR technique). NORs appear as black intranuclear dots while the background is stained yellow-brown.

iv) Image analyzer and morphometry Image analyser is a software system in the computer attached to a microscope which is fitted with an image capture board. The system is used to perform measurement of architectural, cellular and nuclear features of tumour cells. Image analyser can be used for following purposes:

a) *Morphometric study* of tumour cells by measurement of architectural, cellular and nuclear features.

b) *Quantitative nuclear DNA ploidy* measurement.

c) Quantitative valuation of *immunohistochemical staining.*

v) Molecular diagnostic techniques The group of molecular biologic methods in the tumour diagnostic laboratory are a variety of DNA/RNA-based molecular techniques in which the DNA/RNA are extracted (compared from *in situ* above) from the cell and then analysed. These techniques are highly sensitive, specific and rapid and have revolutionised diagnostic pathology in neoplastic as well as non-neoplastic conditions (e.g. in infectious and inherited disorders, and in identity diagnosis). Molecular diagnostic techniques include: DNA analysis by Southern blot, RNA analysis by northern blot, and polymerase chain reaction (PCR). The following techniques of molecular methods in tumour diagnosis have applications in haematologic as well as non-haematologic malignancies:

a) Analysis of molecular cytogenetic abnormalities

b) Mutational analysis

c) Antigen receptor gene rearrangement

d) Study of oncogenic viruses at molecular level.

Besides the application of these molecular techniques for diagnosis of tumour, many of the newer molecular techniques are being applied for predicting prognosis, biologic behaviour of tumour, detection of minimal residual disease and for hereditary predisposition of other family members to develop a particular cancer.

vi) DNA microarray analysis of tumours Currently, it is possible to perform molecular profiling of a tumour by use of gene chip technology which allows measurement of levels of expression of several thousand genes (up-regulation or down-regulation) simultaneously. Fluorescent labels are used to code the cDNA synthesised by trigger from mRNA. The conventional DNA probes are substituted by silicon chip which contains the entire range of genes and high resolution scanners are used for the measurement.

| GIST BOX 20.2 | Pathologic Diagnosis of Cancer |

- Tissue diagnosis of a biopsy or excised specimen by histologic examination is of paramount importance. It includes conventional paraffin-embedding technique and a rapid intraoperative frozen section method.
- Besides routine H & E staining, paraffin-embedded sections can be stained with special stains to demonstrate some cytplasmic constituents, or more importantly by immunohistochemical stains which may localise at the cell membrane, nucleus or the cytoplasm, and accordingly help in identification of the cell of origin of the tumour of uncertain histogenesis and also act as prognostic markers.
- Serum tumour markers are biochemical assays of certain products elaborated by cancers which may help in prognostication of the case e.g. CEA, AFP, hCG, CA-125 etc.
- Besides, a few other modern ancillary techniques which have become available in diagnostic pathology are flow cytometry, *in situ* hybridisation, image analysers, cell proliferation analysis, molecular studies (e.g. PCR) and DNA microarrays for molecular profiling of tumours.

21 Common Specific Tumours

CLASSIFICATION OF TUMOURS

Many types of classification of tumours have been suggested. The most useful and widely accepted classification of tumours is based on the tissue of origin (i.e. histogenesis) and on the anticipated behaviour. In general, on one end are the tumours having expansile growth without stigmata of malignancy; they are essentially *benign tumours*. On the other extreme are tumours having rapidly proliferating growth pattern with local invasion as well as metastatic involvement; they are termed *malignant tumours*. Between the two extremes is, however, another *borderline* or *intermediate group* having localised aggressive growth and invasiveness but seldom having distant metastases e.g. basal cell carcinoma, carcinoid tumour of the appendix, mucoepidermoid tumour of the salivary gland.

As already discussed in chapter 18, the general principle of nomenclature of tumours is to add the suffix *-oma* to the name of tissue of origin. Malignant tumours of epithelial origin are called *carcinomas* while those of mesenchymal origin are termed *sarcomas*.

A classification based on these principles divides all tumours into 2 broad groups: epithelial and mesenchymal (see Table 18.1, page 267). Morphology of some of the common tumours is described below.

EPITHELIAL TUMOURS

Epithelium may be of 2 main types: surface and secretory.

- *Surface epithelium* of squamous type covers the skin, oral cavity, upper part of oesophagus and vagina. The tumours originating from it are called squamous cell papillomas and carcinomas for the benign and malignant tumours respectively. The urinary bladder is lined by transitional epithelium and the tumours in that location are accordingly named transitional cell papilloma and carcinoma. Besides, melanin-containing epithelium in the skin and mucosa is the site for tumours.
- *Secretory epithelium* is present in mucous membranes (e.g. in bowel, gallbladder, uterus) and in glandular structures such as in the breast, salivary glands, liver, kidney, prostate, etc. The tumours arising from secretory and glandular epithelium are termed adenomas and adenocarcinomas.

The prototypes of the epithelial group of benign and malignant tumours are discussed below.

COMMON BENIGN EPITHELIAL TUMOURS

SQUAMOUS PAPILLOMA Squamous papilloma is a benign epithelial tumour of the skin and oral mucosa. Though considered by many authors to include common viral warts (verrucae) (caused by human papilloma viruses HPV types 1,2)) and condyloma acuminate (caused by HPV type 6), true squamous papillomas differ from these viral lesions. If these 'viral tumours' are excluded, squamous papilloma is a rare tumour.

Histologically, squamous papillomas are characterised by hyperkeratosis, acanthosis with elongation of rete ridges and papillomatosis (Fig. 21.1). The *verrucae*, in addition to these features, have foci of vacuolated cells in the acanthotic stratum malpighii, vertical tiers of parakeratosis between the adjacent papillae and irregular clumps of keratohyaline granules in the virus-infected granular cells lying in the valleys between the papillae (Fig. 21.2).

TRANSITIONAL CELL (UROTHELIAL) PAPILLOMA More than 90% of bladder tumours arise from transitional epithelial (urothelium) lining of the bladder in continuity with the epithelial lining of the renal pelvis, ureters, and the major part of the urethra. The WHO and ISUP (International Society of Urologic Pathology), in 1998 have proposed consensus histologic criteria to categorise urothelial tumours into papillomas (exophytic and inverted), carcinoma in situ (CIS), papillary urothelial neoplasms of low malignant potential (PUNLMP), and urothelial carcinoma (low grade and high grade).

Urothelial papillomas may occur singly or may be multiple. These may be exophytic or inverted.

- *Exophytic papillomas* are generally small, less than 2 cm in diameter, having delicate papillae. Each papilla is composed of fibrovascular stromal core covered by normal-looking transitional cells having normal number of layers (up to 6-7) in thickness. The individual cells resemble the normal transitional cells and do not vary in size and shape. Mitoses are absent and basal polarity is retained. Patients of exophytic papillomas may sometimes develop recurrences and require long-term follow up.
- *Inverted papillomas* have an endophytic growth pattern and are benign tumours.

ADENOMA The most common location for adenomas is the bowel, essentially the large intestine. Most of these tumours present as colorectal polyps. Adenomas have 3 main varieties (tubular, villous and tubulovillous), each of which represents a difference in the growth pattern of the same neoplastic process and variable biological behaviour.

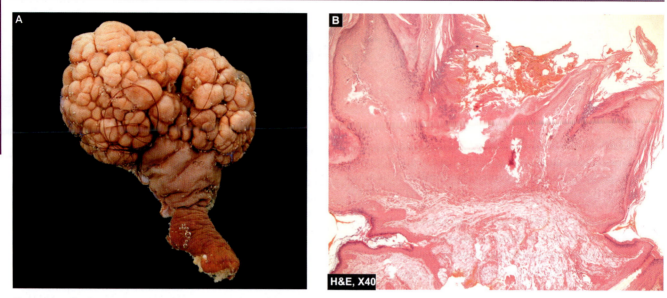

Figure 21.1 ▶ Squamous cell papilloma. A, The skin surface shows a papillary growth with a pedicle while the surface is smooth. B, Microscopy resembles verruca but differs from it by not having vacuolated koilocytic cells in stratum malpighii.

Tubular Adenoma (Adenomatous Polyp) Tubular adenomas or adenomatous polyps are the most common neoplastic polyps (75%). They are common beyond 3rd decade of life and have slight male preponderance. They occur most often in the distal colon and rectum. They may be found singly as sporadic cases, or multiple tubular adenomas as part of familial polyposis syndrome with autosomal dominant inheritance pattern. Tubular adenomas may remain asymptomatic or may manifest by rectal bleeding.

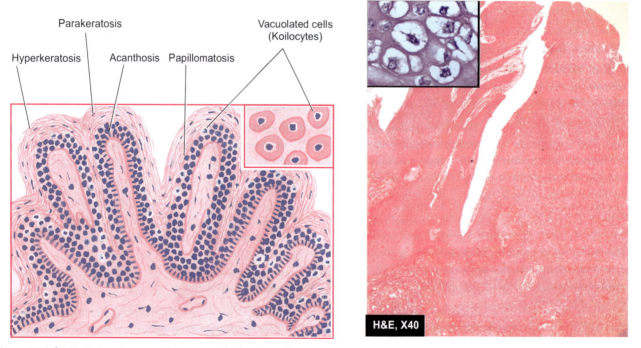

Figure 21.2 ▶ Typical appearance of a verruca. The histologic features include papillomatosis, acanthosis, hyperkeratosis with parakeratosis and elongated rete ridges appearing to point towards the centre. Foci of vacuolated cells (koilocytes) are found in the upper stratum malpighii. *Inset* shows koilocytes and virus-infected keratinocytes containing prominent keratohyaline granules.

Grossly, adenomatous polyps may be single or multiple, sessile or pedunculated, varying in size from less than 1 cm to large, spherical masses with an irregular surface. Usually, the larger lesions have recognisable stalks.

Microscopically, the usual appearance is of benign tumour overlying muscularis mucosa and is composed of branching tubules which are embedded in the lamina propria. The lining epithelial cells are of large intestinal type with diminished mucus secreting capacity, large nuclei and increased mitotic activity (Fig. 21.3,A). However, tubular adenomas may show variable degree of cytologic atypia ranging from atypical epithelium restricted within the glandular basement membrane called as 'carcinoma *in situ*' to invasion into the fibrovascular stromal core termed frank adenocarcinoma.

Malignant transformation is present in about 5% of tubular adenomas; the incidence being higher in larger adenomas.

Villous Adenoma (Villous Papilloma) Villous adenomas or villous papillomas of the colon are much less common than tubular adenomas. The mean age at which they appear is 6th decade of life with approximately equal sex incidence. They are seen most often in the distal colon and rectum, followed in decreasing frequency, by rest of the colon.

Grossly, villous adenomas are round to oval exophytic masses, usually sessile, varying in size from 1 to 10 cm or more in diameter. Their surface may be haemorrhagic or ulcerated.

Microscopically, the characteristic histologic feature is the presence of many slender, finger-like villi, which appear to arise directly from the area of muscularis mucosae. Each of the papillae has fibrovascular stromal core that is covered by epithelial cells varying from apparently benign to anaplastic cells. Excess mucus secretion is sometimes seen (Fig. 21.3,B).

Villous adenomas are invariably symptomatic; rectal bleeding, diarrhoea and mucus being the common features. The presence of severe atypia, carcinoma *in situ* and invasive carcinoma are seen more frequently. Invasive carcinoma has been reported in 30% of villous adenomas.

Tubulovillous Adenoma (Papillary Adenoma, Villoglandular Adenoma) Tubulovillous adenoma is an intermediate form of pattern between tubular adenoma and villous adenoma. It is also known by other names like papillary adenoma and villo-glandular adenoma. The distribution of these adenomas is the same as for tubular adenomas.

Grossly, tubulovillous adenomas may be sessile or pedunculated and range in size from 0.5-5 cm.

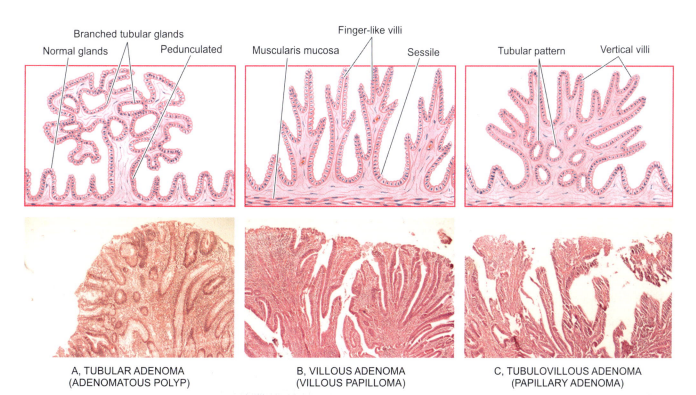

A, TUBULAR ADENOMA (ADENOMATOUS POLYP)

B, VILLOUS ADENOMA (VILLOUS PAPILLOMA)

C, TUBULOVILLOUS ADENOMA (PAPILLARY ADENOMA)

Figure 21.3 ▶ Adenomas (neoplastic polyps)—three main varieties.

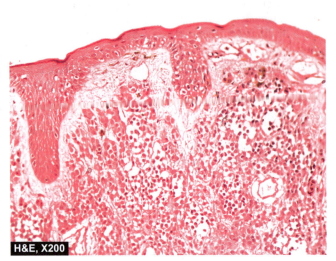

Figure 21.4 ▶ Intradermal naevus showing nests of naevus cells which are typically uniform and present in the dermis. Melanin pigment in naevus cells is coarse and irregular.

Microscopically, they show intermediate or mixed pattern, characteristic vertical villi and deeper part showing tubular pattern (Fig. 21.3,C).

The behaviour of tubulovillous adenoma is intermediate between tubular and villous adenomas.

NAEVOCELLULAR NAEVI Pigmented naevi or moles are extremely common lesions on the skin of most individuals. They are often flat or slightly elevated lesions; rarely they may be papillomatous or pedunculated. Most naevi appear in adolescence and in early adulthood due to hormonal influence but rarely may be present at birth. They are mostly tan to brown and less than 1 cm in size.

Histologically, irrespective of the histologic types, all naevocellular naevi are composed of 'naevus cells' which are actually identical to melanocytes but differ from melanocytes in being arranged in clusters or nests. Naevus cells are cuboidal or oval in shape with homogeneous cytoplasm and contain large round or oval nucleus. Melanin pigment is abundant in the naevus cells present in the lower epidermis and upper dermis, but the cells in the mid-dermis and lower dermis hardly contain any melanin (Fig. 21.4).

The important *histological variants* of naevi are as under:

i) **Lentigo** is the replacement of the basal layer of the epidermis by melanocytes.

ii) **Junctional naevus** is the one in which the naevus cells lie at the epidermal-dermal junction. The naevus cells form well-circumscribed nests.

iii) **Compound naevus** is the commonest type of pigmented naevus. These lesions, in addition to the junctional activity as in junctional naevi, show nests of naevus cells in the dermis to a variable depth.

iv) **Intradermal naevus** shows slight or no junctional activity. The lesion is mainly located in the upper dermis as nests and cords of naevus cells. Multinucleate naevus cells are common.

v) **Spindle cell (epithelioid) naevus or juvenile melanoma** is a compound naevus with junctional activity. The naevus cells are, however, elongated and epithelioid in appearance which may or may not contain melanin. Juvenile melanoma is important since it is frequently confused with malignant melanoma histologically.

vi) **Blue naevus** is characterised by dendritic spindle naevus cells rather than the usual rounded or cuboidal naevus cells. These cells are often quite rich in melanin pigment.

vii) **Dysplastic naevi** are certain atypical naevi which have increased risk of progression to malignant melanoma. These lesions are larger than the usual acquired naevi, are often multiple, and appear as flat macules to slightly elevated plaques with irregular borders and variable pigmentation. Many of the cases are familial and inheritable. Dysplastic naevi have melanocytic proliferation at the epidermo-dermal junction with some cytologic atypia.

COMMON MALIGNANT EPITHELIAL TUMOURS

SQUAMOUS CELL CARCINOMA Squamous cell carcinoma may arise on any part of the skin and mucous membranes lined by squamous epithelium. Most common locations are the face, pinna of the ears, back of hands and mucocutaneous junctions such as on the lips, anal canal and glans penis. Cutaneous squamous carcinoma arising in a pre-existing inflammatory and degenerative lesion has a higher incidence of developing metastases.

Two important factors in the pathogenesis of squamaous cell carcinoma are: *prolonged sun exposure* and *immunosuppression*. In such cases, DNA damage is induced followed by *p53* mutation and other events leading to dysregulation of signaling pathway. Various predisposing conditions include the following:
i) Xeroderma pigmentosum
ii) Epidermodysplasia verruciformis induced by HPV
iii) Solar keratosis
iv) Chronic inflammatory conditions such as chronic ulcers and draining osteomyelitis
v) Old burn scars (Marjolin's ulcers)
vi) Chemical burns
vii) Psoriasis
viii) HIV infection
ix) Ionising radiation
x) Industrial carcinogens (coal tars, oils etc)

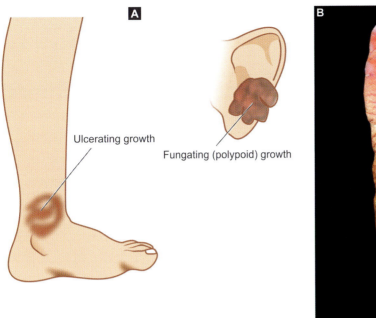
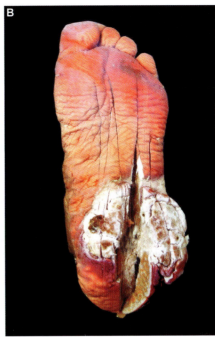

Figure 21.5 ▶ Squamous cell carcinoma. A, Main macroscopic patterns showing ulcerated and fungating polypoid growth. B, The skin surface on the sole of the foot shows a fungating and ulcerated growth. On cutting, the growth is both exophytic and endophytic and is chalky white in colour.

xi) Tobacco smoking in case of lung cancer
xi) Chewing betel nuts and tobacco in case of cancer of oral cavity

Cancer of scrotal skin in chimney-sweeps was the first cancer in which an occupational carcinogen (soot) was implicated. *'Kangari cancer'* of the skin of inner side of thigh and lower abdomen common in natives of Kashmir is another example of skin cancer due to chronic irritation (*Kangari* is an earthenware pot containing glowing charcoal embers used by Kashmiris close to their abdomen to keep them warm).

MORPHOLOGIC FEATURES *Grossly,* squamous carcinoma of the skin and squamous-lined mucosa can have one of the following two patterns **(Fig. 21.5)**:

i) More commonly, an *ulcerated growth* with elevated and indurated margin is seen.

ii) Less often, a raised *fungating or polypoid verrucous* lesion without ulceration is found.

Invasive squamous cell carcinoma of uterine cervix occurs most commonly at the squamo-columnar junction.

Microscopically, squamous cell carcinoma is an invasive carcinoma of the surface epidermis characterised by the following features **(Fig. 21.6)**:

i) There is irregular downward proliferation of epidermal cells into the dermis.

ii) Depending upon the grade of malignancy, the masses of epidermal cells show atypical features such as variation in cell size and shape, nuclear hyperchromatism, absence of intercellular bridges, individual cell keratinisation and occurrence of atypical mitotic figures.

iii) Better-differentiated squamous carcinomas have whorled arrangement of malignant squamous cells forming horn pearls. The centres of these horn pearls may contain laminated, keratin material.

iv) Higher grades of squamous carcinomas, however, have fewer or no horn pearls and may instead have highly atypical cells.

v) An uncommon variant of squamous carcinoma may have spindle-shaped tumour cells *(spindle cell carcinoma)*.

vi) Adenoid changes may be seen in a portion of squamous cell carcinoma *(adenoid squamous cell carcinoma)*.

vii) *Verrucous carcinoma* (Ackerman tumour) is a low-grade variant located most commonly in oral cavity in which the superficial portion of the tumour resembles verruca (hyperkeratosis, parakeratosis, acanthosis and papillomatosis) but differs from it in having downward proliferation as broad masses of well-differentiated squamous epithelium into deeper portion of the tumour. However, there is lack of cellular atypia.

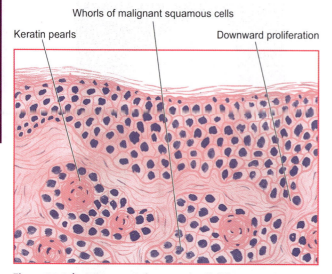 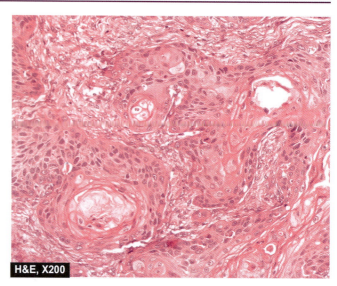

Figure 21.6 ▶ Microscopic features of well-differentiated squamous cell carcinoma. The dermis is invaded by downward proliferating epidermal masses of cells which show atypical features. A few horn pearls with central laminated keratin are present. There is inflammatory reaction in the dermis between the masses of tumour cells.

viii) All variants of squamous cell carcinoma show inflammatory reaction between the collections of tumour cells, while in *pseudocarcinomatous hyperplasia* there is permeation of the epithelial proliferations by inflammatory cells.

It is customary with pathologists to label squamous cell carcinomas with descriptive terms such as: well-differentiated, moderately-differentiated, undifferentiated, keratinising, non-keratinising, spindle cell type etc.

Overall prognosis of squamous cell carcinoma induced by actinic keratosis is excellent. Superficial invasive tumour may metastasise locally. Prognosis of deeply invading tumour depends upon the stage (TNM staging).

BASAL CELL CARCINOMA (RODENT ULCER) Typically, the basal cell carcinoma is a locally invasive, slow-growing tumour of middle-aged that rarely metastasises. It occurs exclusively on hairy skin, the most common location (90%) being the face, usually above a line from the lobe of the ear to the corner of the mouth (Fig. 21.7).

Following conditions predispose an individual to develop basal cell carcinoma:
i) Light-skinned people who have little melanin.
ii) Prolonged exposure to strong sunlight like in those living in Australia and New Zealand.
iii) Inherited defect in DNA repair mechanism in xeroderma pigmentosum.
iv) *Nevoid basal cell carcinoma syndrome* It is an autosomal dominant condition in which multiple basal cell carcinomas appear at a young age (under 20 years). These individuals inherit one defective allele (*PTCH* gene on chromosome 9) while another allele undergoes mutation early in life by sun exposure (Hudson's two hit hypothesis).

***MORPHOLOGIC FEATURES** Grossly*, the most common pattern is a nodulo-ulcerative basal cell carcinoma in which a slow-growing small nodule undergoes central ulceration with pearly, rolled margins. The tumour enlarges in size by burrowing and by destroying the tissues locally like a rodent and hence the name 'rodent ulcer'. However, less frequently non-ulcerated nodular pattern, pigmented basal cell carcinoma and fibrosing variants are also encountered.

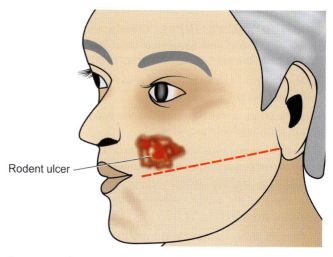

Figure 21.7 ▶ Common location and macroscopic appearance of basal cell carcinoma (rodent ulcer).

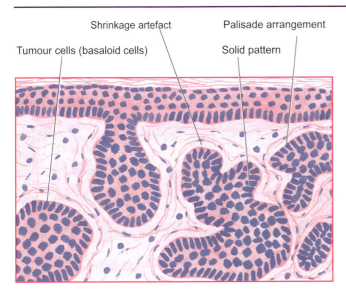 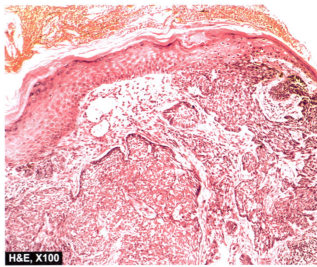

Figure 21.8 ▶ Solid basal cell carcinoma. The dermis is invaded by irregular masses of basaloid cells with characteristic peripheral palisaded appearance. The masses of tumour cells are separated from dermal collagen by a space called shrinkage artefact.

Histologically, the most characteristic feature is the proliferation of basaloid cells (resembling basal layer of epidermis). A variety of patterns of these cells may be seen: solid masses, masses of pigmented cells, strands and nests of tumour cells in morphea pattern, keratotic masses, cystic change with sebaceous differentiation, and adenoid pattern with apocrine or eccrine differentiation. The most common pattern is *solid basal cell carcinoma* in which the dermis contains irregular masses of basaloid cells having characteristic peripheral palisaded appearance of the nuclei (Fig. 21.8). A superficial multicentric variant composed of multiple foci of tumour cells present in the dermis, especially in the trunk, has also been described.

MALIGNANT MELANOMA Malignant melanoma or melanocarcinoma arising from melanocytes is one of the most rapidly spreading malignant tumour of the skin that can occur at all ages. The etiology is unknown but there is role of excessive exposure of white skin to sunlight e.g. higher incidence in New Zealand and Australia where sun exposure in high. Besides the skin, melanomas may occur at various other sites such as oral and anogenital mucosa, oesophagus, conjunctiva, orbit and leptomeninges. The common sites on the skin are the trunk *(in men)*, legs *(in women)*; other locations are face, soles, palms and nail-beds.

Some high risk factors associated with increased incidence of malignant melanoma are as under:
i) Persistent change in appearance of a mole.
ii) Presence of pre-existing naevus (especially dysplastic naevus).
iii) Family history of melanoma in a patient of atypical mole.
iii) Higher age of the patient.
iv) More than 50 moles 2 mm or more in diameter.

Molecular studies in familial and hereditary cases have revealed germline mutation in *CDKN2A* gene which encodes for cyclin-dependent kinase inhibitor, mutational loss of *PTEN* gene and mutation in several other tumour suppressor genes but not *p53*.

Clinically, melanoma often appears as a flat or slightly elevated naevus which has variegated pigmentation, irregular borders and, of late, has undergone secondary changes of ulceration, bleeding and increase in size. Many of the malignant melanomas, however, arise *de novo* rather than from a pre-existing naevus. Malignant melanoma can be differentiated from benign pigmented lesions by subtle clinical and histopathologic features summed up in Table 21.1; contrasting clinical features can be remembered by mnemonic 'ABCD' of melanoma (*A*symmetry, *B*order irregularity, *C*olour change and *D*iameter >6 mm).

MORPHOLOGIC FEATURES *Grossly*, depending upon the clinical course and prognosis, cutaneous malignant melanomas are of the following 5 types:

i) Lentigo maligna melanoma This often develops from a pre-existing lentigo (a flat naevus characterised by replacement of basal layer of epidermis by naevus cells). It is essentially a malignant melanoma *in situ*. It is slow-growing and has good prognosis.

ii) Superficial spreading melanoma This is a slightly elevated lesion with variegated colour and ulcerated surface. It often develops from a superficial spreading melanoma *in situ* (pagetoid melanoma) in 5 to 7 years. The prognosis is worse than for lentigo maligna melanoma.

Section IV: Neoplasia

Table 21.1 Distinguishing features of benign mole and malignant melanoma.

	FEATURE	BENIGN MOLE	MALIGNANT MELANOMA
1.	*Clinical features*		
	i) Symmetry	Symmetrical	A = Asymmetry
	ii) Border	Well-demarcated	B = Border irregularity
	iii) Colour	Uniformly pigmented	C = Colour change
	iv) Diameter	Small, less than 6 mm	D = Diameter more than 6 mm
2.	*Common locations*	Skin of face, mucosa	Skin; mucosa of nose, bowel, anal region
3.	*Histopathology*		
	i) Architecture	Nests of cells	Various patterns: solid sheets, alveoli, nests, islands
	ii) Cell morphology	Uniform looking naevus cells	Malignant cells, atypia, mitoses, nucleoli
	iii) Melanin pigment	Irregular, coarse clumps	Fine granules, uniformly distributed
	iv) Inflammation	May or may not be present	Often present
4.	*Spread*	Remains confined, poses cosmetic problem only	Haematogenous and/or lymphatic spread early

iii) Acral lentigenous melanoma This occurs more commonly on the soles, palms and mucosal surfaces (Fig. 21.9). The tumour often undergoes ulceration and early metastases. The prognosis is worse than that of superficial spreading melanoma.

iv) Nodular melanoma This often appears as an elevated and deeply pigmented nodule that grows rapidly and undergoes ulceration. This variant carries the worst prognosis.

v) Desmoplastic melanoma In this variant, the tumour has a fibrotic stroma, neural invasion and frequent local recurrences.

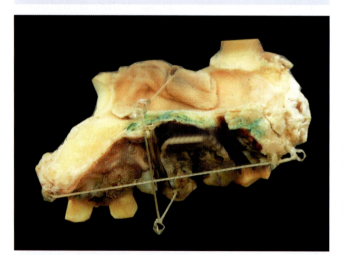

Figure 21.9 ▶ Malignant melanoma of the oral cavity. The hemi-maxillectomy specimen shows an elevated blackish ulcerated area with irregular outlines.

Histologically, irrespective of the type of malignant melanoma, the following characteristics are observed (Fig. 21.10):

i) Origin The malignant melanoma, whether arising from a pre-existing naevus or starting *de novo,* has marked junctional activity at the epidermo-dermal junction and grows downward into the dermis.

ii) Tumour cells The malignant melanoma cells are usually larger than the naevus cells. They may be epithelioid or spindle-shaped, the former being more common. The tumour cells have amphophilic cytoplasm and large, pleomorphic nuclei with conspicuous nucleoli. Mitotic figures are often present and multinucleate giant cells may occur. These tumour cells may be arranged in various patterns such as solid masses, sheets, island, alveoli etc.

iii) Melanin Melanin pigment may be present (melanotic) or absent (amelanotic melanoma) without any prognostic influence. The pigment, if present, tends to be in the form of uniform fine granules (unlike the benign naevi in which coarse irregular clumps of melanin are present). At times, there may be no evidence of melanin in H&E stained sections but Fontana-Masson stain or *dopa reaction* reveals melanin granules in the cytoplasm of tumour cells. Immunohistochemically, melanoma cells are positive for HMB-45 (most specific), S-100 and Melan-A.

iv) Inflammatory infiltrate Some amount of inflammatory infiltrate is present in the invasive melanomas. Infrequently, partial spontaneous regression of the tumour occurs due to destructive effect of dense inflammatory infiltrate.

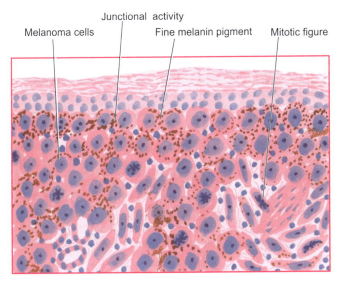 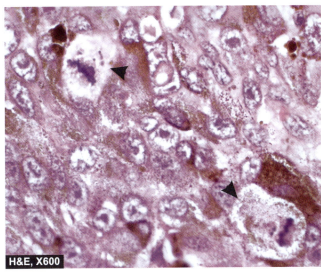

Figure 21.10 ▶ Malignant melanoma shows junctional activity at the dermal-epidermal junction. Tumour cells resembling epithelioid cells with pleomorphic nuclei and prominent nucleoli are seen as solid masses in the dermis. Many of the tumour cells contain fine granular melanin pigment. Photomicrograph shows a prominent atypical mitotic figure (arrow).

Depending upon the depth of invasion into the dermis, *Clark* has described following 5 levels:

Level I: Malignant melanoma cells confined to the epidermis and its appendages.

Level II: Extension into the papillary dermis.

Level III: Extension of tumour cells upto the interface between papillary and reticular dermis.

Level IV: Invasion of reticular dermis.

Level V: Invasion of the subcutaneous fat.

The prognosis for patients with malignant melanoma depends upon the stage at presentation. AJCC staging for melanoma takes into account the microscopic depth of invasion of the primary tumour, ulceration, nodal metastasis and presence of metastatic disease in internal sites. Metastatic spread of malignant melanoma is very common and takes place via lymphatics to the regional lymph nodes and through blood to distant sites like lungs, liver, brain, spinal cord, and adrenals. Just as in breast cancer, sentinel lymph node biopsy is quite helpful in evaluation of regional nodal status.

TRANSITIONAL CELL (UROTHELIAL) CARCINOMA

Transitional cell (or urothelial) carcinoma arises from the epithelial lining of the urinary bladder, renal pelvis, ureters and part of urethra. More than 90% of bladder tumours arise from transitional epithelial (urothelium) lining of the bladder in continuity with the epithelial lining of the renal pelvis, ureters, and the major part of the urethra. Bladder cancer comprises about 3% of all cancers. Most of the cases appear beyond 5th decade of life with 3-times higher preponderance in males than females.

A number of environmental and host factors are implicated in the etiology of the bladder cancer that include: tobacco smoking, industrial occupations (e.g. in workers

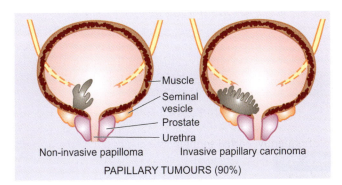 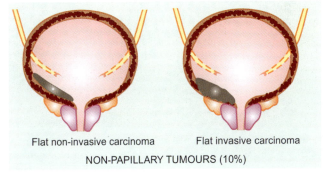

Figure 21.11 ▶ Gross patterns of epithelial bladder tumours.

Section IV: Neoplasia

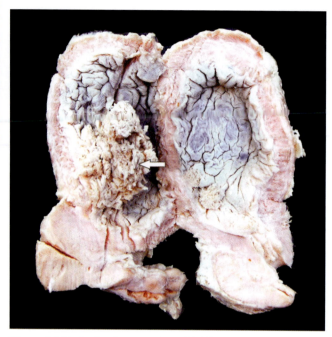

Figure 21.12 ▶ Carcinoma urinary bladder. The mucosal surface shows papillary tumour floating in the lumen (arrow).

engaged in manufacture of aniline dyes, rubber, plastic, textiles and cable), schistosomiasis of the bladder (e.g., in Egypt), long-term immunosuppressive therapy, prior irradiation for pelvic cancer and local lesions such as ectopia vesicae and leukoplakia of the bladder.

Grossly, urothelial tumours may be single or multiple. About 90% of the tumours are papillary (non-invasive or invasive), whereas the remaining 10% are flat indurated (non-invasive or invasive) **(Fig. 21.11).** Most common location in the bladder is lateral walls, followed by posterior wall and region of trigone. The papillary tumours have free floating fern-like arrangement with a broad or narrow pedicle **(Fig. 21.12).** The non-papillary tumours are bulkier with ulcerated surface. More common locations for either of the two types are the trigone, the region of ureteral orifices and on the lateral walls.

Histologically, most common epithelial tumours of the bladder are urothelial (90%); others are squamous cell, glandular, small cell and mixed.

Histologic criteria for categorising these tumours are based on *architecture, cytologic features and invasiveness.*
i) *Architecture* takes into consideration the type of papillae and relationship of cell layers with basement membrane as regards polarity.
ii) *Cytologic criteria* of neoplasm are the extent of resemblance with normal cells, crowding, variation in nuclear size, shape, chromatin, nucleoli (their presence and type), and mitotic figures.
iii) *Criteria for invasion* in papillary as well as non-papillary tumours are penetration of the basement membrane of bladder mucosa and presence or absence of invasion by neoplastic cells in the muscle.

Based on these salient features, urothelial carcinoma can be low-grade or high-grade as under:

Papillary urothelial carcinoma, low grade: These tumours show fused and branching papillary pattern but overall there is an orderly arrangement of layers of cells. These cells are cohesive and show mild variation in polarity, nuclear size, chromatin and shape (round to oval), and inconspicuous small and regular nucleoli. Mitotic figures are infrequent and are seen in lower half **(Fig. 21.13).**

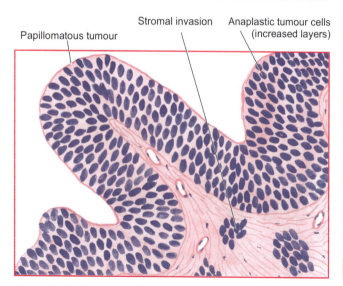
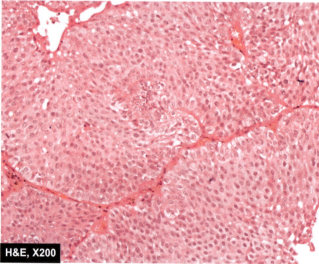

Figure 21.13 ▶ Urothelial (Transitional cell) carcinoma, low grade. There is increase in the number of layers of epithelium in an orderly manner and slight loss of polarity. The cells show slight nuclear enlargement and mild variation in nuclear size and shape and infrequent mitosis.

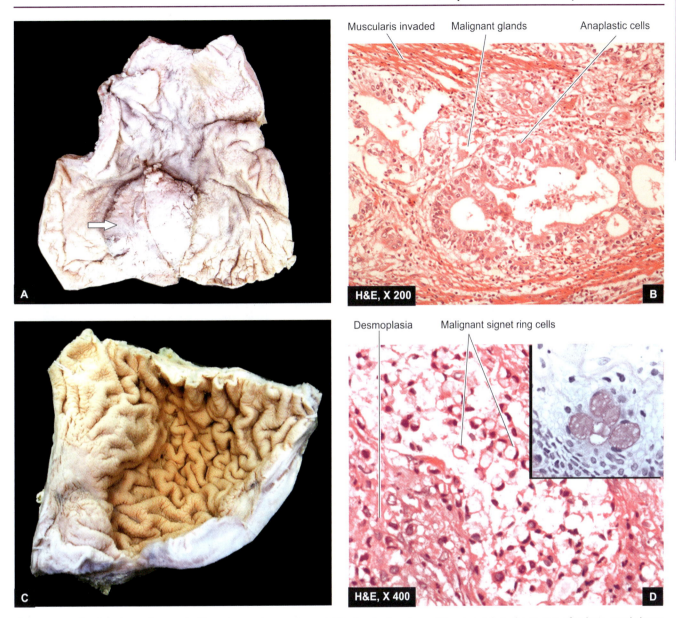

Figure 21.14 ▶ Gastric carcinoma. A, *Ulcerative carcinoma stomach*. The luminal surface of the stomach in the region of pyloric canal shows an elevated irregular growth with ulcerated surface and raised margins. B, Malignant cells forming irregular glands with stratification are seen invading the layers of the stomach wall. C, *Linitis plastica*. The wall of the stomach in the region of pyloric canal is markedly thickened and fibrotic while the mucosal folds are lost. D, Microscopy shows characteristic signet ring tumour cells having abundant mucinous cytoplasm positive for mucicarmine (inbox). The stroma is desmoplastic.

Papillary urothelial carcinoma, high grade: High-grade tumours have increased thickness and have fused and branching papillae which show quite disorderly arrangement. The tumour cells show nuclear enlargement, moderate to marked variation in nuclear size, shape, hyperchromatism, and multiple prominent nucleoli. Mitoses are frequent and atypical and seen at any level in the epithelial layers.

Invasive urothelial carcinoma Any grade of papillary urothelial carcinoma may show invasion into lamina propria or further into muscularis propria (detrusor).

Foci of squamous or glandular metaplasia may be seen in any grade of the tumour.

ADENOCARCINOMA Carcinoma arising from the secretory epithelium of mucosal surfaces and glandular

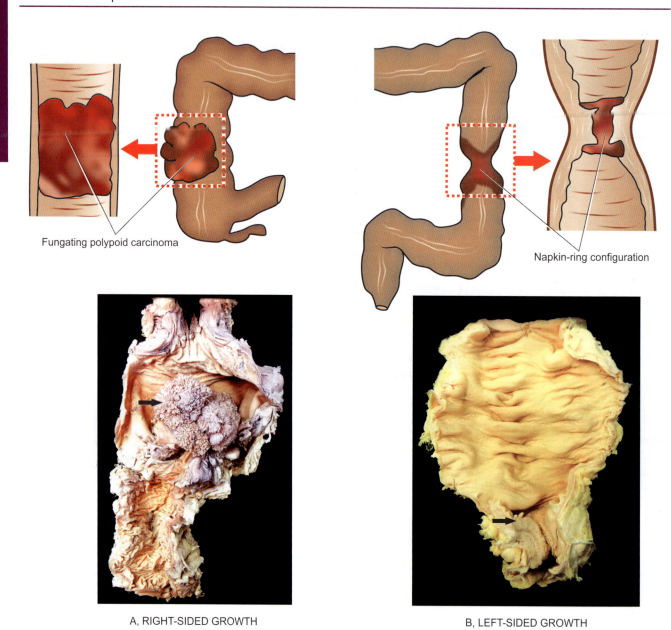

Figure 21.15 ▶ Gross appearance of colorectal carcinoma. A, Right-sided growth—fungating polypoid carcinoma showing cauliflower-like growth projecting into the lumen. B, Left-sided growth—napkin-ring configuration with spread of growth into the bowel wall.

elements is called adenocarcinoma. The common sites are the stomach, large intestine, gallbladder, pancreas, uterus, prostate, breast and other glandular organs. The spread of tumour can occur both by lymphatic and haematogenous routes.

Grossly, appearance of the tumour is variable depending upon its location. The most common patterns, however, observed in hollow viscus are either a *fungating (polypoid)* mass protruding into the lumen or an *infiltrating* type invading the wall. In the case of cancer of the stomach, other gross forms seen are scirrhous (linitis plastica), colloid (mucoid), and ulcer-cancer arising in a pre-existing peptic ulcer (Fig. 21.14). In colorectal cancer, there are distinct differences between the growth on right and left half of the colon: the right-sided growth tending to be large, cauliflower like, soft and friable projecting into the lumen whereas left-sided growths have napkin-ring configuration because the growth encircles the bowel wall circumferentially with increased fibrosis forming annular ring (Fig. 21.15). In the breast, the most common gross

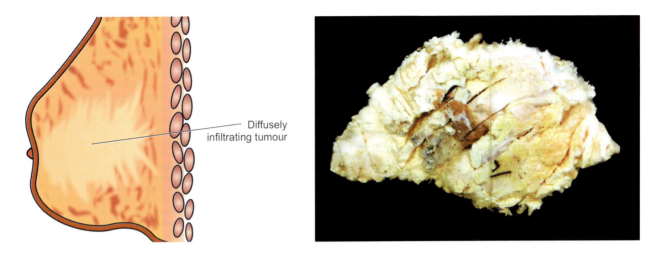

Figure 21.16 ► Infiltrating duct carcinoma—NOS. The breast shows a tumour extending up to nipple and areola. Cut surface shows a grey white firm tumour extending irregularly into adjacent breast parenchyma.

appearance is of a diffuse infiltrating scirrhous mass with cartilaginous consistency that cuts with a grating sound (Fig. 21.16). The malignant prostate is firm and fibrous and in majority of the cases the cancer is located in the peripheral zone as occult or latent growth.

Microscopically, at the margin of tumour there is transition from the normal mucous membrane to the atypical and irregular malignant epithelium and neoplastic glands invading the layers of the wall of viscus (Fig. 21.17). There may be papillary or infiltrating growth pattern.

The tumour may be mucin-secreting or non-mucin-secreting type. Colloid (mucoid) carcinoma is characterised by large pools of mucin in which are present a small number of tumour cells, sometimes having signet-ring appearance. Scirrhous carcinoma (linitis plastica) of the stomach is an adenocarcinoma in which there is pronounced desmoplasia so much so that cancer cells are difficult to find. Depending upon the degree of differentiation, various histological grades of the adenocarcinoma are described: well-differentiated, moderately-differentiated and poorly-differentiated.

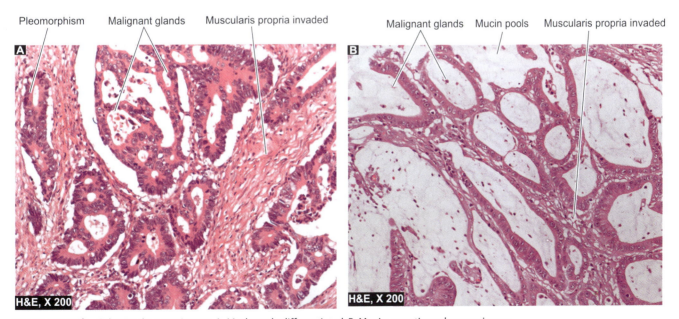

Figure 21.17 ► Colonic adenocarcinoma. A, Moderately differentiated. B, Mucin-secreting adenocarcinoma.

GIST BOX 21.1 — Common Epithelial Tumours

- Epithelial tumours originate from skin or mucosal surface epithelium (squamous, urothelial) or melanin-containing or secretory epithelium.
- Common examples of benign epithelial tumours are squamous papilloma (skin, mucosa), urothelial papilloma (urinary bladder), adenoma (bowel) and naevocellular naevi (moles).
- Squamous cell carcinoma may arise on skin or squamous mucosa. It may be well-differentiated, moderately-differentiated, undifferentiated, keratinising, non-keratinising, spindle cell type.
- Basal cell carcinoma is a locally invasive, slow-growing tumour of middle-aged that rarely metastasises. It occurs exclusively on hairy skin, most commonly on the face.
- Malignant melanoma arising from melanocytes is one of the most rapidly spreading malignant tumour of the skin that can occur at all ages.
- Adenocarcinoma arises from secretory mucosa or from glandular epithelium (e.g. stomach, colorectal region, breast, gallbladder, pancreas, uterus, prostate etc). It may be mucin-secreting or non-mucinous and can be of varying grades.

MESENCHYMAL TUMOURS

GENERAL FEATURES

Mesenchymal or non-epithelial group of tumours includes tumours arising from soft tissues and bones. The soft tissue tumours are considered below while the bone tumours are described in Chapter 30.

As per WHO, soft tissue tumours are defined as all tumours of "non-epithelial extra-skeletal tissues of the body except the reticuloendothelial system, the glia and the supporting tissues of specific organs and viscera". Thus, soft tissues included for the purpose of categorisation of these tumours are: fibrous tissue, adipose tissue, muscle tissue, synovial tissue, blood vessels and neuroectodermal tissues of the peripheral and autonomic nervous system. The lesions of these tissues are embryologically derived from mesoderm, except those of peripheral nerve which are derived from ectoderm. A list of common soft tissue tumours is given in **Table 21.2**.

Benign soft tissue tumours are about 100 times more common than sarcomas. Sarcomas rarely arise from malignant transformation of a pre-existing benign tumour. Instead, sarcomas originate from the primitive mesenchymal cells having the capacity to differentiate along different cell pathways. Soft tissue sarcomas metastasise most frequently by the haematogenous route and disseminate commonly to the lungs, liver, bone and brain. Lymph node metastases are often late and are associated with widespread dissemination

Table 21.2 Classification of common soft tissue tumours.

1. TUMOURS AND TUMOUR-LIKE LESIONS OF FIBROUS TISSUE
    i) Fibromas
    ii) Fibromatosis
        Nodular fasciitis
        Superficial (palmar, plantar)
        Deep (desmoid)
    iii) Fibrosarcoma
2. FIBROHISTIOCYTIC TUMOURS
    i) Benign fibrous histiocytoma
    ii) Dermatofibrosarcoma protuberans
    iii) Malignant fibrous histiocytoma (Pleomorphic sarcoma)
3. TUMOURS OF ADIPOSE TISSUE
    i) Lipoma
    ii) Liposarcoma
4. SKELETAL MUSCLE TUMOURS
    i) Rhabdomyoma
    ii) Rhabdomyosarcoma
5. SMOOTH MUSCLE TUMOURS
    i) Leiomyoma
    ii) Leiomyosarcoma
6. TUMOURS OF BLOOD VESSELS AND LYMPHATICS
    i) Haemangioma, lymphangioma
    ii) Glomus tumour (glomangioma)
    iii) Haemangioendothelioma
    iv) Haemangiopericytoma
    v) Angiosarcoma
    vi) Kaposi's sarcoma
7. TUMOURS OF PERIPHERAL NERVES
    i) Neurofibroma
    ii) Schwannoma
    iii) Malignant peripheral nerve sheath tumour
8. TUMOURS OF UNCERTAIN HISTOGENESIS
    i) Synovial sarcoma
    ii) Alveolar soft part sarcoma
    iii) Granular cell tumour
    iv) Epithelioid sarcoma
    v) Clear cell sarcoma
    vi) Desmoplastic small round cell tumour

of the tumour. Histologic differentiation and grading of soft tissue sarcomas are important because of varying clinical behaviour, prognosis and response to therapy.

Majority of soft tissue tumours have following important general features:

1. *Superficially-located tumours* tend to be benign while *deep-seated lesions* are more likely to be malignant.

2. *Large-sized tumours* are generally more malignant than small ones.

3. *Rapidly-growing tumours* often behave as malignant tumours than those that develop slowly.

4. Malignant tumours have frequently *increased vascularity* while benign tumours are selectively avascular.

5. Although soft tissue tumours may arise anywhere in the body but in general *more common locations* are lower extremity (40%), upper extremity (20%), trunk and retroperitoneum (30%) and head and neck (10%).

6. Generally, *males* are affected more commonly than females.

7. Approximately 15% of soft tissue tumours occur in *children* and include some specific examples of soft tissue sarcomas e.g. rhabdomyosarcoma, synovial sarcoma.

Currently, the WHO classification divides all soft tissue tumours into following 4 categories:

Benign These soft tissue tumours generally do not recur and are cured by complete excision. Common example is lipoma.

Intermediate, locally aggressive These tumours are locally destructive, infiltrative and often recur but do not metastasise. Such tumours are generally treated by wide excision; for example desmoid tumour.

Intermediate, rarely metastasising This category of tumours is also locally destructive, infiltrative and recurrent but in addition about 2% cases may have clinical metastasis which may not be predicted by morphology. Common example in this category is dermatofibrosarcoma protuberans.

Malignant Tumours in this category are clearly malignant—they are locally destructive, infiltrative and they metastasise in a high percent of cases. The metastatic rate in low-grade sarcomas is about 2-10% and in high-grade sarcomas is 20-100%.

Diagnostic Criteria

Accurate pathological diagnosis of soft tissue tumours is based on histogenesis which is important for determining the prognosis and can be made by the following plan:

1. CELL PATTERNS Several morphological patterns in which tumour cells are arranged are peculiar in different tumours e.g.

i) Smooth muscle tumours: interlacing fascicles of pink staining tumour cells.

ii) Fibrohistiocytic tumours: characteristically have storiform pattern in which spindle tumour cells radiate from the centre in a spoke-wheel manner.

iii) Herringbone pattern: is seen in fibrosarcoma in which the tumour cells are arranged like the vertebral column of seafish.

iv) Palisaded arrangement: is characteristically seen in schwannomas in which the nuclei of tumour cells are piled upon each other.

v) Biphasic pattern: is the term used for a combination arrangement of two types—fascicles and epithelial-like e.g. in synovial sarcoma.

2. CELL TYPES After looking at the pattern of cells described above, preliminary categorisation of soft tissue tumours is done on the basis of cell types comprising the soft tissue tumour:

i) Spindle cells: These are the most common cell types in most sarcomas. However, there are subtle differences in different types of spindle cells e.g.

a) Fibrogenic tumours have spindle cells with light pink cytoplasm and tapering-ended nuclei.

b) Neurogenic (Schwann cell) tumours have tumour cells similar to fibrogenic cells but have curved nuclei.

c) Leiomyomatous tumours have spindle cells with blunt-ended (cigar-shaped) nuclei and more intense eosinophilic cytoplasm.

d) Skeletal muscle tumours have spindle cells similar to leiomyomatous cells but in addition have cytoplasmic striations.

ii) Small round cells: Some soft tissue sarcomas are characterised by dominant presence of small round cells or blue cells and are termed by various names such as malignant small round cell tumours, round cell sarcomas, or blue cell tumours (due to presence of lymphocyte-like round nuclear size and dense blue chromatin). Examples of this group of tumours are as under:

a) Rhabdomyosarcoma (embryonal and alveolar types)

b) Primitive neuroectodermal tumour (PNET)

c) Ewing's sarcoma

d) Neuroblastoma

e) Malignant lymphomas.

A few examples of epithelial tumours such as small cell carcinoma and malignant carcinoid tumours enter in the differential diagnosis of small round cell tumours.

iii) Epithelioid cells: Some soft tissue tumours have either epithelioid cells as the main cells (e.g. epithelioid sarcoma) or have epithelial-like cells as a part of biphasic pattern of the tumour (e.g. synovial sarcoma).

3. IMMUNOHISTOCHEMISTRY Soft tissue tumours are distinguished by application of immunohistochemical stains. Antibody stains are available against almost each cell constituent. Based on differential diagnosis made on routine morphology, the panel of antibody stains is chosen for applying on paraffin sections for staining. Some common examples are as under:

i) *Smooth muscle actin (SMA):* for smooth muscle tumours.

ii) *Vimentin:* as common marker to distinguish mesenchymal cells from epithelium.

iii) *Desmin:* for skeletal muscle cells.
iv) *S-100:* for nerve fibres.
v) *Factor VIII:* antigen for vascular endothelium.
vi) *LCA (leucocyte common antigen):* common marker for lymphoid cells.

4. ELECTRON MICROSCOPY EM as such is mainly a research tool and does not have much diagnostic value in soft tissue tumours but can be applied sometimes to look for tonofilaments or cell organelles.

5. CYTOGENETICS Many soft tissue tumours have specific genetic and chromosomal changes which can be done for determining histogenesis, or for diagnosis and prognosis.

Grading

The number of pathological grades of soft tissue tumours may vary according to different grading systems: 2 grade system (grade I-II as low and high grade), 3-grade system (grade I, II, III as low, intermediate and high grade) and 4 grade system (grade I-IV). Pathological grading is based on following 3 features:
i) Tumour differentiation or degree of cytologic atypia
ii) Mitotic count
iii) Tumour necrosis

Staging

Different staging systems for soft tissue sarcomas have been described but two of the most accepted staging systems are *Enneking's staging* and American Joint Committee (AJC) staging system:

Enneking's staging: This staging system is accepted by most oncologists and is based on grade and location of tumour as under:

♦ *According to tumour location*: T1 (intracompartmental) and T2 (extracompartmental) tumours.

♦ *According to tumour grade*: G1 (low grade) and G2 (high grade) tumours.

Accordingly, the stages of soft tissue tumours vary from stage I to stage III as under:

Stage I: G1 and T1-T2 tumours, but no metastases.
Stage II: G2 and T1 -T2 tumours, but without metastases.
Stage III: G1 or G2 , T1 or T2 tumours, but with metastases.

AJC staging: This AJC system of staging is similar to staging for other tumours. It is based on TNM system in which the primary tumour (T), the status of lymph nodes (N) and presence or absence of metastases (M) are taken into consideration for staging, besides the histologic grade of the tumour.

After these brief general comments, some important examples of tumours of different types of mesenchymal tissue origin are described here.

| GIST BOX 21.2 | General Features of Soft Tissue Tumours |

❖ Soft tissue tumours are defined as tumours arising from non-epithelial extra-skeletal tissues of the body except the reticuloendothelial system, the glia and the supporting tissues of specific organs and viscera.
❖ Many of these tumours come to attention after trauma. Many of them have cytogenetic abnormalities. Most occur sporadically; others are part of genetic syndromes.
❖ Soft tissue tumours are divided into benign, intermediate (locally aggressive or rarely metastasising) and malignant.
❖ Their diagnosis rests on a few features: pattern, cellular features and aided by ancillary techniques of immunohistochemistry, EM and molecular profiling.
❖ Based on histologic features, they are divided into low-, intermediate- and high-grade.
❖ Staging of soft tissue tumours is based on either Enneking or AJC method, taking TNM and histologic grade into consideration.

TUMOURS AND TUMOUR-LIKE LESIONS OF FIBROUS TISSUE

Fibromas, reactive proliferations and fibromatosis, and fibrosarcoma are benign, tumour-like, and malignant neoplasms respectively, of fibrous connective tissue.

Fibromas

True fibromas are uncommon tumours in soft tissues. Many fibromas are actually examples of hyperplastic fibrous tissue rather than true neoplasms. On the other hand, combinations of fibrous growth with other mesenchymal tissue elements are more frequent e.g. neurofibroma, fibromyoma etc.

Three types of fibromas are distinguished:

1. Fibroma durum is a benign, often pedunculated and well-circumscribed tumour occurring on the body surfaces and mucous membranes. It is composed of fully matured and richly collagenous fibrous connective tissue **(Fig. 21.18)**.

2. Fibroma molle or fibrolipoma, also termed **soft fibroma,** is similar type of benign growth composed of mixture of mature fibrous connective tissue and adult-type fat.

3. Elastofibroma is a rare benign fibrous tumour located in the subscapular region. It is characterised by association of collagen bundles and branching elastic fibres.

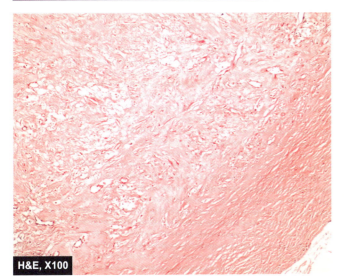

Figure 21.18 ▶ Fibroma of the oral cavity. The circumscribed lesion is composed of mature collagenised fibrous connective tissue.

Reactive Tumour-like Proliferations

These include some of the common examples such as keloid, nodular fasciitis (pseudosarcomatous fasciitis) and myositis ossificans.

KELOID A keloid is a progressive fibrous overgrowth in response to cutaneous injury such as burns, incisions, insect bites, vaccinations and others. Keloids are found more often in blacks and Asians. Their excision is frequently followed by recurrences.

Grossly, the keloid is a firm, smooth, pink, raised patch from which extend claw-like processes (keloid-claw).

Histologically, it is composed of thick, homogeneous, eosinophilic hyalinised bands of collagen admixed with thin collagenous fibres and large active fibroblasts. The adnexal structures are atrophic or destroyed.

There are some differences between a *keloid* and a *hypertrophic scar.* A hypertrophic scar of the skin is more cellular and has numerous fibroblasts than a keloid and is composed of thinner collagenous fibres. A keloid is a progressive lesion and liable to recurrences after surgical excision.

NODULAR FASCIITIS Nodular fasciitis, also called pseudosarcomatous fibromatosis, is a form of benign and reactive fibroblastic growth extending from superficial fascia into the subcutaneous fat, and sometimes into the subjacent muscle. The most common locations are the upper extremity, trunk and neck region of young adults. Local excision is generally curative. Less than 5% cases may have local recurrence.

Grossly, the lesion appears as a solitary well-circumscribed nodule (true to its name) in the superficial fascia. The size may vary from a centimeter to several centimeters in diameter.

Microscopically, various morphologic patterns may be seen but most common is a whorled or S-shaped pattern of fibroblasts present in oedematous background. The individual cells are spindle-shaped, plump fibroblasts showing mild nuclear atypia. Typical mitoses are frequent but atypical mitoses are not present.

MYOSITIS OSSIFICANS Myositis ossificans is a benign, tumour-like lesion characterised by osteoid and heterotopic bone formation in the soft tissues. It is a misnomer since the lesion neither occurs exclusively in the skeletal muscle as the name leads one to believe, nor are the inflammation or ossification always essential.

Myositis ossificans is generally preceded by history of antecedent trauma to a skeletal muscle or its tendon. The trauma may be minor and repetitive e.g. to the adductor muscles of the thigh of a horseman, or may be single injury followed by haemorrhage into the muscle. The patient generally complains of pain, tenderness and swelling. Richly vascularised granulation tissue replaces the affected muscle or tendon. Then follows development of osteoid and bone at the periphery, giving characteristic X-ray appearance.

Grossly, the lesion appears as unencapsulated, gritty mass replacing the muscle.

Histologically, the central region of the mass shows loosely-arranged fibroblasts having high mitotic activity. Towards the periphery, there is presence of osteoid matrix and formation of woven mineralised bone with trapped skeletal muscle fibres and regenerating muscle (myogenic) giant cells. The appearance is sufficiently atypical to suggest osteosarcoma but osteosarcoma lacks maturation phenomena seen in myositis ossificans. This is why the condition is also called *pseudomalignant osseous tumour* of the soft tissues.

Fibromatosis

'Fibromatosis' is the term used for tumour-like lesions of fibrous tissue which continue to proliferate actively and may be difficult to differentiate from sarcomas. These lesions may, therefore, be regarded as non-metastasising fibroblastic tumours which tend to invade locally and recur after surgical excision. In addition, electron microscopy has shown that the cells comprising these lesions have features not only of fibroblasts but of both fibroblasts and smooth muscle cells, so called *myofibroblasts.* Depending upon the anatomic locations and the age group affected, fibromatoses are broadly grouped as under:

A. Infantile or juvenile fibromatoses These include: fibrous hamartoma of infancy, fibromatosis colli, diffuse infantile fibromatosis, juvenile aponeurotic fibroma, juvenile nasopharyngeal angiofibroma and congenital (generalised and solitary) fibromatosis.

B. Adult type of fibromatoses These are: palmar and plantar fibromatosis, nodular fasciitis, cicatricial fibromatosis, keloid, irradiation fibromatosis, penile fibromatosis (Peyronie's disease), abdominal and extra-abdominal desmoid fibromatosis, and retroperitoneal fibromatosis. These are further categorised into *superficial or deep-seated*.

Obviously, it is beyond the scope of the present discussion to cover all these lesions. Some of the important forms of fibromatoses are briefly discussed here.

PALMAR AND PLANTAR (SUPERFICIAL) FIBROMATOSES These fibromatoses, also called Dupuytren-like contractures are the most common form of fibromatoses occurring superficially.

◆ **Palmar fibromatosis** is more common in the elderly males occurring in the palmar fascia and leading to flexion contractures of the fingers (Dupuytren's contracture). It appears as a painless, nodular or irregular, infiltrating, benign fibrous subcutaneous lesion. In almost half the cases, the lesions are bilateral.

◆ **Plantar fibromatosis** is a similar lesion occurring on the medial aspect of plantar arch. However, plantar lesions are less common than palmar type and do not cause contractures as frequently as palmar lesions. They are seen more often in adults and are infrequently multiple and bilateral. Essentially similar lesions occur in the shaft of the penis (*penile fibromatosis* or *Peyronie's disease*) and in the soft tissues of the knuckles (*knuckle pads*).

Histologically, palmar and plantar fibromatoses have similar appearance. The nodules are composed of fibrovascular tissue having plump, tightly-packed fibroblasts which have high mitotic rate. Ultrastructurally, some of the fibroblasts have features of myofibroblasts having contractile nature.

The palmar lesions frequently extend into soft tissues causing contractures. Both palmar and plantar lesions may remain stationary at nodular stage, progress, or regress spontaneously. Recurrence rate after surgical excision in both forms is as high as 50-60%.

DESMOID (DEEP-SEATED) FIBROMATOSES Desmoid fibromatoses or musculo-aponeurotic fibromatoses, commonly referred to as desmoid tumours, are of 2 types: abdominal and extra-abdominal. Both types are, however, histologically similar. Clinically, both types behave in an aggressive manner and have to be distinguished from sarcomas. Recurrences are frequent and multiple. The pathogenesis of these lesions is not known but among the factors implicated are the role of antecedent trauma, genetic influences and relationship to oestrogen as observed by occurrence of these lesions in pregnancy.

◆ **Abdominal desmoids** are locally aggressive infiltrating tumour-like fibroblastic growths, often found in the musculo-aponeurotic structures of the rectus muscle in the anterior abdominal wall in women during or after pregnancy.

◆ **Extra-abdominal desmoids,** on the other hand, are more common in men and are widely distributed such as in the upper and lower extremities, chest wall, back, buttocks, and head and neck region.

◆ **Intra-abdominal desmoids** present at the root of the small bowel mesentery are associated with Gardner's syndrome (consisting of fibromatosis, familial intestinal polyposis, osteomas and epidermal cysts).

Grossly, desmoids are solitary, large, grey-white, firm and unencapsulated tumours infiltrating the muscle locally. Cut surface is whorled and trabeculated.

Microscopically, their appearance is rather misleadingly bland in contrast with aggressive local behaviour. They are composed of uniform-looking fibroblasts arranged in bands and fascicles. Pleomorphism and mitoses are infrequent. The older regions of the tumour have hypocellular hyalinised collagen.

Fibrosarcoma

The number of soft tissue tumours diagnosed as fibrosarcoma has now dropped, partly because of reclassification of fibromatoses which have aggressive and recurrent behaviour, and partly due to inclusion of many of such tumours in the group of fibrous histiocytomas (page 339).

Fibrosarcoma is a slow-growing tumour, affecting adults between 4th and 7th decades of life. Most common locations are the lower extremity (especially thigh and around the knee), upper extremity, trunk, head and neck, and retroperitoneum **(Fig. 21.19)**. The tumour is capable of metastasis, chiefly via the blood stream.

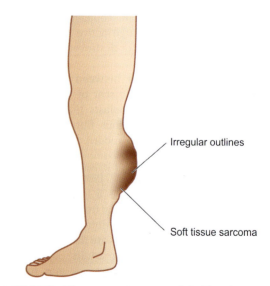

Figure 21.19 ▶ Fibrosarcoma, common clinical location.

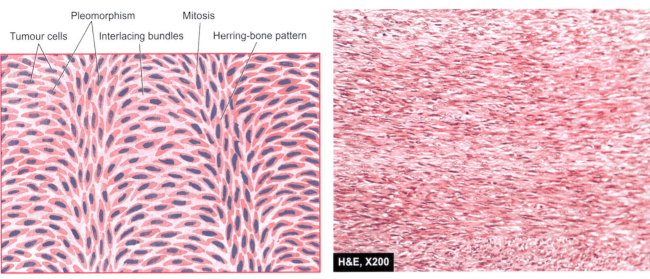

Figure 21.20 ▶ Fibrosarcoma. Microscopy shows a well-differentiated tumour composed of spindle-shaped cells forming interlacing fascicles producing a typical Herring-bone pattern. A few mitotic figures are also seen.

Grossly, fibrosarcoma is a grey-white, firm, lobulated and characteristically circumscribed mass. Cut surface of the tumour is soft, fish flesh-like, with foci of necrosis and haemorrhages.

Histologically, the tumour is composed of uniform, spindle-shaped fibroblasts arranged in intersecting fascicles. In well-differentiated tumours, such areas produce *'herring-bone pattern'* (herring-bone is a sea fish) **(Fig. 21.20).** Poorly-differentiated fibrosarcoma, however, has highly pleomorphic appearance with frequent mitoses and bizarre cells.

 GIST BOX 21.3 | **Tumours and Tumour-like Lesions of Fibrous Tissue**

- True fibromas are uncommon benign tumours in fibrous tissues. Examples are fibroma durum, fibrolipoma and elastofibroma.
- Reactive proliferations of fibrous tissue are tumour-like lesions and include keloid, nodular fasciitis and myositis ossificans.
- Fibromatosis are a group of tumour-like lesions of fibrous tissue which continue to proliferate actively and may be difficult to differentiate from sarcomas. Examples of superficial type are palmar and plantar fibromatosis, and deep-seated desmoid fibromatosis.
- Fibrosarcoma is the malignant counterpart which is generally slow-growing tumour.

FIBROHISTIOCYTIC TUMOURS

The group of fibrohistiocytic tumours is characterised by distinctive light microscopic features that include presence of cells with fibroblastic and histiocytic features in varying proportion and identification of characteristic *cart-wheel or storiform pattern* in which the spindle cells radiate outward from the central focus. The histogenesis of these cells is uncertain but possibly they arise from primitive mesenchymal cells or facultative fibroblasts which are capable of differentiating along different cell lines. The group includes full spectrum of lesions varying from *benign* (benign fibrous histiocytoma) to *malignant* (malignant fibrous histiocytoma), with dermatofibrosarcoma protuberans occupying the *intermediate* (low-grade malignancy) position.

Benign Fibrous Histiocytoma

Depending upon the location and predominant pattern, benign fibrous histiocytomas include a number of diverse entities such as dermatofibroma, sclerosing haemangioma, fibroxanthoma, xanthogranuloma, giant cell tumour of tendon sheath and pigmented villonodular synovitis. All these tumours have mixed composition of benign fibroblastic and histiocytic pattern of cells.

Dermatofibrosarcoma Protuberans

Dermatofibrosarcoma protuberans is a low-grade malignant cutaneous tumour of fibrohistiocytic origin. The tumour recurs locally, and in rare instances gives rise to distant metastases. Most frequent location is the trunk.

Grossly, the tumour forms a firm, solitary or multiple, satellite nodules extending into the subcutaneous fat and having thin and ulcerated skin surface.

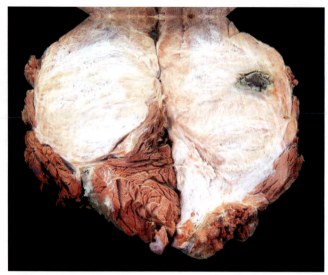

Figure 21.21 ▶ Malignant fibrous histiocytoma. The lobulated tumour infiltrating the skeletal muscle is somewhat circumscribed. Cut surface is grey-white fleshy with areas of haemorrhage and necrosis.

Histologically, the tumour is highly cellular and is composed of fibroblasts arranged in a cart-wheel or storiform pattern.

Malignant Fibrous Histiocytoma (Pleomorphic Sarcoma)

Malignant fibrous histiocytomas (MFH), also called pleomorphic sarcoma now, represent approximately 20-30% of all soft tissue sarcomas. It is the most common soft tissue sarcoma and is the most frequent sarcoma associated with radiotherapy. The tumour occurs more commonly in males and more frequently in the age group of 5th to 7th decades. Most common locations are the lower and upper extremities and retroperitoneum. It begins as a painless, enlarging mass, generally in relation to skeletal muscle, deep fascia or subcutaneous tissue. The tumour is believed to arise from primitive mesenchymal cells which are capable of differentiating towards both fibroblastic and histiocytic cell lines.

Grossly, MFH is a multilobulated, well-circumscribed, firm or fleshy mass, 5-10 cm in diameter. Cut surface is grey-white, soft and myxoid **(Fig. 21.21)**.

Histologically, there is marked variation in appearance from area to area within the same tumour. In general, there is admixture of spindle-shaped *fibroblast-like cells* and mononuclear round to oval *histiocyte-like cells* which may show phagocytic function. There is tendency for the spindle-shaped cells to be arranged in characteristic cart-wheel or storiform pattern. The tumour cells show varying degree of pleomorphism, hyperchromatism, mitotic activity and presence of multinucleate bizarre tumour giant cells. Usually there are numerous blood vessels and some scattered lymphocytes and plasma cells **(Fig. 21.22)**. Important immunohistochemical markers for MFH include vimentin, α-chymotrypsin, CD68 and factor VIII-a.

As per current concept, corresponding WHO categories of MFH as pleomorphic sarcoma are as under:

1. Storifrom-pleomorphic MFH as the prototype of *undifferentiated high-grade pleomorphic sarcoma.*

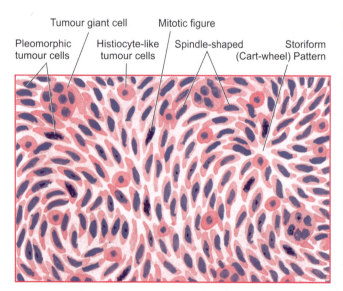
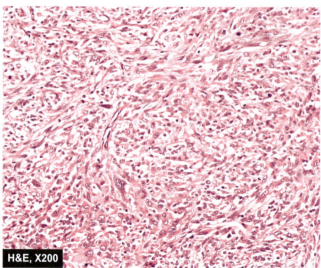

Figure 21.22 ▶ Malignant fibrous histiocytoma (pleomorphic sarcoma). The tumour shows admixture of spindle-shaped pleomorphic cells forming storiform (cart-wheel) pattern and histiocyte-like round to oval cells. Bizarre pleomorphic multinucleate tumour giant cells and some mononuclear inflammatory cells are also present.

2. **Inflammatory MFH** is an undifferentiated high-grade MFH having prominent neutrophilic infiltrate besides the presence of eosinophils, histiocytes and xanthoma cells. Currently, this is termed as *undifferentiated pleomorphic sarcoma with prominent inflammation.*

3. **Giant cell MFH** having prominent presence of tumour giant cells called as *undifferentiated pleomorphic sarcoma with giant cells.*

4. **Myxoid MFH** which shows areas of loose myxoid stroma in the cellular areas and has an overall better prognosis, is now categorised as a specific entity called *myxofiborsarcoma.*

Prognosis of MFH is determined by 2 parameters: depth of location and size of the tumour. Deep-seated and large MFH such as of the retroperitoneum have poorer prognosis than those small in size and located superficially which come to attention earlier. Metastases are frequent, most often to the lungs and regional lymph nodes. Five-year survival rate is approximately 30-50%.

| GIST BOX 21.4 | Fibrohistiocytic Tumours |

- Fibrohistiocytic tumours are characterised by presence of cells with fibroblastic and histiocytic features in varying proportion and identification of characteristic cart-wheel or storiform pattern.
- Benign fibrous histiocytomas include dermatofibroma, sclerosing haemangioma, fibroxanthoma, xanthogranuloma, giant cell tumour of tendon sheath and pigmented villonodular synovitis.
- Dermatofibrosarcoma protuberans is a low-grade malignant cutaneous tumour of fibrohistiocytic origin.
- Malignant fibrous histiocytoma or pleomophic sarcoma is the most common soft tissue sarcoma and has a few variants such as pleomorphic, inflammatory, giant cell type and myxoid.

TUMOURS OF ADIPOSE TISSUE

Lipomas and liposarcomas are the common examples of benign and malignant tumours respectively of adipose tissue. Uncommon varieties of adipose tissue tumours include hibernoma, a benign tumour arising from brown fat, and lipoblastoma (foetal lipoma) resembling foetal fat and found predominantly in children under 3 years of age.

Lipoma

Lipoma is the commonest soft tissue tumour. It appears as a solitary, soft, movable and painless mass which may remain stationary or grow slowly. Lipomas occur most often in 4th to 5th decades of life and are frequent in females. They may be found at different locations in the body but most common sites are the subcutaneous tissues in the neck, back and shoulder **(Fig. 21.23,A)**. A lipoma rarely ever transforms into liposarcoma.

Grossly, a subcutaneous lipoma is usually small, round to oval and encapsulated mass. The cut surface is soft, lobulated, yellowish-orange and greasy **(Fig. 21.23, B)**.

Histologically, the tumour is composed of lobules of mature adipose cells separated by delicate fibrous septa. A thin fibrous capsule surrounds the tumour **(Fig. 21.24)**.

A variety of admixture of lipoma with other tissue components may be seen. These include: fibrolipoma (admixture with fibrous tissue), angiolipoma (combination with proliferating blood vessels) and myelolipoma (admixture with bone marrow elements as seen in adrenals). Infrequently, benign lipoma may infiltrate the striated muscle (infiltrating or intramuscular lipoma). Spindle cell lipoma and pleomorphic (atypical) lipoma are the other unusual variants of lipoma. The latter type may be particularly difficult to distinguish from well-differentiated liposarcoma.

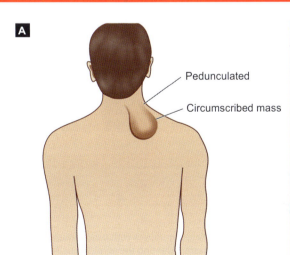
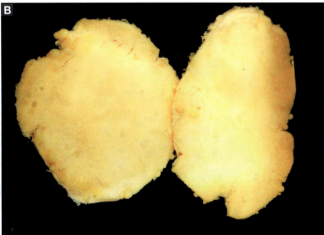

Figure 21.23 ▶ Lipoma. A, Common clinical location. B, The cut surface of the tumour is soft, lobulated, yellowish and greasy.

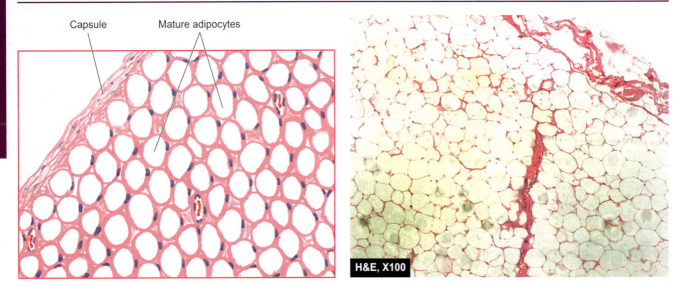

Figure 21.24 ▶ Lipoma. The tumour shows a thin capsule and underlying lobules of mature adipose cells separated by delicate fibrous septa.

Liposarcoma

Liposarcoma is one of the most common soft tissue sarcomas in adults, perhaps next in frequency only to malignant fibrous histiocytoma. Unlike lipoma which originates from mature adipose cells, liposarcoma arises from primitive mesenchymal cells, the *lipoblasts*. The peak incidence is in 5th to 7th decades of life. In contrast to lipomas which are more frequently subcutaneous in location, liposarcomas often occur in the deep tissues. Most frequent sites are intermuscular regions in the thigh, buttocks and retroperitoneum.

Grossly, liposarcoma appears as a nodular mass, 5 cm or more in diameter. The tumour is generally circumscribed but infiltrative. Cut surface is grey-white to yellow, myxoid and gelatinous. Retroperitoneal masses are generally much larger.

Histologically, the hallmark of diagnosis of liposarcoma is the identification of variable number of *lipoblasts* which may be univacuolated or multivacuolated **(Fig. 21.25)**. The vacuoles represent fat in the cytoplasm. Four major histologic varieties of liposarcomas are distinguished: well-differentiated, myxoid, round cell, and pleomorphic:

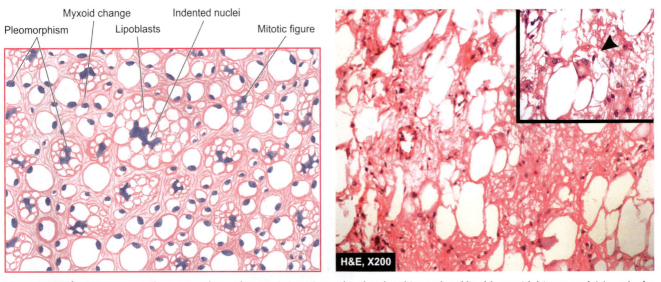

Figure 21.25 ▶ Liposarcoma. The tumour shows characteristic, univacuolated and multivacuolated lipoblasts with bizarre nuclei. Inset in the right photomicrograph shows close-up view of a typical lipoblast having multivacuolated cytoplasm indenting the atypical nucleus.

1. *Well-differentiated liposarcoma* resembles lipoma but contains uni- or multi-vacuolated lipoblasts.
2. *Myxoid liposarcoma* is the most common histologic type. It is composed of monomorphic, fusiform or stellate cells representing primitive mesenchymal cells, lying dispersed in mucopolysaccharide-rich ground substance. Occasional tumour giant cells may be present. Prominent meshwork of capillaries forming chicken-wire pattern is a conspicuous feature.
3. *Round cell liposarcoma* is composed of uniform, round to oval cells having fine multivacuolated cytoplasm with central hyperchromatic nuclei. Round cell liposarcoma may resemble a signet-ring carcinoma but mucin stains help in distinguishing the two.
4. *Pleomorphic liposarcoma* is highly undifferentiated and the most anaplastic type. There are numerous large tumour giant cells and bizarre lipoblasts.

Myxoid and round cell liposarcoma show cytogenetic abnormality of translocation t(12;16) (q13; p11) and molecular profiling of *FUS-DDIT3* fusion gene, features which help in distinguishing these variants from other types.

The *prognosis* of liposarcoma depends upon the location and histologic type. In general, well-differentiated and myxoid varieties have excellent prognosis, while pleomorphic liposarcoma has significantly poorer prognosis. Round cell and pleomorphic variants metastasise frequently to the lungs, other visceral organs and serosal surfaces.

> **GIST BOX 21.5** | **Common Tumours of Adipose Tissue**
>
> ❖ Lipoma is the commonest soft tissue tumour appearing as a solitary, soft, movable and painless mass which may remain stationary or grow slowly.
> ❖ Liposarcoma occurs in 5th to 7th decades of life and arises from primitive mesenchymal cells, the *lipoblasts*. Unlike lipomas, liposarcomas often occur in the deep tissues.
> ❖ Histologic variants of liposarcoma having prognostic significance are well-differentiated, myxoid, round cell and pleomorphic type.

SKELETAL MUSCLE TUMOURS

Rhabdomyoma and rhabdomyosarcoma are the benign and malignant tumours respectively of striated muscle.

Rhabdomyoma

Rhabdomyoma is a rare benign soft tissue tumour. It should not be confused with glycogen-containing lesion of the heart designated as cardiac rhabdomyoma which is probably a hamartomatous lesion and not a true tumour. Soft tissue rhabdomyomas are predominantly located in the head and neck, most often in the upper neck, tongue, larynx and pharynx.

Histologically, the tumour is composed of large, round to oval cells, having abundant, granular, eosinophilic cytoplasm which is frequently vacuolated and contains glycogen. Cross-striations are generally demonstrable in some cells with phosphotungstic acid-haematoxylin (PTAH) stain. The tumour is divided into adult and foetal types, depending upon the degree of resemblance of tumour cells to normal muscle cells.

Rhabdomyosarcoma

Rhabdomyosarcoma is a much more common soft tissue tumour than rhabdomyoma, and is the commonest soft tissue sarcoma in children and young adults. It is a highly malignant tumour arising from rhabdomyoblasts in varying stages of differentiation with or without demonstrable cross-striations. Depending upon the growth pattern and histology, 4 types are distinguished: embryonal, botryoid, alveolar and pleomorphic.

1. **EMBRYONAL RHABDOMYOSARCOMA** The embryonal form is the most common of the rhabdomyosarcomas. It occurs predominantly in children under 12 years of age. The common locations are in the head and neck region, most frequently in the orbit, urogenital tract and the retroperitoneum.

Grossly, the tumour forms a gelatinous mass growing between muscles or in the deep subcutaneous tissues but generally has no direct relationship to the skeletal muscle.

Histologically, the tumour cells have resemblance to embryonal stage of development of muscle fibres. There is considerable variation in cell types. Generally, the tumour consists of a mixture of small, round to oval cells and spindle-shaped strap cells having tapering bipolar cytoplasmic processes in which cross-striations may be evident. The tumour cells form broad fascicles or bands. Mitoses are frequent.

2. **BOTRYOID RHABDOMYOSARCOMA** Botryoid variety is regarded as a variant of embryonal rhabdomyosarcoma occurring in children under 10 years of age. It is seen most frequently in the vagina, urinary bladder and nose.

Grossly, the tumour forms a distinctive grape-like gelatinous mass protruding into the hollow cavity.

Histologically, the tumour grows underneath the mucosal layer, forming the characteristic *cambium layer* of tumour cells. The tumour is hypocellular and myxoid with predominance of small, round to oval tumour cells (Fig. 21.26).

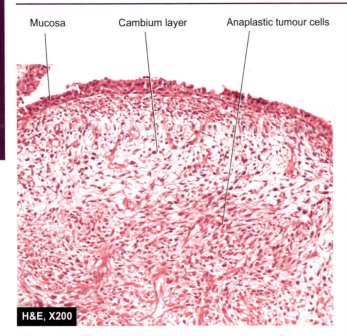

Figure 21.26 ▶ Botryoid rhabdomyosarcoma, nose. The tumour shows the characteristic submucosal Cambium layer of tumour cells. The tumour cells are round to oval and have anaplasia.

3. **ALVEOLAR RHABDOMYOSARCOMA** Alveolar type of rhabdomyosarcoma is more common in older children and young adults under the age of 20 years. The most common locations, unlike the embryonal variety, are the extremities.

Grossly, the tumour differs from embryonal type in arising directly from skeletal muscle and grows rapidly as soft and gelatinous mass.

Histologically, the tumour shows characteristic alveolar pattern resembling pulmonary alveolar spaces. These spaces are formed by fine fibrocollagenous septa. The tumour cells lying in these spaces and lining the fibrous trabeculae are generally small, lymphocyte-like with frequent mitoses and some multinucleate tumour giant cells (Fig. 21.27). Cross-striation can be demonstrated in about a quarter of cases.

4. **PLEOMORPHIC RHABDOMYOSARCOMA** This less frequent variety of rhabdomyosarcoma occurs predominantly in older adults above the age of 40 years. They are most common in the extremities, most frequently in the lower limbs.

Grossly, the tumour forms a well-circumscribed, soft, whitish mass with areas of haemorrhages and necrosis.

Histologically, the tumour cells show considerable variation in size and shape. The tumour is generally composed of highly anaplastic cells having bizarre appearance and numerous multinucleate giant cells. Various shapes include racquet shape, tadpole appearance, large strap cells, and ribbon shapes containing several nuclei in a row.

Conventionally, the cross-striations can be demonstrated with PTAH stain in a few rhabdomyosarcomas. Immunohistochemical stains include: myogenin, Myo-D1, desmin, actin, myosin, myoglobin, and vimentin. Based on cytogenetic and molecular abnormalities, alveolar rhabdomyosarcoma with t(1;13)(q36;q14) and *PAX3-FOXO1A* fusion gene have better prognosis, compared to cases having translocation t(2;13)(p35;q14) and *PAX7-FOXO1A* fusion gene which have worse prognosis.

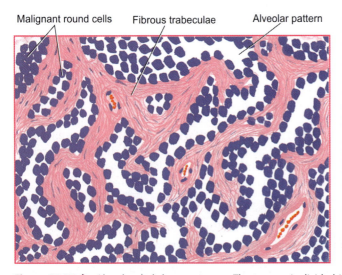
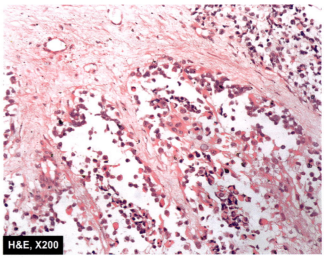

Figure 21.27 ▶ Alveolar rhabdomyosarcoma. The tumour is divided into alveolar spaces composed of fibrocollagenous tissue. The fibrous trabeculae are lined by small, dark, undifferentiated tumour cells, with some cells floating in the alveolar spaces. A few multinucleate tumour giant cells are also present.

> **GIST BOX 21.6** Common Skeletal Muscle Tumours
>
> ❖ Rhabdomyoma is a rare benign soft tissue tumour.
> ❖ Rhabdomyosarcoma is a much more common soft tissue tumour than rhabdomyoma, arising from rhabdomyoblasts. It is the commonest soft tissue sarcoma in children and young adults.
> ❖ Four histologic types are distinguished: embryonal, botryoid, alveolar and pleomorphic. The last named is common in adults while others occur in children.

SMOOTH MUSCLE TUMOURS

Benign and malignant tumours arising from the smooth muscle such as in the uterus, bowel, blood vessel wall etc are called leiomyoma and leiomyosarcoma respectively (*leios* = smooth).

Leiomyoma

Leiomyomas or fibromyomas, commonly called *fibroids* by the gynaecologists, are the most common uterine tumours of smooth muscle origin, often admixed with variable amount of fibrous tissue component. About 20% of women above the age of 30 years harbour uterine myomas of varying size. Vast majority of them are benign and cause no symptoms. Malignant transformation occurs in less than 0.5% of leiomyomas. Symptomatic cases may produce abnormal uterine bleeding, pain, symptoms due to compression of surrounding structures and infertility.

The cause of leiomyomas is unknown but the possible stimulus to their proliferation is oestrogen. This is evidenced by increase in their size in pregnancy **(Fig. 21.28,C)** and high dose oestrogen-therapy and their regression following menopause and castration. Other possible factors implicated in its etiology are human growth hormone and sterility.

Leiomyomas are most frequently located in the uterus where they may occur within the myometrium *(intramural or interstitial)*, the serosa *(subserosal)*, or just underneath the endometrium *(submucosal)*. Subserosal and submucosal leiomyomas may develop pedicles and protrude as pedunculated myomas. Leiomyomas may involve the cervix or broad ligament.

Grossly, irrespective of their location, leiomyomas are often multiple, circumscribed, firm, nodular, grey-white masses of variable size. On cut section, they exhibit characteristic whorled pattern **(Fig. 21.28, A,B)**.

Histologically, they are essentially composed of 2 tissue elements—whorled bundles of smooth muscle cells admixed with variable amount of connective tissue. The smooth muscle cells are uniform in size and shape with abundant cytoplasm and central oval nuclei **(Fig. 21.29)**.

Cellular leiomyoma has preponderance of smooth muscle elements and may superficially resemble leiomyosarcoma but is distinguished from it by the absence of mitoses (see below).

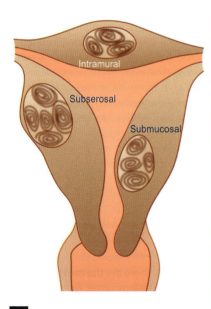
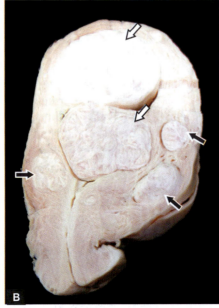
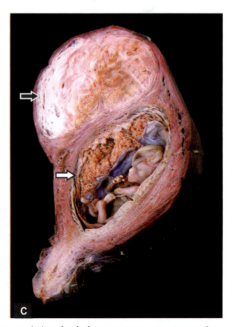

Figure 21.28 ▶ Leiomyomas. **A,** Diagrammatic appearance of common locations and characteristic whorled appearance on cut section. **B,** Sectioned surface of the uterus shows multiple circumscribed, firm nodular masses of variable sizes—submucosal (white arrows) and intramural (black arrows) in location having characteristic whorling. **C,** The opened up uterine cavity shows an intrauterine gestation sac with placenta (white arrow) and a single circumscribed, enlarged, firm nodular mass in intramural location (black arrow) having grey-white whorled pattern.

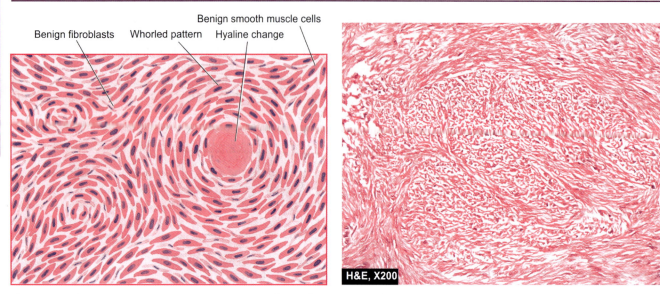

Figure 21.29 ▶ Leiomyoma uterus. Microscopy shows whorls of smooth muscle cells which are spindle-shaped, having abundant cytoplasm and oval nuclei.

The pathologic appearance may be altered by secondary changes in the leiomyomas; these include: hyaline degeneration, cystic degeneration, infarction, calcification, infection and suppuration, necrosis, fatty change, and rarely, sarcomatous change.

Leiomyosarcoma

Leiomyosarcoma is an uncommon malignant tumour as compared to its rather common benign counterpart. The incidence of malignancy in pre-existing leiomyoma is less than 0.5% but primary uterine sarcoma is less common than that which arises in the leiomyoma. The peak age incidence is seen in 4th to 6th decades of life. The symptoms produced are nonspecific such as uterine enlargement and abnormal uterine bleeding.

Grossly, the tumour may form a diffuse, bulky, soft and fleshy mass, or a polypoid mass projecting into lumen.

Histologically, though there are usually some areas showing whorled arrangement of spindle-shaped smooth muscle cells having large and hyperchromatic nuclei, the hallmark of diagnosis and prognosis is the number of mitoses per high power field (HPF). The essential diagnostic criteria are: more than 10 mitoses per 10 HPF with or without cellular atypia, or 5-10 mitoses per 10 HPF with cellular atypia. More the number of mitoses per 10 HPF, worse is the prognosis.

Leiomyosarcoma is liable to recur after removal and eventually metastasises to distant sites such as lungs, liver, bone and brain.

 GIST BOX 21.7 | **Smooth Muscle Tumours**

❖ Leiomyomas or fibroids are the most common benign uterine tumours of smooth muscle origin; other sites include blood vessels wall, bowel.
❖ Leiomyosarcoma is an uncommon malignant tumour.

TUMOURS OF BLOOD VESSELS AND LYMPHATICS

Majority of benign vascular tumours are malformations or hamartomas. A hamartoma is a tumour-like lesion made up of tissues indigenous to the part but lacks the true growth potential of true neoplasms. However, there is no clear-cut distinction between vascular hamartomas and true benign tumours and are often described together. On the other hand, there are true vascular tumours which are of intermediate grade and there are frank malignant tumours.

Haemangioma

Haemangiomas are quite common lesions, especially in infancy and childhood. The most common site is the skin of the face and mucosal surfaces. Amongst the various clinical and histologic types, three important forms are described below.

CAPILLARY HAEMANGIOMA These are the most common type. Clinically, they appear as small or large, flat or slightly elevated, red to purple, soft and lobulated lesions, varying in size from a few millimeters to a few centimeters in diameter. They may be present at birth or appear in early childhood. Strawberry birthmarks and 'port-wine mark' are some good

Chapter 21: Common Specific Tumours 347

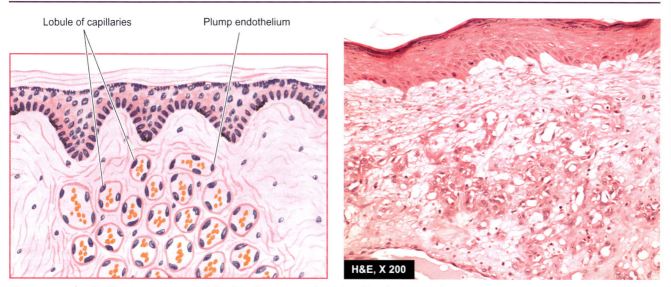

Figure 21.30 ▶ Capillary haemangioma of the skin. There are capillaries lined by plump endothelial cells and containing blood. The intervening stroma consists of scant connective tissue.

examples. The common sites are the skin, subcutaneous tissue and mucous membranes of oral cavity and lips. Less common sites are internal visceral organs like liver, spleen and kidneys.

Histologically, capillary haemangiomas are well-defined but unencapsulated lobules. These lobules are composed of capillary-sized, thin-walled, blood-filled vessels. These vessels are lined by single layer of plump endothelial cells surrounded by a layer of pericytes. The vessels are separated by some connective tissue stroma **(Fig. 21.30)**.

Many of the capillary haemangiomas regress spontaneously within a few years.

CAVERNOUS HAEMANGIOMA Cavernous haemangiomas are single or multiple, discrete or diffuse, red to blue, soft and spongy masses. They are often 1 to 2 cm in diameter. They are most common in the skin (especially of the face and neck); other sites are mucosa of the oral cavity, stomach and small intestine, and internal visceral organs like the liver and spleen.

Histologically, cavernous haemangiomas are composed of thin-walled cavernous vascular spaces, filled partly or completely with blood. The vascular spaces are lined by flattened endothelial cells. They are separated by scanty connective tissue stroma **(Fig. 21.31)**.

Cavernous haemangiomas rarely involute spontaneously.

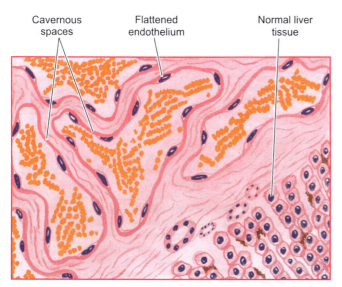
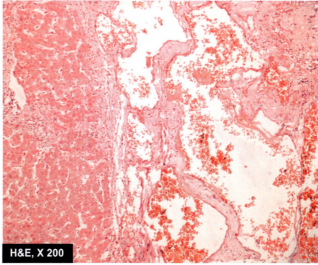

Figure 21.31 ▶ Cavernous haemangioma of the liver. The vascular spaces are large, dilated, many containing blood, and are lined by flattened endothelial cells. Scanty connective tissue stroma is seen between the cavernous spaces.

Section IV: Neoplasia

GRANULOMA PYOGENICUM Granuloma pyogenicum is also referred to as *haemangioma of granulation tissue type*. True to its name, it appears as exophytic, red granulation tissue just like a nodule, commonly on the skin and mucosa of gingiva or oral cavity. *Pregnancy tumour* or *granuloma gravidarum* is a variant occurring on the gingiva during pregnancy and regresses after delivery. Granuloma pyogenicum often develops following trauma and is usually 1 to 2 cm in diameter.

Histologically, it shows proliferating capillaries similar to capillary haemangioma but the capillaries are separated by abundant oedema and inflammatory infiltrate, thus resembling inflammatory granulation tissue.

Lymphangioma

Lymphangiomas are lymphatic counterparts of vascular angiomas. Lymphangiomas are congenital lesions which are classified as capillary, cavernous and cystic hygroma. Combinations are also often seen.

CAPILLARY LYMPHANGIOMA It is also called as lymphangioma simplex. It is a small, circumscribed, slightly elevated lesion measuring 1 to 2 cm in diameter. The common locations are the skin of head and neck, axilla and mucous membranes. Rarely, these may be found in the internal organs.

Histologically, capillary lymphangioma is composed of a network of endothelium-lined, capillary-sized spaces containing lymph and often separated by lymphoid aggregates.

CAVERNOUS LYMPHANGIOMA It is more common than the capillary type. The common sites are in the region of head and neck or axilla. A large cystic variety called *cystic hygroma* occurs in the neck producing gross deformity in the neck.

Histologically, cavernous lymphangioma consists of large dilated lymphatic spaces lined by flattened endothelial cells and containing lymph. Scanty intervening stromal connective tissue is present (Fig. 21.32). These lesions, though benign, are often difficult to remove due to infiltration into adjacent tissues.

Glomus Tumour (Glomangioma)

Glomus tumour is an uncommon true benign tumour arising from contractile glomus cells that are present in the arteriovenous shunts (Sucquet-Hoyer anastomosis). These tumours are found most often in the dermis of the fingers or toes under a nail; other sites are mucosa of the stomach and nasal cavity. These lesions are characterised by extreme pain. They may be single or multiple, small, often less than 1 cm in diameter, flat or slightly elevated, red-blue, painful nodules.

Histologically, the tumours are composed of small blood vessels lined by endothelium and surrounded by aggregates, nests and masses of glomus cells. The glomus cells are round to cuboidal cells with scanty cytoplasm (Fig. 21.33). The intervening connective tissue stroma contains some non-myelinated nerve fibres.

Haemangioendothelioma

Haemangioendothelioma is a true tumour of endothelial cells, the behaviour of which is intermediate between a haemangioma and haemangiosarcoma. It is found most often in the skin and subcutaneous tissue in relation to medium-sized and large veins. *Haemangioblastoma* is

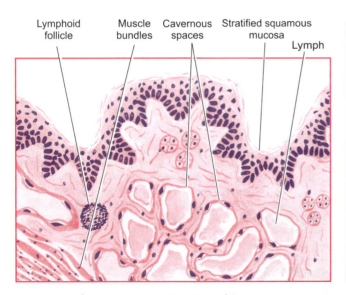
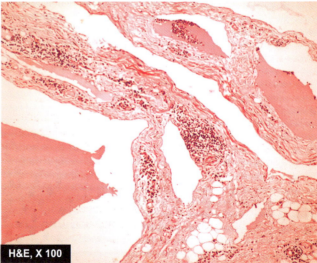

Figure 21.32 ▶ Cavernous lymphangioma of the tongue. Large cystic spaces lined by the flattened endothelial cells and containing lymph are present. Stroma shows scattered collection of lymphocytes.

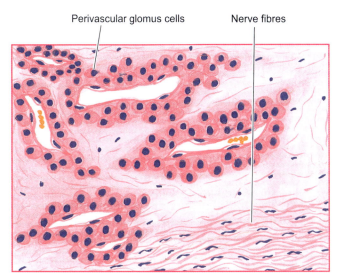
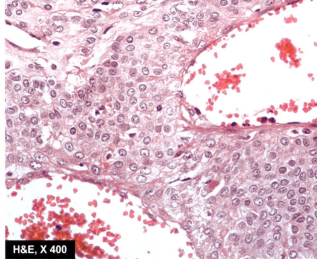

Figure 21.33 ▶ Glomus tumour. There are blood-filled vascular channels lined by endothelial cells and surrounded by nests and masses of glomus cells.

the term used for similar tumour occurring in the cerebellum.

Grossly, the tumour is usually well-defined, grey-red, polypoid mass.

Microscopically, there is an active proliferation of endothelial cells forming several layers around the blood vessels so that vascular lumina are difficult to identify. These cells may have variable mitotic activity. Reticulin stain delineates the pattern of cell proliferation inner to the basement membrane **(Fig. 21.34)**.

Haemangiopericytoma

Haemangiopericytoma is an uncommon tumour arising from pericytes. Pericytes are cells present external to the endothelial cells of capillaries and venules. This is a rare tumour that can occur at any site but is more common in lower extremities and the retroperitoneum. It may occur at any age and may vary in size from 1 to 8 cm.

Microscopically, the tumour is composed of capillaries surrounded by spindle-shaped pericytes outside the vascular basement membrane forming whorled arrangement. These tumour cells may have high mitotic rate and areas of necrosis. Silver impregnation stain (i.e. reticulin stain) is employed to confirm the presence of pericytes outside the basement membrane of capillaries and to distinguish it from haemangioendothelioma **(Fig. 21.35)**.

Local recurrences are common and distant spread occurs in about 20% of cases.

Angiosarcoma

Also known as haemangiosarcoma and malignant haemangioendothelioma, it is a malignant vascular tumour occurring most frequently in the skin, subcutaneous tissue, liver, spleen, bone, lung and retroperitoneal tissues. It can occur in both sexes and at any age. *Hepatic angiosarcomas* are of special interest in view of their association with carcinogens like polyvinyl chloride, arsenical pesticides and radioactive contrast medium, thorotrast, used in the past.

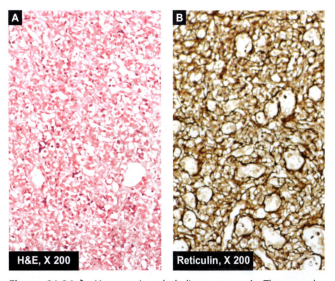

Figure 21.34 ▶ Haemangioendothelioma nose. A, The vascular channels are lined by multiple layers of plump endothelial cells having minimal mitotic activity obliterating the lumina. B, Reticulin stain shows condensation of reticulin around the vessel wall but not between the proliferating cells.

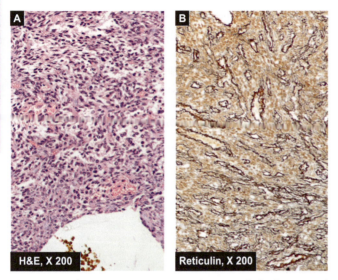

Figure 21.35 ▶ Haemangiopericytoma liver. Spindled cells surround the vascular lumina in a whorled fashion, highlighted by reticulin stain. These tumour cells have bland nuclei and few mitoses.

Grossly, the tumours are usually bulky, pale grey-white, firm masses with poorly-defined margins. Areas of haemorrhage, necrosis and central softening are frequently present.

Microscopically, the tumours may be well-differentiated masses of proliferating endothelial cells around well-formed vascular channels, to poorly-differentiated lesions composed of plump, anaplastic and pleomorphic cells in solid clusters with poorly identifiable vascular channels (Fig. 21.36).

These tumours invade locally and frequently have distant metastases in the lungs and other organs. *Lymphangiosarcoma* is a histologically similar tumour occurring in obstructive lymphoedema of long duration.

Kaposi's Sarcoma

Kaposi's sarcoma is a malignant angiomatous tumour, first described by Kaposi, Hungarian dermatologist, in 1872. However, the tumour has attracted greater attention in the last two decades due to its frequent occurrence in patients with HIV/AIDS.

CLASSIFICATION Presently, four forms of Kaposi's sarcoma are described:

1. **Classic (European) Kaposi's sarcoma** This is the form which was first described by Kaposi. It is more common in men over 60 years of age of Eastern European descent. The disease is slow growing and appears as multiple, small, purple, dome-shaped nodules or plaques in the skin, especially on the legs. Involvement of visceral organs occurs in about 10% cases after many years.

2. **African (Endemic) Kaposi's sarcoma** This form is common in equatorial Africa. It is so common in Uganda that it comprises 9% of all malignant tumours in men. It is found in younger age, especially in boys and in young men and has a more aggressive course than the classic form. The disease begins in the skin but grows rapidly to involve other tissues, especially lymph nodes and the gut.

3. **Epidemic (AIDS-associated) Kaposi's sarcoma** This form is seen in about 30% cases of AIDS, especially in young male homosexuals than the other high-risk groups. The cutaneous lesions are not localised to lower legs but are more extensively distributed involving mucous membranes, lymph nodes and internal organs early in the course of disease.

4. **Kaposi's sarcoma in renal transplant cases** This form is associated with recipients of renal transplants who have been administered immunosuppressive therapy for a long time. The lesions may be localised to the skin or may have widespread systemic involvement.

PATHOGENESIS Pathogenesis of Kaposi's sarcoma is complex. It is an opportunistic neoplasm in immuno-

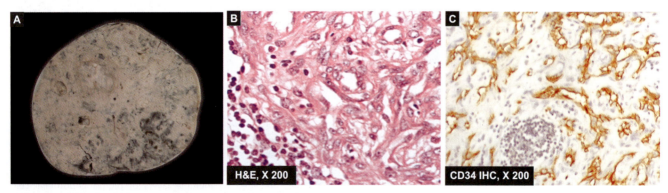

Figure 21.36 ▶ Angiosarcoma spleen. A, Gross appearance of lobulated masses of grey white necrotic and haemorrhagic parenchyma. B, The tumour cells show proliferation of moderately pleomorphic anaplastic cells. C, These tumour cells show positive staining for endothelial marker, CD34.

suppressed patients which has excessive proliferation of spindle cells of vascular origin having features of both endothelium and smooth muscle cells:

i) Epidemiological studies have suggested a *viral association* implicating HIV and human herpesvirus 8 (HSV 8, also called Kaposi's sarcoma-associated herpesvirus or KSHV) (page 307).

ii) Occurrence of Kaposi's sarcoma involves interplay of HIV-1 infection, HHV-8 infection, activation of the immune system and secretion of cytokines (IL-6, TNF-α, GM-CSF, basic fibroblast factor, and oncostatin M). Higher incidence of Kaposi's sarcoma in male homosexuals is explained by increased secretion of cytokines by their activated immune system.

iii) Defective immunoregulation plays a role in its pathogenesis is further substantiated by observation of *second malignancy* (e.g. leukaemia, lymphoma and myeloma) in about one-third of patients with Kaposi's sarcoma.

MORPHOLOGIC FEATURES Pathologically, all forms of Kaposi's sarcoma are similar

Grossly, the lesions in the skin, gut and other organs form prominent, irregular, purple, dome-shaped plaques or nodules.

Histologically, the changes are nonspecific in *the early patch stage* and more characteristic in the *late nodular stage.*

Early patch stage There are irregular vascular spaces separated by interstitial inflammatory cells and extravasated blood and haemosiderin.

Late nodular stage There are slit-like vascular spaces containing red blood cells and separated by spindle-shaped, plump tumour cells. These spindle-shaped tumour cells are probably of endothelial origin **(Fig. 21.37)**.

CLINICAL COURSE The clinical course and biologic behaviour of Kaposi's sarcoma is quite variable. The classic form of Kaposi's sarcoma is largely confined to skin and the course is generally slow and insidious with long survival. The endemic (African) and epidemic (AIDS-associated) Kaposi's sarcoma, on the other hand, has a rapidly progressive course, often with widespread cutaneous as well as visceral involvement, and high mortality.

GIST BOX 21.8 Tumours of Blood Vessels and Lymphatics

- Majority of benign vascular tumours are malformations or hamartomas. True vascular tumours are of intermediate grade and frank malignant tumours.
- Haemangiomas are quite common lesions on the skin and mucosal surfaces. These are of 3 histologic types: capillary, cavernous and lymphangioma.
- Glomus tumour is an uncommon true benign tumour arising from contractile glomus cells and is common in the fingers.
- Haemangioendothelioma is a true tumour of endothelial cells, having an intermediate behaviour. Its common locations are skin and mucosal surfaces.
- Haemangiopericytoma is an uncommon malignant tumour arising from pericytes, occurs commonly in the lower extremities.
- Angiosarcoma is a malignant vascular tumour most frequent in the skin, subcutaneous tissue, liver, spleen, bone, lung and retroperitoneal tissues. It metstasises widely.
- Kaposi's sarcoma is an opportunistic neoplasm seen in immunosuppressed patients and has association with HIV and HHV-8 infection.

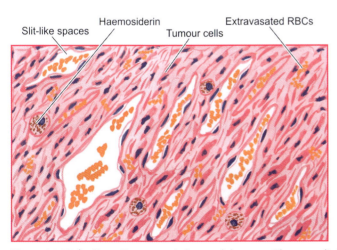
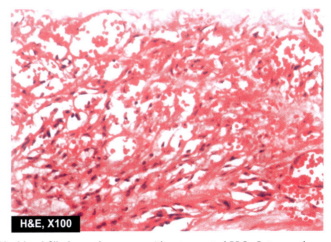

Figure 21.37 ▶ Kaposi's sarcoma in late nodular stage. There are slit-like blood-filled vascular spaces with extravasated RBCs. Between them are present bands of plump spindle-shaped tumour cells.

Section IV: Neoplasia

MESENCHYMAL TUMOURS OF UNCERTAIN HISTOGENESIS

Some soft tissue tumours have a distinctive morphology but their exact histogenesis is unclear. A few examples are described below.

Synovial Sarcoma (Malignant Synovioma)

Whether true benign tumours of synovial tissue exist is controversial. Pigmented villonodular synovitis and giant cell tumours of tendon sheaths, both of which are tumour-like lesions of synovial tissues (page 611). Synovial sarcoma or malignant synovioma, on the other hand, is a distinctive soft tissue sarcoma arising from synovial tissues close to the large joints, tendon sheaths, bursae and joint capsule but almost never arising within joint cavities. Most common locations are the extremities, frequently the lower extremity. However, synovial sarcoma is also found in regions where synovial tissue is not present such as in the anterior abdominal wall, parapharyngeal region and the pelvis. The tumour principally occurs in young adults, usually under 40 years of age. The tumour grows slowly as a painful mass but may metastasise via blood stream, chiefly to the lungs.

The *histogenesis* of tumour is, believed to be from multipotent mesenchymal cells which may differentiate along different cell lines.

Grossly, the tumour is of variable size and is grey-white, round to multilobulated and encapsulated. Cut surface shows fishflesh-like sarcomatous appearance with foci of calcification, cystic spaces and areas of haemorrhages and necrosis.

Microscopically, classic synovial sarcoma shows a characteristic *biphasic cellular pattern* composed of clefts or gland-like structures lined by cuboidal to columnar epithelial-like cells and plump to oval spindle cells (Fig. 21.38). Reticulin fibres are present around spindle cells but absent within the epithelial foci. The spindle cell areas form interlacing bands similar to those seen in fibrosarcoma. Myxoid matrix, calcification and hyalinisation are frequently present in the stroma. Mitoses and multinucleate giant cells are infrequent. Immunohistochemically, both types of tumour cells are positive for cytokeratin.

An uncommon variant of synovial sarcoma is *monophasic pattern* in which the epithelial component is exceedingly rare and thus the tumour may be difficult to distinguish from fibrosarcoma.

Traslocation t(X;18)(p11;q11) and molecular profiling *SS18-SSX1* fusion gene helps in differentiating biphasic from monophasic form of synovial sarcoma.

Alveolar Soft Part Sarcoma

Alveolar soft part sarcoma is a histologically distinct, slow-growing malignant tumour of uncertain histogenesis. The tumour may occur at any age but affects children and young adults more often. Most alveolar soft part sarcomas occur in the deep tissues of the extremities, along the musculofascial planes, or within the skeletal muscles.

Grossly, the tumour is well-demarcated, yellowish and firm.

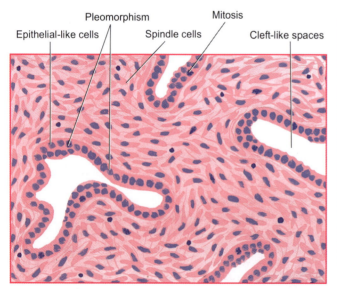
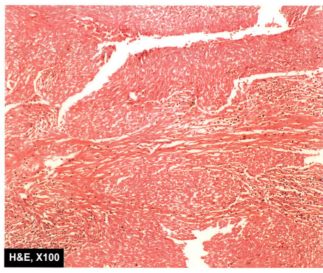

Figure 21.38 ▶ Classic synovial sarcoma, showing characteristic biphasic cellular pattern. The tumour is composed of epithelial-like cells lining cleft-like spaces and gland-like structures, and spindle cell areas forming fibrosarcoma-like growth pattern.

Microscopically, the tumour shows characteristic alveolar pattern. Organoid masses of tumour cells are separated by fibrovascular septa. The tumour cells are large and regular and contain abundant, eosinophilic, granular cytoplasm which contains diastase-resistant PAS-positive material. This feature distinguishes the tumour from paraganglioma, with which it closely resembles.

Translocation t(X;17)(p11;q25) and genetic abnormality *TFE3-ASPL* fusion gene are seen in a large proportion of cases and are helpful in confirming the diagnosis.

Granular Cell Tumour

Granular cell tumour is a benign tumour of unknown histogenesis. It may occur at any age but most often affected are young to middle-aged adults. The most frequent locations are the tongue and subcutaneous tissue of the trunk and extremities.

Grossly, the tumour is generally small, firm, grey-white to yellow-tan nodular mass.

Histologically, the tumour consists of nests or ribbons of large, round or polygonal, uniform cells having finely granular, acidophilic cytoplasm and small dense nuclei. The tumours located in the skin are frequently associated with pseudoepitheliomatous hyperplasia of the overlying skin.

Epithelioid Sarcoma

This soft tissue sarcoma occurring in young adults is peculiar in that it presents as an ulcer with sinuses, often located on the skin and subcutaneous tissues as a small swelling. The tumour is slow growing but metastasising.

Grossly, the tumour is somewhat circumscribed and has nodular appearance with central necrosis.

Microscopically, the tumour cells comprising the nodules have epithelioid appearance by having abundant pink cytoplasm and the centres of nodules show necrosis and thus can be mistaken for a granuloma.

Clear Cell Sarcoma

Clear cell sarcoma, first described by Enginzer, is seen in skin and subcutaneous tissues, especially of hands and feet.

Microscopically, it closely resembles malignant melanoma, and is therefore also called melanoma of the soft tissues.

Clear cell sarcoma can be further distinguished from cutaneous melanoma by translocation t(12;22)(q13;q12) and *EWSR1-ATF1* fusion gene.

Desmoplastic Small Round Cell Tumour

Desmoplastic small round cell tumour (DSRCT) is a rare and highly malignant tumour occurring more commonly in male children and juveniles under 2nd decade of life. The cell of origin is not clear. Some of the common locations are the abdomen, paratesticular region, ovaries, parotid, brain and thorax.

Grossly, the tumour appears as multiple soft to firm masses.

Microscopically, characteristic small and round tumour cells having epithelial, mesenchymal and neural differentiation.

The tumour spreads rapidly to regional lymph nodes and other sites. DSRCT with translocation t(11;22)(p13;q12) and *EWSR1-WT1* fusion gene have particularly poor prognosis.

GIST BOX 21.9 — Mesenchymal Tumours with Uncertain Histogenesis

- Synovial sarcoma arises from synovial tissues close to the large joints, tendon sheaths, bursae and joint capsule. Classic synovial sarcoma shows a biphasic cellular pattern: cuboidal to columnar epithelial-like cells and plump to oval spindle cells.
- Alveolar soft part sarcoma occurs in the deep tissues of the extremities, along the musculofascial planes, or within the skeletal muscles.
- Granular cell tumour is a benign tumour occurring in the tongue and subcutaneous tissue of the trunk and extremities.
- Clear cell sarcoma occurring in the subcutaneous soft tissues has some similarities with cutaneous melanoma.
- Desmoplastic small round cell tumour is a rare and highly malignant tumour occurring in male children and juveniles, most often in the abdomen.

TERATOMAS

Teratomas are complex tumours composed of tissues derived from more than one of the three germ cell layers—endoderm, mesoderm and ectoderm. They are most commonly seen in gonads of males and females (i.e. testis and ovaries). Testicular teratomas are more common in infants and children while ovarian teratomas are more frequent during their active reproductive life. Sometimes, teratomas may be found in combination with other germ cell tumours. AFP levels are slightly raised in teratomas.

Teratomas are classified into 3 types:
1. Mature (differentiated) teratoma
2. Immature teratoma
3. Teratoma with malignant transformation.

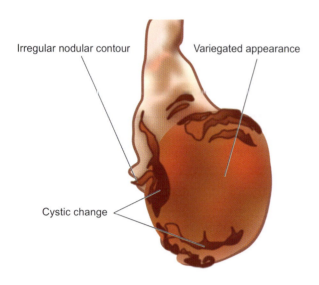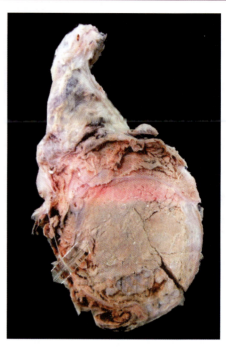

Figure 21.39 ▶ Teratoma testis. The testis is enlarged and nodular distorting the testicular contour. Sectioned surface shows replacement of the entire testis by variegated mass having grey-white solid areas, cystic areas, honey-combed areas and foci of cartilage and bone.

Grossly, most *testicular teratomas* are large, grey-white masses enlarging the involved testis. Cut surface shows characteristic variegated appearance-grey-white solid areas, cystic and honey-combed areas, and foci of cartilage and bone **(Fig. 21.39)**. Dermoid tumours commonly seen in the ovaries are rare in testicular teratomas.

The vast majority of *ovarian teratomas* on the other hand, are benign and cystic and have the predominant ectodermal elements, often termed clinically as dermoid cyst. Benign cystic teratoma or dermoid cyst is characteristically a unilocular cyst, 10-15 cm in diameter, usually lined by skin and hence its name. On sectioning, the cyst is filled with

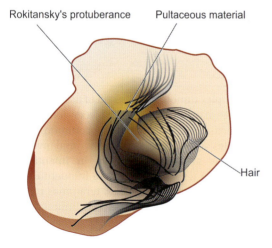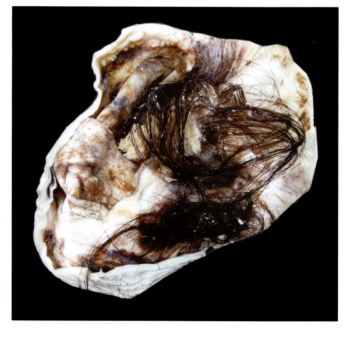

Figure 21.40 ▶ Dermoid cyst of the ovary. The ovary is enlarged and shows a large unilocular cyst containing hair, pultaceous material and bony tissue.

Chapter 21: Common Specific Tumours

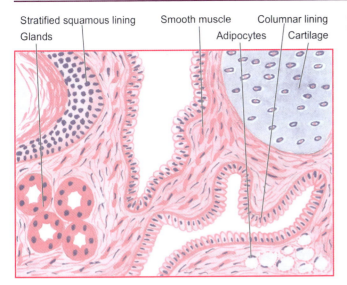
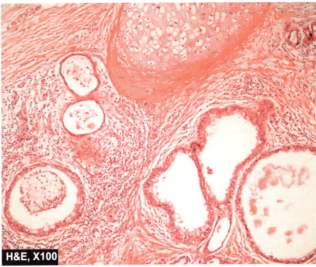

Figure 21.41 ▶ Benign cystic teratoma ovary. Microscopy shows characteristic lining of the cyst wall by epidermis and its appendages. Islands of mature cartilage are also seen.

paste-like sebaceous secretions and desquamated keratin admixed with masses of hair. The cyst wall is thin and opaque grey-white. Generally, in one area of the cyst wall, a solid prominence is seen (Rokitansky's protuberance) where tissue elements such as tooth, bone, cartilage and various other odd tissues are present **(Fig. 21.40)**.

Microscopically, the three categories of teratomas show different appearances:

1. Mature (differentiated) teratoma *Mature testicular teratoma* is composed of disorderly mixture of a variety of well-differentiated structures such as cartilage, smooth muscle, intestinal and respiratory epithelium, mucous glands, cysts lined by squamous and transitional epithelium, neural tissue, fat and bone. This type of mature or differentiated teratoma of the testis is the most common, seen more frequently in infants and children and has favourable prognosis. But similar mature and benign-appearing tumour in adults is invariably associated with small hidden foci of immature elements so that their clinical course in adults is unpredictable. It is believed that all testicular teratomas in the adults are malignant.

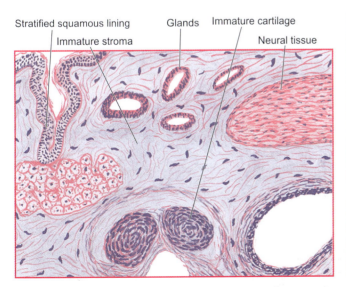
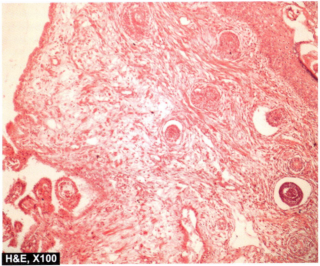

Figure 21.42 ▶ Immature teratoma testis. Microscopy shows a variety of incompletely differentiated tissue elements.

In the case of *mature ovarian teratoma*, the most prominent feature is the lining of the cyst wall by stratified squamous epithelium and its adnexal structures such as sebaceous glands, sweat glands and hair follicles (Fig. 21.41). Though ectodermal derivatives are most prominent features, tissues of mesodermal and endodermal origin are commonly present as in mature testicular teratomas. Thus, viewing a benign teratoma in different microscopic fields reveals a variety of mature differentiated tissue elements, producing *kaleidoscopic patterns*.

2. Immature teratoma Immature teratoma is composed of incompletely differentiated and primitive or embryonic tissues along with some mature elements. Primitive or embryonic tissue commonly present are poorly-formed cartilage, mesenchyme, neural tissues, abortive eye, intestinal, respiratory tissue elements etc (Fig. 21.42). Mitoses are usually frequent.

3. Teratoma with malignant transformation This is an extremely rare form of teratoma in which one or more of the tissue elements show malignant transformation. Such malignant change resembles morphologically with typical malignancies in other organs and tissues and commonly includes rhabdomyosarcoma, squamous cell carcinoma and adenocarcinoma.

GIST BOX 21.10 Teratomas

- Teratomas are composed of tissues derived from three germ cell layers—endoderm, mesoderm and ectoderm. They may be mature, immature and with malignant change.
- They are most commonly seen in gonads of males and females (i.e. testis and ovaries).
- While benign cystic teratomas (commonly called dermoid tumours) are more common in ovaries, testicular teratomas are more often immature and malignant.

Section V ▶ Haematology and Lymphoreticular Tissues

▶ **SECTION CONTENTS**

Chapter 22: Disorders of Erythroid Series: Anaemias
Chapter 23: Platelets and Bleeding Disorders
Chapter 24: Diseases of Leucocytes and Lymphoid Tissues

22 Disorders of Erythroid Series: Anaemias

The section on disorders of the haematopoietic system is concerned with diseases of the blood and the bone marrow. Conventionally, it includes study of constituents of circulating blood and blood-forming organs and thus comprises of discussion on diseases of red blood cells, white blood cells, platelets and bleeding disorders. Since leucocytes are present in blood as 'circulating leucocytes' as well as in lymphoid organs as 'fixed leucocytes', diseases of lymphoid tissues have thus been integrated as diseases of lymphohaematopoietic tissues (Chapter 24).

Besides, the study and understanding of diseases of haematopoietic system involves two phases—laboratory haematology and clinical haematology; therefore learning broad principles of management of common haematological diseases is as desirable for a student of pathology as is the need for a physician to know basic laboratory haematology.

BONE MARROW AND HAEMATOPOIESIS

Haematopoiesis is production of formed elements of the blood. Normally, it takes place in the bone marrow. Circulating blood normally contains 3 main types of mature blood cells—the red cells (erythrocytes), the white cells (leucocytes) and the platelets (thrombocytes). These blood cells perform their respective major physiologic functions: *erythrocytes* largely concerned with oxygen transport, *leucocytes* play various roles in body defense against infection and tissue injury, while *thrombocytes* are primarily involved in maintaining integrity of blood vessels and in preventing blood loss. The lifespan of these cells in circulating blood is variable—neutrophils have a short lifespan of 8-12 hours, followed by platelets with a lifespan of 8-10 days, while the RBCs have the longest lifespan of 90-120 days. The rates of production of these blood cells are normally regulated in healthy individuals in such a way so as to match the rate at which they are lost from circulation. Their concentration is normally maintained within well-defined limits unless the balance is disturbed due to some pathologic processes.

HAEMATOPOIETIC ORGANS

In the human embryo, the *yolk sac* is the main site of haematopoiesis in the first few weeks of gestation. By about 3rd month, however, the *liver and spleen* are the main sites of blood cell formation and continue to do so until about 2 weeks after birth. Haematopoiesis commences in the *bone marrow* by 4th and 5th month and becomes fully active by 7th and 8th month so that at birth practically all the bones contain active marrow. During normal childhood and adult life, therefore, the marrow is the only source of new blood cells. However, during childhood, there is progressive fatty replacement throughout the long bones so that by adult life the haematopoietic marrow is confined to the central skeleton (vertebrae, sternum, ribs, skull, sacrum and pelvis) and proximal ends of femur, tibia and humerus (Fig. 22.1). Even in these haematopoietic areas, about 50% of the marrow consists of fat (Fig. 22.2). Non-haematopoietic marrow in the adult is, however, capable of reverting to active haematopoiesis in certain pathologic conditions. The spleen and liver can also resume their foetal haematopoietic role in certain pathologic conditions and is called *extramedullary haematopoiesis*.

In the bone marrow, developing blood cells are situated outside the marrow sinuses, from where after maturation they enter the marrow sinuses, the marrow microcirculation and then released into circulation.

HAEMATOPOIETIC STEM CELLS

Haematopoiesis involves two stages: mitotic division or proliferation, and differentiation or maturation.

It is known for a few decades that blood cells develop from a small population of common multipotent haematopoietic stem cells (HSC). HSC express a variety of cell surface proteins such as CD34 and adhesion proteins which help these cells to "home" to the bone marrow when infused. HSC have the appearance of small or intermediate-sized lymphocytes

Section V: Haematology and Lymphoreticular Tissues

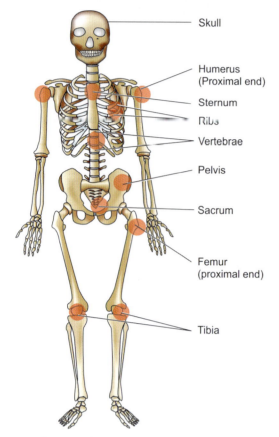

Figure 22.1 ▶ Sites of haematopoiesis in the bone marrow in the adult.

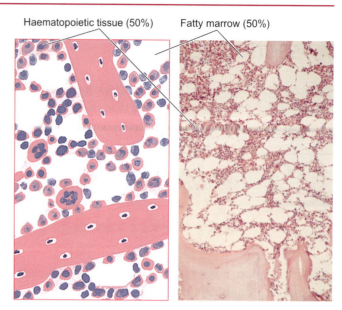

Figure 22.2 ▶ A normal bone marrow in an adult as seen in a section after trephine biopsy. Bony trabeculae support the marrow-containing tissue. Approximately 50% of the soft tissue of the bone consists of haematopoietic tissue and 50% is fatty marrow.

and their presence in the marrow can be demonstrated by cell culture techniques by the growth of colony-forming units (CFU) pertaining to different cell lines. HSC have the capability of maintaining their progeny by self-replication. The bone marrow provides a suitable environment for growth and development of HSC. For instance, if HSC are infused intravenously into a suitably-prepared recipient, they seed the marrow successfully but do not thrive at other sites. This principle forms the basis of bone marrow (or HSC) transplantation performed for various haematologic diseases.

After a series of divisions, HSC differentiate into two types of progenitors—*lymphoid* (immune system) stem cells, and *non-lymphoid or myeloid* (trilineage) stem cells. The former develop into T, B and NK cells while the latter differentiate into 3 types of cell lines—granulocyte-monocyte progenitors (producing neutrophils, eosinophils, basophils and monocytes), erythroid progenitors (producing red cells), and megakaryocytes (as the source of platelets). Monocytes on entering the tissues form a variety of phagocytic macrophages, both of which together constitute mononuclear-phagocyte system (page 123). Lymphopoietic cells in the marrow undergo differentiation to form B, T and natural killer (NK) cells of the immune system. The development of mature cells (*i.e. poiesis*)—red cells (erythropoiesis), granulocytes (granulopoiesis), monocytes, lymphocytes (lymphopoiesis) and platelets (thrombopoiesis) are considered in detail later under relevant headings.

Two cardinal functions of HSC are self-renewal and differentiation of their progenitor cells to produce leucocytes, erythroid cells and platelets **(Fig. 22.3)**. Haematopoiesis or myelopoiesis is regulated by certain endogenous glycoproteins called haematopoietic growth factors, cytokines and hormones. For example:
i) Erythropoietin: for red cell formation
ii) Granulocyte colony-stimulating factor (G-CSF): for production of granulocytes
iii) Granulocyte-macrophage colony-stimulating factor (GM-CSF): for production of granulocytes and monocyte-macrophages
iv) Thrombopoietin; for production of platelets

Each of these growth factors acts on their specific receptors to initiate further cell events as discussed under respective topics later.

BONE MARROW EXAMINATION

Examination of the bone marrow provides an invaluable diagnostic help in some cases, while in others it is of value in confirming a diagnosis suspected on clinical examination or on the blood film. A peripheral blood smear examination, however, must always precede bone marrow examination.

Bone marrow examination may be performed by two methods—*aspiration* and *trephine biopsy*.

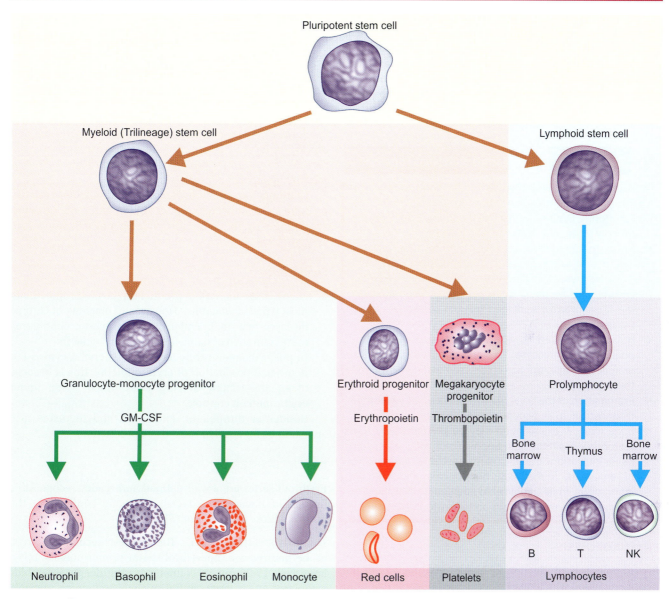

Figure 22.3 ▶ Schematic representation of differentiation of multipotent stem cells into blood cells.

BONE MARROW ASPIRATION The method involves suction of marrow via a strong, wide bore, short-bevelled needle fitted with a stylet and an adjustable guard in order to prevent excessive penetration; for instance *Salah bone marrow aspiration needle*. Smears are prepared immediately from the bone marrow aspirate and are fixed in 95% methanol after air-drying. The usual Romanowsky technique is employed for staining and a stain for iron is performed routinely so as to assess the reticuloendothelial stores of iron.

The marrow film provides assessment of cellularity, details of developing blood cells (i.e. normoblastic or megaloblastic, myeloid, lymphoid, macrophages and megakaryocytic), ratio between erythroid and myeloid cells, storage diseases, and for the presence of cells foreign to the marrow such as secondary carcinoma, granulomatous conditions, fungi (e.g. histoplasmosis) and parasites (e.g. malaria, leishmaniasis, trypanosomiasis). Estimation of the proportion of cellular components in the marrow, however, can be provided by doing a differential count of at least 500 cells termed myelogram. In some conditions, the marrow cells can be used for more detailed special tests such as cytogenetics, microbiological culture, biochemical analysis, and immunological and cytological markers.

TREPHINE BIOPSY Trephine biopsy is performed by a simple *Jamshidi trephine needle* by which a core of tissue from periosteum to bone marrow cavity is obtained. The tissue is then fixed, soft decalcified and processed for histological sections and stained with haematoxylin and eosin and for reticulin. Trephine biopsy is especially useful in cases of dry tap. In addition, trephine is more useful since it provides an excellent view of the overall marrow architecture, cellularity, and presence or absence of infiltrates, but is less valuable than aspiration as far as individual cell morphology is concerned.

GIST BOX 22.1 — Bone Marrow and Haematopoiesis

- Haematopoiesis commences in the bone marrow by 4th and 5th month and becomes fully active by 7th and 8th month. During normal childhood and adult life, the marrow is the only source of new blood cells.
- Haematopoietic stem cells (HSC) in the bone marrow give rise to two types of multipotent stem cells: *non-lymphoid* which differentiate into committed cell lineage, and *lymphoid stem cells* which differentiate in the bone marrow and then migrate to the lymphoid tissues.
- HSC are regulated by a few factors such as erythropoietin, granulocyte colony-stimulating factor, granulocyte-macrophage colony-stimulating factor and thrombopoietin.
- Examination of the bone marrow provides an invaluable diagnostic help and confirming a suspected diagnosis.
- Bone marrow examination may be performed by two methods—aspiration and trephine biopsy.
- Major indications of bone marrow aspiration are typing of anaemias, leukaemias, neutropenia and marrow infiltrations, while trephine has additional advantages in dry aspiration, myelofibrosis and aplastic anaemia.

ERYTHROPOIESIS

Erythropoiesis is production of mature erythrocytes of the peripheral blood which takes place in the bone marrow from morphologically unrecognisable HSC. Red cell production is influenced by growth factors and hormones, notably erythropoietin.

ERYTHROPOIETIN

Erythropoietic activity in the body is regulated by erythropoietin, which is produced in response to anoxia. The principal site of erythropoietin production is the kidney though there is evidence of its extra-renal production in certain unusual circumstances. Its levels are, therefore, lowered in chronic renal diseases, while a case of renal cell carcinoma may be associated with its increased production and erythrocytosis. Erythropoietin acts on the marrow at the various stages of morphologically unidentifiable as well as identifiable erythroid precursors.

Immunoassay of erythropoietin in plasma or serum can be done by sensitive techniques (ELISA and radioimmunoassay) due to its quite low values; normal values are 10-25 U/L.

Significance

1. There is an increased production of erythropoietin in most types of anaemias. However, in anaemia of chronic diseases (e.g. in infections and neoplastic conditions) there is no such enhancement of erythropoietin.
2. In polycythaemia rubra vera, there is erythrocytosis but depressed production of erythropoietin. This is because of an abnormality of HSC class which is not under erythropoietin control.

Besides erythropoietin, androgens and thyroxine also appear to be involved in the red cell production.

ERYTHROID SERIES

Erythroid series are a well-defined and readily recognisable lineage of nucleated red cells normally confined to the marrow. These are as under **(Fig. 22.4)**:

1. **PROERYTHROBLAST** The earliest recognisable cell in the marrow is a proerythroblast or pronormoblast. It is a large cell, 15-20 μm in diameter having deeply basophilic cytoplasm and a large central nucleus containing nucleoli. The deep blue colour of the cytoplasm is due to high content of RNA which is associated with active protein synthesis. As the cells mature, the nuclei lose their nucleoli and become

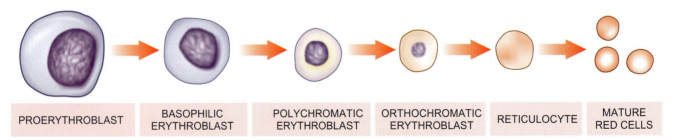

Figure 22.4 ▶ The erythroid series. There is progressive condensation of the nuclear chromatin which is eventually extruded from the cell at the late erythroblast stage. The cytoplasm contains progressively less RNA and more haemoglobin.

smaller and denser, while the cytoplasm on maturation leads to replacement of dense blue colour progressively by pink-staining haemoglobin. Each proerythroblast undergoes 4-5 replications and forms 16-32 mature RBCs.

2. **BASOPHILIC (EARLY) ERYTHROBLAST** It is a round cell having a diameter of 12-16 μm with a large nucleus which is slightly more condensed than the proerythroblast and contains basophilic cytoplasm. Basophilic erythroblast undergoes rapid proliferation.

3. **POLYCHROMATIC (INTERMEDIATE) ERYTHROBLAST** Next maturation stage has a diameter of 12-14 μm. The nucleus at this stage is coarse and deeply basophilic. The cytoplasm is characteristically polychromatic i.e. contains admixture of basophilic RNA and acidophilic haemoglobin. The cell at this stage ceases to undergo proliferative activity.

4. **ORTHOCHROMATIC (LATE) ERYTHROBLAST** The final stage in the maturation of nucleated red cells is the orthochromatic or late erythroblast. The cell at this stage is smaller, 8-12 μm in diameter, containing a small and pyknotic nucleus with dark nuclear chromatin. The cytoplasm is characteristically acidophilic with diffuse basophilic hue due to the presence of large amounts of haemoglobin.

5. **RETICULOCYTE** The nucleus is finally extruded from the late erythroblast within the marrow and a reticulocyte results. The reticulocytes are juvenile red cells devoid of nuclei but contain ribosomal RNA so that they are still able to synthesise haemoglobin. A reticulocyte spends 1-2 days in the marrow and circulates for 1-2 days in the peripheral blood before maturing in the spleen, to become a biconcave red cell. The reticulocytes in the peripheral blood are distinguished from mature red cells by slightly basophilic hue in the cytoplasm similar to that of an orthochromatic erythroblast. Reticulocytes can be counted in the laboratory by *vital staining* with dyes such as new methylene blue or brilliant cresyl blue. The reticulocytes by either of these staining methods contain deep blue reticulofilamentous material (Fig. 22.5). While erythroblasts are not normally present in human peripheral blood, reticulocytes are found normally in the peripheral blood. Normal range of reticulocyte count in health is 0.5-2.5% in adults and 2-6% in infants. Their percentage in the peripheral blood is a fairly accurate reflection of erythropoietic activity. Their proportion is increased in conditions of rapid red cell regeneration e.g. after haemorrhage, haemolysis and haematopoietic response of anaemia to treatment.

THE RED CELL

The mature erythrocytes of the human peripheral blood are non-nucleated cells and lack the usual cell organelles. The normal human erythrocyte is a biconcave disc, 7.2 μm in diameter, and has a thickness of 2.4 μm at the periphery and 1 μm in the centre. The biconcave shape renders the red cells

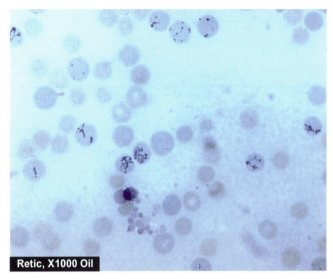

Figure 22.5 ▶ Reticulocytes in blood as seen in blood stained by supravital dye, new methylene blue.

quite flexible so that they can pass through capillaries whose minimum diameter is 3.5 μm. More than 90% of the weight of erythrocyte consists of haemoglobin. The lifespan of red cells is 120 ± 30 days.

RED CELL MEMBRANE The red cell membrane is a trilaminar structure having a bimolecular lipid layer interposed between two layers of proteins.

◆ Important *proteins* in red cell membrane are band 3 protein (named on the basis of the order in which it migrates during electrophoresis), glycophorin and spectrin.

◆ Important *lipids* are glycolipids, phospholipids and cholesterol.

◆ *Carbohydrates* form skeleton of erythrocytes having a lattice-like network which is attached to the internal surface of the membrane and is responsible for biconcave form of the erythrocytes.

NUTRITIONAL REQUIREMENTS FOR ERYTHROPOIESIS

New red cells are being produced each day for which the marrow requires certain essential substances. These substances are as under:

1. **Metals** Iron is essential for red cell production because it forms part of the haem molecule in haemoglobin. Its deficiency leads to iron deficiency anaemia. Cobalt and manganese are certain other metals required for red cell production.

2. **Vitamins** Vitamin B_{12} and folate are essential for biosynthesis of nucleic acids. Deficiency of B_{12} or folate causes megaloblastic anaemia. Vitamin C (ascorbic acid) plays an indirect role by facilitating the iron turnover in the body. Vitamin B_6 (pyridoxine), vitamin E (tocopherol) and riboflavin

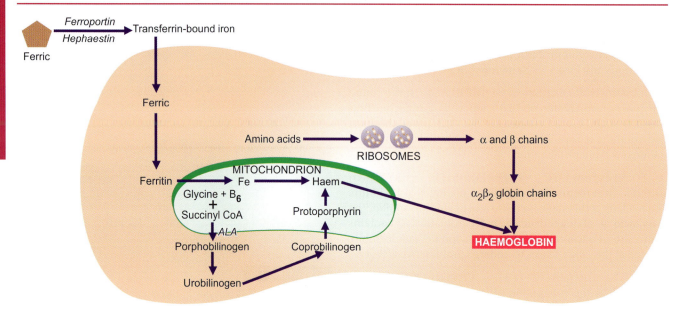

Figure 22.6 ▶ Schematic diagram of haemoglobin synthesis in the developing red cell.

are the other essential vitamins required in the synthesis of red cells.

3. Amino acids Amino acids comprise the globin component of haemoglobin. Severe amino acid deficiency due to protein deprivation causes depressed red cell production.

HAEMOGLOBIN Haemoglobin consists of a basic protein, *globin*, and the iron-porphyrin complex, *haem*. The molecular weight of haemoglobin is 68,000. Normal adult haemoglobin (*HbA*) constitutes 96-98% of the total haemoglobin content and consists of four polypeptide chains, $\alpha_2\beta_2$. Small quantities of 2 other haemoglobins present in adults are: *HbF* containing $\alpha_2\gamma_2$ globin chains comprising 0.5-0.8% of total haemoglobin, and *HbA₂* having $\alpha_2\delta_2$ chains and constituting 1.5-3.5% of total haemoglobin. Most of the haemoglobin (65%) is synthesised by the nucleated red cell precursors in the marrow, while the remainder (35%) is synthesised at the reticulocyte stage.

Synthesis of haem occurs largely in the mitochondria by a series of biochemical reactions summarised in **Fig. 22.6**. Coenzyme, pyridoxal-6-phosphate, derived from pyridoxine (vitamin B_6) is essential for the synthesis of amino levulinic acid (ALA) which is the first step in the biosynthesis of protoporphyrin. The reaction is stimulated by erythropoietin and inhibited by haem. Ultimately, protoporphyrin combines with iron supplied from circulating transferrin to form haem. Each molecule of haem combines with a globin chain synthesised by polyribosomes. A tetramer of 4 globin chains, each having its own haem group, constitutes the haemoglobin molecule **(Fig. 22.7, A)**.

RED CELL FUNCTIONS The essential function of the red cells is to carry oxygen from the lungs to the tissue and to transport carbon dioxide to the lungs. In order to perform these functions, the red cells have the ability to generate energy as ATP by anaerobic glycolytic pathway (Embden-Meyerhof pathway). This pathway also generates reducing power as NADH and NADPH by the hexose monophosphate (HMP) shunt.

1. Oxygen carrying The normal adult haemoglobin, HbA, is an extremely efficient oxygen-carrier. The four units of tetramer of haemoglobin molecule take up oxygen in succession, which, in turn, results in stepwise rise in affinity of haemoglobin for oxygen. This is responsible for the *sigmoid shape* of the oxygen dissociation curve.

The oxygen affinity of haemoglobin is expressed in term of P_{50} value which is the oxygen tension (pO_2) at which 50% of the haemoglobin is saturated with oxygen. Pulmonary capillaries have high pO_2 and, thus, there is virtual saturation of available oxygen-combining sites of haemoglobin. The tissue capillaries, however, have relatively low pO_2 and, thus, part of haemoglobin is in deoxy state. The extent to which oxygen is released from haemoglobin at pO_2, in tissue capillaries depends upon 3 factors—the nature of globin chains, the pH, and the concentration of 2,3-biphosphoglycerate (2,3-BPG) as follows **(Fig. 22.7, B)**:

i) *Normal adult haemoglobin (HbA) has lower affinity for oxygen* than foetal haemoglobin and, therefore, releases greater amount of bound oxygen at pO_2 of tissue capillaries.

ii) A *fall in the pH* (acidic pH) lowers affinity of oxyhaemoglobin for oxygen, so called the Bohr effect, thereby causing enhanced release of oxygen from erythrocytes at the lower pH in tissue capillaries.

iii) *A rise in red cell concentration of 2,3-BPG*, an intermediate product of Embden-Meyerhof pathway, as occurs in anaemia

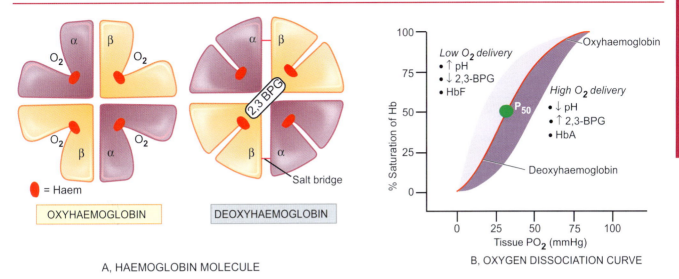

Figure 22.7 ▶ A, Normal adult haemoglobin molecule (HbA) consisting of $α_2β_2$ globin chains, each with its own haem group in oxy and deoxy state. The haemoglobin tetramer can bind up to four molecules of oxygen in the iron containing sites of the haem molecules. As oxygen is bound, salt bridges are broken, and 2,3-BPG and CO_2 are expelled. B, Hb-dissociation curve. On dissociation of oxygen from Hb molecule i.e. on release of oxygen to the tissues, salt bridges are formed again, and 2,3-BPG and CO_2, are bound. The shift of the curve to higher oxygen delivery is affected by acidic pH, increased 2,3-BPG and HbA molecule while oxygen delivery is less with high pH, low 2,3-BPG and HbF.

and hypoxia, causes decreased affinity of HbA for oxygen. This, in turn, results in enhanced supply of oxygen to the tissue.

2. **CO_2 transport** Another important function of the red cells is the CO_2 transport. In the tissue capillaries, the pCO_2 is high so that CO_2 enters the erythrocytes where much of it is converted into bicarbonate ions which diffuse back into the plasma. In the pulmonary capillaries, the process is reversed and bicarbonate ions are converted back into CO_2. Some of the CO_2 produced by tissues is bound to deoxyhaemoglobin forming carbamino-haemoglobin. This compound dissociates in the pulmonary capillaries to release CO_2.

RED CELL DESTRUCTION Red cells have a mean lifespan of 120 days, after which red cell metabolism gradually deteriorates as the enzymes are not replaced. The destroyed red cells are removed mainly by the macrophages of the reticuloendothelial (RE) system of the marrow, and to some extent by the macrophages in the liver and spleen (Fig. 22.8). The breakdown of red cells liberates iron for recirculation via plasma transferrin to marrow erythroblasts, and protoporphyrin which is broken down to bilirubin. Bilirubin circulates to the liver where it is conjugated to its diglucuronide which is excreted in the gut via bile and converted to stercobilinogen and stercobilin excreted in the faeces. Part of stercobilinogen and stercobilin is reabsorbed and excreted in the urine as urobilinogen and urobilin. A small fragment of protoporphyrin is converted to carbon monoxide and excreted in exhaled air from the lungs. Globin chains are broken down to amino acids and reused for protein synthesis in the body.

NORMAL VALUES AND RED CELL INDICES The range of *normal red cell* count in health is $5.5 ± 1.0 × 10^{12}/L$ in men and $4.8 ± 1.0 × 10^{12}/L$ in women. The *packed cell volume* (PCV) or *haematocrit* (HCT) is the volume of erythrocytes per litre of whole blood indicating the proportion of plasma and red cells and ranges $0.47 ± 0.07$ L/L (40-54%) in men and $0.42 ± 0.05$ L/L (37-47%) in women. The *haemoglobin content* in health is $15.5 ± 2.5$ g/dl (13-18 g/dl) in men and $14.0 ± 2.5$ g/dl (11.5-16.5 g/dl) in women. Based on these normal values, a series of *absolute values* or red cell indices can be derived which have diagnostic importance. These are as under:

1. **Mean corpuscular volume (MCV)**

$$\frac{PCV\,(\%)}{RBC\;count\,(millions)} × 10$$

Normal value = $85 ± 8$ fl (77-93 fl)*.

2. **Mean corpuscular haemoglobin (MCH)**

$$\frac{Hb\,(g/dl)}{RBC\;count\,(millions)} × 10$$

Normal range = $29.5 ± 2.5$ pg (27-32 pg)*.

3. **Mean corpuscular haemoglobin concentration (MCHC)**

$$\frac{Hb\,(g/dl)}{PCV\,(\%)} × 100$$

The normal value is $32.5 ± 2.5$ g/dl (30-35 g/dl).

---

*For conversions, the multiples used are as follows: 'deci (d) = 10^{-1}, milli (m) = 10^{-3}, micro (µ) = 10^{-6}, nano (n) = 10^{-9}, pico (p) = 10^{-12}, femto (f) = 10^{-15}

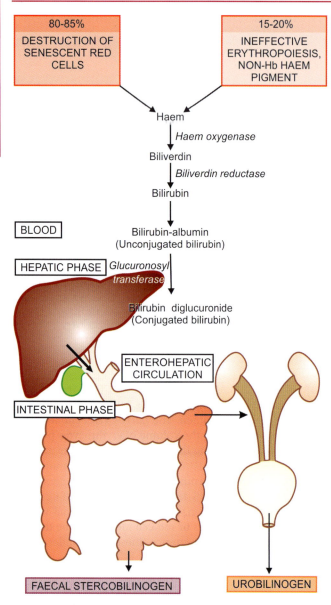

Figure 22.8 ▶ Normal red cell destruction in the RE system.

- in response to anoxia. Its levels are increased in most forms of anaemias.
- ❖ Erythroid series are a series of recognisable nucleated red cells normally seen in the marrow and include proerythroblast, polychromatic erythroblast, orthochromatic erythroblast and reticulocytes.
- ❖ The mature erythrocytes of the human peripheral blood are non-nucleated cells. Red cell membrane is a trilaminar structure having a bimolecular lipid layer interposed between two layers of proteins.
- ❖ Erythropoiesis requires various nutrients, namely iron, vitamins and amino acids.
- ❖ Haemoglobin consists of a basic protein, *globin*, and the iron-porphyrin complex, *haem*.
- ❖ Essential functions performed by red cells are oxygen carrying and carbon dioxide transport.
- ❖ At the end of lifespan, red cells are destroyed and phagocytosed by macrophages.

ANAEMIA—GENERAL CONSIDERATIONS

Anaemia is defined as reduced haemoglobin concentration in blood below the lower limit of the normal range for the age and sex of the individual. As per WHO, the lower extreme of the normal haemoglobin is taken as 13 g/dl for adult males and 12 g/dl for adult females (11 g/dl in pregnant females). At birth, lower limit of normal haemoglobin level is 13 g/dl is taken as the lower limit at birth, whereas at 0-6 months the normal lower level is 10.5 g/dl. Although haemoglobin value is employed as the major parameter for determining whether or not anaemia is present, the red cell counts, haematocrit (PCV) and absolute values (MCV, MCH and MCHC) provide alternate means of assessing anaemia.

PATHOPHYSIOLOGY

Subnormal level of haemoglobin causes lowered oxygen-carrying capacity of the blood. This, in turn, initiates compensatory physiologic adaptations such as follows:
i) Increased release of oxygen from haemoglobin
ii) Increased blood flow to the tissues
iii) Maintenance of the blood volume
iv) Redistribution of blood flow to maintain the cerebral blood supply.

Eventually, however, tissue hypoxia develops causing impaired functions of the affected tissues. The degree of functional impairment of individual tissues is variable depending upon their oxygen requirements. Tissues with high oxygen requirement such as the heart, CNS and the skeletal muscle during exercise, bear the brunt of clinical effects of anaemia.

GENERAL CLINICAL FEATURES

The haemoglobin level at which symptoms and signs of anaemia develop depends upon 4 main factors:

Since MCHC is independent of red cell count and size, it is considered to be of greater clinical significance as compared to other absolute values. It is low in iron deficiency anaemia but is usually normal in macrocytic anaemia.

4. **Red cell distribution width (RDW)** RDW is an assessment of varying volume of red cells based on size of red cells. For example, fragmented red cells have a tiny size while the macrocytes and reticulocytes have large size.

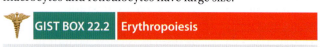

❖ Erythropoietic activity in the body is regulated by erythropoietin, which is produced, mainly from kidneys,

1. *The speed of onset of anaemia:* Rapidly progressive anaemia causes more symptoms than anaemia of slow-onset as there is less time for physiologic adaptation.

2. *The severity of anaemia:* Mild anaemia produces no symptoms or signs but a rapidly developing severe anaemia (haemoglobin below 6.0 g/dl) may produce significant clinical features.

3. *The age of the patient:* The young patients due to good cardiovascular compensation tolerate anaemia quite well as compared to the elderly. The elderly patients develop cardiac and cerebral symptoms more prominently due to associated cardiovascular disease.

4. *The haemoglobin dissociation curve:* In anaemia, the affinity of haemoglobin for oxygen is depressed as 2,3-BPG in the red cells increases. As a result, oxyhaemoglobin is dissociated more readily to release free oxygen for cellular use, causing a shift of the oxyhaemoglobin dissociation curve to the right.

SYMPTOMS In symptomatic cases of anaemia, the presenting features are: tiredness, easy fatiguability, generalised muscular weakness, lethargy and headache. In older patients, there may be symptoms of cardiac failure, angina pectoris, intermittent claudication, confusion and visual disturbances.

SIGNS A few general signs common to all types of anaemias are as under:

1. Pallor Pallor is the most common and characteristic sign which may be seen in the mucous membranes, conjunctivae and skin.

2. Cardiovascular system A hyperdynamic circulation may be present with tachycardia, collapsing pulse, cardiomegaly, midsystolic flow murmur, dyspnoea on exertion, and in the case of elderly, congestive heart failure.

3. Central nervous system The older patients may develop symptoms referable to the CNS such as attacks of faintness, giddiness, headache, tinnitus, drowsiness, numbness and tingling sensations of the hands and feet.

4. Ocular manifestations Retinal haemorrhages may occur if there is associated vascular disease or bleeding diathesis.

5. Reproductive system Menstrual disturbances such as amenorrhoea and menorrhagia and loss of libido are some of the manifestations involving the reproductive system in anaemic subjects.

6. Renal system Mild proteinuria and impaired concentrating capacity of the kidney may occur in severe anaemia.

7. Gastrointestinal system Anorexia, flatulence, nausea, constipation and weight loss may occur.

In addition to the general features, specific signs may be associated with particular types of anaemia which are described later together with discussion of specific types of anaemias.

GENERAL SCHEME OF INVESTIGATIONS OF ANAEMIA

After obtaining the full medical history pertaining to different general and specific signs and symptoms, the patient is examined for evidence of anaemia. Special emphasis is placed on colour of the skin, conjunctivae, sclerae and nails. Changes in the retina, atrophy of the papillae of the tongue, rectal examination for evidence of bleeding, and presence of hepatomegaly, splenomegaly, lymphadenopathy and bony tenderness are looked for.

In order to confirm or deny the presence of anaemia, its type and its cause, the following plan of investigations is generally followed, of which complete blood counts (CBC) with reticulocyte count is the basic test.

A. HAEMOGLOBIN ESTIMATION The first and foremost investigation in any suspected case of anaemia is to carry out a haemoglobin estimation. Several methods are available but most reliable and accurate is the cyanmethaemoglobin (HiCN) method employing Drabkin's solution and a spectrophotometer. If the haemoglobin value is below the lower limit of the normal range for particular age and sex, the patient is said to be anaemic. In pregnancy, there is haemodilution and, therefore, the lower limit in normal pregnant women is less (10.5 g/dl) than in the non-pregnant state.

B. PERIPHERAL BLOOD SMEAR EXAMINATION The haemoglobin estimation is invariably followed by examination of a peripheral blood film for morphologic features after staining it with the Romanowsky dyes (e.g. Leishman's stain, May-Grünwald-Giemsa's stain, Jenner-Giemsa's stain, Wright's stain etc). The blood smear is evaluated in an area where there is neither Rouleaux formation nor so thin as to cause red cell distortion. Such an area can usually be found at junction of the body with the tail of the film, but not actually at the tail. The following abnormalities in erythroid series of cells are particularly looked for in a blood smear:

1. Variation in size (Anisocytosis) Normally, there is slight variation in diameter of the red cells from 6.7-7.7 μm (mean value 7.2 μm). Increased variation in size of the red cell is termed anisocytosis. Anisocytosis may be due to the presence of cells larger than normal (*macrocytosis*) or cells smaller than normal (*microcytosis*). Sometimes both microcytosis and macrocytosis are present (*dimorphic*).

i) *Macrocytes* are classically found in megaloblastic anaemia; other causes are aplastic anaemia, other dyserythropoietic anaemias, chronic liver disease and in conditions with increased erythropoiesis.

ii) *Microcytes* are present in iron deficiency anaemia, thalassaemia and spherocytosis. They may also result from fragmentation of erythrocytes such as in haemolytic anaemia.

2. Variation in shape (Poikilocytosis) Increased variation in shape of the red cells is termed poikilocytosis. The nature of the abnormal shape determines the cause of anaemia. Poikilocytes are produced in various types of abnormal erythropoiesis e.g. in megaloblastic anaemia, iron deficiency anaemia, thalassaemia, myelosclerosis and microangiopathic haemolytic anaemia.

3. **Inadequate haemoglobin formation (Hypochromasia)** Normally, the intensity of pink staining of haemoglobin in a Romanowsky-stained blood smear gradually decreases from the periphery to the centre of the cell. Increased central pallor is referred to as *hypochromasia*. It may develop either from lowered haemoglobin content (e.g. in iron deficiency anaemia, chronic infections), or due to thinness of the red cells (e.g. in thalassaemia, sideroblastic anaemia). Unusually deep pink staining of the red cells due to increased haemoglobin concentration is termed *hyperchromasia* and may be found in megaloblastic anaemia, spherocytosis and in neonatal blood.

4. **Compensatory erythropoiesis** A number of changes are associated with compensatory increase in erythropoietic activity. These are as under:

i) *Polychromasia* is defined as the red cells having more than one type of colour. Polychromatic red cells are slightly larger, generally stained bluish-grey and represent reticulocytes and, thus, correlate well with reticulocyte count.

ii) *Erythroblastaemia* is the presence of nucleated red cells in the peripheral blood film. A small number of erythroblasts (or normoblasts) may be normally found in cord blood at birth. They are found in large numbers in haemolytic disease of the newborn, other haemolytic disorders and in extramedullary erythropoiesis. They may also appear in the blood in various types of severe anaemias except in aplastic anaemia. Erythroblastaemia may also occur after splenectomy.

iii) *Punctate basophilia* or *basophilic stippling* is diffuse and uniform basophilic granularity in the cell which does not stain positively with Perls' reaction (in contrast to Pappenheimer bodies which stain positively). Classical punctate basophilia is seen in aplastic anaemia, thalassaemia, myelodysplasia, infections and lead poisoning.

iv) *Howell-Jolly bodies* are purple nuclear remnants, usually found singly, and are larger than basophilic stippling. They are present in megaloblastic anaemia and after splenectomy.

5. **Red cell morphologic abnormalities** In addition to features of red cells described above, several morphologic abnormalities of red cells may be found in different haematological disorders. Some of these are as follows **(Fig. 22.9)**:

i) *Spherocytosis* is characterised by presence of spheroidal rather than biconcave disc-shaped red cells. Spherocytes are seen in hereditary spherocytosis, autoimmune haemolytic anaemia and in ABO haemolytic disease of the newborn.

ii) *Schistocytosis* is identified by fragmentation of erythrocytes. Schistocytes are found in thalassaemia, hereditary elliptocytosis, megaloblastic anaemia, iron deficiency anaemia, microangiopathic haemolytic anaemia and in severe burns.

iii) *Irregularly contracted red cells* are found in drug and chemical induced haemolytic anaemia and in unstable haemoglobinopathies.

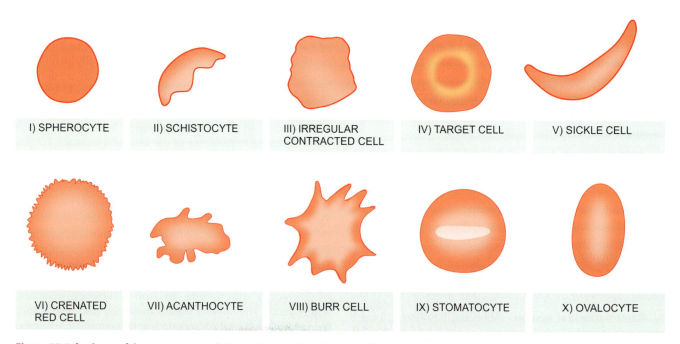

Figure 22.9 ▶ Some of the common morphologic abnormalities of red cells (The serial numbers in the illustrations correspond to the order in which they are described in the text).

iv) *Leptocytosis* is the presence of unusually thin red cells. Leptocytes are seen in severe iron deficiency and thalassaemia. *Target cell* is a form of leptocyte in which there is central round stained area and a peripheral rim of haemoglobin. Target cells are found in thalassaemia, chronic liver disease, and after splenectomy.

v) *Sickle cells or drepanocytes* are sickle-shaped red cells found in sickle cell disease.

vi) *Crenated red cells* are the erythrocytes which develop numerous projections from the surface. They are present in blood films due to alkaline pH, presence of traces of fatty substances on the slides and in cases where the film is made from blood that has been allowed to stand overnight.

vii) *Acanthocytosis* is the presence of coarsely crenated red cells. Acanthocytes are found in large number in blood film made from splenectomised subjects, and in chronic liver disease.

viii) *Burr cells* are cell fragments having one or more spines. They are particularly found in uraemia.

ix) *Stomatocytosis* is the presence of stomatocytes which have central area having slit-like or mouth-like appearance. They are found in hereditary stomatocytosis, or may be seen in chronic alcoholism.

x) *Ovalocytosis* or *elliptocytosis* is the oval or elliptical shape of red cells. Their highest proportion (79%) is seen in hereditary ovalocytosis and elliptocytosis; other conditions showing such abnormal shapes of red cells are megaloblastic anaemia and hypochromic anaemia.

C. RED CELL INDICES An alternative method to diagnose and detect the severity of anaemia is by measuring the red cell indices:

1. In iron deficiency and thalassaemia, MCV, MCH and MCHC are reduced. In early stage of iron deficiency, RDW is increased while in thalassaemia trait RDW is normal (with low MCV) and can be distinguished from iron deficiency.
2. In anaemia due to acute blood loss and haemolytic anaemias, MCV, MCH and MCHC are all within normal limits.
3. In megaloblastic anaemias, MCV is raised above the normal range.

D. LEUCOCYTE AND PLATELET COUNT Measurement of leucocyte and platelet count helps to distinguish pure anaemia from pancytopenia in which red cells, granulocytes and platelets are all reduced. In anaemias due to haemolysis or haemorrhage, the neutrophil count and platelet counts are often elevated. In infections and leukaemias, the leucocyte counts are high and immature leucocytes appear in the blood.

E. RETICULOCYTE COUNT Reticulocyte count (normal 0.5-2.5%) is done in each case of anaemia to assess the marrow erythropoietic activity. In acute haemorrhage and in haemolysis, increased reticulocyte count is indicative of excessive marrow function.

F. ERYTHROCYTE SEDIMENTATION RATE The ESR is a non-specific test used as a screening test for anaemia. It usually gives a clue to the underlying organic disease but anaemia itself may also cause rise in the ESR.

G. BONE MARROW EXAMINATION Bone marrow aspiration is done in cases where the cause for anaemia is not obvious. The procedures involved for marrow aspiration and trephine biopsy and their applications have already been discussed (page 358).

In addition to these general tests, certain specific tests are done in different types of anaemias which are described later under the discussion of specific anaemias.

CLASSIFICATION OF ANAEMIAS

Several types of classifications of anaemias have been proposed. Two of the widely accepted classifications are based on the pathophysiology and morphology **(Table 22.1)**.

PATHOPHYSIOLOGIC CLASSIFICATION Depending upon the pathophysiologic mechanism, anaemias are classified into 3 groups:

I. Anaemia due to blood loss This is further of 2 types:
A. Acute post-haemorrhagic anaemia
B. Anaemia of chronic blood loss

II. Anaemia due to impaired red cell formation A disturbance due to impaired red cell production from various causes may produce anaemia. These are as under:

Table 22.1	Classification of anaemias.

A. PATHOPHYSIOLOGIC
   I. Anaemia due to increased blood loss
      a) Acute post-haemorrhagic anaemia
      b) Chronic blood loss
   II. Anaemias due to impaired red cell production
      a) *Cytoplasmic maturation defects*
         1. Deficient haem synthesis:
            Iron deficiency anaemia
         2. Deficient globin synthesis:
            Thalassaemic syndromes
      b) *Nuclear maturation defects*
         Vitamin B_{12} and/or folic acid deficiency:
         Megaloblastic anaemia
      c) *Defect in stem cell proliferation and differentiation*
         1. Aplastic anaemia
         2. Pure red cell aplasia
      d) *Anaemia of chronic disorders*
      e) *Bone marrow infiltration*
      f) *Congenital anaemia*
   III. Anaemias due to increased red cell destruction (Haemolytic anaemias) (Details in Table 22.7)
      A. *Extrinsic (extracorpuscular) red cell abnormalities*
      B. *Intrinsic (intracorpuscular) red cell abnormalities*
B. MORPHOLOGIC
   I. Microcytic, hypochromic
   II. Normocytic, normochromic
   III. Macrocytic, normochromic

A. *Cytoplasmic maturation defects*
   1. Deficient haem synthesis: iron deficiency anaemia
   2. Deficient globin synthesis: thalassaemic syndromes
B. *Nuclear maturation defects*
   Vitamin B_{12} and/or folic acid deficiency: megaloblastic anaemia
C. *Haematopoietic stem cell proliferation and differentiation abnormality* e.g.
   1. Aplastic anaemia
   2. Pure red cell aplasia
D. *Bone marrow failure due to systemic diseases* (anaemia of chronic disorders) e.g.
   1. Anaemia of inflammation/infections, disseminated malignancy
   2. Anaemia in renal disease
   3. Anaemia due to endocrine and nutritional deficiencies (hypometabolic states)
   4. Anaemia in liver disease
E. *Bone marrow infiltration* e.g.
   1. Leukaemias
   2. Lymphomas
   3. Myelosclerosis
   4. Multiple myeloma
F. *Congenital anaemia* e.g.
   1. Sideroblastic anaemia
   2. Congenital dyserythropoietic anaemia.

The term *hypoproliferative anaemias* is also used to denote impaired marrow proliferative activity and includes 2 main groups: hypoproliferation due to iron deficiency and that due to other hypoproliferative disorders; the latter category includes anaemia of chronic inflammation/infection, renal disease, hypometabolic states, and causes of bone marrow failure.

III. Anaemia due to increased red cell destruction (haemolytic anaemias) This is further divided into 2 groups:
A. Intracorpuscular defect (hereditary and acquired).
B. Extracorpuscular defect (acquired haemolytic anaemias).

MORPHOLOGIC CLASSIFICATION Based on the red cell size, haemoglobin content and red cell indices, anaemias are classified into 3 types:

1. Microcytic, hypochromic MCV, MCH, MCHC are all reduced e.g. in iron deficiency anaemia and in certain non-iron deficient anaemias (sideroblastic anaemia, thalassaemia, anaemia of chronic disorders).

2. Normocytic, normochromic MCV, MCH, MCHC are all normal e.g. after acute blood loss, haemolytic anaemias, bone marrow failure, anaemia of chronic disorders.

3. Macrocytic MCV is raised e.g. in megaloblastic anaemia due to deficiency of vitamin B_{12} or folic acid.

With these general comments on anaemias, a discussion of the specific types of anaemias is given in the following pages.

GIST BOX 22.3 — Anaemias: General Considerations

- Anaemia is reduced haemoglobin concentration in blood below the lower limit of the normal for the age and sex of the individual.
- Anaemia causes lowered oxygen-carrying capacity and eventually tissue hypoxia and impaired function.
- Major symptoms of anaemia are tiredness, weakness and lethargy, and main signs are pallor, hyperdynamic circulation, and impaired functions of CNS and kidneys.
- A suspected case of anaemia is investigated by haemoglobin estimation, peripheral blood smear examination, and complete blood counts including reticulocyte count and ESR.
- Bone marrow aspiration and trephine biopsy are done to confirm and type the anaemia.
- Anaemias are classified based on pathophysiology (into anaemia due to blood loss, impaired red cell production, increased red cell destruction) or morphology (into microcytic hypochromic, macrocytic, normocytic normochromic).

HYPOCHROMIC ANAEMIAS

Hypochromic anaemia due to iron deficiency is the commonest cause of anaemia the world over. It is estimated that about 20% of women in child-bearing age group are iron deficient, while the overall prevalence in adult males is about 2%. It is the most important, though not the sole, cause of microcytic hypochromic anaemia in which all the three red cell indices (MCV, MCH and MCHC) are reduced and occurs due to defective haemoglobin synthesis. Hypochromic anaemias, therefore, are classified into 2 groups:
I. Hypochromic anaemia due to iron deficiency.
II. Hypochromic anaemias other than iron deficiency.

The latter category includes 3 groups of disorders—sideroblastic anaemia, thalassaemia and anaemia of chronic disorders.

IRON DEFICIENCY ANAEMIA

The commonest nutritional deficiency disorder present throughout the world is iron deficiency but its prevalence is higher in the developing countries. The factors responsible for iron deficiency in different populations are variable and are best understood in the context of normal iron metabolism.

Iron Metabolism

The amount of iron obtained from the diet should replace the losses from the skin, bowel and genitourinary tract. These losses together are about 1 mg daily in an adult male or in a non-menstruating female, while in a menstruating woman there is an additional iron loss of 0.5-1 mg daily. The iron required for haemoglobin synthesis is derived from 2 primary sources—ingestion of foods containing iron (e.g.

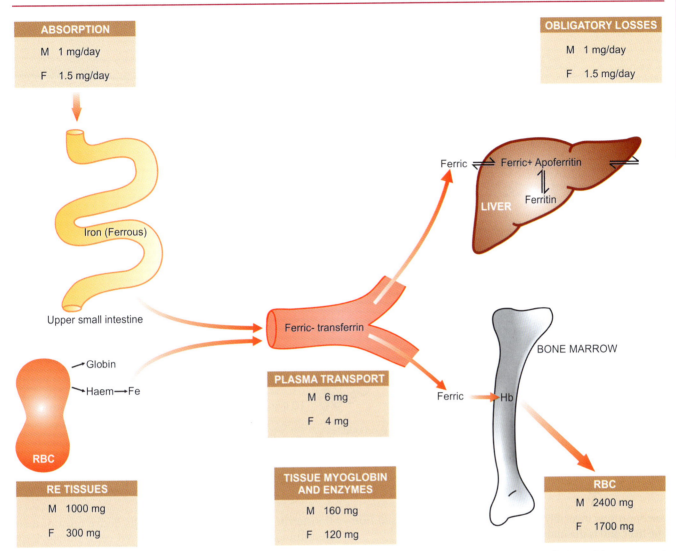

Figure 22.10 ▶ Daily iron cycle. Iron on absorption from upper small intestine circulates in plasma bound to transferrin and is transported to the bone marrow for utilisation in haemoglobin synthesis. The mature red cells are released into circulation, which on completion of their lifespan of 120 days, die. They are then phagocytosed by RE cells and iron stored as ferritin and haemosiderin. Stored iron is mobilised in response to increased demand and used for haemoglobin synthesis, thus completing the cycle (M = males; F = females).

leafy vegetables, beans, meats, liver etc) and recycling of iron from senescent red cells (Fig. 22.10).

ABSORPTION The average Western diet contains 10-15 mg of iron, out of which only 5-10% is normally absorbed. In pregnancy and in iron deficiency, the proportion of absorption is raised to 20-30%. Iron is absorbed mainly in the duodenum and proximal jejunum. The absorption is regulated by *mucosal block mechanism*—when iron stores are low (e.g. during pregnancy, menstruation, periods of growth and various diseases) absorption is enhanced, and when iron stores are increased (e.g. in haemosiderosis) little iron is absorbed or transported. *Iron from diet containing haem is better absorbed than non-haem iron:*

◆ Absorption of **non-haem iron** is enhanced by factors such as ascorbic acid (vitamin C), citric acid, amino acids, sugars, gastric secretions and hydrochloric acid of the stomach. Iron absorption is impaired by factors like medicinal antacids, milk, pancreatic secretions, phytates, phosphates, ethylene diamine tetra-acetic acid (EDTA) and tannates contained in tea. Non-haem iron is released as ferrous or ferric form but is absorbed almost exclusively as ferrous form; reduction of ferric to ferrous form when required takes place at the intestinal brush border by *ferric reductase*. Transport across the membrane is accomplished by divalent metal transporter 1 (DMT 1). Once inside the gut cells, iron may be either stored as ferritin or further transported to transferrin by two vehicle proteins—*ferroportin* and *hephaestin*. The function of

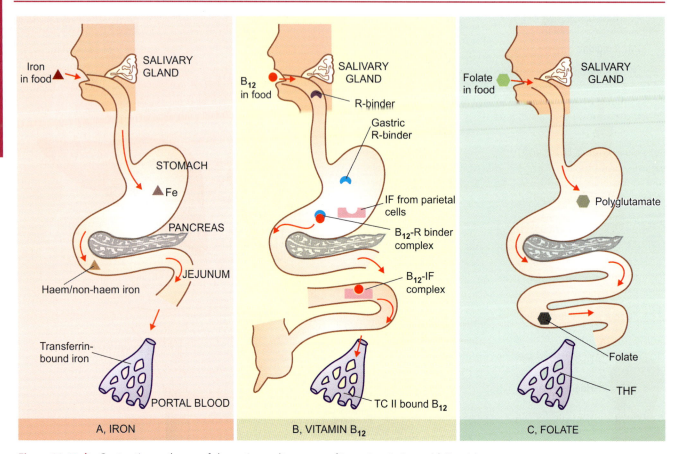

Figure 22.11 ▶ Contrasting pathways of absorption and transport of iron, vitamin B₁₂ and folic acid.

ferroportin is inversely regulated by hepcidin released from the liver and is the main iron regulating hormone.

◈ The mechanism of dietary **haem iron** absorption is not clearly understood yet but it is through a different transport than DMT 1.

After absorption of both non-haem and haem forms of iron, it comes into mucosal pool **(Fig. 22.11, A)**.

TRANSPORT Iron is transported in plasma bound to a β-globulin, *transferrin*, synthesised in the liver. Transferrin-bound iron is made available to the marrow where the developing erythroid cells having *transferrin receptors* utilise iron for haemoglobin synthesis. It may be mentioned here that transferrin receptors are present on cells of many tissues of the body but their number is greatest in the developing erythroblasts. Transferrin is reutilised after iron is released from it. A small amount of transferrin iron is delivered to other sites such as parenchymal cells of the liver. Normally, transferrin is about one-third saturated. But in conditions where transferrin-iron saturation is increased, parenchymal iron uptake is increased. Virtually, no iron is deposited in the mononuclear-phagocyte cells (RE cells) from the plasma transferrin-iron but instead these cells derive most of their iron from phagocytosis of senescent red cells. Storage form of iron (ferritin and haemosiderin) in RE cells is normally not functional but can be readily mobilised in response to increased demands for erythropoiesis. However, conditions such as malignancy, infection and inflammation interfere with the release of iron from iron stores causing ineffective erythropoiesis.

EXCRETION The body is unable to regulate its iron content by excretion alone. The amount of iron lost per day is 0.5-1 mg which is independent of iron intake. This loss is nearly twice more (i.e. 1-2 mg/day) in menstruating women. Iron is lost from the body in both sexes as a result of desquamation of epithelial cells from the gastrointestinal tract, from excretion in the urine and sweat, and loss via hair and nails. Iron excreted in the faeces mainly consists of unabsorbed iron and desquamated mucosal cells.

DISTRIBUTION In an adult, iron is distributed in the body as under:

1. **Haemoglobin**—present in the red cells, contains most of the body iron (65%).

2. **Myoglobin**—comprises a small amount of iron in the muscles (3.5%).
3. **Haem and non-haem enzymes**—e.g. cytochrome, catalase, peroxidases, succinic dehydrogenase and flavoproteins constitute a fraction of total body iron (0.5%).
4. **Transferrin-bound iron**—circulates in the plasma and constitutes another fraction of total body iron (0.5%).

All these forms of iron are in *functional form*.

5. **Ferritin and haemosiderin**—are the *storage forms* of excess iron (30%). They are stored in the mononuclear-phagocyte cells of the spleen, liver and bone marrow and in the parenchymal cells of the liver.

Pathogenesis

Iron deficiency anaemia develops when the supply of iron is inadequate for the requirement of haemoglobin synthesis. Initially, negative iron balance is covered by mobilisation from the tissue stores so as to maintain haemoglobin synthesis. It is only after the tissue stores of iron are exhausted that the supply of iron to the marrow becomes insufficient for haemoglobin formation and thus a state of iron deficiency anaemia develops. The development of iron deficiency depends upon one or more of the following factors:
1. Increased blood loss
2. Increased requirements
3. Inadequate dietary intake
4. Decreased intestinal absorption.

The relative significance of these factors varies with the age and sex of the patient **(Table 22.2)**. Accordingly, certain groups of individuals at increased risk of developing iron deficiency can be identified (*see below*). In general, in developed countries the mechanism of iron deficiency is usually due to chronic occult blood loss, while in the developing countries poor intake of iron or defective absorption are responsible for iron deficiency anaemia.

Etiology

Iron deficiency anaemia is always secondary to an underlying disorder. Correction of the underlying cause, therefore, is essential part of its treatment. Based on the above-mentioned pathogenetic mechanisms, following etiologic factors are involved in development of iron deficiency anaemia at different age and sex **(Table 22.2)**:

1. FEMALES IN REPRODUCTIVE PERIOD OF LIFE The highest incidence of iron deficiency anaemia is in women during their reproductive years of life. It may be from one or more of the following causes:

i) *Blood loss* This is the most important cause of anaemia in women during child-bearing age group. Commonly, it is due to persistent and heavy menstrual blood loss such as occurs in various pathological states and due to insertion of IUCDs. Young girls at the onset of menstruation may develop mild anaemia due to blood loss. Significant blood loss may occur as a result of repeated miscarriages.

Table 22.2 Etiology of iron deficiency anaemia.

I. INCREASED BLOOD LOSS
1. *Uterine* e.g. excessive menstruation in reproductive years, repeated miscarriages, at onset of menarche, post-menopausal uterine bleeding
2. *Gastrointestinal* e.g. peptic ulcer, haemorrhoids hookworm infestation, cancer of stomach and large bowel, oesophageal varices, hiatus hernia, chronic aspirin ingestion, ulcerative colitis, diverticulosis
3. *Renal tract* e.g. haematuria, haemoglobinuria
4. *Nose* e.g. repeated epistaxis
5. *Lungs* e.g. haemoptysis

II. INCREASED REQUIREMENTS
1. Spurts of growth in infancy, childhood and adolescence
2. Prematurity
3. Pregnancy and lactation

III. INADEQUATE DIETARY INTAKE
1. Poor economic status
2. Anorexia e.g. in pregnancy
3. Elderly individuals due to poor dentition, apathy and financial constraints

IV. DECREASED ABSORPTION
1. Partial or total gastrectomy
2. Achlorhydria
3. Intestinal malabsorption such as in coeliac disease

ii) *Inadequate intake* Inadequate intake of iron is prevalent in women of lower economic status. Besides diet deficient in iron, other factors such as anorexia, impaired absorption and diminished bioavailability may act as contributory factors.

iii) *Increased requirements* During pregnancy and adolescence, the demand of body for iron is increased. During a normal pregnancy, about 750 mg of iron may be siphoned off from the mother—about 400 mg to the foetus, 150 mg to the placenta, and 200 mg is lost at parturition and lactation. If several pregnancies occur at short intervals, iron deficiency anaemia certainly follows.

2. POST-MENOPAUSAL FEMALES Though the physiological demand for iron decreases after cessation of menstruation, iron deficiency anaemia may develop in post-menopausal women due to chronic blood loss. Following are among the important causes during these years:

i) *Post-menopausal uterine bleeding* due to carcinoma of the uterus.

ii) *Bleeding from the alimentary tract* such as due to carcinoma of stomach and large bowel and hiatus hernia.

3. ADULT MALES It is uncommon for adult males to develop iron deficiency anaemia in the presence of normal dietary iron content and iron absorption. The vast majority of cases of iron deficiency anaemia in adult males are due to chronic blood loss. The cause for chronic haemorrhage may lie at one of the following sites:

i) *Gastrointestinal tract* is the usual source of bleeding which may be due to peptic ulcer, haemorrhoids, hookworm infestation, carcinoma of stomach and large bowel,

oesophageal varices, hiatus hernia, chronic aspirin ingestion and ulcerative colitis. Other causes in the GIT are malabsorption and following gastrointestinal surgery.
ii) *Urinary tract* e.g. due to haematuria and haemoglobinuria.
iii) *Nose* e.g. in repeated epistaxis.
iv) *Lungs* e.g. in haemoptysis from various causes.

4. **INFANTS AND CHILDREN** Iron deficiency anaemia is fairly common during infancy and childhood with a peak incidence at 1-2 years of age. The principal cause for anaemia at this age is increased demand of iron which is not met by the inadequate intake of iron in the diet. Normal full-term infant has sufficient iron stores for the first 4-6 months of life, while premature infants have inadequate reserves because iron stores from the mother are mainly laid down during the last trimester of pregnancy. Therefore, unless the infant is given supplemental feeding of iron or iron-containing foods, iron deficiency anaemia develops.

Clinical Features

As already mentioned, iron deficiency anaemia is much more common in women between the age of 20 and 45 years than in men; at periods of active growth in infancy, childhood and adolescence; and is also more frequent in premature infants. Initially, there are usually no clinical abnormalities. But subsequently, in addition to features of the underlying disorder causing the anaemia, the clinical consequences of iron deficiency manifest in 2 ways—anaemia itself and epithelial tissue changes.

1. **ANAEMIA** The onset of iron deficiency anaemia is generally slow. The usual symptoms are weakness, fatigue, dyspnoea on exertion, palpitations and pallor of the skin, mucous membranes and sclerae. Older patients may develop angina and congestive cardiac failure. Patients may have unusual dietary cravings such as pica. Menorrhagia is a common symptom in iron deficient women.

2. **EPITHELIAL TISSUE CHANGES** Long-standing chronic iron deficiency anaemia causes epithelial tissue changes in some patients. The changes occur in the nails (koilonychia or spoon-shaped nails), tongue (atrophic glossitis), mouth (angular stomatitis), and oesophagus causing dysphagia from development of thin, membranous webs at the postcricoid area (Plummer-Vinson syndrome).

Laboratory Findings

The development of anaemia progresses in 3 stages:

◆ Firstly, *storage iron depletion* occurs during which iron reserves are lost without compromise of the iron supply for erythropoiesis.
◆ The next stage is *iron deficient erythropoiesis* during which the erythroid iron supply is reduced without the development of anaemia.
◆ The final stage is the development of *frank iron deficiency anaemia* when the red cells become microcytic and hypochromic.

The following laboratory tests can be used to assess the varying degree of iron deficiency (Fig. 22.12):

1. **BLOOD PICTURE AND RED CELL INDICES** The degree of anaemia varies. It is usually mild to moderate but occasionally it may be marked (haemoglobin less than 6 g/dl) due to persistent and severe blood loss. The salient haematological findings in these cases are as under.

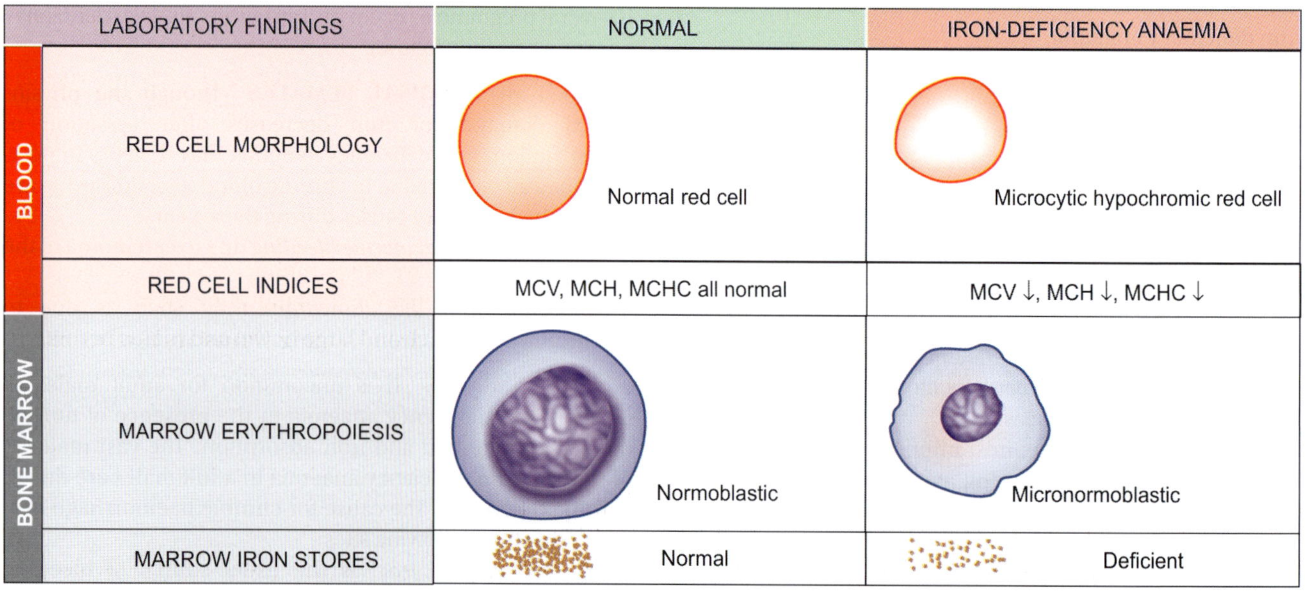

	LABORATORY FINDINGS	NORMAL	IRON-DEFICIENCY ANAEMIA
BLOOD	RED CELL MORPHOLOGY	Normal red cell	Microcytic hypochromic red cell
	RED CELL INDICES	MCV, MCH, MCHC all normal	MCV ↓, MCH ↓, MCHC ↓
BONE MARROW	MARROW ERYTHROPOIESIS	Normoblastic	Micronormoblastic
	MARROW IRON STORES	Normal	Deficient

Figure 22.12 ▶ Laboratory findings in iron deficiency anaemia.

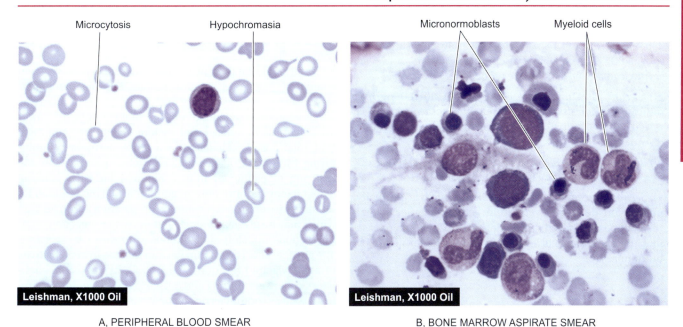

A, PERIPHERAL BLOOD SMEAR   B, BONE MARROW ASPIRATE SMEAR

Figure 22.13 ▶ Iron deficiency anaemia. A, PBF showing microcytic hypochromic anaemia. There is moderate microcytosis and hypochromia. B, Examination of bone marrow aspirate showing micronormoblastic erythropoiesis.

i) Haemoglobin The essential feature is a fall in haemoglobin concentration up to a variable degree.

ii) Red cells The red cells in the blood film are hypochromic and microcytic, and there is anisocytosis and poikilocytosis (Fig. 22.13, A). Hypochromia generally precedes microcytosis. Hypochromia is due to poor filling of the red cells with haemoglobin so that there is increased central pallor. In severe cases, there may be only a thin rim of pink staining at the periphery. Target cells, elliptical forms and polychromatic cells are often present. Normoblasts are uncommon. RBC count is below normal but is generally not proportionate to the fall in haemoglobin value. When iron deficiency is associated with severe folate or vitamin B_{12} deficiency, a *dimorphic* blood picture occurs with dual population of red cells—macrocytic as well as microcytic hypochromic.

iii) Reticulocyte count The reticulocyte count is normal or reduced but may be slightly raised (2-5%) in cases after haemorrhage.

iv) Absolute values The red cell indices reveal a diminished MCV (below 50 fl), diminished MCH (below 15 pg), and diminished MCHC (below 20 g/dl).

v) Leucocytes The total and differential white cell counts are usually normal.

vi) Platelets Platelet count is usually normal but may be slightly to moderately raised in patients who have had recent bleeding.

2. BONE MARROW FINDINGS Bone marrow examination is not essential in such cases routinely but is done in complicated cases so as to distinguish from other hypochromic anaemias. The usual findings are as follows (Fig. 22.13,B):

i) Marrow cellularity The marrow cellularity is increased due to erythroid hyperplasia (myeloid-erythroid ratio decreased).

ii) Erythropoiesis There is normoblastic erythropoiesis with predominance of small polychromatic normoblasts (micronormoblasts). These normoblasts have a thin rim of cytoplasm around the nucleus and a ragged and irregular cell border. The *cytoplasmic maturation lags behind* so that the late normoblasts have pyknotic nucleus but persisting polychromatic cytoplasm (compared from megaloblastic anaemia in which the nuclear maturation lags behind, page 382).

iii) Other cells Myeloid, lymphoid and megakaryocytic cells are normal in number and morphology.

iv) Marrow iron Iron staining (Prussian blue reaction) on bone marrow aspirate smear shows deficient reticuloendothelial iron stores and absence of siderotic iron granules from developing normoblasts.

3. BIOCHEMICAL FINDINGS In addition to blood and bone marrow examination, the following biochemical tests are of value:

i) The *serum iron* level is low (normal 40-140 µg/dl); it is often under 50 µg/dl. When serum iron falls below 15 µg/dl, marrow iron stores are absent.

ii) *Total iron binding capacity (TIBC)* is high (normal 250-450 µg/dl) and rises to give less than 10% saturation (normal 33%). In anaemia of chronic disorders, however, serum iron as well as TIBC are reduced.

iii) *Serum ferritin* is very low (normal 30-250 ng/ml) indicating poor tissue iron stores. The serum ferritin is raised in iron overload and is normal in anaemia of chronic disorders.

iv) *Red cell protoporphyrin* is very low (normal 20-40 µg/dl) as a result of insufficient iron supply to form haem.

v) *Serum transferrin receptor protein* which is normally present on developing erythroid cells and reflects total red cell mass, is raised in iron deficiency due to its release in circulation (normal level 4-9 µg/L as determined by immunoassay).

Principles of Treatment

The management of iron deficiency anaemia consists of 2 essential principles: correction of disorder causing the anaemia, and correction of iron deficiency.

1. CORRECTION OF THE DISORDER The underlying cause of iron deficiency is established after thorough check-up and investigations. Appropriate surgical, medical or preventive measures are instituted to correct the cause of blood loss.

2. CORRECTION OF IRON DEFICIENCY The lack of iron is corrected with iron therapy as under:

i) **Oral therapy** Iron deficiency responds very effectively to the administration of oral iron salts such as ferrous sulfate, ferrous fumarate, ferrous gluconate and polysaccharide iron. These preparations have varying amount of elemental iron in each tablet ranging from 39 mg to 105 mg. Optimal absorption is obtained by giving iron fasting, but if side-effects occur (e.g. nausea, abdominal discomfort, diarrhoea) iron can be given with food or by using a preparation of lower iron content (e.g. ferrous gluconate containing 39 mg elemental iron). Oral iron therapy is continued long enough, both to correct the anaemia and to replenish the body iron stores. The response to oral iron therapy is observed by reticulocytosis which begins to appear in 3-4 days with a peak in about 10 days. Poor response to iron replacement may occur from various causes such as: incorrect diagnosis, non-compliance, continuing blood loss, bone marrow suppression by tumour or chronic inflammation, and malabsorption.

ii) **Parenteral therapy** Parenteral iron therapy is indicated in following types of cases:
a) Intolerance to oral iron therapy
b) In GIT disorders such as malabsorption
c) Post-operative cases
d) Cases requiring a rapid replenishment of iron stores e.g. in women with severe anaemia a few weeks before expected date of delivery.

Parenteral iron therapy is hazardous and expensive when compared with oral administration. The haematological response to parenteral iron therapy is no faster than the administration of adequate dose of oral iron but the stores are replenished much faster. Before giving the parenteral iron, total dose is calculated by a simple formula by multi-plying the grams of haemoglobin below normal with 250 (250 mg of elemental iron is required for each gram of deficit haemoglobin), plus an additional 500 mg is added for building up iron stores. A common preparation is iron dextran which may be given as a single intramuscular injection, or as intravenous infusion after dilution with dextrose or saline. The adverse effects with iron dextran include hypersensitivity or anaphylactoid reactions, haemolysis, hypotension, circu-latory collapse, vomiting and muscle pain. Newer iron comp-lexes such as sodium ferric gluconate and iron sucrose can be administered as repeated intravenous injections with much lesser side effects.

SIDEROBLASTIC ANAEMIA

The sideroblastic anaemias comprise a group of disorders of diverse etiology in which the nucleated erythroid precursors in the bone marrow, show characteristic 'ringed sideroblasts.'

Siderocytes and Sideroblasts

Siderocytes and sideroblasts are erythrocytes and normoblasts respectively which contain cytoplasmic granules of iron (Fig. 22.14).

SIDEROCYTES These are red cells containing granules of non-haem iron. These granules stain positively with Prussian blue reaction as well as stain with Romanowsky dyes when they are referred to as *Pappenheimer bodies*. Siderocytes are normally not present in the human peripheral blood but a small number may appear following splenectomy. This is because the reticulocytes on release from the marrow are finally sequestered in the spleen to become mature red cells. In the absence of spleen, the final maturation step takes place in the peripheral blood and hence siderocytes make their appearance in the blood after splenectomy.

SIDEROBLASTS These are nucleated red cells (normo-blasts) containing siderotic granules which stain positively with Prussian blue reaction. Depending upon the number, size and distribution of siderotic granules, sideroblasts may be normal or abnormal (Fig. 22.15):

Normal sideroblasts contain a few fine, scattered cytoplasmic granules representing iron which has not been utilised for haemoglobin synthesis. These cells comprise 30-50% of normoblasts in the normal marrow but are reduced or absent in iron deficiency.

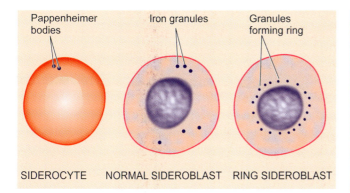

Figure 22.14 ▶ A siderocyte containing Pappenheimer bodies, a normal sideroblast and a ring sideroblast.

Abnormal sideroblasts are further of 2 types:

◈ *One type* is a sideroblast containing numerous, diffusely scattered, coarse cytoplasmic granules and are seen in conditions such as dyserythropoiesis and haemolysis. In this type, there is no defect of haem or globin synthesis but the percentage saturation of transferrin is increased.

◈ The other type is *ringed sideroblast* in which haem synthesis is disturbed as occurs in sideroblastic anaemias. Ringed sideroblasts contain numerous large granules, often forming a complete or partial ring around the nucleus. The ringed arrangement of these granules is due to the presence of iron-laden mitochondria around the nucleus.

Types of Sideroblastic Anaemias

Based on etiology, sideroblastic anaemias are classified into hereditary and acquired types. The acquired type is further divided into primary and secondary forms:

I. HEREDITARY SIDEROBLASTIC ANAEMIA This is a rare X-linked disorder associated with defective enzyme activity of *aminolevulinic acid (ALA) synthetase* required for haem synthesis. The affected males have moderate to marked anaemia while the females are carriers of the disorder and do not develop anaemia. The condition manifests in childhood or in early adult life.

II. ACQUIRED SIDEROBLASTIC ANAEMIA The acquired sideroblastic anaemias are classified into primary and secondary types.

A. Primary acquired sideroblastic anaemia Primary, idiopathic, or refractory acquired sideroblastic anaemia occurs spontaneously in middle-aged and older individuals of both sexes. The disorder has its pathogenesis in disturbed growth and maturation of erythroid precursors at the level of haematopoietic stem cell, possibly due to reduced activity of the enzyme, ALA synthetase. The anaemia is of moderate to severe degree and appears insidiously. The bone marrow cells commonly show chromosomal abnormalities,

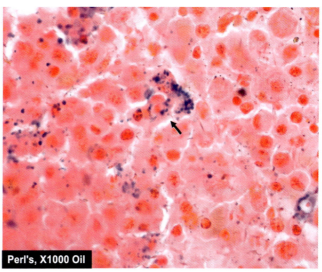

Figure 22.15 Sideroblastic anaemia. Bone marrow aspirate smear in Perls' stain shows marked excess of reticular iron and a ringed sideroblast (arrow) showing Prussian blue granules in the cytoplasm.

neutropenia and thrombocytopenia with associated bleeding diathesis. The spleen and liver may be either normal or mildly enlarged, while the lymph nodes are not enlarged. Unlike other types of sideroblastic anaemia, this type is regarded as a myelodysplastic disorder in the FAB (French-American-British) classification and thus, can be a preleukaemic disorder (page 439). About 10% of individuals with refractory acquired sideroblastic anaemia develop acute myelogenous leukaemia.

B. Secondary acquired sideroblastic anaemia Acquired sideroblastic anaemia may develop secondary to a variety of drugs, chemicals, toxins, haematological and various other diseases.

1. *Drugs, chemicals and toxins:* Isoniazid, an anti-tuberculous drug and a pyridoxine antagonist, is most commonly associated with development of sideroblastic anaemia by producing abnormalities in pyridoxine metabolism. Other drugs occasionally causing acquired sideroblastic anaemia are: cycloserine, chloramphenicol and alkylating agents (e.g. cyclophosphamide). Alcohol and lead also cause sideroblastic anaemia. All these agents cause reversible sideroblastic anaemia which usually resolves following removal of the offending agent.

2. *Haematological disorders:* These include myelofibrosis, polycythaemia vera, acute leukaemia, myeloma, lymphoma and haemolytic anaemia.

3. *Miscellaneous:* Occasionally, secondary sideroblastic anaemia may occur in association with a variety of inflammatory, neoplastic and autoimmune diseases such as carcinoma, myxoedema, rheumatoid arthritis and SLE.

Table 22.3: Laboratory diagnosis of hypochromic anaemias.

	TEST	IRON DEFICIENCY	CHRONIC DISORDERS	THALASSAEMIA MINOR	SIDEROBLASTIC ANAEMIA
1.	MCV, MCH, MCHC	Reduced	Low normal-to-reduced	Very low	Very low (except MCV raised in aquired type)
2.	Serum iron	Reduced	Reduced	Normal	Raised
3.	TIBC	Raised	Low-to-normal	Normal	Normal
4.	Serum ferritin	Reduced	Raised	Normal	Raised (complete saturation)
5.	Marrow-iron stores	Absent	Present	High	High
6.	Iron in normoblasts	Absent	Absent	Present	Ring sideroblasts
7.	Hb electrophoresis	Normal	Normal	Abnormal	Normal

Laboratory Findings

Sideroblastic anaemias usually show the following haematological features:
1. There is generally moderate to severe degree of *anaemia*.
2. The *blood picture* shows hypochromic anaemia which may be microcytic, or there may be some normocytic red cells as well (dimorphic).
3. *Absolute values* (MCV, MCH and MCHC) are reduced in hereditary type but MCV is often raised in acquired type.
4. *Bone marrow examination* shows erythroid hyperplasia with usually macronormoblastic erythropoiesis. Marrow iron stores are raised and pathognomonic ring sideroblasts are present.
5. *Serum ferritin* levels are raised.
6. *Serum iron* is usually raised with almost complete saturation of TIBC.
7. There is increased *iron deposition* in the tissue.

Principles of Treatment

The treatment of secondary sideroblastic anaemia is primarily focussed on removal of the offending agent. No definite treatment is available for hereditary and idiopathic types of sideroblastic anaemias. However, pyridoxine is administered routinely to all cases of sideroblastic anaemia (200 mg per day for 2-3 months). Blood transfusions and other supportive therapy are indicated in all patients.

Differential diagnosis of various types of hypochromic anaemias by laboratory tests is summarised in **Table 22.3**.

ANAEMIA OF CHRONIC DISORDERS

One of the commonly encountered anaemia is in patients of a variety of chronic systemic diseases in which anaemia develops secondary to a disease process but there is no actual invasion of the bone marrow. A list of such chronic systemic diseases is given in **Table 22.4**. In general, anaemia in chronic disorders is usually normocytic normochromic but can have mild degree of microcytosis and hypochromia unrelated to iron deficiency. The severity of anaemia is usually directly related to the primary disease process. The anaemia is corrected only if the primary disease is alleviated.

Pathogenesis

A number of factors may contribute to the development of anaemia in chronic systemic disorders, and in many conditions, the anaemia is complicated by other causes such as iron, B_{12} and folate deficiency, hypersplenism, renal failure with consequent reduced erythropoietic activity, endocrine abnormalities etc. However, in general, 2 factors appear to play significant role in the pathogenesis of anaemia in chronic disorders. These are: *defective red cell production and reduced red cell lifespan*.

1. Defective red cell production Though there is abundance of storage iron in these conditions but the amount of iron available to developing erythroid cells in the marrow is subnormal. The mononuclear phagocyte system is hyperplastic which traps all the available free iron due to the activity of iron binding protein, lactoferrin. A defect in the transfer of iron from macrophages to the developing erythroid cells in the marrow leads to reduced availability

Table 22.4: Anaemias secondary to chronic systemic disorders.

1. ANAEMIA IN CHRONIC INFECTIONS/INFLAMMATION
   a. *Infections* e.g. tuberculosis, lung abscess, pneumonia, osteomyelitis, subacute bacterial endocarditis, pyelonephritis.
   b. *Non-infectious inflammations* e.g. rheumatoid arthritis, SLE, vasculitis, dermatomyositis, scleroderma, sarcoidosis, Crohn's disease.
   c. *Disseminated malignancies* e.g. Hodgkin's disease, disseminated carcinomas and sarcomas.
2. ANAEMIA OF RENAL DISEASE e.g. uraemia, renal failure
3. ANAEMIA OF HYPOMETABOLIC STATE e.g. endocrinopathies (myxoedema, Addison's disease, hyperthyroidism, hypopituitarism, Addison's disease), protein malnutrition, scurvy and pregnancy, liver disease.

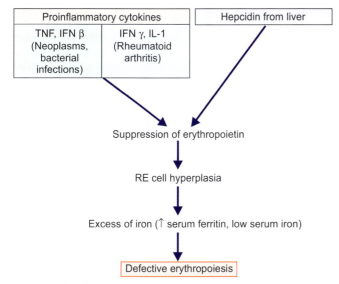

Figure 22.16 ▶ Pathogenesis of anaemia of chronic disorders through suppression of erythropoiesis by cytokines.

of iron for haem synthesis despite adequate iron stores, elevating serum ferritin levels. The defect lies in suppression of erythropoietin by inflammatory cytokines at some stage in erythropoiesis, and hepcidin which is the key iron regulatory hormone. These inflammatory cytokines include TNF and IFN-β released in bacterial infections and tumours, and IL-1 and IFN-γ released in patients of rheumatoid arthritis and autoimmune vasculitis **(Fig. 22.16)**.

2. Reduced red cell lifespan Decreased survival of circulating red cells in chronic renal disease is attributed to hyperplastic mononuclear phagocyte system.

Laboratory Findings

The characteristic features of anaemia in these patients uncomplicated by other deficiencies are as under:

i) Haemoglobin Anaemia is generally mild to moderate. A haemoglobin value of less than 8 g/dl suggests the presence of additional contributory factors.

ii) Blood picture The type of anaemia in these cases is generally normocytic normochromic but may have slight microcytosis and hypochromia.

iii) Absolute values Red cell indices indicate that in spite of normocytic normochromic anaemia, MCHC is slightly low.

iv) Reticulocyte count The reticulocyte count is generally low.

v) Red cell survival Measurement of erythrocyte survival generally reveals mild to moderate shortening of their lifespan.

vi) Bone marrow Examination of the marrow generally reveals normal erythroid maturation. However, the red cell precursors have reduced stainable iron than normal, while macrophages in the marrow usually contain increased amount of iron. Cases of chronic infection often have myeloid hyperplasia and increase in plasma cells.

vii) Serum iron and TIBC Serum iron is characteristically reduced in this group of anaemias while TIBC is low-to-normal (in contrast to iron deficiency where there is reduction in serum iron but high TIBC).

viii) Serum ferritin Serum ferritin levels are increased in these patients and is the most distinguishing feature between true iron-deficiency anaemia and iron-deficient erythropoiesis in anaemia of chronic diseases.

ix) Other plasma proteins In addition, certain other plasma proteins called '*phase reactants*' are raised in patients with chronic inflammation, probably under the stimulus of interleukin-1 released by activated macrophages. These proteins include γ-globulin, C3, haptoglobin, α₁-antitrypsin and fibrinogen. Elevation of these proteins is responsible for raised ESR commonly present in these patients.

 GIST BOX 22.4 | **Hypochromic Anaemias**

- Hypochromic anaemias are classified into 2 groups: due to iron deficiency and from causes other than iron deficiency (i.e. sideroblastic anaemia, thalassaemia and anaemia of chronic disorders).
- The commonest nutritional deficiency throughout the world is iron deficiency but its prevalence is higher in the developing countries.
- The development of iron deficiency may be due to increased blood loss, increased requirement, inadequate dietary intake or decreased intestinal absorption. Accordingly, the causes depend upon age and sex.
- Clinical consequences of iron deficiency manifest as anaemia itself and epithelial tissue changes.
- Laboratory diagnosis of iron deficiency is made by CBC and blood picture showing microcytosis and hypochromia, reduced red cell indices, serum iron and ferritin and bone marrow examination showing micronormoblastic picture with depleted iron stores.
- Sideroblastic anaemia is classified into hereditary and acquired. Marrow iron stores are raised and pathognomonic ring sideroblasts are present. Serum ferritin and serum iron are usually raised.
- Anaemia of chronic disorders is due to chronic systemic diseases, such as inflammatory or infectious and chronic renal diseases. *Serum ferritin* is *increased* and is the most distinguishing feature from true iron-deficiency anaemia.

MEGALOBLASTIC ANAEMIAS—VITAMIN B_{12} AND FOLATE DEFICIENCY

Megaloblastic anaemias are associated with macrocytic blood picture and megaloblastic marrow erythropoiesis. This group is due to deficiency of vitamin B_{12} and/or folate and includes megaloblastic picture from the following two types of etiologies:
1. Nutritional deficiency of vitamin B_{12} or folate, or combined deficiency, most common in developing countries.
2. Deficiency of intrinsic factor, causing impaired absorption of vitamin B_{12} called pernicious anaemia, is rare in India but more prevalent in individuals of European descent.

MEGALOBLASTIC ANAEMIA

The megaloblastic anaemias are disorders caused by impaired DNA synthesis and are characterised by a distinctive abnormality in the haematopoietic precursors in the bone marrow in which the *maturation of the nucleus is delayed relative to that of the cytoplasm*. Since cell division is slow but cytoplasmic development progresses normally, the nucleated red cell precursors tend to be larger which Ehrlich in 1880 termed *megaloblasts*. Megaloblasts are both morphologically and functionally abnormal with the result that the mature red cells formed from them and released into the peripheral blood are also abnormal in shape and size, the most prominent abnormality being *macrocytosis*.

The underlying defect for the asynchronous maturation of the nucleus is defective DNA synthesis due to deficiency of vitamin B_{12} (cobalamin) and/or folic acid (folate). Less common causes are interference with DNA synthesis by congenital or acquired abnormalities of vitamin B_{12} or folic acid metabolism. Before considering the megaloblastic anaemia, an outline of vitamin B_{12} and folic acid metabolism is given for a better understanding of the subject.

The salient nutritional aspects and metabolic functions of vitamin B_{12} and folic acid are summarised in **Table 22.5**.

Table 22.5 Salient features of vitamin B_{12} and folate metabolism.

	FEATURE	VITAMIN B_{12}	FOLATE
1.	Main foods	Animal proteins only	Green vegetables, meats
2.	Cooking	Little effect	Easily destroyed
3.	Daily requirements	2-4 µg	100-200 µg
4.	Daily intake	5-30 µg	100-500 µg
5.	Site of absorption	Ileum	Duodenum and jejunum
6.	Mechanism of absorption	Intrinsic factor	Conversion to methyl-THF
7.	Body stores	2-3 mg (enough for 2-4 yrs)	10-12 mg (enough for 4 months)

Vitamin B_{12} Metabolism

BIOCHEMISTRY Vitamin B_{12} or cobalamin is a complex organometallic compound having a cobalt atom situated within a corrin ring, similar to the structure of porphyrin from which haem is formed. In humans, there are 2 metabolically active forms of cobalamin—methyl-cobalamin and adenosyl-cobalamin, which act as coenzymes. The therapeutic vitamin B_{12} preparation is called cyanocobalamin.

SOURCES The dietary sources of vitamin B_{12} are foods of animal protein origin such as kidney, liver, heart, muscle meats, fish, eggs, cheese and milk. In contrast to folate, fruits and vegetables contain practically no vitamin B_{12} unless contaminated with bacteria. Cooking has little effect on its activity. Vitamin B_{12} is synthesised in the human large bowel by microorganisms but is not absorbed from this site and, thus, the humans are entirely dependent upon dietary sources. The average daily requirement for vitamin B_{12} is 2-4 µg.

ABSORPTION After ingestion, vitamin B_{12} in food is released and forms a stable complex with gastric R-binder. R-binder is a form of glycoprotein found in various secretions (e.g. saliva, milk, gastric juice, bile), phagocytes and plasma. On entering the duodenum, the vitamin B_{12}-R-binder complex is digested releasing vitamin B_{12} which then binds to intrinsic factor (IF). The IF is a glycoprotein of molecular weight 50,000 produced by the parietal cells of the stomach and its secretion roughly parallels that of hydrochloric acid. The vitamin B_{12}-IF complex, on reaching the distal ileum, binds to the specific receptors on the mucosal brush border, thereby enabling the vitamin to be absorbed. The IF, therefore, acts as cell-directed carrier protein similar to transferrin. The receptor-bound vitamin B_{12}-IF complex is taken into the ileal mucosal cells where after several hours the IF is destroyed, vitamin B_{12} released and is transferred to another transport protein, transcobalamin (TC) II. The vitamin B_{12}-TC II complex is finally secreted into the portal circulation from where it is taken by the liver, bone marrow and other cells. There are 2 major vitamin B_{12} binding proteins—TC I and TC II, and a minor protein TC III. TC I is not essential for vitamin B_{12} transport but functions primarily as a storage protein while TC III is similar to TC II and binds a small amount of vitamin B_{12} (see **Fig. 22.11, B**).

TISSUE STORES Normally, the liver is the principal storage site of vitamin B_{12} and stores about 2 mg of the vitamin, while other tissues like the kidney, heart and brain together store about 2 mg. The body stores of vitamin B_{12} are adequate for 2-4 years. Major source of loss is via bile and shedding of intestinal epithelial cells. A major part of the excreted vitamin B_{12} is reabsorbed in the ileum by the IF resulting in enterohepatic circulation.

FUNCTIONS Vitamin B_{12} plays an important role in general cell metabolism, particularly essential for normal

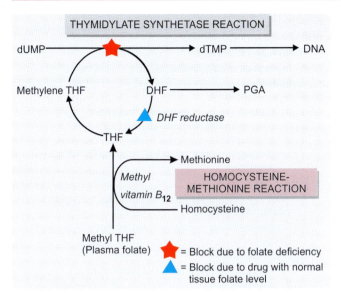

Figure 22.17 ▶ Biochemical basis of megaloblastic anaemia (THF = tetrahydrofolate; DHF = dihydrofolate; PGA = pteroyl glutamic acid; dUMP = deoxy uridylate monophosphate; dTMP = deoxy thymidylate monophosphate).

haematopoiesis and for maintenance of integrity of the nervous system. Vitamin B_{12} acts as a co-enzyme for 2 main biochemical reactions in the body:

❖ *Firstly, as methyl cobalamin (methyl B_{12}) in the methylation of homocysteine to methionine by methyl tetrahydrofolate (THF).* The homocysteine-methionine reaction is closely linked to folate metabolism **(Fig. 22.17)**:

$$\text{Homocysteine} \xrightarrow{\text{Methyl } B_{12}} \text{Methionine}$$

When this reaction is impaired, folate metabolism is deranged and results in defective DNA synthesis responsible for megaloblastic maturation.

❖ *Secondly, as adenosyl cobalamin (adenosyl B_{12}) in propionate metabolism for the conversion of methyl malonyl co-enzyme A to succinyl co-enzyme A:*

$$\text{Propionyl CoA} \xrightarrow{\text{Adenosyl } B_{12}} \text{Methyl malonyl CoA} \rightarrow \text{Succinyl CoA}$$

Lack of adenosyl B_{12} leads to large increase in the level of methyl malonyl CoA and its precursor, propionyl CoA. This results in synthesis of certain fatty acids which are incorporated into the neuronal lipids. This biochemical abnormality may contribute to the neurologic complications of vitamin B_{12} deficiency.

Folate Metabolism

BIOCHEMISTRY Folate or folic acid, a yellow compound, is a member of water-soluble B complex vitamins with the chemical name of *pteroyl glutamic acid (PGA)*. Folic acid does not exist as such in nature but exists as folates in polyglutamate form (conjugated folates). For its metabolic action as co-enzyme, polyglutamates must be reduced to dihydro- and tetrahydrofolate forms.

SOURCES Folate exists in different plants, bacteria and animal tissues. Its main dietary sources are fresh green leafy vegetables, fruits, liver, kidney, and to a lesser extent, muscle meats, cereals and milk. Folate is labile and is largely destroyed by cooking and canning. Some amount of folate synthesised by bacteria in the human large bowel is not available to the body because its absorption takes place in the small intestine. Thus, humans are mainly dependent upon diet for its supply. The average daily requirement is 100-200 μg.

ABSORPTION AND TRANSPORT Folate is normally absorbed from the duodenum and upper jejunum and to a lesser extent, from the lower jejunum and ileum. However, absorption depends upon the form of folate in the diet. Polyglutamate form in the foodstuffs is first cleaved by the enzyme, folate conjugase, in the mucosal cells to mono- and diglutamates which are readily assimilated. Synthetic folic acid preparations in polyglutamate form are also absorbed as rapidly as mono- and diglutamate form because of the absence of natural inhibitors. Mono- and diglutamates undergo further reduction in the mucosal cells to form tetrahydrofolate (THF), a monoglutamate. THF circulates in the plasma as methylated compound, methyl THF, bound to a protein. Once methyl THF is transported into the cell by a carrier protein, it is reconverted to polyglutamate (see **Fig. 22.11, C**).

TISSUE STORES The liver and red cells are the main storage sites of folate, largely as methyl THF polyglutamate form. The total body stores of folate are about 10-12 mg enough for about 4 months. Normally, folate is lost from the sweat, saliva, urine and faeces.

FUNCTIONS Folate plays an essential role in cellular metabolism. It acts as a co-enzyme for 2 important biochemical reactions involving transfer of 1-carbon units (viz. methyl and formyl groups) to various other compounds. These reactions are as under:

❖ *Thymidylate synthetase reaction* Formation of deoxy thymidylate monophosphate (dTMP) from its precursor form, deoxy uridylate monophosphate (dUMP).

❖ *Methylation of homocysteine to methionine* This reaction is linked to vitamin B_{12} metabolism **(Fig. 22.17)**.

These biochemical reactions are considered in detail below together with biochemical basis of the megaloblastic anaemia.

Biochemical Basis of Megaloblastic Anaemia

The basic biochemical abnormality common to both vitamin B_{12} and folate deficiency is a block in the pathway of DNA synthesis and that there is an inter-relationship between vitamin B_{12} and folate metabolism in the methylation reaction of homocysteine to methionine **(Fig. 22.17)**.

As stated above, folate as co-enzyme methylene THF, is required for transfer of 1-carbon moieties (e.g. methyl and formyl) to form building blocks in DNA synthesis. These 1-carbon moieties are derived from serine or formiminoglutamic acid (FIGLU). Two of the important folate-dependent (1-carbon transfer) reactions for formation of building blocks in DNA synthesis are as under:

1. Thymidylate synthetase reaction This reaction involves synthesis of deoxy thymidylate monophosphate (dTMP) from deoxy uridylate monophosphate (dUMP). The methyl group of dUMP → dTMP reaction is supplied by the co-enzyme, methylene-THF. After the transfer of 1-carbon from methylene-THF, dihydrofolate (DHF) is produced which must be reduced to active THF by the enzyme DHF-reductase before it can participate in further 1-carbon transfer reaction. Drugs like methotrexate (anti-cancer) and pyrimethamine (antimalarial) are inhibitory to the enzyme, DHF-reductase, thereby inhibiting the DNA synthesis.

2. Homocysteine-methionine reaction Homocysteine is converted into methionine by transfer of a methyl group from methylene-THF. After transfer of 1-carbon from methylene-THF, THF is produced. This reaction requires the presence of vitamin B_{12} (methyl-B_{12}).

Deficiency of folate from any cause results in reduced supply of the coenzyme, methylene-THF, and thus interferes with the synthesis of DNA. Deficiency of vitamin B_{12} traps folate as its transport form, methyl-THF, thereby resulting in reduced formation of the active form, methylene-THF, needed for DNA synthesis. This is referred to as *methyl-folate trap hypothesis*. An alternative hypothesis of inter-relationship of B_{12} and folate is the *formate-saturation hypothesis*. According to this hypothesis, the active substrate is formyl-THF. Vitamin B_{12} deficiency results in reduced supply of formate to THF causing reduced generation of the active compound, formyl THF.

Etiology and Classification of Megaloblastic Anaemia

The etiology of megaloblastic anaemia varies in different parts of the world. As outlined in Table 22.6, megaloblastic anaemia is classified into 3 broad groups: vitamin B_{12} deficiency, folate deficiency, and deficiency from other causes.

1. VITAMIN B_{12} DEFICIENCY In Western countries, deficiency of vitamin B_{12} is more commonly due to pernicious (Addisonian) anaemia. True vegetarians like traditional Indian Hindus and breast-fed infants have dietary lack of vitamin B_{12}. Gastrectomy by lack of intrinsic factor, and small intestinal lesions involving distal ileum where absorption of vitamin B_{12} occurs, may cause deficiency of the vitamin. Deficiency of vitamin B_{12} takes at least 2 years to develop when the body stores are totally depleted.

2. FOLATE DEFICIENCY Folate deficiency is more often due to poor dietary intake. Other causes include malabsorption, excess folate utilisation such as in pregnancy and in various disease states, chronic alcoholism, and excess urinary folate loss. Folate deficiency arises more rapidly than vitamin B_{12} deficiency since the body's stores of folate are relatively low which can last for up to 4 months only.

Patients with tropical sprue are often deficient in both vitamin B_{12} and folate. Combined deficiency of vitamin B_{12} and folate may occur from severe deficiency of vitamin B_{12} because of the biochemical interrelationship with folate metabolism.

3. OTHER CAUSES In addition to deficiency of vitamin B_{12} and folate, megaloblastic anaemias may occasionally be induced by other factors unrelated to vitamin deficiency. These include many drugs which interfere with DNA synthesis, acquired defects of haematopoietic stem cells, and rarely, congenital enzyme deficiencies.

Clinical Features

Deficiency of vitamin B_{12} and folate may cause following clinical manifestations which may be present singly or in combination and in varying severity:

1. Anaemia Macrocytic megaloblastic anaemia is the cardinal feature of deficiency of vitamin B_{12} and/or folate.

Table 22.6 Etiologic classification of megaloblastic anaemia.

I. VITAMIN B_{12} DEFICIENCY
  A. *Inadequate dietary intake* e.g. strict vegetarians, breast-fed infants.
  B. *Malabsorption*
   1. *Gastric causes:* pernicious anaemia, gastrectomy, congenital lack of intrinsic factor.
   2. *Intestinal causes:* tropical sprue, ileal resection, Crohn's disease, intestinal blind loop syndrome, fish-tapeworm infestation.

II. FOLATE DEFICIENCY
  A. *Inadequate dietary intake* e.g. in alcoholics, teenagers, infants, old age, poverty.
  B. *Malabsorption* e.g. in tropical sprue, coeliac disease, partial gastrectomy, jejunal resection, Crohn's disease.
  C. *Excess demand*
   1. *Physiological:* pregnancy, lactation, infancy.
   2. *Pathological:* malignancy, increased haematopoiesis, chronic exfoliative skin disorders, tuberculosis, rheumatoid arthritis.
  D. *Excess urinary folate loss* e.g. in active liver disease, congestive heart failure.

III. OTHER CAUSES
  A. *Impaired metabolism* e.g. inhibitors of dihydrofolate (DHF) reductase such as methotrexate and pyrimethamine; alcohol, congenital enzyme deficiencies.
  B. *Unknown etiology* e.g. in Di Guglielmo's syndrome, congenital dyserythropoietic anaemia, refractory megaloblastic anaemia.

The onset of anaemia is usually insidious and gradually progressive.

2. **Glossitis** Typically, the patient has a smooth, beefy, red tongue.

3. **Neurologic manifestations** Vitamin B_{12} deficiency, particularly in patients of pernicious anaemia, is associated with significant neurological manifestations in the form of subacute combined, degeneration of the spinal cord and peripheral neuropathy, while folate deficiency may occasionally develop neuropathy only. The underlying pathologic process consists of demyelination of the peripheral nerves, the spinal cord and the cerebrum. Signs and symptoms include numbness, paraesthesia, weakness, ataxia, poor finger coordination and diminished reflexes.

4. **Others** In addition to the cardinal features mentioned above, patients may have various other symptoms. These include: mild jaundice, angular stomatitis, purpura, melanin pigmentation, symptoms of malabsorption, weight loss and anorexia.

Laboratory Findings

The investigations of a suspected case of megaloblastic anaemia are aimed at 2 aspects:

A. *General laboratory investigations of anaemia* which include blood picture, red cell indices, bone marrow findings, and biochemical tests.

B. *Special tests to establish the cause of megaloblastic anaemia* as to know whether it is due to deficiency of vitamin B_{12} or folate.

Based on these principles, the following scheme of investigations is followed:

A. General Laboratory Findings

1. BLOOD PICTURE AND RED CELL INDICES
Estimation of haemoglobin, examination of a blood film and evaluation of absolute values are essential preliminary investigations **(Fig. 22.18)**:

i) Haemoglobin Haemoglobin estimation reveals values below the normal range. The fall in haemoglobin concentration may be of a variable degree.

ii) Red cells Red blood cell morphology in a blood film shows the characteristic macrocytosis. However, *macrocytosis* can also be seen in several other disorders such as: haemolysis, liver disease, chronic alcoholism, hypothyroidism, aplastic anaemia, myeloproliferative disorders and reticulocytosis. In addition, the blood smear demonstrates marked anisocytosis, poikilocytosis and presence of macroovalocytes. Basophilic stippling and occasional normoblast may also be seen **(Fig. 22.19, A)**.

iii) Reticulocyte count The reticulocyte count is generally low to normal in untreated cases.

iv) Absolute values The red cell indices reveal an elevated MCV (above 120 fl) proportionate to the severity of macrocytosis, elevated MCH (above 50 pg) and normal or reduced MCHC.

v) Leucocytes The total white blood cell count may be reduced. Presence of characteristic hypersegmented neutrophils (having more than 5 nuclear lobes) in the blood film should raise the suspicion of megaloblastic anaemia. An occasional myelocyte may also be seen.

vi) Platelets Platelet count may be moderately reduced in severely anaemic patients. Bizarre forms of platelets may be seen.

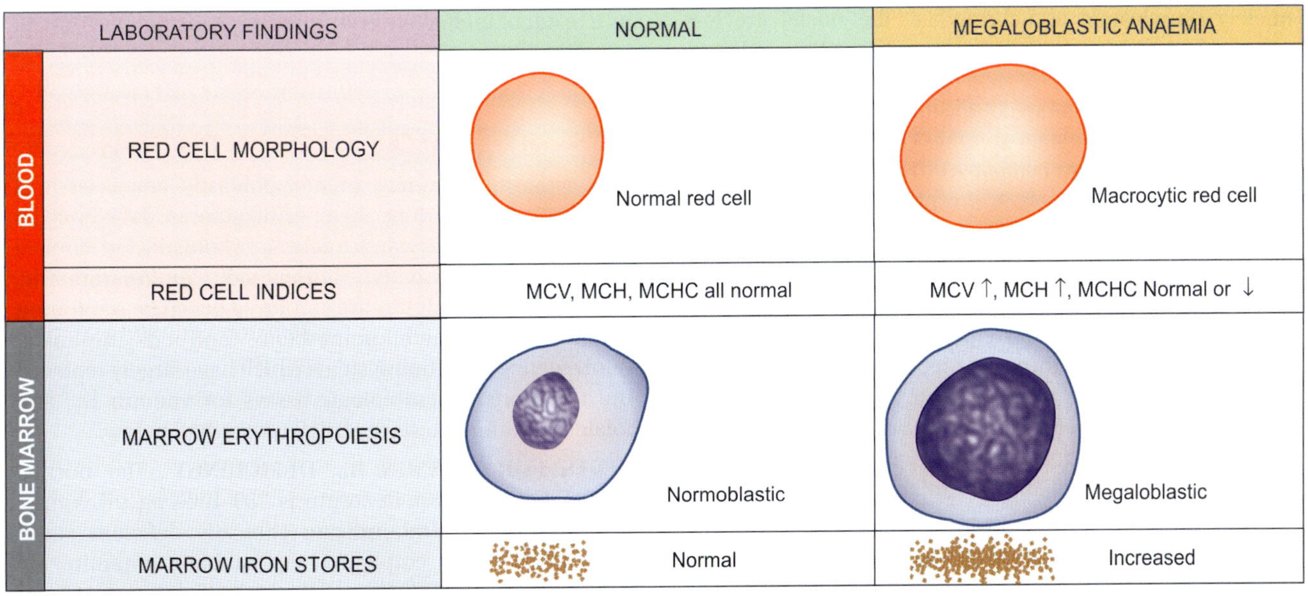

	LABORATORY FINDINGS	NORMAL	MEGALOBLASTIC ANAEMIA
BLOOD	RED CELL MORPHOLOGY	Normal red cell	Macrocytic red cell
	RED CELL INDICES	MCV, MCH, MCHC all normal	MCV ↑, MCH ↑, MCHC Normal or ↓
BONE MARROW	MARROW ERYTHROPOIESIS	Normoblastic	Megaloblastic
	MARROW IRON STORES	Normal	Increased

Figure 22.18 ▶ General laboratory findings in megaloblastic anaemia.

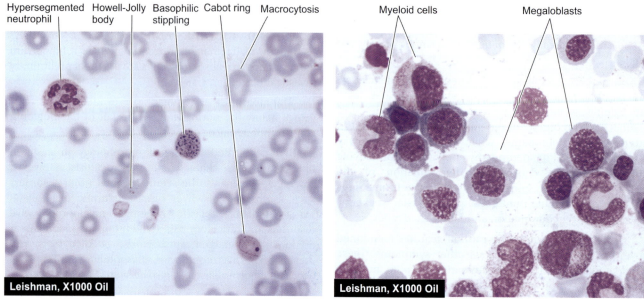

Figure 22.19 ▶ Megaloblastic anaemia. A, PBF showing prominent macrocytosis of red cells and hypersegmented neutrophils. B, Examination of bone marrow aspirate showing megaloblastic erythropoiesis.

2. BONE MARROW FINDINGS The bone marrow examination is very helpful in the diagnosis of megaloblastic anaemia. Significant findings of marrow examination are as under (Fig. 22.19, B):

i) Marrow cellularity The marrow is hypercellular with a decreased myeloid-erythroid ratio.

ii) Erythropoiesis There is erythroid hyperplasia due to characteristic megaloblastic erythropoiesis. *Megaloblasts* are abnormal, large, nucleated erythroid precursors, having nuclear-cytoplasmic asynchrony i.e. the nuclei are less mature than the development of cytoplasm. The nuclei are large, having fine, sieve-like and open chromatin that stains lightly, while the haemoglobinisation of the cytoplasm proceeds normally or at a faster rate i.e. *nuclear maturation lags behind that of cytoplasm* (compared from iron deficiency anaemia in which cytoplasmic maturation lags behind, page 373). Megaloblasts with abnormal mitoses may be seen. Ineffective erythropoiesis such as presence of degenerated erythroid precursors may be present.

iii) Other cells Granulocyte precursors are also affected to some extent. Giant forms of metamyelocytes and band cells may be present in the marrow. Megakaryocytes are usually present in normal number but may occasionally be decreased and show abnormal morphology such as hypersegmented nuclei and agranular cytoplasm.

iv) Marrow iron Prussian blue staining for iron in the marrow shows an increase in the number and size of iron granules in the erythroid precursors. Ring sideroblasts are, however, rare. Iron in the reticulum cells is increased.

v) Chromosomes Marrow cells may show variety of random chromosomal abnormalities such as chromosome breaks, centromere spreading etc.

3. BIOCHEMICAL FINDINGS In addition to the general blood and marrow investigations and specific tests to determine the cause of deficiency (described below), the following biochemical abnormalities are observed in cases of megaloblastic anaemia:

i) There is rise in *serum unconjugated bilirubin and* LDH as a result of ineffective erythropoiesis causing marrow cell breakdown.

ii) The *serum iron and ferritin* may be normal or elevated.

B. Special Tests for Cause of Specific Deficiency

In evaluating a patient of megaloblastic anaemia, it is important to determine the specific vitamin deficiency by assay of vitamin B_{12} and folate. In sophisticated clinical laboratories, currently automated multiparametric, random access analysers are employed based on separation techniques by chemiluminescence and enzyme-linked fluorescence detection systems which have largely replaced the traditional microbiologic assays for vitamin B_{12} and folate. Traditional tests are briefly described below.

TESTS FOR VITAMIN B_{12} DEFICIENCY The normal range of vitamin B_{12} in serum is 280-1000 pg/ml. Values less than 100 pg/ml indicate clinically deficient stage. Traditional tests employed to establish vitamin B_{12} deficiency are serum vitamin B_{12} assay, Schilling (24-hour urinary excretion) test and serum enzyme levels.

1. **SERUM VITAMIN B_{12} ASSAY** Assay of vitamin B_{12} in blood can be done by 2 methods—microbiological assay and radioassay.

i) Microbiological assay In this test, the serum sample to be assayed is added to a medium containing all other essential growth factors required for a vitamin B_{12}-dependent microorganism. The medium along with microorganism is incubated and the amount of vitamin B_{12} is determined turbimetrically which is then compared with the growth produced by a known amount of vitamin B_{12}. Several organisms have been used for this test such as *Euglena gracilis*, *Lactobacillus leichmannii*, *Escherichia coli* and *Ochromonas malhamensis*. *E. gracilis* is, however, considered more sensitive and accurate. The addition of antibiotics to the test interferes with the growth and yields false low result.

ii) Radioassay Assays of serum B_{12} by radioisotope dilution (RID) and radioimmunoassay (RIA) have been developed. These tests are more sensitive and have the advantage over microbiologic assays in that they are simpler and more rapid, and the results are unaffected by antibiotics and other drugs which may affect the living organisms.

2. **SCHILLING TEST (24-HOUR URINARY EXCRETION TEST)** Schilling test is done to detect vitamin B_{12} deficiency as well as to distinguish and detect lack of IF and malabsorption syndrome. The results of test also depend upon good renal function and proper urinary collection. Radioisotope used for labeling B_{12} is either ^{58}Co or ^{57}Co. The test is performed in two stages as under:

Stage I: Without IF The patient after an overnight fasting is administered oral dose of 1 mg of radioactively labelled vitamin B_{12} ('hot' B_{12}) in water. At the same time, 1 mg of unlabelled vitamin B_{12} ('cold' B_{12}) is given by intramuscular route; this 'cold' B_{12} will saturate the serum as well as the tissue binding sites to create excess of circulating vitamin B_{12}. If parenteral administration is not done, whole of orally administered radiolabelled vitamin B_{12} will be taken up by the tissues in the case of dietary vitamin B_{12} deficiency and little will be excreted in the urine. Urine is collected over the next 24 hours and excretion of radioactive-labelled vitamin B_{12} is estimated:

◆ Urinary excretion >10% of the oral dose of 'hot' B_{12} indicates normal absorption of this vitamin and is diagnostic of dietary B_{12} deficiency.

◆ Low urinary excretion of 'hot' B_{12} rules out dietary deficiency and is due to poor absorption of this vitamin, which could be from IF deficiency (stage II) or from malabsorption and therefore, proceed to stage II.

Stage II: With IF If the 24-hour urinary excretion of 'hot' B_{12} is low, the test is repeated using the same procedure as in stage I but concomitantly high oral dose of IF is administered with 'hot' B_{12}.

◆ If the 24-hour urinary excretion of 'hot' B_{12} is now normal or high, it is diagnostic of IF deficiency (i.e. pernicious anaemia). Patients with pernicious anaemia have abnormal test even after treatment with vitamin B_{12} due to IF deficiency.

◆ However, if 24-hour urinary excretion of 'hot' B_{12} remains low, then vitamin B_{12} deficiency is due to other causes in intestinal malabsorption (e.g. pancreatic deficiency, ileal disease, intestinal bacterial overgrowth etc).

3. **SERUM ENZYME LEVELS** Besides Schilling test, another way of distinguishing whether megaloblastic anaemia is due to cobalamine or folate is by serum determination of methylmalonic acid and homocysteine by sophisticated enzymatic assays. Both are elevated in cobalamine deficiency, while in folate deficiency there is only elevation of homocysteine and not of methylmalonic acid.

TESTS FOR FOLATE DEFICIENCY The normal range of serum folate is 6-18 ng/ml. Values of 4 ng/ml or less are generally considered to be diagnostic of folate deficiency. Measurement of *formiminoglutamic acid (FIGLU) urinary excretion* after histidine load was used formerly for assessing folate status but it is less specific and less sensitive than the serum assays. Currently, there are 3 tests used to detect folate deficiency—urinary excretion of FIGLU, serum and red cell folate assay.

1. **URINARY EXCRETION OF FIGLU** Folic acid is required for conversion of formiminoglutamic acid (FIGLU) to glutamic acid in the catabolism of histidine. Thus, on oral administration of histidine, urinary excretion of FIGLU is increased if folate deficiency is present.

2. **SERUM FOLATE ASSAY** The folate in serum can be estimated by 2 methods—microbiological assay and radioassay.

i) Microbiological assay This test is based on the principle that the serum folate acid activity is mainly due to the presence of a folic acid co-enzyme, 5-methyl THF, and that this compound is required for growth of the microorganism, *Lactobacillus casei*. The growth of *L. casei* is inhibited by addition of antibiotics.

ii) Radioassay The principle and method of radioassay by radioisotope dilution (RID) test are similar to that for serum B_{12} assay. The test employs labelled pteroylglutamic acid or methyl-THF. Commercial kits are available which permit simultaneous assay of both vitamin B_{12} and folate.

3. **RED CELL FOLATE ASSAY** Red cells contain 20-50 times more folate than the serum; thus red cell folate assay is more reliable indicator of tissue stores of folate than serum folate assay. Microbiological radioassay and protein-binding assay methods can be used for estimation of red cell folate. Red cell folate values are decreased in patients with megaloblastic anaemia as well as in patients with pernicious anaemia.

Principles of Treatment

Most cases of megaloblastic anaemia need therapy with appropriate vitamin. This includes: hydroxycobalamin as intramuscular injection 1000 µg for 3 weeks and oral folic acid 5 mg tablets daily for 4 months. Severely-anaemic patients in whom a definite deficiency of either vitamin cannot be established with certainty are treated with both vitamins concurrently. Blood transfusion should be avoided since it may cause circulatory overload. Packed cells may, however, be infused slowly.

Treatment of megaloblastic anaemia is quite gratifying. The marrow begins to revert back to normal morphology within a few hours of initiating treatment and becomes normoblastic within 48 hours of start of treatment. Reticulocytosis appears within 4-5 days after therapy is started and peaks at day 7. Haemoglobin should rise by 2-3 g/dl each fortnight. The peripheral neuropathy may show some improvement but subacute combined degeneration of the spinal cord is irreversible.

PERNICIOUS ANAEMIA

Pernicious anaemia (PA) was first described by Addison in 1855 as a chronic disorder of middle-aged and elderly individual of either sex in which intrinsic factor (IF) secretion ceases owing to atrophy of the gastric mucosa. The condition is, therefore, also termed Addisonian megaloblastic anaemia. The average age at presentation is 60 years but rarely it can be seen in children under 10 years of age (juvenile pernicious anaemia). PA is seen most frequently in individuals of northern European descent and African Americans and is uncommon in South Europeans and Orientals.

Pathogenesis

There is evidence to suggest that the atrophy of gastric mucosa in PA resulting in absence or low level of IF is caused by an autoimmune reaction against gastric parietal cells. The evidences in support of immunological abnormalities in pernicious anaemia are as under:
1. The incidence of PA is high in patients with *other autoimmune diseases* such as Graves' disease, myxoedema, thyroiditis, vitiligo, diabetes and idiopathic adrenocortical insufficiency.
2. Patients with PA have abnormal *circulating autoantibodies* such as anti-parietal cell antibody (90% cases) and anti-intrinsic factor antibody (50% cases).
3. *Relatives* of patients with PA have an increased incidence of the disease or increased presence of autoantibodies.
4. *Corticosteroids* have been reported to be beneficial in curing the disease both pathologically and clinically.
5. PA is more common in patients with *agammaglobulinaemia* supporting the role of cellular immune system in destruction of parietal cells.
6. Certain *HLA types* (HLA-DR5) have been reported to be associated with PA.

MORPHOLOGIC FEATURES The most characteristic pathologic finding in PA is gastric atrophy affecting the acid- and pepsin-secreting portion of the stomach and sparing the antrum. Gastric epithelium may show cellular atypia. About 2-3% cases of PA develop carcinoma of the stomach. Other pathologic changes are secondary to vitamin B_{12} deficiency and include megaloblastoid alterations in the gastric and intestinal epithelium and neurologic abnormalities such as peripheral neuropathy and spinal cord damage.

Clinical Features

The disease has insidious onset and progresses slowly. The clinical manifestations are mainly due to vitamin B_{12} deficiency. These include: anaemia, glossitis, neurological abnormalities (neuropathy, subacute combined degeneration of the spinal cord, retrobulbar neuritis), gastrointestinal manifestations (diarrhoea, anorexia, weight loss, dyspepsia), hepatosplenomegaly, congestive heart failure and haemorrhagic manifestations. Other autoimmune diseases such as autoimmune thyroiditis may be associated.

Principles of Treatment

Patients of PA are treated with vitamin B_{12} in the following way:
1. Parenteral vitamin B_{12} replacement therapy.
2. Symptomatic and supportive therapy such as physiotherapy for neurologic deficits and occasionally blood transfusion.
3. Follow-up for early detection of cancer of the stomach.

Most of the abnormalities due to vitamin B_{12} deficiency can be corrected except the irreversible damage to the spinal cord. Corticosteroid therapy can improve the gastric lesion with a return of acid secretion but the higher incidence of gastric polyps and cancer of the stomach in these patients can only be detected by frequent follow-up.

GIST BOX 22.5 — Megaloblastic and Pernicious Anaemias: Vitamin B_{12} and Folate Deficiency

- Megaloblastic anaemias are associated with macrocytic blood picture and megaloblastic marrow erythropoiesis. This group is due to deficiency of vitamin B_{12} and/or folate.
- The only dietary sources of vitamin B_{12} are foods of animal protein origin while folate exists in different plants, bacteria and animal tissues.
- The basic biochemical abnormality in both vitamin B_{12} and folate deficiency is a block in the pathway of DNA synthesis.
- Clinical features of megaloblastic anaemia are anaemia, glossitis, and neurological manifestations.
- Laboratory diagnosis is made by macrocytic blood picture, raised MCV and MCH, and megaloblastic

erythropoiesis in the bone marrow with raised iron stores.
- Specific deficiency of vitamin B_{12} and folate can be made by serum assay and Schilling test.
- Pernicious anaemia is megaloblastic erythropoiesis from impaired absorption of vitamin B_{12} which is due to deficiency of intrinsic factor from atrophic gastritis.

HAEMOLYTIC ANAEMIAS AND ANAEMIA DUE TO BLOOD LOSS

DEFINITION AND CLASSIFICATION

Haemolytic anaemias are defined as anaemias resulting from an increase in the rate of red cell destruction. Normally, effete red cells undergo lysis at the end of their lifespan of 120 ± 30 days within the cells of reticuloendothelial (RE) system in the spleen and elsewhere (extravascular haemolysis), and haemoglobin is not liberated into the plasma in appreciable amounts. The red cell lifespan is shortened in haemolytic anaemia i.e. there is accelerated haemolysis. However, shortening of red cell lifespan does not necessarily result in anaemia. In fact, compensatory bone marrow hyperplasia may cause 6 to 8-fold increase in red cell production without causing anaemia to the patient, so-called *compensated haemolytic disease.*

The premature destruction of red cells in haemolytic anaemia may occur at either of the following 2 sites:

◈ **Firstly,** the red cells undergo lysis in the circulation and release their contents into plasma *(intravascular haemolysis).* In these cases the plasma haemoglobin rises substantially and part of it may be excreted in the urine *(haemoglobinuria).*

◈ **Secondly,** the red cells are taken up by cells of the RE system where they are destroyed and digested *(extravascular haemolysis).* In extravascular haemolysis, plasma haemoglobin level is, therefore, barely raised.

Extravascular haemolysis is more common than the former. One or more factors may be involved in the pathogenesis of various haemolytic anaemias.

Clinically, haemolytic anaemias may be acute or chronic, mild to severe, hereditary or acquired. Haemolytic anaemias are broadly classified into 2 main categories:

I. *Acquired haemolytic anaemias* caused by a variety of extrinsic environmental factors *(i.e. extracorpuscular).*

II. *Hereditary haemolytic anaemias* are usually the result of intrinsic red cell defects *(i.e. intracorpuscular).*

A simplified classification based on these mechanisms is given in **Table 22.7** and diagrammatically represented in **Fig. 22.20**.

GENERAL ASPECTS

A number of clinical and laboratory features are shared by various types of haemolytic anaemias. These are briefly described below:

Table 22.7 Classification of haemolytic anaemias.

I. ACQUIRED
   A. *Antibody:* Immunohaemolytic anaemias
      1. Autoimmune haemolytic anaemia (AIHA)
         i) Warm antibody AIHA
         ii) Cold antibody AIHA
      2. Drug-induced immunohaemolytic anaemia
      3. Isoimmune haemolytic anaemia
   B. *Mechanical trauma:* Microangiopathic haemolytic anaemia
   C. *Direct toxic effects:* Malaria, bacterial, infection and other agents
   D. *Acquired red cell membrane abnormalities:* Paroxysmal nocturnal haemoglobinuria (PNH)
   E. *Splenomegaly*

II. HEREDITARY
   A. Abnormalities of red cell membrane
      1. Hereditary spherocytosis
      2. Hereditary elliptocytosis (hereditary ovalocytosis)
      3. Hereditary stomatocytosis
   B. Disorders of red cell interior
      1. *Red cell enzyme defects (Enzymopathies)*
         i) Defects in the hexose monophosphate shunt: G6PD deficiency
         ii) Defects in the Embden-Meyerhof (or glycolytic) pathway: pyruvate kinase deficiency
      2. *Disorders of haemoglobin (Haemoglobinopathies)*
         i) Structurally abnormal haemoglobins: sickle syndromes, other haemoglobinopathies
         ii) Reduced globin chain synthesis: thalassaemias

General Clinical Features

Some of the general clinical features common to most congenital and acquired haemolytic anaemias are as under:
1. Presence of pallor of mucous membranes.
2. Positive family history with life-long anaemia in patients with congenital haemolytic anaemia.
3. Mild fluctuating jaundice due to unconjugated hyperbilirubinaemia.
4. Urine turns dark on standing due to excess of urobilinogen in urine.
5. Splenomegaly is found in most chronic haemolytic anaemias, both congenital and acquired.
6. Pigment gallstones are found in some cases.

Laboratory Evaluation of Haemolysis

The laboratory findings are conveniently divided into the following 4 groups:

I. Tests of Increased Red Cell Breakdown

1. *Serum bilirubin*—unconjugated (indirect) bilirubin is raised.
2. *Urine urobilinogen* is raised but there is no bilirubinuria.
3. *Faecal stercobilinogen* is raised.
4. *Serum haptoglobin* (α-globulin binding protein) is reduced or absent due to its binding to liberated plasma haemoglobin.

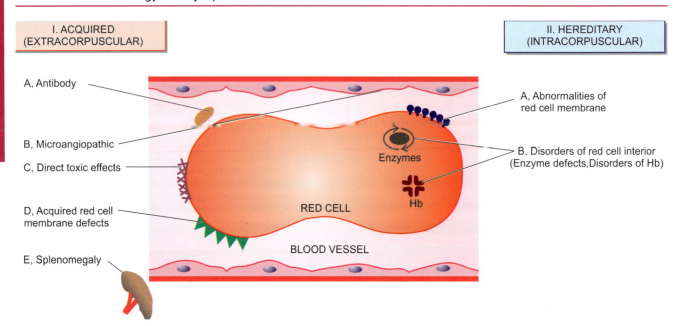

Figure 22.20 ▶ Diagrammatic representation of classification of haemolytic anaemias based on principal mechanisms of haemolysis.

5. *Plasma lactic dehydrogenase* is raised.
6. *Evidences of intravascular haemolysis* in the form of haemoglobinaemia, haemoglobinuria, methaemoglobinaemia and haemosiderinuria.

II. Tests of Increased Red Cell Production

1. *Reticulocyte count* reveals reticulocytosis which is generally early and is hence most useful initial test of marrow erythroid hyperplasia.
2. *Routine blood film* shows macrocytosis, polychromasia and presence of normoblasts.
3. *Bone marrow* shows erythroid hyperplasia with usually raised iron stores.
4. *X-ray of bones* shows evidence of expansion of marrow space, especially in tubular bones and skull.

III. Tests of Damage to Red Cells

1. *Routine blood film* shows a variety of abnormal morphological appearances of red cells described illustrated in **Fig. 22.9**.
2. *Osmotic fragility* is increased (in spherocytosis) or decreased (in thalassaemia).
3. *Autohaemolysis test* with or without addition of glucose.
4. *Coombs' antiglobulin test*.
5. *Electrophoresis* for abnormal haemoglobins.
6. *Estimation of HbA_2* (in β-thalassaemia minor)
7. *Estimation of HbF* by Quick's one stage method
8. *Tests for sickling.*
9. *Screening test for G6PD deficiency* and other enzymes (e.g. Heinz bodies test).

IV. Tests for Shortened Red Cell Lifespan

A shortened red cell survival is best tested by ^{51}Cr labelling method. Normal RBC lifespan of 120 days is shortened to 20-40 days in moderate haemolysis and to 5-20 days in severe haemolysis.

Contrasting features of intravascular and extravascular haemolysis are given in **Table 22.8**.

After these general comments on clinical and laboratory features of haemolysis, we now turn to discuss various types of haemolytic anaemias given in **Table 22.7**.

I. ACQUIRED HAEMOLYTIC ANAEMIAS

Acquired haemolytic anaemias are caused by a variety of extrinsic factors, namely: antibody (immunohaemolytic anaemia), mechanical factors (microangiopathic haemolytic anaemia), direct toxic effect (in malaria, clostridial infection etc), splenomegaly, and certain acquired membrane abnormalities (paroxysmal nocturnal haemoglobinuria). These are briefly discussed below:

A. Immunohaemolytic Anaemias

Immunohaemolytic anaemias are a group of anaemias occurring due to antibody production by the body against its own red cells. Immune haemolysis in these cases may be induced by one of the following three types of antibodies:

1. *Autoimmune haemolytic anaemia (AIHA)* characterised by formation of autoantibodies against patient's own red cells. Depending upon the reactivity of autoantibody, AIHA is further divided into 2 types:

Table 22.8: Contrasting features of extravascular and intravascular haemolysis.

	FEATURE	EXTRAVASCULAR HAEMOLYSIS	INTRAVASCULAR HAEMOLYSIS
1.	Frequency	More common	Less common
2.	Location	RE system organs (spleen, bone marrow, liver)	In peripheral blood
3.	Iron stores	Increased	Decreased
4.	Serum ferritin	Normal to high	Low
5.	Plasma haemoglobin	Absent	Present
6.	Methaemoglobin	Absent	Present
7.	Haemoglobinuria	Absent	Present
8.	Haemosiderinuria	Absent	Present
9.	Unconjugated hyperbilirubinaemia	Markedly elevated	Mildly elevated
10.	Serum LDH	Mildly elevated	Markedly elevated
11.	Serum haptoglobin	Normal	Decreased

i) 'Warm' antibody AIHA in which the autoantibodies are reactive at body temperature (37°C).

ii) 'Cold' antibody AIHA in which the autoantibodies react better with patient's own red cells at 4°C.

2. *Drug-induced immunohaemolytic anaemia.*

3. *Isoimmune haemolytic anaemia* in which the antibodies are acquired by blood transfusions, pregnancies and haemolytic disease of the newborn.

An important diagnostic tool in all cases of immuno-haemolytic anaemias is Coombs' antiglobulin test for detection of incomplete Rh-antibodies in saline directly (direct Coombs') or after addition of albumin (indirect Coombs').

Autoimmune Haemolytic Anaemia (AIHA)

'WARM' ANTIBODY AIHA

Warm antibodies reactive at body temperature and coating the red cells are generally IgG class antibodies and occasionally they are IgA. Human red cells coated with IgG antibodies along with C3 further promote this red cell-RE cell interaction, especially splenic macrophages, accounting for more severe haemolysis. The spleen is particularly efficient in trapping red cells coated with IgG antibodies. It is, thus, the major site of red cell destruction in warm antibody AIHA.

CLINICAL AND LABORATORY FEATURES Warm antibody AIHA may occur at any age and in either sex. The disease may occur without any apparent cause (idiopathic) but about a quarter of patients develop this disorder as a complication of an underlying disease affecting the immune system such as SLE, chronic lymphocytic leukaemia, lymphomas and certain drugs such as methyl DOPA, penicillin etc.

The disease tends to have remissions and relapses. The usual clinical features are as follows:
1. Chronic anaemia of varying severity with remissions and relapses.
2. Splenomegaly.
3. Occasionally hyperbilirubinaemia.

Treatment of these cases consists of removal of the cause whenever present, corticosteroid therapy, and in severe cases blood transfusions. Splenectomy is the second line of therapy in this disorder.

'COLD' ANTIBODY AIHA

Antibodies which are reactive in the cold (4°C) may induce haemolysis under 2 conditions: cold agglutinin disease and paroxysmal cold haemoglobinuria.

1. Cold agglutinin disease In cold agglutinin disease, the antibodies are IgM type which bind to the red cells best at 4°C. These cold antibodies are usually directed against the *I* antigen on the red cell surface. Agglutination of red blood cells by IgM cold agglutinins is most profound at very low temperature but upon warming to 37°C or above, disagglutination occurs quickly. Haemolytic effect is mediated through fixation of C3 to the red blood cell surface and not by agglutination alone. Most cold agglutinins affect juvenile red blood cells. The etiology of cold antibody remains unknown. It is seen in the course of certain infections (e.g. *Mycoplasma* pneumonia, infectious mononucleosis) and in lymphomas.

2. Paroxysmal cold haemoglobinuria (PCH) In PCH, cold antibody is an IgG antibody (Donath-Landsteiner antibody) which is directed against *P* blood group antigen and brings about complement-mediated haemolysis. Attacks of PCH are precipitated by exposure to cold. PCH is uncommon and may be seen in association with tertiary syphilis or as a complication of certain infections such as *Mycoplasma*, pneumonia, flu, measles and mumps.

CLINICAL AND LABORATORY FEATURES The clinical manifestations are due to haemolysis and not due to agglutination. These include the following:
1. Chronic anaemia which is worsened by exposure to cold.
2. Raynaud's phenomenon.
3. Cyanosis affecting the cold exposed regions such as tips of nose, ears, fingers and toes.
4. Haemoglobinaemia and haemoglobinuria occur on exposure to cold.

The haematologic and biochemical findings are somewhat similar to those found in warm antibody AIHA except the thermal amplitude.

Treatment consists of keeping the patient warm and treating the underlying cause.

Drug-induced Immunohaemolytic Anaemia

Drugs may cause immunohaemolytic anaemia by 3 different mechanisms:

1. α-METHYL DOPA TYPE ANTIBODIES A small proportion of patients receiving α-methyl dopa develop immunohaemolytic anaemia which is identical in every respect to warm antibody AIHA described above.

2. PENICILLIN-INDUCED IMMUNOHAEMOLYSIS Patients receiving large doses of penicillin or penicillin-type antibiotics develop antibodies against the red blood cell-drug complex which induces haemolysis.

3. INNOCENT BYSTANDER IMMUNOHAEMOLYSIS Drugs such as quinidine form a complex with plasma proteins to which an antibody forms. This drug-plasma protein-antibody complex may induce lysis of bystanding red blood cells or platelets.

In each type of drug-induced immunohaemolytic anaemia, discontinuation of the drug results in gradual disappearance of haemolysis.

Isoimmune Haemolytic Anaemia

Isoimmune haemolytic anaemias are caused by acquiring isoantibodies or alloantibodies by blood transfusions, pregnancies and in haemolytic disease of the newborn (HDN). HDN results from the passage of IgG antibodies from the maternal circulation across the placenta into the circulation of the foetal red cells.

HDN can occur from incompatibility of ABO or Rh blood group system. ABO incompatibility is much more common but the HDN in such cases is usually mild, while Rh-D incompatibility results in more severe form of the HDN.

HDN due to Rh-D incompatibility Rh incompatibility occurs when a Rh-negative mother is sensitised to Rh-positive blood. This results most often from an Rh-positive foetus by passage of Rh-positive red cells across the placenta into the circulation of Rh-negative mother. Sensitisation is more likely if the mother and foetus are ABO compatible rather than ABO incompatible. Though approximately 95% cases of Rh-HDN are due to anti-D, some cases are due to combination of anti-D with other immune antibodies of the Rh system such as anti-C and anti-E, and rarely anti-C alone.

It must be emphasised here that the risk of sensitisation of a Rh-negative woman married to Rh-positive man is small in first pregnancy but increases during successive pregnancies if prophylactic anti-D immunoglobulin is not given within 72 hours after the first delivery. If both the parents are Rh-D positive (homozygous), all the newborns will be Rh-D positive, while if the father is Rh-D positive (heterozygous), there is a 50% chance of producing a Rh-D negative child.

HDN due to ABO incompatibility About 20% pregnancies with ABO incompatibility between the mother and the foetus develop the HDN. Naturally-occurring anti-A and anti-B antibodies' which are usually of IgM class do not cross the placenta, while immune anti-A and anti-B antibodies which are usually of IgG class may cross the placenta into foetal circulation and damage the foetal red cells. ABO HDN occurs most frequently in infants born to group O mothers who possess anti-A and/or anti-B IgG antibodies. ABO-HDN differs from Rh(D)-HDN, in that it occurs in first pregnancy, Coombs' (antiglobulin) test is generally negative, and is less severe than the latter.

CLINICAL AND LABORATORY FEATURES

i) The HDN due to Rh-D incompatibility in its *severest form* may result in intrauterine death from *hydrops foetalis*.
ii) *Moderate disease* produces a baby born with severe anaemia and jaundice due to unconjugated hyperbilirubinaemia.
iii) When the level of unconjugated bilirubin exceeds 20 mg/dl, it may result in deposition of bile pigment in the basal ganglia of the CNS called *kernicterus* and result in permanent brain damage.
iv) *Mild disease,* however, causes only severe anaemia with or without jaundice.

The course in HDN may range from death, to minimal haemolysis, to mental retardation. The practice of administration of anti-Rh immunoglobulin to the mother before or after delivery has reduced the incidence of HDN as well as protects the mother before the baby's RBCs sensitise the mother's blood. Exchange transfusion of the baby is done to remove the antibodies, remove red cells susceptible to haemolysis and also to lower the bilirubin level.

B. Microangiopathic Haemolytic Anaemia

Microangiopathic haemolytic anaemia is caused by abnormalities in the microvasculature. It is generally due to mechanical trauma to the red cells in circulation and is characterised by red cell fragmentation (schistocytosis). There are 3 different ways by which microangiopathic haemolytic anaemia results:

1. EXTERNAL IMPACT Direct external trauma to red blood cells when they pass through microcirculation, especially over the bony prominences, may cause haemolysis during various activities e.g. in prolonged marchers, joggers, karate players etc. These patients develop haemoglobinaemia, haemoglobinuria (march haemoglobinuria), and sometimes myoglobinuria as a result of damage to muscles.

2. CARDIAC HAEMOLYSIS A small proportion of patients who receive prosthetic cardiac valves or artificial grafts develop haemolysis. This has been attributed to direct mechanical trauma to the red cells or shear stress from turbulent blood flow.

3. FIBRIN DEPOSIT IN MICROVASCULATURE Deposition of fibrin in the microvasculature exposes the red cells to physical obstruction and eventual fragmentation of red cells and trapping of the platelets. Fibrin deposits in the small vessels may occur in the following conditions:

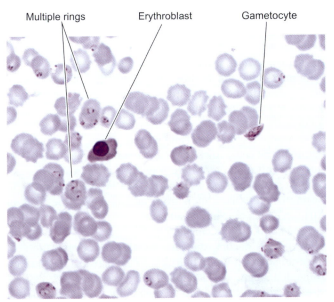

Figure 22.21 ► Malarial parasite, *Plasmodium falciparum*, in the peripheral blood showing numerous ring stages and a crescent of gametocyte. The background shows a normoblast.

i) *Abnormalities of the vessel wall* e.g. in hypertension, eclampsia, disseminated cancers, transplant rejection, haemangioma etc.
ii) *Thrombotic thrombocytopenic purpura*.
iii) *Haemolytic-uraemic syndrome*.
iv) *Disseminated intravascular coagulation* (DIC).
v) *Vasculitis in collagen diseases*.

C. Haemolytic Anaemia From Direct Toxic Effects

Haemolysis may result from direct toxic effects of certain agents. These include the following examples:
1. *Malaria* by direct parasitisation of red cells (black-water fever) **(Fig. 22.21)**.
2. *Bartonellosis* by direct infection of red cells by the microorganisms.
3. *Septicaemia* with *Clostridium welchii* by damaging the red cells.
4. *Other microorganisms* such as pneumococci, staphylococci and *Escherichia coli*.
5. *Copper* by direct haemolytic effect on red cells in Wilson's disease and patients on haemodialysis.
6. *Lead poisoning* shows basophilic stippling of red blood cells.
7. *Snake and spider bites* cause haemolysis by their venoms.
8. *Extensive burns*.

D. Paroxysmal Nocturnal Haemoglobinuria (PNH)

PNH is a rare acquired disorder of red cell membrane in which there is chronic intravascular haemolysis due to undue sensitivity of red blood cells to complement due to defective synthesis of a red cell membrane protein. The defect affects all the cells of myeloid progenitor lineage (RBCs, WBCs, platelets) suggesting a stem cell disorder causing deficient haematopoiesis. The disorder generally presents in adult life.

PATHOGENESIS PNH is considered as an acquired clonal disease of the cell membrane while normal clone also continues to proliferate. The defect is a mutation in the stem cells affecting myeloid progenitor cells that is normally required for the biosynthesis of glycosyl phosphatidyl inositol (GPI) essential for anchoring of the cell; the mutant form of the gene is an X-linked gene called PIG-A (phosphatidyl inositol glycan). Thus, as a result of mutation, there is partial or complete deficiency of anchor protein. Out of about 20 such proteins described so far, the lack of two of the proteins—*decay accelerating factor (DAF, CD55)* and a *membrane inhibitor of reactive lysis (MIRL, CD59)*, makes the RBCs unduly sensitive to the lytic effect of complement.

Since PNH is a stem cell disorder, it may be accompanied with other stem cell disorders such as aplastic anaemia and myelodysplastic syndrome.

CLINICAL AND LABORATORY FEATURES Clinical and laboratory findings are as under:
i) Haemolytic anaemia.
ii) Pancytopenia (mild granulocytopenia and thrombocytopenia frequent).
iii) Intermittent clinical haemoglobinuria; acute haemolytic episodes occur at night identified by passage of brown urine in the morning.
iv) Haemosiderinuria very common.
v) Venous thrombosis as a common complication.

E. Haemolytic Anaemia in Splenomegaly

Haemolytic anaemia is common in splenic enlargement from any cause (page 464). Normally, the spleen acts as a filter and traps the damaged red blood cells, destroys them and the splenic macrophages phagocytose the damaged red cells. A normal spleen poses no risk to normal red blood cells. But splenomegaly exaggerates the damaging effect to which the red cells are exposed. Besides haemolytic anaemia, splenomegaly is usually associated with pancytopenia. Splenectomy or reduction in size of spleen by appropriate therapy relieves the anaemia as well as improves the leucocyte and platelet counts.

II. HEREDITARY HAEMOLYTIC ANAEMIAS

Hereditary haemolytic anaemias are usually the result of intracorpuscular defects. Accordingly, they are broadly classified into 2 groups:
A. Hereditary abnormalities of red cell membrane.
B. Hereditary disorders of the interior of the red cells.

Section V: Haematology and Lymphoreticular Tissues

A. Hereditary Abnormalities of Red Cell Membrane

The abnormalities of red cell membrane are readily identified on blood film examination. There are 3 important types of inherited red cell membrane defects: hereditary spherocytosis, hereditary elliptocytosis (hereditary ovalocytosis) and hereditary stomatocytosis. However, hereditary spherocytosis is more common and discussed below.

Hereditary Spherocytosis

Hereditary spherocytosis (HS) is a common type of hereditary haemolytic anaemia of autosomal dominant inheritance in which the red cell membrane is abnormal. The molecular abnormality in HS is a defect in one of the proteins which anchor the lipid bilayer to the underlying cytoskeleton:

1. **Spectrin deficiency** Spectrin deficiency correlates with the severity of anaemia. Mutation in spectrin by recessive inheritance called α-*spectrin* causes more severe form of anaemia, while mutation by dominant inheritance forming β-*spectrin* results in mild form of the disease.

2. **Ankyrin abnormality** About half the cases of hereditary spherocytosis have defect in ankyrin.

Red cells with such unstable membrane but with normal volume, when released in circulation, lose their membrane further, till they can accommodate the given volume. This results in formation of spheroidal contour and smaller size of red blood cells, termed *microspherocytes*. These deformed red cells are not flexible, unlike normal biconcave red cells. These rigid cells are unable to pass through the spleen, and in the process they lose their surface membrane further. This produces a subpopulation of *hyperspheroidal red cells* in the peripheral blood which are subsequently destroyed in the spleen.

CLINICAL AND LABORATORY FEATURES The disorder may be clinically apparent at any age from infancy to old age and has equal sex incidence. The family history may be present. The major findings are as under:

1. *Anaemia* of mild to moderate degree.
2. *Reticulocytosis*, usually 5-20%.
3. Blood film shows the characteristic abnormality of erythrocytes in the form of microspherocytes (Fig. 22.22).
4. *MCV* is usually normal or slightly decreased but *MCHC* is increased.
5. *Osmotic fragility test* is helpful in testing the spheroidal nature of red cells which lyse more readily in solutions of low salt concentration i.e. *osmotic fragility is increased*.
6. *Direct Coombs' (antiglobulin) test* is negative so as to distinguish this condition from acquired spherocytosis of AIHA in which case it is positive.
7. *Splenomegaly* is a constant feature.
8. *Jaundice* occurs due to increased concentration of unconjugated (indirect) bilirubin in the plasma (also termed congenital haemolytic jaundice).
9. *Pigment gallstones* are frequent due to increased bile pigment production. Splenectomy offers the only reliable mode of treatment.

B. Hereditary Disorders of Red Cell Interior

Inherited disorders involving the interior of the red blood cells are classified into 2 groups:

1. **Red cell enzyme defects (Enzymopathies)** These cause defective red cell metabolism involving 2 pathways:
i) *Defects in the hexose monophosphate shunt:* Common example is glucose-6-phosphate dehydrogenase (G6PD) deficiency.
ii) *Defects in the Embden-Meyerhof (glycolytic) pathway:* Example is pyruvate kinase (PK) deficiency.

2. **Disorders of haemoglobin (haemoglobinopathies)** These are divided into 2 subgroups:

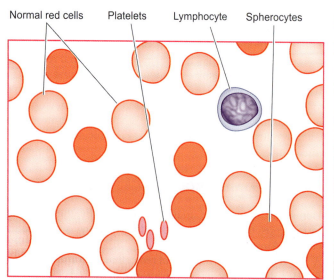
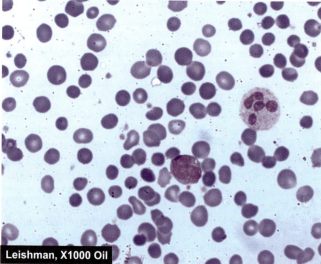

Figure 22.22 ▶ Peripheral blood film findings in hereditary spherocytosis.

i) *Structurally abnormal haemoglobin (Qualitative disorders):* Examples are sickle syndromes and other haemoglobinopathies.

ii) *Reduced globin chain synthesis (Quantitative disorders):* Common examples is various types of thalassaemias.

These disorders are discussed below.

Red Cell Enzyme Defects (Enzymopathies)

G6PD DEFICIENCY

Among the defects in hexose monophosphate shunt, the most common is G6PD deficiency. It affects millions of people throughout the world. G6PD gene is located on the X chromosome and its deficiency is, therefore, a sex (X)-linked trait affecting males, while the females are carriers and are asymptomatic. Several variants of G6PD have been described. The most common and significant clinical variant is A–(negative) type found in black males. Like the HbS gene, the A-type G6PD variant confers protection against malaria. Individuals with A–type G6PD variant have shortened red cell lifespan but without anaemia. However, these individuals develop haemolytic episodes on exposure to oxidant stress such as viral and bacterial infections, certain drugs (antimalarials, sulfonamides, nitrofurantoin, aspirin, vitamin K), metabolic acidosis and on ingestion of fava beans (favism).

Normally, red blood cells are well protected against oxidant stress because of adequate generation of reduced glutathione via the hexose monophosphate shunt. Individuals with inherited deficiency of G6PD, an enzyme required for hexose monophosphate shunt for glucose metabolism, fail to develop adequate levels of reduced glutathione in their red cells. This results in oxidation and precipitation of haemoglobin within the red cells forming Heinz bodies. Besides G6PD deficiency, deficiency of various other enzymes involved in the hexose monophosphate shunt may also infrequently cause clinical problems.

CLINICAL AND LABORATORY FEATURES These are as under:

1. Acute haemolytic anaemia This develops in males, being X-linked disorder, within hours of exposure to oxidant stress. The haemolysis is, however, self-limiting even if the exposure to the oxidant is continued since it *affects the older red cells only*. Haemoglobin level may return to normal when the older population of red cells has been destroyed and only younger cells remain. Formation of Heinz bodies is visualised by means of supravital stains such as crystal violet, also called *Heinz body haemolytic anaemia*. However, Heinz bodies are not seen after the first one or two days since they are removed by the spleen, leading to formation of 'bite cells' and fragmented red cells. Features of intravascular haemolysis such as rise in plasma haemoglobin, haemoglobinuria (seen as darkening of urine), rise in unconjugated bilirubin (jaundice) and fall in plasma haptoglobin (from haemoglobinaemia) are other laboratory findings.

2. Chronic haemolytic anaemia Cases having severe enzyme deficiency have chronic persistent haemolysis throughout life.

3. Between the crises, the affected patient generally has no anaemia. The red cell survival is, however, shortened.

4. Neonatal jaundice Infants born with G6PD deficiency may continue to have unconjugated hyperbilirubinaemia and may even develop kernicterus.

Treatment is directed towards the prevention of haemolytic episodes such as stoppage of offending drug.

Haemoglobinopathies

Haemoglobin in RBCs may be abnormally synthesised due to inherited defects. These disorders may be of two types:

◆ *Qualitative disorders* in which there is structural abnormality in synthesis of haemoglobin e.g. sickle cell syndrome, other haemoglobinopathies.

◆ *Quantitative disorders* in which there quantitatively decreased globin chain synthesis of haemoglobin e.g. thalassaemias.

Both these groups of disorders may occur as *homozygous* state in which both genes coding for that character are abnormal, or *heterozygous* when one gene is abnormal and the other gene is normal. However, there are examples of combined disorders too in which there are two different mutations in loci of two corresponding genes (i.e. double heterozygous) e.g. HbS gene from one parent and β-thal gene from the other parent resulting in $\beta^S\beta^{thal}$. There are geographic variations in the distribution of various haemoglobinopathies world over. These disorders may vary in presentation from asymptomatic laboratory abnormalities to intrauterine death.

Major examples are briefly discussed below.

SICKLE SYNDROMES

The most important and widely prevalent type of haemoglobinopathy is due to the presence of sickle haemoglobin (HbS) in the red blood cells. The red cells with HbS develop 'sickling' when they are exposed to low oxygen tension. Sickle syndromes have the highest frequency in black race and in Central Africa. Patients with HbS are relatively protected against falciparum malaria. Sickle syndromes occur in 3 different forms:

1. *As heterozygous state* for HbS: sickle cell trait (AS).
2. *As homozygous state* for HbS: sickle cell anaemia (SS).
3. *As double heterozygous states* e.g. sickle β-thalassaemia, sickle-C disease (SC), sickle-D disease (SD).

Heterozygous State: Sickle Cell Trait

Sickle cell trait (AS) is a benign heterozygous state of HbS in which only one abnormal gene is inherited. Patients with AS develop no significant clinical problems except when they become severely hypoxic and may develop sickle cell crises. These case may show following laboratory features:

1. *Demonstration of sickling* done under condition of reduced oxygen tension by an oxygen consuming reagent, sodium metabisulfite.
2. *Haemoglobin electrophoresis* reveals 35-40% of the total haemoglobin as HbS.

Homozygous State: Sickle Cell Anaemia

Sickle cell anaemia (SS) is a homozygous state of HbS in the red cells in which an abnormal gene is inherited from each parent. SS is a severe disorder associated with protean clinical manifestations and decreased life expectancy.

1. Basic molecular lesion In HbS, basic genetic defect is the *single point mutation* in one amino acid out of 146 in haemoglobin molecule—there is *substitution of valine for glutamic acid* at 6-residue position of the β-globin, producing Hb $\alpha_2\beta_2^s$.

2. Mechanism of sickling During deoxygenation, the red cells containing HbS change from biconcave disc shape to an elongated crescent-shaped or sickle-shaped cell. This process termed *sickling* occurs both within the intact red cells and *in vitro* in free solution. The mechanism responsible for sickling upon deoxygenation of HbS-containing red cells is the polymerisation of deoxygenated HbS which aggregates to form elongated rod-like polymers. These elongated fibres align and distort the red cell into classic sickle shape.

3. Reversible-irreversible sickling The oxygen-dependent sickling process is usually reversible. However, damage to red cell membrane leads to formation of irreversibly sickled red cells even after they are exposed to normal oxygen tension.

4. Factors determining rate of sickling: Following factors determine the rate at which the polymerisation of HbS and consequent sickling take place:
i) *Presence of non-HbS haemoglobins:* The red cells in patients of SS have predominance of HbS and a small part consists of non-HbS haemoglobins, chiefly HbF (2-20% of the total haemoglobin). HbF-containing red cells are protected from sickling while HbA-containing red cells participate readily in co-polymerisation with HbS.
ii) *Intracellular concentration of HbS.*
iii) *Total haemoglobin concentration.*
iv) *Extent of deoxygenation.*
v) *Acidosis and dehydration.*
vi) *Increased concentration of 2, 3-BPG in the red cells.*

CLINICAL AND LABORATORY FEATURES The clinical manifestations of homozygous sickle cell disease are widespread. The symptoms begin to appear after 6th month of life when most of the HbF is replaced by HbS. Infection and folic acid deficiency result in more severe clinical manifestations (Fig. 22.23):

1. Anaemia There is usually severe chronic haemolytic anaemia (primarily extravascular) with onset of aplastic crisis in between. The symptoms of anaemia are generally

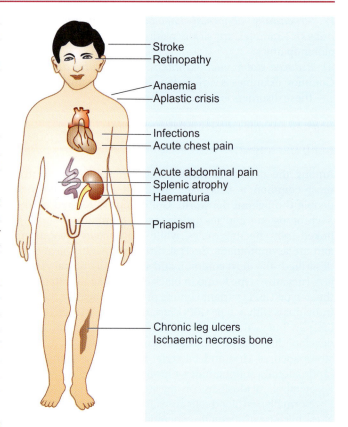

Figure 22.23 ▶ Major clinical manifestations of sickle cell disease.

mild since HbS gives up oxygen more readily than HbA to the tissues.

2. Blood smear PBS shows sickle cells and target cells and features of splenic atrophy such as presence of Howell-Jolly bodies (Fig. 22.24).

3. A positive **sickling test** with a reducing substance such as sodium metabisulfite.

4. Haemoglobin electrophoresis shows no normal HbA but shows predominance of HbS and 2-20% HbF.

5. Vaso-occlusive phenomena Patients of SS develop recurrent vaso-occlusive episodes throughout their lives due to obstruction to capillary blood flow by sickled red cells upon deoxygenation or dehydration. Vaso-obstruction affecting different organs and tissues results in infarcts which may be of 2 types:
i) *Microinfarcts* affecting particularly the abdomen, chest, back and joints and are the cause of recurrent painful crises in SS.
ii) *Macroinfarcts* involving most commonly the spleen (splenic sequestration, autosplenectomy), bone marrow (pains), bones (aseptic necrosis, osteomyelitis), lungs (pulmonary infections), kidneys (renal cortical necrosis), CNS (stroke), retina (damage) and skin (ulcers), and result in anatomic and functional damage to these organs.

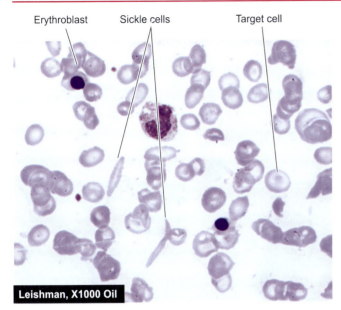

Figure 22.24 ▶ Sickle cell anaemia. PBF shows crescent shaped elongated red blood cells, a few target cells and a few erythroblasts.

6. Constitutional symptoms In addition to the features of anaemia and infarction, patients with SS have impaired growth and development and increased susceptibility to infection due to markedly impaired splenic function.

Double Heterozygous States

Double heterozygous conditions involving combination of HbS with other haemoglobinopathies may occur. Most common among these are sickle-β-thalassaemia ($\beta^S\beta^{thal}$), sickle C disease (SC), and sickle D disease (SD). All these disorders behave like mild form of sickle cell disease.

HBC HAEMOGLOBINOPATHY

HbC haemoglobinopathy is prevalent in West Africa and in American blacks. The molecular lesion in HbC is substitution of lysine for glutamic acid at β-6 globin chain position. The disorder of HbC may occur as benign homozygous HbC disease, or as asymptomatic heterozygous HbC trait, or as double heterozygous combinations such as sickle-HbC disease and HbC-β thalassaemia.

Thalassaemias

The thalassaemias are a diverse group of hereditary disorders in which there is reduced synthesis of one or more of the globin polypeptide chains. Thus, thalassaemias, unlike haemoglobinopathies which are qualitative disorders of haemoglobin, are *quantitative abnormalities of polypeptide globin chain synthesis*. Thalassaemias were first described in people of Mediterranean countries (North Africa, Southern Europe) from where it derives its name 'Mediterranean anaemia.' The condition also occurs in the Middle East, Indian subcontinent, South-East Asia and, in general in blacks. In India, thalassaemia is seen through country and an estimated 35 million have β-thalassaemia major. Its incidence is particularly high in some races such as Punjabis who migrated from Pakistan after partition, Bengalis, Gujaratis and Parsis.

GENETICS AND CLASSIFICATION

Thalassaemias are genetically transmitted disorders. Normally, an individual inherits two β-globin genes located one each on two chromosomes 11, and two α-globin genes one each on two chromosomes 16, from each parent i.e. normal adult haemoglobin (HbA) is $\alpha_2\beta_2$.* Depending upon whether the genetic defect or deletion lies in transmission of α- or β-globin chain genes, thalassaemias are classified into α- and β-thalassaemias. Thus, patients with α-thalassaemia have structurally normal α-globin chains but their production is impaired. Similarly, in β-thalassaemia, β-globin chains are structurally normal but their production is decreased. Each of the two main types of thalassaemias may occur as heterozygous (called *α- and β-thalassaemia minor* or *trait*), or as homozygous state (termed *α- and β-thalassaemia major*). The former is generally asymptomatic, while the latter is a severe congenital haemolytic anaemia.

A classification of various types of thalassaemias along with the clinical syndromes produced and salient laboratory findings are given in **Table 22.9**.

PATHOPHYSIOLOGY OF ANAEMIA IN THALASSAEMIA

A constant feature of all forms of thalassaemia is the presence of anaemia which occurs from following mechanisms:

α-Thalassaemia In α-thalassaemia major, the obvious cause of anaemia is the inability to synthesise adult haemoglobin, while in α-thalassaemia trait there is reduced production of normal adult haemoglobin.

β-Thalassaemia In β-thalassaemia major, the most important cause of anaemia is premature red cell destruction brought about by erythrocyte membrane damage caused by the precipitated α-globin chains. Other contributory factors are: shortened red cell lifespan, ineffective erythropoiesis, and haemodilution due to increased plasma volume. A deficiency of β-globin chains in β-thalassaemia leads to large excess of α-chains within the developing red cells. Part of these excessive α-chains are removed by pairing with γ-globin chains as HbF, while the remainder unaccompanied

---

*In a normal adult, distribution of haemoglobin is as under: HbA ($\alpha_2\beta_2$) = 95-98%, HbA2 ($\alpha_2\delta_2$)(a minor variant of HbA) = 1.5-3.5%, HbF ($\alpha_2\gamma_2$) = less than 1%. But the level of HbF in children under 6 months is slightly higher.

Table 22.9	Classification of thalassaemias.				
	TYPE	HB	HB-ELECTROPHORESIS	GENOTYPE	CLINICAL SYNDROME
α-THALASSAEMIAS					
1.	*Hydrops foetalis*	3-10 gm/dl	Hb Barts (γ_4) (100%)	Deletion of four α-genes	Fatal *in utero* or in early infancy
2.	*Hb-H disease*	2-12 gm/dl	HbF (10%), HbH (2-4%)	Deletion of three α-genes	Haemolytic anaemia
3.	*α-Thalassaemia trait*	10-14 gm/dl	Almost normal	Deletion of two α-genes	Microcytic hypochromic blood picture but no anaemia
β-THALASSAEMIAS					
1.	*β-Thalassaemia major*	< 5 gm/dl	HbA (0-50%), HbF (50-98%)	$\beta^{thal}/\beta^{thal}$	Severe congenital haemolytic anaemia, requires blood transfusions
2.	*β-Thalassaemia intermedia*	5-10 gm/dl	Variable	Multiple mechanisms	Severe anaemia, but regular blood transfusions not required
3.	*β-Thalassaemia minor*	10-12 gm/dl	HbA$_2$ (4-9%), HbF (1-5%)	β^{A}/β^{thal}	Usually asymptomatic

α-chains precipitate rapidly within the red cell as *Heinz bodies*. The precipitated α-chains cause red cell membrane damage. During their passage through the splenic sinusoids, these red cells are further damaged and develop pitting due to removal of the precipitated aggregates. Thus, such red cells are irreparably damaged and are phagocytosed by the RE cells of the spleen and the liver causing anaemia, hepatosplenomegaly, and excess of tissue iron stores. Patients with β-thalassaemia minor, on the other hand, have very mild ineffective erythropoiesis, haemolysis and shortening of red cell lifespan.

α-THALASSAEMIA

α-thalassaemias are disorders in which there is defective synthesis of α-globin chains resulting in depressed production of haemoglobins that contain α-chains i.e. HbA, HbA$_2$ and HbF. The α-thalassaemias are most commonly due to deletion of one or more of the α-chain genes located on short arm of chromosome 16. Since there is a pair of α-chain genes, the clinical manifestations of α-thalassaemia depend upon the number of genes deleted. Accordingly, α-thalassaemias are classified into 4 types:
1. Four α-gene deletion: Hb Bart's hydrops foetalis.
2. Three α-gene deletion: HbH disease.
3. Two α-gene deletion: α-thalassaemia trait.
4. One α-gene deletion: α-thalassaemia trait (carrier).

Hb Bart's Hydrops Foetalis

When there is deletion of all the four α-chain genes (homozygous state) it results in total suppression of α-globin chain synthesis causing the most severe form of α-thalassaemia called Hb Bart's hydrops foetalis. Hb Bart's is a gamma globin chain tetramer (γ_4) which has high oxygen affinity leading to severe tissue hypoxia.

CLINICAL AND LABORATORY FEATURES Hb Bart's hydrops foetalis is incompatible with life due to severe tissue hypoxia. The condition is either fatal *in utero* or the infant dies shortly after birth. If born alive, the features similar to severe Rh haemolytic disease are present. Haemoglobin electrophoresis shows 80-90% Hb-Bart's and a small amount of Hb-H and Hb-Portland but no HbA, HbA$_2$ or HbF.

HbH Disease

Deletion of three α-chain genes produces HbH which is a β-globin chain tetramer (β_4) and markedly impaired α-chain synthesis. HbH is precipitated as Heinz bodies within the affected red cells. An elongated α-chain variant of HbH disease is termed *Hb Constant Spring*.

CLINICAL AND LABORATORY FEATURES HbH disease is generally present as a well-compensated haemolytic anaemia. The features are intermediate between that of β-thalassaemia minor and major. The severity of anaemia fluctuates and may fall to very low levels during pregnancy or infections. Majority of patients have splenomegaly and may develop cholelithiasis. Haemoglobin electrophoresis shows 2-4% HbH and the remainder consists of HbA, HbA$_2$ and HbF.

α-Thalassaemia Trait

α-thalassaemia trait may occur by the following molecular pathogenesis:
◆ By deletion of two of the four α-chain genes in homozygous form called *homozygous α-thalassaemia*, or in double heterozygous form termed *heterozygous α-thalassaemia*.
◆ By deletion of a single α-chain gene causing heterozygous α-thalassaemia trait called *heterozygous α-thalassaemia*.

CLINICAL AND LABORATOY FEATURES α-thalassaemia trait due to two α-chain gene deletion is asymptomatic. It is suspected in a patient of refractory microcytic hypochromic anaemia in whom iron deficiency and β-thalassaemia minor have been excluded and the patient belongs to the high-risk ethnic group. One gene deletion α-thalassaemia trait is a silent carrier state. Haemoglobin electrophoresis reveals small amount of Hb-Bart's in neonatal period (1-2% in α-thalassaemia 2 and 5-6% in α-thalassaemia 1) which gradually disappears by adult life. HbA_2 is either normal or slightly decreased (contrary to the elevated HBA_2 levels in β-thalassaemia trait).

β-THALASSAEMIAS

β-thalassaemias are caused by decreased rate of β-chain synthesis resulting in reduced formation of HbA in the red cells. The molecular pathogenesis of the β-thalassaemias is more complex than that of α-thalassaemias. In contrast to α-thalassaemia, gene deletion rarely ever causes β-thalassaemia and is only seen in an entity called *hereditary persistence of foetal haemoglobin (HPFH)*. Instead, most of β-thalassaemias arise from different types of mutations of β-globin gene resulting from single base changes. The symbol β° is used to indicate the complete absence of β-globin chain synthesis while β+ denotes partial synthesis of the β-globin chains. More than 100 such mutations have been described affecting the preferred sites in the coding sequences. Some of the important ones having effects on β-globin chain synthesis are as under:

i) *Transcription defect:* Mutation affecting transcriptional promoter sequence causing reduced synthesis of β-globin chain. Hence the result is partially preserved synthesis i.e. β+ *thalassaemia*.

ii) *Translation defect:* Mutation in the coding sequence causing stop codon (chain termination) interrupting β-globin messenger RNA. This would result in no synthesis of β-globin chain i.e. β° *thalassaemia*.

iii) *mRNA splicing defect:* Mutation leads to defective mRNA processing forming abnormal mRNA that is degraded in the nucleus. Depending upon whether part of splice site remains intact or is totally degraded, it may result in β+ *thalassaemia* or β° *thalassaemia*.

Depending upon the extent of reduction in β-chain synthesis, there are 3 types of β-thalassaemia:

1. **Homozygous form: β-Thalassaemia major** It is the most severe form of congenital haemolytic anaemia. It is further of 2 types:
   i) *β° thalassaemia major* characterised by complete absence of β-chain synthesis.
   ii) *β+ thalassaemia major* having incomplete suppression of β-chain synthesis.

2. **β-Thalassaemia intermedia** It is β-thalassaemia of intermediate degree of severity that does not require regular blood transfusions. These cases are genetically heterozygous (β°/β or β+/β).

3. **Heterozygous form: β-thalassaemia minor (trait)** It is a mild asymptomatic condition in which there is moderate suppression of β-chain synthesis.

An individual may inherit one β-chain gene from each parent and produce heterozygous, homozygous, or double heterozygous states. Statistically, 25% of offsprings born to two heterozygotes (i.e. β-thalassaemia trait) will have the homozygous state i.e. β-thalassaemia major.

β-*Thalassaemia Major*

β-thalassaemia major, also termed Mediterranean or Cooley's anaemia is the most common form of congenital haemolytic anaemia. β-thalassaemia major is a homozygous state with either complete absence of β-chain synthesis (β° *thalassaemia major*) or only small amounts of β-chains are formed (β+ thalassaemia major). These result in excessive formation of alternate haemoglobins, HbF ($α_2γ_2$) and HbA_2 ($α_2δ_2$).

CLINICAL AND LABORATORY FEATURES The condition appears insidiously and has following features:

1. Anaemia starts appearing within the first 4-6 months of life when the switch over from γ-chain to β-chain production occurs. It is generally severe.
2. Marked hepatosplenomegaly occurs due to excessive red cell destruction, extramedullary haematopoiesis and iron overload.
3. Expansion of bones occurs due to marked erythroid hyperplasia leading to thalassaemic facies and malocclusion of the jaw.
4. Iron overload due to repeated blood transfusions causes damage to the endocrine organs resulting in slow rate of growth and development, delayed puberty, diabetes mellitus and damage to the liver and heart **(Fig. 22.25)**.
5. *Blood film* shows severe microcytic hypochromic red cell morphology, marked anisopoikilocytosis, basophilic stippling, presence of many target cells, tear drop cells and normoblasts **(Fig. 22.26)**.
6. *Serum bilirubin* (unconjugated) is generally raised.
7. *Reticulocytosis* is generally present.
8. *MCV, MCH and MCHC* are significantly reduced.
9. Osmotic fragility characteristically reveals increased resistance to saline haemolysis i.e. *decreased osmotic fragility*.
10. *Haemoglobin electrophoresis* shows presence of increased amounts of HbF, increased amount of HbA_2, and almost complete absence or presence of variable amounts of HbA. The increased level of HbA_2 has not been found in any other haemoglobin abnormality except β-thalassaemia. The increased synthesis of HbA_2 is probably due to increased activity at both δ-chain loci.
10. *Bone marrow aspirate examination* shows normoblastic erythroid hyperplasia with predominance of intermediate and late normoblasts which are generally smaller in size than normal. Iron staining demonstrates siderotic granules in the

Section V: Haematology and Lymphoreticular Tissues

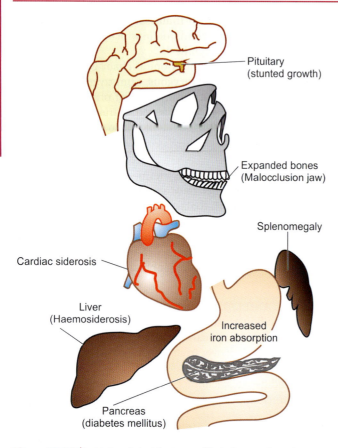

Figure 22.25 ▶ Major clinical features of β-thalassaemia major.

cytoplasm of normoblasts, increased reticuloendothelial iron but ring sideroblasts are only occasionally seen.

Since these patients require multiple blood transfusions, they are at increased risk of developing AIDS. In general, patients with β-thalassaemia major have short life expectancy. The biggest problem is iron overload and consequent myocardial siderosis leading to cardiac arrhythmias, congestive heart failure, and ultimately death.

β-*Thalassaemia Minor*

The β-thalassaemia minor or β-thalassaemia trait, a heterozygous state, is a common entity characterised by moderate reduction in β-chain synthesis.

CLINICAL AND LABORATORY FEATURES Clinically, the condition is usually asymptomatic and the diagnosis is generally made when the patient is being investigated for mild chronic anaemia. The spleen may be palpable. Osmotic fragility test shows increased resistance to haemolysis i.e. *decreased osmotic fragility. Haemoglobin electrophoresis* is confirmatory for the diagnosis and shows about two-fold increase in HbA_2 and a slight elevation in HbF (2-3%).

ANAEMIA DUE TO BLOOD LOSS

Depending upon the rate of blood loss due to haemorrhage, the effects of post-haemorrhagic anaemia appear.

ACUTE BLOOD LOSS When the loss of blood occurs suddenly, the following events take place:
i) Immediate threat to life due to hypovolaemia which may result in shock and death.
ii) If the patient survives, shifting of interstitial fluid to intravascular compartment with consequent haemodilution with low haematocrit.
iii) Hypoxia stimulates production of erythropoietin resulting in increased marrow erythropoiesis.

CHRONIC BLOOD LOSS When the loss of blood is slow and insidious, the effects of anaemia will become apparent

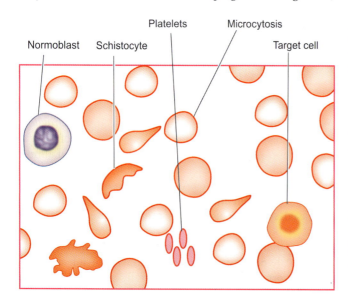

Figure 22.26 ▶ Peripheral blood film findings in β-thalassaemia major.

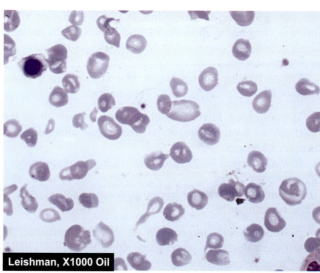

only when the rate of loss is more than rate of production and the iron stores are depleted. This results in iron deficiency anaemia (page 371).

| GIST BOX 22.6 | Haemolytic Anaemias and Anaemia Due to Blood Loss |

- Haemolytic anaemias (HA) result from an increased rate of red cell destruction and premature destruction of red cells either at intravascular or extravascular locations, the latter is more common.
- HA are divided into hereditary and acquired, the former are more common.
- Immune HA are due to antibody production in the body against own red cells. These may be autoimmune (warm and cold antibody), drug-induced or isoimmune (haemolytic disease of the newborn, HDN).
- Microangiopathic HA are caused due to abnormalities in the microvasculature.
- PNH is a chronic acquired HA due to defect in the stem cells and hence affects all cells in myeloid progenitor lineage.
- Hereditary defects in the red cell membrane are spherocytosis (spectrin deficiency or ankyrin defect), elliptocytosis (spectrin or protein 4.1 defect) and stomatocytosis.
- Inherited defects in red cell enzymes are deficiency of G6PD and pyruvate kinase.
- Haemoglobinopathies may be qualitative (structural e.g. sickle cell syndrome) or quantitative (reduced globin synthesis e.g. thalassaemia) disorders of haemoglobin.
- Sickle cell syndrome is widely prevalent and is due to genetic defect of a single point mutation. Red cells have sickle haemoglobin which undergo sickling when they are exposed to low oxygen tension. There is vasoocclusive phenomenon.
- Thalassaemias are hereditary defects of reduced synthesis of either α-(α-thalassaemia) or β-(β-thalassaemia) globin chains which are structurally normal.
- β-thalassaemia is more common and may occur as a trait (heterozygous) or major (homozygous) form of disease.
- β-thalassaemia major has high foetal haemoglobin, anaemia, hepatosplenomegaly and iron overload.
- β-thalassaemia trait cases have mild persistent anaemia and high HbA2.

APLASTIC ANAEMIA AND OTHER PRIMARY BONE MARROW DISORDERS

'Bone marrow failure' is the term used for primary disorders of the bone marrow which result in impaired formation of the erythropoietic precursors and consequent anaemia. It includes the following disorders:
1. *Aplastic anaemia*, most importantly.

2. *Other primary bone marrow disorders* e.g. myelophthisic anaemia, pure red cell aplasia, and myelodysplastic syndromes.

These disorders are examples of hypoproliferative anaemias in which anaemia is not the only finding but the major problem is pancytopenia i.e. anaemia, leucopenia and thrombocytopenia. While myelodysplastic syndromes are discussed in Chapter 24 (page 439), other conditions are considered below.

APLASTIC ANAEMIA

Aplastic anaemia is defined as pancytopenia (i.e. simultaneous presence of anaemia, leucopenia and thrombocytopenia) resulting from aplasia of the bone marrow. The underlying defect in all cases appears to be sufficient reduction in the number of haematopoietic pluripotent stem cells which results in decreased or total absence of these cells for division and differentiation.

Etiology and Classification

More than half the cases of aplastic anaemia are idiopathic. Cases with known etiology are classified into 2 main types (Table 22.10): primary and secondary:

A. PRIMARY APLASTIC ANAEMIA Primary aplastic anaemia includes 2 entities: a congenital form called Fanconi's anaemia and an immunologically-mediated acquired form.

1. Fanconi's anaemia This has an autosomal recessive inheritance and is often associated with other congenital anomalies such as skeletal and renal abnormalities, and sometimes mental retardation.

2. Immune causes In many cases, suppression of haematopoietic stem cells by immunologic mechanisms

| Table 22.10 | Causes of aplastic anaemia. |

A. PRIMARY APLASTIC ANAEMIA
 1. Fanconi's anaemia (congenital)
 2. Immunologically-mediated (acquired)
B. SECONDARY APLASTIC ANAEMIA
 1. Drugs
  i) Dose-related aplasia e.g. with antimetabolites (methotrexate), mitotic inhibitors (daunorubicin), alkylating agents (busulfan), nitroso urea, anthracyclines.
  ii) Idiosyncratic aplasia e.g. with chloramphenicol, sulfa drugs, oxyphenbutazone, phenylbutazone, chlorpromazine, gold salts.
 2. Toxic chemicals e.g. benzene derivatives, insecticides, arsenicals.
 3. Infections e.g. infectious hepatitis, EB virus infection, AIDS, other viral illnesses.
 4. Miscellaneous e.g. association with SLE and therapeutic X-rays

may cause aplastic anaemia. The observations in support of autoimmune mechanisms are the clinical response to immunosuppressive therapy and *in vitro* marrow culture experiments.

B. SECONDARY APLASTIC ANAEMIA Secondary causes are more common than primary and include a variety of industrial, physical, chemical, iatrogenic and infectious causes:

1. Drugs A number of drugs are cytotoxic to the marrow and cause aplastic anaemia. The association of a drug with aplastic anaemia may be either predictably dose-related or an idiosyncratic reaction.

i) *Dose-related aplasia* of the bone marrow occurs with antimetabolites (e.g. methotrexate), mitotic inhibitors (e.g. daunorubicin), alkylating agents (e.g. busulfan), nitroso urea and anthracyclines. In such cases, withdrawal of the drug usually allows recovery of the marrow elements.

ii) *Idiosyncratic aplasia* is depression of the bone marrow due to qualitatively abnormal reaction of an individual to a drug when first administered. The most serious and most common example of idiosyncratic aplasia is associated with chloramphenicol. Other such common drugs are sulfa drugs, oxyphenbutazone, phenylbutazone, chlorpromazine, gold salts etc.

2. Toxic chemicals These include examples of industrial, domestic and accidental use of substances such as benzene derivatives, insecticides, arsenicals etc.

3. Infections Aplastic anaemia may occur following viral hepatitis, Epstein-Barr virus infection, AIDS and other viral illnesses.

4. Miscellaneous Lastly, aplastic anaemia has been reported in association with certain other illnesses such as SLE, and with therapeutic X-rays.

Clinical Features

The onset of aplastic anaemia may occur at any age and is usually insidious. The clinical manifestations include the following:
1. Anaemia and its symptoms like mild progressive weakness and fatigue.
2. Haemorrhage from various sites due to thrombocytopenia such as from the skin, nose, gums, vagina, bowel, and occasionally in the CNS and retina.
3. Infections of the mouth and throat are commonly present.
4. The lymph nodes, liver and spleen are generally not enlarged.

Laboratory Findings

The diagnosis of aplastic anaemia is made by a thorough laboratory evaluation and excluding other causes of pancytopenia (Table 22.11). The following haematological features are found:

Table 22.11 Causes of pancytopenia.

I. Aplastic anaemia (Table 22.10)
II. Pancytopenia with normal or increased marrow cellularity e.g.
  1. Myelodysplastic syndromes
  2. Hypersplenism
  3. Megaloblastic anaemia
III. Paroxysmal nocturnal haemoglobinuria (page 389)
IV. Bone marrow infiltrations e.g.
  1. Haematologic malignancies (leukaemias, lymphomas, myeloma)
  2. Non-haematologic metastatic malignancies
  3. Storage diseases
  4. Osteopetrosis
  5. Myelofibrosis

1. Anaemia Haemoglobin levels are moderately reduced. The blood picture generally shows normocytic normochromic anaemia but sometimes macrocytosis may be present. The reticulocyte count is reduced or zero.

2. Leucopenia The absolute granulocyte count is particularly low (below 1500/µl) with relative lymphocytosis. The neutrophils are morphologically normal but their alkaline phosphatase score is high.

3. Thrombocytopenia Platelet count is always reduced.

4. Bone marrow examination A bone marrow aspirate may yield a 'dry tap'. A trephine biopsy is generally essential for making the diagnosis which reveals patchy cellular areas in a hypocellular or aplastic marrow due to replacement by fat. There is usually a severe depression of myeloid cells, megakaryocytes and erythroid cells so that the marrow chiefly consists of lymphocytes and plasma cells **(Fig. 22.27)**. Haematopoietic stem cells bearing CD34 marker are markedly reduced or absent.

Severe aplastic anaemia is a serious disorder terminating in death within 6-12 months in 50-80% of cases. Death is usually due to bleeding and/or infection.

OTHER PRIMARY BONE MARROW DIORDERS
MYELOPHTHISIC ANAEMIA

MYELOPHTHISIC ANAEMIA Development of severe anaemia may result from infiltration of the marrow termed as myelophthisic anaemia. The causes for marrow infiltrations include the following **(Table 22.11)**:
1. Haematologic malignancies (e.g. leukaemia, lymphoma, myeloma).
2. Metastatic deposits from non-haematologic malignancies (e.g. cancer breast, stomach, prostate, lung, thyroid).
3. Advanced tuberculosis.
4. Primary lipid storage diseases (Gaucher's and Niemann-Pick disease).
5. Osteopetrosis and myelofibrosis may rarely cause myelophthisis.

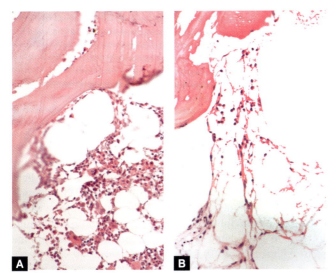

Figure 22.27 ▶ Bone marrow trephine biopsy in aplastic anaemia contrasted against normal cellular marrow. A, normal marrow biopsy shows about 50% fatty spaces and about 50% is haematopoietic marrow which contains a heterogeneous mixture of myeloid, erythroid and lymphoid cells. B, In aplastic anaemia, the biopsy shows suppression of myeloid and erythroid cells and replacement of haematopoietic elements by fat. There are scanty foci of cellular components composed chiefly of lymphoid cells.

Treatment consists of reversing the underlying pathologic process.

PURE RED CELL APLASIA Pure red cell aplasia (PRCA) is a rare syndrome involving a selective failure in the production of erythroid elements in the bone marrow but with normal granulopoiesis and megakaryocytopoiesis. Patients have normocytic normochromic anaemia with normal granulocyte and platelet count. Reticulocytes are markedly decreased or are absent.

PRCA exists in the following forms:

1. **Transient self-limited PRCA** It is due to temporary marrow failure in aplastic crisis in haemolytic anaemias and in acute B19 parvovirus infection and in transient erythroblastopenia in normal children.

2. **Acquired PRCA** It is seen in middle-aged adults in association with some other diseases, most commonly thymoma; others are connective tissue diseases (SLE, rheumatoid arthritis), lymphoid malignancies (lymphoma, T-cell chronic lymphocytic leukaemia) and solid tumours.

3. **Chronic B19 parvovirus infections** PRCA may occur from chronic B19 parvovirus infection in children and is common and treatable. B19 parvovirus produces cytopathic effects on the marrow erythroid precursor cells and are characteristically seen as giant pronormoblasts.

4. **Congenital PRCA (Blackfan-Diamond syndrome)** It is a rare chronic disorder detected at birth or in early childhood. It occurs due to mutation in a ribosomal RNA processing gene termed as *RPS19*.

> **GIST BOX 22.7 Aplastic Anaemia and Other Primary Bone Marrow Disorders**
>
> ❖ Aplastic anaemia is pancytopenia due to aplasia of bone marrow. It may be primary (inherited) or secondary (acquired). Secondary causes are more common and may be due to drugs, toxic chemicals or viral infections.
> ❖ Other primary bone marrow failure disorders are myelophthisic anaemia (from marrow infiltration), pure red cell aplasia (selective failure of marrow erythropoiesis) and myelodysplastic syndromes.

23 Platelets and Bleeding Disorders

PLATELETS

THROMBOPOIESIS

As illustrated in Fig. 22.3, the trilineage myeloid stem cells in the bone marrow differentiate into erythroid progenitor, granulocyte-monocyte progenitor, and megakaryocyte progenitor cells. Platelets are formed in the bone marrow by a process of fragmentation of the cytoplasm of megakaryocytes. Platelet production is under the control of thrombopoietin, the nature and origin of which are not yet established. The stages in platelet production are: megakaryoblast, promegakaryocyte, megakaryocyte, and discoid platelets (Fig. 23.1).

MEGAKARYOBLAST The earliest precursor of platelets in the bone marrow is megakaryoblast. It arises from haematopoietic stem cell by a process of differentiation.

PROMEGAKARYOCYTE A megakaryoblast undergoes endo-reduplication of nuclear chromatin i.e. nuclear chromatin replicates repeatedly in multiples of two without division of the cell. Ultimately, a large cell containing up to 32 times the normal diploid content of nuclear DNA (polyploidy) is formed when further nuclear replication ceases and cytoplasm becomes granular.

MEGAKARYOCYTE A mature megakaryocyte is a large cell, 30-90 μm in diameter, and contains 4-16 nuclear lobes having coarsely clumped chromatin. The cytoplasm is abundant, light blue in colour and contains red-purple granules. Platelets are formed from pseudopods of megakaryocyte cytoplasm which get detached into the blood stream. Each megakaryocyte may form up to 4000 platelets. The formation of platelets from the stem cell takes about 10 days.

PLATELETS Platelets are small (1-4 μm in diameter), discoid, non-nucleate structures containing red-purple granules. The normal platelet count ranges from 150,000-400,000/μl and the lifespan of platelets is 7-10 days. About 70% of platelets are in circulation while remaining 30% lie sequestered in the spleen. Newly-formed platelets spend 24-36 hours in the spleen before being released into circulation but splenic stasis does not cause any injury to the platelets normally. Factors such as stress, epinephrine and exercise stimulate platelet production.

The main *functions* of platelets is in haemostasis which includes two closely linked processes:

1. Primary haemostasis This term is used for platelet plug formation at the site of injury. It is an immediate phenomenon appearing within seconds of injury and is responsible for cessation of bleeding from microvasculature. Primary

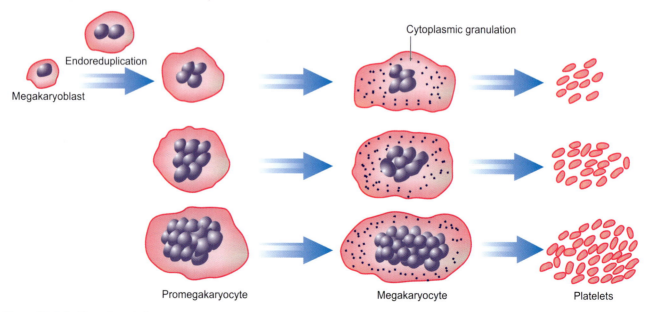

Figure 23.1 ▶ Thrombopoiesis.

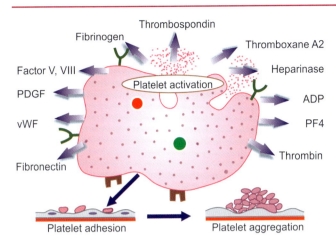

Figure 23.2 ▶ Main events in primary haemostasis—platelet adhesion, release (activation) and aggregation.

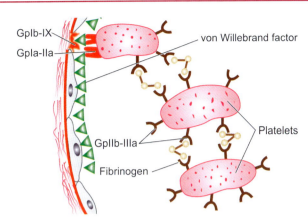

Figure 23.3 ▶ Molecular mechanisms in platelet adhesion and release reaction (Gp = glycoprotein).

haemostasis involves three steps: platelet adhesion, platelet granule release and platelet aggregation which are regulated by changes in membrane phospholipids, and calcium **(Fig. 23.2)**. At molecular level, these important events are depicted diagrammatically in **Fig. 23.3** and briefly outlined below:

i) *Platelet adhesion:* Platelets adhere to collagen in the subendothelium due to presence of receptor on platelet surface, glycoprotein (Gp) Ia-IIa which is an integrin. The adhesion to the vessel wall is further stabilised by von Willebrand factor, an adhesion glycoprotein. This is achieved by formation of a link between von Willebrand factor and another platelet receptor, GpIb-IX complex.

ii) *Platelet release:* After adhesion, platelets become activated and release three types of granules from their cytoplasm: dense granules, α-granules and lysosomal vesicles. Important products released from these granules are: ADP, ATP, calcium, serotonin, platelet factor 4, factor V, factor VIII, thrombospondin, platelet-derived growth factor (PDGF), von Willebrand factor (vWF), fibronectin, fibrinogen, plasminogen activator inhibitor –1 (PAI-1) and thromboxane A2.

iii) *Platelet aggregation:* This process is mediated by fibrinogen which forms bridge between adjacent platelets via glycoprotein receptors on platelets, GpIIb-IIIa.

2. Secondary haemostasis This involves plasma coagulation system resulting in fibrin plug formation and takes several minutes for completion. This is discussed in detail in Chapter 17.

> **GIST BOX 23.1**   **Thrombopoiesis**
>
> ❖ The stages in platelet production are megakaryoblast, promegakaryocyte, megakaryocyte, and discoid platelets.
> ❖ The major functions of platelets are haemostasis by platelet adhesion, release reaction, and aggregation.

INVESTIGATIONS OF HAEMOSTATIC FUNCTION

In general, the haemostatic mechanisms have 2 primary functions:
1. To promote *local haemostasis* at the site of injured blood vessel.
2. To ensure that the circulating blood remains in *fluid state* while in the vascular bed i.e. to prevent the occurrence of generalised thrombosis.

Formation of haemostatic plug is a complex mechanism and involves maintenance of a delicate balance among at least 5 components **(Fig. 23.4)**. Accordingly, there are specific tests for assessing each of these components:

A. *Blood vessel wall:* Tests for disordered vascular haemostasis
B. *Platelets:* Tests for platelets and their functions
C. *Plasma coagulation factors:* Tests for blood coagulation
D. *Fibrinolytic system:* Tests or fibrinolysis
E. *Inhibitors:* Tests for coagulation inhibitors

Anything that interferes with any of these components results in defective haemostasis with abnormal bleeding. In general, in order to establish a definite diagnosis in any case suspected to have abnormal haemostatic functions, the following scheme is followed:

1. Comprehensive *clinical evaluation,* including the patient's history, family history and details of the site, frequency and character of haemostatic defect.
2. Series of *screening tests* for assessing the abnormalities in various components involved in maintaining haemostatic balance.
3. *Specific tests* to pinpoint the cause.

A brief review of general principles of tests used to investigate haemostatic abnormalities is presented below and summarised in **Table 23.1**.

A. Investigation of Disordered Vascular Haemostasis

Disorders of vascular haemostasis may be due to increased vascular permeability, reduced capillary strength and failure

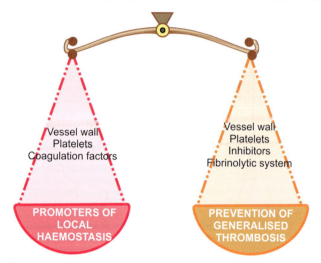

Figure 23.4 ▶ The haemostatic balance.

to contract after injury. Tests of defective vascular function are as under:

1. BLEEDING TIME This simple test is based on the principle of formation of haemostatic plug following a standard incision on the volar surface of the forearm and the time the incision takes to stop bleeding is measured. The test is dependent upon capillary function as well as on platelet number and ability of platelets to adhere to form aggregates. Normal range is 3-8 minutes. A prolonged bleeding time may be due to following causes:
i) Thrombocytopenia.
ii) Disorders of platelet function.
iii) von Willebrand's disease.
iv) Vascular abnormalities (e.g. in Ehlers-Danlos syndrome).
v) Severe deficiency of factor V and XI.

2. HESS CAPILLARY RESISTANCE TEST (TOURNIQUET TEST) This test is done by tying sphygmomanometer cuff to the upper arm and raising the pressure in it between diastolic and systolic for 5 minutes. After deflation, the number of petechiae appearing in the next 5 minutes in 3 cm^2 area over the cubital fossa are counted. Presence of more than 20 petechiae is considered a positive test. The test is positive in increased capillary fragility as well as in thrombocytopenia.

B. Investigation of Platelets and Platelet Function

Haemostatic disorders are commonly due to abnormalities in platelet number, morphology or function.

1. SCREENING TESTS The screening tests carried out for assessing platelet-related causes are as under:
i) Peripheral blood platelet count.
ii) Skin bleeding time.
iii) Examination of fresh blood film to see the morphologic abnormalities of platelets.

2. SPECIAL TESTS If these screening tests suggest a disorder of platelet function, the following platelet function tests may be carried out:
i) *Platelet adhesion tests* such as retention in a glass bead column, and other sophisticated techniques.
ii) *Aggregation tests* which are turbidometric techniques using ADP, collagen or ristocetin.
iii) *Granular content* of the platelets and their release can be assessed by electron microscopy or by measuring the substances released.
iv) *Platelet coagulant activity* is measured indirectly by prothrombin consumption index.

Table 23.1 Screening tests for haemostasis (coagulation tests).

LABORATORY TEST	FACTOR/FUNCTION MEASURED	ASSOCIATED DISORDERS
1. Bleeding time	Platelet function, vascular integrity	i) Qualitative disorders of platelets ii) von Willebrand's disease iii) Quantitative disorders of platelets iv) Acquired vascular disorders
2. Platelet count	Quantification of platelets	i) Thrombocytopenia ii) Thrombocytosis
3. Prothrombin time	Evaluation of extrinsic and common pathway (deficiency of factors I, II, V, VII, X)	i) Oral anticoagulant therapy ii) DIC iii) Liver disease
4. Partial thromboplastin time	Evaluation of intrinsic and common pathway (deficiency of factors I, II, V, VIII, IX, X, XI, XII)	i) Parenteral heparin therapy ii) DIC iii) Liver disease
5. Thrombin time	Evaluation of common pathway	i) Afibrinogenaemia ii) DIC iii) Parenteral heparin therapy

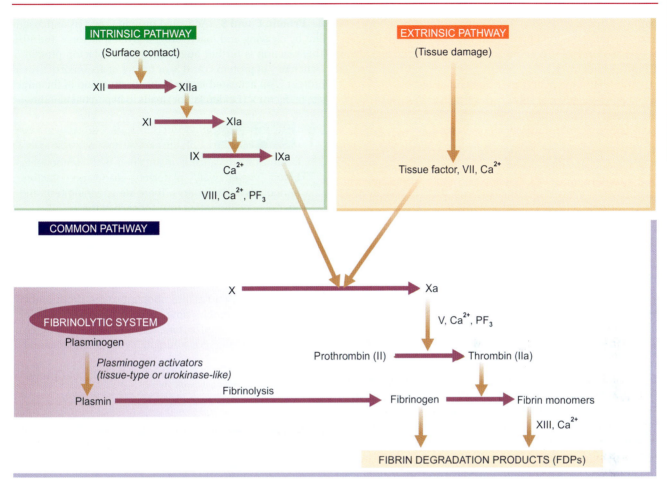

Figure 23.5 ▶ Pathways of blood coagulation, fibrinolytic system and participation of platelets in activation of the cascade and their role in haemostatic plug formation.

C. Investigation of Blood Coagulation

The normal blood coagulation system consists of cascade of activation of 13 coagulation factors. These form intrinsic, extrinsic and common pathways which culminate in formation of thrombin that acts on fibrinogen to produce fibrin. Fibrin clot so formed is strengthened by factor XIII which itself gets activated by thrombin. The process of fibrinolysis or clot dissolution and the role of platelets in activation of cascade and formation of haemostatic plug is illustrated in Fig. 23.5. Coagulation tests include screening and confirmatory special tests as under:

SCREENING TESTS Tests for blood coagulation system include a battery of screening tests. These are as under:

1. Whole blood coagulation time The estimation of whole blood coagulation time done by various capillary and tube methods is of limited value since it is an insensitive and nonspecific test. Normal range is 4-9 minutes at 37°C.

2. Activated partial thromboplastin time (APTT) or partial thromboplastin time with kaolin (PTTK) This test is used to measure the intrinsic system factors* (VIII, IX, XI and XII) as well as factors common to both intrinsic and extrinsic systems (factors X, V, prothrombin and fibrinogen). The test consists of addition of 3 substances to the plasma—calcium, phospholipid and a surface activator such as kaolin. The normal range is 30-40 seconds. The common causes of a prolonged PTTK (or APTT) are as follows:
i) Parenteral administration of heparin.
ii) Disseminated intravascular coagulation.
iii) Liver disease.
iv) Circulating anticoagulants.

3. One-stage prothrombin time (PT) PT measures the extrinsic system* factor VII as well as factors in the common

---

*PTT is mainly used for assessment of factors in 'intrinsic pathway' while PT is used for testing factors in 'extrinsic pathway' of coagulation. *Easy way to remember*: P**I**TT for PTT (**I** for intrinsic); P**E**T for PT (**E** for extrinsic).

pathway. In this test, tissue thromboplastin (e.g. brain extract) and calcium are added to the test. The normal PT in this test is 10-14 seconds. The common causes of prolonged one-stage PT are as under:
i) Administration of oral anticoagulant drugs.
ii) Liver disease, especially obstructive liver disease.
iii) Vitamin K deficiency.
iv) Disseminated intravascular coagulation.

4. Measurement of fibrinogen The *screening tests* for fibrinogen deficiency are semiquantitative fibrinogen titre and thrombin time (TT). The normal value of thrombin time is under 20 seconds, while a fibrinogen titre in plasma dilution up to 32 is considered normal. Following are the common causes for higher values in both these tests:
i) Hypofibrinogenaemia (e.g. in DIC).
ii) Raised concentration of FDP.
iii) Presence of heparin.

SPECIAL TESTS In the presence of an abnormality in screening tests, detailed investigations for the possible cause are carried out. These include the following:

1. Coagulation factor assays These bioassays are based on results of PTTK or PT tests and employ the use of substrate plasma that contains all other coagulation factors except the one to be measured. The unknown level of the factor activity is compared with a standard control plasma with a known level of activity. Results are expressed as percentage of normal activity.

2. Quantitative assays The coagulation factors can be quantitatively assayed by immunological and other chemical methods.

D. Investigation of Fibrinolytic System

Increased levels of circulating plasminogen activator are present in patients with hyperfibrinolysis. Following *screening tests* are done to assess these abnormalities in fibrinolytic system:
1. Estimation of fibrinogen.
2. Fibrin degradation products (FDP) in the serum.
3. Ethanol gelation test.
4. Euglobin or whole blood lysis time.

More *specific tests* include: functional assays, immunological assays by ELISA, and chromogenic assays of plasminogen activators, plasminogen, plasminogen activator inhibitor, and FDP.

E. Investigation of Coagulation Inhibitors

There is an inbuilt system in the body by which coagulation remains confined as per need and does not become generalised. Important inhibitors are as under:

1. Antithrombin III This binds to thrombin and forms thrombin-antithrombin complex which does not permit coagulation.

2. Protein C and S Activated protein C acts as anticoagulant by cleaving and inactivating activated factor V and VIII. This reaction is further augmented by a cofactor, protein S. Deficiency of protein C and S, or failure of action of activated protein C on activated factor V due to mutation of the target site on factor V (Leiden factor) leads to hypercoagulability.

> **GIST BOX 23.2 Investigations of Haemostatic Function**
>
> ❖ Haemostatic balance is maintained by 5 components: blood vessel wall, platelets, coagulation factors, fibrinolysis and inhibitors. There are screening tests and special or confirmatory tests for each of these.
> ❖ Tests for vessels wall are bleeding time and Hess capillary test.
> ❖ Platelets tests are counts, and tests for adhesion, aggregation and release.
> ❖ Screening tests for coagulation factors are coagulation test, activated partial thromboplastin time, prothrombin time and thrombin time. Special tests are assay of various coagulation factors.
> ❖ Tests for fibrinolysis are euglobinlysis test and measurement of FDPs.
> ❖ Tests for inhibitors are for antithrombin and protein C and S.

BLEEDING DISORDERS (HAEMORRHAGIC DIATHESIS)

Bleeding disorders or haemorrhagic diatheses are a group of disorders characterised by defective haemostasis with abnormal bleeding. The tendency to bleeding may be *spontaneous* in the form of small haemorrhages into the skin and mucous membranes (e.g. petechiae, purpura, ecchymoses), or there may be excessive external or internal bleeding *following trivial trauma* and surgical procedure (e.g. haematoma, haemarthrosis etc).

The causes of haemorrhagic diatheses may or may not be related to platelet abnormalities. These causes are broadly divided into the following groups:
I. Haemorrhagic diathesis due to vascular abnormalities
II. Haemorrhagic diathesis related to platelet abnormalities
III. Disorders of coagulation factors
IV. Haemorrhagic diathesis due to fibrinolytic defects
V. Combination of all these as occurs in disseminated intravascular coagulation (DIC).

Besides, a brief comment of hypercoagulable state is also made.

I. HAEMORRHAGIC DIATHESES DUE TO VASCULAR DISORDERS

Vascular bleeding disorders, also called non-thrombocytopenic purpuras or vascular purpuras, are normally mild and characterised by petechiae, purpuras or ecchymoses confined to the skin and mucous membranes. The pathogenesis of bleeding is poorly understood since majority of the standard screening tests of haemostasis including the bleeding time, coagulation time, platelet count and platelet function, are usually normal. Vascular purpuras arise from damage to the capillary endothelium, abnormalities in the subendothelial matrix or extravascular connective tissue that supports the blood vessels, or from formation of abnormal blood vessels.

Vascular bleeding disorders may be *inherited* or *acquired*.

A. Inherited Vascular Bleeding Disorders

A few examples of hereditary vascular disorders are given below:

1. **Hereditary haemorrhagic telangiectasia (Osler-Weber-Rendu disease)** This is an uncommon inherited autosomal dominant disorder. The condition begins in childhood and is characterised by abnormally telangiectatic (dilated) capillaries due to vascular malformations in the skin and mucosal surfaces, especially on lips, tongue, nose and palms and soles. Clinically, patients present with bleeding from stomach, epistaxis or from other mucosal surfaces.

2. **Inherited disorders of connective tissue matrix** These include Marfan's syndrome, Ehlers-Danlos syndrome and pseudoxanthoma elasticum, all of which have inherited defect in the connective tissue matrix and, thus, have fragile skin vessels and easy bruising.

B. Acquired Vascular Bleeding Disorders

Several acquired conditions are associated with vascular purpuras. These are as under:

1. **Henoch-Schönlein purpura** The salient features of Henoch-Schönlein or anaphylactoid purpura are as under:
i) It is a self-limited type of hypersensitivity vasculitis occurring in children and young adults.
ii) The hypersensitivity vasculitis produces purpuric rash on the extensor surfaces of arms, legs and on the buttocks, as well as haematuria, colicky abdominal pain due to bleeding into the GIT, polyarthralgia and acute nephritis.
iii) In spite of these haemorrhagic features, all coagulation tests are normal.
iv) The vessel wall shows leucocytoclastic vasculitis as seen by viable and necrotic neutrophils.
v) Circulating immune complexes are deposited in the vessel wall consisting of IgA, C3 and fibrin, and in some cases, properdin suggesting activation of alternate complement pathway as the trigger event.

2. **Haemolytic-uraemic syndrome** Haemolytic-uraemic syndrome is a disease of infancy and early childhood in which there is bleeding tendency and varying degree of acute renal failure (page 408). The disorder remains confined to the kidney where hyaline thrombi are seen in the glomerular capillaries.

3. **Simple easy bruising (Devil's pinches)** Easy bruising of unknown cause is a common phenomenon in women of child-bearing age group.

4. **Infection** Many infections cause vascular haemorrhages either by causing toxic damage to the endothelium or by DIC. These are especially prone to occur in septicaemia and severe measles.

5. **Drug reactions** Certain drugs form antibodies and produce hypersensitivity (or leucocytoclastic) vasculitis responsible for abnormal bleeding.

6. **Steroid purpura** Long-term steroid therapy or Cushing's syndrome may be associated with vascular purpura due to defective vascular support.

7. **Senile purpura** Atrophy of the supportive tissue of cutaneous blood vessels in old age may cause senile atrophy, especially in the dorsum of forearm and hand.

8. **Scurvy** Deficiency of vitamin C causes defective collagen synthesis which causes skin bleeding as well as bleeding into muscles, and occasionally into the gastrointestinal and genitourinary tracts.

> **GIST BOX 23.3** Haemorrhagic Diathesis due to Vascular Disorders
>
> ❖ These are commonly called vascular purpuras because the cause lies in the vascular wall—damaged endothelium, abnormality in subendothelial matrix, abnormal formation of blood vessels.
> ❖ Examples of inherited vascular purpuras are hereditary haemorrhagic telangiectasia, connective tissue matrix disorders.
> ❖ Acquired causes are Henoch-Schönlein purpura, haemolytic-uraemic syndrome, simple easy bruising, certain bacterial and viral infection, intake of some drugs and steroids, senility, scurvy etc.

II. HAEMORRHAGIC DIATHESES DUE TO PLATELET DISORDERS

Disorders of platelets produce bleeding disorders by one of the following 3 mechanisms:
A. *Due to reduction in the number of platelets* i.e. various forms of thrombocytopenias.
B. *Due to rise in platelet count* i.e. thrombocytosis.
C. *Due to defective platelet functions.*

A. Thrombocytopenias

Thrombocytopenia is defined as a reduction in the peripheral blood platelet count below the lower limit of normal i.e. below 150,000/μl. Thrombocytopenia is associated with abnormal bleeding that includes spontaneous skin purpura and mucosal haemorrhages as well as prolonged bleeding

Table 23.2	Causes of thrombocytopenia.

I. IMPAIRED PLATELET PRODUCTION

1. *Generalised bone marrow failure e.g.*

    Aplastic anaemia, leukaemia, myelofibrosis, megaloblastic anaemia, marrow infiltrations (carcinomas, lymphomas, multiple myeloma, storage diseases).

2. *Selective suppression of platelet production e.g.*

    Drugs (quinine, quinidine, sulfonamides, PAS, rifampicin, anticancer drugs, thiazide diuretics), (heparin, diclofenac, acyclovir), alcohol intake.

II. ACCELERATED PLATELET DESTRUCTION

1. *Immunologic thrombocytopenias e.g.*

    ITP (acute and chronic), neonatal and post-transfusion (isoimmune), drug-induced, secondary immune thrombocytopenia (post-infection, SLE, AIDS, CLL, lymphoma).

2. *Increased consumption e.g.*

    DIC, TTP, giant haemangiomas, microangiopathic haemolytic anaemia.

III. SPLENIC SEQUESTRATION

   Splenomegaly

IV. DILUTIONAL LOSS

   Massive transfusion of old stored blood to bleeding patients

after trauma. However, spontaneous haemorrhagic tendency may become clinically evident only after severe depletion of the platelet count to level below 20,000/μl.

Thrombocytopenia may result from 4 main groups of causes:
1. Impaired platelet production
2. Accelerated platelet destruction
3. Splenic sequestration
4. Dilutional loss

A list of causes of thrombocytopenia is given in **Table 23.2**. Three of the common and important causes—drug-induced thrombocytopenia, idiopathic thrombocytopenic purpura (ITP), and thrombotic thrombocytopenic purpura (TTP), are discussed below.

Drug-induced Thrombocytopenia

Many commonly used drugs cause thrombocytopenia by depressing megakaryocyte production. In most cases, an immune mechanism by formation of drug-antibody complexes is implicated in which the platelet is damaged as an 'innocent bystander'. Drug-induced thrombocytopenia is associated with many commonly used drugs and includes: chemotherapeutic agents (alkylating agents, anthracyclines, antimetabolites), certain antibiotics (sulfonamides, PAS, rifampicin, penicillins), drugs used in cardiovascular diseases (digitoxin, thiazide diuretics), diclofenac, acyclovir, heparin and excessive consumption of ethanol.

Clinically, the patient presents with acute purpura. The platelet count is markedly lowered, often below 10,000/μl and the bone marrow shows normal or increased number of megakaryocytes.

The immediate treatment is to stop or replace the suspected drug with instruction to the patient to avoid taking the offending drug in future. Occasional patients may require temporary support with glucocorticoids, plasmapheresis or platelet transfusions.

Heparin-induced Thrombocytopenia

Thrombocytopenia due to administration of heparin is distinct from that caused by other drugs in following ways:

i) Thrombocytopenia is generally not so severe to fall to level below 20,000/μl.

ii) Unlike drug-induced thrombocytopenia, heparin-induced thrombocytopenia is not associated with bleeding but instead these patients are more prone to develop thrombosis.

The underlying mechanism of heparin-induced thrombocytopenia is formation of antibody against platelet factor 4 (PF-4)-heparin complex. This specific antibody activates the endothelial cells and initiates thrombus formation. It occurs in a small proportion of cases after the patient has received heparin for 5-10 days.

Diagnosis is made by a combination of laboratory and clinical features with 4 *Ts*: thrombocytopenia, thrombosis, time of fall of platelet count, absence of other causes of thrombocytopenia.

Immune Thrombocytopenic Purpura (ITP)

Idiopathic (now called immune) thrombocytopenic purpura (ITP) is characterised by immunologic destruction of platelets and normal or increased megakaryocytes in the bone marrow.

PATHOGENESIS On the basis of duration of illness, ITP is classified into acute and chronic forms, both of which have different pathogenesis.

Acute ITP This is a self-limited disorder, seen most frequently in children following recovery from a viral illness (e.g. hepatitis C, infectious mononucleosis, CMV infection, HIV infection) or an upper respiratory illness. The onset of acute ITP is sudden and severe thrombocytopenia but recovery occurs within a few weeks to 6 months. The mechanism of acute ITP is by formation of *immune complexes* containing viral antigens, and by formation of *antibodies* against viral antigens which cross react with platelets and lead to their immunologic destruction.

Chronic ITP Chronic ITP occurs more commonly in adults, particularly in women of child-bearing age (20-40 years). The disorder develops insidiously and persists for several years. Though chronic ITP is idiopathic, similar immunologic thrombocytopenia may be seen in association with SLE, AIDS and autoimmune thyroiditis. The pathogenesis of chronic ITP is explained by formation of *anti-platelet autoantibodies*, usually by platelet-associated IgG humoral antibodies synthesised mainly in the spleen. These antibodies are directed against target antigens on the platelet glycoproteins, GpIIb-IIIa and GpIb-IX complex. Some of the antibodies directed against platelet surface also interfere in their function. The mechanism of platelet destruction is similar to that seen in autoimmune haemolytic anaemias. Sensitised platelets are destroyed mainly in the spleen and rendered susceptible to phagocytosis by cells of the reticuloendothelial system.

CLINICAL FEATURES The clinical manifestation of ITP may develop abruptly in cases of acute ITP, or the onset may be insidious as occurs in majority of cases of chronic ITP. The usual manifestations are petechial haemorrhages, easy bruising, and mucosal bleeding such as menorrhagia in women, nasal bleeding, bleeding from gums, melaena and haematuria. Intracranial haemorrhage is, however, rare. Splenomegaly and hepatomegaly may occur in cases with chronic ITP but lymphadenopathy is quite uncommon in either type of ITP.

LABORATORY FINDINGS The diagnosis of ITP can be suspected on clinical features after excluding the known causes of thrombocytopenia and is supported by the following haematologic findings:
1. *Platelet count* is markedly reduced, usually in the range of 10,000-50,000/μl.
2. *Blood film* shows only occasional platelets which are often large in size (Fig. 23.6, A).

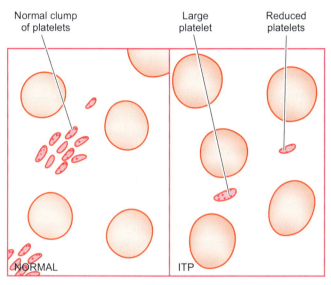

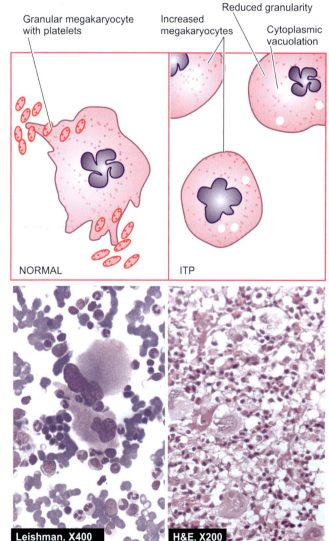

Figure 23.6 ▶ Laboratory findings of ITP contrasted with those found in a normal individual. A, Peripheral blood in ITP shows presence of reduced number of platelets which are often large. B, C, Bone marrow aspirate and trephine in ITP show characteristically increased number of megakaryocytes with single non-lobulated nuclei and reduced cytoplasmic granularity.

3. *Bone marrow* shows increased number of megakaryocytes which have large non-lobulated single nuclei and may have reduced cytoplasmic granularity and presence of vacuoles (Fig. 23.6, B).
4. With sensitive techniques, *anti-platelet IgG antibody* can be demonstrated on platelet surface or in the serum of patients.
5. *Platelet survival studies* reveal markedly reduced platelet lifespan, sometimes less than one hour, as compared with normal lifespan of 7-10 days.

PRINCIPLES OF TREATMENT Spontaneous recovery occurs in 90% cases of acute ITP, while only less than 10% cases of chronic ITP recover spontaneously. Treatment is directed at reducing the level and source of autoantibodies and reducing the rate of destruction of sensitised platelets. This is possible by corticosteroid therapy, immunosuppressive drugs (e.g. vincristine, cyclophosphamide and azathioprine) and splenectomy. Beneficial effects of splenectomy in chronic ITP are due to both removal of the major site of platelet destruction and the major source of autoantibody synthesis. Platelet transfusions are helpful as a palliative measure only in patients with severe haemorrhage.

Thrombotic Thrombocytopenic Purpura (TTP) and Haemolytic-Uraemic Syndrome (HUS)

Thrombotic thrombocytopenic purpura (TTP) and haemolytic-uraemic syndrome (HUS) are a group of thrombotic microangiopathies which are essentially characterised by triad of *thrombocytopenia, microangiopathic haemolytic anaemia and formation of hyaline fibrin microthrombi* within the microvasculature throughout the body. These are often fulminant and lethal disorders occurring in young adults. The intravascular microthrombi are composed predominantly of platelets and fibrin. The widespread presence of these platelet microthrombi is responsible for thrombocytopenia due to increased consumption of platelets, microangiopathic haemolytic anaemia and protean clinical manifestations involving different organs and tissues throughout the body.

PATHOGENESIS Unlike DIC, a clinicopathologically related condition, activation of the clotting system is not the primary event in formation of microthrombi. TTP is initiated by endothelial injury followed by release of von Willebrand factor and other procoagulant material from endothelial cells, leading to the formation of microthrombi. Trigger for the endothelial injury comes from immunologic damage by diverse conditions such as in pregnancy, metastatic cancer, high-dose chemotherapy, HIV infection, and mitomycin C.

CLINICAL FEATURES The clinical manifestations of TTP are due to microthrombi in the arterioles, capillaries and venules throughout the body. Besides features of thrombocytopenia and microangiopathic haemolytic anaemia, characteristic findings include fever, transient neurologic deficits and renal failure. The spleen may be palpable.

LABORATORY FINDINGS The diagnosis can be made from the following findings:
1. Thrombocytopenia.
2. Microangiopathic haemolytic anaemia with negative Coombs' test.
3. Leucocytosis, sometimes with leukaemoid reaction.
4. Bone marrow examination reveals normal or slightly increased megakaryocytes accompanied with some myeloid hyperplasia.
5. Diagnosis is, however, established by examination of biopsy (e.g. from gingiva) which demonstrates typical microthrombi in arterioles, capillaries and venules, unassociated with any inflammatory changes in the vessel wall.

B. Thrombocytosis

Thrombocytosis is defined as platelet count in excess of 4,00,000/μl. While essential or primary thrombocytosis or thrombocythaemia is discussed under myeloproliferative disorders in the next chapter, secondary or reactive thrombocytosis can occur following massive haemorrhage, iron deficiency, severe sepsis, marked inflammation, disseminated cancers, haemolysis, or following splenectomy. Thrombocytosis causes bleeding or thrombosis but how it produces is not clearly known.

As such, transitory and secondary thrombocytosis does not require any separate treatment other than treating the cause.

C. Disorders of Platelet Functions

Defective platelet function is suspected in patients who show skin and mucosal haemorrhages and have prolonged bleeding time but a normal platelet count. These disorders may be hereditary or acquired.

Hereditary Disorders

Depending upon the predominant functional abnormality, inherited disorders of platelet functions are classified into the following 3 groups:

1. DEFECTIVE PLATELET ADHESION These are as under:
i) *Bernard-Soulier syndrome* is an autosomal recessive disorder with inherited deficiency of a platelet membrane glycoprotein which is essential for adhesion of platelets to vessel wall.
ii) *In von Willebrand's disease,* there is defective platelet adhesion as well as deficiency of factor VIII (page 410).

2. DEFECTIVE PLATELET AGGREGATION In *thrombasthenia (Glanzmann's disease),* there is failure of primary platelet aggregation with ADP or collagen due to inherited deficiency of two of platelet membrane glycoproteins.

3. DISORDERS OF PLATELET RELEASE REACTION These disorders are characterised by normal initial aggregation of platelets with ADP or collagen but the subsequent release of ADP, prostaglandins and 5-HT is defective due to complex intrinsic deficiencies.

Acquired Disorders

Acquired defects of platelet functions include the following clinically significant examples:

1. ASPIRIN THERAPY Prolonged use of aspirin leads to easy bruising and abnormal bleeding time. This is because aspirin inhibits the enzyme cyclooxygenase, and thereby suppresses the synthesis of prostaglandins which are involved in platelet aggregation as well as release reaction. The anti-platelet effect of aspirin is clinically applied in preventing major thromboembolic disease in recurrent myocardial infarction.

2. OTHERS Several other acquired disorders are associated with various abnormalities in platelet functions at different levels. These include: uraemia, liver disease, multiple myeloma, Waldenström's macroglobulinaemia and various myeloproliferative disorders.

> **GIST BOX 23.4 Haemorrhagic Diathesis due to Platelet Disorders**
>
> ❖ Platelet disorders may be due to reduction or increased number, or defective functions.
> ❖ Thrombocytopenia may result from impaired production, accelerated destruction, splenic sequestration or dilutional loss.
> ❖ Idiopathic (or immune) thrombocytopenic purpura (ITP), is characterised by immunologic destruction of platelets and normal or increased megakaryocytes in the bone marrow. It may be acute or chronic.
> ❖ Thrombotic thrombocytopenic purpura (TTP) and haemolytic-uraemic syndrome have thrombocytopenia and hyaline fibrin microthrombi within the microvasculature throughout the body.
> ❖ Defective platelet functions may be hereditary (platelet adhesion, aggregation, release reaction) or acquired (aspirin, uraemia, liver disease etc).

III. COAGULATION DISORDERS

The physiology of normal coagulation is described in Chapter 17 together with relatively more common coagulation disorders of arterial and venous thrombosis and embolism. A deficiency of each of the thirteen known plasma coagulation factors has been reported, which may be inherited or acquired. In general, coagulation disorders are less common as compared with other bleeding disorders. The type of bleeding in coagulation disorders is different from that seen in vascular and platelet abnormalities. Instead of spontaneous appearance of petechiae and purpuras, the plasma coagulation defects manifest more often in the form of large ecchymoses, haematomas and bleeding into muscles, joints, body cavities, GIT and urinary tract. For establishing the diagnosis, *screening tests for coagulation* (whole blood coagulation time, bleeding time, activated partial thromboplastin time and prothrombin time) are carried out, followed by *coagulation factor assays.*

Disorders of plasma coagulation factors may have hereditary or acquired origin.

Hereditary coagulation disorders Most of the inherited plasma coagulation disorders are due to qualitative or quantitative defect in a single coagulation factor. Out of defects in various coagulation factors, two of the most common inherited coagulation disorders are the sex-(X)-linked disorders—*classic haemophilia or haemophilia A* (due to inherited deficiency of factor VIII), and *Christmas disease or haemophilia B* (due to inherited deficiency of factor IX). Another common and related coagulation disorder, *von Willebrand's disease* (due to inherited defect of von Willebrand's factor), is also discussed here.

Acquired coagulation disorders These disorders, on the other hand, are usually characterised by deficiencies of multiple coagulation factors. The most common acquired clotting abnormalities are: vitamin K deficiency, coagulation disorder in liver diseases, fibrinolytic defects and disseminated intravascular coagulation (DIC).

Common hereditary and acquired coagulation disorders are discussed below.

1. Classic Haemophilia (Haemophilia A)

Classic haemophilia or haemophilia A is the most common hereditary coagulation disorder occurring due to deficiency or reduced activity of factor VIII (anti-haemophilic factor). The disorder is inherited as a sex-(X-) linked recessive trait and, therefore, manifests clinically in males, while females are usually the carriers. However, rarely there may be true female haemophilics (homozygous state) arising from consanguinity within the family e.g. daughter born to haemophiliac father and carrier mother. The chances of a proven carrier mother passing on the abnormality to her children are 50:50 for each son and 50:50 for each daughter. A haemophilic father cannot transmit the disorder to his sons (as they inherit his Y chromosome only that does not carry the genetic abnormality) while all his daughters will be asymptomatic carriers. However, cases without family history of haemophilia are due to spontaneous somatic mutations of gene coding for factor VIII.

The disease has been known since ancient times but Schönlein in 1839 gave this bleeder's disease its present name haemophilia. In 1952, it was found that haemophilia was not always due to deficiency of factor VIII as was previously considered but instead blood of some patients was deficient in factor IX (Christmas factor or plasma thromboplastin component). Currently, *haemophilia A (classic haemophilia)* is inherited deficiency of factor VIII due to mutation in F8 gene, and *haemophilia B (Christmas disease)* is inherited deficiency of factor IX due to mutation in F9 gene.

The frequency of haemophilia varies in different races, the highest incidence being in populations of Britain, Northern Europe and Australia. Haemohilia A comprises about 80% cases. Western literature reports give an overall incidence of haemophilia A in 1 in 10,000 male births. Another interesting facet of the haemophilia which has attracted investigators and researchers is the prevalence of this disorder in the blood of royal families in Great Britain and some European countries.

PATHOGENESIS Haemophilia A is caused by quantitative reduction of factor VIII in 90% of cases, while 10% cases have normal or increased level of factor VIII with reduced activity. Factor VIII is synthesised in hepatic parenchymal cells and regulates the activation of factor X in intrinsic coagulation pathway. Factor VIII circulates in blood complexed to another larger protein, von Willebrand's factor (vWF), which comprises 99% of the factor VIII-vWF complex. The genetic coding, synthesis and functions of vWF are different from those of factor VIII and are considered separately below under von Willebrand's disease. Normal haemostasis requires 25% factor VIII activity. Though occasional patients with 25% factor VIII level may develop bleeding, most symptomatic haemophilic patients have factor VIII levels below 5%.

CLINICAL FEATURES Patients of haemophilia suffer from bleeding for hours or days after the injury. The clinical severity of the disease correlates well with plasma level of factor VIII activity. Haemophilic bleeding can involve any organ but occurs most commonly as recurrent painful haemarthroses and muscle haematomas, and sometimes as haematuria. Spontaneous intracranial haemorrhage and oropharyngeal bleeding are rare, but when they occur they are the most feared complications.

> *LABORATORY FINDINGS* The following tests are abnormal:
> i) Whole blood coagulation time is prolonged in severe cases only.
> ii) Prothrombin time is usually normal.
> iii) Activated partial thromboplastin time (APTT or PTTK) is typically prolonged.
> iv) Specific assay for factor VIII shows lowered activity. The diagnosis of *female carriers* is made by the findings of about half the activity of factor VIII, while the *manifest disease* is associated with factor VIII activity below 25%.

PRINCIPLES OF TREATMENT Symptomatic patients with bleeding episodes are treated with factor VIII replacement therapy, consisting of factor VIII concentrates or plasma cryoprecipitates. With the availability of this treatment, the life expectancy of even severe haemophilic patients was approaching normal but the occurrence of AIDS in multitransfused haemophilic patients has adversely affected the life expectancy.

2. Christmas Disease (Haemophilia B)

Inherited deficiency of factor IX (Christmas factor or plasma thromboplastin component) produces Christmas disease or haemophilia B. Haemophilia B is rarer than haemophilia A constituting about 20% cases; its estimated incidence is 1 in 100,000 male births. The inheritance pattern and clinical features of factor IX deficiency are indistinguishable from those of classic haemophilia but accurate laboratory diagnosis is critical since haemophilia B requires treatment with different plasma fraction. The usual screening tests for coagulation are similar to those in classic haemophilia but bioassay of factor IX reveals lowered activity.

PRINCIPLES OF TREATMENT Therapy in symptomatic haemophilia B consists of infusion of either fresh frozen plasma or a plasma enriched with factor IX. Besides the expected possibilities of complications of hepatitis, chronic liver disease and AIDS, the replacement therapy in factor IX deficiency may activate the coagulation system and cause thrombosis and embolism.

3. von Willebrand's Disease

DEFINITION AND PATHOGENESIS von Willebrand's disease (vWD) is the most common hereditary coagulation disorder occurring due to qualitative or quantitative defect in von Willebrand's factor (vWF). Its incidence is estimated to be 1 in 1,000 individuals of either sex. The vWF comprises the larger fraction of factor VIII-vWF complex which circulates in the blood. Though the two components of factor VIII-vWF complex circulate together as a unit and perform the important function in clotting and facilitate platelet adhesion to subendothelial collagen, vWF differs from factor VIII in the following respects:

i) The *gene* for vWF is located at chromosome 12, while that of factor VIII is in X-chromosome. Thus, vWD is inherited as an autosomal dominant trait which may occur in either sex, while factor VIII deficiency (haemophilia A) is a sex (X-)-linked recessive disorder.

ii) The vWF is *synthesised* in the endothelial cells, megakaryocytes and platelets but not in the liver cells, while the principal site of synthesis of factor VIII is the liver.

iii) The main *function* of vWF is to facilitate the adhesion of platelets to subendothelial collagen, while factor VIII is involved in activation of factor X in the intrinsic coagulation pathway.

CLINICAL FEATURES Clinically, the patients of vWD are characterised by spontaneous bleeding from mucous membranes and excessive bleeding from wounds. There are 3 major types of vWD:

Type I disease is the most common and is characterised by mild to moderate decrease in plasma vWF (50% activity). The synthesis of vWF is normal but the release of its multimers is inhibited.

Type II disease is much less common and is characterised by normal or near normal levels of vWF which is functionally defective.

Type III disease is extremely rare and is the most severe form of the disease. These patients have no detectable vWF activity and may have sufficiently low factor VIII levels.

Bleeding episodes in vWD are treated with cryoprecipitates or factor VIII concentrates.

LABORATORY FINDINGS These are as under:
i) Prolonged bleeding time.
ii) Normal platelet count.
iii) Reduced plasma vWF concentration.
iv) Defective platelet aggregation with ristocetin, an antibiotic.
v) Reduced factor VIII activity.

4. Vitamin K Deficiency

Vitamin K is a fat-soluble vitamin which plays important role in haemostasis since it serves as a cofactor in the formation of 6 prothrombin complex proteins *(vitamin K-dependent coagulation factors)* synthesised in the liver: factor II, VII, IX, X, protein C and protein S. Vitamin K is obtained from green vegetables, absorbed in the small intestine and stored in the liver (page 102). Some quantity of vitamin K is endogenously synthesised by the bacteria in the colon.

Vitamin K deficiency may present in the newborn or in subsequent childhood or adult life:

i) **Neonatal vitamin K deficiency** Deficiency of vitamin K in the newborn causes haemorrhagic disease of the newborn. Liver cell immaturity, lack of gut bacterial synthesis of the vitamin and low quantities in breast milk, all contribute to vitamin K deficiency in the newborn and may cause haemorrhage on 2nd to 4th day of life. Routine administration of vitamin K to all newly born infants has led to disappearance of neonatal vitamin K deficiency.

ii) **Vitamin K deficiency in children and adult** There are 3 major causes of vitamin K deficiency in childhood or adult life:
a) Inadequate dietary intake.
b) Intestinal malabsorption.
c) Loss of storage site due to hepatocellular disease.

With the onset of vitamin K deficiency, the plasma levels of all the 6 vitamin K-dependent factors (prothrombin complex proteins) fall. This, in turn, results in prolonged PT and PTTK. Parenteral administration of vitamin K rapidly restores vitamin K levels in the liver.

5. Coagulation Disorders in Liver Disease

Since liver is the major site for synthesis and metabolism of coagulation factors, liver disease often leads to multiple haemostatic abnormalities. The liver also produces inhibitors of coagulation such as antithrombin III and protein C and S and plays a role in the clearance of activated factors and fibrinolytic enzymes. Thus, patients with liver disease may develop hypercoagulability and are predisposed to develop DIC and systemic fibrinolysis.

The major causes of bleeding in liver diseases are as under:

A. Morphologic lesions:
i) Portal hypertension e.g. varices, splenomegaly with secondary thrombocytopenia
ii) Peptic ulceration
iii) Gastritis

B. Hepatic dysfunctions:
i) Impaired hepatic synthesis of coagulation factors
ii) Impaired hepatic synthesis of coagulation inhibitors: protein C, protein S and antithrombin III
iii) Impaired absorption and metabolism of vitamin K
iv) Failure to clear activated coagulation factors causing DIC and systemic fibrinolysis

C. Complications of therapy:
i) Following massive transfusion leading to dilution of platelets and coagulation factors.
ii) Infusion of activated coagulation proteins.
iii) Following heparin therapy.

Many a times, the haemostatic abnormality in liver disease is complex but most patients have prolonged PT and PTTK, mild thrombocytopenia, normal fibrinogen level and decreased hepatic stores of vitamin K.

| GIST BOX 23.5 | Coagulation Disorders |

- Disorders of coagulation factors may be hereditary or acquired.
- Common hereditary coagulation disorders are haemophilia A (due to deficiency or reduced activity of factor VIII), haemophilia B (due to deficiency of factor IX), and von Willebrand disease (due to qualitative or quantitative defect in von Willebrand's factor (vWF)
- Common acquired causes are vitamin K deficiency in different ages and liver diseases causing reduced synthesis of coagulation factors.

IV. OTHER BLEEDING AND COAGULATION DISORDERS

Haemorrhagic Diatheses Due to Fibrinolytic Defects

Normally, fibrinolysis consisting of plasminogen-plasmin and fibrin degradation products (FDPs) is an essential protective physiologic mechanism to limit the blood coagulation in the

body. However, unchecked and excessive fibrinolysis may sometimes be the cause of bleeding. The causes of *primary pathologic fibrinolysis* leading to haemorrhagic defects are as under:
1. Deficiency of α_2-plasmin inhibitor following trauma or surgery.
2. Impaired clearance of tissue plasminogen activator such as in cirrhosis of liver.

At times, it may be difficult to distinguish primary pathologic fibrinolysis from secondary fibrinolysis accompanying DIC.

Hypercoagulable State

As discussed in Chapter 17, hypercoagulability or thrombophilia is a state of increased risk of thrombosis due to abnormality in haemostatic equilibrium i.e. reverse of abnormal bleeding (page 250). It may occur due to inherited or acquired disorders as under:

I. Inherited factors:
1. Antithrombin III deficiency
2. Protein C deficiency
3. Protein S deficiency
4. Activated protein C resistance (Factor V Leiden)
5. Inherited disorders of fibrinolytic pathways e.g. dysfibrinogenaemia, dysplasminogenaemia
6. Increased prothrombin production

II. Acquired factors:
1. Antiphospholipid antibodies (APLA) e.g. lupus anticoagulant, anticardiolipin antibodies
2. Impaired venous return due to stasis
3. Oral contraceptives
4. Disseminated malignancy
5. Nephrotic syndrome
6. Postoperative cases

Disseminated Intravascular Coagulation (DIC)

Disseminated intravascular coagulation (DIC), also termed defibrination syndrome or consumption coagulopathy, is a complex thrombo-haemorrhagic disorder (intravascular coagulation and haemorrhage) occurring as a secondary complication in some systemic diseases.

Etiology

Although there are numerous conditions associated with DIC, most frequent causes are listed below:

1. Massive tissue injury In obstetrical syndromes (e.g. abruptio placentae, amniotic fluid embolism, retained dead foetus), massive trauma, metastatic malignancies, surgery.

2. Infections Especially endotoxaemia, gram-negative and meningococcal septicaemia, certain viral infections, malaria, aspergillosis.

3. Widespread endothelial damage In aortic aneurysm, haemolytic-uraemic syndrome, severe burns, acute glomerulonephritis.

4. Miscellaneous: Snake bite, shock, acute intravascular haemolysis, heat stroke.

Pathogenesis

Although in each case, a distinct triggering mechanism has been identified, the sequence of events, in general, can be summarised as under **(Fig. 23.7)**:

1. Activation of coagulation The etiologic factors listed above initiate widespread activation of coagulation pathway by release of tissue factor.

2. Thrombotic phase Endothelial damage from the various thrombogenic stimuli causes generalised platelet aggregation and adhesion with resultant deposition of small thrombi and emboli throughout the microvasculature.

3. Consumption phase The early thrombotic phase is followed by a phase of consumption of coagulation factors and platelets.

4. Secondary fibrinolysis As a protective mechanism, fibrinolytic system is secondarily activated at the site of intravascular coagulation. Secondary fibrinolysis causes breakdown of fibrin resulting in formation of FDPs in the circulation.

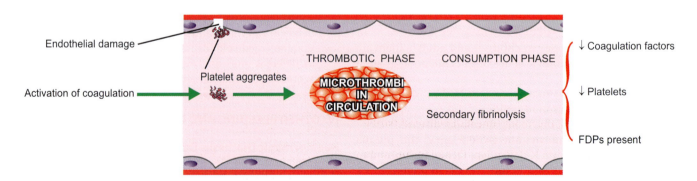

Figure 23.7 ▶ The pathogenesis of disseminated intravascular coagulation.

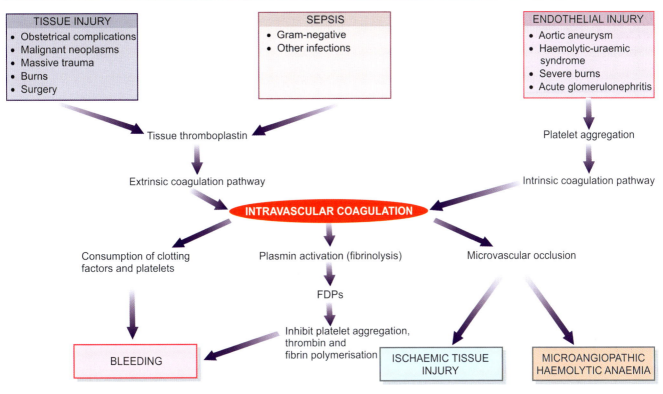

Figure 23.8 ▶ Pathophysiology of disseminated intravascular coagulation.

Pathophysiology of DIC is summed up schematically in **Fig. 23.8**.

Clinical Features

There are 2 main features of DIC—*bleeding* as the most common manifestation, and *organ damage* due to ischaemia caused by the effect of widespread intravascular thrombosis such as in the kidney and brain. Less common manifestations include: microangiopathic haemolytic anaemia and thrombosis in larger arteries and veins.

Laboratory Findings

The laboratory investigations include the following:
1. The platelet count is low.
2. Blood film shows the features of microangiopathic haemolytic anaemia. There is presence of schistocytes and fragmented red cells due to damage caused by trapping and passage through the fibrin thrombi.
3. Prothrombin time, thrombin time and activated partial thromboplastin time, are all prolonged.
4. Plasma fibrinogen levels are reduced due to consumption in microvascular coagulation.
5. Fibrin degradation products (FDPs) are raised due to secondary fibrinolysis.

A summary of important laboratory findings in common causes of haemostatic abnormalities is summed up in **Table 23.3**.

> **GIST BOX 23.6** **Other Bleeding and Coagulation Disorders**
>
> ❖ Uncontrolled and excessive fibrinolysis may sometimes be the cause of bleeding.
> ❖ Excessive fibrinolysis may sometimes be the cause of bleeding.
> ❖ Hypercoagulability or thrombophilia is increased risk of thrombosis due to abnormality in haemostatic equilibrium i.e. reverse of abnormal bleeding. It may be from inherited or acquired disorders.
> ❖ Disseminated intravascular coagulation (DIC) is a complex of intravascular coagulation and haemorrhage. It may occur from various causes e.g. massive bleeding, fulminant infections etc.
> ❖ DIC passes through phases of activation of coagulation, thrombotic phase, consumptive phase and secondary fibrinolysis.
> ❖ Major findings in DIC are thrombocytopenia, prolonged prothrombin time, reduced fibrinogen, and presence of FDPs.

Table 23.3 Major laboratory findings in common haemostatic disorders.

DISORDER	PLATELET COUNT	BT	PT	APTT	TT	FDPS	F-VIII	F-IX
I. VASCULAR DISORDERS								
Vascular purpuras	N	N	N	N	N	Absent	N	N
II. PLATELET DISORDERS								
1. ITP	↓	↑	N	N	N	Absent	N	N
2. Heparin	↓	↑	N	↑	↑	Absent	N	N
3. TTP	↓	↑	N	N	N	Absent	N	N
III. COAGULATION DISORDERS								
1. Haemophilia A	N	↑	N	↑	↑	Absent	↓	N
2. Haemophilia B	N	↑	N	↑	↑	Absent	N	↓
3. von Willebrand's	N	↑	N	↑	↑	Absent	↓	N
4. Vit. K deficiency	N	↑	↑	↑	↑	Absent	N	N
5. Liver disease	N	↑	↑	↑	N	Absent	N	N
IV. DIC	↓	↑	↑	↑	↑	Present	↓	↓

24 Diseases of Leucocytes and Lymphoid Tissues

As illustrated in Fig. 22.3, haematopoietic stem cells in the bone marrow differentiate into two types of progenitors—*lymphoid* (immune system) stem cells, and *non-lymphoid or myeloid* (trilineage) stem cells. The former develop into T, B and NK cells while the latter differentiate into 3 types of cell lines—granulocyte-monocyte progenitors (producing neutrophils, eosinophils, basophils and monocytes), erythroid progenitors (producing red cells, discussed in Chapter 22), and megakaryocytes (as the source of platelets, discussed in Chapter 23). In this chapter, we will discuss the abnormalities pertaining to leucocyte pool of two cell lines (granulocyte-monocyte cell line and the lymphoid cell lines), besides discussion on all haematopoietic and lymphoid neoplasms.

Leucocyte pool in the body lies at two distinct locations: in circulating blood and in the tissues. This concept holds more true for lymphoid cells in particular, which are present in circulation as well as are distributed in the lymphoid tissues of the body (lymph nodes, spleen, mucosa-associated lymphoid tissue—MALT, pharyngeal lymphoid tissue). B, T and NK lymphoid cells are formed after differentiation from lymphopoietic precursor cells in the bone marrow undergo further maturation in peripheral lymphoid organs and thymus (Chapter 14). Thus, relationship of haematopoietic tissues and lymphoreticular tissues is quite close. In fact, current WHO classification of lymphoma-leukaemia does not consider diseases of lymphocytes in the blood and in the lymphoid tissues as separate disorders; instead these diseases are seen to represent different stages of the same biologic process. Thus, in current times, diseases of leucocytes are studied together with diseases of lymphoreticular tissues of the body.

Accordingly, following topics have been covered in this chapter:
1. Lymph nodes: Normal and reactive hyperplasia
2. While blood cells: Normal and reactive proliferations
3. Lymphohaematopoietic malignancies (Leukaemias-lymphomas): General
4. Myeloid neoplasms
5. Lymphoid neoplasms: General
6. Hodgkin's disease
7. Non-Hodgkin's lymphomas-leukaemias
8. Plasma cell disorders
9. Histiocytic neoplasms (Langerhans cell histiocytosis)
10. Spleen

LYMPH NODES: NORMAL AND REACTIVE HYPERPLASIA

Normal Structure

The lymph nodes are bean-shaped or oval structures varying in length from 1 to 2 cm and form the part of lymphatic network distributed throughout the body. Each lymph node is covered by a connective tissue *capsule*. At the convex surface of the capsule several *afferent lymphatics* enter which drain into the peripheral *subcapsular sinus,* branch into the lymph node and terminate at the concavity (hilum) as a single *efferent lymphatic* vessel. These lymphatic vessels are lined by mononuclear phagocytic cells.

The inner structure of the lymph node is divided into a peripheral cortex and central medulla. The *cortex* consists of several rounded aggregates of lymphocytes called *lymphoid follicles.* The follicle has a pale-staining germinal centre surrounded by small dark-staining lymphocytes called the mantle zone. The deeper region of the cortex or *paracortex* is the zone between the peripheral cortex and the inner medulla. The *medulla* is predominantly composed of cords of plasma cells and some lymphocytes. The capsule and the structure within the lymph node are connected by supportive delicate reticulin framework **(Fig. 24.1, A).**

Functionally, the lymph node is divided into T and B lymphocyte zones:
◈ *B-cell zone* lies in the follicles in the cortex, the mantle zone and the interfollicular space, while *plasma cells* are also present in the interfollicular zone.
◈ *T-cell zone* is predominantly present in the medulla.

There are two main functions of the lymph node—to mount immune response in the body, and to perform the function of active phagocytosis for particulate material. Besides T- and B-cells, the follicular centre has *dendritic histiocytes* and antigen-presenting *Langerhans' histiocytes* (formerly together called tingible body macrophages due to engulfment of particulate material by them) and *endothelial cells.* The follicular centre is a very active zone where lymphocytes from peripheral blood continuously enter and leave, interact with macrophage-histiocytes and endothelial cells and undergo maturation and transformation. Lymphocytes and endothelial cells have surface molecules which interact and serve as 'addresses' so that endothelial cells can direct the lymphocytes; these molecules are appropriately termed as *addressins* or *homing receptors.* Peripheral blood B and T lymphocytes on entering the lymph node are stimulated

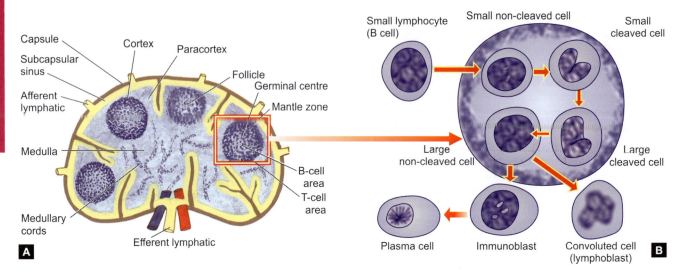

Figure 24.1 ▶ Normal lymph node. A, The anatomic structure and functional zones of a lymph node. B, Maturation of lymphoid cells in the follicle.

immunologically which transforms them to undergo cytoplasmic and nuclear maturation which may be in the follicular centre or paracortex as per following sequence and schematically depicted in **Fig. 24.1, B**:
i) Follicular centre, small non-cleaved cells or centroblasts
ii) Follicular centre, small cleaved cells or centrocytes
iii) Follicular centre, large cleaved cells
iv) Follicular centre, large non-cleaved cells
v) Immunoblasts (in paracortex)
vi) Convoluted cells or lymphoblasts (in paracortex)
vii) Plasma cells.

Lymph nodes are secondarily involved in a variety of systemic diseases, local injuries and infections, and are also the site for some important primary neoplasms. Many of these diseases such as tuberculosis, sarcoidosis, histoplasmosis, typhoid fever, viral infections etc. have been considered elsewhere in the textbook along with description of these primary diseases. Reactive lymphadenitis is discussed below while the subject of lymphoid neoplasms including plasma cell disorders and Langerhans' cell histiocytosis is discussed later under haematologic neoplasms.

REACTIVE LYMPHADENITIS

Lymph nodes undergo reactive changes in response to a wide variety of stimuli which include microbial infections, drugs, environmental pollutants, tissue injury, immune-complexes and malignant neoplasms. However, the most common causes of lymph node enlargement are inflammatory and immune reactions, aside from primary malignant neoplasms and metastatic tumour deposits. Those due to primary inflammatory reaction are termed *reactive lymphadenitis,* and those due to primary immune reactions are referred to as *lymphadenopathy.*

Reactive lymphadenitis is a nonspecific response and is categorised into acute and chronic types, each with a few variant forms.

Acute Nonspecific Lymphadenitis

All kinds of acute inflammations may cause acute nonspecific lymphadenitis in the nodes draining the area of inflamed tissue. Most common causes are microbiologic infections or their breakdown products, and foreign bodies in the wound or into the circulation etc. Most frequently involved lymph nodes are: *cervical* (due to infections in the oral cavity), *axillary* (due to infection in the arm), *inguinal* (due to infection in the lower extremities), and *mesenteric* (due to acute appendicitis, acute enteritis etc).

Acute lymphadenitis is usually mild and transient but occasionally it may be more severe. Acutely inflamed nodes are enlarged, tender, and if extensively involved, may be fluctuant. The overlying skin is red and hot. After control of infection, majority of cases heal completely without leaving any scar. If the inflammation does not subside, acute lymphadenitis changes into chronic lymphadenitis.

> **MORPHOLOGIC FEATURES Grossly,** the affected lymph nodes are enlarged 2-3 times their normal size and may show abscess formation if the involvement is extensive.
>
> **Microscopically,** the sinusoids are congested, widely dilated and oedematous and contain numerous neutrophils. The lymphoid follicles are prominent with presence of many mitoses and phagocytosis. In more severe cases, necrosis may occur and neutrophil abscesses may form.

Chronic Nonspecific Lymphadenitis

Chronic nonspecific lymphadenitis, commonly called *reactive lymphoid hyperplasia,* is a common form of inflammatory reaction of draining lymph nodes as a response to antigenic stimuli such as repeated attacks of acute lymphadenitis and lymph from malignant tumours.

Depending upon the pattern in chronic nonspecific lymphadenitis, three types are distinguished, each having its own set of causes. These are: *follicular hyperplasia, paracortical hyperplasia* and *sinus histiocytosis.* However, mixed patterns may also be seen in which case one of the patterns predominates over the others.

MORPHOLOGIC FEATURES   Grossly, the affected lymph nodes are usually enlarged, firm and non-tender.

Microscopically, the features of 3 patterns of reactive lymphoid hyperplasia are as under:

1. Follicular hyperplasia This is the most frequent pattern, particularly encountered in children. Besides nonspecific stimulation, a few specific causes are: rheumatoid arthritis, toxoplasmosis, syphilis and AIDS. The microscopic features are as follows (Fig. 24.2):
i) There is marked enlargement and prominence of the germinal centres of lymphoid follicles (proliferation of B-cell areas) due to the presence of numerous mitotically active lymphocytes and proliferation of phagocytic cells containing phagocytosed material.
ii) Parafollicular and medullary regions are more cellular and contain plasma cells, histiocytes, and some neutrophils and eosinophils.
iii) There is hyperplasia of mononuclear phagocytic cells lining the lymphatic sinuses in the lymph node.

A clinicopathologic variant of follicular hyperplasia is *angiofollicular lymphoid hyperplasia* or *Castleman's disease.* This condition may occur at any age and possibly has an association with Epstein-Barr virus infection.

2. Paracortical lymphoid hyperplasia This is due to hyperplasia of T-cell-dependent area of the lymph node. Amongst the important causes are immunologic reactions due to drugs (e.g. dilantin), vaccination, viruses (e.g. infectious mononucleosis) and autoimmune disorders. Its histologic features are as under:
i) Expansion of the paracortex (T-cell area) with increased number of T-cell transformed immunoblasts.
ii) Encroachment by the enlarged paracortex on the lymphoid follicles, sometimes resulting in their effacement.
iii) Hyperplasia of the mononuclear phagocytic cells in the lymphatic sinuses.

Variants of paracortical lymphoid hyperplasia are angio-immunoblastic lymphadenopathy, dermatopathic lymphadenopathy, dilantin lymphadenopathy and post-vaccinal lymphadenopathy.

3. Sinus histiocytosis or sinus hyperplasia This is a very common type found in regional lymph nodes draining inflammatory lesions, or as an immune reaction of the host to a draining malignant tumour or its products. The hallmark of histologic diagnosis is the expansion of the sinuses by proliferating large histiocytes containing phagocytosed material (Fig. 24.3). The presence of sinus histiocytosis in the draining lymph nodes of carcinoma such as in breast carcinoma has been considered by some workers to confer better prognosis in such patients due to good host immune response.

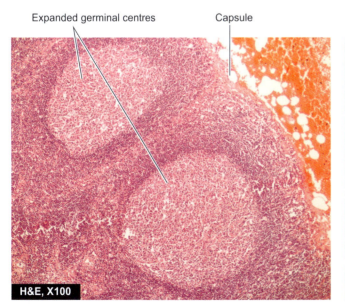

Figure 24.2 ▶ Reactive lymphadenitis, follicular hyperplasia type.

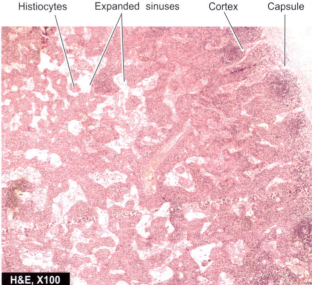

Figure 24.3 ▶ Reactive lymphadenitis, sinus histiocytosis type.

A variant form, *sinus histiocytosis with massive lymphadenopathy,* is characterised by marked enlargement of lymph nodes, especially of the neck, in young adolescents. It is associated with characteristic clinical features of painless but massive lymphadenopathy with fever and leucocytosis and usually runs a benign and self-limiting course.

HIV-related Lymphadenopathy

HIV infection and AIDS have already been discussed in Chapter 14; here one of the frequent finding in early cases of AIDS, **persistent generalised lymphadenopathy (PGL)**, is described. The presence of enlarged lymph nodes of more than 1 cm diameter at two or more extra-inguinal sites for more than 3 months without any other obvious cause is frequently the earliest symptom of primary HIV infection.

Histologically, the findings at biopsy of involved lymph node vary depending upon the stage of HIV infection:
1. *In the early stage* marked follicular hyperplasia is the dominant finding and reflects the polyclonal B-cell proliferation.
2. *In the intermediate stage,* there is a combination of follicular hyperplasia and follicular involution. However, adenopathic form of Kaposi's sarcoma too may develop at this stage (page 350).
3. *In the last stage,* there is decrease in the lymph node size indicative of prognostic marker of disease progression. Microscopic findings of node at this stage reveal follicular involution and lymphocyte depletion. At this stage, other stigmata of AIDS in the lymph node may also appear e.g. lymphoma, mycobacterial infection, toxoplasmosis, systemic fungal infections etc.

| GIST BOX 24.1 | Lymph Nodes—Normal and Reactive Hyperplasia |

- A normal lymph node has T-cell zone in the medulla and B-cell zone in the follicles of cortex.
- Reactive lymphadenitis is enlargement of lymph node in response to stimuli e.g. microbes, drugs, pollutants, immune complexes etc.
- Reactive lymphadentitis may be acute or chronic.
- Chronic reactive lymphadenitis is more common and may be follicular hyperplasia or sinus histiocytosis type.

WHITE BLOOD CELLS: NORMAL AND REACTIVE PROLIFERATIONS

The leucocytes of the peripheral blood are of 2 main varieties, distinguished by the presence or absence of granules: *granulocytes* and *nongranular leucocytes.* The granulocytes, according to the appearance of nuclei, are subdivided into polymorphonuclear leucocytes and monocytes. Further, depending upon the colour and content of granules, polymorphonuclear leucocytes are of 3 types: neutrophils, eosinophils and basophils. The nongranular leucocytes are 3 types of lymphocytes: T, B and natural killer (NK) cells.

GRANULOPOIESIS

Site of Formation and Kinetics

All forms of granulocytes are produced in the bone marrow and are termed, *'myeloid series.'* Myeloid series include maturing stages: myeloblast (most primitive precursor), promyelocyte, myelocyte, metamyelocyte, band forms and segmented granulocyte (mature form). It takes about 12 days for formation of mature granulocytes from the myeloblast. These maturing cells are further divided into:
◆ *'proliferative or mitotic pool'* comprised by myeloblast, promyelocyte and myelocyte; and
◆ *'mature or post-mitotic pool'* composed of metamyelocyte, band forms and segmented granulocytes).

Normally the bone marrow contains more myeloid cells than the erythroid cells in the ratio of 2:1 to 15:1 (average 3:1), the largest proportion being that of metamyelocytes, band forms and segmented neutrophils. The bone marrow storage compartment contains about 10-15 times the number of granulocytes found in the peripheral blood. Following their release from the bone marrow, granulocytes spend about 10 hours in the circulation before they move into the tissues, where they perform their respective functions. The blood pool of granulocytes consists of 2 components of about equal size—the *circulating pool* that is included in the blood count, and the *marginating pool* that is not included in the blood count. Granulocytes spend about 4-5 days in the tissues before they are either destroyed during phagocytosis or die due to senescence. To control the various compartments of granulocytes, a 'feed-back system' exists between the circulating and tissue granulocytes on one side, and the marrow granulocytes on the other. The presence of a humoral regulatory substance, 'granulopoietin' analogous to erythropoietin has also been identified by *in vitro* studies of colony-forming units (CFU) and is characterised as G-CSF (granulocyte colony-stimulating factor) and GM-CSF (granulocyte-monocyte colony-stimulating factor).

The kinetics of monocytes is less well understood than that of other myeloid cells. Monocytes spend about 20-40 hours in the circulation after which they leave the blood to enter extravascular tissues where they perform their main function of active phagocytosis. The extravascular lifespan of tissue macrophages which are the transformed form of blood monocytes, may vary from a few months to a few years.

Myeloid Series

The development of myeloid cells from myeloblast takes place in the following sequence **(Fig. 24.4)**:

1. **MYELOBLAST** The myeloblast is the earliest recognisable precursor of the granulocytes, normally comprising

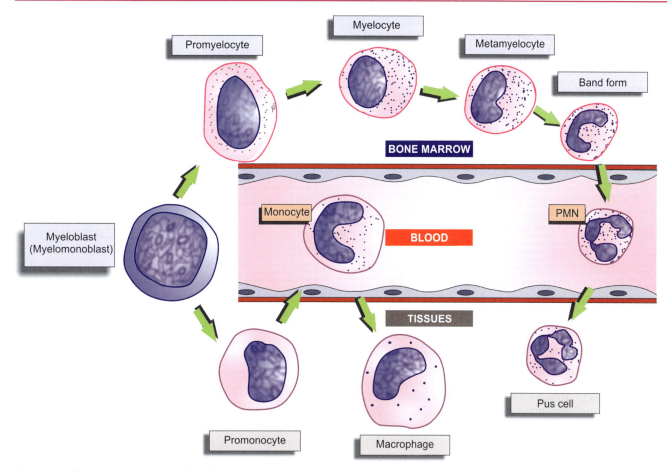

Figure 24.4 ▶ Granulopoiesis and the cellular compartments of myeloid cells in the bone marrow, blood and tissues.

about 2% of the total marrow cells. The myeloblast varies considerably in size (10-18 μm in diameter), having a large round to oval nucleus nearly filling the cell, has fine nuclear chromatin and contains 2-5 well-defined pale nucleoli. The thin rim of cytoplasm is deeply basophilic and devoid of granules. The myeloblasts of acute myeloid leukaemia may, however, show the presence of rod-like cytoplasmic inclusions called *Auer's rods* which represent abnormal derivatives of primary azurophilic granules.

The nuclei of successive stages during their development from myeloblast become progressively coarser and lose their nucleoli and the cytoplasm loses its blue colour. As the cells become mature lysosomal granules appear; firstly non-specific primary or azurophilic granules appear which are followed by specific or secondary granules that differentiate the neutrophils, eosinophils and basophils.

2. PROMYELOCYTE The promyelocyte is slightly larger than the myeloblast (12-18 μm diameter). It possesses a round to oval nucleus, having fine nuclear chromatin which is slightly condensed around the nuclear membrane. The nucleoli are present but are less prominent and fewer than those in the myeloblast. The main distinction of promyelocyte from myeloblast is in the cytoplasm which contains azurophilic (primary or non-specific) granules.

3. MYELOCYTE The myelocyte is the stage in which specific or secondary granules appear in the cytoplasm, and accordingly, the cell can be identified at this stage as belonging to the neutrophilic, eosinophilic or basophilic myelocyte. Primary granules also persist at this stage but formation of new primary granules stops. The nucleus of myelocyte is eccentric, round to oval, having somewhat coarse nuclear chromatin and no visible nucleoli. The myeloid cells up to the myelocyte stage continue to divide and, therefore, are included in *mitotic or proliferative pool*.

4. METAMYELOCYTE The metamyelocyte stage is 10-18 μm in diameter and is characterised by a clearly indented or horseshoe-shaped nucleus without nucleoli. The nuclear chromatin is dense and clumped. The cytoplasm contains both primary and secondary granules. The metamyelocytes are best distinguished from the monocytes by the clumped nuclear chromatin while the latter have fine chromatin.

5. BAND FORMS Band form is juvenile granulocyte, 10-16 µm in diameter, characterised by further condensation of nuclear chromatin and transformation of nuclear shape into band configuration of uniform thickness.

6. SEGMENTED GRANULOCYTES The mature polymorphonuclear leucocytes, namely: the neutrophils, eosinophils and basophils, are described separately below.

Common surface markers for all stages of myeloid series of cells are CD33, CD13 and CD15. However, stages from myelocytes to mature neutrophils also carry CD11b and CD14. Band forms and mature neutrophils have further CD 10 and CD16.

Monocyte-Macrophage Series

The monocyte-macrophage series of cells, though comprise a part of myeloid series along with other granulocytic series, but are described separately here in view of different morphologic stages in their maturation **(Fig. 24.4)**.

1. MONOBLAST The monoblast is the least mature of the recognisable cell of monocyte-macrophage series. It is very similar in appearance to myeloblast except that it has ground-glass cytoplasm with irregular border and may show phagocytosis as indicated by the presence of engulfed red cells in the cytoplasm. However, differentiation from myeloblast at times may be difficult even by electron microscopy and, therefore, it is preferable to call the earliest precursor of granulocytic series as *myelomonoblast*.

2. PROMONOCYTE The promonocyte is a young monocyte, about 20 µm in diameter and possesses a large indented nucleus containing a nucleolus. The cytoplasm is basophilic and contains no azurophilic granules but may have fine granules which are larger than those in the mature monocyte.

3. MONOCYTE The mature form of monocytic series is described below, while the transformed stages of these cells in various tissues (i.e. macrophages) are a part of RE system.

Monocyte-macrophage series having specialised function of phagocytosis secrete active products such as lysozyme, neutral proteases, acid hydrolases, components of complement, transferrin, fibronectin, nucleosides and several cytokines (TNF-α, IL-1, IL-8, IL-12, IL-18). They express lineage-specific molecules CD14, cell surface LPS receptors etc.

LYMPHOPOIESIS

Sites of Formation and Kinetics

The lymphocytes and the plasma cells are immunocompetent cells of the body. In humans, the bone marrow and the thymus are the *primary lymphopoietic organs* where lymphoid stem cells undergo spontaneous division independent of antigenic stimulation. The *secondary or reactive lymphoid tissue* is comprised by the lymph nodes, spleen and gut-associated lymphoid tissue (GALT). These sites actively produce lymphocytes from the germinal centres of lymphoid follicles as a response to antigenic stimulation. Lymphocytes pass through a series of developmental changes in the course of their evolution into lymphocyte subpopulations and subsets. It includes migration of immature lymphocytes to other organs such as the thymus where locally-produced factors act on them.

Functionally, the lymphocytes are divided into T, B and natural killer (NK) cells depending upon whether they are immunologically active in cell-mediated immunity (T cells), in humoral antibody response (B cells) or form part of the natural or innate immunity and act as killer of some viruses (NK cells). In human beings, the B cells are derived from the bone marrow stem cells, while in birds they mature in the bursa of Fabricius. After antigenic activation, B cells proliferate and mature into plasma cells which secrete specific immunoglobulin antibodies. The T cells are also produced in the bone marrow and possibly in the thymus. NK cells do not have B or T cell markers, nor are these cells dependent upon thymus for development. The concept of T, B and NK cells along with lymphocyte subpopulations and their functions is discussed in Chapter 14.

Lymphoid Series

The maturation stages in production of lymphocytes are illustrated in **Fig. 24.5** and are as under:

1. LYMPHOBLAST The lymphoblast is the earliest identifiable precursor of lymphoid cells and is a rapidly dividing cell. It is a large cell, 10-18 µm in diameter, containing a large round to oval nucleus having slightly clumped or stippled nuclear chromatin. The nuclear membrane is denser and the number of nucleoli is fewer (1-2) as compared with those in myeloblast (2-5). The cytoplasm is scanty, basophilic and non-granular.

The distinguishing morphologic features between the myeloblast and lymphoblast are summarised in **Table 24.1**.

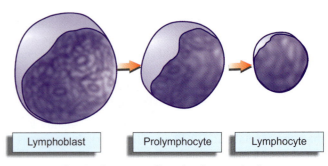

Figure 24.5 ▶ The formation of lymphoid series of cells.

Chapter 24: Diseases of Leucocytes and Lymphoid Tissues

Table 24.1 Morphologic characteristics of the blast cells in Romanowsky stains.

FEATURE	MYELOBLAST	LYMPHOBLAST
1. Size	10-18 μm	10-18 μm
2. Nucleus	Round or oval	Round or oval
3. Nuclear chromatin	Fine meshwork	Slightly clumped
4. Nuclear membrane	Very fine	Fairly dense
5. Nucleoli	2-5	1-2
6. Cytoplasm	Scanty, blue, agranular, Auer rods may be seen	Scanty, clear blue, agranular

Table 24.2 Normal white blood cell counts in health.

	ABSOLUTE COUNT
TLC	
Adults	4,000–11,000/μl
Infants (Full term, at birth)	10,000–25,000/μl
Infants (1 year)	6,000–16,000/μl
Children (4–7 years)	5,000–15,000/μl
Children (8–12 years)	4,500–13,500/μl
DLC IN ADULTS	
Polymorphs (neutrophils) 40–75%	2,000–7,500/μl
Lymphocytes 20–50%	1,500–4,000/μl
Monocytes 2–10%	200–800/μl
Eosinophils 1–6%	40–400/μl
Basophils <1%	10–100/μl

2. **PROLYMPHOCYTE** This stage is an intermediate stage between the lymphoblast and mature lymphocyte. These young lymphocytes are 9-18 μm in diameter, contain round to indented nucleus with slightly stippled or coarse chromatin and may have 0-1 nucleoli.

3. **LYMPHOCYTE** The mature lymphocytes are described below.

MATURE LEUCOCYTES IN HEALTH AND REACTIVE PROLIFERATION IN DISEASE

Normally, only mature leucocytes namely: polymorphs, lymphocytes, monocytes, eosinophils and basophils, are found in the peripheral blood. The normal range of total and differential leucocyte count (TLC and DLC expressed sequentially as P, L, M, E, B) in health in adults and children is given in **Table 24.2**. White cell count tends to be higher in infants and children than in adults. It also normally undergoes minor degree of diurnal variation with a slight rise in the afternoon. The total white cell count is normally high in pregnancy and following delivery, usually returning to normal within a week. Pathological variations in white cell values together with brief review of their morphology and functions are considered below **(Fig. 24.6)**:

Polymorphs (Neutrophils)

MORPHOLOGY A polymorphonuclear neutrophil (PMN), commonly called polymorph or neutrophil, is 12-15 μm in diameter. It consists of a characteristic dense nucleus, having 2-5 lobes and pale cytoplasm containing numerous fine violet-pink granules. These lysosomal granules contain several enzymes and are of 2 types:

Primary or azurophilic granules are large and coarse and appear early at the promyelocyte stage. These granules contain hydrolases, elastase, myeloperoxidase, cathepsin-G, cationic proteins, permeability increasing protein, and microbicidal protein called defensins.

Secondary or specific granules are smaller and more numerous. These appear later at myelocyte stage, are MPO-negative and contain lactoferrin, NADPH oxidase, histaminase, vitamin B_{12} binding protein, and receptors for chemoattractants and for laminin.

The normal **functions** of neutrophils are as under:

1. *Chemotaxis* or cell mobilisation in which the cell is attracted towards bacteria or at the site of inflammation.

2. *Phagocytosis* in which the foreign particulate material of tiny sizes is phagocytosed by actively motile neutrophils; thus PMNs act as microphages compared to function of monocytes as macrophages.

3. *Killing* of the microorganism is mediated by oxygen-dependent and oxygen-independent pathways (page 112).

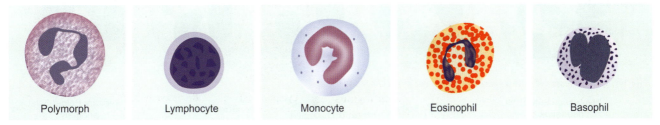

Figure 24.6 ▶ Morphology of normal mature leucocytes in peripheral blood.

PATHOLOGIC VARIATIONS Pathologic variations in neutrophils include variations in count, morphology and defective function.

VARIATION IN COUNT An increase in neutrophil count (*neutrophil leucocytosis* or *neutrophilia*) or a decrease in count (*neutropenia*) may occur in various diseases.

Neutrophil leucocytosis An increase in circulating neutrophils above 7,500/µl is the commonest type of leucocytosis and occurs most commonly as a response to acute bacterial infections. Some common causes of neutrophilia are as under:

1. *Acute infections, local or generalised,* especially by cocci but also by certain bacilli, fungi, spirochaetes, parasites and some viruses. For example: pneumonia, cholecystitis, salpingitis, meningitis, diphtheria, plague, peritonitis, appendicitis, actinomycosis, poliomyelitis, abscesses, furuncles, carbuncles, tonsillitis, otitis media, osteomyelitis etc.

2. *Other inflammations* e.g. tissue damage resulting from burns, operations, ischaemic necrosis (such as in MI), gout, collagen-vascular diseases, hypersensitivity reactions etc.

3. *Intoxication* e.g. uraemia, diabetic ketosis, eclampsia, poisonings by chemicals and drugs.

4. *Acute haemorrhage,* internal or external.

5. *Acute haemolysis.*

6. *Disseminated malignancies.*

7. *Myeloproliferative disorders* e.g. myeloid leukaemia, polycythaemia vera, myeloid metaplasia.

8. *Miscellaneous* e.g. following corticosteroid therapy, idiopathic neutrophilia.

Neutropenia When the absolute neutrophil count falls below 2,500/µl, the patient is said to have neutropenia and is prone to develop recurrent infections. Some common causes of neutropenia (and hence leucopenia) are as follows:

1. *Certain infections* e.g. typhoid, paratyphoid, brucellosis, influenza, measles, viral hepatitis, malaria, kala-azar etc.

2. *Overwhelming bacterial infections* especially in patients with poor resistance e.g. miliary tuberculosis, septicaemia.

3. *Drugs, chemicals and physical agents* which induce aplasia of the bone marrow cause neutropenia, e.g. antimetabolites, nitrogen mustards, benzene, ionising radiation. Occasionally, certain drugs produce neutropenia due to individual sensitivity such as: anti-inflammatory (amidopyrine, phenylbutazone), antibacterial (chloramphenicol, cotrimoxazole), anticonvulsants, antithyroids, hypoglycaemics and antihistaminics.

4. *Certain haematological and other diseases* e.g. pernicious anaemia, aplastic anaemia, cirrhosis of the liver with splenomegaly, SLE, Gaucher's disease.

5. *Cachexia and debility.*

6. *Anaphylactoid shock.*

7. *Certain rare hereditary, congenital or familial disorders* e.g. cyclic neutropenia, primary splenic neutropenia, idiopathic benign neutropenia.

VARIATIONS IN MORPHOLOGY Some of the common variations in neutrophil morphology are shown in Fig. 24.7. These are as under:

1. **Granules** Heavy, dark staining, coarse toxic granules are characteristic of bacterial infections.

2. **Vacuoles** In bacterial infections such as in septicaemia, cytoplasmic vacuolation may develop.

3. **Döhle bodies** These are small, round or oval patches, 2-3 µm in size, in the cytoplasm. They are mostly seen in bacterial infections.

4. **Nuclear changes** These include the following:

i) *Sex chromatin* is a normal finding in 2-3% of neutrophils in female sex. It consists of a drumstick appendage of chromatin, about 1 µm across, and attached to one of the nuclear lobes by a thin chromatin strand. Their presence in more than 20% of PMNs is indicative of female sex chromosomes.

ii) A *'shift-to-left'* is the term used for appearance of neutrophils with decreased number of nuclear lobes in the peripheral blood e.g. presence of band and stab forms and

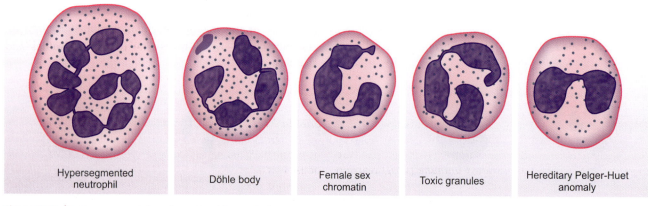

Figure 24.7 ▶ Common variations in neutrophil morphology.

a few myelocytes in the peripheral blood. It is seen in severe infections, leucoerythroblastic reaction or leukaemia.

iii) A *'shift-to-right'* is appearance of hypersegmented (more than 5 nuclear lobes) neutrophils in the peripheral blood such as in megaloblastic anaemia, uraemia, and sometimes in leukaemia.

iv) *Pelger-Huët anomaly* is an uncommon autosomal dominant inherited disorder in which nuclei in majority of neutrophils are distinctively bilobed (spectacle-shaped) and coarsely staining chromatin. Acquired pseudo-Pelger-Huët abnormality may occur in acute infections or in MDS. However, the physiologic role of multilobed nucleus of neutrophils is unknown and the bilobed anomaly is an innocuous condition.

DEFECTIVE FUNCTIONS The following abnormalities in neutrophil function may sometimes be found:

1. Defective chemotaxis e.g. in a rare congenital abnormality called lazy-leucocyte syndrome; following corticosteroid therapy, aspirin ingestion, alcoholism, and in myeloid leukaemia.

2. Defective phagocytosis due to lack of opsonisation e.g. in hypogammaglobulinaemia, hypocomplementaemia, after splenectomy, in sickle cell disease.

3. Defective killing e.g. in chronic granulomatous disease, Chédiak-Higashi syndrome, myeloid leukaemias.

Lymphocytes

MORPHOLOGY Majority of lymphocytes in the peripheral blood are *small* (9-12 μm in diameter) but *large* lymphocytes (12-16 μm in diameter) are also found. Both small and large lymphocytes have round or slightly indented nucleus with coarsely-clumped chromatin and scanty basophilic cytoplasm. Plasma cells are derived from B lymphocytes under the influence of appropriate stimuli. The nucleus of plasma cell is eccentric and has cart-wheel pattern of clumped nuclear chromatin. The cytoplasm is characteristically deeply basophilic with a pale perinuclear zone. Plasma cells are normally not present in peripheral blood but their pathological proliferation occurs in myelomatosis. Reactive lymphocytes (or Turk cells or plasmacytoid lymphocytes) are seen in certain viral infections and have sufficiently basophilic cytoplasm that they resemble plasma cells.

As discussed in Chapter 14, functionally, there are 3 types of lymphocytes and possess distinct surface markers called clusters of differentiation (CD) which aid in identification of stage of their differentiation (page 196):

T lymphocytes i.e. thymus-dependent lymphocytes, which mature in the thymus and are also known as thymocytes. They are mainly involved in direct action on antigens and are therefore involved in *cell-mediated immune (CMI)* reaction by its subsets such as cytotoxic (killer) T cells (CD3+), CD8+ T cells, and *delayed hypersensitivity reaction* by CD4+ T cells.

B lymphocytes i.e. bone marrow-dependent or bursa-equivalent lymphocytes as well as their derivatives, plasma cells, are the source of specific immunoglobulin antibodies. They are, therefore, involved in *humoral immunity (HI) or circulating immune reactions.*

NK cells i.e. natural killer cells are those lymphocytes which morphologically have appearance of lymphocytes but do not possess functional features of T or B cells. As the name indicates they are identified with *'natural'* or innate immunity and bring about direct *'killing'* of microorganisms (particularly certain viruses) or lysis of foreign body.

Stages of immunolgic differentiation of lymphoid cells is again discussed on page 442.

PATHOLOGIC VARIATIONS A rise in the absolute count of lymphocytes exceeding the upper limit of normal (above 4,000/μm) is termed *lymphocytosis,* while absolute lymphocyte count below 1,500/μm is referred to as *lymphopenia.*

Lymphocytosis Some of the common causes of lymphocytosis are as under:

1. *Certain acute infections* e.g. pertussis, infectious mononucleosis, viral hepatitis, infectious lymphocytosis.
2. *Certain chronic infections* e.g. brucellosis, tuberculosis, secondary syphilis.
3. *Haematopoietic disorders* e.g. lymphocytic leukaemias, lymphoma, heavy chain disease.
4. *Relative lymphocytosis* is found in viral exanthemas, convalescence from acute infections, thyrotoxicosis, conditions causing neutropenia.

Lymphopenia Lymphopenia is uncommon and occurs in the following conditions:

1. Most acute infections.
2. Severe bone marrow failure.
3. Corticosteroid and immunosuppressive therapy.
4. Widespread irradiation.

Monocytes

MORPHOLOGY The monocyte is the largest mature leucocyte in the peripheral blood measuring 12-20 μm in diameter. It possesses a large, central, oval, notched or indented or horseshoe-shaped nucleus which has characteristically fine reticulated chromatin network. The cytoplasm is abundant, pale blue and contains many fine dust-like granules and vacuoles.

The main **functions** of monocytes are as under:

1. *Phagocytosis* of antigenic material or microorganisms.
2. Immunologic function as *antigen-presenting cells* and present the antigen to lymphocytes to deal with further.
3. As *mediator of inflammation*, they are involved in release of prostaglandins, stimulation of the liver to secrete acute phase reactants.

Tissue macrophages of different types included in RE system are derived from blood monocytes (page 123).

PATHOLOGIC VARIATIONS A rise in the blood monocytes above 800/μl is termed *monocytosis*. Some common causes of monocytosis are as follows:
1. *Certain bacterial infections* e.g. tuberculosis, subacute bacterial endocarditis, syphilis.
2. *Viral infections.*
3. *Protozoal and rickettsial infections* e.g. malaria, typhus, trypanosomiasis, kala-azar.
4. *Convalescence from acute infection.*
5. *Haematopoietic disorders* e.g. monocytic leukaemia, lymphomas, myeloproliferative disorders, multiple myeloma, lipid storage disease.
6. *Malignancies* e.g. cancer of the ovary, stomach, breast.
7. *Granulomatous diseases* e.g. sarcoidosis, inflammatory bowel disease.
8. *Collagen-vascular diseases.*

Eosinophils

MORPHOLOGY Eosinophils are similar to segmented neutrophils in size (12-15 μm in diameter), and have coarse, deep red staining granules in the cytoplasm and have usually two nuclear lobes. Granules in eosinophils contain basic protein and stain more intensely for peroxidase than granules in the neutrophils. In addition, eosinophils also contain cell adhesion molecules, cytokines (IL-3, IL-5), and a protein that precipitates Charcot-Leyden crystals in lung tissues in asthmatic patients.

Eosinophils are involved in reactions to foreign proteins and to antigen-antibody reactions.

PATHOLOGIC VARIATIONS An increase in the number of eosinophilic leucocytes above 400/μl is referred to as *eosinophilia* and below 40/μl is termed as *eosinopenia*.

Eosinophilia. The causes are as under:
1. *Allergic disorders* e.g. bronchial asthma, urticaria, angioneurotic oedema, hay fever, drug hypersensitivity.
2. *Parasitic infestations* e.g. trichinosis, echinococcosis, intestinal parasitism.
3. *Skin diseases* e.g. pemphigus, dermatitis herpetiformis, erythema multiforme.
4. *Löeffler's syndrome.*
5. *Pulmonary infiltration with eosinophilia* (PIE) syndrome.
6. *Tropical eosinophilia.*
7. *Haematopoietic diseases* e.g. CML, polycythaemia vera, pernicious anaemia, Hodgkin's disease, following splenectomy.
8. *Malignant diseases* with metastases.
9. *Irradiation.*
10. *Miscellaneous disorders* e.g. polyarteritis nodosa, rheumatoid arthritis, sarcoidosis.

Eosinopenia Adrenal steroids and ACTH induce eosinopenia in man.

Basophils

MORPHOLOGY Basophils resemble the other mature granulocytes but are distinguished by coarse, intensely basophilic granules which usually fill the cytoplasm and often overlie and obscure the nucleus.

The granules of circulating basophils (as well as their tissue counterparts as mast cells) contain heparin, histamine and 5 HT. Mast cells or basophils on degranulation are associated with histamine release.

PATHOLOGIC VARIATIONS Basophil leucocytosis or *basophilia* refers to an increase in the number of basophilic leucocytes above 100/μl. Basophilia is unusual and is found in the following conditions:
1. Chronic myeloid leukaemia
2. Polycythaemia vera
3. Myelosclerosis
4. Myxoedema
5. Ulcerative colitis
6. Following splenectomy
7. Hodgkin's disease
8. Urticaria pigmentosa.

INFECTIOUS MONONUCLEOSIS

Infectious mononucleosis (IM) or glandular fever is a benign, self-limiting lymphoproliferative disease caused by Epstein-Barr virus (EBV), one of the herpesviruses. Infection may occur from childhood to old age but the classical acute infection is more common in teenagers and young adults. The infection is transmitted by person-to-person contact such as by kissing with transfer of virally-contaminated saliva. Groups of cases occur particularly in young people living together in boarding schools, colleges, camps and military institutions. Primary infection in childhood is generally asymptomatic, while 50% of adults develop clinical manifestations. The condition is so common that by the age of 40, most people have been infected and developed antibodies. It may be mentioned here that EBV is oncogenic as well and is strongly implicated in the African (endemic) Burkitt's lymphoma and nasopharyngeal carcinoma (page 306).

Pathogenesis

EBV, the etiologic agent for IM, is a B lymphotropic herpesvirus. The disease is characterised by fever, generalised lymphadenopathy, hepatosplenomegaly, sore throat, and appearance in blood of atypical 'mononucleosis cells'. The pathogenesis of these pathologic features is outlined below:
1. In a susceptible sero-negative host who lacks antibodies, the virus in the contaminated saliva *invades and replicates within epithelial cells* of the salivary gland and then enters B cells in the lymphoid tissues which possess receptors for EBV. The infection spreads throughout the body via bloodstream or by infected B cells.

2. Viraemia and death of infected B cells cause an acute febrile illness and appearance of specific humoral antibodies which peak about 2 weeks after the infection and persist throughout life. The appearance of antibodies marks the *disappearance of virus from the blood.*

3. Though the viral agent has disappeared from the blood, the EBV-infected B cells continue to be present in the circulation as latent infection. *EBV-infected B cells undergo polyclonal activation and proliferation.* These cells perform two important roles which are the characteristic diagnostic features of IM:

i) They secrete *antibodies*—initially IgM but later IgG class antibodies appear. IgM antibody is the heterophile anti-sheep antibody used for diagnosis of IM while IgG antibody persists for life and provides immunity against re-infection.

ii) They *activate CD8+T lymphocytes*—also called cytotoxic T cells (or CTL) or suppressor T cells. CD8+ T cells bring about killing of B cells and are pathognomonic atypical lymphocytes seen in blood in IM.

4. The proliferation of these cells is responsible for *generalised lymphadenopathy and hepatosplenomegaly.*

5. The *sore throat* in IM may be caused by either necrosis of B cells or due to viral replication within the salivary epithelial cells in early stage.

Besides the involvement of EBV in the pathogenesis of IM, its role in neoplastic transformation in nasopharyngeal carcinoma and Burkitt's lymphoma is discussed in Chapter 19 and diagrammatically depicted in **Fig. 24.8**.

Clinical Features

The incubation period of IM is 30-50 days in young adults, while children have shorter incubation period. A prodromal period of 3-5 days is followed by frank clinical features lasting for 1-3 weeks, and subsequently complete recovery occurs after 2 months. The usual clinical features are as under:

1. **During prodromal period (first 3-5 days),** the symptoms are mild such as malaise, myalgia, headache and fatigue.

2. **Frank clinical features (next 7-21 days)** seen commonly are fever (90%), sore throat (80%) and bilateral cervical lymphadenopathy (95%). Other features are splenomegaly (50% patients), hepatomegaly (10% cases), transient erythematous maculopapular rash on the trunk and extremities (10%), periorbital oedema (10%) and jaundice (5%).

3. **Complications** Although most cases of IM run a self-limited course, complications may develop in some cases as under:

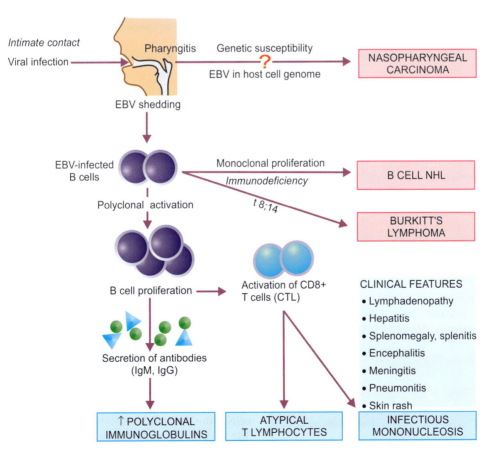

Figure 24.8 ▶ The role of EBV in the pathogenesis of infectious mononucleosis, nasopharyngeal carcinoma and Burkitt's lymphoma.

i) Neurologic manifestations in children.
ii) Splenic rupture due to splenitis.
iii) Upper airway obstruction due to hypertrophied adenotonsillitis.
iv) Autoimmune haemolytic anaemia, cold antibody type.
v) Bacterial superinfection.
vi) Rarely, myocarditis, hepatitis, pneumonia.

Laboratory Findings

The diagnosis of IM is made by characteristic haematologic and serologic findings.

1. HAEMATOLOGIC FINDINGS Major abnormalities in blood are as under:

i) TLC There is a moderate rise in total white cell count (10,000-20,000/μl) during 2nd to 3rd week after infection.

ii) DLC There is an absolute lymphocytosis. The lymphocytosis is due to rise in normal as well as atypical T lymphocytes. There is relative neutropenia.

iii) Atypical T cells Essential to the diagnosis of IM is the presence of at least 10-12% *atypical T cells (or mononucleosis cells)* lying in peripheral blood lymphocytosis **(Fig. 24.9)**. The mononucleosis cells are variable in appearance and are classed as Downey type I, II and III, of which Downey type I are found most frequently. These atypical T lymphocytes are usually of the size of large lymphocytes (12-16 μm diameter). The nucleus, rather than the usual round configuration, is oval, kidney-shaped or slightly lobate due to indentation of nuclear membrane and contains relatively fine chromatin without nucleoli, suggesting an immature pattern but short of leukaemic features. The cytoplasm is more abundant, basophilic and finely granular and may contain vacuoles.

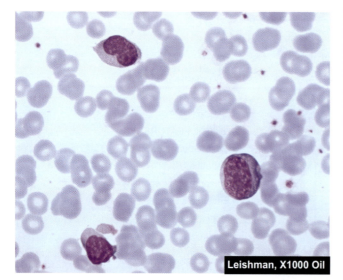

Figure 24.9 ▶ Peripheral blood film showing atypical lymphocytes in infectious mononucleosis.

The greatest number of atypical lymphocytes is found between 7th to 10th day of the illness and these cells may persist in the blood for up to 2 months.

iv) CD4+ and CD8+ T cell counts There is reversal of CD4+/CD8+ T cell ratio. There is marked decrease in CD4+ T cells while there is substantial rise in CD8+ T cells.

v) Platelets There is generally thrombocytopenia in the first 4 weeks of illness.

2. SEROLOGIC DIAGNOSIS The second characteristic laboratory finding is the demonstration of antibodies in the serum of infected patient. These are as under:

i) Test for heterophile antibodies Heterophile antibody test (Paul-Bunnell test) is used for making the diagnosis of IM. In this test, patient's serum is absorbed with guinea pig kidney. Serum dilutions are prepared which are used for agglutination of red cells of sheep, horse or cow and are reported as heterophile titer of test serum. A high serum titer of 40 or more times is diagnostic of acute IM infection in symptomatic case in the first week. Heterophile antibodies peak during the 3rd week in 80-90% cases. The test remains positive for about 3 months after the illness started. Thus, the test has to be repeatedly performed. Similar antibody is also produced in patients suffering from serum sickness and has to be distinguished by differential absorption studies. Heterophile antibodies are not demonstrable in children under 5 years of age or in quite elderly. Currently, more sensitive and rapid kit-based test for heterophile antibodies, monospot, is also available.

ii) EBV-specific antibodies tests Specific antibodies against the viral capsid and nucleus of EBV can be demonstrated in patients who are negative for heterophile antibody test:

a) Specific antibodies against EBV capsid antigen show elevated titers in over 90% cases during acute infection. IgM class antibody appears early and is thus most useful for diagnosis of acute infection. IgG class antibody appears later and persists throughout life; thus it does not have diagnostic value but is instead used for assessing the past exposure to EBV infection.

b) Antibodies against EBV nuclear antigen are detected 3 to 6 weeks after infection and, like IgG class antibodies, persist throughout life.

c) Antibodies to early antigens may be elevated but are less useful for making diagnosis of IM. However, titers of these antibodies remain elevated for 3 to 6 months and their levels are high in cases of nasopharyngeal carcinoma and African Burkitt's lymphoma.

d) IgA antibodies to EBV antigen are seen in patients of nasopharyngeal carcinoma or those who are at high risk of developing this EBV-induced cancer.

iii) EBV antigen detection Detection of EBV DNA or proteins can be done in blood or CSF by PCR method.

Chapter 24: Diseases of Leucocytes and Lymphoid Tissues

3. LIVER FUNCTION TESTS In addition, abnormalities of the liver function test are found in about 90% of cases. These include elevated serum levels of transaminases (SGOT and SGPT), rise in serum alkaline phosphatase and mild elevation of serum bilirubin.

LEUKAEMOID REACTIONS

Leukaemoid reaction is defined as a reactive excessive leucocytosis in the peripheral blood resembling that of leukaemia in a subject who does not have leukaemia. In spite of confusing blood picture, the clinical features of leukaemia such as splenomegaly, lymphadenopathy and haemorrhages are usually absent and the features of underlying disorder causing the leukaemoid reaction are generally obvious.

Leukaemoid reaction may be myeloid or lymphoid; the former is much more common.

Myeloid Leukaemoid Reaction

CAUSES Majority of leukaemoid reactions involve the granulocyte series. It may occur in association with a wide variety of diseases. These are as under:

1. *Infections* e.g. staphylococcal pneumonia, disseminated tuberculosis, meningitis, diphtheria, sepsis, endocarditis, plague, infected abortions etc.

2. *Intoxication* e.g. eclampsia, mercury poisoning, severe burns.

3. *Malignant diseases* e.g. multiple myeloma, myelofibrosis, Hodgkin's disease, bone metastases.

4. *Severe haemorrhage and severe haemolysis.*

LABORATORY FINDINGS Myeloid leukaemoid reaction is characterised by the following laboratory features:

1. *Leucocytosis,* usually moderate, not exceeding 100,000/µl.

2. Proportion of *immature cells* mild to moderate, comprised by metamyelocytes, myelocytes (5-15%), and blasts fewer than 5% i.e. the blood picture simulates somewhat with that of CML **(Fig. 24.10, A)**.

3. Infective cases may show *toxic granulation and Döhle bodies* in the cytoplasm of neutrophils.

4. *Neutrophil (or Leucocyte) alkaline phosphatase (NAP or LAP) score* in the cytoplasm of mature neutrophils in leukaemoid reaction is characteristically high and is very useful to distinguish it from chronic myeloid leukaemia in doubtful cases **(Fig. 24.10, B)**.

5. *Cytogenetic studies* may be helpful in exceptional cases which reveal negative Philadelphia chromosome i.e. t (9; 22) or BCR-ABL fusion gene in myeloid leukaemoid reaction but positive in cases of CML.

6. *Additional features* include anaemia, normal-to-raised platelet count, myeloid hyperplasia of the marrow and absence of infiltration by immature cells in organs and tissues.

Table 24.3 sums up the features to distinguish myeloid leukaemoid reaction from chronic myeloid leukaemia.

Lymphoid Leukaemoid Reaction

CAUSES Lymphoid leukaemoid reaction may be found in the following conditions:

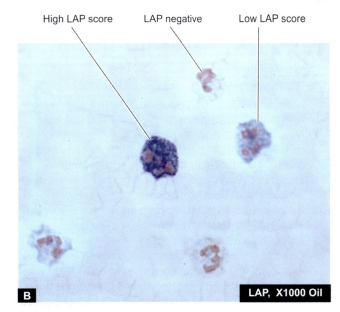

Figure 24.10 ▶ Leukaemoid reaction. A, Peripheral blood film showing marked neutrophilic leucocytosis accompanied with late precursors of myeloid series. B, Neutrophil (or leucocyte) alkaline phosphatase (NAP or LAP) activity is higher as demonstrated by this cytochemical stain.

Section V: Haematology and Lymphoreticular Tissues

Table 24.3 Contrasting features of leukaemoid reaction and chronic myeloid leukaemia.

	FEATURE	LEUKAEMOID REACTION	CML
1.	TLC	25,000-100,000/µl	≥ 100,000/µl
2.	DLC	i) Dominant cells PMNs ii) Immature cells predominantly metamyelocytes and myelocytes (5-15%), myeloblasts and promyelocytes ≥ 5% iii) Basophils normal	i) All maturation stages ii) Immature cells all stages, myeloblasts and promyelocytes ≤ 10% iii) Basophilia present
3.	NAP score	Elevated	Reduced
4.	Philadelphia chromosome	Absent	Present
5.	ABL-BCR fusion gene	Absent	Present
6.	Major etiology	Infections, intoxication, disseminated malignancy, severe haemorrhage	RNA viruses, HTLV oncogenesis, genetic factors, radiations, certain drugs and chemicals
7.	Additional haematologic findings	i) Anaemia ii) Normal to raised platelet count iii) Myeloid hyperplasia in bone marrow	Anaemia Normal to raised platelet count Myeloid hyperplasia in bone marrow
8.	Organ infiltration	Absent	May be present
9.	Massive splenomegaly	Absent	Present

1. *Infections* e.g. infectious mononucleosis, cytomegalovirus infection, pertussis (whooping cough), chickenpox, measles, infectious lymphocytosis, tuberculosis.
2. *Malignant diseases* may rarely produce lymphoid leukaemoid reaction.

LABORATORY FINDINGS The blood picture is characterised by the following findings:
1. Leucocytosis not exceeding 100,000/µl.
2. The differential white cell count reveals mostly mature lymphocytes simulating the blood picture found in cases of CLL.

 GIST BOX 24.2 White Blood Cells—Normal and Reactive Proliferations

- Granulopoiesis occurs under the influence of regulatory hormone granulopoietin having G-CSF and GM-CSF.
- Myeloid series of cells include myeloblasts, promyelocyte, myelocyte, metamyelocyte, band form and mature granulocytes (polymorph, eosinophil, basophil).
- Monocytic series are formed from monoblast and lymphoid cells from lymphoblasts.
- Peripheral blood normally contains mature leucocytes expressed as total and differential cell counts which remain within normal range.
- Pathologic variation in count of leucocytes is given as leucocytosis and may be due to neutrophilia (e.g. acute bacterial infections), lymphocytosis (e.g. viral infections), monocytosis (e.g. chronic bacterial or viral infections), eosinophilia (e.g. allergic disorders) and basophilia (e.g. CML).

- Infectious mononucleosis or glandular fever is a self-limited viral infection caused by EB virus producing fever, soar throat, lymphadenopathy and abnormal atypical T lymphocytes.
- Leukaemoid reaction is due to reactive proliferation of leucocytes, which may be myeloid or lymphoid. Myeloid leukaemoid reaction is more common and is due to an underlying cause. It requires distinction from CML—myeloid leukaemoid reaction has high LAP scores and is Philadelphia chromosome negative.

LYMPHOHAEMATOPOIETIC MALIGNANCIES (LEUKAEMIAS-LYMPHOMAS): GENERAL

CLASSIFICATION: HISTORY AND CURRENT CONCEPTS

Neoplastic proliferations of white blood cells are termed leukaemias and lymphomas and are the most important group of leucocyte disorders.

Historically, **leukaemias** have been classified on the basis of cell types predominantly involved into *myeloid* and *lymphoid,* and on the basis of natural history of the disease, into *acute* and *chronic.* Thus, the main types of leukaemias are: *acute myeloblastic leukaemia* and *acute lymphoblastic leukaemia* (AML and ALL), and *chronic myeloid leukaemia* and *chronic lymphocytic leukaemias* (CML and CLL); besides there are some other uncommon variants. In general, acute leukaemias are characterised by predominance of undifferentiated leucocyte precursors or leukaemic blasts and have a rapidly downhill course. Chronic leukaemias, on the other hand, have easily recognisable late precursor series of leucocytes circulating in large number as the predominant leukaemic cell type and the patients tend to have more indolent behaviour. The incidence of both acute and chronic leukaemias is higher in men than in women. ALL is primarily a disease of children and young adults, whereas AML occurs at all ages. CLL tends to occur in the elderly, while CML is found in middle age.

Similarly, over the years, **lymphomas** which are malignant tumours of lymphoreticular tissues have been categorised into two distinct clinicopathologic groups: *Hodgkin's lymphoma* or *Hodgkin's disease (HD)* characterised by pathognomonic presence of Reed-Sternberg cells, and a heterogeneous group of *non-Hodgkin's lymphomas (NHL)*.

Over the last 50 years, several classification systems have been proposed for leukaemias and lymphomas—clinicians favouring an approach based on clinical findings while pathologists have been interested in classifying them on morphologic features. Newer classification schemes have been based on cytochemistry, immunophenotyping, cytogenetics and molecular markers which have become available to pathologists and haematologists. The last classification scheme proposed by the World Health Organization (WHO) in 2008 combines all tumours of haematopoietic and lymphoid tissues together. The basis of the WHO classification is the *cell type of the neoplasm* as identified by combined approach of clinical features and morphologic, cytogenetic and molecular characteristics, *rather than location of the neoplasm* (whether in blood or in tissues) because of the fact that haematopoietic cells are present in circulation as well as in tissues in general, and lymphoreticular tissues in particular.

As per WHO classification scheme, neoplasms of haematopoietic and lymphoid tissues are considered as a unified group and are divided into 3 broad categories:

I. Myeloid neoplasms This group includes neoplasms of myeloid cell lineage and therefore includes neoplastic proliferations of red blood cells, platelets, granulocytes and monocytes. There are 5 categories under myeloid series of neoplasms: myeloproliferative disorders, myeloproliferative/myelodysplastic diseases, myelodysplastic syndromes (MDS), and acute myeloid leukaemia (AML), acute biphenotypic leukaemias.

II. Lymphoid neoplasms Neoplasms of lymphoid lineage include leukaemias and lymphomas of B, T or NK cell origin. This group is thus divided into Hodgkin's disease and non-Hodgkin's lymphomas; the latter includes B cell neoplasms (including plasma cell disorders), T cell neoplasms, and rarely NK cell neoplasms.

III. Histiocytic neoplasms This group is of interest mainly due to neoplastic proliferations of histiocytes in Langerhans cell histiocytosis.

Besides the WHO classification, another widely used classification is the French-American-British (FAB) Cooperative Group classification of lymphomas and leukaemias based on morphology and cytochemistry.

These as well as other classification schemes have been tabulated and discussed later under separate headings of myeloid and lymphoid malignancies.

ETIOLOGY OF LYMPHOHAEMATOPOIETIC MALIGNANCIES

The exact etiology of leukaemias and lymphomas is not known. However, a number of factors have been implicated:

1. HEREDITY There is evidence to suggest that there is role of family history, occurrence in identical twins and predisposition of these malignancies in certain genetic syndromes:

i) Identical twins There is high concordance rate among identical twins if acute leukaemia develops in the first year of life. Hodgkin's disease is 99 times more common in identical twin of an affected case compared with general population, implicating genetic origin strongly.

ii) Family history Families with excessive incidence of leukaemia have been identified.

iii) Genetic disease association Acute leukaemia occurs with increased frequency with a variety of congenital disorders such as Down's, Bloom's, Klinefelter's and Wiskott-Aldrich's syndromes, Fanconi's anaemia and ataxia telangiectasia. Hodgkin's disease has familial incidence and with certain HLA type.

2. INFECTIONS There is evidence to suggest that certain infections, particularly viruses, are involved in development of lymphomas and leukaemias (Chapter 19):

i) Human T cell leukaemia-lymphoma virus I (HTLV-I) implicated in etiology of adult T cell leukaemia-lymphoma (ATLL).

ii) HTLV II for T cell variant of hairy cell leukaemia.

iii) Epstein-Barr virus (EBV) implicated in the etiology of Hodgkin's disease (mixed cellularity type and nodular sclerosis type), endemic variety of Burkitt's lymphoma, post-transplant lymphoma.

iv) HIV in diffuse large B-cell lymphoma and Burkitt's lymphoma.

v) Hepatitis C virus (HCV) in lymphoplasmacytic lymphoma.

vi) Human herpes virus 8 (HHV-8) in primary effusion lymphoma.

vii) Helicobacter pylori bacterial infection of gastric mucosa in MALT lymphoma of the stomach.

3. ENVIRONMENTAL FACTORS Certain environmental factors are known to play a role in the etiology of leukaemias and lymphomas:

i) Ionising radiation Damage due to radiation exposure has been linked to development of leukaemias and lymphomas. Individuals exposed to occupational radiation exposure, patients receiving radiation therapy, and Japanese survivors of the atomic bomb explosions have been found to be at higher risk of developing haematopoietic malignancies, particularly prone to development of CML, AML and ALL but not to CLL or hairy cell leukaemia.

ii) Chemical carcinogens Benzene, tobacco smoking, alcohol, use of certain hair dyes and exposure to agriculture chemicals are associated with increased risk of development of haematopoietic malignancies.

iii) Certain drugs Long-term exposure to certain drugs such as phenytoin, alkylating agents and other chemotherapeutic agents is associated with increased incidence of leukaemias and lymphomas. Patients treated for Hodgkin's disease can develop NHL.

4. ASSOCIATION WITH DISEASES OF IMMUNITY Since lymphoid cells are the immune cells of the body, diseases with derangements of the immune system have higher incidence of haematopoietic malignancies:

i) Immunodeficiency diseases Various inherited and acquired immunodeficiency diseases including AIDS and iatrogenic immunosuppression induced by chemotherapy or radiation, are associated with subsequent development of lymphomatous transformation.

ii) Autoimmune disease association A few autoimmune diseases such as Sjögren's syndrome, nontropical sprue, rheumatoid arthritis and SLE are associated with higher incidence of NHL.

PATHOGENESIS

It needs to be emphasised that since haematopoietic cells have a rapid turnover, they are more vulnerable to chromosomal damages and cytogenetic changes under influence of various etiologic factors listed above.

1. Genetic damage to single clone of target cells Leukaemias and lymphomas arise following malignant transformation of a single clone of cells belonging to myeloid or lymphoid series, followed by proliferation of the transformed clone. Basic mechanism of malignant transformation is genetic damage to the DNA of the target white cells followed by proliferation, disrupting normal growth and differentiation. The heritable genetic damage may be induced by various etiologic agents listed above (e.g. RNA viruses HTLV-I, EBV etc) and causes insertional mutagenesis for which oncogenes may play a role (page 309). The evolution of leukaemia is a multi-step process, and in many cases, acute leukaemia may develop after a pre-existing myelodysplastic or myeloproliferative disorder.

2. Chromosomal translocations A number of cytogenetic abnormalities have been detected in cases of leukaemias-

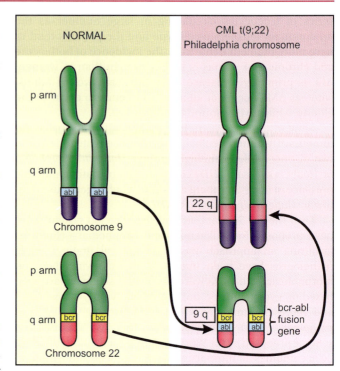

Figure 24.11 ▶ The Philadelphia (Ph) chromosome. There is reciprocal translocation of the part of the long arms of chromosome 22 to the long arms of chromosome 9 written as t(9;22).

lymphomas, most consistent of which are chromosomal translocations. In NHL, translocation involving antigen receptor genes, immunoglobulin genes, or overexpression of *BCL*-2 protein may be seen. The most consistent chromosomal abnormality in various forms of acute and chronic leukaemias is Philadelphia (Ph) chromosome seen in 70-90% cases with CML, involving reciprocal translocation of parts of long arm of chromosome 22 to the long arm of chromosome 9 i.e. t(9;22) **(Fig. 24.11)**.

3. Maturation defect In acute leukaemia, the single most prominent characteristic of the leukaemic cells is a defect in maturation beyond the myeloblast or promyelocyte level in AML, and the lymphoblast level in ALL. It needs to be emphasised that it is the maturation defect in leukaemic blasts rather than rapid proliferation of leukaemic cells responsible for causing acute leukaemia. In fact, the generation time of leukaemic blasts is somewhat prolonged rather than shortened.

4. Myelosuppression As the leukaemic cells accumulate in the bone marrow, there is suppression of normal haematopoietic stem cells, partly by physically replacing the normal marrow precursors, and partly by inhibiting normal haematopoiesis via cell-mediated or humoral mechanisms. This is based on the observation that some patients with acute leukaemia have a hypocellular marrow indicating that marrow failure is not due to overcrowding by leukaemic cells alone. Nevertheless, some normal haematopoietic stem cells do remain in the marrow which are capable of proliferating and restoring normal haematopoiesis after effective anti-leukaemic treatment.

5. **Organ infiltration** The leukaemic cells proliferate primarily in the bone marrow, circulate in the blood and infiltrate into other tissues such as lymph nodes, liver, spleen, skin, viscera and the central nervous system.

6. **Cytokines** Presence of reactive inflammatory cells in the Hodgkin's disease is due to secretion of cytokines from the Reed Sternberg cells e.g. IL-5 (growth factor for eosinophils), IL-13 (for autocrine stimulation of RS cells) and transforming growth factor-β (for fibrogenesis).

GIST BOX 24.3 — Lymphohaematopoietic Malignancies (Leukaemias-Lymphomas)—General

- As per current concepts, neoplasms of haematopoietic and lymphoid tissues are considered as a unified group and are divided into neoplasms of myeloid, lymphoid and histiocytic cells.
- Although the exact etiology of leukaemias and lymphomas is not known, a number of factors have been implicated e.g. heredity, viral and certain bacterial infections, ionising radiations, chemical carcinogens, certain drugs, immunodeficiency, and autoimmune diseases.
- Pathogenesis of these cancers evolves through genetic damage to single clone of target cells, chromosomal translocations, maturation defect and myelosuppression and secretion of certain cytokines.

MYELOID NEOPLASMS

Based on the cell line of differentiation of the pluripotent stem cell, the WHO classification divides all haematopoieitc neoplasms into 2 groups: myeloid and lymphoid neoplasms. Since myeloid trilineage stem cells further differentiate into 3 series of progenitor cells: erythroid, granulocyte-monocyte, and megakaryocytic series, therefore all examples of myeloid neoplasms fall into these three categories of cell-lines. Based on this concept, myeloid neoplasms have following 5 groups (Fig. 24.12):

I. Myeloproliferative diseases
II. Myelodysplastic/myeloproliferative diseases
III. Myelodysplastic syndrome (MDS)
IV. Acute myeloid leukaemia (AML)
V. Acute biphenotypic leukaemia

Each of these groups is subclassified into further types as shown in Table 24.4. Important examples within each group are discussed here.

Table 24.4 WHO classification of myeloid neoplasms.

I. MYELOPROLIFERATIVE DISEASES
1. Chronic myeloid leukaemia (CML), {Ph chromosome t(9;22)(q34; q11), BCR/ABL-positive}
2. Chronic neutrophilic leukaemia
3. Chronic eosinophilic leukaemia/ hypereosinophilic syndrome
4. Chronic idiopathic myelofibrosis
5. Polycythaemia vera (PV)
6. Essential thrombocythaemia (ET)
7. Chronic myeloproliferative disease, unclassifiable

II. MYELODYSPLASTIC/MYELOPROLIFERATIVE DISEASES
1. Chronic myelomonocytic leukaemia (CMML)

III. MYELODYSPLASTIC SYNDROME (MDS)
1. Refractory anaemia (RA)
2. Refractory anaemia with ring sideroblasts (RARS)
3. Refractory cytopenia with multilineage dysplasia (RCMD)
4. RCMD with ringed sideroblasts (RCMD-RS)
5. Refractory anaemia with excess blasts (RAEB-1)
6. RAEB-2
7. Myelodysplastic syndrome unclassified (MDS-U)
8. MDS with isolated del 5q

IV. ACUTE MYELOID LEUKAEMIA (AML)
1. Acute myeloid leukaemias with recurrent genetic abnormalities
   i. AML with t(8;21)(q22;q22); RUNX1-RUNX1T1
   ii. AML with inv(16)(p13.1;q22) or t(16;16)(p13.1;q22); CBF & β-MYH11
   iii. Acute promyelocytic leukaemia (M3) with t(15;17)(q22;q12); PML/RAR-α and variants
   iv. AML with t(9;11)(p22;q23); MLLT3-MLL
   v. AML with t(6;9)(p23;q34); DEK-NUP214
   vi. AML with inv(3)(q21q26.2) or t(3;3)(q21;q26.2); RPN1-EVI1
   vii. AML (megakaryoblastic) with t(1;22)(p13;q13); RBM15-MKL1
   viii. AML with mutated NPM1
   ix. AML with mutated CEBPA
2. Acute myeloid leukaemia with myelodysplasia related changes
3. Therapy related acute myeloid leukaemia
   i. Alkylating agent related
   ii. Topoisomerase II inhibitor related (some may be lymphoid)
4. Acute myeloid leukaemia, not otherwise categorised
   i. AML minimally differentiated (M0)
   ii. AML without maturation (M1)
   iii. AML with maturation (M2)*
   iv. Acute myelomonocytic leukaemia (M4)
   v. Acute monoblastic and monocytic leukaemia (M5a, M5b)
   vi. Acute erythroid leukaemia (M6)
   vii. Acute megakaryoblastic leukaemia (M7)
   viii. Acute basophilic leukaemia
   ix. Acute panmyelosis with myelofibrosis
5. Myeloid sarcoma
6. Myeloid proliferations related to Down's syndrome
   i. Transient abnormal myelopoiesis
   ii. Myeloid leukaemia associated with Down's syndrome
7. Blastic plasmacytoid dentritic cell neoplasm

V. ACUTE BIPHENOTYPIC LEUKAEMIA

*AML (M3) or acute promyelocytic leukaemia is listed at IV (iii) in the same table above.

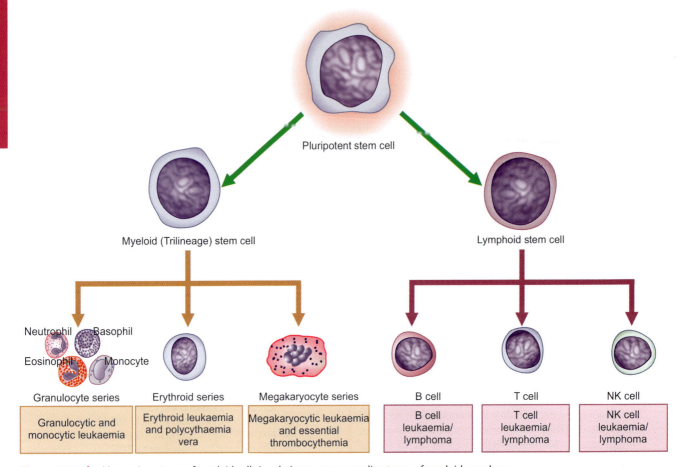

Figure 24.12 ▶ Maturation stages of myeloid cells in relation to corresponding types of myeloid neoplasms.

MYELOPROLIFERATIVE DISEASES

The myeloproliferative disorders are a group of neoplastic proliferation of multipotent haematopoietic stem cells. Besides their common stem cell origin, these disorders are closely related, occasionally leading to evolution of one entity into another during the course of the disease.

The WHO classification of myeloproliferative disorders includes 7 types as shown in **Table 24.4**. Classic and common examples are chronic myeloid leukaemia (CML), polycythaemia vera (PV), and essential thrombocytosis (ET), each one representing corresponding excess of granulocytes, red blood cells, and platelets, respectively. The group as a whole has slow and insidious onset of clinical features and indolent clinical behaviour.

Chronic Myeloid Leukaemia (CML)

Definition and Pathophysiology

By WHO definition, CML is established by identification of the clone of haematopoietic stem cell that possesses the balanced reciprocal translocation between chromosomes 9 and 22, forming Philadelphia chromosome **(Fig. 24.11)**. The t(9;22) involves fusion of BCR (breakpoint cluster region) gene on chromosome 22q11 with ABL (named after Abelson murine leukaemia virus) gene located on chromosome 9q34. The fusion product so formed is termed "Ph chromosome t(9;22)(q34;q11)/ BCR-ABL1" which should be positive for making the diagnosis of CML. This identification may be done by PCR or by FISH. The underlying pathophysiologic mechanism of human CML is based on the observation that BCR-ABL fusion product proteins are capable of transforming haematopoietic progenitor cells *in vitro* and form malignant clone. BCR-ABL fusion product brings about following functional changes:

i) ABL protein is activated to function as a tyrosine kinase enzyme that in turn activates other kinases which *inhibits apoptosis*.
ii) Ability of ABL to act as *DNA-binding protein* is altered.
iii) Binding of ABL to *actin microfilaments* of the cytoskeleton is increased.

Exact mechanism of progression of CML to the blastic phase is unclear but following mechanisms may be involved:
i) Structural alterations in tumour suppressor *p53* gene.
ii) Structural alterations in tumour suppressor *RB* gene.

iii) Alterations in *RAS* oncogene.
iv) Alterations in *MYC* oncogene.
v) Release of cytokine *IL-1β*.
vi) Functional inactivation of tumour suppressor protein, *phosphatase A2*.

Clinical Features

Chronic myeloid (myelogenous, granulocytic) leukaemia comprises about 20% of all leukaemias and its peak incidence is seen in 3rd and 4th decades of life. A distinctive variant of CML seen in children is called *juvenile CML*. Both sexes are affected equally. The onset of CML is generally insidious. Some of the common presenting manifestations are as under:
1. Features of *anaemia* such as weakness, pallor, dyspnoea and tachycardia.
2. Symptoms due to *hypermetabolism* such as weight loss, lassitude, anorexia, night sweats.
3. *Splenomegaly* is almost always present and is frequently massive. In some patients, it may be associated with acute pain due to splenic infarction.
4. *Bleeding tendencies* such as easy bruising, epistaxis, menorrhagia and haematomas may occur.
5. Less *common* features include gout, visual disturbance, neurologic manifestations and priapism.
6. *Juvenile CML* is more often associated with lymph node enlargement than splenomegaly. Other features are frequent infections, haemorrhagic manifestations and facial rash.

Laboratory Findings

The diagnosis of CML is generally possible on blood picture alone. However, bone marrow, cytochemical stains and other investigations are of help.

I. **BLOOD PICTURE** The typical blood picture in a case of CML at the time of presentation shows the following features (Fig. 24.13):

1. Anaemia Anaemia is usually of moderate degree and is normocytic normochromic in type. Occasional normoblasts may be present.

2. White blood cells Characteristically, there is marked leucocytosis (approximately 200,000/μl or more at the time of presentation). The natural history of CML consists of 3 phases—chronic, accelerated, and blastic.

◈ *Chronic phase of CML* begins as a myeloproliferative disorder and consists of excessive proliferation of myeloid cells of intermediate grade (i.e. myelocytes and metamyelocytes) and mature segmented neutrophils. Myeloblasts usually do not exceed 10% of cells in the peripheral blood and bone marrow. An increase in the proportion of basophils up to 10% is a characteristic feature of CML. A rising *basophilia* is indicative of impending blastic transformation. An *accelerated phase of CML* is also described in which there is progressively rising leucocytosis associated with thrombocytosis or thrombocytopenia and splenomegaly. Accelerated phase has increasing degree of anaemia, blast count in blood or marrow between 10-20%, marrow basophils 20% or more, and platelet count falling below 1,00,000/μl.

◈ *Blastic phase or blast crisis in CML* fulfills the definition of acute leukaemia in having blood or marrow blasts ≥20%. These blast cells may be myeloid, lymphoid, erythroid or undifferentiated and are established by morphology, cytochemistry, or immunophenotyping. Myeloid blast crisis in CML is more common and resembles AML. However, unlike AML, Auer rods are not seen in myeloblasts of CML in blast crisis.

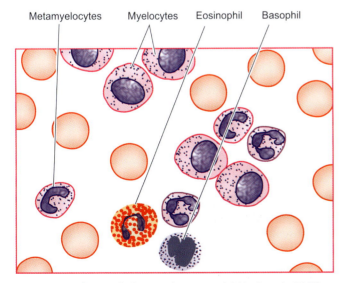
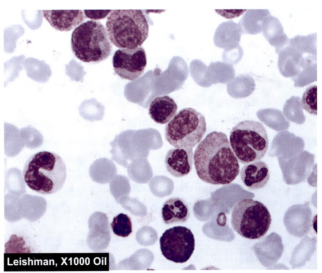

Figure 24.13 ▶ PBF findings in chronic myeloid leukaemia (CML).

3. Platelets Platelet count may be normal but is raised in about half the cases.

II. BONE MARROW EXAMINATION Examination of marrow aspiration yields the following results:

1. Cellularity Generally, there is hypercellularity with total or partial replacement of fat spaces by proliferating myeloid cells.

2. Myeloid cells The myeloid cells predominate in the bone marrow with increased myeloid-erythroid ratio. The differential counts of myeloid cells in the marrow show similar findings as seen in the peripheral blood with predominance of myelocytes.

3. Erythropoiesis Erythropoiesis is normoblastic but there is reduction in erythropoietic cells.

4. Megakaryocytes Megakaryocytes are conspicuous but are usually smaller in size than normal.

5. Cytogenetics Cytogenetic studies on blood and bone marrow cells show the characteristic chromosomal abnormality called Philadelphia (Ph) chromosome seen in 90-95% cases of CML. Ph chromosome is formed by reciprocal balanced translocation between part of long arm of chromosome 22 and part of long arm of chromosome 9{(t(9;22) (q34;q11)} forming product of fusion gene, BCR-ABL1 (*see* **Fig. 24.11**).

III. CYTOCHEMISTRY The only significant finding on cytochemical stains is reduced scores of *neutrophil alkaline phosphatase (NAP)* which helps to distinguish CML from myeloid leukaemoid reaction in which case NAP scores are elevated (*see* **Fig. 24.10,B, and Table 24.3**). However, NAP scores in CML return to normal with successful therapy, corticosteroid administration and in infections.

IV. OTHER INVESTIGATIONS A few other accompanying findings are seen in CML:

1. Elevated serum B_{12} and vitamin B_{12} binding capacity.
2. Elevated serum uric acid (hyperuricaemia).

General Principles of Treatment and Prognosis

Insight into molecular mechanism of CML has brought about major changes in its therapy. The approach of modern therapy in CML is targetted at removal of all malignant clones of cells bearing BCR-ABL fusion protein, so that patient reverts back to prolonged non-clonal haematopoiesis i.e. molecular remission from disease. This is achievable by the following approaches:

1. Imatinib oral therapy The basic principle underlying imatinib oral treatment is to competitively inhibit ATP binding site of the ABL kinase, which in turn, inhibits signal transduction BCR-ABL fusion protein. Imatinib induces apoptosis in BCR-ABL positive cells and thus eliminates them. Imatinib is found more effective in newly diagnosed cases of CML. Complete haematologic remission is achieved for 18 months in 97% cases treated with imatinib.

2. Allogenic bone marrow (stem cell) transplantation Although this treatment modality offers proven cure, it is complicated with mortality due to procedure and development of post-transplant graft-versus-host disease (GVHD) and, therefore, post-transplant immunosuppressive treatment has to be continued.

3. Interferon-α Prior to imatinib and allogenic transplantation, chronic phase of CML used to be treated with interferon-α and was the drug of choice.

4. Chemotherapy Chemotherapeutic agents are used in treatment of CML for lowering the total population of WBCs. These include use of busulfan, cyclophosphamide (melphalan) and hydroxyurea.

5. Others Besides above, other forms of treatment include splenic irradiation, splenectomy and leucopheresis.

The most common cause of death (in 80% cases) in CML is disease acceleration and blastic transformation.

Polycythaemia Vera

Definition and Pathophysiology

Polycythaemia vera (PV) is a clonal disorder characterised by increased production of all myeloid elements resulting in pancytosis (i.e increased red cells, granulocytes, platelets) in the absence of any recognisable cause.

◈ The term 'polycythaemia vera' or 'polycythaemia rubra vera' is used for *primary or idiopathic polycythaemia* only and is the most common of all the myeloproliferative disorders.

◈ *Secondary polycythaemia or erythrocytosis,* on the other hand, may occur secondary to several causes e.g.
i) High altitude.
ii) Cardiovascular disease.
iii) Pulmonary disease with alveolar hypoventilation.
iv) Heavy smoking.
v) Inappropriate increase in erythropoietin (renal cell carcinoma, hydronephrosis, hepatocellular carcinoma, cerebellar haemangioblastoma, massive uterine leiomyoma).
vi) Sometimes relative or spurious polycythaemia may result from plasma loss such as in burns and in dehydration from vomiting or water deprivation.

None of the secondary causes of polycythaemia is associated with splenic enlargement or increased leucocytes and platelets which are typical of PV.

The exact etiology of PV is not known but about a third of cases show inconsistent and varied chromosomal abnormalities such as 20q, trisomy 8 and 9p. Major pathogenetic mechanism is a tyrosine kinase JAK2 mutation which removes the autoinhibitory control and activates the kinases.

Clinical Features

PV is a disease of late middle life and is slightly more common in males. The disease generally runs a chronic but slowly progressive course. Clinical features are the result of hyperviscosity, hypervolaemia, hypermetabolism and decreased cerebral perfusion. These are as under:
1. Headache, vertigo, tinnitus, visual alterations, syncope or even coma.
2. Increased risk of thrombosis due to accelerated atherosclerosis.
3. Increased risk of haemorrhages due to increased blood volume and intrinsic platelet dysfunction e.g. epistaxis, peptic ulcer disease.
4. Splenomegaly producing abdominal fullness.
5. Pruritus, especially after a bath.
6. Increased risk of urate stones and gout due to hyperuricaemia.

Laboratory Findings

PV is diagnosed by the following haematologic findings:
1. *Raised haemoglobin* concentration (above 17.5 g/dl in males and 15.5 g/dl in females).
2. *Erythrocytosis* (above 6 million/μl in males and 5.5 million/μl in females).
3. Haematocrit (PCV) above 55% in males and above 47% in females.
4. Mild to moderate *leucocytosis* (15,000-25,000/μl) with basophilia and raised neutrophil alkaline phosphatase scores.
5. *Thrombocytosis* with defective platelet function.
6. Bone marrow examination reveals erythroid hyperplasia or *panhyperplasia*.
7. *Cytogenetic abnormalities* such as 20q, trisomy 8 and 9p are found in 30% cases of PV.
8. In PV, unlike secondary polycythaemia, *erythropoietin* levels in serum and urine are reduced.

General Principles of Treatment and Prognosis

Since PV runs an indolent course, therapy is aimed at maintaining normal blood counts and relieve the patient of symptoms.
1. *Phlebotomy* (venesection) by blood letting is done at regular interval to reduce total blood cell mass and to induce a state of iron deficiency.
2. *Anticoagulant therapy* is administered in case thrombosis has occurred.
3. *Chemotherapy* may be indicated to induce myelosuppression.
4. Hyperuricaemia is treated with *uricosuric drugs*.
5. Interferon-α is associated with good results because it reduces JAK2 expression in these patients which is the underlying cytogenetic abnormality.

Patients receiving phlebotomy alone may survive for 10-12 years. About 25% patients progress to myelofibrosis. A small proportion of patients develop secondary haematologic malignancies such as AML, non-Hodgkin's lymphoma and multiple myeloma. Major complication and cause of death in PV is vascular thrombosis.

Essential Thrombocythaemia

Definition and Pathophysiology

Essential thrombocythaemia (ET), also termed essential thrombocytosis or primary (idiopathic) thrombocythaemia is a clonal disorder characterised by markedly elevated platelet count in the absence of any recognisable stimulus. *Secondary or reactive thrombocytosis,* on the other hand, occurs in response to known stimuli such as: chronic infection, haemorrhage, postoperative state, chronic iron deficiency, malignancy, rheumatoid arthritis and postsplenectomy.

ET is an uncommon disorder and represents an overproduction of platelets from megakaryocyte colonies without any added stimulus but no clonal marker is available to distinguish primary from secondary thrombocytosis. Though an elevated platelet count is the dominant feature, other cell lines may also be involved in the expansion of neoplastic clone.

The underlying pathophysiologic mechanism in ET is the absence of control by thrombopoietin that regulates endomitosis in the megakaryocytes to produce platelets. The result is uncontrolled proliferation of not only megakaryocytes but also of the platelets. There is a probable role of heredity in ET since families with ET have been reported.

Clinical Features

The condition has an insidious onset and is more frequent in older people. Haemorrhagic and thrombotic events are common. These include the following:
1. Arterial or venous thrombosis.
2. Easy bruisability following minor trauma.
3. Spontaneous bleeding.
4. Transient ischaemic attack or frank stroke due to platelet aggregation in microvasculature of the CNS.

Laboratory Findings

The prominent laboratory features pertain to platelets. These include the following:
1. Sustained elevation in platelet count (above 400,000 μl).
2. Blood film shows many large platelets, megakaryocyte fragments and hypogranular forms.
3. Consistently abnormal platelet functions, especially abnormality in platelet aggregation.
4. Bone marrow examination reveals a large number of hyperdiploid megakaryocytes and variable amount of increased fibrosis.

Section V: Haematology and Lymphoreticular Tissues

General Principles of Treatment and Prognosis

ET runs a benign course and may not require any therapy. Treatment is given only if platelet count is higher than one million. Complications of ET are occurrence of acquired von Willebrand's disease and bleeding but incidence of thrombosis is not higher than matched controls.

> **GIST BOX 24.4 — Myeloproliferative Diseases**
>
> ❖ These are a group of closely-related disorders having common origin from stem cells.
> ❖ CML is identified by identification of clone of cells having reciprocal t(9;22) forming fusion gene complex BCR-ABL or Philadelphia chromosome. Clinically, CML cases have anaemia, splenomegaly and bleeding tendencies. It has a chronic phase and a more aggressive blastic phase.
> ❖ Polycythaemia vera is a clonal disorder characterised by increased production of all myeloid elements resulting in pancytosis (i.e increased red cells, granulocytes, platelets) in the absence of any recognisable cause.
> ❖ Essential thrombocythaemia is uncommon and has overproduction of platelets.

ACUTE MYELOID LEUKAEMIA

Definition and Pathophysiology

Acute myeloid leukaemia (AML) is a heterogeneous disease characterised by infiltration of malignant myeloid cells into the blood, bone marrow and other tissues. AML is mainly a disease of adults (median age 50 years), while children and older individuals may also develop it sometimes.

AML develops due to inhibition of maturation of myeloid stem cells due to mutations. These mutations may be induced by several etiologic factors—heredity, radiation, chemical carcinogens (tobacco smoking, rubber, plastic, paint, insecticides etc) and long-term use of anticancer drugs but viruses do not appear to have role in the etiology of AML. The defect induced by mutations causes accumulation of precursor myeloid cells of the stage at which the myeloid maturation and differentiation is blocked. A few important examples of chromosomal mutations in AML are translocations {t(8;21)(q22q22)} and {t(15;17)(q22;q12)} and inversions {inv(16)(p13;q22)}.

Classification

Currently, two main classification schemes for AML are followed:

FAB CLASSIFICATION According to revised FAB classification system, a leukaemia is acute if the bone marrow consists of more than 30% blasts. Based on morphology and cytochemistry, FAB classification divides AML into 8 subtypes (M0 to M7) **(Table 24.5)**.

WHO CLASSIFICATION WHO classification for AML differs from revised FAB classification in the following 2 ways:
◆ **Firstly**, it places limited reliance on blast morphology and cytochemistry for making the diagnosis of subtype of AML

Table 24.5 Revised FAB classification of acute myeloblastic leukaemias.

FAB CLASS	OLD NAME	PERCENT CASES	MORPHOLOGY	CYTOCHEMISTRY
M0:	Minimally differentiated AML	5	Blasts lack definite cytologic and cytochemical features but have myeloid lineage antigens	Myeloperoxidase –
M1:	AML without maturation	20	Myeloblasts predominate; few if any granules or Auer rods	Myeloperoxidase +
M2:	AML with maturation	30	Myeloblasts with promyelocytes predominate; Auer rods may be present	Myeloperoxidase +++
M3:	Acute promyelocytic leukaemia	10	Hypergranular promyelocytes; often with multiple Auer rods per cell	Myeloperoxidase +++
M4:	Acute myelomonocytic leukaemia (Naegeli type)	20	Mature cells of both myeloid and monocytic series in peripheral blood; myeloid cells resemble M2	Myeloperoxidase ++ Non-specific esterase +
M5:	Acute monocytic leukaemia (Schilling type)	10	Two subtypes: M5a shows poorly-differentiated monoblasts, M5b shows differentiated promonocytes and monocytes	Non-specific esterase ++
M6:	Acute erythroleukaemia (Di Guglielmo's syndrome)	4	Erythroblasts predominate (>50%); myeloblasts and promyelocytes also increased	Erythroblasts:PAS + Myeloblasts: myeloperoxidase +
M7:	Acute megakaryocytic leukaemia	1	Pleomorphic undifferentiated blasts predominate; react with antiplatelet antibodies	Platelet peroxidase +

but instead takes into consideration *clinical, cytogenetic and molecular abnormalities* in different types. These features can be studied by multiparametric flow cytometry.

◆ **Secondly**, WHO classification for AML has revised and lowered the cut-off percentage of *marrow blasts to 20%* from 30% in the FAB classification for making the diagnosis of AML. Latest WHO classification of AML is given in Table 24.4.

Both FAB as well as WHO classification schemes for AML are followed in different settings depending upon the laboratory facilities available in various centres. Moreover, most of the current clinical and laboratory data are based on FAB groupings. Hence detailed morphologic and cytochemical features of various AML groups are required to be understood well (Table 24.5).

Clinical Features

AML and ALL share many clinical features and the two are difficult to distinguish on clinical features alone. In approximately 25% of patients with AML, a preleukaemic syndrome with anaemia and other cytopenias may be present for a few months to years prior to the development of overt leukaemia.

Clinical manifestations of AML are divided into 2 groups: those *due to bone marrow failure,* and those *due to organ infiltration.*

I. DUE TO BONE MARROW FAILURE   These are as under:
1. *Anaemia* producing pallor, lethargy, dyspnoea.
2. *Bleeding manifestations* due to thrombocytopenia causing spontaneous bruises, petechiae, bleeding from gums and other bleeding tendencies.
3. *Infections* are quite common and include those of mouth, throat, skin, respiratory, perianal and other sites.
4. *Fever* is generally attributed to infections in acute leukaemia but sometimes no obvious source of infection can be found and may occur in the absence of infection.

II. DUE TO ORGAN INFILTRATION   The clinical manifestations of AML are more often due to replacement of the marrow and other tissues by leukaemic cells. These features are as under:
1. *Pain and tenderness of bones* (e.g. sternal tenderness) are due to bone infarcts or subperiosteal infiltrates by leukaemic cells.
2. *Lymphadenopathy* and enlargement of the *tonsils* may occur.
3. *Splenomegaly* of moderate grade may occur. Splenic infarction, subcapsular haemorrhages, and rarely, splenic rupture may occur.
4. *Hepatomegaly* is frequently present due to leukaemic infiltration but the infiltrates usually do not interfere with the function of the liver.
5. *Leukaemic infiltration of the kidney* may be present and ordinarily does not interfere with its function unless secondary complications such as haemorrhage or blockage of ureter supervene.
6. *Gum hypertrophy* due to leukaemic infiltration of the gingivae is a frequent finding in myelomonocytic (M4) and monocytic (M5) leukaemias.
7. *Chloroma or granulocytic sarcoma* is a localised tumour-forming mass occurring in the skin or orbit due to local infiltration of the tissues by leukaemic cells. The tumour is greenish in appearance due to the presence of myeloperoxidase.
8. *Meningeal involvement* manifested by raised intracranial pressure, headache, nausea and vomiting, blurring of vision and diplopia are seen more frequently in ALL during haematologic remission. Sudden death from massive intracranial haemorrhage as a result of leucostasis may occur.
9. *Other organ infiltrations* include testicular swelling and mediastinal compression.

Laboratory Findings

The diagnosis of AML is made by a combination of routine blood picture and bone marrow examination, coupled with cytochemical stains and other special laboratory investigations.

I. BLOOD PICTURE   Findings of routine haematologic investigations are as under (Fig. 24.14):

1. Anaemia   Anaemia is almost always present in AML. It is generally severe, progressive and normochromic. A moderate reticulocytosis up to 5% and a few nucleated red cells may be present.

2. Thrombocytopenia   The platelet count is usually moderately to severely reduced (below 50,000/µl) but occasionally it may be normal. Bleeding tendencies in AML are usually correlated with the level of thrombocytopenia but most serious spontaneous haemorrhagic episodes develop in patients with fewer than 20,000/µl platelets. Acute promyelocytic leukaemia (M3) may be associated with a serious coagulation abnormality, disseminated intravascular coagulation (DIC).

3. White blood cells   The total WBC count ranges from subnormal-to-markedly elevated values. In 25% of patients, the total WBC count at presentation is reduced to 1,000-4,000/µl. More often, however, there is progressive rise in white cell count which may exceed 100,000/µl in more advanced disease. Majority of leucocytes in the peripheral blood are blasts and there is often neutropenia due to marrow infiltration by leukaemic cells. The basic morphologic features of myeloblasts and lymphoblasts are summed up in Table 24.1. Typical characteristics of different forms of AML (M0 to M7) are given in Table 24.5. In general, the *identification of blast cells is greatly aided by the company they keep* i.e. by more mature and easily identifiable leucocytes in the company of blastic cells of myeloid series. Some *'smear cells'* in the peripheral blood representing degenerated leucocytes may be seen.

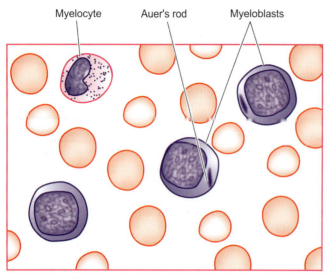 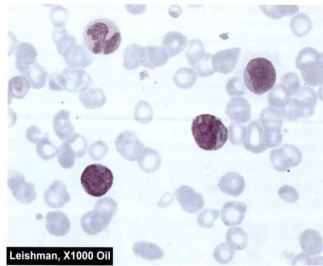

Figure 24.14 ▶ PBF findings in a case of acute myeloblastic leukaemia (AML).

II. BONE MARROW EXAMINATION An examination of bone marrow aspirate or trephine reveals the following features:

1. Cellularity Typically, the marrow is hypercellular but sometimes a 'blood tap' or 'dry tap' occurs. A dry tap in AML may be due to pancytopenia, but sometimes even when the marrow is so much packed with leukaemic cells that they cannot be aspirated because the cells are adhesive and enmeshed in reticulin fibres. In such cases, trephine biopsy is indicated.

2. Leukaemic cells The bone marrow is generally tightly packed with leukaemic blast cells. The diagnosis of the type of leukaemic cells, according to FAB classification, is generally possible with routine Romanowsky stains but cytochemical stains may be employed as an adjunct to Romanowsky staining for determining the type of leukaemia. The essential criteria for diagnosis of AML, as per FAB classification, was the presence of at least 30% blasts in the bone marrow. However, as per WHO classification, these criteria have been revised and lowered to 20% blasts in the marrow for labelling and treating a case as AML.

3. Erythropoiesis Erythropoietic cells are reduced. Dyserythropoiesis, megaloblastic features and ring sideroblasts are commonly present.

4. Megakaryocytes They are usually reduced or absent.

5. Cytogenetics Chromosomal analysis of dividing leukaemic cells in the marrow shows karyotypic abnormalities in 75% of cases which may have a relationship to prognosis. WHO classification emphasises on the categorisation of AML on the basis of cytogenetic abnormalities.

Two of the most consistent cytogenetic abnormalities in specific FAB groups are as under:

i) *M3* cases have $t(15;17)(q22;q12)$.

ii) *M4E0* (E for abnormal eosinophils in the bone marrow) cases have $inv(16)(p13q22)$.

6. Immunophenotyping AML cells express CD13 and CD33 antigens. M7 shows CD41 and CD42 positivity.

III. CYTOCHEMISTRY Some of the commonly employed cytochemical stains, as an aid to classify the type of AML are as under (also see Table 24.5):

1. Myeloperoxidase Positive in immature myeloid cells containing granules and Auer rods but negative in M0 myeloblasts.

2. Sudan Black Positive in immature cells in AML.

3. Periodic acid-Schiff (PAS) Positive in immature lymphoid cells and in erythroleukaemia (M6).

4. Non-specific esterase (NSE) Positive in monocytic series (M4 and M5).

5. Acid phosphatase Focal positivity in leukaemic blasts in ALL and diffuse reaction in monocytic cells (M4 and M5).

IV. BIOCHEMICAL INVESTIGATIONS These may be of some help:

1. Serum muramidase Serum levels of lysozyme (i.e. muramidase) are elevated in myelomonocytic (M4) and monocytic (M5) leukaemias.

2. Serum uric acid Because of rapidly growing number of leukaemic cells, serum uric acid level is frequently increased. The levels are further raised after treatment with cytotoxic drugs because of increased cell breakdown.

General Principles of Treatment and Prognosis

The management of acute leukaemia involves the following aspects:

I. TREATMENT OF ANAEMIA AND HAEMORRHAGE
Anaemia and haemorrhage are managed by fresh blood transfusions and platelet concentrates. Patients with severe thrombocytopenia (platelet count below 20,000/µl) require regular platelet transfusions since haemorrhage is an important cause of death in these cases.

II. TREATMENT AND PROPHYLAXIS OF INFECTION
Neutropenia due to bone marrow replacement by leukaemic blasts and as a result of intensive cytotoxic therapy renders these patients highly susceptible to infection. The infections are predominantly bacterial but viral, fungal, and protozoal infections also occur. For prophylaxis against infection in such cases, the patient should be isolated and preferably placed in laminar airflow rooms. Efforts are made to reduce the gut and other commensal flora which are the usual source of infection. This is achieved by bowel sterilisation and by topical antiseptics. If these fail to achieve the desired results, systemic antibiotics and leucocyte concentrates are considered for therapy.

III. CYTOTOXIC DRUG THERAPY The aims of cytotoxic therapy are firstly to induce remission, and secondly to continue therapy to reduce the hidden leukaemic cell population by repeated courses of therapy. Most commonly, cyclic combinations of 2, 3 and 4 drugs are given with treatment-free intervals to allow the bone marrow to recover.

The most effective treatment of AML is a combination of 3 drugs: cytosine arabinoside, anthracyclines (daunorubicin, adriamycin) and 6-thioguanine. Another addition is amsacrine (m-AMSA) administered with cytosine arabinoside, with or without 6-thioguanine. Following remission-induction therapy, various drug combinations are given intermittently for maintenance. However, promyelocytic leukaemia (M3) is treated with tretinoin orally that reduces the leukaemic cells bearing t(15;17)(q22;q21) but development of DIC due to liberation of granules of dying cells is a problem.

IV. BONE MARROW TRANSPLANTATION Bone marrow (or stem cell) transplantation from suitable allogenic or autologous donor (HLA and mixed lymphocytes culture-matched) is increasingly being used for treating young adults with AML in first remission. The basic principle of marrow transplantation is to reconstitute the patient's haematopoietic system after total body irradiation and intensive chemotherapy have been given so as to kill the remaining leukaemic cells. Bone marrow transplantation has resulted in cure in about half the cases.

Remission rate with AML is lower (50-70%) than in ALL, often takes longer to achieve remission, and disease-free intervals are shorter. AML is most malignant of all leukaemias; median survival with treatment is 12-18 months.

GIST BOX 24.5 | Acute Myeloid Leukaemia

- AML is a disease of adults characterised by infiltration of malignant myeloid cells into the blood, bone marrow and other tissues.
- According to revised FAB classification system, bone marrow in AML has more than 30% blasts. Based on morphology and cytochemistry, FAB classification divides AML into 8 subtypes (M0 to M7).
- WHO classification takes into account genetic and molecular features and marrow blast count of >20% is taken for diagnosis of AML. Accordingly, WHO classification has several newer entities.
- AML is characterised by anaemia, thrombocytopenia, and leucocytosis with blasts in blood. Bone marrow shows myeloblasts in excess of 20% and reduced megakaryocytes.

MYELODYSPLASTIC SYNDROMES

Definition and Classification

Myelodysplastic syndromes (MDS) are a heterogeneous group of haematopoietic clonal stem cell disorders having abnormal development of different marrow elements (i.e. dysmyelopoiesis), usually characterised by cytopenias, associated with cellular marrow and ineffective blood cell formation. These conditions are, therefore, also termed as preleukaemic syndromes or dysmyelopoietic syndromes.

There have been two main classification schemes for MDS:

FAB CLASSIFICATION OF MDS As per FAB (French-American-British) Cooperative Group, the marrow may contain <30% myeloblasts in MDS and this was considered as the dividing line for distinguishing cases of AML (blasts >30%) from MDS. FAB classified MDS into the following 5 groups:

1. *Refractory anaemia (RA)* Blood blasts <1%, marrow blasts <5%.

2. *Refractory anaemia with ringed sideroblasts (RARS) (primary acquired sideroblastic anaemia)* Blood blast <1%; marrow blasts <5%; ring sideroblsts ≥15%.

3. *Refractory anaemia with excess blasts (RAEB)* Blood blasts 5%, marrow blasts 5-20%.

4. *Refractory anaemia with excess of blasts in transformation (RAEB-t)* Blood blasts 5%, marrow blasts 21-30%.

5. *Chronic myelomonocytic leukaemia (CMML)* Blood blasts, 5%, monocytosis.

WHO CLASSIFICATION OF MDS WHO classification differs from FAB classification in following ways:

i) Marrow blast count for making the diagnosis of AML has been revised and brought down to 20%.

ii) FAB category of RAEB-*t* (group 4 above) cases have prognosis similar to patients of AML and thus included in AML.

iii) CMML category of FAB (category 4) has been excluded from WHO classification of MDS since these cases behave like a myeloproliferative disorder and thus CMML has been put in the hybrid category of myelodysplastic/myeloproliferative disorder.

Thus, the WHO classification of MDS consists of following 8 categories:

1. Refractory anaemia (RA) Same as FAB type 1 MDS. Incidence 5-10%; characterised by anaemia without any blasts in blood; marrow may show <5% blasts.

2. Refractory anaemia with ringed sideroblasts (RARS) Same as FAB type 2 MDS; Incidence 10-12%.

3. Refractory cytopenia with multilineage dysplasia (RCMD) New entity. Incidence 24%; blood shows cytopenia of 2 or 3 cell lineage and monocytosis but no blasts; marrow shows <5% blasts.

4. RCMD with ringed sideroblasts (RCMD-RS) New entity. Incidence 15%; all blood and marrow findings similar to RCMD plus in addition ≥15% ringed sideroblasts in marrow.

5. Refractory anaemia with excess blasts (RAEB-1) In WHO classification, RAEB of FAB category 3 has been divided into 2 subtypes with combined incidence of 40%. RAEB-1 has blood cytopenia with <5% blasts and monocytosis; and marrow blast count 5-9%.

6. RAEB-2 Findings of blood and marrow similar to RAEB-1 but marrow blast count is 10-19%.

7. Myelodysplastic syndrome unclassified (MDS-U) New entity in MDS. Blood cytopenia without any blasts; marrow shows dysplasia of myeloid and thrombocytic cell lineage and marrow blast count <5%.

8. MDS with isolated del (5q) New entity in MDS. Anaemia in blood and blasts <5%; marrow blasts <5%, normal or increased megakaryocytes which may be hypolobated and characteristic isolated deletion of 5q.

Pathophysiology

i) Primary MDS is idiopathic but factors implicated in etiology are radiation exposure and benzene carcinogen.

ii) Secondary (therapy-related) MDS may occur following earlier anti-cancer treatment, aplastic anaemia treated with immunosuppressive therapy and in Fanconi's anaemia.

iii) Several cytogenetic abnormalities are seen in about 50% of MDS which include trisomy, translocations and deletions. Cases evolving into leukaemia more often have aneuploidy.

iv) At molecular level, mutations are seen in *N-RAS* oncogene and *p53* anti-oncogene, which together with suppressed immunity, accelerate apoptosis in the bone marrow. Mutations in the mitochondrial genes probably account for occurrence of sideroblastic anaemia in MDS and consequently disordered iron metabolism and ineffective erythropoiesis.

Clinical Features

In general, MDS is found more frequently in older people past 6th decade of life, with slight male preponderance. Therapy-related MDS is generally not age-related and may occur about a decade after anti-cancer therapy. Clinical features are quite non-specific and MDS may be discovered during routine CBC examination done for some other cause. At presentation, the patient may have following features:

1. Anaemia appreciated by pallor, fatigue and weakness.
2. Fever.
3. Weight loss.
4. Sweet syndrome having neutrophilic dermatosis seen in some cases.
5. Splenomegaly seen in 20% cases of MDS.

Laboratory Findings

Various combinations of features are seen in different types of MDS. In general, laboratory findings are as under:

BLOOD FINDINGS There is cytopenia affecting two (bicytopenia) or all the three blood cell lines (pancytopenia):

1. Anaemia: Generally macrocytic or dimorphic.

2. TLC: Usually normal; cases of CMML may have high TLC but these cases in WHO classification of myeloid neoplasms have been put in a separate group of myelodysplastic/myeloproliferative diseases and not in MDS.

3. DLC: Neutrophils are hyposegmented and hypogranulated. Myeloblasts may be seen in PBF and their number correlates with marrow blasts count.

4. Platelets: Thrombocytopenia with large agranular platelets.

BONE MARROW FINDINGS There is constellation of findings in the marrow as under:

1. Cellularity: Normal to hypercellular to hypocellular.

2. Erythroid series: Dyserythropoiesis as seen by abnormally appearing nuclei and ring sideroblasts. Megaloblasts may be seen.

3. Myeloid series: Hypogranular and hyposegmented myeloid precursor cells. Myeloblasts increased depending upon the type of MDS.

4. Megakaryocyte series: Reduced in number and having abnormal nuclei.

General Principles of Treatment and Prognosis

MDS is difficult to treat and may not respond to cytotoxic chemotherapy. Stem cell transplantation offers cure and longer survival. Survival rates vary depending upon the type of MDS: cases of refractory anaemia with or without sideroblasts (RA and RARS) and 5q syndrome survive for years, while cases of refractory anaemia with excess blasts (RAEB-1 and 2) have poor survival for a few months only. Patients generally either succumb to infections or develop into acute myeloid leukaemia.

> **GIST BOX 24.6 Acute Myeloid Leukaemia**
>
> ❖ As per WHO classification of MDS, since marrow blast count for making the diagnosis of AML has been put at 20% or more, cases of MDS have blast count below 20%.
> ❖ FAB category of RAEB-*t* cases have been included in AML in WHO classification of MDS.
> ❖ FAB category of CMML has been included in myeloproliferative disorder in WHO scheme of MDS.
> ❖ WHO has thus divided MDS into 8 types: refractory anaemia, refractory anaemia with ring sideroblasts, refractory cytopenia with multilineage dysplasia (RCMD), RCMD with ring sideroblasts, RAEB-1 and RAEB-2, MDS unclassified, and MDS with isolated del (5q).

LYMPHOID NEOPLASMS: GENERAL

HISTORY AND CLASSIFICATION

Lymphoid cells constitute the immune system of the body. These cells circulate in the blood and also lie in the lymphoid tissues and undergo differentiation and maturation in these organs. The haematopoietic stem cells which form myeloid and lymphoid series, undergo further differentiation of lymphoid cells into B cells (including formation of plasma cells), T cells and NK cells. Lymphoid malignancies can be formed by malignant transformation of each of these cell lines. These lymphoid malignancies can range from indolent to highly aggressive human cancers.

Conventionally, malignancies of lymphoid cells in blood have been termed as lymphatic leukaemias and those of lymphoid tissues as lymphomas. Just like myeloid leukaemias discussed earlier, lymphoid leukaemias have been classified on the basis of survival and biologic course, into chronic and acute *(CLL and ALL)*. Similarly, two clinicopathologically distinct groups of lymphomas are distinguished: *Hodgkin's lymphoma* or *Hodgkin's disease (HD)* and *non-Hodgkin's lymphomas (NHL)*.

However, while HD can be identified by the pathognomonic presence of Reed-Sternberg cells, there have been controversies and confusion in classification of other lymphoid cancers (i.e. NHL and lymphoid leukaemias). In order to resolve the issue, over the years several classification schemes have emerged for lymphoid cancers due to following two main reasons:

1. **Biologic course of lymphoma-leukaemia** While some of the lymphoid malignancies initially present as leukaemias (i.e. in the blood and bone marrow), many others present as solid masses in the lymphoid tissues or in various other tissues, especially in the spleen, liver, bone marrow and other tissues. Still others may have initial presentation as either leukaemia or lymphomas. In fact, the line of demarcation for lymphoid malignancies is so blurred that during the biologic course of the disease, lymphoid leukaemia or lymphoma may spill over and transform to the other.

2. **Technological advances** In recent times, modern diagnostic tools have become available to pathologists and haematologists which go much beyond making the diagnosis of lymphomas and leukaemias on clinical grounds and based on morphology and cytochemical stains alone. The additional tools include immunophenotyping, cytogenetics and molecular markers for the stage of differentiation of the cell of origin rather than location of the cell alone.

These aspects form the basis of current concept for WHO classification of malignancies of lymphoid cells of blood and lymphoreticular tissues as 'lymphoid neoplasms' as a unified group. However, it needs to be appreciated that in several centres in developing countries of the world, limited laboratory facilities are available. Thus, judiciously speaking, some of the older classification schemes for lymphoid malignancies need to be retained, while others can be dumped as historical. In view of this, a balanced approach of middle path has been followed in this textbook retaining relevant good points of old classification and adding new classification schemes of lymphoid malignancies:

I. HISTORICAL CLASSIFICATIONS These classifications can be traced as under:

Morphologic classification *Rappaport classification (1966)* proposed a clinically relevant morphologic classification based on two main features: *low-power microscopy* of the overall pattern of the lymph node architecture, and *high-power microscopy* revealing the cytology of the neoplastic cells. Based on these two features, Rappaport divided NHL into two major subtypes:

1. *Nodular or follicular lymphomas* which retain some of the features of normal lymph node in that the neoplastic cells form lymphoid 'nodules' rather than lymphoid follicles with germinal centres.

2. *Diffuse lymphomas,* on the other hand, are characterised by effacement of the normal lymph node architecture and there may be infiltration of neoplastic cells outside the capsule of the involved lymph node.

NHL was further classified according to the degree of differentiation of neoplastic cells into: *well-differentiated, poorly-differentiated,* and *histiocytic (large cells) types* of both nodular and diffuse lymphomas.

Immunologic classifications *Lukes-Collins classification (1974)* was proposed to correlate the type of NHL with the immune system because the identification of T and B-cells and their subpopulations had become possible in early 70s.

Table 24.6 FAB classification of ALL.

A. MORPHOLOGIC CRITERIA

FAB CLASS		PERCENT CASES	MORPHOLOGY	CYTOCHEMISTRY
L1:	Childhood-ALL (B-ALL, and T-ALL)	More common in children	Homogeneous small lymphoblasts; scanty cytoplasm, regular round nuclei, inconspicuous nucleoli	PAS ± Acid phosphatase ±
L2:	Adult-ALL (mostly T-ALL)	More frequent in adults	Heterogeneous lymphoblasts; variable amount of cytoplasm, irregular or cleft nuclei, large nucleoli	PAS ± Acid phosphatase ±
L3:	Burkitt type-ALL (B-ALL)	Uncommon	Large homogeneous lymphoblasts; round nuclei, prominent nucleoli, cytoplasmic vacuolation	PAS – Acid phosphatase –

B. CYTOGENETIC AND IMMUNOLOGIC CRITERIA

SUBTYPE	INCIDENCE	MARKERS	FAB SUBTYPE	CYTOGENETIC ABNORMALITIES
Pre-B ALL	75%	CD10+ (90%), TdT+	L1, L2	t(9;22) i.e. Philadelphia+ALL
B cell ALL	5%	CD10+ (50%), TdT–	L3	t(8;14) (Burkitt's leukaemia)
T cell ALL	20%	CD10+ (30%), TdT+	L1, L2	14q11

(TdT= terminal deoxynucleotidyl transferase)

Its subsequent modification was *Kiel classification (1981)*. Both these classifications employed immunologic markers for tumour cells, and divided all malignant lymphomas of either B-cell or T-cell origin, and rarely of macrophages. The B and T-cell tumours were further subdivided on the basis of their light microscopic characteristics. The majority of NHLs were B lymphocyte derivatives and arise from follicular centre cells (FCC). The FCC in the germinal centre undergo transformation to become large immunoblasts and pass through the four stages—*small cleaved cells* and *large cleaved cells, small non-cleaved cells* and *large non-cleaved cells.*

Though these classification schemes were immunologically correct, they were unclear about varying prognosis of different clinical types of NHL of either B-cell or T-cell origin.

II. OLD CLINICOPATHOLOGIC CLASSIFICATIONS In view of the objections to above pure morphologic and immunologically correct classifications, following three clinically relevant classifications were proposed which cannot be readily abandoned:

FAB classification of lymphoid leukaemia Although old FAB classification for lymphoid leukaemia based on morphology and cytochemistry divided ALL into 3 types (L1 to L3), but it was subsequently revised to include cytogenetic and immunologic features as well **(Table 24.6)**. FAB classification is still followed in many centres where both pathologists and clinicians stick to labelling lymphoid leukaemia separate from lymphomas.

Working Formulations for Clinical Usage (1982) This classification proposed by a panel of experts from National Cancer Institute of the US incorporates the best features of all previous classification systems, and as the name implies, has strong clinical relevance. Based on the natural history of disease and long-term survival studies, Working Formulations divides all NHLs into following 3 prognostic groups:

◆ *Low-grade NHL:* 5-year survival 50-70%
◆ *Intermediate-grade NHL:* 5-year survival 35-45%
◆ *High-grade NHL:* 5-year survival 25-35%.

In this classification, no attempt is made to determine whether the tumour cells have origin from B-cells, T-cells or macrophages. Each prognostic group includes a few morphologic subtypes, and lastly, a miscellaneous group is also described.

Working Formulations classification still has many takers in several centres and is retained in **Table 24.7**.

REAL classification (1994) International Lymphoma Study Group (Harris et al) proposed another classification called *r*evised *E*uropean-*A*merican classification of *l*ymphoid neoplasms abbreviated as REAL classification. This classification was based on the hypothesis that all forms of lymphoid malignancies (NHLs as well as lymphoblastic leukaemias) represent malignant counterparts of normal population of immune cells (B-cells, T-cells and histiocytes) present in the lymph node and bone marrow. It is believed that lymphoid malignancies arise due to arrest at the various differentiation stages of B and T-cells since tumours of histiocytic origin are quite uncommon. Accordingly, it is considered essential to understand and correlate the differentiation stages of B and T-cells with various lymphoid malignancies **(Fig. 24.15)**. REAL classification divides all lymphoid malignancies into two broad groups, each having further subtypes:

Chapter 24: Diseases of Leucocytes and Lymphoid Tissues

Table 24.7	Classification of NHL-Working Formulations for Clinical Usage (1982).

I. LOW-GRADE

    A) Small lymphocytic
    B) Follicular, predominantly small cleaved cell
    C) Follicular, mixed small and large cleaved cell

II. INTERMEDIATE-GRADE

    D) Follicular, predominantly large cell
    E) Diffuse, small cleaved cell
    F) Diffuse, mixed small and large cell
    G) Diffuse, large, cell

III. HIGH-GRADE

    H) Large cell, immunoblastic
    I) Lymphoblastic
    J) Small non-cleaved cell (Burkitt's)

IV. MISCELLANEOUS

    1. Adult T-cell leukaemia/lymphoma
    2. Cutaneous T-cell lymphoma
    3. Histiocytic (Histiocytic medullary reticulosis)

◆ *Leukaemias and lymphomas of B-cell origin:* B-cell derivation comprises 80% cases of lymphoid leukaemias and 90% cases of NHLs. Based upon these phenotypic and genotypic features, B-cell neoplasms are of pre-B and mature B-cell origin. Based on their biologic behaviour, B-cell malignancies are further subclassified into indolent and aggressive. All these tumours express Pan-B (CD19) antigen besides other markers.

◆ *Leukaemias and lymphomas of T-cell origin:* T-cell malignancies comprise the remainder 20% cases of lymphoid leukaemia and 10% cases of NHLs. T-cell malignancies reflect the stages of T-cell ontogeny. Like B-cell malignancies, T-cell derivatives too are further categorised into indolent and aggressive T-cell malignancies. The most widely expressed T-cell antigens are CD2 and CD7.

REAL classification subsequently merged into WHO classification described below.

III. WHO CLASSIFICATION OF LYMPHOID NEOPLASMS (2008)

In view of confusion surrounding the classification

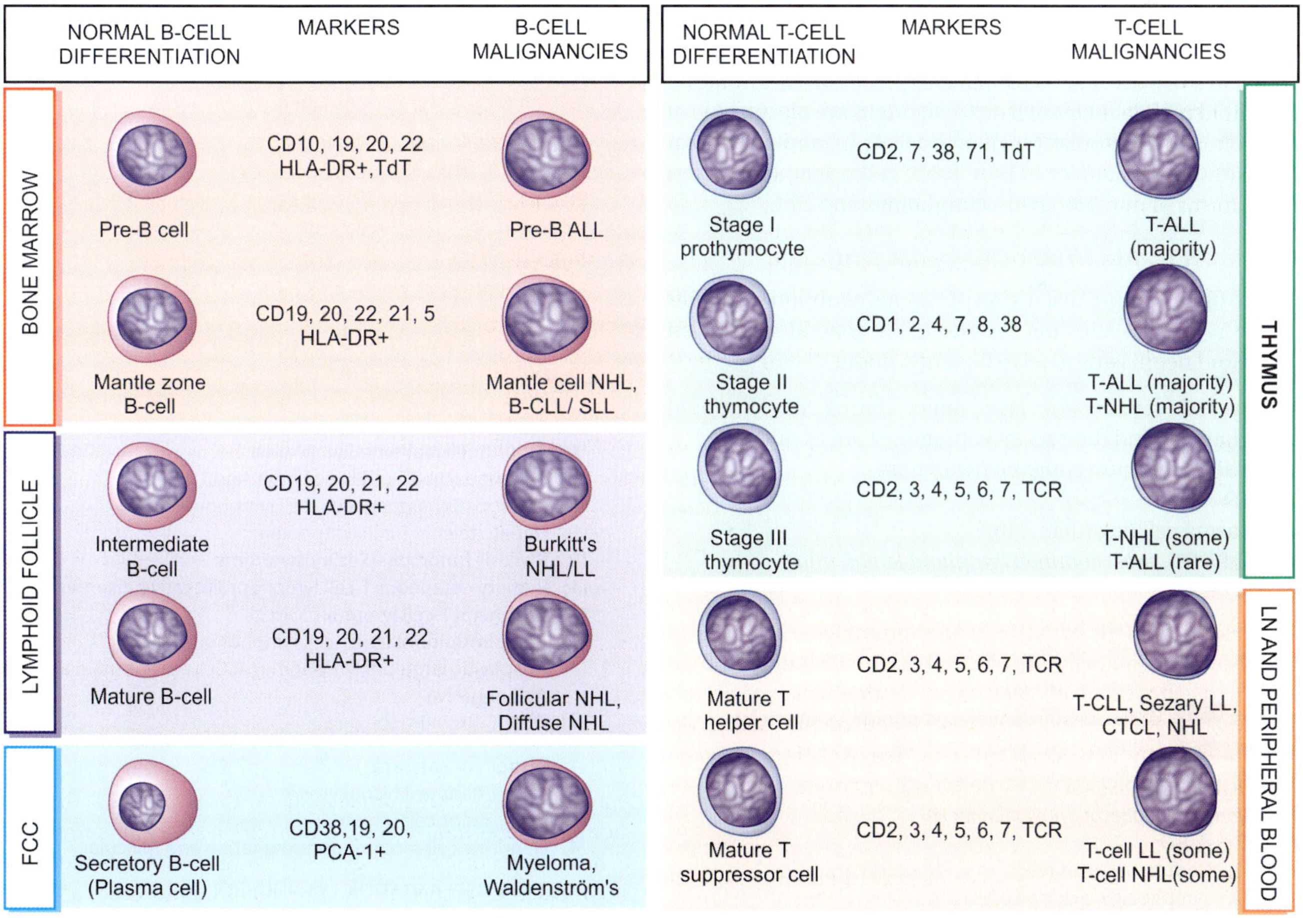

	NORMAL B-CELL DIFFERENTIATION	MARKERS	B-CELL MALIGNANCIES	NORMAL T-CELL DIFFERENTIATION	MARKERS	T-CELL MALIGNANCIES	
BONE MARROW	Pre-B cell	CD10, 19, 20, 22 HLA-DR+, TdT	Pre-B ALL	Stage I prothymocyte	CD2, 7, 38, 71, TdT	T-ALL (majority)	THYMUS
	Mantle zone B-cell	CD19, 20, 22, 21, 5 HLA-DR+	Mantle cell NHL, B-CLL/ SLL	Stage II thymocyte	CD1, 2, 4, 7, 8, 38	T-ALL (majority) T-NHL (majority)	
LYMPHOID FOLLICLE	Intermediate B-cell	CD19, 20, 21, 22 HLA-DR+	Burkitt's NHL/LL	Stage III thymocyte	CD2, 3, 4, 5, 6, 7, TCR	T-NHL (some) T-ALL (rare)	LN AND PERIPHERAL BLOOD
	Mature B-cell	CD19, 20, 21, 22 HLA-DR+	Follicular NHL, Diffuse NHL	Mature T helper cell	CD2, 3, 4, 5, 6, 7, TCR	T-CLL, Sezary LL, CTCL, NHL	
FCC	Secretory B-cell (Plasma cell)	CD38,19, 20, PCA-1+	Myeloma, Waldenström's	Mature T suppressor cell	CD2, 3, 4, 5, 6, 7, TCR	T-cell LL (some) T-cell NHL(some)	

(PCA = Plasma cell antigen; TCR = T cell receptor; FCC = Follicular centre B cells; LN = Lymph node; LL = Lymphoid leukaemia; CTCL=Cutaneous T-cell leukaemia-lymphoma)

Figure 24.15 ▶ Schematic representation of WHO-REAL classification of lymphoid neoplasms. Various immunophenotypes of B and T-cell malignancies are correlated with normal immunophenotypic differentiation/maturation stages of B and T-cells in the bone marrow, lymphoid tissue, peripheral blood and thymus.

schemes of lymphoid cancer, Harris et al, who described REAL classification, evolved a consensus international classification of all lymphoid neoplasms together as a unified group (lymphoid leukaemias-lymphomas) under the aegis of the WHO. Although this classification has many similarities with REAL classification as regards identification of B and T cell types (Fig. 24.15), WHO classification has more classes. WHO classification takes into account morphology, clinical features, immunophenotyping, and cytogenetic of the tumour cells. Hence, on this basis, it is possible to know the stage of maturity of the neoplastic cell and thus it has a better clinical and therapeutic relevance.

As per current WHO classification, all lymphoid neoplasms (i.e. lymphoid leukaemias and lymphomas) fall into following 5 categories (Table 24.8):
I. Hodgkin's disease
II. B-cell malignancies: Precursor (or immature), and peripheral (or mature)
III. T-cell/NK cell malignancies: Precursor (or immature), and peripheral (or mature)
IV. Histiocytic and dendritic cell neoplasms
V. Post-transplant lymphoproliferative disorders (PTLDs).

Thus, in the WHO classification of lymphoid neoplasms, Hodgkin's disease stands distinctive; precursor or immature lymphoid malignancies of B or T-cell origin are blastic type of leukaemias-lymphomas (i.e. B or T-cell ALL), and peripheral or mature malignancies of B or T/NK cell origin are various other forms of non-Hodgkin's lymphomas and CLL.

COMMON TO ALL LYMPHOID MALIGNANCIES

Before plunging into discussion of various common examples in the WHO classification system, a few general aspects on lymphoid neoplasms need to be understood:

1. Overall frequency Five major forms of lymphoid malignancies and their relative frequency are as under:
i) NHL= 62%, *most common lymphoma*
ii) HD= 8%
iii) Plasma cell disorders = 16%
iv) CLL= 9%, *most common lymphoid leukaemia*
v) ALL= 4%

2. Incidence of B, T, NK cell malignancies Majority of lymphoid malignancies are of B cell origin (75% of lymphoid

Table 24.8 WHO Classification of Lymphoid Malignancies (2008).

I) HODGKIN'S DISEASE
Nodular lymphocytic predominant HD
Classic HD
  1. Nodular sclerosis HD
  2. Lymphocytic rich classic HD
  3. Mixed cellularity
  4. Lymphocytic depletion HD

II) B CELL MALIGNANCIES
Precursor (Immature) B-cell malignancies
Precursor B lymphoblastic leukaemia/lymphoma (precursor B-cell ALL)

Peripheral (Mature) B-cell malignancies
  1. Chronic lymphocytic leukemia/small lymphocytic lymphoma (B-cell CLL/SLL)
  2. B-cell prolymphocytic leukemia
  3. Splenic marginal zone lymphoma
  4. Hairy cell leukemia and variant
  5. Splenic lymphoma/leukemia
  6. Lymphoplasmacytic lymphoma
  7. Waldenström macroglobulinemia
  8. Heavy chain diseases (α,γ,μ)
  9. Plasma cell myeloma and plasmacytoma
  10. Extranodal marginal zone lymphoma of mucosa-associated lymphoid tissue (MALT lymphoma)
  11. Nodal marginal zone lymphoma
  12. Follicular lymphoma
  13. Mantle cell lymphoma
  14. Diffuse large B-cell lymphoma (DLBCL), NOS
  15. T-cell/histiocyte rich large B-cell lymphoma
  16. Primary mediastinal (thymic) large B-cell lymphoma
  17. Intravascular and ALK-positive large B-cell lymphoma
  18. Plasmablastic lymphoma
  19. Primary effusion lymphoma
  20. Burkitt lymphoma/leukaemia

III) T CELL/NK CELL MALIGNANCIES
Precursor (Immature) T-cell malignancies
Precursor T lymphoblastic lymphoma/leukaemia (Precursor T-cell ALL)

Peripheral (Mature) T-cell and NK-cell malignancies
  1. T-cell prolymphocytic leukemia
  2. T-cell large granular lymphocytic leukemia
  3. Chronic lymphoproliferative disorder of NK cells
  4. Aggressive NK-cell leukemia
  5. Systemic EBV-positive T-cell lymphoproliferative disease of childhood
  6. Adult T-cell leukemia/lymphoma
  7. Extranodal NK/T-cell lymphoma, nasal type
  8. Enteropathy-associated T-cell lymphoma
  9. Hepatosplenic T-cell lymphoma
  10. Mycosis fungoides/Sézary syndrome
  11. Primary cutaneous T-cell lymphoproliferative disorders
  12. Peripheral T-cell lymphoma, NOS
  13. Angioimmunoblastic T-cell lymphoma
  14. Anaplastic large cell lymphoma (ALCL), ALK-positive and ALK-negative

IV) HISTIOCYTIC AND DENDRITIC CELL NEOPLASMS
  1. Histiocytic sarcoma
  2. Langerhans cell histiocytosis
  3. Langerhans cell sarcoma
  4. Dendritic cell sarcoma, interdigitating and follicular

V) POST-TRANSPLANTATION LYMPHOPROLIFERATIVE DISORDERS (PTLDS)

Modified from Campo et al. Blood 2011.

leukaemias and 90% of lymphomas) while remaining are T cell malignancies; NK-cell lymphomas-leukaemias are rare.

Relative frequency of subtypes within various common NHLs listed in Table 24.8 is as under:
i) Diffuse large B cell lymphoma = 31%
ii) Follicular lymphoma = 22%
iii) MALT lymphoma = 8%
iv) Mature T cell lymphoma = 8%
v) Small lymphocytic lymphoma (SLL/CLL) = 7%
vi) Mantle cell lymphoma = 6%
vii) Mediastinal large B cell lymphoma = 2.5%
viii) Anaplastic large cell lymphoma (ALCL) = 2.5%
ix) Burkitt's lymphoma = 2.5%
x) Others = ~10%

3. Diagnosis The diagnosis of lymphoma (both Hodgkin's and non-Hodgkin's) can only be reliably made on examination of lymph node biopsy. While the initial diagnosis of ALL and CLL can be made on CBC examination, bone marrow biopsy is done for genetic and immunologic studies. Subsequently, clinical chemistry, electrophoresis and tests for organ involvement including CSF examination if CNS involvement is suspected, need to be carried out.

4. Staging In both HD and NHL, Ann Arbor staging system is followed for proper evaluation and planning treatment.

5. Ancillary studies CT scan, PET scan and gallium scan are additional imaging modalities which can be used in staging HD and NHL cases.

6. Immune abnormalities Since lymphoid neoplasms arise from immune cells of the body, immune derangements pertaining to the cell of origin may accompany these cancers. This is particularly so in B-cell malignancies and include occurrence of autoimmune haemolytic anaemia, autoimmune thrombocytopenia and hypogammaglobulinaemia.

| GIST BOX 24.7 | Lymphoid Neoplasms: General |

- Conventionally, malignancies of lymphoid cells in blood have been termed as lymphatic leukaemias and those of lymphoid tissues as lymphomas. However, recent WHO classification has categorised these together because these neoplasms may present initially in blood and infiltrate tissues, and vice versa.
- FAB classification, Working Formulation for Clinical Usage, and REAL classification are the other systems of classifying these malignancies, which are based on morphology, cytochemistry, clinical features and prognosis.
- WHO classification is based on immunophenotyping and cytogenetics and molecular markers.
- While CLL is the most common lymphoid leukaemia, NHL is more common than Hodgkin's disease.

HODGKIN'S DISEASE

Hodgkin's disease (HD) primarily arises within the lymph nodes and involves the extranodal sites secondarily. This group comprises about 8% of all cases of lymphoid neoplasms. The incidence of the disease has bimodal peaks—one in young adults between the age of 15 and 35 years and the other peak after 5th decade of life. The HD is more prevalent in young adult males than females. The classical diagnostic feature is the presence of *Reed-Sternberg (RS) cell (or Dorothy-Reed-Sternberg cell)* (described later).

CLASSIFICATION

The diagnosis of HD requires accurate microscopic diagnosis by biopsy, usually from lymph node, and occasionally from other tissues. Unlike NHL, there is only one universally accepted classification of HD i.e. *Rye classification* adopted since 1966. Rye classification divides HD into the following 4 subtypes:
1. Lymphocyte-predominance type
2. Nodular-sclerosis type
3. Mixed-cellularity type
4. Lymphocyte-depletion type.

However, the WHO classification of lymphoid neoplasms has modified Rye classification and divides HD into 2 main groups as under:
I. Nodular lymphocyte-predominant HD (a new type).
II. Classic HD (includes all the 4 above subtypes in the Rye classification).

Central to the diagnosis of HD is the essential identification of *Reed-Sternberg cell* though this is not the sole criteria (see below).

The salient features of the 4 histologic subtypes of HD are summarised in Table 24.9.

REED-STERNBERG CELL

The diagnosis of Hodgkin's disease rests on identification of RS cells, though uncommonly similar cells can occur in infectious mononucleosis and other forms of lymphomas. Therefore, additional cellular and architectural features of the biopsy must be given due consideration for making the histologic diagnosis.

There are several morphologic variants of RS cells which characterise different histologic subtypes of HD (Fig. 24.16):

1. Classic RS cell This is a large cell which has characteristically a bilobed nucleus appearing as mirror image of each other but occasionally the nucleus may be multilobed. Each lobe of the nucleus contains a prominent, eosinophilic, inclusion-like nucleolus with a clear halo around it, giving an owl-eye appearance. The cytoplasm of cell is abundant and amphophilic.

2. Lacunar type RS cell It is smaller and in addition to above features has a pericellular space or lacuna in which

Section V: Haematology and Lymphoreticular Tissues

Table 24.9 Modified WHO classification of Hodgkin's disease.

HISTOLOGIC SUBTYPE	INCIDENCE	MAIN PATHOLOGY	RS CELLS	PROGNOSIS
I. CLASSIC HD				
Lymphocyte-predominance	5%	Proliferating lymphocytes, a few histiocytes	Few, classic and polyploid type, CD15–, CD30–, CD20+	Excellent
Nodular sclerosis	70%	Lymphoid nodules, collagen bands	Frequent, lacunar type, CD15+, CD30+	Very good
Mixed cellularity	22%	Mixed infiltrate	Numerous, classic type, CD15+, CD30+	Good
Lymphocyte-depletion (Diffuse fibrotic and reticular variants)	1%	Scanty lymphocytes, atypical histiocytes, fibrosis	Numerous, pleomorphic type, CD15+, CD30+	Poor
II. NODULAR LYMPHOCYTE-PREDOMINANT HD				
	2%	Proliferation of small lymphocytes, nodular pattern of growth	Sparse number of RS cells, CD45+, EMA+, CD15-, CD30-	Chronic relapsing, may transform into large B cell NHL

it lies, which is due to artefactual shrinkage of the cell cytoplasm. It is characteristically found in nodular sclerosis variety of HD.

3. **Polyploid type (or popcorn or lymphocytic-histiocytic i.e. L and H) RS cells** These are seen in lymphocyte predominance type of HD. This type of RS cell is larger with lobulated nucleus in the shape of popcorn.

4. **Pleomorphic RS cells** These are a feature of lymphocyte depletion type. These cells have pleomorphic and atypical nuclei.

The nature and origin of RS cells, which are the real neoplastic cells in HD, have been a matter of considerable debate. One main reason for this difficulty in their characterisation is that in HD, unlike most other malignancies, the number of neoplastic cells (i.e. RS cells) is very small (less than 5%) which are interspersed in the predominant reactive cells. In general, the number of RS cells is inversely proportional to the number of lymphocytes in a particular histologic subtype of HD.

Immunophenotyping of RS cells reveals monoclonal lymphoid cell origin of RS cell from B-cells of the germinal centre in most subtypes of Hodgkin's disease. RS cells in all types of Hodgkin's disease, except in lymphocyte predominance type, express immunoreactivity for CD15 and CD30 **(Fig. 24.17)**. RS cells in lymphocyte predominance type, however, are negative for both CD15 and CD30, but positive for CD20.

RS cells are invariably accompanied by variable number of *atypical Hodgkin cells* which are believed to be precursor RS cells but are not considered diagnostic of HD. Hodgkin cells are large mononuclear cells (rather than mirror image nuclei) having nuclear and cytoplasmic similarity to that of RS cell.

MORPHOLOGIC FEATURES

Grossly, the gross appearance of Hodgkin's and non-Hodgkin's lymphoma is much the same. Any lymph node group may be involved but most commonly affected are the cervical, supraclavicular and axillary groups. Initially, the lymph nodes are discrete and separate from one another but later the lymph nodes form a large matted mass due to infiltration into the surrounding connective tissue. Extranodal involvements produce either a discrete tumour or diffuse enlargement of the affected organ. The sectioned surface of the involved lymph nodes or extranodal organ involved appears grey-white and fishflesh-like. *Nodular sclerosis type HD* may show formation of nodules due to scarring while *mixed cellularity* and *lymphocyte depletion types HD* may show abundance of necrosis. Lymphomatous involvement of the liver, spleen and other organs may be diffuse or may form spherical masses similar to metastatic carcinoma.

Microscopically, the criteria for diagnosis of histologic subtypes of HD are as under:

I. CLASSIC HD

As per WHO classification, classic group of HD includes 4 types of HD of older Rye classification:

1. **Lymphocyte-predominance type (Fig. 24.16,A)** The lymphocyte-predominance type of HD is characterised by proliferation of small lymphocytes admixed with a varying number of histiocytes forming nodular or diffuse pattern.

i) *Nodular form* is characterised by replacement of nodal architecture by numerous large neoplastic nodules.

ii) *Diffuse form* does not have discernible nodules but instead there is diffuse proliferation of cells.

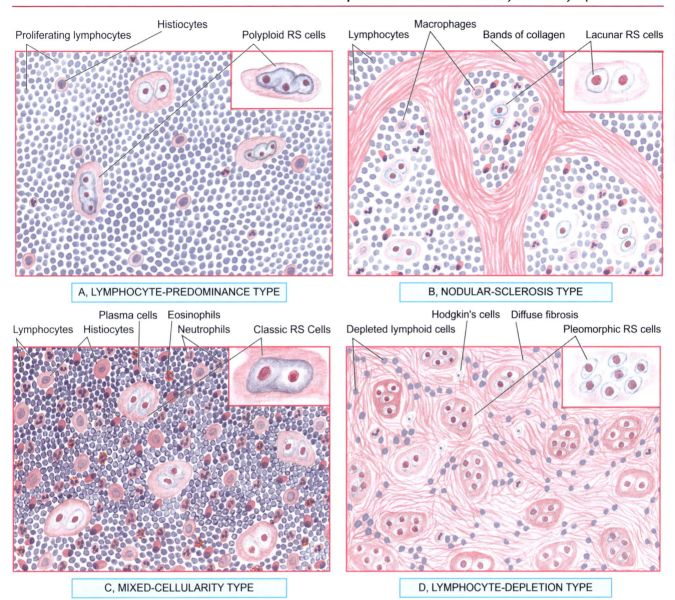

Figure 24.16 ▶ Microscopic features of 4 forms of Hodgkin's disease of lymph node. The inset on right side of each type shows the morphologic variant of RS cell seen more often in particular histologic type.

However, currently nodular form of lymphocyte predominent HD has been categorised separately due to its distinct immunophenotyping features and prognosis (discussed below).

For making the diagnosis, definite demonstration of RS cells is essential which are few in number, requiring a thorough search. In addition to typical RS cells, *polyploid variant* having polyploid, and twisted nucleus (popcornlike) may be found in some cases. This type of HD usually does not show other cells like plasma cells, eosinophils and neutrophils, nor are necrosis or fibrosis seen.

2. Nodular-sclerosis type (Fig. 24.16,B) Nodular sclerosis is the most frequent type of HD, seen more commonly in women than in men. It is characterised by two essential features (Fig. 24.18, A):

i) *Bands of collagen:* Variable amount of fibrous tissue is characteristically present in the involved lymph nodes. Occasionally, the entire lymph node may be replaced by dense hyalinised collagen.

ii) *Lacunar type RS cells:* Characteristic lacunar type of RS cells with distinctive pericellular halo are present. These

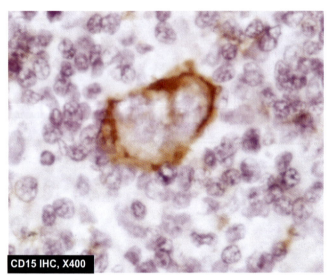

Figure 24.17 ► RS cells showing positive immunostaining for CD15, a B-cell marker.

cells appear lacunar due to the shrinkage of cytoplasm in formalin-fixed tissue. The pericellular halo is not seen if the tissue is fixed in Zenker's fluid.

In addition to these 2 characteristics, the nodules between the fibrous septa consist predominantly of lymphocytes and macrophages, sometimes with foci of necrosis.

3. Mixed-cellularity type (Fig. 24.16,C) This form of HD generally replaces the entire affected lymph nodes by heterogeneous mixture of various types of apparently normal cells. These include proliferating lymphocytes, histiocytes, eosinophils, neutrophils and plasma cells. Some amount of fibrosis and focal areas of necrosis are generally present. Typical RS cells are frequent (Fig. 24.18, B).

4. Lymphocyte-depletion type (Fig. 24.16,D) In this type of HD, the lymph node is depleted of lymphocytes. There are two variants of lymphocyte-depletion HD:

i) *Diffuse fibrotic variant* is hypocellular and the entire lymph node is replaced by diffuse fibrosis, appearing as homogeneous, fibrillar hyaline material. The area of hyalinosis contains some lymphocytes, atypical histiocytes (Hodgkin cells), and numerous typical and atypical (pleomorphic) RS cells.

ii) *Reticular variant* is much more cellular and consists of large number of atypical pleomorphic histiocytes, scanty lymphocytes and a few typical RS cells.

II. NODULAR LYMPHOCYTE-PREDOMINANT HD

This is a newly described entity which is distinct from the classic HD described above. This type was previously included in lymphocyte predominant type of HD. Its peculiarities are as under:

i) These cases of HD have a nodular growth pattern (similar to nodular sclerosis type).

ii) Like lymphocyte-predominant pattern of classic type, there is predominance of small lymphocytes with sparse number of RS cells.

iii) These cases of HD have distinctive immunophenotyping—CD45 positive, epithelial membrane antigen (EMA) positive but negative for the usual markers for RS cells (CD15 and CD30 negative).

iv) Though generally it has a chronic relapsing course, but some cases of this type of HD may transform into large B-cell NHL.

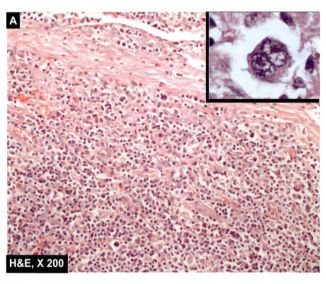
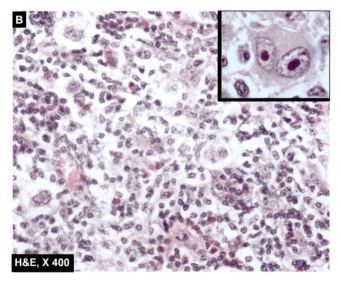

Figure 24.18 ► Hodgkin's disease. A, Nodular sclerosis type. There are bands of collagen forming nodules and characteristic lacunar RS cells (inbox in left figure). B, Mixed cellularity type. There is admixture of mature lymphocytes, plasma cells, neutrophils and eosinophils and classic RS cells in the centre of the field (inbox in right figure).

OTHER LABORATORY FINDINGS

Besides clinical and pathologic findings, there are some haematologic and immunologic abnormalities in HD.

Haematologic abnormalities

1. A moderate, normocytic and normochromic *anaemia* is often present.
2. *Serum iron and TIBC* are low but marrow iron stores are normal or increased.
3. *Marrow infiltration* by the disease may produce marrow failure with leucoerythroblastic reaction.
4. *Routine blood counts* reveal moderate leukaemoid reaction. Cases with pruritus frequently show peripheral eosinophilia. Advanced disease is associated with absolute lymphopenia.
5. *Platelet count* is normal or increased.
6. *ESR* is invariably elevated.

Immunologic abnormalities

1. There is progressive fall in immunocompetent T-cells with *defective cellular immunity.* There is reversal of CD4: CD8 ratio and anergy to routine skin tests.
2. *Humoral antibody production* is normal in untreated patients until late in the disease.

CLINICAL FEATURES

Hodgkin's disease is particularly frequent among young and middle-aged adults. All histologic subtypes of HD, except the nodular sclerosis variety, are more common in males. The disease usually begins with superficial lymph node enlargement and subsequently spreads to other lymphoid and non-lymphoid structures.

1. Most commonly, patients present with painless, movable and firm *lymphadenopathy.* The cervical and mediastinal lymph nodes are involved most frequently. Other lymph node groups like axillary, inguinal and abdominal are involved sometimes.
2. Approximately half the patients develop *splenomegaly* during the course of the disease. *Liver enlargement* too may occur.
3. *Constitutional symptoms* (type B symptoms) are present in 25-40% of patients. The most common is low-grade fever with night sweats and weight loss. Other symptoms include fatigue, malaise, weakness and pruritus.

STAGING

Following biopsy and histopathologic classification of HD, the extent of involvement of the disease (i.e. staging) is studied in order to select proper treatment and assess the prognosis. *Ann Arbor staging classification* takes into account both clinical and pathologic stage of the disease.

Table 24.10 Ann Arbor staging classification of Hodgkin's disease.

Stage		Description
Stage I (A or B)	I	Involvement of a single lymph node region.
	I$_E$	Involvement of a single extra-lymphatic organ or site.
Stage II (A or B)	II	Involvement of two or more lymph node regions on the same side of the diaphragm.
	II$_E$	(or) with localised contiguous involvement of an extranodal organ or site.
Stage III (A or B)	III	Involvement of lymph node regions on both sides of the diaphragm.
	III$_E$	(or) with localised contiguous involvement of an extranodal organ or site.
	III$_S$	(or) with involvement of spleen.
	III$_{ES}$	(or) both features of III$_E$ and III$_S$.
Stage IV (A or B)	IV	Multiple or disseminated involvement of one or more extra-lymphatic organs or tissues with or without lymphatic involvement.

(A = Asymptomatic; B = Presence of constitutional symptoms; E = Extranodal involvement; S = Splenomegaly).

The suffix *A* or *B* are added to the above stages depending upon whether the three constitutional symptoms (fever, night sweats and unexplained weight loss exceeding 10% of normal) are absent (A) or present (B). The suffix *E* or *S* are used for extranodal involvement and splenomegaly respectively **(Table 24.10)**.

For complete staging, a number of other *essential diagnostic studies* are recommended. These are as under:

1. Detailed physical examination including sites of nodal involvement and splenomegaly.
2. Chest radiograph to exclude mediastinal, pleural and lung parenchymal involvement.
3. CT scan of abdomen and pelvis.
4. Documentation of constitutional symptoms (B symptoms).
5. Laboratory evaluation of complete blood counts, liver and kidney function tests.
6. Bilateral bone marrow biopsy.
7. Finally, histopathologic documentation of the type of Hodgkin's disease.

More invasive investigations include *lymphangiography of lower extremities* and *staging laparotomy.* Staging laparotomy includes biopsy of selected lymph nodes in the retroperitoneum, splenectomy and wedge biopsy of the liver.

PROGNOSIS

With use of aggressive radiotherapy and chemotherapy, the outlook for Hodgkin's disease has improved significantly.

Although several factors affect the prognosis, two important considerations in evaluating its outcome are the *extent of involvement by the disease (i.e. staging)* and the *histologic subtype*.

With appropriate treatment, the overall 5 years survival rate for *stage I and II A* is as high as about 100%, while the advanced stage of the disease may have upto 50% 5-year survival rate.

◆ Patients with *lymphocyte-predominance type* of HD tend to have localised form of the disease and have excellent prognosis.

◆ *Nodular sclerosis* variety too has very good prognosis but those patients with larger mediastinal mass respond poorly to both chemotherapy and radiotherapy.

◆ *Mixed cellularity type* occupies intermediate clinical position between the lymphocyte predominance and the lymphocyte-depletion type, but patients with disseminated disease and systemic manifestations do poorly.

◆ *Lymphocyte-depletion type* is usually disseminated at the time of diagnosis and is associated with constitutional symptoms. These patients usually have the most aggressive form of the disease.

The salient features to distinguish Hodgkin's disease and non-Hodgkin's lymphoma are summarised in **Table 24.11**.

Table 24.11 Contrasting features of Hodgkin's disease and non-Hodgkin's lymphoma.

	FEATURE	HODGKIN'S	NON-HODGKIN'S
1.	Cell derivation	B-cell mostly	90% B 10% T
2.	Nodal involvement	Localised, may spread to contiguous nodes	Disseminated nodal spread
3.	Extranodal spread	Uncommon	Common
4.	Bone marrow involvement	Uncommon	Common
5.	Constitutional symptoms	Common	Uncommon
6.	Chromosomal defects	Aneuploidy	Translocations, deletions
7.	Spill-over	Never	May spread to blood
8.	Prognosis	Better (75-85% cure)	Bad (30-40% cure)

GIST BOX 24.8 Hodgkin's Disease

❖ Hodgkin's disease (HD) primarily arises within the lymph nodes and involves the extranodal sites secondarily.
❖ Based on microscopy, HD is divided into classic and nodular lymphocyte predominant. Classic type has further 4 types: lymphocyte predominance, nodular sclerosis (most common), mixed cellularity, and lymphocyte depletion type (least common).
❖ Prognosis of lymphocyte predominance HD is excellent followed by nodular sclerosis and mixed cellularity. Lymphocyte-depletion HD has worst outcome.
❖ Clinically, patients of HD have lymphadenopathy, and may have splenomegaly, hepatomegaly and constitutional symptoms.
❖ Ann Arbor staging is followed for HD. Nodular sclerosis type has the best prognosis while lymphocyte depletion type has the worst prognosis.
❖ Various types of HD are diagnosed by biopsy and characteristic Reed-Strernberg cells.

NON-HODGKIN'S LYMPHOMAS-LEUKAEMIAS

Non-Hodgkin's lymphomas (NHLs) and lymphoid leukaemias comprise a large group of heterogeneous of neoplasms of lymphoid tissues and blood. As outlined in **Table 24.8**, NHLs have several types and are far more common (62%) than HD (8%). As per WHO classification give in **Table 24.8**, some common and important examples are discussed below.

PRECURSOR (IMMATURE) B- AND T-CELL LEUKAEMIA/LYMPHOMA (*SYNONYM:* ACUTE LYMPHOBLASTIC LEUKAEMIA)

Lymphoid malignancy originating from precursor series of B or T cell (i.e. pre-B and pre-T) is the most common form of cancer of children under 4 years of age, together constituting 4% of all lymphoid malignancies. Pre-B cell ALL constitutes 90% cases while pre-T cell lymphoid malignancies comprise the remaining 10%. This group of lymphoid malignancies arises from more primitive stages of B or T cells but the stage of differentiation is not related to aggressiveness. Both these are presented together because of morphologic similarities.

Clinical Features

PRECURSOR B-CELL LYMPHOBLASTIC LEUKAEMIA/LYMPHOMA Most often, it presents as ALL in children; rarely presentation may be in the form of lymphoma in children or adults and it rapidly transforms into leukaemia. In cases having leukaemic presentation, extranodal site involvement is early such as lymphadenopathy accompanied with hepatomegaly, splenomegaly, CNS infiltration, testicular enlargement, and at times cutaneous infiltration. Infections due to cytopenia are present.

PRECURSOR T-CELL LYMPHOBLASTIC LEUKAEMIA/LYMPHOMA As the name implies, these cases may present as ALL or as lymphoma. Since the precursor T-cells differentiate in the thymus, this tumour often presents as mediastinal mass and pleural effusion and progresses rapidly to develop leukaemia in the blood and bone marrow. Clinically, features of bone marrow failure are present which include anaemia, neutropenia and thrombocytopenia. Lymphadenopathy, hepatosplenomegaly and CNS involvement are frequent.

Precursor T-cell lymphoma-leukaemia is, however, more aggressive than its B-cell counterpart.

Laboratory Findings

Precursor B and T-cell ALL/lymphoma are indistinguishable on routine morphology. The diagnosis is made by following investigations:

1. Blood examination Peripheral blood generally shows anaemia and thrombocytopenia, and may show leucopenia-to-normal TLC to leucocytosis. DLC shows large number of circulating lymphoblasts (generally in excess of 20%) having round to convoluted nuclei, high nucleo-cytoplasmic ratio and absence of cytoplasmic granularity. It is important to distinguish AML from ALL; the morphologic features of myeloblasts and lymphoblasts are contrasted in Table 24.1. Typical characteristics of different forms of ALL (L1 to L3) are given in Table 24.6. It is usual to find some *'smear cells'* in the peripheral blood which represent degenerated leucocytes (Fig. 24.19).

2. Bone marrow examination Marrow examination shows 20-95% malignant undifferentiated cells of precursor B or T cell origin as demonstrated by immunophenotyping. Megakaryocytes are usually reduced or absent.

3. Cytochemistry Cytochemical stains may be employed as an adjunct to Romanowsky staining for determining the type of leukaemia. Some of the commonly employed cytochemical stains in characterisation of leukaemic blasts in ALL are as under:

i) Periodic acid-Schiff (PAS): Positive in immature lymphoid cells in ALL.

ii) Acid phosphatase: Focal positivity in leukaemic blasts in ALL.

iii) Myeloperoxidase: Negative in immature cells in ALL.

iv) Sudan Black: Negative in immature cells in ALL.

v) Non-specific esterase (NSE): Negative in ALL.

Immunophenotyping TdT (terminal deoxynucleotidyl transferase) is expressed by the nuclei of both pre-B and pre-T stages of differentiation of lymphoid cells. Specific diagnosis is eastablished by following immunophenotyping:

Pre-B-cell type: Typically positive for pan-B cell markers CD19, CD10, CD9a.

Pre-T-cell type: Typically positive for CD1, CD2, CD3, CD5, CD7.

Cytogenetic analysis Leukaemic blasts in pre-B-cell ALL show characteristic cytogenetic abnormality of t(9;22) i.e. Philadelphia positive-ALL.

Principles of Treatment and Prognosis

Treatment plan for children with pre-B or pre-T cell ALL is intensive remission induction with combination therapy. Patients presenting with pre-B or pre-T cell lymphoma are treated as a case of ALL.

CHEMOTHERAPY The most useful drugs in the treatment of ALL are combination of vincristine, prednisolone, anthracyclines (daunorubicin, adriamycin) and L-asparaginase. Other agents used are cytosine arabinoside and methotrexate. Though 90% of children with ALL show remission with this therapy, patients with T cell ALL and those with meningeal involvement carry a less favourable prognosis. CNS involvement is beyond the reach of most of the cytotoxic drugs used in the therapy of ALL. CNS prophylaxis in such cases is considered after the initial remission has been obtained

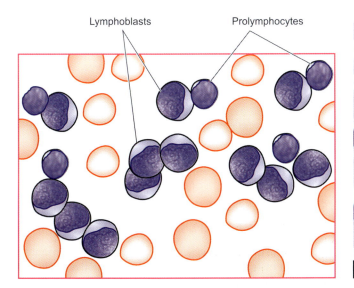
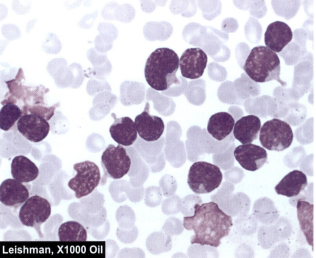

Figure 24.19 ▶ PBF findings in acute lymphoblastic leukaemia (ALL). The cells are large, with round to convoluted nuclei having high N/C ratio and no cytoplasmic granularity. A few degenerated cells (smear cells) are also seen.

	FEATURE	AML	ALL
1.	Common age	Adults between 15-40 years; comprise 20% of childhood leukaemias	Children under 15 years; comprise 80% of childhood leukaemias
2.	Physical findings	Splenomegaly + Hepatomegaly + Lymphadenopathy + Bony tenderness + Gum hypertrophy +	Splenomegaly ++ Hepatomegaly ++ Lymphadenopathy ++ Bony tenderness + CNS involvement +
3.	Laboratory findings	Low-to-high TLC Predominance of myeloblasts and promyelocytes in blood and bone marrow Thrombocytopenia moderate to severe.	Low-to-high TLC Predominance of lymphoblasts in blood and bone marrow Thrombocytopenia moderate to severe.
4.	Diagnostic criteria	FAB types M0-M7 WHO criteria = >20% blasts	FAB types L1-L3, WHO types Pre B (90%) Pre T (10%) WHO criteria = >20% blasts
5.	Cytochemical stains	Myeloperoxidase +, Sudan black +, NSE + in M4 and M5, acid phosphatase (diffuse) + in M4 and M5	PAS +, acid phosphatase (focal) +
6.	Specific therapy	Cytosine arabinoside, anthracyclines (daunorubicin, adriamycin) and 6-thioguanine	Vincristine, prednisolone, anthracyclines and L-asparaginase
7.	Immunophenotyping	CD13, 33, 41, 42	Both B and T cell ALL TdT +ve Pre-B: CD19, 20 Pre-T: CD1, 2, 3, 5, 7
8.	Cytogenetics	M3: t(15;17) M4: in(16)	Pre B: t(9;21)
9.	Response to therapy	Remission rate low, duration of remission shorter	Remission rate high, duration of remission prolonged
10.	Median survival	12-18 months	Children without CNS prophylaxis 33 months, with CNS prophylaxis 60 months; adults 12-18 months

and includes cranial irradiation and course of intrathecal methotrexate or cytosine arabinoside.

BONE MARROW TRANSPLANTATION Bone marrow (Stem cell) transplantation from suitable allogenic or autologous donor (HLA and mixed lymphocytes culture-matched) is used in pre-B and pre-T cell ALL in adults with relapses. Bone marrow transplantation has resulted in cure in about half the cases.

Prognosis and disease-free survival of children with both pre-B cell and pre-T cell ALL is better than in adults. Mean survival with treatment in children without CNS prophylaxis is 33 months, while with CNS prophylaxis is 60 months or more. Adult pre-T cell ALL, however, is as grave as AML and median survival is 12-18 months. Patients having limited disease confined to lymph nodes in both pre-B and pre-T cell type have a higher cure rate and better prognosis.

The salient differences between the two main forms of acute leukaemia (AML and ALL) are summarised in **Table 24.12**.

GIST BOX 24.9 ALL (Precursor B- and T-Cell Leukaemia/Lymphoma)

❖ ALL is lymphoid malignancy of precursor series of B or T cells and is the most common cancer in children under 4 years of age; T cell type being more aggressive.
❖ It may have leukaemic presentation or as lymphoma with involvement of extranodal sites.
❖ As per FAB classification, ALL is further of 3 types: L1 (B/T cell childhood type), L2 (adult T cell type) and L3 (Burkitt type B cell) leukaemia.
❖ Blood examination shows leucocytosis, large number of undifferentiated lymphoblasts (20-95%) and thrombocytopenia.

PERIPHERAL (MATURE) B-CELL MALIGNANCIES

Peripheral or mature B-cell cancers are the most common lymphoid malignancies. These arise from the stage of lymphoid cells at which they become committed to B cell development, acquire surface characteristics and begin to secrete immunoglobulins. This group includes following common examples.

Chronic Lymphocytic Leukaemia/ Small Lymphocytic Lymphoma (B-cell CLL/SLL)

As the name implies, this subtype may present as leukaemia or lymphoma constituting 9% of all lymphoid neoplasms. As lymphoid leukaemia (CLL), this is the most common form while as SLL it constitutes 7% of all NHLs. B-cell CLL/SLL occurs more commonly in middle and older age groups (over 50 years of age) with a male preponderance (male-female ratio 2:1).

Clinical Features

The condition may remain asymptomatic, or may have an insidious onset and may present with nonspecific clinical features. Common presenting manifestations are as under:
1. Features of *anaemia* such as gradually increasing weakness, fatigue and dyspnoea.
2. Enlargement of superficial *lymph nodes* is a very common finding. The lymph nodes are usually symmetrically enlarged, discrete and non-tender.
3. *Splenomegaly* and *hepatomegaly* are usual.
4. *Haemorrhagic manifestations* are found in case of CLL with thrombocytopenia.
5. *Susceptibility to infections,* particularly of respiratory tract, is common in CLL.
6. *Less common findings* are: mediastinal pressure, tonsillar enlargement, disturbed vision, and bone and joint pains.

Laboratory Findings

The diagnosis of CLL can usually be made on the basis of physical findings and blood smear examination (Fig. 24.20):

I. BLOOD PICTURE The findings of routine blood picture are as under:

1. Anaemia Anaemia is usually mild to moderate and normocytic normochromic in type. Mild reticulocytosis may be present. About 20% cases develop a Coombs'-positive autoimmune haemolytic anaemia.

2. White blood cells Typically, there is marked leucocytosis but less than that seen in CML (50,000-200,000/μl). Usually, more than 90% of leucocytes are mature small lymphocytes. Smudge or basket cells (degenerated forms) are present due to damaged nuclei of fragile malignant lymphocytes. The absolute neutrophil count is, however, generally within normal range. Granulocytopenia occurs when disease is fairly advanced.

3. Platelets The platelet count is normal or moderately reduced as an autoimmune phenomenon.

II. BONE MARROW EXAMINATION The typical findings are as under:
1. Increased lymphocyte count (25-95%).
2. Reduced myeloid precursors.
3. Reduced erythroid precursors.

III. LYMPH NODE BIOPSY Cases with lymphadenopathy at presentation show replacement of the lymph node by diffuse proliferation of well-differentiated, mature, small and uniform lymphocytes without any cytologic atypia

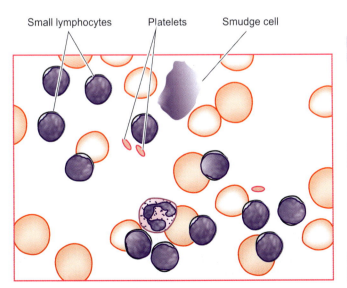
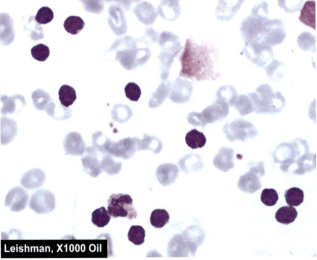

Figure 24.20 ▶ PBF in chronic lymphocytic leukaemia (CLL). There is large excess of mature and small differentiated lymphocytes and some degenerated forms appearing as bare smudged nuclei.

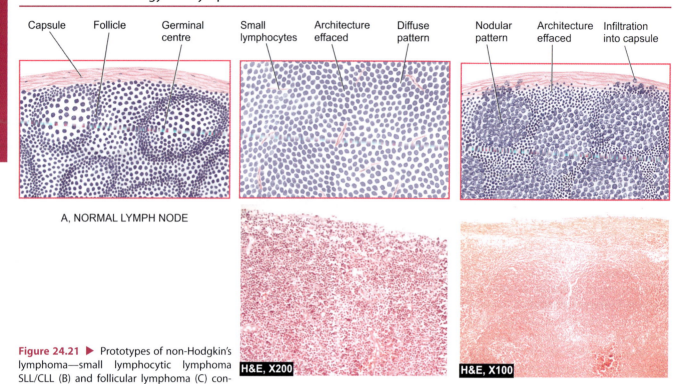

Figure 24.21 ▶ Prototypes of non-Hodgkin's lymphoma—small lymphocytic lymphoma SLL/CLL (B) and follicular lymphoma (C) contrasted with structure of normal lymph node (A).

or significant mitoses (Fig. 24.21,B). These cells are of monoclonal B-cell origin having immunologic features of mantle zone B-cells.

IV. OTHER INVESTIGATIONS These include the following:
1. *Erythrocyte rosette test* with mouse red cells is positive in more than 95% of cases indicating that CLL is a monoclonal B cell neoplasm.
2. *Positive for B-cell markers* e.g. typically CD5 positive; other pan-B cell markers are CD19, CD20, CD23, surface immunoglobulins of various classes, monoclonal light chains (λ or κ type).
3. *Serum immunoglobulin levels* are generally reduced.
4. *Coombs' test* is positive in 20% cases.
5. *Cytogenetic abnormalities*, most commonly trisomy 12 seen in about 25% cases.

Treatment Plan and Prognosis

Unlike other leukaemias, none of the available drugs and radiation therapy are capable of eradicating CLL and induce true complete remission. Treatment is, therefore, palliative and symptomatic, and with optimal management patient can usually lead a relatively normal life for several years. These approaches include: alkylating drugs (e.g. chlorambucil, cyclophosphamide), corticosteroids and radiotherapy. Splenectomy is indicated in cases of CLL with autoimmune haemolytic anaemia.

Prognosis of CLL/SLL is generally better than CML since *blastic transformation seldom occurs*. Prognosis correlates with the stage of disease as under:

Stage A: characterised by lymphocytosis alone, or with limited lymphadenopathy, has a good prognosis (median survival more than 10 years).

Stage B: having lymphocytosis with associated significant lymphadenopathy and hepatosplenomegaly has intermediate prognosis (median survival about 5 years).

Stage C: having lymphocytosis with associated anaemia and thrombocytopenia has a worse prognosis (median survival of less than 2 years).

Generally, the course is indolent. However, some cases of SLL may transform into more aggressive diffuse large B-cell lymphoma, or may be associated with occurrence of an IgM monoclonal gammopathy called Waldenström's macroglobulinaemia (page 458).

Follicular Lymphoma

In the earlier classification schemes, follicular lymphoma was known as nodular (poorly-differentiated) or follicular lymphoma (predominantly small/large cleaved cell type). Follicular lymphomas comprise approximately 22% of all NHLs. Follicular lymphomas occur in older individuals, most frequently presenting with painless peripheral lymphadenopathy which is usually waxing and waning type.

In contrast to diffuse lymphomas, extranodal involvement is also infrequent.

MORPHOLOGIC FEATURES Following features are seen:

Lymph node biopsy As the name suggests, follicular lymphoma is characterised by follicular or nodular pattern of growth. The nuclei of tumour cells may vary from predominantly small cleaved (or indented) to predominantly large cleaved variety (Fig. 24.21,C). The former is more common, has infrequent mitoses and the rate of growth slow (low grade), while the patients with large cell lymphoma have high proliferation and progress rapidly (high grade). In all follicular lymphomas, the tumour cells are positive for pan-B markers such as CD19 and CD20 along with expression of *BCL-2* protein (for distinction from normal germinal centre which is *BCL-2* negative). Cytogenetic studies show characteristic translocation *t*(14;18) in tumour cells.

Blood and bone marrow Peripheral blood involvement as occurs in SLL is uncommon in this variety. Infiltration in the bone marrow is typically paratrabecular.

About half the cases of low-grade follicular lymphomas, during their indolent biologic course, may evolve into diffuse large B-cell lymphoma. Median survival for patients with low grade follicular lymphoma is 7-9 years.

Diffuse Large B-Cell Lymphoma (DLBCL)

Diffuse large B-cell lymphoma (DLBCL), earlier termed as diffuse poorly-differentiated lymphocytic lymphoma or follicular centre cell diffuse large, cleaved/non-cleaved lymphoma, is the most common comprising about 31% of all NHLs. It occurs in older patients with mean age of 60 years. It may present primarily as a lymph node disease or at extranodal sites. About half the cases have extranodal involvement at the time of presentation, particularly in the bone marrow and the alimentary tract. Primary diffuse large B-cell lymphoma of CNS may also occur.

A few subtypes of diffuse large B-cell lymphoma are described in distinct clinicopathologic settings:

i) *Epstein-Barr virus (EBV)* infection has been etiologically implicated in diffuse large B-cell lymphoma in *immunosuppressed patients* of AIDS and organ transplant cases.

ii) *Human herpes virus type 8 (HHV-8)* infection along with presence of immunosuppression is associated with a subtype of diffuse large B-cell lymphoma presenting with effusion, termed *primary effusion lymphoma*.

iii) *Mediastinal large B-cell lymphoma* is diagnosed in patients with prominent involvement of mediastinum, occurs in young females and frequently spreads to CNS and abdominal viscera.

In general, DLBCL is aggressive tumour and disseminates widely.

Burkitt's Lymphoma/Leukaemia

Burkitt's lymphoma/leukaemia is an uncommon tumour in adults but comprises about 30% of childhood NHLs. Burkitt's leukaemia corresponds to L3 ALL of FAB grouping and is uncommon. Three subgroups of Burkitt's lymphoma are recognised: *African endemic, sporadic and immunodeficiency-associated*:

i) *African endemic Burkitt's lymphoma* was first described in African children, predominantly presenting as jaw tumour that spreads to extranodal sites such as the bone marrow and meninges. The relationship of this tumour with oncogenic virus, Epstein-Barr virus (EBV), has been discussed in Chapter 19.

ii) *Sporadic Burkitt's lymphoma* is a related tumour in which the tumour cells are similar to those of Burkitt's lymphoma but are more pleomorphic and may sometimes be multinucleated. Sporadic variety has a propensity to infiltrate the CNS and is more aggressive than true Burkitt's lymphoma.

iii) *Immunodeficiency-associated Burkitt's lymphoma* includes cases seen in association with HIV infection.

MORPHOLOGIC FEATURES **Histologically,** all three types of Burkitt's lymphoma are similar. Tumour cells are intermediate in size, non-cleaved, and homogeneous in size and shape. The nuclei are round to oval and contain 2-5 nucleoli. The cytoplasm is basophilic and contains lipid vacuolation. The tumour cells have a very high mitotic rate, and therefore high cell death. This feature accounts for presence of numerous macrophages in the background of this tumour containing phagocytosed tumour debris giving it a 'starry sky' appearance (Fig. 24.22).

Burkitt's leukaemia is identified by classical appearance of monomorphic medium-sized cells having round nuclei, frequent mitoses, multiple nucleoli, and basophilic cytoplasm with vacuoles.

Immunophenotypically, the tumour cells are positive for CD19 and CD10 and surface immunoglobulin IgM. Typical cytogenetic abnormalities in the tumour cells are *t*(8;14) and *t*(8;22) involving *MYC* gene on chromosome 8, with overexpression of MYC protein having transforming activity.

Burkitt's lymphoma is a high-grade tumour and is a very rapidly progressive human tumour.

Extranodal Marginal Zone B-Cell Lymphoma of MALT Type (*Synonym: Maltoma*)

MALT refers to mucosa-associated lymphoid tissue. This type comprises about 8% of all NHLs. In the earlier classification, maltoma was included under SLL, but in the WHO scheme it is categorised separately for 2 reasons:

i) *Etiologic association with H. pylori infection:* Most frequent is gastric lymphoma of MALT type with its characteristic etiologic association with *H. pylori*.

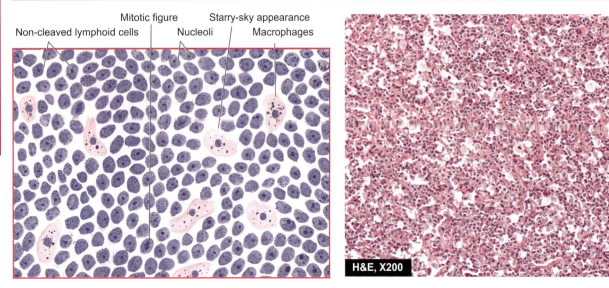

Figure 24.22 ▶ Burkitt's lymphoma. The tumour shows uniform cells having high mitotic rate. Scattered among the tumour cells are benign macrophages surrounded by a clear space giving 'starry sky' appearance.

ii) *Occurrence at extranodal sites:* Besides stomach, other extranodal sites for this subtype of NHL are intestine, orbit, lung, thyroid, salivary glands and CNS.

About half the cases of gastric MALT lymphoma show genetic mutation *t*(11;18). Median age for this form of NHL is 60 years and often remains localised to the organ of origin but may infiltrate the regional lymph nodes.

MALT lymphoma has a good prognosis. Rarely, it may be more aggressive and may metastasise, or transform into diffuse large B-cell lymphoma.

Hairy Cell Leukaemia (HCL)

Hairy cell leukaemia (HCL) is an unusual and uncommon form of B-cell malignancy characterised by presence of hairy cells in the blood and bone marrow and splenomegaly. It occurs in the older males. HCL is characterised clinically by the manifestations due to infiltration of reticuloendothelial organs (bone marrow, liver and spleen) and, hence, its previous name as *leukaemic reticuloendotheliosis*. Patients have susceptibility to infection with *M. avium intercellulare*.

MORPHOLOGIC FEATURES Laboratory diagnosis is made by the presence of pancytopenia due to marrow failure and splenic sequestration, and identification of characteristic hairy cells in the blood and bone marrow. Hairy cells are abnormal mononuclear cells with hairy cytoplasmic projections which are seen in the bone marrow, peripheral blood and spleen. These cells are best recognised under phase contrast microscopy but may also be visible in routine blood smears (Fig. 24.23). These leukaemic 'hairy cells' have characteristically positive cytochemical staining for *tartrate-resistant acid phosphatase (TRAP)*.

The controversy on the origin of hairy cells whether these cells represent neoplastic T cells, B cells or monocytes, is settled with the molecular analysis of these cells which assigns them *B cell origin* expressing CD19, CD20 and CD22 antigen. In addition to B cell markers, hairy cells are also positive for CD11, CD25 and CD103.

The disease often runs a chronic course requiring supportive care. The mean survival is 4-5 years. Patients respond to splenectomy, α-interferon therapy and 2-chlorodeoxyadenosine (2-CDA).

 GIST BOX 24.10 | **Peripheral Mature B-Cell Malignancies**

- B-cell CLL-SLL may appear as leukaemia or lymphoma, presenting with anaemia, lymphadenopathy and hepatosplenomegaly.
- Blood examination in CLL shows leucocytosis with marked lymphocytosis and basket or smear cells.
- Lymph node biopsy in CLL-SLL shows diffuse infiltration by well-differentiated nature uniform lymphocytes.
- Follicular lymphoma occurring in older patients is nodular replacement of nodal architecture.
- Burkitt's lymphoma/leukaemia is an uncommon B cell malignancy that occurs as African endemic, sporadic and immunodeficiency associated.
- Maltoma is a lymphoma arising in lymphoid tissues of the stomach, intestine and other mucosal sites and has *H. pylori* association.
- Hairy cell leukaemia is B cell malignancy characterised by hairy cells in the blood, bone marrow and spleen.

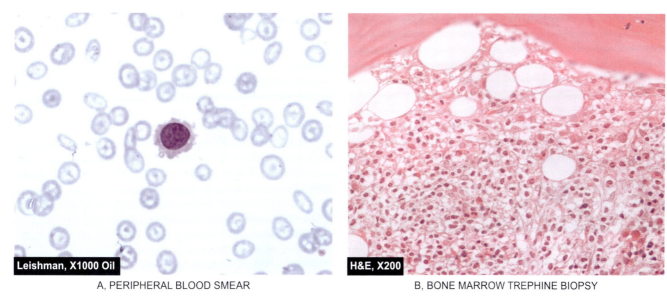

Figure 24.23 ▶ Hairy cell leukaemia. A, Peripheral blood shows presence of a leukaemic cells with hairy cytoplasmic projections. B, Trephine biopsy shows replacement of marrow spaces with abnormal mononuclear cells.

PERIPHERAL (MATURE) T-CELL MALIGNANCIES

Peripheral or mature T-cell lymphoid malignancies are relatively less common compared to mature B cell cancers. These arise at the stage when the lymphoid cells migrate to thymus and become committed to T-cell differentiation by acquiring T cell antigen receptor genes. A few common examples are discussed here.

Mycosis Fungoides/Sézary Syndrome

Mycosis fungoides is a slowly evolving cutaneous T-cell lymphoma occurring in middle-aged adult males.

> ***MORPHOLOGICAL FEATURES*** The condition is often preceded by eczema or dermatitis for several years (*premycotic stage*). This is followed by infiltration by CD4+ T-cells in the epidermis and dermis as a plaque (*plaque stage*) and eventually as *tumour stage*. The disease may spread to viscera and to peripheral blood as a leukaemia characterised by Sézary cells having cerebriform nuclei termed as Sézary syndrome.

Mycosis fungoides/Sézary syndrome is an indolent NHL and has a median survival of 8 to 9 years.

Adult T-cell Lymphoma/Leukaemia (ATLL)

This is an uncommon T-cell malignancy but has gained much prominence due to association with retrovirus, human T-cell lymphotropic virus-I (HTLV-I) (page 309). The infection is acquired by blood transfusion, breast milk, sexual route or transplacentally. ATLL is common in Japan, the Caribbean and parts of the US but is rare in rest of the world.

The patients have usually widespread lymphadenopathy with leukaemia, hepatosplenomegaly and involvement of skin and leptomeninges. This disease runs a fulminant course.

Anaplastic Large T/NK Cell Lymphoma (ALCL)

ALCL is the T-cell counterpart of diffuse large B-cell lymphoma (DLBCL) and was previously included under malignant histiocytosis or diagnosed as anaplastic carcinoma. ALCL is defined by:
i) documentation of *t*(2;5);
ii) overexpression of ALK (anaplastic lymphoma kinase) protein.

Accordingly, depending upon presence or absence of rearrangmement of ALK gene located on chromosome 2p23, it is categorised into ALK positive and ALK negative.

Clinically, ALCL occurs in young patients and is more common in males. Cutaneous involvement is frequent and produces an indolent cutaneous large T/null cell lymphoma. But bone marrow and other organ infiltration is rare.

LYMPH NODE METASTATIC TUMOURS

The regional lymph nodes draining the site of a primary malignant tumour are commonly enlarged. This enlargement may be due to benign *reactive hyperplasia* or *metastatic tumour deposits*.

1. Benign reactive hyperplasia, as already discussed (page 416), is due to immunologic reaction by the lymph node in response to tumour-associated antigens. It may be expressed as sinus histiocytosis, follicular hyperplasia, plasmacytosis and occasionally may show non-caseating granulomas.

Section V: Haematology and Lymphoreticular Tissues

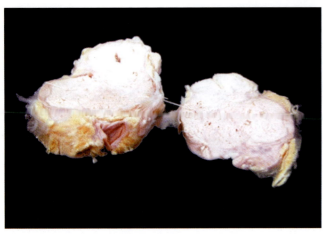

Figure 24.24 ▶ Metastatic carcinomatous deposits in the matted mass of lymph nodes. There are areas of necrosis in the circumscribed nodular areas.

2. **Metastatic deposits** in regional lymph nodes occur most commonly from carcinomas and malignant melanoma. Sarcomas often disseminate via haematogenous route but uncommonly may metastasise to the regional lymph nodes. Metastatic tumour cells from the primary malignant tumour are drained via lymphatics into the subcapsular sinuses initially but subsequently the lymph node stroma is also invaded. The pushing margins of advancing metastatic tumour in stroma of lymph node are characteristically well demarcated. Areas of necrosis are frequent in metastatic carcinomas **(Fig. 24.24)**.

The morphologic features of primary malignant tumour are recapitulated in metastatic tumour in lymph nodes.

 GIST BOX 24.11 — **Peripheral Mature T-Cell Malignancies, Metastatic Tumours**

- Mycosis fungoides-Sezary's syndrome is a slow growing cutaneous T cell lymphoma-leukaemia.
- Adult T-cell lymphoma leukaemia is etiologically linked to human T-cell lymphotropic virus.
- Anaplastic large cell lymphoma (ALCL) of T/NK cells is a diffuse large cell lymphoma similar to its B-cell counterpart, DLBCL.
- Other peripheral T cell lymphomas are angioimmunoblastic type, extranodal nasal type, enteropathy type and hepatosplenic type.
- Regional lymph nodes draining the site of a primary malignant tumour may be enlarged due to benign reactive hyperplasia or metastatic tumour deposits.

PLASMA CELL DISORDERS

The plasma cell disorders are characterised by abnormal proliferation of immunoglobulin-producing cells and result in accumulation of monoclonal immunoglobulin in serum and urine. The group as a whole is known by various synonyms such as *plasma cell dyscrasias, paraproteinaemias, dysproteinaemias and monoclonal gammopathies*. The group comprises the following six disease entities:

1. Multiple myeloma
2. Localised plasmacytoma
3. Lymphoplasmacytic lymphoma (discussed above)
3. Waldenström's macroglobulinaemia
4. Heavy chain disease
5. Primary amyloidosis (Chapter 7)
6. Monoclonal gammopathy of undetermined significance (MGUS).

The feature common to all plasma cell disorders is the neoplastic proliferation of cells derived from B-lymphocyte lineage. These disorders constitute 16% of all B-cell malignancies. Normally B lymphocytes have surface immunoglobulin molecules of both M and G chains. Under normal circumstances, B-cells are stimulated by exposure to surface immunoglobulin-specific antigen and mature to form IgG-producing plasma cells. However, in plasma cell disorders, the control over this process is lost and results in abnormal production of immunoglobulin that appears in the blood and urine. These disorders differ from other B-cell lymphoid malignancies in having monoclonal synthesis of immunoglobulins and lack of prominent lymphadenopathy. In addition to the rise in complete immunoglobulins, plasma cell disorders synthesise excess of light chains (kappa or lambda), or heavy chains of a single class (alpha, gamma, or mu). Bence-Jones proteins are free light chains present in blood and excreted in urine of some plasma cell disorders.

After these brief general comments, we now turn to the discussion of the specific plasma cell disorders.

MULTIPLE MYELOMA

Multiple myeloma is a multifocal malignant proliferation of plasma cells derived from a single clone of cells (i.e. monoclonal). The term multiple myeloma is used interchangeably with myeloma. The tumour, its products (M component), and the host response result in the most important and most common syndrome in the group of plasma cell disorders that produces osseous as well as extraosseous manifestations. Multiple myeloma primarily affects the elderly (peak incidence in 5th-6th decades) and increases in incidence with age. It is rare under the age of 40. Myeloma is more common in males than females.

Etiology and Pathogenesis

Myeloma is a monoclonal proliferation of B-cells. The etiology of myeloma remains unknown. However, following factors and abnormalities have been implicated:

1. **Radiation exposure** Large dose exposure to radiation with a long latent period has been seen in myeloma. For instance, survivors of nuclear attack in World War-II developed myeloma about 20 years later.

2. **Epidemiologic factors** Myeloma has higher incidence in blacks. Occupational exposure to petroleum products has been associated with higher incidence. Certain occupations such as farmers, wood workers and leather workers are more prone.

3. **Karyotypic abnormalities** Several chromosomal alterations have been observed in cases of myeloma, which include following translocations and deletions:
i) Translocations t(11;14)(q13;q32) and t(4;14)(p16;q32).
ii) Deletion of 13q.

4. **Oncogenes-antioncogenes** Overexpression and mutations in following genes have been noted in proliferation of tumour cells in myeloma:
i) Overexpression of *MYC* and *RAS* growth promoting oncogenes in some cases.
ii) Mutation in *p53* and *RB* growth-suppressing antioncogene in some cases.

Based on above, **molecular pathogenesis** of multiple myeloma and its major manifestations can be summed up as under and is schematically illustrated in **Fig. 24.25**:

1. Cell-surface *adhesion molecules* bind myeloma cells to bone marrow stromal cells and extracellular matrix proteins.
2. This binding triggers *adhesion-mediated signaling* and mediates *production of several cytokines* by fibroblasts and macrophages of the marrow. These include: IL-6, VEGF, TGF-β, TNF-α IL-1, lymphotoxin, macrophage inhibitory factor-1α (MIP-1α) and receptor activator of nuclear factor-κB (RANK) ligand.
3. Adhesion-mediated signalling affects the cell cycle via cyclin-D and p21 causing abnormal production of *myeloma (M) proteins*.
4. *IL-6 cytokine* plays a central role in cytokine-mediated signalling and causes proliferation as well as cell survival of tumour cells via its antiapoptotic effects on tumour cells.
5. Certain cytokines produced by myeloma cells bring about bony destruction by acting as *osteoclast-activating factor (OAF)*. These are: IL-1, lymphotoxin, VEGF, macrophage inhibitory factor-1α (MIP-1α), receptor activator of NF-κB ligand, and tumour necrosis factor (TNF).
6. Other effects of adhesion-mediated and cytokine-mediated signaling are development of *drug resistance and migration* of tumour cells in the bone marrow milieu.

Morphologic Features

Myeloma affects principally the bone marrow though during the course of the disease other organs are also involved. Therefore, the pathologic findings are described below under two headings—*osseous (bone marrow) lesions* and *extraosseous lesions*.

A. OSSEOUS (BONE MARROW) LESIONS In more than 95% of cases, multiple myeloma begins in the bone marrow. In majority of cases, the disease involves multiple bones. By the time the diagnosis is made, most of the bone marrow is involved. Most commonly affected bones are those with red marrow i.e. skull, spine, ribs and pelvis, but later long bones of the limbs are also involved **(Fig. 24.26)**. The lesions begin in the medullary cavity, erode the cancellous bone and ultimately cause destruction of the bony cortex. Radiographically, these lesions appear as punched out, rounded, 1-2 cm sized defects in the affected bone.

Grossly, the normal bone marrow is replaced by soft, gelatinous, reddish-grey tumours. The affected bone usually shows focal or diffuse osteoporosis.

Microscopically, the diagnosis of multiple myeloma can be usually established by examining bone marrow aspiration from an area of bony rarefaction. However, if the bone marrow aspiration yields dry tap or negative results, biopsy of radiologically abnormal or tender site is usually diagnostic. The following features characterise a case of myeloma:

i) **Cellularity** There is usually hypercellularity of the bone marrow.

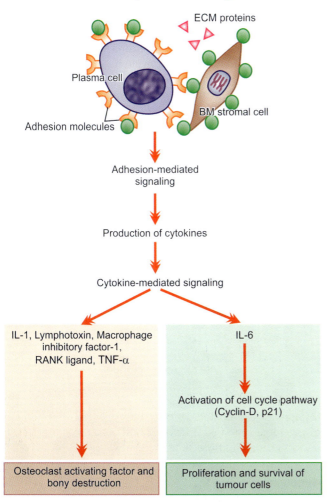

Figure 24.25 ▶ Schematic diagram showing molecular pathogenesis of multiple myeloma and its major manifestations.

460 **Section V:** Haematology and Lymphoreticular Tissues

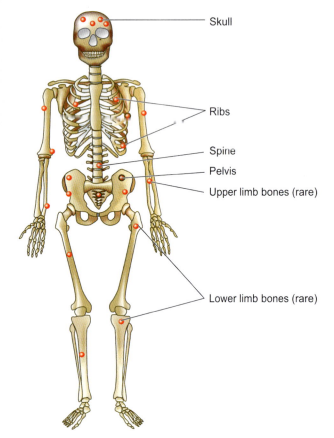

Figure 24.26 ▶ The major sites of lesions in multiple myeloma.

ii) Myeloma cells Myeloma cells constitute ≥10% of the marrow cellularity. These cells may form clumps or sheets, or may be scattered among the normal haematopoietic cells. Myeloma cells may vary in size from small, differentiated cells resembling normal plasma cells to large, immature and undifferentiated cells. Binucleate and multinucleate cells are sometimes present. The nucleus of myeloma cell is commonly eccentric similar to plasma cells but usually lacks the cart-wheel chromatin pattern seen in classical plasma cells. Nucleoli are frequently present. The cytoplasm of these cells is abundant and basophilic with perinuclear halo, vacuolisation and contains Russell bodies consisting of hyaline globules composed of synthesised immunoglobulin (Fig. 24.27).

In addition to neoplastic proliferation of plasma cells in multiple myeloma, *reactive plasmacytosis* in the bone marrow can occur in some other disorders; these include: aplastic anaemia, rheumatoid arthritis, SLE, cirrhosis of liver, metastatic cancer and chronic inflammation and infections such as tuberculosis. However, in all these conditions the plasma cells are mature and they do not exceed 10% of the total marrow cells.

B. EXTRAOSSEOUS LESIONS Late in the course of disease, lesions at several extraosseous sites become evident. Some of the commonly involved sites are as under:

1. Blood Approximately 50% of patients with multiple myeloma have a few atypical plasma cells in the blood. Other changes in the blood in myeloma are the presence of anaemia (usually normocytic normochromic type), marked red cell rouleaux formation due to hyperviscosity of blood, and an elevated ESR.

2. Myeloma kidney Renal involvement in myeloma called myeloma nephrosis occurs in many cases. The main mechanism of myeloma kidney is by filtration of light chain proteins (Bence Jones proteins) which are precipitated in the distal convoluted tubules in combination with Tamm-Horsfall proteins as tubular casts. The casts may be

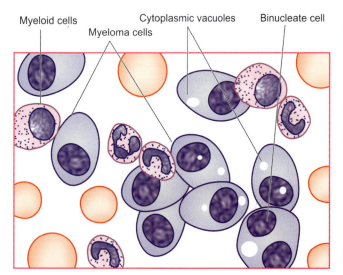
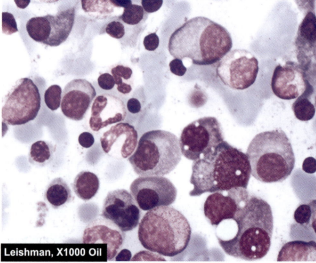

Figure 24.27 ▶ Bone marrow aspirate in myeloma showing numerous plasma cells, many with abnormal features.

surrounded by some multinucleate giant-cells and a few inflammatory cells.

3. Myeloma neuropathy Infiltration of the nerve trunk roots by tumour cells produces nonspecific polyneuropathy. Pathologic fractures, particularly of the vertebrae, may occur causing neurologic complications.

4. Systemic amyloidosis Systemic primary generalised amyloidosis (AL amyloid) may occur in 10% cases of multiple myeloma and involve multiple organs and systems.

5. Liver, spleen involvement Involvement of the liver and spleen by myeloma cells sufficient to cause hepatomegaly, and splenomegaly occurs in a small percentage of cases.

Clinical Features

The clinical manifestations of myeloma result from the effects of infiltration of the bones and other organs by neoplastic plasma cells and from immunoglobulin synthesis. The principal clinical features are as under:

1. *Bone pain* is the most common symptom. The pain usually involves the back and ribs. Pathological fractures may occur causing persistent localised pain. Bone pain results from the proliferation of tumour cells in the marrow and activation of osteoclasts which destroy the bones.

2. *Susceptibility to infections* is the next most common clinical feature. Particularly common are bacterial infections such as pneumonias and pyelonephritis. Increased susceptibility to infection is related mainly to hypogammaglobulinaemia, and partly to granulocyte dysfunction and neutropenia.

3. *Renal failure* occurs in about 25% of patients, while renal pathology occurs in 50% of cases. Causes of renal failure in myeloma are hypercalcaemia, glomerular deposits of amyloid, hyperuricaemia and infiltration of the kidney by myeloma cells.

4. *Anaemia* occurs in about 80% of patients of myeloma and is related to marrow replacement by the tumour cells (myelophthisis) and inhibition of haematopoiesis.

5. *Bleeding tendencies* may appear in some patients due to thrombocytopenia, deranged platelet function and interaction of the M component with coagulation factors.

6. *Hyperviscosity syndrome* owing to hyperglobulinaemia may produce headache, fatigue, visual disturbances and haemorrhages.

7. *Neurologic symptoms* occur in a minority of patients and are explained by hyperviscosity, cryoglobulins and amyloid deposits.

8. *Biochemical abnormalities*. These include the following:
i) hypercalcaemia due to destruction of bone;
ii) hyperuricaemia from necrosis of tumour mass and from uraemia related to renal failure; and
iii) increased β-2 microglobulins and other globulins in urine and serum.

9. *POEMS syndrome* is seen in about 1% cases of myeloma and includes simultaneous manifestations of *p*olyneuropathy, *o*rganomegaly, *e*ndocrinopathy, *m*ultiple myeloma and *s*kin changes.

Diagnosis

The diagnosis of myeloma is made by classic *triad* of features:
1. *Marrow plasmacytosis* of more than 10%
2. Radiologic evidence of *lytic bony lesions*
3. Demonstration of serum and/or urine *M component*.

There is rise in the total serum protein concentration due to *paraproteinaemia* but normal serum immunoglobulins (IgG, IgA and IgM) and albumin are depressed. Paraproteins are abnormal immunoglobulins or their parts circulating in plasma and excreted in urine. About two-third cases of myeloma excrete Bence Jones (light chain) proteins in the urine, consisting of either kappa (κ) or lambda (λ) light chains, along with presence of Bence Jones paraproteins in the serum. On serum electrophoresis, the paraprotein usually appears as a single narrow homogeneous *M-band* component, most commonly in the region of γ-globulin **(Fig. 24.28)**. Most frequent paraprotein is *IgG* seen in about 50% cases of myeloma, *IgA* in 25%, and IgD in 1%, while about 20% patients have only light chains in serum and urine (*light chain myeloma*). *Non-secretory myeloma* is absence of M-band on serum and/or electrophoresis but presence of other two features out of triad listed above. Though the commonest cause of paraproteinaemias is multiple myeloma, certain other conditions which may produce serum paraproteins need to be distinguished.

LOCALISED PLASMACYTOMA

Two variants of myeloma which do not fulfil the criteria of classical triad are the localised form of *solitary bone plasmacytoma* and *extramedullary plasmacytoma*. Both these are associated with M component in about a third of cases and occur in young individuals. Solitary bone plasmacytoma is a lytic bony lesion without marrow plasmacytosis. Extramedullary plasmacytoma involves most commonly the submucosal lymphoid tissue of nasopharynx or paranasal sinuses. Both variants have better prognosis than the classic multiple myeloma. *Plasma cell granuloma*, on the other hand, is an inflammatory condition having admixture of other inflammatory cells with mature plasma cells, which can be easily distinguished by a discernible observer.

The management of the patients is similar to that of myeloma. Patients respond to chemotherapy with a median survival of 3-5 years.

MONOCLONAL GAMMOPATHY OF UNDETERMINED SIGNIFICANCE (MGUS)

Due to longevity, monoclonal gammopathy of undetermined significance (MGUS) is now increasingly diagnosed in

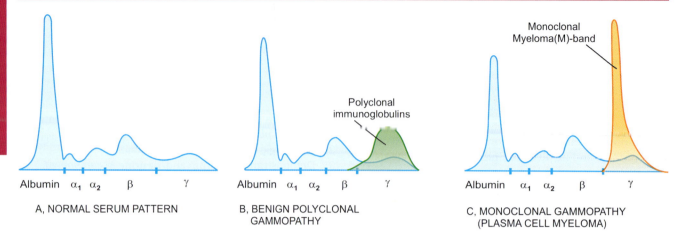

Figure 24.28 ▶ Serum electrophoresis showing normal serum pattern (A), as contrasted with that in benign polyclonal gammopathy (B) and in monoclonal gammopathy (C), typical of plasma cell myeloma.

asymptomatic healthy ageing population—1% at 50 years of age and in 10% individuals older than 75 years. This makes it the most common form of plasma cell dyscrasia. The defining criteria for MGUS are as under:

i) M-protein in serum <3 gm/dl
ii) Marrow plasmacytosis <10%
iii) No evidence of other B-cell proliferative disorder
iv) Absence of myeloma-related end-organ tissue damage (i.e. absence of lytic bone lesions, high calcium level, anaemia).

The condition needs to be cautiously distinguished from myeloma and long term follow-up is required. In fact, MGUS has been considered as a forerunner of multiple myeloma in many studies because MGUS has been found to have the same chromosomal abnormalities as in myeloma.

 GIST BOX 24.12 | **Plasma Cell Disorders**

❖ Multiple myeloma is a multifocal malignant proliferation of plasma cells derived from a single clone of B cells (i.e. monoclonal).
❖ Prolonged radiation exposure and black race are some of the factors implicated in its etiology.
❖ The diagnosis of myeloma is made by osteolytic punched out osseous lesions, marrow plasmacytosis and demonstration of M band in serum or urine electrophoresis.
❖ Localised plasmacytoma may be solitary bone lesion or extramedullary. It is generally not associated with marrow plasmacytosis.
❖ While Waldenstrom's macroglobulinaemia is an uncommon malignant proliferation of B cells, heavy chain diseases are rare and are due to malignant proliferation of B cells with monoclonal excess of one of heavy chains.

❖ Monoclonal gammopathy of undetermined significance (MGUS) is common and is now increasingly diagnosed in asymptomatic healthy ageing population.

HISTIOCYTIC NEOPLASMS: LANGERHANS CELL HISTIOCYTOSIS

The term histiocytosis is used for a group of proliferations of dendritic cells, Langerhans cells or macrophages and includes both benign and malignant examples. While histiocytic sarcoma, Langerhans cell sarcoma and dendritic cell sarcoma are clearly malignant lymphomas and are uncommon, monoclonal proliferation of Langerhans cells are grouped under Langerhans cell histiocytosis (LCH) and are somewhat more common. LCH includes three clinicopathologically related conditions occurring in children: eosinophilic granuloma, Hand-Schüller-Christian disease and Letterer-Siwe syndrome. As a group, all the three conditions are associated with proliferation of 3 types of cells: histiocytes, lymphocytes and eosinophils.

Earlier, this group was referred to as histiocytosis-X but now following facts about this group are known:

◆ *Firstly,* histiocytosis-X are not proliferations of unknown origin (X-for unknown) but proliferating cells are actually Langerhans' cells of marrow origin. Langerhans' cells are normally present mainly in the epidermis of the skin but also in some other organs.

◆ *Secondly,* the three conditions included under histiocytosis-X are actually different expression of the same basic disorder. This concept has emerged from 2 features:

i) Demonstration of common antigens on these cells by *immunohistochemical stains* for S-100 protein (Fig. 24.29), CD1a and HLA-DR.

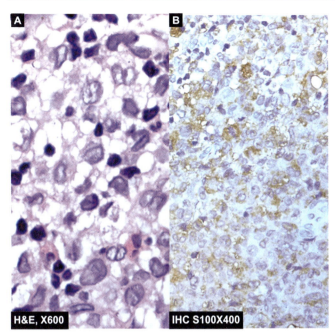

Figure 24.29 ▶ Langerhans cell histiocytosis—eosinophilic granuloma. A, Bone biopsy shows presence of infiltrate by collections of histiocytes having vesicular nuclei admixed with eosinophils. B, Immunohistochemical stain with S-100 shows cytoplasmic and nuclear positivity.

ii) Electron microscopic demonstration of *histiocytosis-X bodies* or *Birbeck granules* in the cytoplasm. These are rod-shaped structures having dilated tennis-racket like terminal end. Their function is not known but they arise from receptor-mediated endocytosis of langerin found in human epidermal cells, a protein involved in Birbeck granule biosynthesis.

The three disorders included in the group are briefly considered below.

EOSINOPHILIC GRANULOMA

Unifocal eosinophilic granuloma is more common (60%) than the multifocal variety which is often a component of Hand-Schüller-Christian disease (described below). Most of the patients are children and young adults, predominantly males. The condition commonly presents as a solitary osteolytic lesion in the femur, skull, vertebrae, ribs and pelvis. The diagnosis requires biopsy of the lytic bone lesion.

Microscopically, the lesion consists largely of closely-packed aggregates of macrophages admixed with variable number of eosinophils (Fig. 24.29). The macrophages contain droplets of fat or a few granules of brown pigment indicative of phagocytic activity. A few multinucleate macrophages may also be seen. The cytoplasm of these macrophages may contain rod-shaped inclusions called *histiocytosis-X bodies or* Birbeck granules, best seen by electron microscopy.

Clinically, unifocal eosinophilic granuloma is a benign disorder. The bony lesion remains asymptomatic until the erosion of the bone causes pain or fracture. Spontaneous fibrosis or healing may occur in some cases, while others may require curettage or radiotherapy.

HAND-SCHÜLLER-CHRISTIAN DISEASE

A triad of features consisting of *multifocal bony defects, diabetes insipidus* and *exophthalmos* is termed Hand-Schüller-Christian disease. The disease develops in children under 5 years of age. The multifocal lytic bony lesions may develop at any site. Orbital lesion causes exophthalmos, while involvement of the hypothalamus causes diabetes insipidus. Multiple spherical lesions in the lungs are frequently present. Half the patients have involvement of the liver, spleen and lymph nodes.

Microscopically, the lesions are indistinguishable from those of unifocal eosinophilic granuloma.

Clinically, the affected children frequently have fever, skin lesions, recurrent pneumonitis and other infections. Though the condition is benign, it is more disabling than the unifocal eosinophilic granuloma. The lesions may resolve spontaneously or may require chemotherapy or radiation.

LETTERER-SIWE DISEASE

Letterer-Siwe disease is an acute disseminated form of LCH occurring in infants and children under 2 years of age. The disease is characterised by hepatosplenomegaly, lymphadenopathy, thrombocytopenia, anaemia and leucopenia. There is generalised hyperplasia of tissue macrophages in various organs.

Microscopically, the involved organs contain aggregates of macrophages which are pleomorphic and show nuclear atypia. The cytoplasm of these cells contains vacuoles and rod-shaped *histiocytosis-X bodies.*

Clinically, the child has acute symptoms of fever, skin rash, loss of weight, anaemia, bleeding disorders and enlargement of lymph nodes, liver and spleen. Cystic bony lesions may be apparent in the skull, pelvis and long bones. Intense chemotherapy helps to control Letterer-Siwe disease but intercurrent infections result in fatal outcome in many cases. The condition is currently regarded as an unusual form of malignant lymphoma.

 GIST BOX 24.13 | **Langerhans Cell Histiocytosis**

❖ Monoclonal proliferation of Langerhans cells are grouped under Langerhans cell histiocytosis (LCH) and includes three clinicopathologically related conditions ocurring in children: eosinophilic granuloma, Hand-Schüller-Christian disease and Letterer-Siwe syndrome.

- As a group, all the three conditions are associated with proliferation of 3 types of cells: histiocytes, lymphocytes and eosinophils.
- Unifocal eosinophilic granuloma is a benign disorder.
- A triad of features consisting of *multifocal bony defects, diabetes insipidus* and *exophthalmos* is termed Hand-Schüller-Christian disease.
- Letterer-Siwe disease is an acute disseminated form of LCH and behaves like a lymphoma.

SPLEEN

NORMAL STRUCTURE

The spleen is the largest lymphoid organ of the body. Under normal conditions, the average weight of the spleen is about 150 gm in the adult. Normally, the organ lies well protected by the 9th, 10th and 11th ribs in the upper left quadrant. The surface of the spleen is covered by a layer of peritoneum underneath which the organ is ensheathed by a thin *capsule*. From the capsule extend connective tissue *trabeculae* into the pulp of the organ and serve as supportive network. Blood enters the spleen by the splenic artery which divides into branches that penetrate the spleen via trabeculae. From the trabeculae arise small branches called *central arterioles*. Blood in the central arterioles empties partly into splenic venules and from there into splenic vein, but largely into vascular sinuses of the red pulp and thence into the splenic venous system.

Grossly, the spleen consists of homogeneous, soft, dark red mass called the *red pulp* and long oval grey-white nodules called the *white pulp (malpighian bodies)*.

Microscopically, the red pulp consists of a network of thin-walled venous sinuses and adjacent blood spaces. The blood spaces contain blood cells, lymphocytes and macrophages and appear to be arranged in cords called *splenic cords* or *cords of Billroth*. The white pulp is made up of lymphocytes surrounding an eccentrically placed arteriole. The periarteriolar lymphocytes are mainly T-cells, while at other places the lymphocytes have a germinal centre composed principally of B-cells surrounded by densely packed lymphocytes.

The spleen is a lymphoreticular organ that performs at least the following four *functions:*
1. Like other lymphoid tissues, it is an organ of the immune system where B and T lymphocytes multiply and help in *immune responses.*
2. The spleen plays an active role in *sequestering* and removing normal and abnormal blood cells.
3. The vasculature of the spleen plays a role in *regulating portal blood flow.*
4. Under pathologic conditions, the spleen may become the site of *extramedullary haematopoiesis.*

The spleen is rarely the primary site of disease. Being the largest lymphoreticular organ, it is involved secondarily in a wide variety of systemic disorders which manifest most commonly as splenic enlargement (splenomegaly) described below. A few other systemic involvements such as splenic infarcts (page 263) and chronic venous congestion (CVC) of spleen (page 237) have already been discussed.

SPLENIC ENLARGEMENT AND EFFECTS ON FUNCTION

Splenomegaly

Enlargement of the spleen termed splenomegaly, occurs in a wide variety of disorders which increase the cellularity and vascularity of the organ. Many of the causes are exaggerated forms of normal splenic function. Splenic enlargement may occur as a result of one of the following pathophysiologic mechanisms:
I. Infections
II. Disordered immunoregulation
III. Altered splenic blood flow
IV. Lymphohaematogenous malignancies
V. Diseases with abnormal erythrocytes
VI. Storage diseases
VII. Miscellaneous causes.

Based on these mechanisms, an abbreviated list of causes of splenomegaly is given in **Table 24.13**.

The **degree of splenomegaly** varies with the disease entity:

◈ *Mild enlargement (up to 5 cm)* occurs in CVC of spleen in CHF, acute malaria, typhoid fever, bacterial endocarditis, SLE, rheumatoid arthritis and thalassaemia minor.

◈ *Moderate enlargement (up to umbilicus)* occurs in hepatitis, cirrhosis, lymphomas, infectious mononucleosis, haemolytic anaemia, splenic abscesses and amyloidosis.

◈ *Massive enlargement (below umbilicus)* occurs in CML, myeloid metaplasia with myelofibrosis, storage diseases, thalassaemia major, chronic malaria, leishmaniasis and portal vein obstruction.

Mild to moderate splenomegaly is usually symptomless, while a massively enlarged spleen may cause dragging sensation in the left hypochondrium. Spleen becomes palpable only when it is enlarged.

Hypersplenism

The term hypersplenism is used for conditions which cause excessive removal of erythrocytes, granulocytes or platelets from the circulation. The mechanism for excessive removal could be due to increased sequestration of cells in the spleen

Table 24.13	Causes of splenomegaly.

I. INFECTIONS
   1. Malaria
   2. Leishmaniasis
   3. Typhoid
   4. Infectious mononucleosis
   5. Bacterial septicaemia
   6. Bacterial endocarditis
   7. Tuberculosis
   8. Syphilis
   9. Viral hepatitis
   10. AIDS

II. DISORDERS OF IMMUNOREGULATION
   1. Rheumatoid arthritis
   2. SLE
   3. Immune haemolytic anaemias
   4. Immune thrombocytopenias
   5. Immune neutropenias

III. ALTERED SPLENIC BLOOD FLOW
   1. Cirrhosis of liver
   2. Portal vein obstruction
   3. Splenic vein obstruction
   4. Congestive heart failure

IV. LYMPHO-HAEMATOGENOUS MALIGNANCIES
   1. Hodgkin's disease
   2. Non-Hodgkin's lymphomas
   3. Multiple myeloma
   4. Leukaemias
   5. Myeloproliferative disorders (e.g. CML, polycythaemia vera, myeloid metaplasia with myelofibrosis)

V. DISEASES WITH ABNORMAL ERYTHROCYTES
   1. Thalassaemias
   2. Spherocytosis
   3. Sickle cell disease
   4. Ovalocytosis

VI. STORAGE DISEASES
   1. Gaucher's disease
   2. Niemann-Pick's disease

VII. MISCELLANEOUS
   1. Amyloidosis
   2. Primary and metastatic splenic tumours
   3. Idiopathic splenomegaly

by altered splenic blood flow or by production of antibodies against respective blood cells. The criteria for hypersplenism are as under:
1. Splenomegaly.
2. Splenic destruction of one or more of the cell types in the peripheral blood causing anaemia, leucopenia, thrombocytopenia, or pancytopenia.
3. Bone marrow cellularity is normal or hyperplastic.
4. Splenectomy is followed by improvement in the severity of blood cytopenia.

EFFECTS OF SPLENECTOMY

In view of the prominent role of normal spleen in sequestration of blood cells, splenectomy in a normal individual is followed by significant haematologic alterations. Induction of similar haematologic effects is made use in the treatment of certain pathologic conditions. For example, in autoimmune haemolytic anaemia or thrombocytopenia, the respective blood cell counts are increased following splenectomy. The blood changes following splenectomy are as under:

1. Red cells There is appearance of target cells in the blood film. Howell-Jolly bodies are present in the red cells as they are no longer cleared by the spleen. Osmotic fragility test shows increased resistance to haemolysis. There may be appearance of normoblasts.

2. White cells There is leucocytosis reaching its peak in 1-2 days after splenectomy. There is shift-to-left of the myeloid cells with appearance of some myelocytes.

3. Platelets Within hours after splenectomy, there is rise in platelet count up to 3-4 times normal.

SPLENIC RUPTURE

The most common cause of splenic rupture or laceration is blunt trauma. The trauma may be direct or indirect. Non-traumatic or spontaneous rupture occurs in an enlarged spleen but almost never in a normal spleen. In acute infections, the spleen can enlarge rapidly to 2 to 3 times its normal size causing acute splenic enlargement termed *acute splenic tumour* e.g. in pneumonias, septicaemia, acute endocarditis etc. Some of the other common causes of spontaneous splenic rupture are splenomegaly due to chronic malaria, infectious mononucleosis, typhoid fever, splenic abscess, thalassaemia and leukaemias.

Rupture of spleen is an acute surgical emergency due to rapid blood loss and haemoperitoneum. Sometimes fragments of splenic tissue are autotransplanted within the peritoneal cavity and grow into tiny spleens there *(splenosis)*.

TUMOURS

◆ **Primary tumours** of the spleen are extremely rare. The only notable benign tumours are haemangiomas and lymphangioma, while examples of primary malignant neoplasms of haematopoietic system i.e. Hodgkin's disease and non-Hodgkin's lymphomas. Non-haematopoietic tumours of the spleen such as angiosarcoma are rare.

◆ **Secondary tumours** occur late in the course of disease and represent haematogenous dissemination of the malignant tumour. Splenic metastases appear as multiple nodules. The most frequent primary sites include: lung, breast, prostate, colon and stomach. Rarely, direct extension from an adjacent malignant neoplasm may occur.

> **GIST BOX 24.14 — Splenic Enlargement and Other Splenic Disorders**
>
> - Enlargement of the spleen, splenomegaly, may result from a variety of causes and may produce mild, moderate and marked enlargement.
> - Hypersplenism is a condition which causes excessive removal of red cells, granulocytes and platelets. Thus, there is pancytopenia.
> - Removal of spleen may cause appearance of target cells, leucocytosis, and thrombocytosis.
> - Splenic rupture may occur from blunt trauma, especially if it is enlarged.
> - Spleen may be the site of primary (e.g. haemangioma, lymphoma) and metastatic tumours.

Section VI ▶ Selected Topics from Systemic Pathology

▶ **SECTION CONTENTS**

Chapter 25: Diseases of Cardiovascular System
Chapter 26: Diseases of Oral Cavity and Salivary Glands
Chapter 27: Jaundice, Hepatitis and Cirrhosis
Chapter 28: Hypertension and its Consequences
Chapter 29: Diabetes Mellitus and its Complications
Chapter 30: Common Diseases of Bones, Cartilage and Joints

25 Diseases of Cardiovascular System

NORMAL STRUCTURE

The blood vessels are closed circuits for the transport of blood from the left heart to the metabolising cells, and then back to the right heart. The blood containing oxygen, nutrients and metabolites is routed through arteries, arterioles, capillaries, venules and veins. These blood vessels differ from each other in their structure and function.

THE HEART

The heart is a muscular pump that ejects blood into the vascular tree with sufficient pressure to maintain optimal circulation. Average weight of the heart in an adult male is 300-350 gm while that of an adult female is 250-300 gm. Heart is divided into four chambers: a right and a left atrium both lying superiorly, and a right and a left ventricle both lying inferiorly and are larger. The atria are separated by a thin interatrial partition called *interatrial septum*, while the ventricles are separated by thick muscular partition called *interventricular septum*. The thickness of the right ventricular wall is 0.3 to 0.5 cm while that of the left ventricular wall is 1.3 to 1.5 cm. The blood in the heart chambers moves in a carefully prescribed pathway: venous blood from systemic circulation → right atrium → right ventricle → pulmonary arteries → lungs → pulmonary veins → left atrium → left ventricle → aorta → systemic arterial supply **(Fig. 25.1)**.

The transport of blood is regulated by cardiac valves: two loose flap-like atrioventricular valves, tricuspid on the right and mitral (bicuspid) on the left; and two semilunar valves with three leaflets each, the pulmonary and aortic valves, guarding the outflow tracts. The normal circumference of the valvular openings measures about 12 cm in tricuspid, 8.5 cm in pulmonary, 10 cm in mitral and 7.5 cm in aortic valve.

Wall of the heart consists mainly of the *myocardium* which is covered externally by thin membrane, the *epicardium* or visceral pericardium, and lined internally by another thin layer, the *endocardium*.

◆ The **myocardium** is the muscle tissue of the heart composed of syncytium of branching and anastomosing, transversely striated muscle fibres arranged in parallel fashion. The space between myocardial fibres contains a rich capillary network and loose connective tissue. The

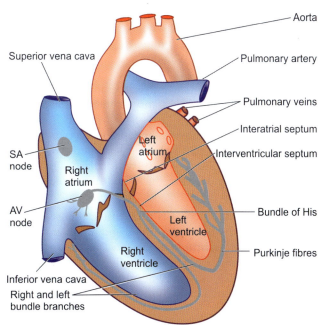

Figure 25.1 ▶ Normal structure of the heart.

myocardial fibres are connected to each other by irregular joints called as *intercalated* discs. They represent apposed cell membranes of individual cells which act as tight junctions for free transport of ions and action potentials. The cardiac myocyte is very rich in mitochondria which are the source of large amount of ATP required for cardiac contraction. The cardiac muscle fibre has abundant sarcoplasmic reticulum corresponding to endoplasmic reticulum of other cells. Transverse lines divide each fibre into *sarcomeres* which act as structural and functional subunits. Each sarcomere consists of prominent central *dark A-band* attributed to thick myosin filaments and flanked on either side by *light I-bands* consisting of thin actin filament. The actin bands are in the form of twisted rods overlying protein molecules called *tropomyosin*. These protein molecules are of 3 types: *troponin-I, troponin-T, and troponin-C*. Troponin molecules respond to calcium ions in cyclical contraction-relaxation of myocardial fibres. Myocardial fibres are terminally differentiated cells and do not regenerate but there is recent evidence that new cardiac myocytes can be formed from stem cells recruited from the circulation.

❖ The **conduction system** of the heart located in the myocardium is responsible for regulating rate and rhythm of the heart. It is composed of specialised Purkinje fibres which contain some contractile myofilaments and conduct action potentials rapidly. The conduction system consists of 4 major components:

1. The *sinoatrial (SA) node* is located in the posterior wall of the right atrium adjacent to the point at which the superior vena cava enters the heart. It is also called cardiac pacemaker since it is responsible for determining the rate of contraction for all cardiac muscle.
2. The *atrioventricular (AV) bundle* conducts the impulse from the SA node to the AV node.
3. The *atrioventricular (AV) node* is located on the top of the interventricular septum and receives impulses from the SA node via AV bundle and transmits them to the bundle of His.
4. The *bundle of His* extends through the interventricular septum and divides into right and left bundle branches which arborise in the respective ventricular walls. These fibres transmit impulses from the AV node to the ventricular walls.

❖ The **pericardium** consists of a closely apposed layer, *visceral pericardium or epicardium,* and an outer fibrous sac, the *parietal pericardium*. The two layers enclose a narrow pericardial cavity which is lined by mesothelial cells and normally contains 10-30 ml of clear, watery serous fluid. This fluid functions as lubricant and shock absorbent to the heart.

❖ The **endocardium** is the smooth shiny inner lining of the myocardium that covers all the cardiac chambers, the cardiac valves, the chordae tendineae and the papillary muscles. It is lined by endothelium with connective tissue and elastic fibres in its deeper part.

❖ The **valve cusps and semilunar leaflets** are delicate and translucent structures. The valves are strengthened by collagen and elastic tissue and covered by a layer of endothelium (valvular endocardium).

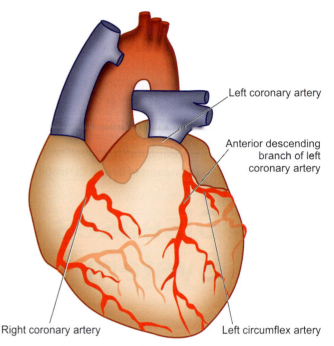

Figure 25.2 ▶ Distribution of blood supply to the heart.

Myocardial Blood Supply

The cardiac muscle, in order to function properly, must receive adequate supply of oxygen and nutrients. Blood is transported to myocardial cells by the coronary arteries which originate immediately above the aortic semilunar valve. Most of blood flow to the myocardium occurs during diastole. There are three major coronary trunks, each supplying blood to specific segments of the heart **(Fig. 25.2)**:

1. The **anterior descending branch of the left coronary artery,** commonly called **LAD** (left anterior descending coronary) supplies most of the apex of the heart, the anterior surface of the left ventricle, the adjacent third of the anterior wall of the right ventricle, and the anterior two-third of the interventricular septum.
2. The **circumflex branch of the left coronary artery,** commonly called **LCX** (left circumflex coronary) supplies the left atrium and a small portion of the lateral aspect of the left ventricle.
3. The **right coronary artery,** abbreviated as **RCA** supplies the right atrium, the remainder of the anterior surface of the right ventricle, the adjacent half of the posterior wall of the left ventricle and the posterior third of the interventricular septum.

Coronary veins run parallel to the major coronary arteries to collect blood after the cellular needs of the heart are met. Subsequently, these veins drain into the *coronary sinus*.

ARTERIES

Depending upon the calibre and certain histologic features, arteries are divided into 3 types: large (elastic) arteries, medium-sized (muscular) arteries and the smallest arterioles.

Histologically, all major arteries of the body have 3 layers in their walls: the tunica intima, the tunica media and the tunica adventitia. These layers progressively decrease with diminution in the size of the vessels.

1. Tunica intima This is the inner coat of the artery. It is composed of the lining endothelium, subendothelial connective tissue and bounded externally by internal elastic lamina.

❖ *Endothelium* is a layer of flattened cells adjacent to the flowing blood. Narrow junctions exist between the adjoining endothelial cells through which certain materials pass. The integrity of the endothelial layer is of paramount importance in maintenance of vascular functions since damage to it is the most important event in the initiation of thrombus formation at the site.

❖ *Subendothelial tissue* consists of loose meshwork of connective tissue that includes myointimal cells, collagen, proteoglycans, elastin and matrix glycoproteins.

❖ *Internal elastic lamina* is a layer of elastic fibres having minute fenestrations.

2. Tunica media Tunica media is the middle coat of the arterial wall, bounded internally by internal elastic lamina and externally by external elastic lamina. This layer is the thickest and consists mainly of smooth muscle cells and elastic fibres. The *external elastic lamina* consisting of condensed elastic tissue is less well defined than the *internal elastic lamina*.

3. Tunica adventitia The outer coat of arteries is the tunica adventitia. It consists of loose mesh of connective tissue and some elastic fibres that merge with the adjacent tissues. This layer is rich in lymphatics and autonomic nerve fibres.

The layers of arterial wall receive nutrition and oxygen from 2 sources:
1. Tunica intima and inner third of the media are nourished by *direct diffusion* from the blood present in the lumen.
2. Outer two-thirds of the media and the adventitia are supplied by *vasa vasora (i.e. vessels of vessels)*, the nutrient vessels arising from the parent artery.

As the calibre of the artery decreases, the three layers progressively diminish. Thus, there are structural variations in three types of arteries:

❖ *Large, elastic arteries* such as the aorta, innominate, common carotid, major pulmonary, and common iliac arteries have very high content of elastic tissue in the media and thick elastic laminae and hence the name.

❖ *Medium-sized, muscular arteries* are the branches of elastic arteries. All the three layers of arterial wall are thinner than in the elastic arteries. The internal elastic lamina appears as a single wavy line while the external elastic lamina is less prominent. The media primarily consists of smooth muscle cells and some elastic fibres **(Fig. 25.3)**.

❖ *Arterioles* are the smallest branches with internal diameter 20-100 μm. Structurally, they consist of three layers as in muscular arteries but are much thinner and cannot be distinguished. The arterioles consist of a layer of endothelial cells in the intima, one or two smooth muscle cells in the media and small amount of collagen and elastic tissue comprising the adventitia. The elastic laminae are virtually lost.

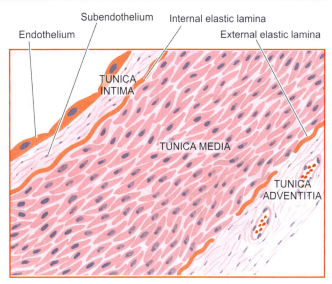

Figure 25.3 ▶ The structure of a medium-sized muscular artery.

VEINS

The structure of normal veins is basically similar to that of arteries. The walls of the veins are thinner, the three tunicae (intima, media and adventitia) are less clearly demarcated, elastic tissue is scanty and not clearly organised into internal and external elastic laminae. The media contains very small amount of smooth muscle cells with abundant collagen. All veins, except vena cavae and common iliac veins, have valves best developed in veins of the lower limbs. The valves are delicate folds of intima, located every 1-6 cm, often next to the point of entry of a tributary vein. They prevent any significant retrograde venous blood flow.

CAPILLARIES

Capillaries are about the size of an RBC (7-8 μm) and have 1-2 endothelial cells but no media. Blood from capillaries returns to the heart via *post-capillary venules* and from there into venules and then drained into veins.

In the following pages, diseases of cardiovascular system discussed are as under:
1. Cardiac failure
2. Congenital heart disease
3. Atherosclerosis
4. Ischaemic heart disease
5. Rheumatic heart disease
6. Non-rheumatic endocarditis
7. Pathology of cardiovascular interventions.

| GIST BOX 25.1 | Normal Structure of Heart and Blood Vessels |

- Average weight of the heart is 300-350 gm in adult male and 250-300 gm in adult female.
- The thickness of the right ventricular wall is 0.3 to 0.5 cm while that of the left ventricular wall is 1.3 to 1.5 cm.
- The normal circumference of the valvular openings measures about 12 cm in tricuspid, 8.5 cm in pulmonary, 10 cm in mitral and 7.5 cm in aortic valve.
- Wall of the heart consists mainly of the *myocardium* which is covered externally by the epicardium, and lined internally by the *endocardium*.
- There are three major coronary trunks, each supplying blood to specific segments of the heart: left anterior descending coronary (LAD), left circumflex coronary (LCX) and right coronary artery (RCA).
- Arteries are of 3 types: large (elastic) arteries, medium-sized (muscular) arteries and the smallest arterioles.
- Major arteries of the body have 3 layers in their walls: the tunica intima, the tunica media and the tunica adventitia. Internal and external elastic laminae bounding the media are well developed in arteries.
- The walls of the veins are thinner, three tunicae (intima, media and adventitia) are less clearly demarcated, elastic tissue is scanty and not clearly organised into internal and external elastic laminae.
- Capillaries are tiny of the size of a red cell and have 1-2 endothelial cells only in their wall.

CARDIAC FAILURE

Cardiac failure is defined as the pathophysiologic state in which impaired cardiac function is unable to maintain an adequate circulation for the metabolic needs of the tissues of the body. It may be *acute* or *chronic*. The term congestive heart failure (CHF) is used for the chronic form of heart failure in which the patient has evidence of congestion of peripheral circulation and of lungs (page 236). CHF is the end-result of various forms of serious heart diseases.

ETIOLOGY

Heart failure may be caused by one of the following factors, either singly or in combination:

1. INTRINSIC PUMP FAILURE The most common and most important cause of heart failure is weakening of the ventricular muscle due to disease so that the heart fails to act as an efficient pump. The various diseases which may culminate in pump failure by this mechanism are as under:
i) Ischaemic heart disease
ii) Myocarditis
iii) Cardiomyopathies
iv) Metabolic disorders e.g. beriberi
v) Disorders of the rhythm e.g. atrial fibrillation and flutter.

2. INCREASED WORKLOAD ON THE HEART Increased mechanical load on the heart results in increased myocardial demand resulting in myocardial failure. Increased load on the heart may be in the form of pressure load or volume load.

i) Increased pressure load may occur in the following states:
a) Systemic and pulmonary arterial hypertension.
b) Valvular disease e.g. mitral stenosis, aortic stenosis, pulmonary stenosis.
c) Chronic lung diseases.

ii) Increased volume load occurs when a ventricle is required to eject more than normal volume of the blood resulting in cardiac failure. This is seen in the following conditions:
a) Valvular insufficiency
b) Severe anaemia
c) Thyrotoxicosis
d) Arteriovenous shunts
e) Hypoxia due to lung diseases.

3. IMPAIRED FILLING OF CARDIAC CHAMBERS Decreased cardiac output and cardiac failure may result from extra-cardiac causes or defect in filling of the heart:
a) Cardiac tamponade e.g. haemopericardium, hydropericardium
b) Constrictive pericarditis.

TYPES OF HEART FAILURE

Heart failure may be acute or chronic, right-sided or left-sided, and forward or backward failure.

Acute and Chronic Heart Failure

Depending upon whether the heart failure develops rapidly or slowly, it may be acute or chronic.

Acute heart failure Sudden and rapid development of heart failure occurs in the following conditions:
i) Larger myocardial infarction
ii) Valve rupture
iii) Cardiac tamponade
iv) Massive pulmonary embolism
v) Acute viral myocarditis
vi) Acute bacterial toxaemia.

In acute heart failure, there is sudden reduction in cardiac output resulting in systemic hypotension but oedema does not occur. Instead, a state of cardiogenic shock and cerebral hypoxia develops.

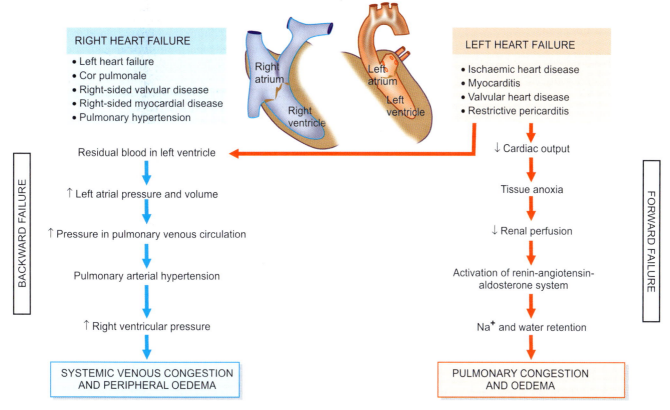

Figure 25.4 ▶ Schematic evolution of congestive heart failure and its effects.

Chronic heart failure More often, heart failure develops slowly as observed in the following states:
i) Myocardial ischaemia from atherosclerotic coronary artery disease
ii) Multivalvular heart disease
iii) Systemic arterial hypertension
iv) Chronic lung diseases resulting in hypoxia and pulmonary arterial hypertension
v) Progression of acute into chronic failure.

In chronic heart failure, compensatory mechanisms like tachycardia, cardiac dilatation and cardiac hypertrophy try to make adjustments so as to maintain adequate cardiac output. This often results in well-maintained arterial pressure and there is accumulation of oedema.

Left-sided and Right-sided Heart Failure

Though heart as an organ eventually fails as a whole, but functionally, the left and right heart act as independent units. From clinical point of view, therefore, it is helpful to consider failure of the left and right heart separately. The clinical manifestations of heart failure result from accumulation of excess fluid *upstream* to the left or right cardiac chamber whichever is initially affected **(Fig. 25.4)**:

Left-sided heart failure It is initiated by stress to the left heart. The major causes are as follows:
i) Systemic hypertension
ii) Mitral or aortic valve disease (stenosis)
iii) Ischaemic heart disease
iv) Myocardial diseases e.g. cardiomyopathies, myocarditis.
v) Restrictive pericarditis.

The clinical manifestations of left-sided heart failure result from decreased left ventricular output and hence there is accumulation of fluid *upstream* in the lungs. Accordingly, the major pathologic changes are as under:
i) Pulmonary congestion and oedema causes dyspnoea and orthopnoea (page 236).
ii) Decreased left ventricular output causing hypoperfusion and diminished oxygenation of tissues e.g. in kidneys causing ischaemic acute tubular necrosis, in brain causing hypoxic encephalopathy, and in skeletal muscles causing muscular weakness and fatigue.

Right-sided heart failure Right-sided heart failure occurs more often as a consequence of left-sided heart failure. However, some conditions affect the right ventricle primarily, producing right-sided heart failure. These are as follows:
i) As a consequence of left ventricular failure.
ii) Cor pulmonale in which right heart failure occurs due to lung parenchymal diseases.
iii) Pulmonary or tricuspid valvular disease.
iv) Pulmonary hypertension secondary to pulmonary thromboembolism.

v) Myocardial disease affecting right heart.
vi) Congenital heart disease with left-to-right shunt.

Whatever be the underlying cause, the clinical manifestations of right-sided heart failure are *upstream* of the right heart such as systemic (due to caval blood) and portal venous congestion, and reduced cardiac output. Accordingly, the pathologic changes are as under:

i) Systemic venous congestion in different tissues and organs e.g. subcutaneous oedema on dependent parts, passive congestion of the liver, spleen, and kidneys (page 236), ascites, hydrothorax, congestion of leg veins and neck veins.

ii) Reduced cardiac output resulting in circulatory stagnation causing anoxia, cyanosis and coldness of extremities.

In summary, in early stage the left heart failure manifests with features of pulmonary congestion and decreased left ventricular output, while the right heart failure presents with systemic venous congestion and involvement of the liver and spleen. CHF, however, combines the features of both left and right heart failure.

Backward and Forward Heart Failure

The mechanism of clinical manifestations resulting from heart failure can be explained on the basis of mutually interdependent backward and forward failure.

Backward heart failure According to this concept, either of the ventricles fails to eject blood normally, resulting in rise of end-diastolic volume in the ventricle and increase in volume and pressure in the atrium which is transmitted *backward* producing elevated pressure in the veins.

Forward heart failure According to this hypothesis, clinical manifestations result directly from failure of the heart to pump blood causing diminished flow of blood to the tissues, especially diminished renal perfusion and activation of renin-angiotensin-aldosterone system.

COMPENSATORY MECHANISMS: CARDIAC HYPERTROPHY AND DILATATION

In order to maintain normal cardiac output, several compensatory mechanisms play a role as under:

◆ Compensatory enlargement in the form of *cardiac hypertrophy, cardiac dilatation, or both.*

◆ *Tachycardia* (i.e. increased heart rate) due to activation of neurohumoral system e.g. release of norepinephrine and atrial natruretic peptide, activation of renin-angiotensin-aldosterone mechanism.

According to *Starling's law* on pathophysiology of heart, the failing dilated heart, in order to maintain cardiac performance, increases the myocardial contractility and thereby attempts to maintain stroke volume. This is achieved by increasing the length of sarcomeres in dilated heart. Ultimately, however, dilatation decreases the force of contraction and leads to residual volume in the cardiac chambers causing volume overload resulting in cardiac failure that ends in death **(Fig. 25.5)**.

Cardiac Hypertrophy

Hypertrophy of the heart is defined as an increase in size and weight of the myocardium. It generally results from increased pressure load while increased volume load (e.g. valvular

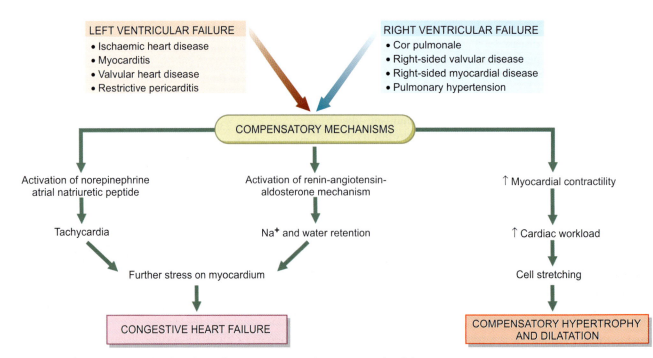

Figure 25.5 ▶ Schematic pathophysiology of compensatory mechanisms in cardiac failure.

incompetence) results in hypertrophy with dilatation of the affected chamber due to regurgitation of the blood through incompetent valve. The atria may also undergo compensatory changes due to increased workload.

The basic factors that stimulate the hypertrophy of the myocardial fibres are not known. It appears that stretching of myocardial fibres in response to stress induces the cells to increase in length. The elongated fibres receive better nutrition and thus increase in size. Other factors which may stimulate increase in size of myocardial fibres are anoxia (e.g. in coronary atherosclerosis) and influence of certain hormones (e.g. catecholamines, pituitary growth hormone).

CAUSES Hypertrophy with or without dilatation may involve predominantly the left or the right heart, or both sides.

Left ventricular hypertrophy The common causes are as under:
i) Systemic hypertension
ii) Aortic stenosis and insufficiency
iii) Mitral insufficiency
iv) Coarctation of the aorta
v) Occlusive coronary artery disease
vi) Congenital anomalies like septal defects and patent ductus arteriosus
vii) Conditions with increased cardiac output e.g. thyrotoxicosis, anaemia, arteriovenous fistulae.

Right ventricular hypertrophy Most of the causes of right ventricular hypertrophy are due to pulmonary arterial hypertension. These are as follows:
i) Pulmonary stenosis and insufficiency
ii) Tricuspid insufficiency
iii) Mitral stenosis and/or insufficiency
iv) Chronic lung diseases e.g. chronic emphysema, bronchiectasis, pneumoconiosis, pulmonary vascular disease etc.
v) Left ventricular hypertrophy and failure of the left ventricle.

Cardiac Dilatation

Quite often, hypertrophy of the heart is accompanied by cardiac dilatation. Stress leading to accumulation of excessive volume of blood in a chamber of the heart causes increase in length of myocardial fibres and hence cardiac dilatation as a compensatory mechanism.

CAUSES Accumulation of excessive volume of blood within the cardiac chambers from the following causes may result in dilatation of the respective ventricles or both:
i) Valvular insufficiency (mitral and/or aortic insufficiency in left ventricular dilatation, tricuspid and/or pulmonary insufficiency in right ventricular dilatation)
ii) Left-to-right shunts e.g. in VSD
iii) Conditions with high cardiac output e.g. thyrotoxicosis, arteriovenous shunt
iv) Myocardial diseases e.g. cardiomyopathies, myocarditis
v) Systemic hypertension.

MORPHOLOGIC FEATURES

Hypertrophy of the myocardium without dilatation is referred to as *concentric,* and when associated with dilatation is called *eccentric* **(Fig. 25.6)**. The weight of the heart is increased above normal, often over 500 gm. However, excessive epicardial fat is not indicative of true hypertrophy.

Grossly, thickness of the left ventricular wall (excluding trabeculae carneae and papillary muscles) above 15 mm is indicative of significant hypertrophy. In concentric hypertrophy, the lumen of the chamber is smaller than usual, while in eccentric hypertrophy the lumen is dilated **(Fig. 25.7)**. In pure hypertrophy, the papillary muscles and trabeculae carneae are rounded and enlarged, while in hypertrophy with dilatation these are flattened.

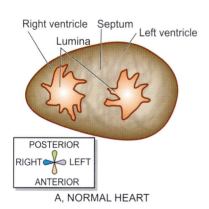
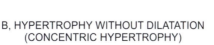
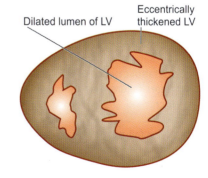

Figure 25.6 ▶ Schematic diagram showing transverse section through the ventricles with left ventricular hypertrophy (concentric and eccentric).

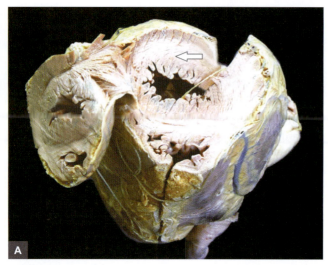 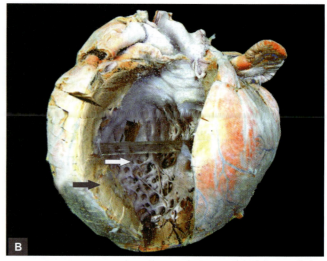

Figure 25.7 ▶ A, Concentric cardiac hypertrophy. Weight of the heart is increased. The chambers opened up at the apex show concentric thickening of left ventricular wall (white arrow) with obliterated lumen (hypertrophy without dilatation). B, Eccentric cardiac hypertrophy. The heart is heavier. The free left ventricular wall is thickened (black arrow) while the lumen is dilated (white arrow) (hypertrophy with dilatation).

Microscopically, there is increase in size of individual muscle fibres. There may be multiple minute foci of degenerative changes and necrosis in the hypertrophied myocardium (see Fig. 3.5). These changes appear to arise as a result of relative hypoxia of the hypertrophied muscle as the blood supply is inadequate to meet the demands of the increased fibre size. Ventricular hypertrophy renders the inner part of the myocardium more liable to ischaemia.

Electron microscopy reveals increase in the number of myofilaments comprising myofibrils, mitochondrial changes and multiple intercalated discs which are active sites for the formation of new sarcomeres. Besides, the nucleic acid content determinations have shown increase in total RNA and increased ratio of RNA to DNA content of the hypertrophied myocardial fibres.

 GIST BOX 25.2 | Heart Failure

- Heart failure is a pathophysiologic state of impaired cardiac function when it is unable to maintain the metabolic needs of the tissues of the body.
- Heart failure may be caused by intrinsic pump failure, increased pressure or volume overload, or impaired filling.
- Heart failure may be acute or chronic, left-sided or right-sided, backward or forward failure.
- Compensatory mechanisms in heart failure are its enlargement in the form of cardiac hypertrophy (concentric or eccentric), cardiac dilatation, or both.

CONGENITAL HEART DISEASE

Congenital heart disease is the abnormality of the heart present from birth. It is the most common and important form of heart disease in the early years of life and is present in about 0.5% of newborn children. The incidence is higher in premature infants. The cause of congenital heart disease is unknown in majority of cases. It is attributed to multifactorial inheritance involving genetic and environmental influences. Other factors like rubella infection to the mother during pregnancy, drugs taken by the mother and heavy alcohol drinking by the mother, have all been implicated in causing *in utero* foetal injury resulting in congenital malformations of the heart.

CLASSIFICATION Congenital anomalies of the heart may be either *shunts* (left-to-right or right-to-left), or defects causing *obstructions* to flow. However, complex anomalies involving *combinations* of shunts and obstructions are also often present.

A simple classification of important and common examples of these groups is given in **Table 25.1**.

I. MALPOSITIONS OF THE HEART

Dextrocardia is the condition when the apex of the heart points to the right side of the chest. It may be accompanied by situs inversus so that all other organs of the body are also transposed in similar way and thus heart is in normal position in relation to them. However, isolated dextrocardia is associated with major anomalies of the heart such as transposition of the atria in relation to ventricles or transposition of the great arteries.

Table 25.1	Classification of congenital heart diseases.	
I.	MALPOSITIONS OF THE HEART	
II.	SHUNTS (CYANOTIC CONGENITAL HEART DISEASE)	
	A. *Left-to-right shunts* *(Acyanotic or late cyanotic group)*	
	1. Ventricular septal defect (VSD)	25-30%
	2. Atrial septal defect (ASD)	10-15%
	3. Patent ductus arteriosus (PDA)	10-20%
	B. *Right-to-left shunts (Cyanotic group)*	
	1. Tetralogy of Fallot	6-15%
	2. Transposition of great arteries	4-10%
	3. Persistent truncus arteriosus	2%
	4. Tricuspid atresia and stenosis	1%
III.	OBSTRUCTIONS (OBSTRUCTIVE CONGENITAL HEART DISEASE)	
	1. Coarctation of aorta	5-7%
	2. Aortic stenosis and atresia	4-6%
	3. Pulmonary stenosis and atresia	5-7%

II. SHUNTS (CYANOTIC CONGENITAL HEART DISEASE)

A shunt may be left-to-right side or right-to-left side of the circulation.

A. Left-to-Right Shunts (Acyanotic or Late Cyanotic Group)

In conditions where there is shunting of blood from left-to-right side of the heart, there is volume overload on the right heart producing pulmonary hypertension and right ventricular hypertrophy. At a later stage, the pressure on the right side is higher than on the left side creating late cyanotic heart disease. The important conditions included in this category are described below:

VENTRICULAR SEPTAL DEFECT (VSD) VSD is the most common congenital anomaly of the heart and comprises about 30% of all congenital heart diseases. The condition is recognised early in life. The smaller defects often close spontaneously, while larger defects remain patent and produce significant effects.

Depending upon the location of the defect, VSD may be of the following types:
1. In 90% of cases, the defect involves *membranous septum* and is very close to the bundle of His (Fig. 25.8).
2. The remaining 10% cases have VSD immediately below the pulmonary valve (*subpulmonic*), below the aortic valve (*subaortic*), or exist in the form of multiple defects in the muscular septum.

MORPHOLOGIC FEATURES The *effects* of VSD are produced due to left-to-right shunt at the ventricular level, increased pulmonary flow and increased volume in the left side of the heart. These effects are as under:
i) Volume hypertrophy of the right ventricle.
ii) Enlargement and haemodynamic changes in the tricuspid and pulmonary valves.
iii) Endocardial hypertrophy of the right ventricle.

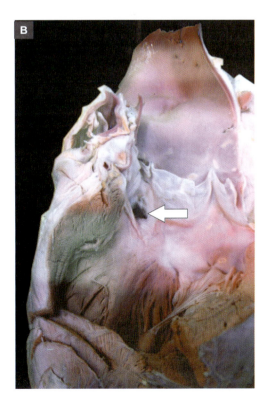

Figure 25.8 ▶ Ventricular septal defect. A, Schematic representation (LA = Left atrium; LV = Left ventricle; AO = Aorta; PV = Pulmonary valve; PT = Pulmonary trunk; RA = Right atrium; RV = Right ventricle; SVC = Superior vena cava; IVC = Inferior vena cava). B, The opened up chambers of the heart show a communication in the inter-ventricular septum superiorly (white arrow).

iv) Pressure hypertrophy of the right atrium.
v) Volume hypertrophy of the left atrium and left ventricle.
vi) Enlargement and haemodynamic changes in the mitral and aortic valves.

ATRIAL SEPTAL DEFECT (ASD) Isolated ASD comprises about 10% of congenital heart diseases. The condition remains unnoticed in infancy and childhood till pulmonary hypertension is induced causing late cyanotic heart disease and right-sided heart failure.

Depending upon the location of the defect, there are 3 types of ASD:

i) Fossa ovalis type or ostium secundum type is the most common form comprising about 90% cases of ASD. The defect is situated in the region of the fossa ovalis **(Fig. 25.9)**.

ii) Ostium primum type comprises about 5% cases of ASD. The defect lies low in the interatrial septum adjacent to atrioventricular valves. There may be cleft in the aortic leaflet of the mitral valve producing mitral insufficiency.

iii) Sinus venosus type accounts for about 5% cases of ASD. The defect is located high in the interatrial septum near the entry of the superior vena cava.

MORPHOLOGIC FEATURES The *effects* of ASD are produced due to left-to-right shunt at the atrial level with increased pulmonary flow. These effects are as follows:

i) Volume hypertrophy of the right atrium and right ventricle.

ii) Enlargement and haemodynamic changes of tricuspid and pulmonary valves.
iii) Focal or diffuse endocardial hypertrophy of the right atrium and right ventricle.
iv) Volume atrophy of the left atrium and left ventricle.
v) Small-sized mitral and aortic orifices.

PATENT DUCTUS ARTERIOSUS (PDA) The ductus arteriosus is a normal vascular connection between the aorta and the bifurcation of the pulmonary artery. Normally, the ductus closes functionally within the first or second day of life. Its persistence after 3 months of age is considered abnormal. The cause for patency of ductus arteriosus is not known but possibly it is due to continued synthesis of PGE2 after birth which keeps it patent as evidenced by association of PDA with respiratory distress syndrome in infants and pharmacologic closure of PDA with administration of indomethacin to suppress PGE2 synthesis. PDA constitutes about 10% of congenital malformations of the heart and great vessels. In about 90% of cases, it occurs as an isolated defect, while in the remaining cases it may be associated with other anomalies like VSD, coarctation of aorta and pulmonary or aortic stenosis. A patent ductus may be up to 2 cm in length and up to 1 cm in diameter **(Fig. 25.10)**.

MORPHOLOGIC FEATURES The *effects* of PDA on heart occur due to left-to-right shunt at the level of ductus resulting in increased pulmonary flow and increased volume in the left heart. These effects are as follows:

i) Volume hypertrophy of the left atrium and left ventricle.

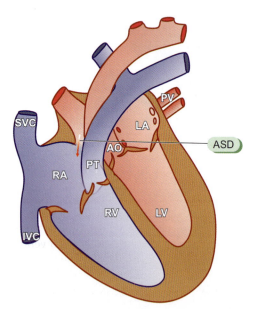

Figure 25.9 ▶ Atrial septal defect fossa ovalis type, a schematic representation (LA = Left atrium; LV = Left ventricle; PV = Pulmonary vein; AO = Aorta; PT = Pulmonary trunk; RA = Right atrium; RV = Right ventricle; SVC = Superior vena cava; IVC = Inferior vena cava).

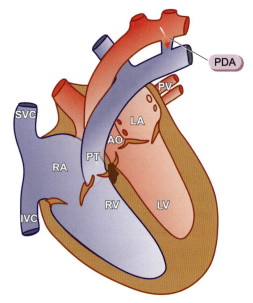

Figure 25.10 ▶ Patent ductus arteriosus, a schematic representation (LA = Left atrium; LV = Left ventricle; PT = Pulmonary trunk; PV = Pulmonary vein, AO = Aorta; RA = Right atrium; RV = Right ventricle; SVC = Superior vena cava; IVC = Inferior vena cava).

ii) Enlargement and haemodynamic changes of the mitral and pulmonary valves.
iii) Enlargement of the ascending aorta.

B. Right-to-Left Shunts (Cyanotic Group)

In conditions where there is shunting of blood from right side to the left side of the heart, there is entry of poorly-oxygenated blood into systemic circulation resulting in early cyanosis. The examples described below are not pure shunts but are combinations of shunts with obstructions but are described here since there is functional shunting of blood from one to the other side of circulation.

TETRALOGY OF FALLOT Tetralogy of Fallot is the most common cyanotic congenital heart disease, found in about 10% of children with anomalies of the heart.

MORPHOLOGIC FEATURES The four features of tetralogy are as under **(Fig. 25.11)**:
i) Ventricular septal defect (VSD) (*'shunt'*).
ii) Displacement of the aorta to right so that it overrides the VSD.
iii) Pulmonary stenosis (*'obstruction'*).
iv) Right ventricular hypertrophy.

The severity of the clinical manifestations is related to two factors: extent of pulmonary stenosis and the size of VSD. Accordingly, there are two forms of tetralogy: cyanotic and acyanotic:

a) Cyanotic tetralogy Pulmonary stenosis is greater and the VSD is mild so that there is more resistance to the outflow of blood from right ventricle resulting in right-to-left shunt at the ventricular level and cyanosis. The *effects* on the heart are as follows:
i) Pressure hypertrophy of the right atrium and right ventricle.
ii) Smaller and abnormal tricuspid valve.
iii) Smaller left atrium and left ventricle.
iv) Enlarged aortic orifice.

b) Acyanotic tetralogy The VSD is larger and pulmonary stenosis is mild so that there is mainly left-to-right shunt with increased pulmonary flow and increased volume in the left heart but no cyanosis. The *effects* on the heart are as under:
i) Pressure hypertrophy of the right ventricle and right atrium.
ii) Volume hypertrophy of the left atrium and left ventricle.
iii) Enlargement of mitral and aortic orifices.

TRANSPOSITION OF GREAT ARTERIES The term transposition is used for complex malformations as regards position of the aorta, pulmonary trunk, atrioventricular orifices and the position of atria in relation to ventricles.

MORPHOLOGIC FEATURES There are several forms of transpositions. The common ones are described below:

i) Regular transposition is the most common type. In this, the aorta which is normally situated to the right and posterior with respect to the pulmonary trunk, is instead displaced anteriorly and to right. In regular complete transposition, the aorta emerges from the right ventricle and the pulmonary trunk from the left ventricle so that there is cyanosis from birth.

ii) Corrected transposition is an uncommon anomaly. There is complete transposition of the great arteries with aorta arising from the right ventricle and the pulmonary trunk from the left ventricle, as well as transposition of the great veins so that the pulmonary veins enter the right atrium and the systemic veins drain into the left atrium. This results in a physiologically corrected circulation.

PERSISTENT TRUNCUS ARTERIOSUS Persistent truncus arteriosus (PTA) is a rare anomaly.

MORPHOLOGIC FEATURES In PTA, the arch that normally separates the aorta from the pulmonary artery fails to develop. This results in a single large common vessel receiving blood from the right as well as left ventricle. The orifice may have 3 to 6 cusps. There is often an associated VSD. There is left-to-right shunt and frequently early systemic cyanosis. The prognosis is generally poor.

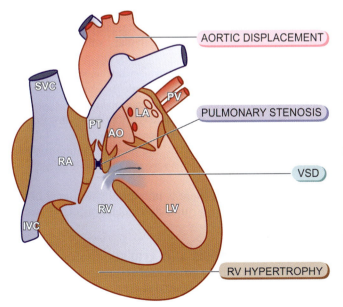

Figure 25.11 ▶ Tetralogy of Fallot, a schematic representation (LA = Left atrium; LV = Left ventricle; PT = Pulmonary trunk; PV = Pulmonary vein; AO = Aorta; RA = Right atrium; RV = Right ventricle; SVC = Superior vena cava; IVC = Inferior vena cava).

TRICUSPID ATRESIA AND STENOSIS Tricuspid atresia and stenosis are rare anomalies. There is often associated pulmonary stenosis or pulmonary atresia.

MORPHOLOGIC FEATURES In tricuspid atresia, there is absence of tricuspid orifice and instead there is a dimple in the floor of the right atrium. In tricuspid stenosis, the tricuspid ring is small and the valve cusps are malformed. In both the conditions, there is often an interatrial defect through which right-to-left shunt of blood takes place. Children are cyanotic since birth and live for a few weeks or months.

III. OBSTRUCTIONS (OBSTRUCTIVE CONGENITAL HEART DISEASE)

Congenital obstruction to blood flow may result from obstruction in the aorta due to narrowing (*coarctation of aorta*), obstruction to outflow from the left ventricle (*aortic stenosis and atresia*), and obstruction to outflow from the right ventricle (*pulmonary stenosis and atresia*).

COARCTATION OF AORTA The word 'coarctation' means contracted or compressed. Coarctation of aorta is localised narrowing in any part of aorta, but the constriction is more often just distal to ductus arteriosus (*postductal or adult*), or occasionally proximal to the ductus arteriosus (*preductal or infantile type*) in the region of transverse aorta:

MORPHOLOGIC FEATURES The two common forms of coarctation of the aorta are as under:

i) Postductal or adult type The obstruction is just distal to the point of entry of ductus arteriosus which is often closed **(Fig. 25.12)**. In the stenotic segment, the aorta is drawn in as if a suture has been tied around it. The aorta is dilated on either side of the constriction. The condition is recognised in adulthood, characterised by hypertension in the upper extremities, weak pulses and low blood pressure in the lower extremities and effects of arterial insufficiency such as claudication and coldness. In time, there is development of collateral circulation between pre-stenotic and post-stenotic arterial branches so that intercostal arteries are enlarged and palpable and may produce erosions on the inner surface of the ribs.

ii) Preductal or infantile type The manifestations are produced early in life. The narrowing is proximal to the ductus arteriosus which usually remains patent. The narrowing is generally gradual and involves larger segment of the proximal aorta. There is often associated interatrial septal defect. Preductal coarctation results in right ventricular hypertrophy while the left ventricle is small. Cyanosis develops in the lower half of the body while the upper half remains unaffected since it is supplied by vessels originating proximal to the coarctation. Children with this defect have poor prognosis.

AORTIC STENOSIS AND ATRESIA The most common congenital anomaly of the aorta is bicuspid aortic valve which

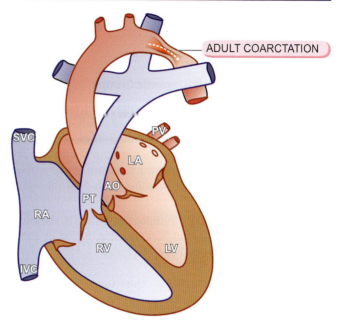

Figure 25.12 ▶ Postductal or adult type coarctation of the aorta, a schematic representation (LA = Left atrium; LV = Left ventricle; PT = Pulmonary trunk; PV = Pulmonary vein; AO = Aorta; RA = Right atrium; RV = Right ventricle; SVC = Superior vena cava; IVC = Inferior vena cava).

does not have much functional significance but predisposes it to calcification. Congenital aortic atresia is rare and incompatible with survival. Aortic stenosis may be acquired (e.g. in rheumatic heart disease, calcific aortic stenosis) or congenital.

MORPHOLOGIC FEATURES Congenital aortic stenosis may be of three types: valvular, subvalvular and supravalvular.
i) Valvular stenosis The aortic valve cusps are malformed and are irregularly thickened. The aortic valve may have one, two or three such maldeveloped cusps.
ii) Subvalvular stenosis There is thick fibrous ring under the aortic valve causing subaortic stenosis.
iii) Supravalvular stenosis The most uncommon type, there is fibrous constriction above the sinuses of Valsalva.

In all these cases, there is pressure hypertrophy of the left ventricle and left atrium, and dilatation of the aortic root.

PULMONARY STENOSIS AND ATRESIA Isolated pulmonary stenosis and atresia do not cause cyanosis and hence are included under acyanotic heart diseases.

MORPHOLOGIC FEATURES The changes in these conditions are as under:

Pulmonary stenosis It is the commonest form of obstructive congenital heart disease comprising about 7% of all congenital heart diseases. It may occur as a component of tetralogy of Fallot or as an isolated defect. Pulmonary stenosis is caused by fusion of cusps of the pulmonary valve forming a diaphragm-like obstruction to the outflow of blood from the right ventricle and dilatation of the pulmonary trunk.

Pulmonary atresia There is no communication between the right ventricle and lungs so that the blood bypasses the right ventricle through an interatrial septal defect. It then enters the lungs via patent ductus arteriosus.

> **GIST BOX 25.3 Congenital Heart Disease**
>
> ❖ Congenital anomalies of the heart may be either shunts (left-to-right or right-to-left), or defects causing obstructions to flow.
> ❖ Left-to-right shunts are acyanotic group of heart diseases; e.g. ventricular and atrial septal defects, and patent ductus arteriosus.
> ❖ Right-to-left shunts are cyanotic group of heart disease. Examples are tetralogy of Fallot, transposition of great arteries, persistent truncus arteriosus and tricuspid atresia and stenosis.
> ❖ Obstructive congenital heart diseases are coarctation of aorta, and stenosis and atresia of aorta or pulmonary artery.

ATHEROSCLEROSIS

Atherosclerosis is a thickening and hardening of large and medium-sized muscular arteries, primarily due to involvement of tunica intima and is characterised by fibrofatty plaques or atheromas.

The term atherosclerosis is derived from *athero* (meaning porridge) referring to the soft lipid-rich material in the centre of atheroma, and *sclerosis* (scarring) referring to connective tissue in the plaques.

Atherosclerosis is the commonest and the most important of the arterial diseases. Though any large and medium-sized artery may be involved in atherosclerosis, the most commonly affected are the aorta, the coronaries and the cerebral arterial systems. Therefore, the major clinical syndromes resulting from ischaemia due to atherosclerosis are as under:
1. Heart (angina and myocardial infarcts or *heart attacks*)
2. Brain (transient cerebral ischaemia and cerebral infarcts or *strokes*)
3. Other sequelae are: peripheral vascular disease, aneurysmal dilatation due to weakened arterial wall, chronic ischaemic heart disease, ischaemic encephalopathy and mesenteric arterial occlusion.

ETIOLOGY

Atherosclerosis is widely prevalent in industrialised countries. However, majority of the data on etiology are based on the animal experimental work and epidemiological studies. The incidence for atherosclerosis quoted in the literature is based on the major clinical syndromes produced by it, the most important interpretation being that death from myocardial infarction is related to underlying atherosclerosis. Cardiovascular disease, mostly related to atherosclerotic coronary heart disease or ischaemic heart disease (IHD) is the most common cause of premature death in the developed countries of the world. It is estimated that by the year 2020, cardiovascular disease, mainly atherosclerosis, will become the leading cause of total global disease burden.

Systematic large-scale studies of investigations on living populations have revealed a number of *risk factors* which are associated with increased risk of developing clinical atherosclerosis. Often, they are acting in combination rather than singly. These risk factors are divided into two groups (Table 25.2):

I. Major risk factors These are further considered under 2 headings:

A) *Major risk factors modifiable by life style and/or therapy*: This includes major risk factors which can be controlled by modifying life style and/or by pharmacotherapy and includes: dyslipidaemias, hypertension, diabetes mellitus and smoking.

B) *Constitutional risk factors:* These are non-modifiable major risk factors that include: increasing age, male sex, genetic abnormalities, and familial and racial predisposition.

II. Non-traditional emerging risk factors This group includes a host of factors whose role in atherosclerosis is minimal, and in some cases, even uncertain.

Table 25.2	Risk factors in atherosclerosis.
I. MAJOR RISK FACTORS	II. EMERGING RISK FACTORS
A) Modifiable	1. Environmental influences
1. Dyslipidaemia	2. Obesity
2. Hypertension	3. Hormones: oestrogen deficiency, oral contraceptives
3. Diabetes mellitus	
4. Smoking	4. Physical inactivity
B) Constitutional	5. Stressful life
1. Age	6. Homocystinuria
2. Sex	7. Role of alcohol
3. Genetic factors	8. Prothrombotic factors
4. Familial and racial factors	9. Infections (*C. pneumoniae*, Herpesvirus, CMV)
	10. High CRP

Section VI: Selected Topics from Systemic Pathology

Apparently, a combination of etiologic risk factors have additive effect in producing the lesions of atherosclerosis.

Major Risk Factors Modifiable By Life Style and/or Therapy

There are four major risk factors in atherogenesis—lipid disorders, hypertension, cigarette smoking and diabetes mellitus.

1. DYSLIPIDAEMIAS Virchow in 19th century first identified cholesterol crystals in the atherosclerotic lesions. Since then, extensive information on lipoproteins and their role in atherosclerotic lesions has been gathered. Abnormalities in plasma lipoproteins have been firmly established as the most important major risk factor for atherosclerosis. It has been firmly established that hypercholesterolaemia has directly proportionate relationship with atherosclerosis and IHD. The following evidences are cited in support of this:

i) The atherosclerotic plaques contain cholesterol and cholesterol esters, largely derived from the lipoproteins in the blood.

ii) The lesions of atherosclerosis can be induced in experimental animals by feeding them with diet rich in cholesterol.

iii) Individuals with hypercholesterolaemia due to various causes such as in diabetes mellitus, myxoedema, nephrotic syndrome, von Gierke's disease, xanthomatosis and familial hypercholesterolaemia have increased risk of developing atherosclerosis and IHD.

iv) Populations having hypercholesterolaemia have higher mortality from IHD. Dietary regulation and administration of cholesterol-lowering drugs have beneficial effect on reducing the risk of IHD.

The concentration of total cholesterol in the serum reflects the concentrations of different lipoproteins in the serum. The lipoproteins are divided into classes according to the density of solvent in which they remain suspended on centrifugation at high speed. The major classes of lipoprotein particles are *chylomicrons, very-low density lipoproteins (VLDL), low-density lipoproteins (LDL),* and *high-density lipoproteins (HDL)*. Lipids are insoluble in blood and therefore are carried in circulation and across the cell membrane by carrier proteins called *apoproteins*. Different apoproteins are named by letter A, B, C, D etc while their subfractions are numbered serially.

The major fractions of lipoproteins tested in blood lipid profile and their varying effects on atherosclerosis and IHD are as under (Table 25.3):

i) **Total cholesterol** Desirable normal serum level is 140-199 mg/dl, while levels between 200-240 mg/dl are considered borderline high. An elevation of total serum cholesterol levels above 260 mg/dl in men and women between 30 and 50 years of age has three times higher risk of developing IHD as compared with people with total serum cholesterol levels within normal limits.

ii) **Triglycerides** Normal serum level is below 150 mg/dl.

iii) **Low-density lipoproteins (LDL) cholesterol** Optimal serum level of LDL is <100 mg/dl. LDL is richest in cholesterol and has the *maximum association* with atherosclerosis.

iv) **Very-low-density lipoprotein (VLDL)** VLDL carries much of the triglycerides and its blood levels therefore parallel with that of triglycerides; VLDL has *less marked* effect than LDL.

v) **High-density lipoproteins (HDL) cholesterol** Normal desirable serum level is <50 mg/dl. HDL is *protective* ('good cholesterol') against atherosclerosis.

Many studies have demonstrated the harmful effect of diet containing larger quantities of saturated fats (e.g. in eggs, meat, milk, butter etc) and trans fats (i.e. unsaturated fats produced by artificial hydrogenation of polyunsaturated fats) which raise the plasma cholesterol level. This type of diet is consumed more often by the affluent societies who are at greater risk of developing atherosclerosis. On the contrary, a diet low in saturated fats and high in poly-unsaturated fats and having omega-3 fatty acids (e.g. in fish, fish oils etc) lowers the plasma cholesterol levels. Aside from lipid-rich diet, high intake of the total number of calories from carbohydrates, proteins, alcohol and sweets has adverse effects.

Besides above, *familial hypercholesterolaemia*, an autosomal codominant disorder, is characterised by elevated LDL cholesterol and normal triglycerides and occurrence of xanthomas and premature coronary artery disease. It occurs due to mutations in LDL receptor gene.

Table 25.3 Fractions of lipoproteins in serum.

CLASSES	SITES OF SYNTHESIS	NORMAL SERUM LEVELS*	ROLE IN ATHEROSCLEROSIS
1. HDL cholesterol	Liver, intestine	> 50 mg/dl	Protective
2. LDL cholesterol	Liver	< 100 mg/dl	Maximum
3. VLDL triglycerides	Intestine, liver	< 150 mg/dl	Less marked
4. Total cholesterol	Liver, intestine	< 200 mg/dl	Maximum
5. Chylomicrons	Liver, intestine, macrophage	—	Indirect

*Easy way to remember optimum desirable cut off levels of serum lipids in mg/dl is a multiple of 50: <200 for cholesterol, <150 for LDL, <100 for triglycerides (or VLDL), and >50 for HDL.
Lipids can also be measured in plasma (EDTA blood); plasma values are 3% lower than in serum.

Currently, management of dyslipidaemia is directed at *lowering LDL* in particular, and total cholesterol in general, by use of statins, and for *raising HDL* by weight loss, exercise and use of nicotinic acid. Thus currently, preferred term for hyperlipidaemia is dyslipidaemia because one risky plasma lipoprotein (i.e. LDL) is elevated and needs to be brought down, while the other good plasma lipoprotein (i.e. HDL) when low requires to be raised.

How hypercholesterolaemia and various classes of lipoproteins produce atherosclerosis is described under 'pathogenesis'.

2. HYPERTENSION Hypertension is a risk factor for all clinical manifestations of atherosclerosis. Hypertension doubles the risk of all forms of cardiovascular disease. It acts probably by mechanical injury to the arterial wall due to increased blood pressure. Elevation of systolic pressure of over 160 mmHg or a diastolic pressure of over 95 mmHg is associated with five times higher risk of developing IHD than in people with blood pressure within normal range (140/90 mmHg or less) (Chapter 28).

3. SMOKING The extent and severity of atherosclerosis are much greater in smokers than in non-smokers. Cigarette smoking is associated with higher risk of atherosclerotic IHD and sudden cardiac death. Men who smoke a pack of cigarettes a day are 3-5 times more likely to die of IHD than non-smokers. The increased risk and severity of atherosclerosis in smokers is due to reduced level of HDL, deranged coagulation system and accumulation of carbon monoxide in the blood that produces carboxyhaemoglobin and eventually hypoxia in the arterial wall favouring atherosclerosis.

4. DIABETES MELLITUS Clinical manifestations of atherosclerosis are far more common and develop at an early age in people with both type 1 and type 2 diabetes mellitus. In particular, association of type 2 diabetes mellitus characterised by metabolic (insulin resistance) syndrome and abnormal lipid profile termed 'diabetic dyslipidaemia' is common and heightens the risk of cardiovascular disease (Chapter 29). The risk of developing IHD is doubled, tendency to develop cerebrovascular disease is high, and frequency to develop gangrene of foot is about 100 times increased. The causes of increased severity of atherosclerosis are complex and numerous which include endothelial dysfunction, increased aggregation of platelets, increased LDL and decreased HDL.

Constitutional Risk Factors

Age, sex and genetic influences, race and family do affect the appearance of lesions of atherosclerosis.

1. AGE Atherosclerosis is an age-related disease. Though early lesions of atherosclerosis may be present in childhood, clinically significant lesions are found with increasing age. Fully-developed atheromatous plaques usually appear in the 4th decade and beyond. Evidence in support comes from the high death rate from IHD in this age group.

2. SEX The incidence and severity of atherosclerosis are more in men than in women and the changes appear a decade earlier in men (≥ 45 years) than in women (≥ 55 years). The prevalence of atherosclerotic IHD is about three times higher in men in 4th decade than in women and the difference slowly declines with age but remains higher at all ages in men. The lower incidence of IHD in women, especially in premenopausal age, is probably due to high levels of oestrogen and high-density lipoproteins, both of which have anti-atherogenic influence.

3. GENETIC FACTORS Genetic factors play a significant role in atherogenesis. Hereditary derangements of lipoprotein metabolism predispose the individual to high blood lipid level and familial hypercholesterolaemia.

4. FAMILIAL AND RACIAL FACTORS The familial predisposition to atherosclerosis may be related to other risk factors like diabetes, hypertension and hyperlipoproteinaemia. Racial differences too exist; Blacks have generally less severe atherosclerosis than Whites.

Emerging Risk Factors

There are a number of nontraditional newly emerging risk factors for which the role in the etiology of atherosclerosis is yet not fully supported. These factors are as under:

1. Higher incidence of atherosclerosis in developed countries and low prevalence in underdeveloped countries, suggesting the role of *environmental influences.*
2. *Metabolic syndrome* characterised by abdominal obesity along with glucose intolerance, insulin resistance and dyslipidaemia and hypertension, is associated with increased risk.
3. Use of *exogenous hormones* (e.g. oral contraceptives) by women or *endogenous oestrogen deficiency* (e.g. in postmenopausal women) has been shown to have an increased risk of developing myocardial infarction or stroke.
4. *Physical inactivity* and lack of exercise are associated with the risk of developing atherosclerosis and its complications.
5. *Stressful life style,* termed as 'type A' behaviour pattern, characterised by aggressiveness, competitive drive, ambitiousness and a sense of urgency, is associated with enhanced risk of IHD compared with 'type B' behaviour of relaxed and happy-go-lucky type.
6. *Hypercystinaemia* due to elevated serum homocysteine level from low folate and vitamin B_{12} have a relationship with coronary artery disease and its consequences.
7. Patients with *homocystinuria,* an uncommon inborn error of metabolism, having hypercystinaemia have also been reported to have early atherosclerosis and coronary artery disease.
8. *Prothrombotic factors* and elevated fibrinogen levels favour formation of thrombi which is the gravest complication of atherosclerosis.
9. Role of *infections,* particularly of *Chlamydia pneumoniae* and viruses such as herpesvirus and cytomegalovirus,

has been found in coronary atherosclerotic lesions by causing inflammation. Possibly, infections may be acting in combination with some other factors.

10. Markers of inflammation such as *elevated C reactive protein*, an acute phase reactant, correlate with risk of developing atherosclerosis.

However, there are some reports in the literature which suggest that moderate consumption of *alcohol* has slightly beneficial effect by raising the level of HDL cholesterol.

PATHOGENESIS

As stated above, atherosclerosis is not caused by a single etiologic factor but is a multifactorial process whose exact pathogenesis is still not known. Since the times of Virchow, a number of theories have been proposed.

❖ **Insudation hypothesis** The concept hypothesised by *Virchow in 1856* that atherosclerosis is a form of cellular proliferation of the intimal cells resulting from increased imbibing of lipids from the blood came to be called the *'lipid theory.'* Modified form of this theory is currently known as *'response to injury hypothesis'* and is now-a-days the most widely accepted theory.

❖ **Encrustation hypothesis** The proposal put forth by *Rokitansky in 1852* that atheroma represented a form of encrustation on the arterial wall from the components in the blood forming thrombi composed of platelets, fibrin and leucocytes, was named as *'encrustation theory'* or *'thrombogenic theory.'* Since currently it is believed that encrustation or thrombosis is not the sole factor in atherogenesis but the components of thrombus (platelets, fibrin and leucocytes) have a role in atheromatous lesions, this theory has now been incorporated into the response-to-injury hypothesis mentioned above.

Though, there is no consensus regarding the origin and progression of lesion of atherosclerosis, the role of four key factors—arterial smooth muscle cells, endothelial cells, blood monocytes and dyslipidaemia, is accepted by all. However, the areas of disagreement exist in the mechanism and sequence of events involving these factors in initiation, progression and complications of disease. Currently, pathogenesis of atherosclerosis is explained on the basis of the following two theories:

1. *Reaction-to-injury hypothesis*, first described in 1973, and modified in 1986 and 1993 by Ross.
2. *Monoclonal theory*, based on neoplastic proliferation of smooth muscle cells, postulated by Benditt and Benditt in 1973.

1. Reaction-to-Injury Hypothesis

This theory is most widely accepted and incorporates aspects of two older historical theories of atherosclerosis—the lipid theory of Virchow and thrombogenic (encrustation) theory of Rokitansky.

❖ The *original response to injury theory* was first described in 1973 according to which the initial event in atherogenesis was considered to be endothelial injury followed by smooth muscle cell proliferation so that the early lesions, according to this theory, consist of smooth muscle cells mainly.

❖ The *modified response-to-injury hypothesis* described subsequently in 1993 implicates lipoprotein entry into the intima as the initial event followed by lipid accumulation in the macrophages (foam cells now) which according to modified theory, are believed to be the dominant cells in early lesions.

Both these theories—original and modified, have attracted support and criticism. However, following is the generally accepted role of key components involved in atherogenesis, diagrammatically illustrated in Fig. 25.13.

i) Endothelial injury It has been known for many years that endothelial injury is the initial triggering event in the development of lesions of atherosclerosis. Actual endothelial denudation is not an essential requirement, but endothelial dysfunction may initiate the sequence of events. Numerous causes ascribed to endothelial injury in experimental animals are: mechanical trauma, haemodynamic forces, immunological and chemical mechanisms, metabolic agent as chronic dyslipidaemia, homocysteine, circulating toxins from systemic infections, viruses, hypoxia, radiation, carbon monoxide and tobacco products.

In humans, two of the major risk factors which act together to produce endothelial injury are: *haemodynamic stress from hypertension and chronic dyslipidaemia*. The role of haemodynamic forces in causing endothelial injury is further supported by the distribution of atheromatous plaques at points of bifurcation or branching of blood vessels which are under greatest shear stress.

ii) Intimal smooth muscle cell proliferation Endothelial injury causes adherence, aggregation and platelet release reaction at the site of exposed subendothelial connective tissue and infiltration by inflammatory cells. Proliferation of intimal smooth muscle cells and production of extracellular matrix are stimulated by various cytokines such as IL-1 and TNF-α released from invading monocyte-macrophages and by activated platelets at the site of endothelial injury. These cytokines lead to local synthesis of following growth factors having distinct roles in plaque evolution:

Platelet-derived growth factor *(PDGF)* and fibroblast growth factor *(FGF)* stimulate proliferation and migration of smooth muscle cells from their usual location in the media into the intima.

Transforming growth factor-β *(TGF-β)* and interferon (IFN)-γ derived from activated T lymphocytes within lesions regulate the synthesis of collagen by smooth muscle cells.

Smooth muscle cell proliferation is also facilitated by biomolecules such as nitric oxide and *endothelin* released from endothelial cells. Intimal proliferation of smooth

Chapter 25: Diseases of Cardiovascular System

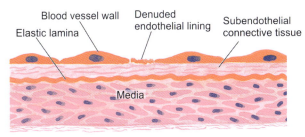

A, ENDOTHELIAL INJURY

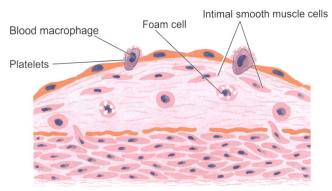

B, PLATELET ADHESION AND MONOCYTE MIGRATION

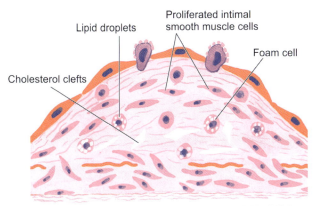

C, INTIMAL SMOOTH MUSCLE CELL PROLIFERATION

Figure 25.13 ▶ Diagrammatic representation of pathogenesis of atherosclerosis as explained by 'reaction-to-injury' hypothesis. A, Endothelial injury. B, Adhesion of platelets and migration of blood monocytes from blood stream. C, Smooth muscle cell proliferation into the intima and ingrowth of new blood vessels.

muscle cells is accompanied by synthesis of matrix proteins—collagen, elastic fibre proteins and proteoglycans.

iii) Role of blood monocytes Though blood monocytes do not possess receptors for normal LDL, LDL does appear in the monocyte cytoplasm to form foam cell by mechanism illustrated in Fig. 25.14. Plasma LDL on entry into the intima undergoes oxidation. The 'oxidised LDL' formed in the intima performs the following all-important functions on monocytes and endothelium:

a) For monocytes: Oxidised LDL acts to attract, proliferate, immobilise and activate them as well as is readily taken up by scavenger receptor on the monocyte to transform it to a lipid-laden foam cell.

b) For endothelium: Oxidised LDL is cytotoxic.

Death of foam cell by apoptosis releases lipid to form lipid core of plaque.

iv) Role of dyslipidaemia As stated already, chronic dyslipidaemia in itself may initiate endothelial injury and dysfunction by causing increased permeability. In particular, hypercholesterolaemia with increased serum concentration of LDL promotes formation of foam cells, while high serum concentration of HDL has anti-atherogenic effect.

v) Thrombosis As apparent from the foregoing, endothelial injury exposes subendothelial connective tissue resulting in formation of small platelet aggregates at the site and causing proliferation of smooth muscle cells. This causes mild inflammatory reaction which together with foam cells is incorporated into the atheromatous plaque. The lesions enlarge by attaching fibrin and cells from the blood so that thrombus becomes a part of atheromatous plaque.

2. Monoclonal Hypothesis

This hypothesis is based on the postulate that proliferation of smooth muscle cells is the primary event and that this proliferation is monoclonal in origin similar to cellular proliferation in neoplasms (e.g. in uterine leiomyoma, page 285). The evidence cited in support of monoclonal hypothesis is the observation on proliferated smooth muscle cells in atheromatous plaques which have only one of the two forms of glucose-6-phosphate dehydrogenase (G6PD) isoenzymes, suggesting monoclonality in origin. The monoclonal proliferation of smooth muscle cells in atherosclerosis may be initiated by mutation caused by exogenous chemicals (e.g. cigarette smoke), endogenous metabolites (e.g. lipoproteins) and some viruses (e.g. Marek's disease virus in chickens, herpesvirus).

MORPHOLOGIC FEATURES

Early lesions in the form of diffuse intimal thickening, fatty streaks and gelatinous lesions are often the forerunners in the evolution of atherosclerotic lesions. However, the clinical disease states due to luminal narrowing in atherosclerosis are caused by fully developed atheromatous plaques and complicated plaques (Fig. 25.15).

1. FATTY STREAKS AND DOTS Fatty streaks and dots on the intima by themselves are harmless but may be the precursor lesions of atheromatous plaques. They are seen in all races of the world and begin to appear in the first year of life. However, they are uncommon in older persons and are probably absorbed. They are especially prominent in the aorta and other major arteries, more often on the posterior wall than the anterior wall.

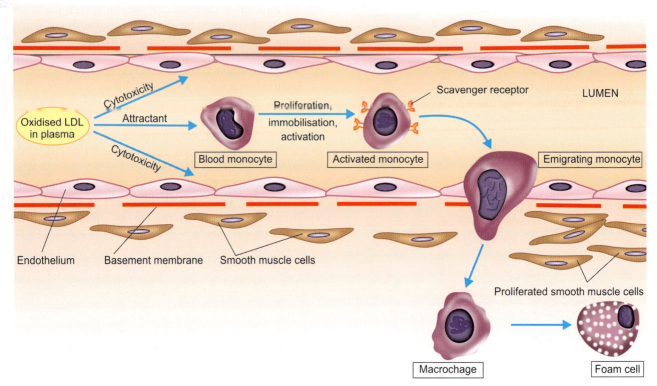

Figure 25.14 ▶ Mechanism of foam cell formation.

Grossly, the lesions may appear as flat or slightly elevated and yellow. They may be either in the form of small, multiple dots, about 1 mm in size, or in the form of elongated, beaded streaks.

Microscopically, fatty streaks lying under the endothelium are composed of closely-packed foam cells, lipid-containing elongated smooth muscle cells and a few lymphoid cells. Small amount of extracellular lipid, collagen and proteoglycans are also present.

2. GELATINOUS LESIONS Gelatinous lesions develop in the intima of the aorta and other major arteries in the first few months of life. Like fatty streaks, they may also be precursors of plaques. They are round or oval, circumscribed grey elevations, about 1 cm in diameter.

Microscopically, gelatinous lesions are foci of increased ground substance in the intima with thinned overlying endothelium.

3. ATHEROMATOUS PLAQUES A fully developed atherosclerotic lesion is called atheromatous plaque, also called *fibrous plaque, fibrofatty plaque or atheroma*. Unlike fatty streaks, atheromatous plaques are selective in different geographic locations and races and are seen in advanced age. These lesions may develop from progression of early lesions of the atherosclerosis just described. *Most often and most severely affected is the abdominal aorta,* though smaller lesions may be seen in descending thoracic aorta and aortic arch. The major branches of the aorta around the ostia are often severely involved, especially the iliac, femoral, carotid, coronary, and cerebral arteries.

Grossly, atheromatous plaques are white to yellowish-white lesions, varying in diameter from 1-2 cm and raised on the surface by a few millimetres to a centimetre in thickness **(Fig. 25.16)**. Cut section of the plaque reveals the luminal surface as a firm, white *fibrous cap* and a *central core* composed of yellow to yellow-white, soft, porridge-like material and hence the name atheroma.

Microscopically, the appearance of plaque varies depending upon the age of the lesion. However, the following features are invariably present **(Fig. 25.17)**:

i) Superficial luminal part of the *fibrous cap* is covered by endothelium, and is composed of smooth muscle cells, dense connective tissue and extracellular matrix containing proteoglycans and collagen.
ii) *Cellular area* under the fibrous cap is comprised by a mixture of macrophages, foam cells, lymphocytes and a few smooth muscle cells which may contain lipid.
iii) Deeper *central soft core* consists of extracellular lipid material, cholesterol clefts, fibrin, necrotic debris and lipid-laden foam cells.

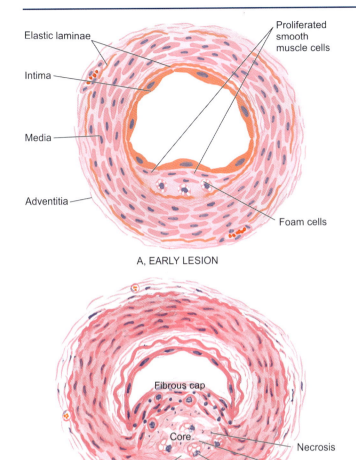

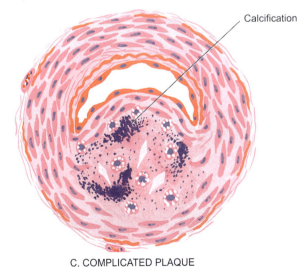

Figure 25.15 ▶ Schematic evolution of lesions in atherosclerosis.

iv) In older and *more advanced lesions,* the collagen in the fibrous cap may be dense and hyalinised, smooth muscle cells may be atrophic and foam cells are fewer.

4. COMPLICATED PLAQUES Various pathologic changes that occur in fully-developed atheromatous plaques are called the complicated lesions. These account for the most serious harmful effects of atherosclerosis and even death. These changes include calcification, ulceration, thrombosis, haemorrhage and aneurysmal dilatation. It is not uncommon to see more than one form of complication in a plaque.

i) Calcification Calcification occurs more commonly in advanced atheromatous plaques, especially in the aorta and coronaries. The diseased intima cracks like an egg-shell when the vessel is incised and opened.

Microscopically, the calcium salts are deposited in the vicinity of necrotic area and in the soft lipid pool deep in the thickened intima **(Fig. 25.18)**. This form of atherosclerotic *intimal* calcification differs from Mönckeberg's *medial* calcific arteriosclerosis that affects only the tunica media.

ii) Ulceration The layers covering the soft pultaceous material of an atheroma may ulcerate as a result of haemodynamic forces or mechanical trauma. This results in discharge of emboli composed of lipid material and debris into the blood stream, leaving a shallow, ragged ulcer with yellow lipid debris in the base of the ulcer. Occasionally, atheromatous plaque in a coronary artery may suddenly rupture into the arterial lumen forcibly and cause thromboembolic occlusion.

iii) Thrombosis The ulcerated plaque and the areas of endothelial damage are vulnerable sites for formation of superimposed thrombi. These thrombi may get dislodged to become emboli and lodge elsewhere in the circulation, or may get organised and incorporated into the arterial wall as mural thrombi. Mural thrombi may become occlusive thrombi which may subsequently recanalise.

iv) Haemorrhage Intimal haemorrhage may occur in an atheromatous plaque either from the blood in the vascular lumen through an ulcerated plaque, or from rupture of thin-walled capillaries that vascularise the atheroma from adventitial vasa vasorum. Haemorrhage is particularly a common complication in coronary arteries. The haematoma formed at the site contains numerous haemosiderin-laden macrophages.

v) Aneurysm formation Though atherosclerosis is primarily an intimal disease, advanced lesions are associated with secondary changes in the media and adventitia. The changes in media include atrophy and thinning of the media and fragmentation of internal elastic lamina. The adventitia undergoes fibrosis and some inflammatory changes. These changes cause weakening in the arterial wall resulting in aneurysmal dilatation.

Section VI: Selected Topics from Systemic Pathology

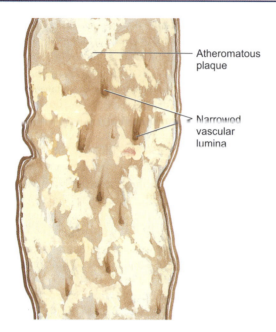
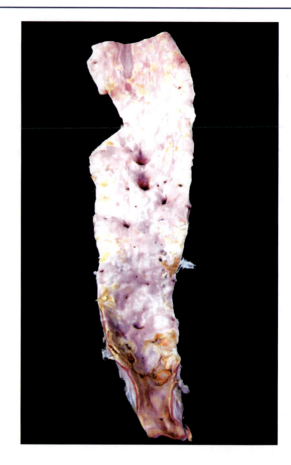

Figure 25.16 ▶ Structure of a fully-developed atheroma. The opened up inner surface of the abdominal aorta shows a variety of atheromatous lesions. While some are raised yellowish-white lesions raised above the surface, a few have ulcerated surface. Orifices of some of the branches coming out of the wall are narrowed by the atherosclerotic process.

CLINICAL EFFECTS

The clinical effects of atherosclerosis depend upon the size and type of arteries affected. In general, the clinical effects result from the following:

1. Slow luminal narrowing causing ischaemia and atrophy.
2. Sudden luminal occlusion causing infarction necrosis.
3. Propagation of plaque by formation of thrombi and emboli.
4. Formation of aneurysmal dilatation and eventual rupture.

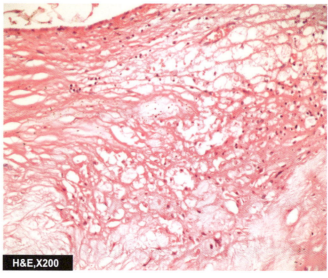

Figure 25.17 ▶ Histologic appearance of a fully-developed atheroma.

Chapter 25: Diseases of Cardiovascular System

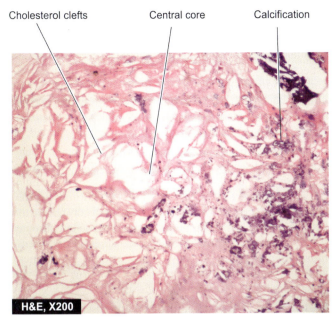

Figure 25.18 ▶ Complicated atheromatous plaque lesion. There is narrowing of the lumen of coronary due to fully developed atheromatous plaque which has dystrophic calcification in its core.

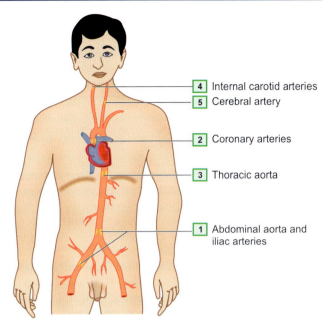

Figure 25.19 ▶ Major sites of atherosclerosis (serially numbered) in descending order of frequency.

Large arteries affected most often are the aorta, renal, mesenteric and carotids, whereas the medium- and small-sized arteries frequently involved are the coronaries, cerebrals and arteries of the lower limbs. Accordingly, the symptomatic atherosclerotic disease involves most often the heart, brain, kidneys, small intestine and lower extremities (Fig. 25.19). The effects pertaining to these organs are described in relevant chapters later while the major effects are listed below (Fig. 25.20):

i) *Heart*—Myocardial infarction, ischaemic heart disease.

ii) *Brain*—Chronic ischaemic brain damage, cerebral infarction and stroke.

iii) *Aorta*—Aneurysm formation, thrombosis and embolisation to other organs.

iv) *Small intestine*—Ischaemic bowel disease, infarction.

v) *Lower extremities*—Intermittent claudication, gangrene.

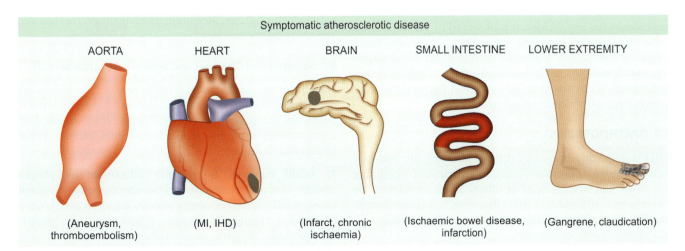

Figure 25.20 ▶ Major forms of symptomatic atherosclerotic disease.

> **GIST BOX 25.4 | Atherosclerosis**
>
> - Atherosclerosis is thickening and hardening of large and medium-sized muscular arteries, primarily due to involvement of tunica intima and is characterised by fibrofatty plaques or atheromas.
> - Major risk factors are modifiable by life style and/or therapy and include: dyslipidaemias, hypertension, diabetes mellitus and smoking.
> - Constitutional risk factors are advancing age, male sex, and genetic influences, familial predisposition and white race.
> - Atherogenesis is explained commonly by reaction to injury hypothesis that involves: endothelial injury, intimal smooth muscle cell proliferation, circulating monocytes, dyslipidaemia and thrmbosis.
> - The lesions of atherosclerosis begin with fatty streaks and gelatinous lesions.
> - Full blown atheromatous lesions or fibrofatty plaques have a superficial cap and cellular or soft centre.
> - Complicated atheromas may have dystrophic calcification, ulceration, thrombosis, haemorrhage and aneurysm formation.
> - Major clinical effects of atherosclerosis are on the heart (coronary artery disease), brain (stroke), aorta (aneurysmal dilatation), intestine (ischaemia) and lower extremities (gangrene).

ISCHAEMIC HEART DISEASE

Ischaemic heart disease (IHD) is defined as acute or chronic form of cardiac disability arising from imbalance between the myocardial supply and demand for oxygenated blood. Since narrowing or obstruction of the coronary arterial system is the most common cause of myocardial anoxia, the alternate term *'coronary artery disease (CAD)'* is used synonymously with IHD. IHD or CAD is the leading cause of death in most developed countries (about one-third of all deaths) and somewhat low incidence is observed in the developing countries. Men develop IHD earlier than women and death rates are also slightly higher for men than for women until the menopause. As per rising trends of IHD worldwide, it is estimated that by the year 2020 it would become the most common cause of death throughout world.

ETIOPATHOGENESIS

IHD is invariably caused by disease affecting the coronary arteries, the most prevalent being atherosclerosis accounting for more than 90% cases, while other causes are responsible for less than 10% cases of IHD. Therefore, it is convenient to consider the etiology of IHD under three broad headings:
i) coronary atherosclerosis;
ii) superadded changes in coronary atherosclerosis; and
iii) non-atherosclerotic causes.

I. Coronary Atherosclerosis

Coronary atherosclerosis resulting in 'fixed' obstruction is the major cause of IHD in more than 90% cases. The general aspects of atherosclerosis as regards its etiology, pathogenesis and the morphologic features of atherosclerotic lesions have already been dealt with at length above. Here, a brief account of the specific features in pathology of lesions in *atherosclerotic coronary artery disease* in particular is presented.

1. Distribution Atherosclerotic lesions in coronary arteries are distributed in one or more of the three major coronary arterial trunks, the highest incidence being in the anterior descending branch of the left coronary (LAD), followed in decreasing frequency, by the right coronary artery (RCA) and still less in circumflex branch of the left coronary (CXA). About one-third of cases have *single-vessel disease*, most often left anterior descending arterial involvement; another one-third have *two-vessel disease,* and the remainder has *three major vessel disease.*

2. Location Almost all adults show atherosclerotic plaques scattered throughout the coronary arterial system. However, significant stenotic lesions that may produce chronic myocardial ischaemia show more than 75% (three-fourth) reduction in the cross-sectional area of a coronary artery or its branch. The area of severest involvement is about 3 to 4 cm from the coronary ostia, more often at or near the bifurcation of the arteries, suggesting the role of haemodynamic forces in atherogenesis.

3. Fixed atherosclerotic plaques The atherosclerotic plaques in the coronaries are more often eccentrically located bulging into the lumen from one side **(Fig. 25.21)**. Occasionally, there may be concentric thickening of the wall of the artery. Atherosclerosis produces gradual luminal narrowing that may eventually lead to 'fixed' coronary obstruction. The general features of atheromas of coronary arteries are similar to those affecting elsewhere in the body and may develop similar complications like calcification, coronary thrombosis, ulceration, haemorrhage, rupture and aneurysm formation.

II. Superadded Changes in Coronary Atherosclerosis

The attacks of *acute coronary syndromes,* which include acute myocardial infarction, unstable angina and sudden ischaemic death, are precipitated by certain changes superimposed on a pre-existing fixed coronary atheromatous plaque. These changes are as under:

1. Acute changes in chronic atheromatous plaque Though chronic fixed obstructions are the most frequent cause of IHD, acute coronary episodes are often precipitated by sudden changes in chronic plaques such as plaque haemorrhage, fissuring, or ulceration that results in thrombosis and embolisation of atheromatous debris. Acute plaque changes are brought about by factors such as sudden

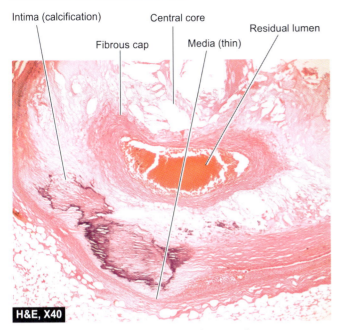

Figure 25.21 ▶ Left anterior descending (LAD) coronary artery showing critical narrowing with eccentric luminal obliteration due to complicated atheromatous plaque.

coronary artery spasm, tachycardia, intraplaque haemorrhage and hypercholesterolaemia.

2. Coronary artery thrombosis Transmural acute myocardial infarction is often precipitated by partial or complete coronary thrombosis. The initiation of thrombus occurs due to surface ulceration of fixed chronic atheromatous plaque, ultimately causing complete luminal occlusion. The lipid core of plaque, in particular, is highly thrombogenic. Small fragments of thrombotic material are then dislodged which are embolised to terminal coronary branches and cause microinfarcts of the myocardium.

3. Local platelet aggregation and coronary artery spasm Some cases of acute coronary episodes are caused by local aggregates of platelets on the atheromatous plaque, short of forming a thrombus. The aggregated platelets release vasospasmic mediators such as thromboxane A2 which may probably be responsible for coronary vasospasm in the already atherosclerotic vessel.

Based on progressive pathological changes and clinical correlation, American Heart Association (1995) has classified human coronary atherosclerosis into 6 sequential types in ascending order of grades of lesions as shown in Table 25.4.

III. Non-atherosclerotic Causes

Several other coronary lesions may cause IHD in less than 10% of cases. These are as under:

1. Vasospasm It has been possible to document vasospasm of one of the major coronary arterial trunks in patients with no significant atherosclerotic coronary narrowing which may cause angina or myocardial infarction.

2. Stenosis of coronary ostia Coronary ostial narrowing may result from extension of syphilitic aortitis or from aortic atherosclerotic plaques encroaching on the opening.

3. Arteritis Various types of inflammatory involvements of coronary arteries or small branches like in rheumatic arteritis, polyarteritis nodosa, thromboangiitis obliterans (Buerger's disease), Takayasu's disease, Kawasaki's disease, tuberculosis and other bacterial infections may contribute to myocardial damage.

4. Embolism Rarely, emboli originating from elsewhere in the body may occlude the left coronary artery and its branches and produce IHD. The emboli may originate from bland thrombi, or from vegetations of bacterial endocarditis; rarely fat embolism and air embolism of coronary circulation may occur.

Table 25.4 Classification of human atherosclerosis proposed by American Heart Association.

TYPES	MAIN HISTOLOGY	MAIN PATHOGENESIS	AGE AT ONSET	CLINICAL EFFECTS
Type I: Initial lesions	Macrophages, occasional foam cell	Accumulation of lipoprotein	1st decade	Asymptomatic
Type II: Fatty streaks	Many layers of macrophages and foam cells	Accumulation of lipoprotein	1st decade	Asymptomatic
Type III: Intermediate lesions	Many lipid-laden cells and scattered extracellular lipid droplets	Accumulation of lipoprotein	3rd decade	Asymptomatic
Type IV: Atheromatous lesions	Intra- as well as extracellular lipid pool	Accumulation of lipid	3rd decade	Asymptomatic or manifest symptoms
Type V: Fibrofatty lesions	Fibrotic cap and lipid core (V a), may have calcification (V b)	Smooth muscle cell proliferation and increased collagen	4th decade	Asymptomatic or manifest symptoms
Type VI: Complicated lesions	Ulceration, haemorrhage, haematoma, thrombosis	Haemodynamic stress, thrombosis, haematoma	4th decade	Asymptomatic or manifest symptoms

5. Thrombotic diseases Another infrequent cause of coronary occlusion is from hypercoagulability of the blood such as in shock, polycythaemia vera, sickle cell anaemia and thrombotic thrombocytopenic purpura.

6. Trauma Contusion of a coronary artery from penetrating injuries may produce thrombotic occlusion.

7. Aneurysms Extension of dissecting aneurysm of the aorta into the coronary artery may produce thrombotic coronary occlusion. Rarely, congenital, mycotic and syphilitic aneurysms may occur in coronary arteries and produce similar occlusive effects.

8. Compression Compression of a coronary from outside by a primary or secondary tumour of the heart may result in coronary occlusion.

EFFECTS OF MYOCARDIAL ISCHAEMIA

Development of lesions in the coronaries is not always accompanied by cardiac disease. Depending upon the suddenness of onset, duration, degree, location and extent of the area affected by myocardial ischaemia, the range of changes and clinical features may range from an asymptomatic state at one extreme to immediate mortality at the other (Fig. 25.22):

A. Asymptomatic state
B. Angina pectoris (AP)
C. Acute myocardial infarction (MI)
D. Chronic ischaemic heart disease (CIHD)/Ischaemic cardiomyopathy/ Myocardial fibrosis
E. Sudden cardiac death

The term *acute coronary syndromes* include a triad of acute myocardial infarction, unstable angina and sudden cardiac death.

Angina Pectoris

Angina pectoris is a clinical syndrome of IHD resulting from transient myocardial ischaemia. It is characterised by paroxysmal pain in the substernal or precordial region of the chest which is aggravated by an increase in the demand of the heart and relieved by a decrease in the work of the heart. Often, the pain radiates to the left arm, neck, jaw or right arm. It is more common in men past 5th decade of life.

There are 3 overlapping clinical patterns of angina pectoris with some differences in their pathogenesis:
i) Stable or typical angina
ii) Prinzmetal's variant angina
iii) Unstable or crescendo angina

STABLE OR TYPICAL ANGINA This is the most common pattern. Stable or typical angina is characterised by attacks of pain following physical exertion or emotional excitement and is relieved by rest. The pathogenesis of condition lies in *chronic stenosing coronary atherosclerosis* that cannot perfuse the myocardium adequately when the workload on the heart increases. During the attacks, there is depression of ST segment in the ECG due to poor perfusion of the subendocardial region of the left ventricle but there is no elevation of enzymes in the blood as there is no irreversible myocardial injury.

PRINZMETAL'S VARIANT ANGINA This pattern of angina is characterised by pain at rest and has no relationship with physical activity. The exact pathogenesis of Prinzmetal's angina is not known. It may occur due to *sudden vasospasm* of a coronary trunk induced by coronary atherosclerosis, or may be due to release of humoral vasoconstrictors by mast cells in the coronary adventitia. ECG shows ST segment elevation due to transmural ischaemia. These patients respond well to vasodilators like nitroglycerin.

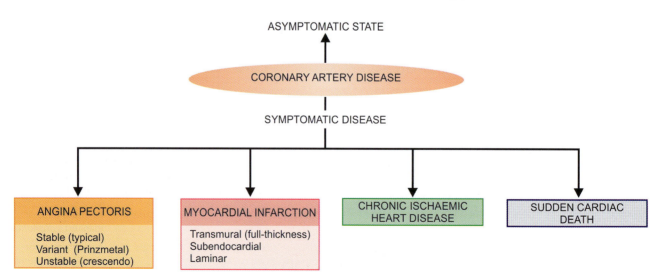

Figure 25.22 ▶ Spectrum of coronary ischaemic manifestations.

UNSTABLE OR CRESCENDO ANGINA Also referred to as 'pre-infarction angina' or 'acute coronary insufficiency', this is the most serious pattern of angina. It is characterised by more frequent onset of pain of prolonged duration and occurring often at rest. It is thus indicative of an impending acute myocardial infarction. Distinction between unstable angina and acute MI is made by ST segment changes on ECG— acute MI characterised by ST segment elevation while unstable angina may have non-ST segment elevation MI. *Multiple factors* are involved in the pathogenesis of unstable angina which include: stenosing coronary atherosclerosis, complicated coronary plaques (e.g. superimposed thrombosis, haemorrhage, rupture, ulceration etc), platelet thrombi over atherosclerotic plaques and vasospasm of coronary arteries. More often, the lesions lie in a branch of the major coronary trunk so that collaterals prevent infarction.

Acute Myocardial Infarction

Acute myocardial infarction (MI) is the most important and feared consequence of coronary artery disease. Many patients may die within the first few hours of the onset, while remainder suffer from effects of impaired cardiac function. A significant factor that may prevent or diminish the myocardial damage is the development of collateral circulation through anastomotic channels over a period of time. A regular and well-planned exercise programme encourages good collateral circulation and improved cardiac performance.

INCIDENCE In developed countries, acute MI accounts for 10-25% of all deaths. Due to the dominant etiologic role of coronary atherosclerosis in acute MI, the incidence of acute MI correlates well with the incidence of atherosclerosis in a geographic area.

Age Acute MI may virtually occur at all ages, though the incidence is higher in the elderly. About 5% of heart attacks occur in young people under the age of 40 years, particularly in those with major risk factors to develop atherosclerosis like hypertension, diabetes mellitus, cigarette smoking and dyslipidaemia including familial hypercholesterolaemia.

Sex Males throughout their life are at a significantly higher risk of developing acute MI as compared to females. Women during reproductive period have remarkably low incidence of acute MI, probably due to the protective influence of oestrogen. The use of oral contraceptives is associated with high risk of developing acute MI. After menopause, this gender difference gradually declines but the incidence of disease among women never reaches that among men of the same age.

ETIOPATHOGENESIS The etiologic role of severe coronary atherosclerosis (more than 75% compromise of lumen) of one or more of the three major coronary arterial trunks in the pathogenesis of about 90% cases of acute MI is well documented by autopsy studies as well as by coronary angiographic studies. A few notable features in the development of acute MI are as under:

1. Myocardial ischaemia Myocardial ischaemia is brought about by one or more of the following mechanisms:
i) Diminished coronary blood flow e.g. in coronary artery disease, shock.
ii) Increased myocardial demand e.g. in exercise, emotions.
iii) Hypertrophy of the heart without simultaneous increase of coronary blood flow e.g. in hypertension, valvular heart disease.

2. Role of platelets Rupture of an atherosclerotic plaque exposes the subendothelial collagen to platelets which undergo aggregation, activation and release reaction. These events contribute to the build-up of the platelet mass that may give rise to emboli or initiate thrombosis.

3. Acute plaque rupture In general, slowly-developing coronary ischaemia from stenosing coronary atherosclerosis of high-grade may not cause acute MI but continue to produce episodes of angina pectoris. But acute complications in coronary atherosclerotic plaques in the form of superimposed coronary thrombosis due to plaque rupture and plaque haemorrhage is frequently encountered in cases of acute MI:
i) *Superimposed coronary thrombosis* due to disruption of plaque is seen in about half the cases of acute MI. Infusion of intracoronary fibrinolysins in the first half an hour of development of acute MI in such cases restores blood flow in the blocked vessel in majority of cases.
ii) *Intramural haemorrhage* is found in about one-third cases of acute MI.
  Plaque haemorrhage and thrombosis may occur together in some cases.

4. Non-atherosclerotic causes About 10% cases of acute MI are caused by non-atherosclerotic factors such as coronary vasospasm, arteritis, coronary ostial stenosis, embolism, thrombotic diseases, trauma and outside compression as already described.

5. Transmural *versus* subendocardial infarcts There are some differences in the pathogenesis of the *transmural infarcts* involving the full thickness of ventricular wall and the *subendocardial (laminar) infarcts* affecting the inner subendocardial one-third to half. These are as under **(Table 25.5)**:
i) *Transmural (full thickness) infarcts* are the most common type seen in 95% cases. Critical coronary narrowing (more than 75% compromised lumen) is of great significance in the causation of such infarcts. Atherosclerotic plaques with superimposed thrombosis and intramural haemorrhage are significant in about 90% cases, and non-atherosclerotic causes in the remaining 10% cases.
ii) *Subendocardial (laminar) infarcts* have their genesis in reduced coronary perfusion due to coronary atherosclerosis but without critical stenosis (not necessarily 75% compromised lumen), aortic stenosis or haemorrhagic shock. This

	FEATURE	TRANSMURAL INFARCT	SUBENDOCARDIAL INFARCT
1.	Definition	Full-thickness, solid	Inner third to half, patchy
2.	Frequency	Most frequent (95%)	Less frequent
3.	Distribution	Specific area of coronary supply	Circumferential
4.	Pathogenesis	> 75% coronary stenosis	Hypoperfusion of myocardium
5.	Coronary thrombosis	Common	Rare
6.	Epicarditis	Common	None

Table 25.5 Contrasting features of subendocardial and transmural infarcts.

is because subendocardial myocardium is normally least well perfused by coronaries and thus is more vulnerable to any reduction in the coronary flow. Superimposed coronary thrombosis is frequently encountered in these cases too, and hence the beneficial role of fibrinolytic treatment in such patients.

TYPES OF INFARCTS Infarcts have been classified in a number of ways by the physicians and the pathologists:
1. *According to the anatomic region of the left ventricle involved*, they are called anterior, posterior (inferior), lateral, septal and circumferential, and their combinations like anterolateral, posterolateral (or inferolateral) and anteroseptal.
2. *According to the degree of thickness of the ventricular wall involved*, infarcts are of two types (Fig. 25.23):
i) Full-thickness or transmural, when they involve the entire thickness of the ventricular wall.
ii) Subendocardial or laminar, when they occupy the inner subendocardial half of the myocardium.
3. *According to the age of infarcts,* they are of two types:
i) Newly-formed infarcts called as acute, recent or fresh.
ii) Advanced infarcts called as old, healed or organised.

LOCATION OF INFARCTS Infarcts are most frequently located in the left ventricle. Right ventricle is less susceptible to infarction due to its thin wall, having less metabolic requirements and is thus adequately nourished by the thebesian vessels. Atrial infarcts, whenever present, are more often in the right atrium, usually accompanying the infarct of the left ventricle. Left atrium is relatively protected from infarction because it is supplied by the oxygenated blood in the left atrial chamber.

The region of infarction depends upon the area of obstructed blood supply by one or more of the three coronary arterial trunks. Accordingly, there are three regions of myocardial infarction (Fig. 25.24):
1. *Stenosis of the left anterior descending coronary artery* is the most common (40-50%). The region of infarction is the anterior part of the left ventricle including the apex and the anterior two-thirds of the interventricular septum.
2. *Stenosis of the right coronary artery* is the next most frequent (30-40%). It involves the posterior part of the left ventricle and the posterior one-third of the interventricular septum.
3. *Stenosis of the left circumflex coronary artery* is seen least frequently (15-20%). Its area of involvement is the lateral wall of the left ventricle.

MORPHOLOGIC FEATURES The gross and microscopic changes in the myocardial infarction vary according to the age of the infarct and are therefore described sequentially (Table 25.6).

Grossly, most infarcts occur singly and vary in size from 4 to 10 cm. As explained above, they are found most often in the left ventricle. Less often, there are multifocal lesions. The transmural infarcts, which by definition involve the entire thickness of the ventricular wall, usually have a thin rim of preserved subendocardial myocardium which is perfused directly by the blood in the ventricular chamber. The subendocardial infarcts which affect the inner subendocardial half of the myocardium produce less well-defined gross changes than the transmural infarcts. The sequence of macroscopic changes in all myocardial infarcts is as under:

1. *In 6 to 12 hours old infarcts,* no striking gross changes are discernible except that the affected myocardium is slightly paler and drier than normal. However, the early infarcts (3 to 6 hours old) can be detected by histochemical staining for *dehydrogenases* on unfixed slice of the heart. This consists of immersing a slice of unfixed heart in the solution of triphenyltetrazolium chloride (TTC) which

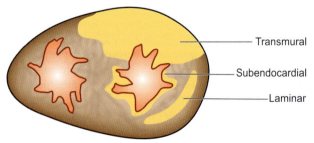

Figure 25.23 ▶ Diagrammatic representation of extent of myocardial infarction in the depth of myocardium.

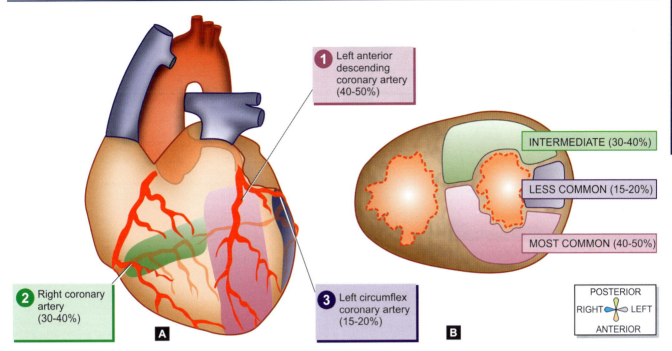

Figure 25.24 ▶ Common locations and the regions of involvement in myocardial infarction. The figure shows region of myocardium affected by stenosis of three respective coronary trunks in descending order shown as: 1) left anterior descending coronary, 2) right coronary and 3) left circumflex coronary artery. A, As viewed from anterior surface. B, As viewed on transverse section at the apex of the heart.

imparts red brown colour to the normal heart muscle, while the area of infarcted muscle fails to stain due to lack of dehydrogenases. Another stain for viability of cardiac muscle is nitroblue tetrazolium (NBT) dye which imparts blue colour to unaffected cardiac muscle while infarcted myocardium remains unstained.

Table 25.6	Sequential pathologic changes in myocardial infarction.	
TIME	GROSS CHANGES	LIGHT MICROSCOPY
FIRST WEEK		
0-6 hours	No change or pale; TTC/ NBT test negative in infarcted area	No change; (?) stretching and waviness of fibres
6-12 hours	-do-	Coagulative necrosis begins; neutrophilic infiltration begins; oedema and haemorrhages present
24 hours	Cyanotic red-purple area of haemorrhage	Coagulative necrosis progresses; marginal neutrophilic infiltrate
48-72 hours	Pale, hyperaemic	Coagulative necrosis complete, neutrophilic infiltrate well developed
3rd -7th day	Hyperaemic border, centre yellow and soft	Neutrophils are necrosed and gradually disappear, beginning of resorption of necrosed fibres by macrophages, onset of fibrovascular response
SECOND WEEK		
10th day	Red-purple periphery	Most of the necrosed muscle in a small infarct removed; fibrovascular reaction more prominent; pigmented macrophages, eosinophils, lymphocytes, plasma cells present
14th day	—	Necrosed muscle mostly removed; neutrophils disappear; fibrocollagenic tissue at the periphery
THIRD WEEK	—	Necrosed muscle fibres from larger infarcts removed; more ingrowth of fibrocollagenic tissue
FOURTH TO SIXTH WEEK	Thin, grey-white, hard, shrunken fibrous scar	Increased fibrocollagenic tissue, decreased vascularity; fewer pigmented macrophages, lymphocytes and plasma cells

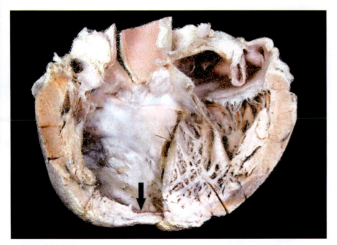

Figure 25.25 ▶ Myocardial infarction, healed. Opened up left heart shows grey white thinning of myocardium at the apex (arrow) due to healed fibrous scarring.

2. *By about 24 hours,* the infarct develops cyanotic, red-purple, blotchy areas of haemorrhage due to stagnation of blood.

3. *During the next 48 to 72 hours,* the infarct develops a yellow border due to neutrophilic infiltration and thus becomes more well-defined.

4. *In 3-7 days,* the infarct has hyperaemic border while the centre is yellow and soft.

5. *By 10 days,* the periphery of the infarct appears reddish-purple due to growth of granulation tissue. With the passage of time, further healing takes place; the necrotic muscle is resorbed and the infarct shrinks and becomes pale grey.

6. *By the end of 6 weeks,* the infarcted area is replaced by a thin, grey-white, hard, shrunken fibrous scar which is well developed in about 2 to 3 months. However, the time taken by an infarct to heal by fibrous scar may vary depending upon the size of the infarct and adequacy of collateral circulation (Fig. 25.25).

Microscopically, the changes are similar in both transmural and subendocardial infarcts. As elsewhere in the body, myocardial ischaemia induces ischaemic coagulative necrosis of the myocardium which eventually heals by fibrosis. However, sequential light microscopic changes are observed as described here and diagrammatically shown in Fig. 25.26.

1. **First week** The progression of changes takes place in the following way:

i) In the *first 6 hours* after infarction, usually no detectable histologic change is observed in routine light microscopy. However, some investigators have described stretching and waviness of the myocardial fibres within one hour of the onset of ischaemia.

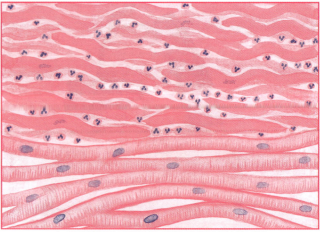

A, CHANGES DURING THE FIRST 24 HOURS

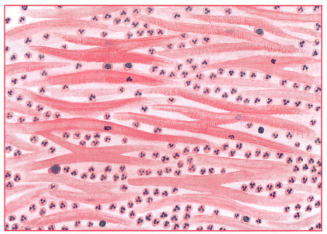

B, CHANGES DURING THE FIRST 48-72 HOURS

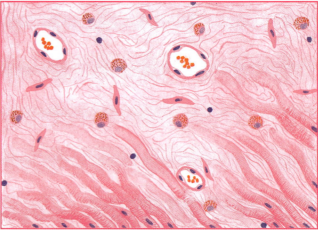

C, CHANGES BY THE END OF FIRST WEEK

Figure 25.26 ▶ Sequence of light microscopic changes in myocardial infarction (For details, consult the text).

ii) *After 6 hours,* there is appearance of some oedema fluid between the myocardial fibres. The muscle fibres at the margin of the infarct show vacuolar degeneration called myocytolysis.

iii) By *12 hours,* coagulative necrosis of the myocardial fibres sets in and neutrophils begin to appear at the margin of the infarct. Coagulative necrosis of fibres is characterised by loss of striations and intense eosinophilic, hyaline appearance and may show nuclear changes like karyolysis, pyknosis and karyorrhexis. Haemorrhages and oedema are present in the interstitium.

iv) During *first 24 hours,* coagulative necrosis progresses further as evidenced by shrunken eosinophilic cytoplasm and pyknosis of the nuclei. The neutrophilic infiltrate at the margins of the infarct is slight.

v) During *first 48 to 72 hours,* coagulative necrosis is complete with loss of nuclei. The neutrophilic infiltrate is well developed and extends centrally into the interstitium.

vi) *In 3-7 days,* neutrophils are necrosed and gradually disappear. The process of resorption of necrosed muscle fibres by macrophages begins. Simultaneously, there is onset of proliferation of capillaries and fibroblasts from the margins of the infarct (Fig. 25.27).

2. Second week The changes are as under:

i) By *10th day,* most of the necrosed muscle at the periphery of infarct is removed. The fibrovascular reaction at the margin of infarct is more prominent. Many pigmented macrophages containing yellow-brown lipofuscin (derived from breakdown of myocardial cells) and golden brown haemosiderin (derived from lysed erythrocytes in haemorrhagic areas) are seen. Also present are a few other inflammatory cells like eosinophils, lymphocytes and plasma cells.

ii) By the *end of the 2nd week,* most of the necrosed muscle in small infarcts is removed, neutrophils have almost disappeared, and newly laid collagen fibres replace the periphery of the infarct.

3. Third week Necrosed muscle fibres from larger infarcts continue to be removed and replaced by ingrowth of newly formed collagen fibres. Pigmented macrophages as well as lymphocytes and plasma cells are prominent while eosinophils gradually disappear.

4. Fourth to sixth week With further removal of necrotic tissue, there is increase in collagenous connective tissue, decreased vascularity and fewer pigmented macrophages, lymphocytes and plasma cells. Thus, at the end of 6 weeks, a contracted fibrocollagenic scar with diminished vascularity is formed. The pigmented macrophages may persist for a long duration in the scar, sometimes for years.

A summary of the sequence of gross and microscopic changes in myocardial infarction of varying duration is presented in Table 25.6.

SALVAGE IN EARLY INFARCTS AND REPERFUSION INJURY In vast majority of cases of acute MI, occlusive coronary artery thrombosis has been demonstrated superimposed on fibrofatty plaque. The ischaemic injury to myocardium is reversible if perfusion is restored within the first 30 minutes of onset of infarction failing which irreversible ischaemic necrosis of myocardium sets in. The salvage in early infarcts can be achieved by the following interventions:

1. Institution of *thrombolytic therapy* with thrombolytic agents such as streptokinase and tissue plasminogen activator (door-to-needle time ≤30 minutes).
2. *Percutaneous transluminal coronary angioplasty (PTCA).*
3. *Coronary artery stenting.*
4. *Coronary artery bypass surgery.*

However, late attempt at reperfusion is fraught with the risk of ischaemic reperfusion injury (page 32). Further myonecrosis during reperfusion occurs due to rapid influx of calcium ions and generation of toxic oxygen free radicals.

Grossly, the myocardial infarct following reperfusion injury appears *haemorrhagic* rather than pale.

Microscopically, myofibres show *contraction band necrosis* which are transverse and thick eosinophilic bands.

CHANGES IN EARLY INFARCTS By special techniques like electron microscopy, chemical and histochemical studies, changes can be demonstrated in early infarcts before detectable light microscopic alterations appear.

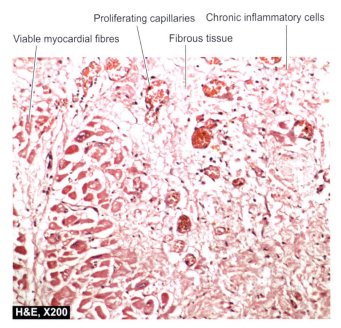

Figure 25.27 ▶ Old myocardial infarct. The infarcted area shows ingrowth of inflammatory granulation tissue.

1. **Electron microscopic changes** Changes by EM examination are evident in less than half an hour on onset of infarction. These changes are as under:
i) Disappearance of perinuclear glycogen granules within 5 minutes of ischaemia.
ii) Swelling of mitochondria in 20 to 30 minutes.
iii) Disruption of sarcolemma.
iv) Nuclear alterations like peripheral clumping of nuclear chromatin.

2. **Chemical and histochemical changes** Analysis of tissues from early infarcts by chemical and histochemical techniques has shown a number of findings. These are as follows:
i) Glycogen depletion in myocardial fibres within 30 to 60 minutes of infarction.
ii) Increase in lactic acid in the myocardial fibres.
iii) Loss of K^+ from the ischaemic fibres.
iv) Increase of Na^+ in the ischaemic cells.
v) Influx of Ca^{++} into the cells causing irreversible cell injury.
Based on the above observations and on leakage of enzymes from the ischaemic myocardium, alterations in the concentrations of various enzymes are detected in the blood of these patients.

DIAGNOSIS The diagnosis of acute MI is made on the observations of 3 types of features—clinical features, ECG changes, and serum enzyme determinations.

1. **Clinical features** Typically, acute MI has a sudden onset. The following clinical features usually characterise a case of acute MI.
i) *Pain:* Usually sudden, severe, crushing and prolonged, substernal or precordial in location, unrelieved by rest or nitroglycerin, often radiating to one or both the arms, neck and back.
ii) *Indigestion:* Pain is often accompanied by epigastric or substernal discomfort interpreted as 'heartburn' with nausea and vomiting.
iii) *Apprehension:* The patient is often terrified, restless and apprehensive due to great fear of death.

iv) *Shock:* Systolic blood pressure is below 80 mmHg; lethargy, cold clammy limbs, peripheral cyanosis, weak pulse, tachycardia or bradycardia are often present.
v) *Oliguria:* Urine flow is usually less than 20 ml per hour.
vi) *Low grade fever:* Mild rise in temperature occurs within 24 hours and lasts up to one week, accompanied by leucocytosis and elevated ESR.
vii) *Acute pulmonary oedema:* Some cases develop severe pulmonary congestion due to left ventricular failure and develop suffocation, dyspnoea, orthopnoea and bubbling respiration.

2. **ECG changes** The ECG changes are one of the most important parameters. Most characteristic ECG change is ST segment elevation in acute MI (termed as STEMI); other changes inlcude T wave inversion and appearance of wide deep Q waves **(Fig. 25.28)**.

3. **Serum cardiac markers** Certain proteins and enzymes are released into the blood from necrotic heart muscle after acute MI. Measurement of their levels in serum is helpful in making a diagnosis and plan management. Rapid assay of some more specific cardiac proteins is available rendering the estimation of non-specific estimation of SGOT of historical importance only in current practice. Important myocardial markers in use nowadays are as under **(Fig. 25.29)**:

i) *Creatine phosphokinase (CK) and CK-MB* CK has three forms—
a) CK-MM derived from skeletal muscle;
b) CK-BB derived from brain and lungs; and
c) CK-MB, mainly from cardiac muscles and insignificant amount from extracardiac tissue.

Thus, total CK estimation lacks specificity while elevation of CK-MB isoenzyme is considerably specific for myocardial damage. CK-MB has further 2 forms—CK-MB2 is the myocardial form while CK-MB1 is extracardiac form. A ratio of CK-MB2: CK-MB1 above 1.5 is highly sensitive for the diagnosis of acute MI after 4-6 hours of onset of myocardial ischaemia. CK-MB disappears from blood by 48 hours.

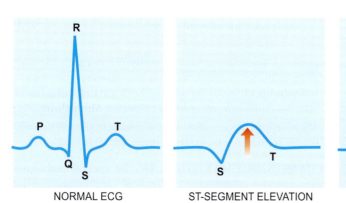
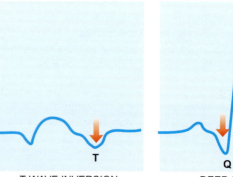

Figure 25.28 ▶ Some common ECG changes in acute myocardial infarction.

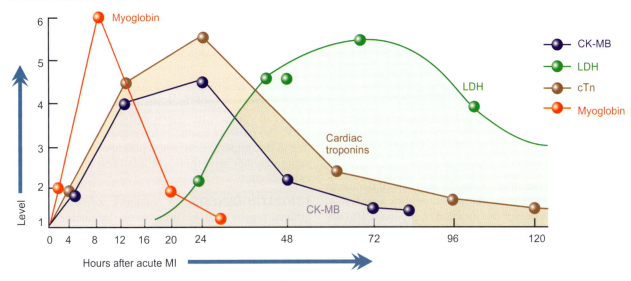

Figure 25.29 ▶ Time course of serum cardiac markers for the diagnosis of acute MI.

ii) *Lactate dehydrogenase (LDH)* Total LDH estimation also lacks specificity since this enzyme is present in various tissues besides myocardium such as in skeletal muscle, kidneys, liver, lungs and red blood cells. However, like CK, LDH too has two isoforms of which LDH-1 is myocardial-specific. Estimation of ratio of LDH-1 : LDH-2 above 1 is reasonably helpful in making a diagnosis. LDH levels begin to rise after 24 hours, reach peak in 3 to 6 days and return to normal in 14 days.

iii) *Cardiac-specific troponins (cTn)* Immunoassay of cTn as a serum cardiac marker has rendered LDH estimation obsolete. Troponins are contractile muscle proteins present in human cardiac and skeletal muscle but cardiac troponins are specific for myocardium. There are two types of cTn:
a) cardiac troponin T (cTnT); and
b) cardiac troponin I (cTnI).

Both cTnT and cTnI are not found in the blood normally, but after myocardial injury their levels rise very high around the same time when CK-MB is elevated (i.e. after 4-6 hours). Both troponin levels remain high for much longer duration; cTnI for 7-10 days and cTnT for 10-14 days.

iv) *Myoglobin* Though myoglobin is the first cardiac marker to become elevated after myocardial infarction, it lacks cardiac specificity and is excreted in the urine rapidly. Its levels, thus, return to normal within 24 hours of attack of acute MI.

COMPLICATIONS Following an attack of acute MI, only 10-20% cases do not develop major complications and recover. The remainder 80-90% cases develop one or more major complications, some of which are fatal. The immediate mortality from acute MI (sudden cardiac death) is about 25%. The important complications which may develop following acute MI are as follows:

1. **Arrhythmias** Arrhythmias (or abnormalities in the normal heart rhythm) are the most common complication in acute MI. These occur due to ischaemic injury or irritation to the conduction system, resulting in abnormal rhythm. Other causes of arrhythmias include leakage of K^+ from ischaemic muscle cells and increased concentration of lactate and free fatty acids in the tissue fluid. Arrhythmias may be in the form of sinus tachycardia or sinus bradycardia, atrial fibrillation, premature systoles, and the most serious ventricular fibrillation responsible for many sudden cardiac deaths.

2. **Congestive heart failure** About half the patients with MI develop CHF which may be in the form of right ventricular failure, left ventricular failure or both. CHF is responsible for about 40% of deaths from acute MI. If the patient survives, healing may restore normal cardiac function but in some CHF may persist and require regular treatment later.

3. **Cardiogenic shock** About 10% of patients with acute MI develop cardiogenic shock characterised by hypotension with systolic blood pressure of 80 mmHg or less for many days. Shock may be accompanied by peripheral circulatory failure, oliguria and mental confusion.

4. **Mural thrombosis and thromboembolism** The incidence of thromboembolism from intracardiac thrombi and from thrombosis in the leg veins is 15-45% in cases of acute MI and is the major cause of death in 12% cases. Mural thrombosis in the heart develops due to involvement of the endocardium and subendocardium in the infarct and due to slowing of the heart rate. Mural thrombi often form thromboemboli. Another source of thromboemboli is the venous thrombosis in the leg veins due to prolonged bed rest. Thromboemboli from either source may cause occlusion of the pulmonary,

renal, mesenteric, splenic, pancreatic or cerebral arteries and cause infarcts in these organs.

5. Rupture Rupture of the heart occurs in up to 5% cases of acute MI causing death. Rupture occurs most often from the infarcted ventricular wall into the pericardial cavity causing haemopericardium and tamponade. Other sites of rupture are through interventricular septum and rupture of a papillary muscle in infarct of the left ventricle. Rupture at any of these sites occurs usually in the first week and is often fatal.

6. Cardiac aneurysm Another 5% of patients of acute MI develop aneurysm, often of the left ventricle. It occurs in healed infarcts through thin, fibrous, non-elastic scar tissue. Cardiac aneurysms impair the function of the heart and are the common sites for mural thrombi. Rarely, calcification of the wall of aneurysm may occur.

7. Pericarditis Sterile pericarditis appearing on about the second day is common over transmural infarcts. It is characterised by fibrinous pericarditis and may be associated with pericardial effusion. Often, it is of no functional significance and resolves spontaneously.

8. Postmyocardial infarction syndrome About 3 to 4% of patients who suffered from acute MI develop postmyocardial infarction syndrome or *Dressler's syndrome* subsequently. It usually occurs 1 to 6 weeks after the attack of MI. It is characterised by pneumonitis. The symptoms are usually mild and disappear in a few weeks. The exact pathogenesis of this syndrome is not known. It may be due to autoimmune reaction as evidenced by circulating anti-heart antibodies in the serum of these patients. But these antibodies are also present in some patients with acute MI who do not develop this syndrome.

Chronic Ischaemic Heart Disease

Chronic ischaemic heart disease, ischaemic cardiomyopathy or myocardial fibrosis, are the terms used for focal or diffuse fibrosis in the myocardium characteristically found in elderly patients of progressive IHD. Such small areas of fibrous scarring are commonly found in the heart of patients who have history of episodes of angina and attacks of MI some years back. The patients generally have gradually developing CHF due to decompensation over a period of years. Occasionally, serious cardiac arrhythmias or infarction may supervene and cause death.

ETIOPATHOGENESIS In majority of cases, coronary atherosclerosis causes progressive ischaemic myocardial damage and replacement by myocardial fibrosis. A small percentage of cases may result from other causes such as emboli, coronary arteritis and myocarditis.

The mechanism of development of myocardial fibrosis can be explained by one of the following concepts:
i) Myocardial fibrosis represents healing of minute infarcts involving small scattered groups of myocardial fibres.
ii) An alternate concept of development of myocardial fibrosis is healing of minute areas of focal myocytolysis—the myocardial fibres in a small area undergo slow degeneration due to myocardial ischaemia. These fibres lose their myofibrils but nuclei remain intact. These foci are infiltrated by macrophages and eventually are replaced by proliferating fibroblasts and collagen.

> *MORPHOLOGIC FEATURES Grossly,* the heart may be normal in size or hypertrophied. The left ventricular wall generally shows foci of grey-white fibrosis in brown myocardium. Healed scars of previous MI may be present.

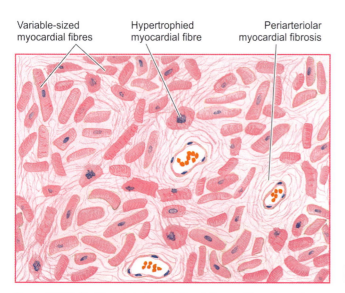
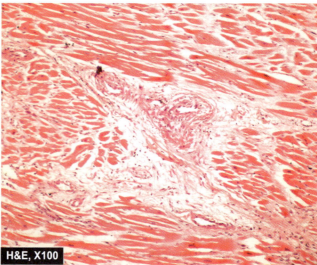

Figure 25.30 ▶ Chronic ischaemic heart disease. There is patchy myocardial fibrosis, especially around small blood vessels in the interstitium. The intervening single cells and groups of myocardial cells show myocytolysis.

Valves of the left heart may be distorted, thickened and show calcification. Coronary arteries invariably show moderate to severe atherosclerosis.

Microscopically, the characteristic features are as follows **(Fig. 25.30)**:

i) There are scattered areas of diffuse myocardial fibrosis, especially around the small blood vessels in the interstitial tissue of the myocardium.
ii) Intervening single fibres and groups of myocardial fibres show variation in fibre size and foci of myocytolysis.
iii) Areas of brown atrophy of the myocardium may also be present.
iv) Coronary arteries show atherosclerotic plaques and may have complicated lesions in the form of superimposed thrombosis.

Sudden Cardiac Death

Sudden cardiac death is defined as sudden death within 24 hours of the onset of cardiac symptoms. The most important cause is coronary atherosclerosis; less commonly it may be due to coronary vasospasm and other non-ischaemic causes. These include: calcific aortic stenosis, myocarditis of various types, hypertrophic cardiomyopathy, mitral valve prolapse, endocarditis, and hereditary and acquired defects of the conduction system. The mechanism of sudden death by myocardial ischaemia is almost always by fatal arrhythmias, chiefly ventricular asystole or fibrillation.

MORPHOLOGIC FEATURES At autopsy, such cases reveal most commonly critical atherosclerotic coronary narrowing (more than 75% compromised lumen) in one or more of the three major coronary arterial trunks with superimposed thrombosis or plaque-haemorrhage. Healed and new myocardial infarcts are found in many cases.

Table 25.7 lists the important forms of coronary artery pathology in various types of IHD.

| GIST BOX 25.5 | Ischaemic Heart Disease |

- Ischaemic heart disease (IHD) is acute or chronic cardiac disability arising from imbalance between the myocardial supply and demand for oxygenated blood.
- Atherosclerotic coronary artery disease (CAD) is the most common cause of IHD, most commonly of LAD, others are RCA and CXA. Often, there are superimposed changes on the plaque.
- *Acute coronary syndromes* include a triad of acute myocardial infarction, unstable angina and sudden cardiac death
- Angina pectoris results from transient myocardial ischaemia and is characterised by paroxysmal pain in the substernal or precordial region.
- Acute myocardial infarction (MI) is the most important and feared consequence of coronary artery disease.

Table 25.7 Lesions in coronary artery in various forms of IHD.

	TYPES OF IHD	CORONARY LESION	MORPHOLOGY	CLINICAL EFFECTS
1.	Stable angina	• Critical coronary narrowing (3/4th)	A, Normal	Nil
2.	Chronic IHD	• Chronic progressive coronary atherosclerosis	B, Severe, fixed 3/4th narrowing	Stable angina, CIHD
3.	Unstable (pre-infarction) angina	• Plaque rupture, haemorrhage, ulceration • Mural thrombosis with thromboembolism		
4.	Myocardial infarction	• Plaque haemorrhage • Fissuring and ulceration • Complete mural thrombosis	C, Thrombosis with haemorrhage	Plaque haemorrhage, unstable angina
5.	Sudden ischaemic death	• Severe multivessel disease • Acute changes in plaque • Thrombosis with thromboembolism	D, Occlusive thrombosis	Acute coronary syndromes

- Early thrombolyitc therapy within 30 minutes of occurrence may help in restoration of blood supply.
- ❖ The gross and microscopic changes in the myocardial infarction, most often in the left ventricle, vary according to the age of the infarct.
- ❖ The diagnosis of acute MI is made by clinical features, ECG changes, and serum enzyme determinations.
- ❖ Chronic ischaemic heart disease is focal or diffuse fibrosis in the myocardium characteristically found in elderly patients of progressive IHD.
- ❖ Sudden death by myocardial ischaemia is almost always by fatal arrhythmias, chiefly ventricular asystole or fibrillation.

RHEUMATIC HEART DISEASE

Rheumatic fever (RF) is a systemic, post-streptococcal, non-suppurative inflammatory disease, principally affecting the heart, joints, central nervous system, skin and subcutaneous tissues. The chronic stage of RF involves all the layers of the heart (pancarditis) causing major cardiac sequelae referred to as rheumatic heart disease (RHD). In spite of its name suggesting an acute arthritis migrating from joint to joint, it is well known that it is the heart rather than the joints which is first and major organ affected. Decades ago, William Boyd gave the dictum *'rheumatism licks the joint, but bites the whole heart.'*

INCIDENCE

The disease appears most commonly in children between the age of 5 to 15 years when the streptococcal infection is most frequent and intense. Both the sexes are affected equally, though some investigators have noted a slight female preponderance.

The geographic distribution, incidence and severity of RF and RHD are generally related to the frequency and severity of streptococcal pharyngeal infection. The disease is seen more commonly in poor socioeconomic strata of the society living in damp and overcrowded places which promote interpersonal spread of the streptococcal infection. Its incidence has declined in the developed countries as a result of improved living conditions and early use of antibiotics in streptococcal infection. But it is still common in the developing countries of the world, particularly prevalent in Indian subcontinent (India, Pakistan, Bangladesh, Nepal, Afghanistan), some Arab countries, sub-Saharan Africa and some South American countries. In India, RHD and RF continue to be a major public health problem. In a multicentric survey in school-going children by the Indian Council of Medical Research, an incidence of 1 to 5.5 per 1000 children has been reported.

ETIOPATHOGENESIS

After a long controversy, the etiologic role of preceding throat infection with β-haemolytic streptococci of group A in RF is now well accepted. However, the mechanism of lesions in the heart, joints and other tissues is not by direct infection but by induction of hypersensitivity or autoimmunity in a susceptible host. Thus, there are 3 types of factors in the etiology and pathogenesis of RF and RHD: *environmental factors, host susceptibility* and *immunologic evidences.*

A. ENVIRONMENTAL FACTORS There is sufficient clinical and epidemiological evidence to support the concept that RF occurs following infection of the throat and upper respiratory tract with β-haemolytic streptococci of Lancefield group A. These evidences are as under:

1. There is often a *history* of infection of the pharynx, upper respiratory tract with this microorganism about 2 to 3 weeks prior to the attack of RF. This period is usually the latent period required for sensitisation to the bacteria.
2. *Subsequent or ongoing attacks* of streptococcal infection are generally associated with recurrent episodes of acute RF.
3. A higher incidence of RF has been observed after outbreaks and *epidemics* of streptococcal infection of throat in children from schools or in young men from training camps.
4. Administration of *antibiotics* leads to lowering of the incidence as well as severity of RF and its recurrences.
5. Cardiac lesions similar to those seen in RHD have been produced in experimental animals by *induction* of repeated infection with β-haemolytic streptococci of group A.
6. *Socioeconomic factors* like poverty, poor nutrition, density of population, overcrowding in quarters for sleeping etc are associated with spread of infection, lack of proper medical attention, and hence higher incidence of RF.
7. The *geographic distribution* of the disease, as already pointed out, shows higher frequency and severity of the disease in the developing countries of the world where the living conditions in underprivileged populations are substandard and medical facilities are insufficient. Children in these regions develop recurrent throat infections which remain untreated and have higher incidence of RF.
8. The role of *climate* in the development of RF has been reported by some workers. The incidence of the disease is higher in subtropical and tropical regions with cold, damp climate near the rivers and waterways which favour the spread of infection.

Despite all these evidences, only a small proportion of patients with streptococcal pharyngeal infection develop RF—the attack rate is less than 3%. There is a suggestion that a *concomitant virus* enhances the effect of streptococci in individuals who develop RF.

B. HOST SUSCEPTIBILITY Since all individuals with streptococcal infections do not develop RF, role of inherited characteristic for the disease has been reported:

1. Clustering of disease in *families.*
2. Occurrence in *identical twins.*
3. Individuals with *HLA class II* alleles have strong association with RF.

4. First-degree relatives of patients with RF and RHD have increased expression of a particular alloantigen, *D8-17*, on B cells, which may act as a marker for *inherited susceptibility* for the disease.

C. IMMUNOLOGIC EVIDENCE It has been observed that though throat of patients during acute RF may contain streptococci, the clinical symptoms of RF appear after a delay of 2-3 weeks and the organisms cannot be grown from the lesions in the target tissues. This has led to the concept that lesions have immune pathogenesis. Evidences in support are as under:

1. Patients with RF have *elevated titres* of antibodies to the antigens of β-haemolytic streptococci of group A such as anti-streptolysin O (ASO) and S, anti-streptokinase, anti-streptohyaluronidase and anti-DNAase B.
2. *Cell wall polysaccharide* of group A *Streptococcus* forms antibodies which are reactive against cardiac valves. This is supported by observation of persistently elevated corresponding autoantibodies in patients who have cardiac valvular involvement than those without cardiac valve involvement.
3. *Hyaluronatecapsule* of group A *Streptococcus* is identical to human hyaluronate present in joint tissues and thus these tissues are the target of attack.
4. *Membrane antigens* of group A *Streptococcus* react with sarcolemma of smooth and cardiac muscle, dermal fibroblasts and neurons of caudate nucleus.

SUMMARY OF ORGANISM-HOST SUSCEPTIBILITY-IMMUNITY HYPOTHESIS Combining the three types of evidences given above, pathogenesis of RF-RHD can be summed up as under **(Fig. 25.31)**:

1. A susceptible host, on being encountered with group A *Streptococcus* infection, mounts an *autoimmune reaction* by formation of autoantibodies against bacteria.
2. These autoantibodies cause damage to human tissues due to *cross-reactivity* between epitopes in the components of bacteria and the host.
3. Streptococcal epitopes present on the bacterial cell wall, cell membrane and the *streptococcal M protein*, are immunologically identical to human molecules on myosin, keratin, actin, laminin, vimentin and N-acetylglucosamine.
4. *Molecular mimicry and cross-reactivity* between streptococcal M protein in particular and the human molecules forms the basis of autoimmune damage to human target tissues in RHD i.e. cardiac muscle, valves, joints, skin, neurons etc.

MORPHOLOGIC FEATURES

RF is generally regarded as an autoimmune focal inflammatory disorder of the connective tissues throughout the body. The *cardiac lesions* of RF in the form of pancarditis, particularly the valvular lesions, are its major manifestations. However, supportive connective tissues at other sites like the synovial membrane, periarticular tissue, skin and subcutaneous tissue, arterial wall, lungs, pleura and the CNS are all affected (*extracardiac lesions*).

A. Cardiac Lesions

The cardiac manifestations of RF are in the form of focal inflammatory involvement of the interstitial tissue of all the three layers of the heart, the so-called *pancarditis*. The pathognomonic feature of pancarditis in RF is the presence of distinctive *Aschoff nodules* or *Aschoff bodies*.

THE ASCHOFF NODULES OR BODIES The Aschoff nodules or the Aschoff bodies are spheroidal or fusiform distinct tiny structures, 1-2 mm in size, occurring in the interstitium of the heart in RF and may be visible to naked eye. They are especially found in the vicinity of small blood vessels in the myocardium and endocardium and

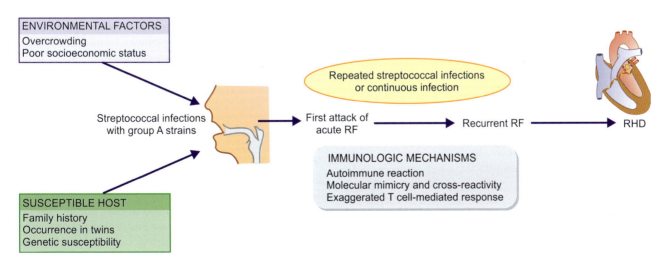

Figure 25.31 ▶ Pathogenesis of RHD, schematic evolution.

occasionally in the pericardium and the adventitia of the proximal part of the aorta. Lesions similar to the Aschoff nodules may be found in the extracardiac tissues.

Evolution of fully-developed Aschoff bodies occurs through 3 stages all of which may be found in the same heart at different stages of development. These are as follows:

1. **Early (exudative or degenerative) stage** The earliest sign of injury in the heart in RF is apparent by about 4th week of illness. Initially, there is oedema of the connective tissue and increase in acid mucopolysaccharide in the ground substance. This results in separation of the collagen fibres by accumulating ground substance. Eventually, the collagen fibres are fragmented and disintegrated and the affected focus takes the appearance and staining characteristics of fibrin. This change is referred to as *fibrinoid degeneration*.

2. **Intermediate (proliferative or granulomatous) stage** It is this stage of the Aschoff body which is pathognomonic of rheumatic conditions (Fig. 25.32). This stage is apparent in 4th to 13th week of illness. The early stage of fibrinoid change is followed by proliferation of cells that includes infiltration by lymphocytes (mostly T cells), plasma cells, a few neutrophils and the characteristic *cardiac histiocytes (Anitschkow cells)* at the margin of the lesion. Cardiac histiocytes or Anitschkow cells are present in small numbers in normal heart but their number is increased in the Aschoff bodies; therefore they are not characteristic of RHD. These are large mononuclear cells having central round nuclei and contain moderate amount of amphophilic cytoplasm. The nuclei are vesicular and contain prominent central chromatin mass which in longitudinal section appears serrated or caterpillar-like, while in cross-section the chromatin mass appears as a small rounded body in the centre of the vesicular nucleus, just like an owl's eye. Some of these modified cardiac histiocytes become multinucleate cells containing 1 to 4 nuclei and are called *Aschoff cells* and are pathognomonic of RHD.

3. **Late (healing or fibrous) stage** The stage of healing by fibrosis of the Aschoff nodule occurs in about *12 to 16 weeks* after the illness. The nodule becomes oval or fusiform in shape, about 200 μm wide and 600 μm long. The Anitschkow cells in the nodule become spindle-shaped with diminished cytoplasm and the nuclei stain solidly rather than showing vesicular character. These cells tend to be arranged in a palisaded manner. With passage of months and years, the Aschoff body becomes less cellular and the collagenous tissue is increased. Eventually, it is replaced by a small fibrocollagenous scar with little cellularity, frequently in perivascular location.

RHEUMATIC PANCARDITIS Although all the three layers of the heart are affected in RF, the intensity of their involvement is variable.

1. RHEUMATIC ENDOCARDITIS Endocardial lesions of RF may involve the valvular and mural endocardium, causing *rheumatic valvulitis* and *mural endocarditis*, respectively. Rheumatic valvulitis is chiefly responsible for the major cardiac manifestations in chronic RHD.

RHEUMATIC VALVULITIS *Grossly*, the valves in **acute RF** show thickening and loss of translucency of the valve leaflets or cusps. This is followed by the formation of characteristic, small (1 to 3 mm in diameter), multiple, warty *vegetations* or *verrucae*, chiefly along the line of closure of the leaflets and cusps. These tiny vegetations are almost continuous so that the free margin of the cusps or leaflets appears as a rough and irregular ridge. The vegetations in RF appear grey-brown, translucent and are firmly attached so that they are not likely to get detached to form emboli, unlike the friable vegetations of infective endocarditis (page 509).

Though all the four heart valves are affected, their frequency and severity of involvement varies: mitral valve alone being the most common site, followed in decreasing order of frequency, by combined mitral and aortic valve (Fig. 25.33). The tricuspid and pulmonary valves usually show infrequent and slight involvement. The higher incidence of vegetations on left side of the heart is possibly because of the greater mechanical stresses on the valves of the left heart, especially along the line of closure of the valve cusps (Fig. 25.34, A). The occurrence of vegetations on the atrial surfaces of the atrioventricular valves (mitral and tricuspid) and on the ventricular surface of the semilunar

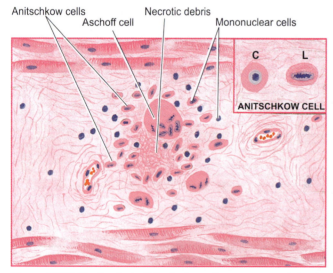

Figure 25.32 ▶ An Aschoff body (granulomatous stage) in the myocardium. *Inbox* shows Anitschkow cell in longitudinal section (LS) with caterpillar-like serrated nuclear chromatin, while cross section (CS) shows owl-eye appearance of central chromatin mass and perinuclear halo.

Chapter 25: Diseases of Cardiovascular System

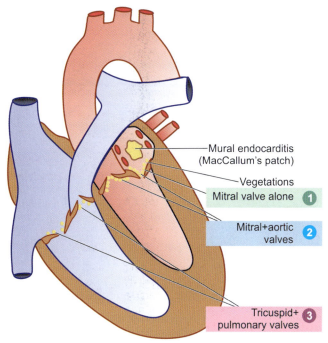

Figure 25.33 ▶ Schematic representation of the anatomic regions of involvement and location of vegetations in rheumatic endocarditis (both valvular and mural). Serial numbers 1, 2 and 3 are denoted for the frequency of valvular involvement.

The **chronic stage of RHD** is characterised by permanent deformity of one or more valves, especially the mitral (in 98% cases alone or along with other valves) and aortic. The approximate frequency of deformity of various valves is as under:

- Mitral alone = 37% cases.
- Mitral + aortic = 27% cases.
- Mitral + aortic + tricuspid = 22% cases.
- Mitral + tricuspid = 11% cases.
- Aortic alone = 2%.
- Mitral + aortic + tricuspid + pulmonary = less than 1% cases.

Thus, mitral valve is almost always involved in RHD. Gross appearance of chronic healed mitral valve in RHD is characteristically *'fish mouth'* or *'button hole'* stenosis. Mitral stenosis and insufficiency are commonly combined in chronic RHD; calcific aortic stenosis may also be found. These healed chronic valvular lesions in RHD occur due to diffuse fibrocollagenous thickening and calcification of the valve cusps or leaflets which cause adhesions between the lateral portions, especially in the region of the commissures. Thickening, shortening and fusion of the chordae tendineae further contribute to the chronic valvular lesions **(Fig. 25.34, B)**.

Microscopically, the inflammatory changes begin in the region of the valve rings (where the leaflets are attached to the fibrous annulus) and then extend throughout the entire leaflet, whereas vegetations are usually located on the free margin of the leaflets and cusps.

valves (aortic and pulmonary) further lends support to the role of mechanical pressure on the valves in the pathogenesis of vegetations.

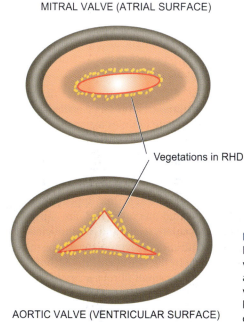

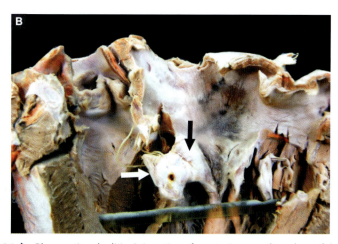

Figure 25.34 ▶ Rheumatic valvulitis. A, Location of vegetations on the valves of the left heart. The location of vegetations on mitral valve (left upper diagram) is shown as viewed from the left atrium, while the vegetations on aortic valve (left lower diagram) are shown as seen from the left ventricular surface. B, Opened up chambers and valves of the left heart show irregularly scarred mitral valve leaving a fish-mouth or buttonhole opening between its two cusps (black arrow). The free surface and margin of the mitral valve shows tiny firm granular vegetations (white arrow).

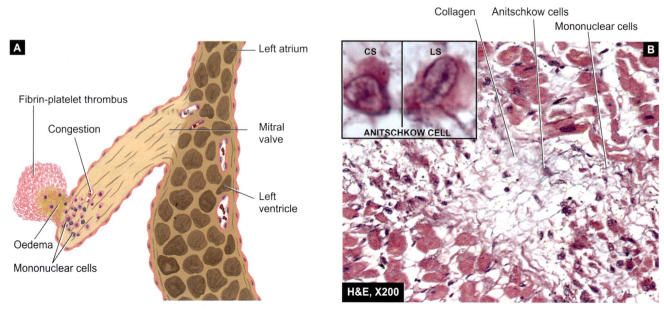

Figure 25.35 ▶ Rheumatic heart disease. A, Microscopic structure of the rheumatic valvulitis and a vegetation on the cusp of mitral valve in sagittal section. B, Section of the myocardium shows a healed Aschoff nodule in the interstitium having collagen, sparse cellularity, a multinucleate giant cell and Anitschkow cells. Inbox shows an Anitschkow cell in cross section (CS) and in longitudinal section (LS).

i) In the **early (acute) stage,** the histological changes are oedema of the valve leaflet, presence of increased number of capillaries and infiltration with lymphocytes, plasma cells, histiocytes with many Anitschkow cells and a few polymorphs. Occasionally, Aschoff bodies with central foci of fibrinoid necrosis and surrounded by palisade of cardiac histiocytes are seen, but more often the cellular infiltration is diffuse in acute stage of RF. Vegetations present at the free margins of cusps appear as eosinophilic, tiny structures mainly consisting of fibrin with superimposed platelet-thrombi and do not contain bacteria **(Fig. 25.35, A)**.

ii) In the **healed (chronic) stage,** the vegetations have undergone organisation. The valves show diffuse thickening as a result of fibrous tissue with hyalinisation, and often calcification. Vascularisation of the valve cusps may still be evident in the form of thick-walled blood vessels with narrowed lumina **(Fig. 25.35, B)**. Typical Aschoff bodies are rarely seen in the valves at this stage.

RHEUMATIC MURAL ENDOCARDITIS Mural endocardium may also show features of rheumatic carditis though the changes are less conspicuous as compared to valvular changes.

Grossly, the lesions are seen most commonly as *MacCallum's patch* which is the region of endocardial surface in the posterior wall of the left atrium just above the posterior leaflet of the mitral valve. MacCallum's patch appears as a map-like area of thickened, roughened and wrinkled part of the endocardium *(see Fig. 25.33)*.

Microscopically, the appearance of MacCallum's patch is similar to that seen in rheumatic valvulitis. The affected area shows oedema, fibrinoid change in the collagen, and cellular infiltrate of lymphocytes, plasma cells and macrophages with many Anitschkow cells. Typical Aschoff bodies may sometimes be found.

2. RHEUMATIC MYOCARDITIS *Grossly*, in the *early (acute) stage*, the myocardium, especially of the left ventricle, is soft and flabby. In the *intermediate stage,* the interstitial tissue of the myocardium shows small foci of necrosis. Later, tiny pale foci of the Aschoff bodies may be visible throughout the myocardium.

Microscopically, the most characteristic feature of rheumatic myocarditis is the presence of distinctive Aschoff bodies. These diagnostic nodules are scattered throughout the interstitial tissue of the myocardium and are most frequent in the interventricular septum, left ventricle and left atrium. Derangements of the conduction system may, thus, be present. The Aschoff bodies are best identified in the intermediate stage when they appear as granulomas with central fibrinoid necrosis and are surrounded by palisade of Anitschkow cells and multinucleate Aschoff cells. There is infiltration by lymphocytes, plasma cells and some neutrophils. In the late stage, the Aschoff bodies are gradually replaced by small fibrous scars in the vicinity of blood vessels and the inflammatory infiltrate subsides. Presence of active Aschoff bodies along with old healed lesions is indicative of rheumatic activity.

3. RHEUMATIC PERICARDITIS Inflammatory involvement of the pericardium commonly accompanies RHD.

Grossly, the usual finding is fibrinous pericarditis in which there is loss of normal shiny pericardial surface due to deposition of fibrin on its surface and accumulation of slight amount of fibrinous exudate in the pericardial sac. If the parietal pericardium is pulled off from the visceral pericardium, the two separated surfaces are shaggy due to thick fibrin covering them. This appearance is often likened to *'bread and butter appearance'* i.e. resembling the buttered surfaces of two slices in a sandwich when they are gently pulled apart. If fibrinous pericarditis fails to resolve and, instead, undergoes organisation, the two layers of the pericardium form fibrous adhesions resulting in chronic adhesive pericarditis.

Microscopically, fibrin is identified on the surfaces. The subserosal connective tissue is infiltrated by lymphocytes, plasma cells, histiocytes and a few neutrophils. Characteristic Aschoff bodies may be seen which later undergo organisation and fibrosis. Organisation of the exudate causes fibrous adhesions between the visceral and parietal surfaces of the pericardial sac and obliterates the pericardial cavity.

B. Extracardiac Lesions

Patients of the syndrome of acute rheumatism develop lesions in connective tissue elsewhere in the body, chiefly the joints, subcutaneous tissue, arteries, brain and lungs.

1. POLYARTHRITIS Acute and painful inflammation of the synovial membranes of some of the joints, especially the larger joints of the limbs, is seen in about 90% cases of RF in adults and less often in children. As pain and swelling subside in one joint, others tend to get involved, producing the characteristic *'migratory polyarthritis'* involving two or more joints at a time.

Histologically, the changes are transitory. The synovial membrane and the periarticular connective tissue show hyperaemia, oedema, fibrinoid change and neutrophilic infiltration. Sometimes, focal lesions resembling Aschoff bodies are observed. A serous effusion into the joint cavity is commonly present.

2. SUBCUTANEOUS NODULES The subcutaneous nodules of RF occur more often in children than in adult. These nodules are small (0.5 to 2 cm in diameter), spherical or ovoid and painless. They are attached to deeper structures like tendons, ligaments, fascia or periosteum and therefore often remain unnoticed by the patient. Characteristic locations are extensor surfaces of the wrists, elbows, ankles and knees.

Histologically, the subcutaneous nodules of RF are representative of giant Aschoff bodies of the heart. They consist of 3 distinct zones: a central area with fibrinoid changes, surrounded by a zone of histiocytes and fibroblasts forming a palisade arrangement, and the outermost zone of connective tissue which is infiltrated by non-specific chronic inflammatory cells and proliferating blood vessels.

It may be mentioned here that histologically similar but clinically different subcutaneous lesions appear in rheumatoid arthritis; they are larger, painful and tender and persist for months to years.

3. ERYTHEMA MARGINATUM This non-pruritic erythematous rash is characteristic of RF. The lesions occur mainly on the trunk and proximal parts of the extremities. The erythematous area develops central clearing and has slightly elevated red margins. The erythema is transient and migratory.

4. RHEUMATIC ARTERITIS Arteritis in RF involves not only the coronary arteries and the aorta but also occurs in arteries of various other organs such as renal, mesenteric and cerebral arteries. The lesions in the coronaries are seen mainly in the small intramyocardial branches.

Histologically, the lesions may be like those of hypersensitivity angiitis, or sometimes may resemble polyarteritis nodosa. Occasionally, foci of fibrinoid necrosis or ill-formed Aschoff bodies may be present close to the vessel wall.

5. CHOREA MINOR Chorea minor or Sydenham's chorea or Saint Vitus' dance is a delayed manifestation of RF as a result of involvement of the central nervous system. The condition is characterised by disordered and involuntary jerky movements of the trunk and the extremities accompanied by some degree of emotional instability. The condition occurs more often in younger age, particularly in girls.

Histologically, the lesions are located in the cerebral hemispheres, brainstem and the basal ganglia. They consist of small haemorrhages, oedema and perivascular infiltration of lymphocytes. There may be endarteritis obliterans and thrombosis of cortical and meningeal vessels.

6. RHEUMATIC PNEUMONITIS AND PLEURITIS Involvement of the lungs and pleura occurs rarely in RF. Pleuritis is often accompanied with serofibrinous pleural effusion but definite Aschoff bodies are not present. In rheumatic pneumonitis, the lungs are large, firm and rubbery.

Histologically, the changes are oedema, capillary haemorrhages and focal areas of fibrinous exudate in the alveoli. Aschoff bodies are generally not found.

PROGNOSIS

If the heart is spared in a case of acute RF, the patient may have complete recovery without any sequelae. However, once the heart is involved, it is often associated with reactivation and recurrences of the disease. Myocarditis, in particular, is the most life-threatening due to involvement of the conduction system of the heart and results in serious arrhythmias. The long-term sequelae or **stigmata** are the chronic valvular deformities, especially the mitral stenosis, as already just explained. Initially, a state of compensation occurs, while later decompensation of the heart leads to full-blown cardiac failure. Currently, surgical replacement of the damaged valves can alter the clinical course of the disease.

The major **causes of death** in RHD are cardiac failure, bacterial endocarditis and embolism:
1. *Cardiac failure* is the most common cause of death from RHD. In young patients, cardiac failure occurs due to the chronic valvular deformities, while in older patients coronary artery disease may be superimposed on the old RHD.
2. *Bacterial endocarditis* of both acute and subacute type may supervene due to inadequate use of antibiotics.
3. *Embolism* in RHD originates most commonly from mural thrombi in the left atrium and its appendages, in association with mitral stenosis. The organs most frequently affected are the brain, kidneys, spleen and lungs.
4. *Sudden death* may occur in RHD as a result of ball thrombus in the left atrium or due to acute coronary insufficiency in association with aortic stenosis.

GIST BOX 25.6 — Rheumatic Heart Disease

- Rheumatic fever is a systemic, post-streptococcal, non-suppurative inflammatory disease, principally affecting the heart, joints, central nervous system, skin and subcutaneous tissues.
- The chronic stage of RF involves all the layers of the heart (pancarditis) causing major cardiac sequelae referred to as rheumatic heart disease (RHD).
- The disease is more common in children between the age of 5 to 15 years.
- There are 3 types of factors in the etiology and pathogenesis of RF and RHD: environmental factors, host susceptibility and immunologic evidences.
- The pathognomonic feature of pancarditis in RF is the presence of distinctive Aschoff nodules or Aschoff bodies.
- The chronic stage of RHD is characterised by permanent deformity of one or more valves, especially the mitral (alone or with other valves) and aortic.
- Patients of RF-RHD develop extra-cardiac lesions in connective tissue elsewhere in the body, chiefly the joints, subcutaneous tissue, arteries, brain and lungs.

NON-RHEUMATIC ENDOCARDITIS

Inflammatory involvement of the endocardial layer of the heart is called endocarditis. Though in common usage, if not specified endocarditis would mean inflammation of the valvular endocardium, several workers designate endocarditis on the basis of anatomic area of the involved endocardium such as: *valvular* for valvular endocardium, *mural* for inner lining of the lumina of cardiac chambers, *chordal* for the endocardium of the chordae tendineae, *trabecular* for the endocardium of trabeculae carneae, and *papillary* for the endocardium covering the papillary muscles. Endocarditis can be broadly grouped into *non-infective* and *infective* types **(Table 25.8)**. Most types of endocarditis are characterised by the presence of 'vegetations' or 'verrucae' which have distinct features.

ATYPICAL VERRUCOUS (LIBMAN-SACKS) ENDOCARDITIS

Libman and Sacks, two American physicians, described a form of endocarditis in 1924 that is characterised by sterile endocardial vegetations which are distinguishable from the vegetations of RHD and bacterial endocarditis.

ETIOPATHOGENESIS Atypical verrucous endocarditis is one of the manifestations of 'collagen diseases'. Characteristic lesions of Libman-Sacks endocarditis are seen in *50%* cases of *acute systemic lupus erythematosus (SLE)*; other diseases associated with this form of endocarditis are systemic sclerosis, thrombotic thrombocytopenic purpura (TTP) and other collagen diseases.

MORPHOLOGIC FEATURES **Grossly**, characteristic vegetations occur most frequently on the mitral and tricuspid valves. The vegetations of atypical verrucous endocarditis are small (1 to 4 mm in diameter), granular, multiple and tend to occur on both surfaces of affected valves, in the valve pockets and on the adjoining ventricular and atrial endocardium. The vegetations are sterile unless superimposed by bacterial endocarditis.

Table 25.8 — Classification of endocarditis.

A. NON-INFECTIVE
 1. Rheumatic endocarditis (page 502)
 2. Atypical verrucous (Libman-Sacks) endocarditis
 3. Non-bacterial thrombotic (cachectic, marantic) endocarditis

B. INFECTIVE
 1. Bacterial endocarditis
 2. Other infective types (tuberculous, syphilitic, fungal, viral, rickettsial)

Unlike vegetations of RHD, the healed vegetations of Libman-Sacks endocarditis do not produce any significant valvular deformity. Frequently, fibrinous or serofibrinous pericarditis with pericardial effusion is associated.

Microscopically, the verrucae of Libman-Sacks endocarditis are composed of fibrinoid material with superimposed fibrin and platelet thrombi. The endocardium underlying the verrucae shows characteristic histological changes which include fibrinoid necrosis, proliferation of capillaries and infiltration by histiocytes, plasma cells, lymphocytes, neutrophils and the pathognomonic *haematoxylin bodies of Gross* which are counterparts of LE cells of the blood. Similar inflammatory changes may be found in the interstitial connective tissue of the myocardium. The Aschoff bodies are never found in the endocardium or myocardium.

NON-BACTERIAL THROMBOTIC (CACHECTIC, MARANTIC) ENDOCARDITIS

Non-bacterial thrombotic, cachectic, marantic or terminal endocarditis or endocarditis simplex is an involvement of the heart valves by sterile thrombotic vegetations.

ETIOPATHOGENESIS The exact pathogenesis of lesions in non-bacterial thrombotic endocarditis (NBTE) is not clear. Vegetations are found at autopsy in 0.5 to 5% of cases. Following diseases and conditions are frequently associated with their presence:
1. In patients having *hypercoagulable state* from various etiologies e.g. advanced cancer (in 50% case of NBTE) especially mucinous adenocarcinomas, chronic tuberculosis, renal failure and chronic sepsis. In view of its association with chronic debilitating and wasting diseases, alternate names for NBTE such as 'cachectic', 'marantic' and 'terminal' endocarditis are used synonymously.
2. Occurrence of these lesions in young and well-nourished patients is explained on the basis of *alternative hypothesis* such as allergy, vitamin C deficiency, deep vein thrombosis, and endocardial trauma (e.g. due to catheter in pulmonary artery and haemodynamic trauma to the valves).

MORPHOLOGIC FEATURES ***Grossly,*** the verrucae of NBTE are located on cardiac valves, chiefly mitral, and less often aortic and tricuspid valve. These verrucae are usually small (1 to 5 mm in diameter), single or multiple, brownish and occur along the line of closure of the leaflets but are more friable than the vegetations of RHD. Organised and healed vegetations appear as fibrous nodules. Normal age-related appearance of tag-like appendage at the margin of the valve cusps known as 'Lambl's excrescences' is an example of such healed lesions.

Microscopically, the vegetations in NBTE are composed of fibrin along with entangled RBCs, WBCs and platelets. Vegetations in NBTE are sterile, bland and do not cause tissue destruction. The underlying valve shows swollen collagen, fibrinoid change and capillary proliferation but does not show any inflammatory infiltrate.

Embolic phenomenon is seen in many cases of NBTE and results in infarcts in the brain, lungs, spleen and kidneys. The bland vegetations of NBTE on infection may produce bacterial endocarditis.

INFECTIVE (BACTERIAL) ENDOCARDITIS

DEFINITION Infective or bacterial endocarditis (IE or BE) is serious infection of the valvular and mural endocardium caused by different forms of microorganisms and is characterised by typical infected and friable vegetations. A few specific forms of IE are named by the microbial etiologic agent causing them e.g. tubercle bacilli, fungi etc. Depending upon the severity of infection, BE is subdivided into 2 clinical forms:

1. **Acute bacterial endocarditis (ABE)** is fulminant and destructive acute infection of the endocardium by highly virulent bacteria in a previously normal heart and almost invariably runs a rapidly fatal course in a period of 2-6 weeks.

2. **Subacute bacterial endocarditis (SABE) or endocarditis lenta** (*lenta* = slow) is caused by less virulent bacteria in a previously diseased heart and has a gradual downhill course in a period of 6 weeks to a few months and sometimes years.

Although classification of bacterial endocarditis into acute and subacute forms has been largely discarded because the clinical course is altered by antibiotic treatment, still a few important distinguishing features are worth noting (Table 25.9). However, features of the vegetations in the two forms of BE are difficult to distinguish.

INCIDENCE Introduction of antibiotic drugs has helped greatly in lowering the incidence of BE as compared with its

Table 25.9 Distinguishing features of acute and subacute bacterial endocarditis.

	FEATURE	ACUTE	SUBACUTE
1.	Duration	<6 weeks	>6 weeks
2.	Most common organisms	Staph. aureus, β-streptococci	Streptococcus viridans
3.	Virulence of organisms	Highly virulent	Less virulent
4.	Previous condition of valves	Usually previously normal	Usually previously damaged
5.	Lesion on valves	Invasive, destructive, suppurative	Usually not invasive or suppurative
6.	Clinical features	Features of acute systemic infection	Splenomegaly, clubbing of fingers, petechiae

incidence in the pre-antibiotic era. Though BE may occur at any age, most cases of ABE as well as SABE occur over 50 years of age. Males are affected more often than females.

ETIOLOGY All cases of BE are caused by *infection with microorganisms* in patients having certain *predisposing factors*.

A. Infective agents About 90% cases of BE are caused by streptococci and staphylococci.

◆ *In ABE,* the most common causative organisms are virulent strains of staphylococci, chiefly *Staphylococcus aureus*. Others are pneumococci, gonococci, β-streptococci and enterococci.

◆ *In SABE,* the commonest causative organisms are the streptococci with low virulence, predominantly *Streptococcus viridans*, which forms part of normal flora of the mouth and pharynx. Other less common etiologic agents include other strains of streptococci and staphylococci (e.g. *Streptococcus bovis* which is the normal inhabitant of gastrointestinal tract, *Streptococcus pneumoniae*, and *Staphylococcus epidermidis* which is a commensal of the skin), gram-negative enteric bacilli (e.g. *E. coli, Klebsiella, Pseudomonas* and *Salmonella*), pneumococci, gonococci and *Haemophilus influenzae*.

B. Predisposing factors There are 3 main types of factors which predispose to the development of both forms of BE:

◆ Conditions initiating transient bacteraemia, septicaemia and pyaemia.
◆ Underlying heart disease.
◆ Impaired host defenses.

1. *Bacteraemia, septicaemia and pyaemia:* Bacteria gain entry to the blood stream causing transient and clinically silent bacteraemia in a variety of day-to-day procedures as well as from other sources of infection. Some of the common examples are:

i) Periodontal infections such as trauma from vigorous brushing of teeth, hard chewing, tooth extraction and other dental procedures.
ii) Infections of the genitourinary tract such as in catheterisation, cystoscopy, obstetrical procedures including normal delivery and abortions.
iii) Infections of gastrointestinal and biliary tract.
iv) Surgery of the bowel, biliary tract and genitourinary tracts.
v) Skin infections such as boils, carbuncles and abscesses.
vi) Upper and lower respiratory tract infections including bacterial pneumonias.
vii) Intravenous drug abuse.
viii) Cardiac catheterisation and cardiac surgery for implantation of prosthetic valves.

2. *Underlying heart disease:* SABE occurs much more frequently in previously diseased heart valves, whereas the ABE is common in previously normal heart. Amongst the commonly associated underlying heart diseases are the following:

i) Chronic rheumatic valvular disease in about 50% cases.

ii) Congenital heart diseases in about 20% cases. These include VSD, subaortic stenosis, pulmonary stenosis, bicuspid aortic valve, coarctation of the aorta, and PDA.
iii) Other causes are syphilitic aortic valve disease, atherosclerotic valvular disease, floppy mitral valve, and prosthetic heart valves.

3. *Impaired host defenses.* All conditions in which there is depression of specific immunity, deficiency of complement and defective phagocytic function, predispose to BE. Following are some of the examples of such conditions:
i) Impaired specific immunity in lymphomas.
ii) Leukaemias.
iii) Cytotoxic therapy for various forms of cancers and transplant patients.
iv) Deficient functions of neutrophils and macrophages.

PATHOGENESIS Bacteria causing BE on entering the blood stream from any of the above-mentioned routes are implanted on the cardiac valves or mural endocardium because they have surface adhesion molecules which mediate their adherence to injured endocardium. There are several predisposing conditions which explain the development of bacterial implants on the valves:

1. The circulating bacteria are lodged much more frequently on *previously damaged valves* from diseases, chiefly RHD, congenital heart diseases and prosthetic valves, than on healthy valves.
2. Conditions producing *haemodynamic stress* on the valves are liable to cause damage to the endothelium, favouring the formation of platelet-fibrin thrombi which get infected from circulating bacteria.
3. Another alternative hypothesis is the occurrence of *nonbacterial thrombotic endocarditis* from prolonged stress which is followed by bacterial contamination.

MORPHOLOGIC FEATURES The characteristic pathologic feature in both ABE and SABE is the presence of typical vegetations or verrucae on the valve cusps or leaflets, and less often, on mural endocardium, which are quite distinct for other types. A summary of the distinguishing features of the principal types of vegetations is presented in Table 25.10.

Grossly, the lesions are found commonly on the valves of the left heart, most frequently on the mitral, followed in descending frequency, by the aortic, simultaneous involvement of both mitral and aortic valves, and quite rarely on the valves of the right heart. The vegetations in SABE are more often seen on previously diseased valves, whereas the vegetations of ABE are often found on previously normal valves. Like in RHD, the vegetations are often located on the atrial surface of atrioventricular valves and ventricular surface of the semilunar valves. They begin from the contact areas of the valve and may extend along the surface of the valves and on to the adjacent endocardium (Fig. 25.36).

Chapter 25: Diseases of Cardiovascular System

Table 25.10 Distinguishing features of vegetations in major forms of endocarditis.

FEATURE	RHEUMATIC	LIBMAN-SACKS	NON-BACTERIAL THROMBOTIC	BACTERIAL (INFECTIVE)
1. Valves commonly affected	Mitral alone; mitral and aortic combined	Mitral, tricuspid	Mainly mitral; less often aortic and tricuspid	Mitral; aortic; combined mitral and aortic
2. Location on valve cusps or leaflets	Occur along the line of closure, atrial surface of atrioventricular valves and ventricular surface of semilunar valves	Occur on both surfaces of valve leaflets or cusps, in the valve pockets	Occur along the line of closure	SABE more often on diseased valves: ABE on previously normal valves; location same as in RHD
3. Macroscopy	Small, multiple, warty, grey brown, translucent, firmly attached, generally produce permanent valvular deformity	Medium-sized, multiple, generally do not produce significant valvular deformity	Small but larger than those of rheumatic, single or multiple, brownish, firm, but more friable than those of rheumatic	Often large, grey-tawny to greenish, irregular, single or multiple, typically friable
4. Microscopy	Composed of fibrin with superimposed platelet thrombi and no bacteria, Adjacent and underlying endocardium shows oedema, proliferation of capillaries, mononuclear inflammatory infiltrate and occasional Aschoff bodies.	Composed of fibrinoid material with superimposed fibrin and platelet thrombi and no bacteria. The underlying endocardium shows fibrinoid necrosis, proliferation of capillaries and acute and chronic inflammatory infiltrate including the haematoxylin bodies of Gross.	Composed of degenerated valvular tissue, fibrin-platelets thrombi and no bacteria. The underlying valve shows swelling of collagen, fibrinoid change, proliferation of capillaries but no significant inflammatory cell infiltrate.	Composed of outer eosinophilic zone of fibrin and platelets, covering colonies of bacteria and deeper zone of non-specific acute and chronic inflammatory cells. The underlying endocardium may show abscesses in ABE and inflammatory granulation tissue in the SABE.

The *vegetations* of BE vary in size from a few millimeters to several centimeters, grey-tawny to greenish, irregular, single or multiple, and typically *friable*. They may appear flat, filiform, fungating or polypoid. The vegetations in ABE tend to be bulkier and globular than those of SABE and are located more often on previously normal valves, may cause ulceration or perforation of the underlying valve leaflet, or may produce myocardial abscesses.

Microscopically, the vegetations of BE consist of 3 zones (Fig. 25.37):
i) The *outer layer or cap* consists of eosinophilic material composed of fibrin and platelets.
ii) Underneath this layer is the *basophilic zone* containing colonies of bacteria. However, bacterial component of the vegetations may be lacking in treated cases.
iii) The *deeper zone* consists of non-specific inflammatory reaction in the cusp itself, and in the case of SABE there may be evidence of repair.

In the acute fulminant form of the disease, the inflammatory cell infiltrate chiefly consists of neutrophils and is accompanied with tissue necrosis and abscesses in the valve rings and in the myocardium. In the subacute form, there is healing by granulation tissue, mononuclear inflammatory cell infiltration and fibroblastic proliferation. Histological evidence of pre-existing valvular disease such as RHD may be present in SABE.

COMPLICATIONS AND SEQUELAE Most cases of BE present with fever. The acute form of BE is characterised by high grade fever, chills, weakness and malaise while the subacute form of the disease has non-specific manifestations like slight fever, fatigue, loss of weight and flu-like symptoms. In the early stage, the lesions are confined to the heart, while subsequent progression of the disease leads to involvement of extra-cardiac organs. In general, severe complications develop early in ABE than in SABE. Complications and sequelae of BE are divided into cardiac and extracardiac (Fig. 25.38):

A. Cardiac complications These include the following:
i) Valvular stenosis or insufficiency
ii) Perforation, rupture, and aneurysm of valve leaflets
iii) Abscesses in the valve ring

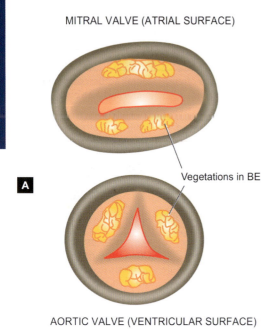

Figure 25.36 ▶ Infective endocarditis. A, Location of vegetations on the valves of the left heart. The vegetations are shown on the mitral valve (left upper diagram) as viewed from the left atrium, while those on the aortic valve (left lower diagram) are shown as seen from the left ventricle. B, Vegetations on valves in infective endocarditis. Opened up chambers and valves of the left heart show presence of irregular, soft, elevated grey white friable vegetations on the atrial (superior) surface of the mitral valve (arrow).

iv) Myocardial abscesses
v) Suppurative pericarditis
vi) Cardiac failure from one or more of the foregoing complications.

B. Extracardiac complications Since the vegetations in BE are typically friable, they tend to get dislodged due to rapid stream of blood and give rise to embolism which is responsible for very common and serious extra-cardiac complications. These are as follows:

i) Emboli originating from the *left side of the heart* and entering the systemic circulation affect organs like the spleen, kidneys, and brain causing infarcts, abscesses and mycotic aneurysms.

ii) Emboli arising from *right side of the heart* enter the pulmonary circulation and produce pulmonary abscesses.

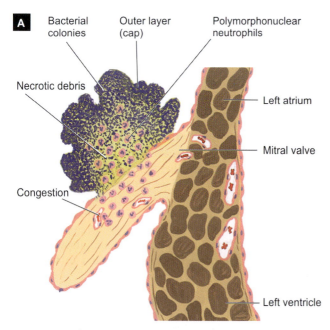
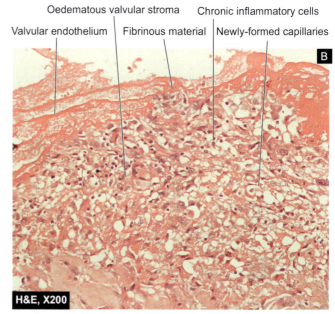

Figure 25.37 ▶ Infective endocarditis. A, Microscopic structure of a vegetation of BE on the surface of mitral valve in sagittal section. B, Section of the mitral valve shows fibrin cap on luminal surface, layer of bacteria, and deeper zone of inflammatory cells, with prominence of neutrophils.

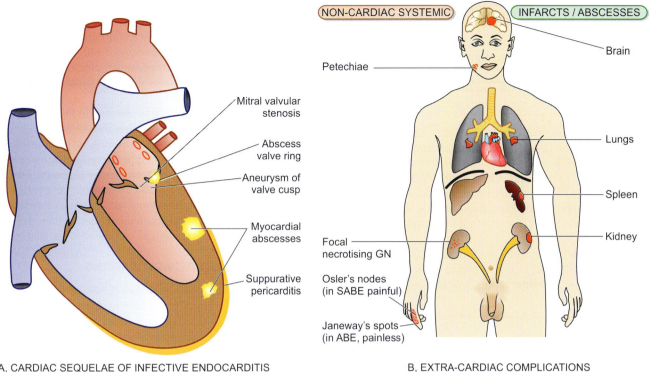

Figure 25.38 ▶ Complications and sequelae of infective endocarditis.

iii) *Petechiae* may be seen in the skin and conjunctiva due to either emboli or toxic damage to the capillaries.

iv) In SABE, there are painful, tender nodules on the finger tips of hands and feet called *Osler's nodes,* while in ABE there is appearance of painless, non-tender subcutaneous maculopapular lesions on the pulp of the fingers called *Janeway's spots.* In either case, their origin is due to toxic or allergic inflammation of the vessel wall.

v) *Focal necrotising glomerulonephritis* is seen more commonly in SABE than in ABE. Occasionally diffuse glomerulonephritis may occur. Both these have their pathogenesis in circulating immune complexes (hypersensitivity phenomenon).

Treatment of BE with antibiotics in adequate dosage kills the bacteria but complications and sequelae of healed endocardial lesions may occur even after successful therapy. The *causes of death* are cardiac failure, persistent infection, embolism to vital organs, renal failure and rupture of mycotic aneurysm of cerebral arteries.

Specific Types of Infective Endocarditis

Besides BE, various other microbes may occasionally produce infective endocarditis which are named according to the etiologic agent causing it. These include the following:

1. **Tuberculous endocarditis** Though tubercle bacilli are bacteria, tuberculous endocarditis is described separate from the bacterial endocarditis due to specific granulomatous inflammation found in tuberculosis. It is characterised by presence of typical tubercles on the valvular as well as mural endocardium and may form tuberculous thromboemboli.

2. **Syphilitic endocarditis** The endocardial lesions in syphilis have already been described in relation to syphilitic aortitis on page 151. The severest manifestation of cardiovascular syphilis is aortic valvular incompetence.

3. **Fungal endocarditis** Rarely, endocardium may be infected with fungi such as from *Candida albicans, Histoplasma capsulatum, Aspergillus, Mucor,* coccidioidomycosis, cryptococcosis, blastomycosis and actinomycosis. Opportunistic fungal infections like candidiasis and aspergillosis are seen more commonly in patients receiving long-term antibiotic therapy, intravenous drug abusers and after prosthetic valve replacement. Fungal endocarditis produces an appearance similar to that in BE but the vegetations are bulkier in fungal endocarditis.

4. **Viral endocarditis** There is only experimental evidence of existence of this entity.

5. **Rickettsial endocarditis** Another rare cause of endocarditis is from infection with rickettsiae in Q fever.

> **GIST BOX 25.7 Non-rheumatic Endocarditis**
>
> - Endocarditis can be non-infective and infective types; most types are characterised by the presence of 'vegetations' or 'verrucae'.
> - Atypical verrucous endocarditis is a manifestation of collagen diseases. Vegetations are small, granular and multiple.
> - Non-bacterial thrombotic endocarditis is an involvement of the heart valves by sterile thrombotic vegetations, often preceded by hypercoagulable state.
> - Infective or bacterial endocarditis occurs following conditions initiating transient bacteraemia, septicaemia and pyaemia, underlying heart disease and impaired host defenses. It is characterised by typical infected and friable vegetations.
> - Since vegetations in BE are typically friable, they tend to get dislodged due to rapid stream of blood and give rise to embolism and cause serious extra-cardiac complications.

PATHOLOGY OF CARDIOVASCULAR INTERVENTIONS

Nowadays, with the development of surgical and non-surgical coronary revascularisation procedures in coronary artery disease in conjunction with lifestyle changes for modifying the risk factors, it has become possible to study the pathology of native as well as grafted vessel. Besides, the myocardial tissue by endomyocardial biopsy is also accessible for histopathologic study.

ENDOMYOCARDIAL BIOPSY

Endomyocardial biopsy (EMB) is done for making a final histopathologic diagnosis in certain cardiac diseases. The main *indications* for EMB are: myocarditis, cardiac transplant cases, restrictive heart disease, infiltrative heart diseases such as in amyloidosis, storage disorders etc.

EMB is done by biopsy forceps introduced via cardiac catheter into either of the ventricles but preferably right ventricle is biopsied for its relative ease and safety. The route for the catheter may be through internal jugular vein or femoral vein for accessing the right ventricle.

BALLOON ANGIOPLASTY

Balloon angioplasty or percutaneous coronary intervention (PCI) is a non-surgical procedure that employs percutaneous insertion and manipulation of a balloon catheter into the occluded coronary artery. The balloon is inflated to dilate the stenotic artery which causes endothelial damage, plaque fracture, medial dissection and haemorrhage in the affected arterial wall. PCI is accompanied with insertion of coronary stents in the blocked coronaries with a success rate of symptoms in over 95% cases. However, case selection for PCI is important and major indications are 2 or 3 vessel block but blockage of left main coronary is a contraindication for PCI. Unstable angioplasty may be associated with acute coronary syndromes. PCI is followed by administration of anti-platelet (oral aspirin) and antithrombin therapy to avoid occurrence of coronary thrombosis.

Recurrent stenosis after metal stenting in PCI may occur within 6 months in about 20% patients, more often in patients of diabetes mellitus. Restenosis is multifactorial in etiology that includes smooth muscle cell proliferation, extracellular matrix and local thrombosis. However, widespread use of drug-delivering stents has made it possible to overcome several long-term complications of coronary stenting. Currently, stents with anti-proliferative, anti-inflammatory, cytotoxic and cytostatic agents are commercially available.

CORONARY ARTERY BYPASS GRAFTING

Coronary artery bypass grafting (CABG) employs the use of autologous grafts to replace or bypass the blocked coronary arteries. Most frequently used is autologous graft of saphenous vein which is reversed (due to valves in the vein) and transplanted, or left internal mammary artery may be used being in the operative area of the heart. Long-term follow-up of CABG surgery has yielded following observations on pathology of grafted vessel:

1. In a reversed saphenous vein graft, long-term luminal patency is 50% after 10 years. Pathologic changes which develop in grafted vein include thrombosis in early stage, intimal thickening and graft atherosclerosis with or without complicated lesions.
2. Internal mammary artery graft, however, has a patency of more than 90% after 10 years.
3. Atherosclerosis with superimposed complications may develop in native coronary artery distal to the grafted vessel as well as in the grafted vessel.

CARDIAC TRANSPLANTATION

Since the first human-to-human cardiac transplant was carried out successfully by South African surgeon Dr Christian Barnard in 1967, cardiac transplantation and prolonged assisted circulation is being done in many countries in end-stage cardiac diseases, most often in idiopathic dilated cardiomyopathy, heart failure and IHD. Worldwide, about 3,000 cardiac transplants are performed annually. The survival following heart transplants is reported as: 1 year in 85%, 5 years in 65% and 10 years in 45% cases. Major complications are: transplant rejection reaction, infections (particularly with *Toxoplasma gondii* and cytomegaloviruses), graft coronary atherosclerosis and higher incidence of malignancy due to long-term administration of immunosuppressive therapy. One of the main problems in cardiac transplant centres is the availability of donors.

The concept of cardiac stem cells resident in the heart, and possibly of bone marrow stem cells transdifferentiating into cardiac myocyte, has generated interest in treatment of patients of IHD with transplantation of these stem cells. Preliminary studies in IHD cases have yielded encouraging results in clinical improvement and reduction in infarct size and holds promise for future.

> **GIST BOX 25.8** **Pathology of Cardiovascular Interventions**
>
> ❖ Endomyocardial biopsy (EMB) from right venricle is done for making a final histopathologic diagnosis in certain cardiac diseases.
> ❖ Balloon angioplasty is percutaneous insertion and manipulation of a balloon catheter into the occluded coronary artery.
> ❖ Coronary artery bypass grafting (CABG) employs the use of autologous grafts to replace or bypass the blocked coronary arteries. Most frequently used is autologous graft of saphenous vein.
> ❖ Following CABG, atherosclerosis with superimposed complications may develop in native coronary artery distal to the grafted vessel as well as in the grafted vessel.

26 Diseases of Oral Cavity and Salivary Glands

ORAL SOFT TISSUES

NORMAL STRUCTURE

The oral cavity is the point of entry for digestive and respiratory tracts. The mucous membrane of the mouth consists of squamous epithelium covering vascularised connective tissue. The epithelium is keratinised over the hard palate, lips and gingiva, while elsewhere it is non-keratinised. Mucous glands (minor salivary glands) are scattered throughout the oral mucosa. Sebaceous glands are present in the region of the lips and the buccal mucosa only. Lymphoid tissue is present in the form of tonsils and adenoids.

The oral cavity is the site of numerous congenital and acquired diseases. Besides, many systemic diseases have oral manifestations. Some of the commonly occurring conditions are discussed here.

DEVELOPMENTAL ANOMALIES

1. FACIAL CLEFTS *Cleft upper lip (harelip) and cleft palate*, alone or in combination, are the commonest developmental anomalies of the face. These occur from the failure of fusion of facial processes.

2. FORDYCE'S GRANULES Fordyce's granules are symmetric, small, light yellow macular spots on the lips and buccal mucosa and represent collections of sebaceous glands. They remain undeveloped until puberty but occur quite commonly in adults.

3. LEUKOEDEMA This is an asymptomatic condition occurring in children and is characterised by symmetric, grey-white areas on the buccal mucosa. Histologically, there is pronounced intracellular oedema. There is no increased malignant potential compared to leukoplakia discussed below.

4. DEVELOPMENTAL DEFECTS OF THE TONGUE These are as under:

i) **Macroglossia** is the enlargement of the tongue, usually due to lymphangioma or haemangioma, and sometimes due to amyloid tumour.

ii) **Microglossia and aglossia** are rare congenital anomalies representing small-sized and absence of tongue respectively.

iii) **Fissured tongue (scrotal, furrowed or grooved tongue)** is a genetically-determined condition characterised by numerous small furrows or grooves on the dorsum of the tongue. It is often associated with mild glossitis.

iv) **Bifid tongue** is a rare condition occurring due to failure of the two lateral halves of the tongue to fuse in the midline.

v) **Tongue tie** occurs when the lingual fraenum is quite short, or when the fraenum is attached near the tongue tip.

vi) **Hairy tongue** is not a true developmental defect, but is mentioned here because of its similarity with other conditions discussed here. The filiform papillae are hypertrophied and elongated. These 'hairs' (papillae) are stained black, brown or yellowish-white by food, tobacco, oxidising agents or by oral flora.

MUCOCUTANEOUS LESIONS

Lesions of the oral mucosa occur in many diseases of the skin and they are similar in morphology. Some of these are listed as under:

LICHEN PLANUS Characteristically, oral lichen planus appears as interlacing network of whitening or keratosis on the buccal mucosa but other oral tissues such as gingiva, tongue and palate may also be involved.

VESICULAR LESIONS A number of vesicular or bullous diseases of the skin have oral lesions.

i) **Pemphigus vulgaris** Vesicular oral lesions appear invariably in all cases at some time in the course of pemphigus vulgaris. In about half the cases oral lesions are the initial manifestations.

ii) **Pemphigoid** Vesicles or bullae appear on oral mucosa as well as on conjunctiva in pemphigoid and are seen more often in older women.

iii) **Erythema multiforme** Subepithelial vesicles may occur on the skin as well as mucosae.

iv) **Stevens-Johnson syndrome** It is a rather fatal and severe form of erythema multiforme involving oral and other mucous membranes occurring following ingestion of sulfa drugs.

v) **Epidermolysis bullosa** It is a hereditary condition having subepidermal bullae on the skin as well as has oral lesions.

INFLAMMATORY AND PIGMENTARY DISEASES

STOMATITIS Inflammation of the mucous membrane of the mouth is called stomatitis. It can occur in the course of several different diseases.

i) **Aphthous, ulcers (Canker sores)** These are the commonest form of oral ulcerations. The etiology is unknown but may be precipitated by emotional factors, stress, allergy, hormonal imbalance, nutritional deficiencies, gastrointestinal disturbances, trauma etc. The condition is characterised by painful oral ulcers, 1 cm or more in size. Recurrent *aphthae* may form a part of Behçet's syndrome and inflammatory bowel disease.

ii) Herpetic stomatitis It is an acute disease occurring in infants and young children. It is the most common manifestation of primary infection with herpes simplex virus. The lesions are in the form of vesicles around the lips. Similar lesions may appear on the genital skin. Recurrent attacks occur due to stress, emotional upsets and upper respiratory infections.

iii) Necrotising stomatitis (Noma or Cancrum oris) This occurs more commonly in poorly-nourished children like in kwashiorkor; infectious diseases such as measles, immunodeficiencies and emotional stress. The lesions are characterised by necrosis of the marginal gingiva and may extend on to oral mucosa, causing cellulitis of the tissue of the cheek. The condition may progress to gangrene of the cheek.

iv) Mycotic infections Fungal infections commonly involving the oral mucosa are actinomycosis and candidiasis.
❖ *Cervicofacial actinomycosis* is the commonest form of the disease developing at the angle of the mandible (page 151).
❖ *Candidiasis (moniliasis or thrush)* is caused by *Candida albicans* which is a commensal in the mouth (page 182). It appears as an opportunistic infection in immuno-compromised host. There are erythematous lesions on the palate and angular cheilitis.

GLOSSITIS **Acute glossitis** characterised by swollen papillae occurs in eruptions of measles and scarlet fever. In **chronic glossitis,** the tongue is raw and red without swollen papillae and is seen in malnutrition such as in pellagra, ariboflavinosis and niacin deficiency. In iron deficiency anaemia, pernicious anaemia and sprue, there is *chronic atrophic glossitis* characterised by atrophied papillae and smooth raw tongue.

SYPHILITIC LESIONS Oral lesions may occur in primary, secondary, tertiary and congenital syphilis (page 149).
i) Extragenital chancre of *primary syphilis* occurs most commonly on the lips.
ii) *Secondary syphilis* shows maculopapular eruptions and mucous patches in the mouth.
iii) In the *tertiary syphilis,* gummas or diffuse fibrosis may be seen on the hard palate and tongue.
iv) Oral lesions of the *congenital syphilis* are fissures at the angles of mouth and characteristic peg-shaped notched Hutchinson's incisors.

TUBERCULOUS LESIONS Involvement of the mouth in tuberculosis is rare. The lesions are in the form of ulcers or elevated nodules.

HIV INFECTION HIV infection of low grade as well as full-blown acquired immunodeficiency syndrome (AIDS) are

Table 26.1	Oral manifestations of AIDS.
A.	**OPPORTUNISTIC INFECTIONS**
Fungal :	Candidiasis (oral thrush)
	Histoplasmosis
	Cryptococcosis
Bacterial :	Dental caries and periodontitis
	Mycobacterial infections
Viral :	Herpetic stomatitis
	Cytomegalovirus
	Human papillomavirus
B.	**TUMOURS**
	Kaposi's sarcoma
	Squamous cell carcinoma
	Non-Hodgkin's lymphoma
C.	**OTHERS**
	Hairy leukoplakia
	Recurrent aphthous ulcers

associated with oral manifestations such as opportunistic infections, malignancy, hairy leukoplakia and others; these are listed in **Table 26.1**. About half the cases of Kaposi's sarcoma have intraoral lesions as part of systemic involvement (page 350).

PIGMENTARY LESIONS Oral and labial melanotic pigmentation may be observed in certain systemic and metabolic disorders such as Addison's disease, Albright syndrome, Peutz-Jeghers syndrome and haemochromatosis. All types of pigmented naevi as well as malignant melanoma can occur in oral cavity. Exogenous pigmentation such as due to deposition of lead sulfide can also occur.

TUMOURS AND TUMOUR-LIKE LESIONS

Benign and malignant tumours as also a number of tumour-like lesions and premalignant lesions are encountered in the oral soft tissues. A list of such lesions is presented in **Table 26.2**.

A. Tumour-like Lesions

A number of proliferative lesions arising from the oral tissues are tumour-like masses which clinically may resemble neoplasms. Some of these are as under:

FIBROUS GROWTHS Fibrous growths of the oral soft tissues are very common. These are not true tumours (unlike intraoral fibroma and papilloma), but are instead inflammatory or irritative in origin. A few common varieties are as under:

i) Fibroepithelial polyps occur due to irritation or chronic trauma. These are composed of reparative fibrous tissue, covered by a thin layer of stratified squamous epithelium.

ii) Fibrous epulis is a lesion occurring on the gingiva and is localised hyperplasia of the connective tissue following

Section VI: Selected Topics from Systemic Pathology

Table 26.2 Classification of tumours and tumour-like lesions of the oral soft tissues.

A. **TUMOUR-LIKE LESIONS**
   1. Fibrous growths
      (Fibroepithelial polyps, fibrous epulis, denture hyperplasia)
   2. Pyogenic granuloma
   3. Mucocele
   4. Ranula
   5. Dermoid cyst

B. **BENIGN TUMOURS**
   1. Squamous papilloma
   2. Haemangioma
   3. Lymphangioma
   4. Fibroma
   5. Fibromatosis gingivae
   6. Tumours of minor salivary glands
      (e.g. Pleomorphic adenoma)
   7. Granular cell myoblastoma
   8. Other rare benign tumours

C. **PREMALIGNANT LESIONS**
   1. Hyperkeratotic leukoplakia
   2. Dysplastic leukoplakia

D. **MALIGNANT TUMOURS**
   1. Squamous cell (Epidermoid) carcinoma
   2. Other malignant tumours

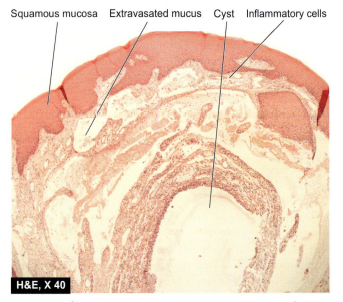

Figure 26.2 ▶ Mucous retention cyst (mucocele). There is inflammatory reaction around extravasated mucus.

trauma or inflammation in the area (Fig. 26.1). *Giant cell epulis* is a variant seen more commonly in females as reactive change to trauma; the lesion shows numerous osteoclast-like giant cells and vascular stroma.

iii) Denture hyperplasia occurs in edentulous or partly edentulous patients. The lesion is an inflammatory hyperplasia in response to local irritation by ill-fitting denture or an elongated tooth.

PYOGENIC GRANULOMA This is an elevated, bright red swelling of variable size occurring on the lips, tongue, buccal mucosa and gingiva. It is a vasoproliferative inflammatory lesion. *Pregnancy tumour* is a variant of pyogenic granuloma.

MUCOCELE Also called mucous cyst or retention cyst, it is a cystic dilatation of the mucous glands of the oral mucosa. The cyst often ruptures on distension and incites inflammatory reaction due to mucous extravasation (Fig. 26.2).

RANULA It is a large mucocele located on the floor of the mouth. The cyst is lined by true epithelial lining.

DERMOID CYST This tumour-like mass in the floor of the mouth represents a developmental malformation. The cyst is lined by stratified squamous epithelium. The cyst wall contains sebaceous glands, sweat glands, hair follicles and other mature tissues.

B. Benign Tumours

Different parts of the mouth have a variety of mesodermal tissues and keratinising and non-keratinising epithelium. Therefore, majority of neoplasms arising from the oral tissues are just like their counterparts in other parts of the body. Some of the common benign tumours of the mouth are as under:

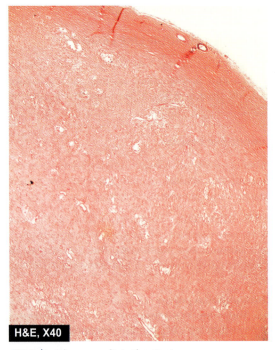

Figure 26.1 ▶ Fibrous epulis in the gingiva.

SQUAMOUS PAPILLOMA Papilloma can occur anywhere in the mouth and has the usual papillary or finger-like projections (page 321).

Microscopically, each papilla is composed of vascularised connective tissue covered by squamous epithelium.

HAEMANGIOMA Haemangioma can occur anywhere in the mouth; when it occurs on the tongue it may cause macroglossia. It is most commonly capillary type, although cavernous and mixed types may also occur (page 346).

LYMPHANGIOMA Lymphangioma may develop most commonly on the tongue producing macroglossia; on the lips producing macrocheilia, and on the cheek. *Cystic hygroma* is a special variety of lymphangioma occurring in children on the lateral side of neck (page 348).

Microscopically, lymphangioma is characterised by large lymphatic spaces lined by endothelium and containing lymph.

FIBROMA Although most common benign oral mucous membrane mass is fibroma appearing as a discrete superficial pedunculated mass, it appears to be non-neoplastic in nature. It probably arises as a response to physical trauma.

Microscopically, fibroma is composed of collagenic fibrous connective tissue covered by stratified squamous epithelium (page 336).

FIBROMATOSIS GINGIVAE This is a fibrous overgrowth of unknown etiology involving the entire gingiva. Sometimes the fibrous overgrowth is so much that the teeth are covered by fibrous tissue.

TUMOURS OF MINOR SALIVARY GLANDS Minor salivary glands present in the oral cavity may sometimes be the site of origin of salivary tumours similar to those seen in the major salivary glands (page 516). Pleomorphic adenoma is a common example.

GRANULAR CELL TUMOUR Earlier called as granular cell myoblastoma, it is benign tumour which now by electron microscopic studies is known to be mesenchymal in origin than odontogenic. The most common location is the tongue but may occur in any other location on the oral cavity. It occurs exclusively in females. A similar lesion seen in infants is termed as congenital epulis.

Microscopically, the tumour is composed of large polyhedral cells with granular, acidophilic cytoplasm. The covering epithelium usually shows pronounced pseudo-epitheliomatous hyperplasia.

OTHER RARE BENIGN TUMOURS Some other rare benign tumours which can occur in the oral soft tissues are: neurilemmoma, neurofibroma, lipoma, giant cell granuloma, rhabdomyoma, leiomyoma, solitary plasmacytoma, osteoma, chondroma, naevi and vascular oral lesions seen in hereditary haemorrhagic telangiectasia (Osler-Rendu-Weber syndrome) and encephalofacial angiomatosis (Sturge-Weber syndrome).

C. Oral Leukoplakia (White Lesions)

DEFINITION Leukoplakia *(white plaque)* may be clinically defined as a white patch or plaque on the oral mucosa, exceeding 5 mm in diameter, which cannot be rubbed off nor can be classified into any other diagnosable disease. A number of other lesions are characterised by the formation of white patches listed in Table 26.3. However, from the pathologist's point of view, the term 'leukoplakia' is reserved for epithelial thickening which may range from completely benign to atypical and to premalignant cellular changes.

INCIDENCE It occurs more frequently in males than females. The lesions may be of variable size and appearance. The sites of predilection, in descending order of frequency, are: cheek mucosa, angles of mouth, alveolar mucosa, tongue, lip, hard and soft palate, and floor of the mouth. In about 4-6% cases of leukoplakia, carcinomatous change is reported. However, it is difficult to decide which white lesions may undergo malignant transformation, but speckled or nodular form is more likely to progress to malignancy. Therefore, it is desirable that all oral white patches be biopsied to exclude malignancy.

ETIOLOGY The etiological factors are similar to those suggested for carcinoma of the oral mucosa (discussed below). *It has the strongest association with the use of tobacco in various forms,* e.g. in heavy smokers (especially in pipe and cigar smokers) and improves when smoking is discontinued, and in those who chew tobacco containing products e.g. *paan, paan masaala, zarda, gutka* etc. The condition is also known by other names such as *smokers' keratosis* and *stomatitis nicotina.* Other etiological factors implicated are chronic friction such as with ill-fitting dentures or jagged teeth, and local irritants like excessive consumption of alcohol and

Table 26.3	Causes of white lesions in the oral mucosa.
A.	BENIGN
	1. Fordyce's granules
	2. Hairy tongue
	3. Leukoedema
	4. Lupus erythematosus
	5. White sponge naevus
B.	PREMALIGNANT
	1. Leukoplakia
	2. Oral lichen planus
C.	MALIGNANT
	Squamous cell carcinoma

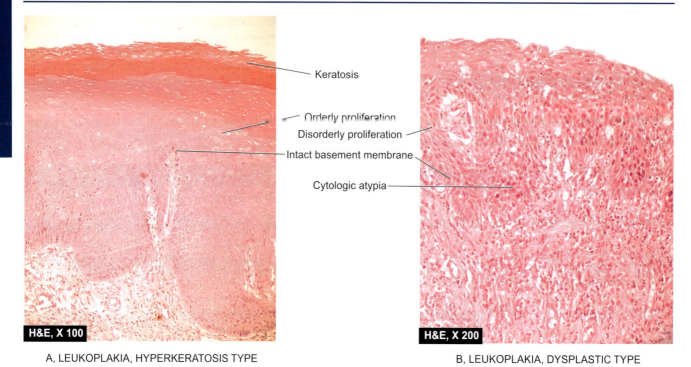

Figure 26.3 ▶ Leukoplakia oral mucosa. A, *Hyperkeratosis type*. There is keratosis and orderly arrangement of increased number of layers of stratified mucosa. B, *Dysplastic type*. The number of layers is increased and the individual cells in layers show features of cytologic atypia and mitosis but there is no invasion across the basement membrane.

very hot and spicy foods and beverages. A special variety of leukoplakia called *'hairy leukoplakia'* has been described in patients of AIDS and has hairy or corrugated surface but is not related to development of oral cancer.

MORPHOLOGIC FEATURES *Grossly,* the lesions of leukoplakia may appear white, whitish-yellow, or red-velvety of more than 5 mm diameter and variable in appearance. They are usually circumscribed, slightly elevated, smooth or wrinkled, speckled or nodular.

Histologically, leukoplakia is of 2 types:

1. Hyperkeratotic type This is characterised by an orderly and regular hyperplasia of squamous epithelium with hyperkeratosis on the surface **(Fig. 26.3, A)**.

2. Dysplastic type When the changes such as irregular stratification of the epithelium, focal areas of increased and abnormal mitotic figures, hyperchromatism, pleomorphism, loss of polarity and individual cell keratinisation are present, the lesion is considered as epithelial dysplasia. The subepithelial tissues usually show an inflammatory infiltrate composed of lymphocytes and plasma cells. The extent and degree of the epithelial changes indicate the degree of severity of the epithelial dysplasia. Usually, mild dysplasia may revert back to normal if the offending etiologic factor is removed, whereas severe dysplasia indicates that the case may progress to carcinoma. *Erythroplasia* is a form of dysplastic leukoplakia in which the epithelial atypia is more marked and thus has higher risk of developing malignancy. If the epithelial dysplasia is extensive so as to involve the entire thickness of the epithelium, the lesion is called carcinoma *in situ* which may progress to invasive carcinoma **(Fig. 26.3, B)**.

D. Malignant Tumours

Squamous Cell (Epidermoid) Carcinoma

Oral cancer is a disease with very poor prognosis because it is not recognised and treated when small and early.

INCIDENCE Squamous cell (epidermoid) carcinoma comprises 90% of all oral malignant tumours and 5% of all human malignancies. The peak incidence in the UK and the USA is from 55 to 75 years of age, whereas in India it is seen at a relatively younger age (40 to 45 years). Oral cancer is a very frequent malignancy in India, Sri Lanka and some Eastern countries, probably related to habits of betel-nut chewing and reversed smoking (page 300). There is a definite male preponderance. It can occur anywhere in the mouth but certain sites are more commonly involved. These sites, in descending order of frequency, are: the lips (more commonly lower), tongue, anterior floor of mouth, buccal mucosa in the region of alveolar lingual sulcus, and palate **(Fig. 26.4)**.

Chapter 26: Diseases of Oral Cavity and Salivary Glands

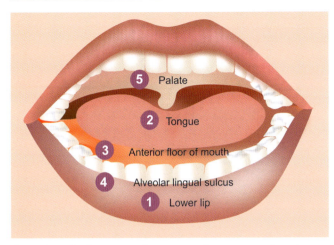

Figure 26.4 ▶ Frequency of occurrence of squamous cell carcinomas in the oral cavity.

ETIOLOGY As with other forms of cancer, the etiology of squamous cell carcinoma is unknown. But a number of etiological factors have been implicated:

Strong association
i) Tobacco smoking and tobacco chewing causing leukoplakia is the most important factor as discussed above.
ii) Chronic alcohol consumption.
iii) Human papilloma virus infection, particularly HPV 16, 18 and 33 types.

Weak association
i) Chronic irritation from ill-fitting denture or jagged teeth.
ii) Submucosal fibrosis as seen in Indians consuming excess of chillies.
iii) Poor orodental hygiene.
iv) Nutritional deficiencies.
v) Exposure to sunlight (in relation to lip cancer).
vi) Exposure to radiation.
vii) Plummer-Vinson syndrome, characterised by atrophy of the upper alimentary tract.

The most common molecular alterations in oncogenes seen in squamous cell carcinoma of the oral cavity are in *p16, p53, p63, cyclin D, PTEN*, and *EGFR*.

MORPHOLOGIC FEATURES *Grossly,* squamous cell carcinoma of oral cavity may have the following types (Fig. 26.5):

i) **Ulcerative type**—is the most frequent type and is characterised by indurated ulcer and firm everted or rolled edges.

ii) **Papillary or verrucous type**—is soft and wart-like growth.

iii) **Nodular type**—appears as a firm, slow growing submucosal nodule.

iv) **Scirrhous type**—is characterised by infiltration into deeper structures.

All these types may appear on a background of leukoplakia or erythroplasia of the oral mucosa. Enlarged cervical lymph nodes may sometimes be present.

Histologically, squamous cell carcinoma ranges from well-differentiated keratinising carcinoma to highly-undifferentiated neoplasm (page 324). Changes of epithelial dysplasia are often present in the surrounding areas of the lesion. Carcinoma of the lip and intraoral squamous carcinoma are usually always well-differentiated (Fig. 26.6).

Carcinoma of the lip has a more favourable prognosis due to visible and easily accessible location and less frequent metastasis to the regional lymph nodes. However, intraoral squamous carcinomas have poor prognosis because they are detected late and metastasis to regional lymph nodes occur early, especially in the case of carcinoma of tongue and soft palate.

Verrucous carcinoma, on the other hand, is composed of very well-differentiated squamous epithelium with minimal atypia and hence has very good prognosis.

Other Malignant Tumours

Other less common malignant neoplasms which may be encountered in the oral cavity are: malignant melanoma, lymphoepithelial carcinoma, malignant lymphoma, malignant tumours of minor salivary glands, and various sarcomas like rhabdomyosarcoma, liposarcoma, alveolar soft part

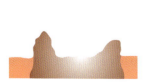
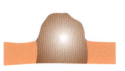
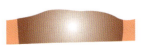

A, ULCERATIVE TYPE   B, PAPILLARY (VERRUCOUS) TYPE   C, NODULAR TYPE   D, SCIRRHOUS TYPE

Figure 26.5 ▶ Squamous cell (Epidermoid) carcinoma of oral cavity, patterns of gross appearance.

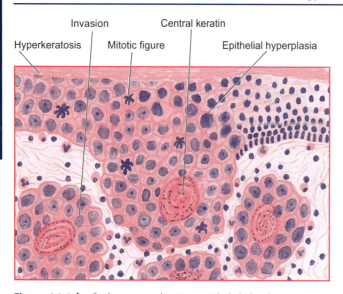
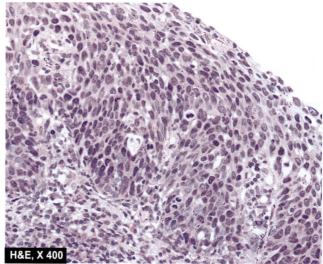

Figure 26.6 ▶ Oral mucosa showing epithelial dysplasia progressing to invasive squamous cell carcinoma. There is keratosis, irregular stratification, cellular pleomorphism, increased and abnormal mitotic figures and individual cell keratinisation, while a few areas show superficial invasive islands of malignant cells in the subepithelial soft tissues.

sarcoma, Kaposi's sarcoma and fibrosarcoma. Metastatic tumours can also occur in the soft tissues of the mouth.

 GIST BOX 26.1 | **Diseases of Oral Soft Tissues**

❖ Benign lesions of the oral soft tissues are fibrous growths, pyogenic granuloma, haemangioma, lymphangioma etc.
❖ Oral leukoplakia is white patch, commonly due to use of tobacco, and may be hyperkeratotic or dysplastic type.
❖ Squamous cell carcinoma is the most common oral malignant tumour. Its locations, in descending order of frequency, are the lower lip, tongue, anterior floor of mouth, buccal mucosa and palate.
❖ Intraoral cancer has a bad prognosis while that of lip has a favourable outcome.

TEETH AND PERIODONTAL TISSUES

NORMAL STRUCTURE

The teeth are normally composed of 3 calcified tissues, namely: *enamel, dentin* and *cementum*; and the *pulp* which is composed of connective tissue. The teeth are peculiar than other calcified tissues of the body by being surrounded by the portion of oral mucosa called the gingiva or gum, and that they are part of a highly specialised odontogenic apparatus; other parts of this apparatus being the mandible and maxilla.

Embryologically, odontogenic development takes place from primitive structure, the *dental lamina* or primitive oral cavity, as follows:

◈ Inner epithelial layer of the dental lamina is ectoderm-derived columnar to cuboidal oral epithelium called **ameloblasts** which secrete enamel matrix, also called enamel organ.
◈ Mesoderm-derived connective tissue gives rise to structures in the **dental papilla** (i.e. dental pulp or core of loose connective tissue, blood vessels and nerves).
◈ Outer margin of the dental papilla differentiates into **odontoblasts**, which continue with ameloblastic epithelium; odontoblasts secrete dentin.

The normal structure of tooth in an adult is as follows (Fig. 26.7, A):

Enamel is the outer covering of teeth composed almost entirely of inorganic material (as in bone) which can be demonstrated in ground sections only because it is lost in decalcified section.

Dentin lies under the enamel and comprises most of the tooth substance. It is composed of organic material in the form of collagen fibrils as well as inorganic material in the form of calcium phosphates as in bone. Dentin is composed of odontoblasts or dentin cells which are counterparts of osteocytes in bone but differ from the latter in having odontoblast processes. Dentin in the crown of tooth is covered with thicker layer of enamel.

Cementum is the portion of tooth which covers the dentin at the root of tooth and is the site where periodontal ligament is attached. Cementum is similar to bone in morphology and composition.

Dental pulp is inner to dentine and occupies the pulp cavity and root canal. It consists of connective tissue, blood vessels and nerves.

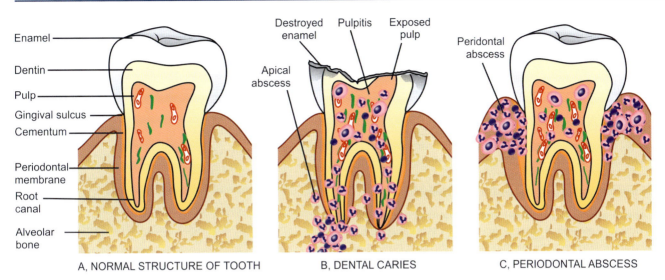

Figure 26.7 ▶ The normal structure of molar tooth in longitudinal section embedded in the jaw (A) contrasted with dental caries (B) and periodontal disease (C). In caries, there is complete destruction of enamel, deposition of secondary dentine and evidence of pulpitis (B), while there is formation of abscess in the periodontal tissue in chronic marginal gingivitis (C).

Nests of odontogenic epithelium are normally present in the jaw and may develop into cysts and tumours.

INFLAMMATORY DISEASES

Dental Caries

Dental caries is the most common disease of dental tissues, causing destruction of the calcified tissues of the teeth.

ETIOPATHOGENESIS Dental caries is essentially a disease of modern society, associated with diet containing high proportion of refined carbohydrates. It has been known for almost 100 years that mixture of sugar or bread with saliva in the presence of acidogenic bacteria of the mouth, especially streptococci, produces organic acids which can decalcify enamel and dentin. Enamel is largely composed of inorganic material which virtually disintegrates. Dentin contains organic material also which is left after decalcification. Bacteria present in the oral cavity cause proteolysis of the remaining organic material of dentin, completing the process of destruction. Diets rich in carbohydrates do not require much chewing and thus the soft and sticky food gets clung to the teeth rather than being cleared away, particularly in the areas of occlusal pits and fissures. 'Bacterial plaques' are formed in such stagnation areas. If these plaques are not removed by brushing or by vigorous chewing of fibrous foods, the process of tooth decay begins. There is evidence that consumption of water containing one part per million (ppm) fluoride is sufficient to reduce the rate of tooth decay in children.

MORPHOLOGIC FEATURES Caries occurs chiefly in the areas of pits and fissures, mainly of the molars and premolars, where food retention occurs, and in the cervical part of the tooth.

Grossly, the earliest change is the appearance of a small, chalky-white spot on the enamel which subsequently enlarges and often becomes yellow or brown and breaks down to form carious cavity. Eventually, the cavity becomes larger due to fractures of enamel. Once the lesion reaches enamel-dentin junction, destruction of dentine also begins.

Microscopically, inflammation (pulpitis) and necrosis of pulp take place. There is evidence of reaction of the tooth to the carious process in the form of *secondary dentin,* which is a layer of odontoblasts laid down under the original dentin **(Fig. 26.7, B)**.

SEQUELAE OF CARIES Carious destruction of dental hard tissues frequently produces pulpitis and other inflammatory lesions like apical granuloma and apical abscess. Less common causes of these lesions are fracture of tooth and accidental exposure of pulp by the dentist.

1. **Pulpitis** Pulpitis may be acute or chronic.

a) *Acute pulpitis* is accompanied by severe pain which may be continuous, throbbing or dull, and is accentuated by heat or cold. It is often accompanied by mild fever and leucocytosis.

b) *Chronic pulpitis* occurs when pulp is exposed widely. It is often not associated with pain. Chronically inflamed pulp tissue may protrude through the cavity forming polyp of the pulp. It may be partly covered by implanted squamous epithelium.

2. Apical granuloma Pulpitis may lead to spread of infection through the apical foramen into the tissues surrounding the root of the tooth.

Histologically, there is chronic inflammatory reaction with formation of granulation tissue and inclusion of nests or strands of squamous epithelium derived from remnants of odontogenic epithelium normally present in the periodontal membrane. An apical granuloma may develop into a dental (radicular) cyst as discussed below.

3. Apical abscess An apical granuloma or acute pulpitis may develop into apical abscess. Acute abscess is very painful, while pus in chronic abscess may escape through root canal and cause further complications like osteomyelitis, cellulitis, cerebral abscess, meningitis and cavernous sinus thrombosis.

Periodontal Disease

Chronic inflammation and degeneration of the supporting tissues of teeth resulting in teeth loss is a common condition. Besides inflammation, other diseases associated with gingival swelling are leukaemia, scurvy, fibrous hyperplasia and epulis.

The inflammatory periodontal disease affects adults more commonly. Pregnancy, puberty and use of drugs like dilantin are associated with periodontal disease more often. The disease begins as *chronic marginal gingivitis,* secondary to bacterial plaques around the teeth such as due to calculus (tartar) on the tooth surface, impacted food, uncontrolled diabetes, tooth-decay and ill-fitting dental appliances. The gingival sulcus acts as convenient site for lodgement of food debris and bacterial plaque leading to formation of periodontal pocket from which purulent discharge can be expressed by digital pressure.

Microscopically, chronic marginal gingivitis is characterised by heavy chronic inflammatory cell infiltrate, destruction of collagen, and epithelial hyperplasia so as to line the pocket (Fig. 26.7, C). Untreated chronic marginal gingivitis slowly progresses to *chronic periodontitis* or *pyorrhoea* in which there is inflammatory destruction of deeper tissues. At this stage, progressive resorption of alveolar bone occurs and the tooth ultimately gets detached.

EPITHELIAL CYSTS OF THE JAW

The epithelium-lined cysts of dental tissue can have inflammatory or developmental origin. A classification of such cysts is given in Table 26.4.

Table 26.4 Classification of epithelial cysts of jaw.

A. INFLAMMATORY
Radicular (apical, periodontal, dental) cyst

B. DEVELOPMENTAL
1. Odontogenic cysts
   (i) Dentigerous (follicular) cyst
   (ii) Eruption cyst
   (iii) Gingival cyst
   (iv) Primordial cyst (odontogenic keratocyst)
2. Non-odontogenic and fissural cysts
   (i) Nasopalatine duct (Incisive canal, Median anterior maxillary) cyst
   (ii) Nasolabial (nasoalveolar) cyst
   (iii) Globulomaxillary cyst
   (iv) Dermoid cyst

A. Inflammatory Cysts

Radicular Cyst

Radicular cyst, also called as apical, periodontal or simply dental cyst, is the most common cyst originating from the dental tissues. It arises consequent to inflammation following destruction of dental pulp such as in dental caries, pulpitis, and apical granuloma. The epithelial cells of Malassez, which are nests of odontogenic epithelium embedded in the periodontium, proliferate within apical granuloma under the influence of inflammation, leading to the formation of an epithelium-lined cystic cavity. Most often, radicular cyst is observed at the apex of an erupted tooth and sometimes contains thick pultaceous material.

Histologically, the radicular cyst is lined by nonkeratinised squamous epithelium. Epithelial rete processes may penetrate the underlying connective tissues. Radicular cyst of the maxilla may be lined by respiratory epithelium. The cyst wall is fibrous and contains chronic inflammatory cells (lymphocytes, plasma cells with Russell bodies and macrophages) hyaline bodies and deposits of cholesterol crystals which may be associated with foreign body giant cells (Fig. 26.8).

B. Developmental Cysts

Odontogenic Cysts

DENTIGEROUS (FOLLICULAR) CYST Dentigerous cyst arises from enamel of an unerupted tooth. The mandibular

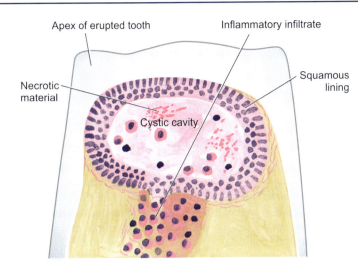

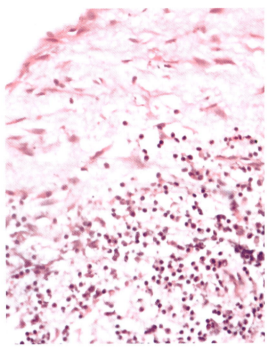

Figure 26.8 ▶ Dental (Radicular) cyst. The cyst wall is composed of fibrous tissue and is lined by non-keratinised squamous epithelium. The cyst wall is densely infiltrated by chronic inflammatory cells, chiefly lymphocytes, plasma cells and macrophages.

third molars and the maxillary canines are most often involved. Dentigerous cysts are less common than radicular cysts and occur more commonly in children and young individuals. These cysts are more significant because of reported occurrence of ameloblastoma and carcinoma in them.

Histologically, dentigerous cyst is composed of a thin fibrous tissue wall lined by stratified squamous epithelium. Thus, the cyst may resemble radicular cyst, except that chronic inflammatory changes so characteristic of radicular cyst, are usually absent in dentigerous cyst (Fig. 26.9).

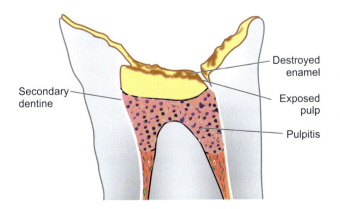

Figure 26.9 ▶ Dentigerous (Follicular) cyst. The cyst is composed of thin fibrous tissue wall and is lined by stratified squamous epithelium. A partly formed unerupted tooth is also seen in the wall. Inflammatory changes are conspicuously absent.

ERUPTION CYST This is a cyst lying over the crown of an unerupted tooth and is lined by stratified squamous epithelium. It is thus a form of dentigerous cyst.

GINGIVAL CYST It arises from the epithelial rests in the gingiva and is lined by keratinising squamous epithelium.

PRIMORDIAL CYST (ODONTOGENIC KERATOCYST) Primordial cyst, like dentigerous cyst, also arises from tooth-forming epithelium. The common location is mandibular third molar. Multiple primordial cysts occur in association with naevoid basal cell carcinoma syndrome. Primordial cysts have a marked tendency to recur (50%).

Histologically, the cyst wall is thin and is lined by regular layer of keratinising stratified squamous epithelium. Inflammatory changes are generally absent.

Non-odontogenic and Fissural Cysts

NASOPALATINE DUCT (INCISIVE CANAL, MEDIAN, ANTERIOR MAXILLARY) CYST This is the most common non-odontogenic (fissural) cyst and arises from the epithelial remnants of the nasopalatine duct.

Histologically, the cyst is lined by stratified squamous epithelium, respiratory epithelium, or both.

NASOLABIAL (NASOALVEOLAR) CYST This cyst is situated in the soft tissues at the junction of median nasal, lateral nasal and maxillary processes, at the ala of the nose, and sometimes extending into the nostril.

Histologically, the cyst is lined by squamous or respiratory epithelium, or both.

GLOBULOMAXILLARY CYST This is an intraosseous cyst and is rare.

DERMOID CYST The dermoid cyst is common in the region of head and neck, especially in the floor of the mouth. The cyst arises from remains in the midline during closure of mandibular and branchial arches.

ODONTOGENIC TUMOURS

Odontogenic tumours are a group of uncommon lesions of the jaw derived from the odontogenic apparatus. These tumours are usually benign but some have malignant counterparts. An abbreviated WHO classification is presented in Table 26.5.

A. Benign Odontogenic Tumours

Ameloblastoma

Ameloblastoma is the most common benign but locally invasive epithelial odontogenic tumour. It is most frequent in the 3rd to 5th decades of life. Preferential sites are the mandible in the molar-ramus area and the maxilla. The tumour originates from dental epithelium of the enamel itself or its epithelial residues. Sometimes, the tumour may arise from the epithelial lining of a dentigerous cyst or from basal layer of oral mucosa. Radiologically, typical picture is of a multilocular destruction of the bone. Rare instances of an extraosseous example, presence of an embedded tooth, or unilocular ameloblastoma can occur. Tumour with histologic resemblance to ameloblastoma can occur occasionally in the long bone, like adamantinoma of the tibia.

Grossly, the tumour is greyish-white, usually solid, sometimes cystic, replacing and expanding the affected bone.

Histologically, ameloblastoma can show different patterns as follows:

i) Follicular pattern is the most common. The tumour consists of follicles of variable size and shape and separated from each other by fibrous tissue. The structure of follicles is similar to that of enamel organ consisting of central area of stellate cells resembling stellate reticulum, and peripheral layer of cuboidal or columnar cells resembling epithelium. The central stellate areas may show cystic changes (Fig. 26.10).

ii) Plexiform pattern is the next common pattern after follicular pattern. The tumour epithelium is seen to form irregular plexiform masses or network of strands. The stroma is usually scanty. Microcyst formation can occur in the stroma.

iii) Acanthomatous pattern is squamous metaplasia within the islands of tumour cells.

iv) Basal cell pattern of ameloblastoma is similar to basal cell carcinoma of the skin.

v) Granular cell pattern is characterised by appearance of acidophilic granularity in the cytoplasm of tumour cells.

Combination of more than one morphologic pattern may also be seen.

Tumour cells in ameloblastoma exhibit positive immunostaining for cytokeratin and laminin as are seen in developing tooth.

Odontogenic Adenomatoid Tumour (Adeno-ameloblastoma)

This is a benign tumour seen more often in females in their 2nd decade of life. The tumour is commonly associated with an unerupted tooth and thus closely resembles dentigerous cyst radiologically. Unlike ameloblastoma, adenomatoid odontogenic tumour is not invasive nor does it recur after enucleation.

Histologically, the lesion has extensive cyst formations. The wall of cyst contains scanty fibrous connective tissue in which are present characteristic tubule-like structures composed of epithelial cells and hence the name 'adenomatoid' (gland-like).

Calcifying Epithelial Odontogenic Tumour

This is a rare lesion which is locally invasive and recurrent like ameloblastoma. It is seen commonly in 4th and 5th decades and occurs more commonly in the region of mandible.

Table 26.5 Classification of odontogenic tumours.

- A. **BENIGN**
    - a) *Epithelial origin*
        1. Ameloblastoma
        2. Adenomatoid odontogenic tumour (Adenoameloblastoma)
        3. Calcifying epithelial odontogenic tumour
    - b) *Mesenchymal origin*
        1. Odontogenic myxoma
        2. Odontogenic fibroma
        3. Cementoma
    - c) *Mixed epithelial-mesenchymal origin*
        1. Ameloblastic fibroma
        2. Ameloblastic fibro-odontoma
        3. Complex odontomas
- B. **MALIGNANT**
    - a) *Epithelial origin*
        1. Malignant ameloblastoma
        2. Ameloblastic carcinoma
    - b) *Mesenchymal origin*
        - Ameloblastic fibrosarcoma

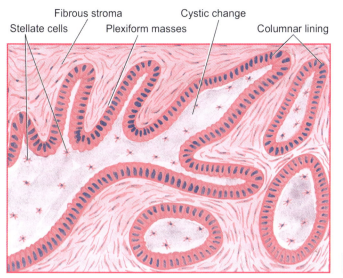
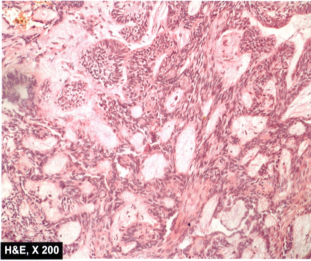

Figure 26.10 ▶ Ameloblastoma, follicular and plexiform patterns. Epithelial follicles are composed of central area of stellate cells and peripheral layer of cuboidal or columnar cells. Plexiform areas show irregular plexiform masses and network of strands of epithelial cells. A few areas show central cystic change.

Histologically, the tumour consists of closely packed polyhedral epithelial cells having features of nuclear pleomorphism, giant nuclei and rare mitotic figures. The stroma is often scanty and appears homogeneous and hyalinised in which small calcified deposits are seen which are a striking feature of this tumour.

Odontogenic Myxoma (Myxofibroma)

Odontogenic myxoma is a locally invasive and recurring tumour.

Microscopically, it is characterised by abundant mucoid stroma and loose stellate cells in which are seen a few strands of odontogenic epithelium.

Ameloblastic Fibroma

This is a benign tumour consisting of epithelial and connective tissues derived from odontogenic apparatus. It resembles ameloblastoma but can be distinguished from it because ameloblastic fibroma occurs in younger age group (below 20 years) and the clinical behaviour is always benign.

Histologically, it consists of epithelial follicles similar to those of ameloblastoma, set in a very cellular connective tissue stroma.

Odontomas

Odontomas are hamartomas that contain both epithelial and mesodermal dental tissue components. There are 3 subtypes:

i) **Complex odontoma** is always benign and consists of enamel, dentin and cementum which are not differentiated, so that the structure of actual tooth is not identifiable.

ii) **Compound odontoma** is also benign and is comprised of differentiated dental tissue elements forming a number of denticles in fibrous tissue.

iii) **Ameloblastic fibro-odontoma** is a lesion that resembles ameloblastic fibroma with odontoma formation.

Cementomas

Cementomas are a variety of benign lesions which are characterised by the presence of cementum or cementum-like tissue. Five types of cementomas are described:

i) **Benign cementoblastoma (true cementoma)** is a solitary lesion of jaw, characterised by features comparable to those of osteoid osteoma and osteoblastoma.

ii) **Cementifying fibroma** consists of cellular fibrous tissue containing calcified masses of cementum-like tissue.

iii) **Periapical cemental dysplasia (Periapical fibrous dysplasia)** is most common and resembles cementifying fibroma except that it contains more fibrous tissue as well as cementum-like tissue.

iv) **Multiple apical cementomas** are found on the apical region of teeth and detected incidentally in postmenopausal women.

v) **Gigantiform cementoma** is a large lobulated mass of cementum-like tissue. Sometimes, there are multiple such masses in the jaw.

B. Malignant Odontogenic Tumours

Malignant odontogenic tumours are rare.

Odontogenic Carcinoma

i) *Malignant ameloblastoma* is the term used for the uncommon metastasising ameloblastoma.

ii) *Ameloblastic carcinoma* is the term employed for the ameloblastic tumour having cytologic features of malignancy in the primary tumour.

iii) *Primary intraosseous carcinoma* may develop within the jaw from the rests of odontogenic epithelium.

iv) Rarely, carcinomas may arise from the odontogenic epithelium lining the *odontogenic cysts*.

Odontogenic Sarcomas

The only example of odontogenic sarcoma is a rare ameloblastic fibrosarcoma. This tumour resembles ameloblastic fibroma but the mesodermal component in it is malignant (sarcomatous) whereas the ameloblastic epithelium remains differentiated and benign.

| GIST BOX 26.2 | Diseases of Teeth and Periodontal Tissues |

- Normal tooth is composed of enamel, dentin and cementum and central pulp.
- In dental caries, there is destruction of enamel and occurrence of pulpitis.
- Chronic periodontal inflammation causes periodontitis and pyorrhea.
- Common inflammatory cyst of the jaw is radicular cyst while common developmental cyst is dentigerous cyst.
- Benign odontogenic tumours of the jaw originate from epithelium (e.g. ameloblastoma) or mesenchyme (e.g. myxoma).
- Odontogenic carcinoma and sarcoma are uncommon malignant tumours.

SALIVARY GLANDS

NORMAL STRUCTURE

There are two main groups of salivary glands—major and minor. The major salivary glands are the three paired glands: parotid, submandibular and sublingual. The minor salivary glands are numerous and are widely distributed in the mucosa of oral cavity. The main duct of the parotid gland drains into the oral cavity opposite the second maxillary molar, while the ducts of submandibular and sublingual glands empty in the floor of the mouth. At times, heterotopic salivary gland tissue may be present in lymph nodes near or within the parotid gland.

Histologically, the salivary glands are tubuloalveolar glands and may contain mucous cells, serous cells, or both. The parotid gland is purely serous. The submandibular gland is mixed type but is predominantly serous, whereas the sublingual gland, though also a mixed gland, is predominantly mucous type. Similarly, minor salivary glands may also be serous, mucous or mixed type.

The secretory acini of the major salivary glands are drained by ducts lined by:
- low cuboidal epithelium in the intercalated portion,
- tall columnar epithelium in the intralobular ducts, and
- simpler epithelium in the secretory ducts.

The product of major salivary glands is *saliva* which performs various functions such as lubrication for swallowing and speech, and has enzyme amylase and antibacterial properties too.

INFLAMMATORY AND SALIVARY FLOW DISEASES

Sialorrhoea (Ptyalism)

Increased flow of saliva is termed sialorrhoea or ptyalism. It occurs commonly due to: stomatitis, teething, mentally retarded state, schizophrenia, neurological disturbances, increased gastric secretion and sialosis (i.e. uniform, symmetric, painless hypertrophy of salivary glands).

Xerostomia

Decreased salivary flow is termed xerostomia. It is associated with the following conditions: Sjögren's syndrome, sarcoidosis, mumps parotitis, Mikulicz's syndrome, megaloblastic anaemia, dehydration, drug intake (e.g. antihistamines, antihypertensives, antidepressants).

Sialadenitis

Inflammation of salivary glands, sialadenitis, may be acute or chronic; the latter being more common.

ETIOLOGY Sialadenitis can occur due to the following causes:

1. Viral infections The most common inflammatory lesion of the salivary glands particularly of the parotid glands, is mumps occurring in children of school-age. It is characterised by triad of pathological involvement—*epidemic parotitis (mumps), orchitis-oophoritis, and pancreatitis* (Fig. 26.11). Involvement of the testis and pancreas may lead to their atrophy. Less commonly, cytomegalovirus infection may occur in parotid glands of infants and young children.

2. Bacterial and mycotic infections Bacterial infections may cause acute sialadenitis more often. Sometimes there are recurrent attacks of acute parotitis when parotitis becomes chronic.

Chapter 26: Diseases of Oral Cavity and Salivary Glands

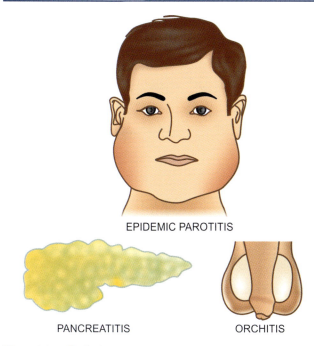

Figure 26.11 ▶ Lesions in mumps.

i) *Acute sialadenitis* The causes are as follows:
a) Acute infectious fevers
b) Acute postoperative parotitis (ascent of microorganisms up the parotid duct from the mouth)
c) General debility
d) Old age
e) Dehydration.

ii) *Chronic sialadenitis* This may result from the following causes:
a) *Recurrent obstructive type.* Recurrent obstruction due to calculi (sialolithiasis), stricture, surgery, injury etc. may cause repeated attacks of acute sialadenitis by ascending infection and then chronicity.
b) *Recurrent non-obstructive type.* Recurrent mild ascending infection of the parotid gland may occur due to non-obstructive causes which reduce salivary secretion like due to intake of drugs causing hyposalivation (e.g. antihistamines, antihypertensives, antidepressants), effect of irradiation and congenital malformations of the duct system.
c) *Chronic inflammatory diseases.* Tuberculosis, actinomycosis and other mycoses may rarely occur in the salivary glands.

3. **Autoimmune disease** Inflammatory changes are seen in salivary glands in 2 autoimmune diseases:
i) *Sjögren's syndrome* characterised by triad of dry eyes (keratoconjunctivitis sicca), dry mouth (xerostomia) and rheumatoid arthritis (page 220).
ii) *Mikulicz's syndrome* is the combination of inflammatory enlargement of salivary and lacrimal glands with xerostomia.

MORPHOLOGIC FEATURES Irrespective of the underlying etiology of sialadenitis, there is swelling of the affected salivary gland, usually restricted by the fibrous capsule. Acute stage is generally associated with local redness, pain and tenderness with purulent ductal discharge. Late chronic cases may be replaced by firm fibrous swelling.

Microscopically, acute viral sialadenitis in mumps shows swelling and cytoplasmic vacuolation of the acinar epithelial cells and degenerative changes in the ductal epithelium. There is interstitial oedema, fibrinoid degeneration of the collagen and dense infiltration by mononuclear cells (lymphocytes, plasma cells and macrophages). *Chronic and recurrent sialadenitis* is characterised by increased lymphoid tissue in the interstitium, progressive loss of secretory tissue and replacement by fibrosis.

TUMOURS OF SALIVARY GLANDS

The major as well as minor salivary glands can give rise to a variety of benign and malignant tumours (Table 26.6). The major glands, particularly the parotid glands (85%), are the most common sites. Majority of parotid gland tumour (65-85%) are benign, while in the other major and minor salivary glands 35-50% of the tumours are malignant. Most of the salivary gland tumours originate from the ductal lining epithelium and the underlying myoepithelial cells; a few arise from acini. Recurrent tumours of the parotid glands, due to

Table 26.6 — Classification of salivary gland tumours.

A.	**BENIGN**	
1.	Adenomas	
	i) Pleomorphic adenoma (Mixed tumour) (50%)	
	ii) Monomorphic adenoma	
		(a) Warthin's tumour (Papillary cystadenoma lymphomatosum, Adenolymphoma) (8%)
		(b) Oxyphil adenoma (Oncocytomas) (1%)
		(c) Other types (Myoepithelioma, Basal cell adenoma, Clear cell adenoma) (uncommon)
2.	Mesenchymal tumours (rare)	
B.	**MALIGNANT**	
1.	Mucoepidermoid carcinoma (15%)	
2.	Malignant mixed tumour	
	i) Carcinoma in pleomorphic adenoma (3-5%)	
	ii) Carcinosarcoma (rare)	
	iii) Metastasising mixed salivary tumour (rare)	
3.	Adenoid cystic carcinoma (cylindroma) (5%)	
4.	Acinic cell carcinoma (5%)	
5.	Adenocarcinoma (10%)	
6.	Epidermoid carcinoma (1%)	
7.	Undifferentiated carcinoma (< 1%)	
8.	Miscellaneous (2%)	

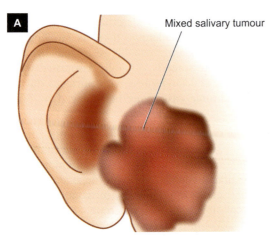
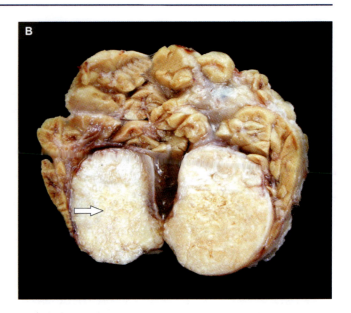

Figure 26.12 ▶ Pleomorphic adenoma (mixed salivary tumour) of the parotid gland. A, Diagrammatic location. B, Sectioned surface of the parotid gland shows lobules of grey-white circumscribed tumour having semitranslucent parenchyma (arrow).

their location, are often associated with facial palsy and obvious scarring following surgical treatment.

A. Benign Salivary Gland Tumours

Adenomas

The adenomas of the salivary glands are benign epithelial tumours. They are broadly classified into 2 major groups—pleomorphic and monomorphic adenomas.

Pleomorphic Adenoma (Mixed Salivary Tumour)

This is the most common tumour of major (60-75%) and minor (50%) salivary glands. Pleomorphic adenoma is the commonest tumour in the parotid gland and occurs less often in other major and minor salivary glands. The tumour is commoner in women and is seen more frequently in 3rd to 5th decades of life. The tumour is solitary, smooth-surfaced, sometimes nodular, painless and slow-growing. It is often located below and in front of the ear **(Fig. 26.12)**.

MORPHOLOGIC FEATURES **Grossly,** pleomorphic adenoma is a circumscribed, pseudoencapsulated, rounded, at times multilobulated, firm mass, 2-5 cm in diameter, with bosselated surface. The cut surface is grey-white and bluish, variegated, semitranslucent, usually solid but occasionally may show small cystic spaces. The consistency is soft and mucoid.

Microscopically, the pleomorphic adenoma is characterised by pleomorphic or 'mixed' appearance in which there are epithelial elements present in a stromal matrix of mucoid, myxoid and chondroid tissue **(Fig. 26.13)**:

◈ **Epithelial component** may form various patterns like ducts, acini, tubules, sheets and strands of cells of ductal or myoepithelial origin. The ductal cells are cuboidal or columnar, while the underlying myoepithelial cells may be polygonal or spindle-shaped resembling smooth muscle cells. The material found in the lumina of duct-like structures is PAS-positive epithelial mucin. Focal areas of squamous metaplasia and keratinisation may be present.

Immunohistochemically, the tumour cells are immunoreactive for epithelial (cytokeratin, EMA, CEA) as well as myoepithelial (actin, vimentin and S-100) antibodies.

◈ **Stromal elements** are present as loose connective tissue, and as myxoid, mucoid and chondroid matrix, which simulates cartilage *(pseudocartilage)*. However, true cartilage and even bone may also be observed in a small proportion of these tumours.

Based on morphology, immunohistochemistry, ultra-structure and molecular characteristics, the mesenchymal matrix of the tumour has been assigned as a product of epithelial origin and are actually modified myoepithelial cells as seen by S-100 immunostain positivity.

The epithelial and mesenchymal elements are intermixed and either of the two components may be dominant in any tumour.

PROGNOSIS Pleomorphic adenoma is notorious for recurrences, sometimes after many years. The main factors responsible for the tendency to recur are incomplete surgical removal due to proximity to the facial nerve, multiple foci of tumour, pseudoencapsulation, and implantation in the surgical field. Although the tumour is entirely benign, under exceptionally rare circumstances, an ordinary pleomorphic

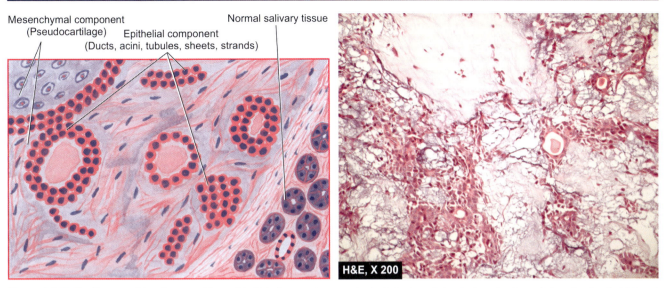

Figure 26.13 ▶ Pleomorphic adenoma. The epithelial element is comprised of ducts, acini, tubules, sheets and strands of cuboidal and myoepithelial cells. These are seen randomly admixed with mesenchymal elements composed of pseudocartilage which is the matrix of myxoid, chondroid and mucoid material.

adenoma may metastasise to distant sites which too will have benign appearance as the original tumour. However, actual malignant transformation can also occur in a pleomorphic adenoma *(discussed below)*.

Monomorphic Adenomas

These are benign epithelial tumours of salivary glands without any evidence of mesenchyme-like tissues. Their various forms are as under:

WARTHIN'S TUMOUR (PAPILLARY CYSTADENOMA LYMPHOMATOSUM, ADENOLYMPHOMA) It is a benign tumour of the parotid gland comprising about 8% of all parotid neoplasms, seen more commonly in men from 4th to 7th decades of life. Rarely, it may arise in the submandibular gland or in minor salivary glands. *Histogenesis* of the tumour has been much debated; most accepted theory is that the tumour develops from parotid ductal epithelium present in lymph nodes adjacent to or within parotid gland.

MORPHOLOGIC FEATURES **Grossly,** the tumour is encapsulated, round or oval with smooth surface. The cut surface shows characteristic slit-like or cystic spaces, containing milky fluid and having papillary projections.
Microscopically, the tumour shows 2 components: epithelial parenchyma and lymphoid stroma **(Fig. 26.14)**:

◈ **Epithelial parenchyma** is composed of glandular and cystic structures having papillary arrangement and is lined by characteristic eosinophilic epithelium. Variants of epithelial patterns include presence of mucous goblet cells and sebaceous differentiation.

◈ **Lymphoid stroma** is present under the epithelium in the form of prominent lymphoid tissue, often with germinal centres.

OXYPHIL ADENOMA (ONCOCYTOMA) It is a benign slow-growing tumour of the major salivary glands. The tumour consists of parallel sheets, acini or tubules of large cells with glandular eosinophilic cytoplasm (oncocytes). It is also called as mitochondrioma because of cytoplasmic granularity due to mitochondria.

OTHER TYPES OF MONOMORPHIC ADENOMAS There are some uncommon forms of monomorphic adenomas:
i) *Myoepithelioma* is an adenoma composed exclusively of myoepithelial cells which may be arranged in tubular, alveolar or trabecular pattern.
ii) *Basal cell adenoma* is characterised by the type and arrangement of cells resembling basal cell carcinoma of the skin.
iii) *Clear cell adenoma* has spindle-shaped or polyhedral cells with clear cytoplasm.

Miscellaneous Benign Tumours

A number of mesenchymal tumours can rarely occur in salivary glands. These include: fibroma, lipoma, neurilemmomas, neurofibroma, haemangioma and lymphangioma.

B. Malignant Salivary Gland Tumours

Mucoepidermoid Carcinoma

The status of 'mucoepidermoid tumour' as an intermediate grade tumour in the older classification has undergone

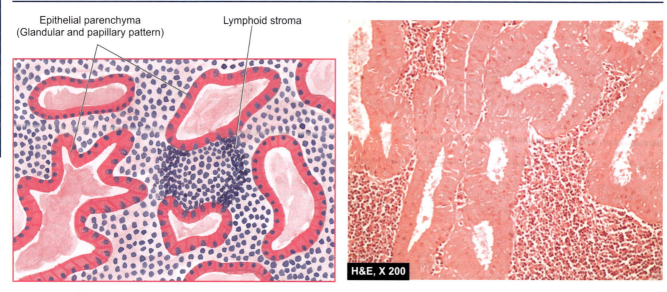

Figure 26.14 ▶ Warthin's tumour, showing eosinophilic epithelium forming glandular and papillary, cystic pattern with intervening stroma of lymphoid tissue.

upgradation to mucoepidermoid carcinoma now having the following peculiar features:
1. It is the most *common malignant* salivary gland tumour (both in the major and minor glands).
2. The *parotid gland* amongst the major salivary glands and the minor salivary glands in the *palate* are the most common sites.
3. Common age group affected is 30-60 years but it is also the most common malignant salivary gland tumour affecting *children and adolescents.*
4. It is the most common example of *radiation-induced* malignant tumour, especially therapeutic radiation.

> **MORPHOLOGIC FEATURES** **Grossly,** the tumour is usually circumscribed but not encapsulated. It varies in size from 1 to 4 cm.
>
> *Microscopically*, the tumour is classified into low, intermediate and high grade depending upon the degree of differentiation and tumour invasiveness. The tumour is composed of combination of 4 types of cells: mucin-producing, squamous, intermediate and clear cells. Well-differentiated tumours have predominance of mucinous cells, while poorly differentiated have more solid and infiltrative pattern (Fig. 26.15).

Malignant Mixed Tumour

Malignant mixed tumour comprises three distinct clinicopathologic entities:
1. Carcinoma arising in benign mixed salivary gland tumour (carcinoma *ex* pleomorphic adenoma)
2. Carcinosarcoma
3. Metastasising mixed salivary tumour.

Carcinoma *ex* pleomorphic adenoma is more common (3-5%) while the other two are rare tumours. The slow-growing adenoma may have been present for a number of years when suddenly it undergoes rapid increase in its size, becomes painful and the individual may develop facial palsy. Malignant transformation occurs in later age (6th decade) than the usual age for pleomorphic adenoma (4th to 6th

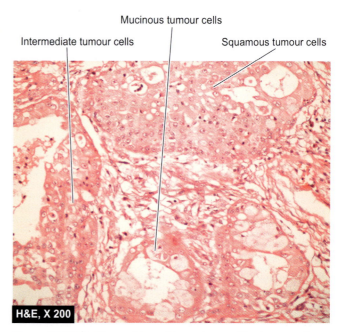

Figure 26.15 ▶ Mucoepidermoid carcinoma. The tumour shows combination of mucinous, squamous and intermediate cells and having infiltrative border.

decades). It may occur in primary tumour but more often occurs in its recurrences.

MORPHOLOGIC FEATURES **Grossly,** the tumour is poorly-circumscribed with irregular infiltrating margin. Cut section may show haemorrhages, necrosis and cystic degeneration.

Microscopically, besides the typical appearance of pleomorphic adenoma, malignant areas show cytologic features of carcinoma such as anaplasia, nuclear hyperchromatism, large nucleolisation, mitoses and evidence of invasive growth. All types of usual salivary gland carcinomas (described below) may develop in pleomorphic adenoma.

Adenoid Cystic Carcinoma (Cylindroma)

This is a highly malignant tumour due to its typical infiltrative nature, especially along the nerve sheaths.

Histologically, adenoid cystic carcinoma is characterised by cribriform appearance i.e. the epithelial tumour cells of duct-lining and myoepithelial cells are arranged in duct-like structures or masses of cells, having typical fenestrations or cyst-like spaces and hence the name 'adenoid cystic'. These cystic spaces contain PAS-positive basophilic material (Fig. 26.16).

Acinic Cell Carcinoma

This is a rare tumour composed of acinic cells resembling serous cells of normal salivary gland. These cells are arranged in sheets or acini and have characteristic basophilic granular cytoplasm. The degree of atypia may vary from a benign cytologic appearance to cellular features of malignancy.

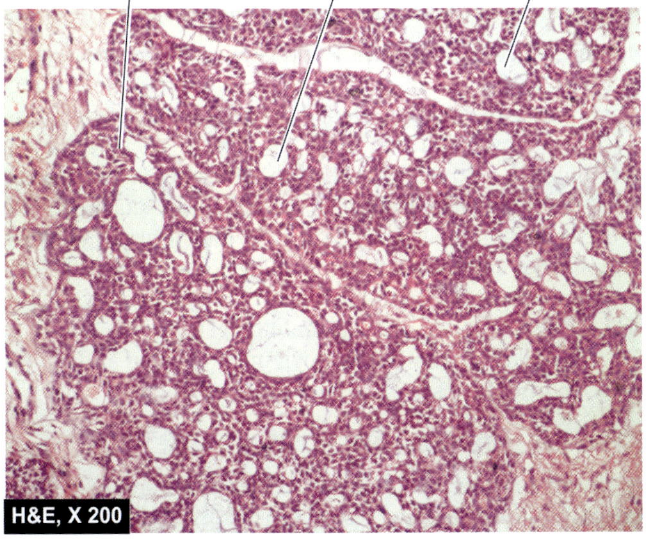

Adenocarcinoma

Adenocarcinoma of the salivary gland does not differ from adenocarcinoma elsewhere in the body. It may have some variants such as mucoid adenocarcinoma, clear-cell adenocarcinoma and papillary cystadenocarcinoma.

Epidermoid Carcinoma

This rare tumour has features of squamous cell carcinoma with keratin formation and has intercellular bridges similar to its appearance elsewhere in the body. The tumour commonly infiltrates the skin and involves the facial nerve early.

Undifferentiated Carcinoma

This highly malignant tumour consists of anaplastic epithelial cells which are too poorly differentiated to be placed in any other known category.

Miscellaneous Malignant Tumours

Some rare malignant tumours of epithelial and mesenchymal origin are melanoma, sebaceous carcinoma, undifferentiated carcinoma, lymphoma, fibrosarcoma and leiomyosarcoma. All these tumours are similar in morphology to such tumours elsewhere in the body.

Besides, metastatic involvement of major salivary glands or the adjacent lymph nodes is common, especially from epidermoid carcinoma and malignant melanoma.

| GIST BOX 26.3 | Diseases of Salivary Glands |

- Salivary flow disturbances include sialorrhoea (hypersalivation) and xerostomia (decreased salivation).
- Sialadentitis is inflammation of the parotid glands, commonly due to mumps in children, and may be accompanied with orchitis-oophoritis and pancreatitis.
- Most common benign tumour of the salivary glands is pleomorphic adenoma. It is composed of epithelial and stromal elements.
- Warthin's tumour is a monomorphic adenoma and has cystic spaces lined by papillary arrangement lined by epithelial cells with eosinophilic cytoplasm and lymphoid stroma.
- About 5% of mixed salivary tumours show malignant change.
- Mucoepidermoid carcinoma, adenoid cystic carcinoma, and acinic cell carcinoma are some of the other malignant salivary gland tumours.

Figure 26.16 ▶ Adenoid cystic carcinoma. It shows nests of tumour cells having fenestrations containing basophilic material.

27 Jaundice, Hepatitis and Cirrhosis

JAUNDICE

Jaundice or icterus refers to the yellow pigmentation of the skin or sclerae by bilirubin (page 58). Bilirubin pigment has high affinity for elastic tissue and hence jaundice is particularly noticeable in tissues rich in elastin content. Jaundice is the result of elevated levels of bilirubin in the blood termed hyperbilirubinaemia. Normal serum bilirubin concentration ranges from 0.3-1.3 mg/dl, about 80% of which is unconjugated. Jaundice becomes clinically evident when the total serum bilirubin exceeds 2 mg/dl. A rise of serum bilirubin between the normal and 2 mg/dl is generally not accompanied by visible jaundice and is called *latent jaundice*.

Before considering the features and types of jaundice, it is essential to review the normal bilirubin metabolism.

NORMAL BILIRUBIN METABOLISM

Normal metabolism of bilirubin can be conveniently described under 4 main headings—source, transport, hepatic phase and intestinal phase as illustrated schematically earlier (*see* Fig. 22.8, page 364).

1. SOURCE OF BILIRUBIN About 80-85% of the bilirubin is derived from the catabolism of haemoglobin present in senescent red blood cells. The destruction of effete erythrocytes at the end of their normal lifespan of 120 days takes place in the reticuloendothelial system in the bone marrow, spleen and liver. The remaining 15-20% of the bilirubin comes partly from non-haemoglobin haem-containing pigments such as myoglobin, catalase and cytochromes, and partly from ineffective erythropoiesis. In either case, haem moiety is formed which is converted to biliverdin by microsomal haem oxygenase for which oxygen and NADPH are essential requirements. Bilirubin is formed from biliverdin by biliverdin reductase.

2. TRANSPORT OF BILIRUBIN Bilirubin on release from macrophages circulates as unconjugated bilirubin in plasma tightly bound to albumin. Certain drugs such as sulfonamides and salicylates compete with bilirubin for albumin binding and displace bilirubin from albumin, thus facilitating bilirubin to enter into the brain in neonates and increase the risk of *kernicterus*. Bilirubin is found in body fluids in proportion to their albumin content such as in CSF, joint effusions, cysts etc.

3. HEPATIC PHASE On coming in contact with the hepatocyte surface, unconjugated bilirubin is preferentially metabolised which involves 3 steps: hepatic uptake, conjugation and secretion in bile.

i) Hepatic uptake Albumin-bound unconjugated bilirubin upon entry into the hepatocyte, is dissociated into bilirubin and albumin. The bilirubin gets bound to cytoplasmic protein *glutathione-S-transferase (GST)* (earlier called ligandin).

ii) Conjugation Unconjugated bilirubin is not water-soluble but is alcohol-soluble and is converted into water-soluble compound by conjugation. Conjugation occurs in endoplasmic reticulum and involves conversion to bilirubin mono- and diglucuronide by the action of microsomal enzyme, *bilirubin-UDP-glucuronosyl transferase* (Fig. 27.1). The process of conjugation can be induced by drugs like phenobarbital.

Conjugated bilirubin is bound to albumin in two forms: reversible and irreversible. Reversible binding is similar to that of unconjugated bilirubin. However, when present in serum for a long time (e.g. in cholestasis, long-standing biliary obstruction, chronic active hepatitis), conjugated bilirubin is bound to albumin irreversibly and is termed *delta bilirubin* or *biliprotein*. This irreversible conjugated delta bilirubin is not excreted by the kidney, and remains detectable in serum for sufficient time after recovery from the diseases listed above.

iii) Secretion into bile Conjugated (water-soluble) bilirubin is rapidly transported directly into bile canaliculi by energy-dependent process and then excreted into the bile.

4. INTESTINAL PHASE Appearance of conjugated bilirubin in the intestinal lumen is followed by either direct excretion in the stool as stercobilinogen which imparts the normal yellow colour to stool, or may be metabolised to urobilinogen by the action of intestinal bacteria. Conjugated bilirubin is normally not reabsorbable whereas its metabolic product, urobilinogen, is reabsorbed from the small intestine and reaches enterohepatic circulation. Some of the absorbed urobilinogen in resecreted by the liver into the bile while the rest is excreted in the urine as urobilinogen.

The major differences between unconjugated and conjugated bilirubin are summarised in Table 27.1.

TYPES OF LIVER CELL NECROSIS

All forms of injury to the liver such as microbiologic, toxic, circulatory or traumatic, result in necrosis of liver cells. The extent of involvement of hepatic lobule in necrosis varies (Fig. 27.2). Accordingly, liver cell necrosis is divided into 3 types: *diffuse* (submassive to massive), *zonal* and *focal*.

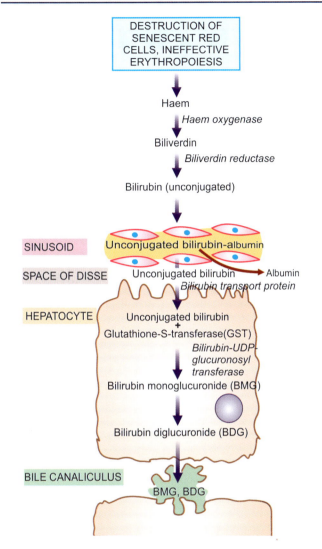

Figure 27.1 ▶ Schematic representation of hepatic phase of bilirubin transport.

Table 27.1	Major differences between unconjugated and conjugated bilirubin.		
	FEATURE	UNCONJUGATED BILIRUBIN	CONJUGATED BILIRUBIN
1.	Normal serum level	More	Less (less than 0.25 mg/dl)
2.	Water solubility	Absent	Present
3.	Affinity to lipids (alcohol solubility)	Present	Absent
4.	Serum albumin binding	High	Low
5.	van den Bergh reaction	Indirect (Total minus direct)	Direct
6.	Renal excretion	Absent	Present
7.	Bilirubin albumin covalent complex formation	Absent	Present
8.	Affinity to brain tissue	Present (Kernicterus)	Absent

1. DIFFUSE (SUBMASSIVE TO MASSIVE) NECROSIS When there is extensive and diffuse necrosis of the liver involving all the cells in groups of lobules, it is termed diffuse, or submassive to massive necrosis. It is most commonly caused by viral hepatitis or drug toxicity.

2. ZONAL NECROSIS Zonal necrosis is necrosis of hepatocytes in 3 different zones of the hepatic lobule. Accordingly, it is of 3 types; each type affecting respective zone is caused by different etiologic factors:

i) Centrilobular necrosis is the commonest type involving hepatocytes in zone 3 (i.e. located around the central vein). Centrilobular necrosis is characteristic feature of ischaemic injury such as in shock and CHF since zone 3 is farthest from the blood supply. Besides, it also occurs in poisoning with chloroform, carbon tetrachloride and certain drugs.

ii) Midzonal necrosis is uncommon and involves zone 2 of the hepatic lobule. This pattern of necrosis is seen in yellow fever and viral hepatitis. In viral hepatitis, some of the necrosed hepatocytes of the mid-zone are transformed into acidophilic, rounded Councilman bodies.

iii) Periportal (peripheral) necrosis is seen in zone 1 involving the parenchyma closest to the arterial and portal blood supply. Since zone 1 is most well perfused, it is most vulnerable to the effects of circulating hepatotoxins e.g. in phosphorus poisoning and eclampsia.

3. FOCAL NECROSIS This form of necrosis involves small groups of hepatocytes irregularly distributed in the hepatic lobule. Focal necrosis is most often caused by microbiologic infections. These include viral hepatitis, miliary tuberculosis, typhoid fever and various other forms of bacterial, viral and fungal infections. Focal necrosis may also occur in drug-induced hepatitis.

CLASSIFICATION AND FEATURES OF JAUNDICE

Based on pathophysiology, jaundice may result from one or more of the following mechanisms:
1. Increased bilirubin production
2. Decreased hepatic uptake
3. Decreased hepatic conjugation
4. Decreased excretion of bilirubin into bile

Accordingly, a simple age-old classification of jaundice was to divide it into 3 predominant types: *pre-hepatic (haemolytic), hepatic,* and *post-hepatic cholestatic.* However, hyperbilirubinaemia due to first three mechanisms is *mainly unconjugated* while the last variety yields *mainly conjugated* hyperbilirubinaemia. Hence, currently pathophysiologic

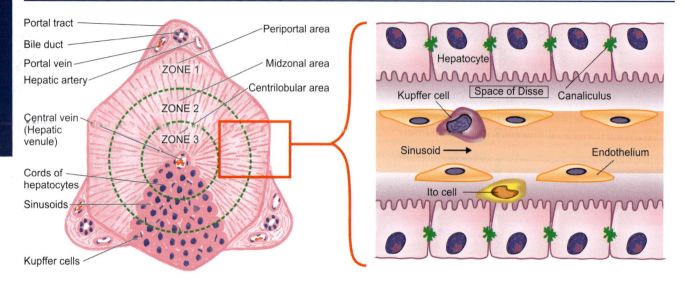

Figure 27.2 ▶ Histology of hepatic lobule. The hexagonal or pyramidal structure with central vein and peripheral 4 to 5 portal triads is termed the classical lobule. The figure on left shows functional divisions of the lobule into 3 zones shown by circles. The figure on right shows hepatic sinusoid perisinusoidal space and cords of hepatocytes.

classification of jaundice is based on predominance of the type of hyperbilirubinaemia. A simple test to determine whether hyperbilirubinaemia is of unconjugated or conjugated variety is to determine whether bilirubin is present in urine or not; its absence in urine suggests unconjugated hyperbilirubinaemia since unconjugated bilirubin is not filtered by the glomerulus. The presence of bilirubin in the urine is evidence of conjugated hyperbilirubinaemia.

Based on these mechanisms, the pathogenesis and main features of the two predominant forms of hyperbilirubinaemia are discussed below **(Table 27.2)**.

I. Predominantly Unconjugated Hyperbilirubinaemia

This form of jaundice can result from the following three sets of conditions:

1. INCREASED BILIRUBIN PRODUCTION (HAEMO-LYTIC, ACHOLURIC OR PREHEPATIC JAUNDICE) This results from excessive red cell destruction as occurs in intra- and extravascular haemolysis or due to ineffective erythropoiesis. There is increased release of haemoglobin from excessive breakdown of red cells that leads to over-production of bilirubin. Hyperbilirubinaemia develops when the capacity of the liver to conjugate large amount of bilirubin is exceeded. In premature infants, the liver is deficient in enzyme necessary for conjugation while the rate of red cell destruction is high. This results in *icterus neonatorum* which is particularly severe in haemolytic disease of the newborn due to maternal isoantibodies (page 388). Since there is predominantly unconjugated

Table 27.2	Pathophysiologic classification of jaundice.
I.	PREDOMINANTLY UNCONJUGATED HYPERBILIRUBINAEMIA
1.	Increased bilirubin production (Haemolytic, acholuric or prehepatic jaundice)
	i) Intra- and extravascular haemolysis
	ii) Ineffective erythropoiesis
2.	Decreased hepatic uptake
	i) Drugs
	ii) Prolonged starvation
	iii) Sepsis
3.	Decreased bilirubin conjugation
	i) Hereditary disorders (e.g. Gilbert's syndrome, Crigler-Najjar syndrome)
	ii) Acquired defects (e.g. drugs, hepatitis, cirrhosis)
	iii) Neonatal jaundice
II.	PREDOMINANTLY CONJUGATED HYPERBILIRUBINAEMIA (CHOLESTASIS)
1.	Intrahepatic cholestasis (Impaired hepatic excretion)
	i) Hereditary disorders or 'pure cholestasis' (e.g. Dubin-Johnson syndrome, Rotor's syndrome, fibrocystic disease of pancreas, benign familial recurrent cholestasis, intrahepatic atresia, cholestatic jaundice of pregnancy)
	ii) Acquired disorders or 'hepatocellular cholestasis' (e.g. viral hepatitis, drugs, alcohol-induced injury, sepsis, cirrhosis)
2.	Extrahepatic cholestasis (Extrahepatic biliary obstruction)
	Mechanical obstruction (e.g. gallstones, inflammatory strictures, carcinoma head of pancreas, tumours of bile ducts, sclerosing cholangitis, congenital atresia of extrahepatic ducts)

hyperbilirubinaemia in such cases, there is danger of permanent brain damage in these infants from kernicterus when the serum level of unconjugated bilirubin exceeds 20 mg/dl.

Laboratory data in haemolytic jaundice, in addition to predominant unconjugated hyperbilirubinaemia, reveal normal serum levels of transaminases, alkaline phosphatase and proteins. Bile pigment being unconjugated type is absent from urine (acholuric jaundice). However, there is dark brown colour of stools due to excessive faecal excretion of bile pigment and there is increased urinary excretion of urobilinogen.

2. DECREASED HEPATIC UPTAKE The uptake of bilirubin by the hepatocyte that involves dissociation of the pigment from albumin and its binding to cytoplasmic protein, GST or ligandin, may be deranged in certain conditions e.g. due to drugs, prolonged starvation and sepsis.

3. DECREASED BILIRUBIN CONJUGATION This mechanism involves deranged hepatic conjugation due to defect or deficiency of the enzyme, glucuronosyl transferase. This can occur in certain inherited disorders of the enzyme (e.g. Gilbert's syndrome and Crigler-Najjar syndrome), or acquired defects in its activity (e.g. due to drugs, hepatitis, cirrhosis). However, hepatocellular damage causes deranged excretory capacity of the liver more than its conjugating capacity. The physiologic neonatal jaundice is also partly due to relative deficiency of UDP-glucuronosyl transferase in the neonatal liver and is partly as a result of increased rate of red cell destruction in neonates.

II. Predominantly Conjugated Hyperbilirubinaemia (Cholestasis)

This form of hyperbilirubinaemia is defined as failure of normal amounts of bile to reach the duodenum. Morphologically, cholestasis means accumulation of bile in liver cells and biliary passages. The defect in excretion may be within the biliary canaliculi of the hepatocyte and in the microscopic bile ducts *(intrahepatic cholestasis or medical jaundice)*, or there may be mechanical obstruction to the extrahepatic biliary excretory apparatus *(extrahepatic cholestasis or obstructive jaundice)*. It is important to distinguish these two forms of cholestasis since extrahepatic cholestasis or obstructive jaundice is often treatable with surgery, whereas the intrahepatic cholestasis or medical jaundice cannot be benefitted by surgery but may in fact worsen by the operation. Prolonged cholestasis of either of the two types may progress to biliary cirrhosis.

1. INTRAHEPATIC CHOLESTASIS Intrahepatic cholestasis is due to impaired hepatic excretion of bile and may occur from hereditary or acquired disorders.

i) Hereditary disorders producing intrahepatic obstruction to biliary excretion are characterised by *'pure cholestasis'* e.g. in Dubin-Johnson syndrome, Rotor syndrome, fibrocystic disease of pancreas, benign familial recurrent cholestasis, intrahepatic atresia and cholestatic jaundice of pregnancy.

ii) Acquired disorders with intrahepatic excretory defect of bilirubin are largely due to hepatocellular diseases and hence are termed *'hepatocellular cholestasis'* e.g. in viral hepatitis, alcoholic hepatitis, and drug-induced cholestasis such as from administration of chlorpromazine and oral contraceptives.

The **features** of intrahepatic cholestasis include: predominant conjugated hyperbilirubinaemia due to regurgitation of conjugated bilirubin into blood, bilirubinuria, elevated levels of serum bile acids and consequent pruritus, elevated serum alkaline phosphatase, hyperlipidaemia and hypoprothrombinaemia. 'Pure cholestasis' can be distinguished from 'hepatocellular cholestasis' by elevated serum levels of transaminases in the latter due to liver cell injury.

◈ **Liver biopsy** in cases with intrahepatic cholestasis reveals milder degree of cholestasis than the extrahepatic disorders **(Fig. 27.3, A)**. The biliary canaliculi of the hepatocytes are dilated and contain characteristic elongated green-brown *bile plugs*. The cytoplasm of the affected hepatocytes shows feathery degeneration. Canalicular bile stasis eventually causes proliferation of intralobular ductules followed by periportal fibrosis and produces a picture resembling biliary cirrhosis.

2. EXTRAHEPATIC CHOLESTASIS Extrahepatic cholestasis results from mechanical obstruction to large bile ducts outside the liver or within the porta hepatis. The common causes are gallstones, inflammatory strictures, carcinoma head of pancreas, tumours of bile duct, sclerosing cholangitis and congenital atresia of extrahepatic ducts. The obstruction may be complete and sudden with eventual progressive obstructive jaundice, or the obstruction may be partial and incomplete resulting in intermittent jaundice.

The **features** of extrahepatic cholestasis (obstructive jaundice), like in intrahepatic cholestasis, are: predominant conjugated hyperbilirubinaemia, bilirubinuria, elevated serum bile acids causing intense pruritus, high serum alkaline phosphatase and hyperlipidaemia. However, there are certain features which help to distinguish extrahepatic from intrahepatic cholestasis. In extrahepatic cholestasis, there is malabsorption of fat-soluble vitamins (A, D, E and K) and steatorrhoea resulting in vitamin K deficiency. Prolonged prothrombin time in such cases shows improvement following parenteral administration of vitamin K, whereas hypoprothrombinaemia due to hepatocellular disease (intrahepatic cholestasis) shows no such improvement in prothrombin time with vitamin K administration. The stools of such patients are clay-coloured due to absence of bilirubin metabolite, stercobilin, in faeces and there is virtual disappearance of urobilinogen from the urine. These patients may have fever due to high incidence of ascending bacterial infections (ascending cholangitis).

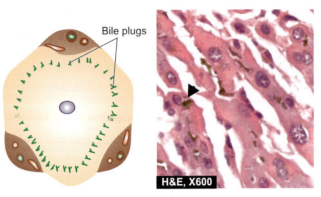 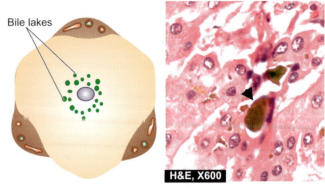

A, INTRAHEPATIC CHOLESTASIS   **B, EXTRAHEPATIC CHOLESTASIS**

Figure 27.3 ▶ Salient features in morphology of liver in intra- and extrahepatic cholestasis. A, Intrahepatic cholestasis is characterised by elongated bile plugs in the canaliculi of hepatocytes at the periphery of the lobule. B, Extrahepatic cholestasis shows characteristic bile lakes due to rupture of canaliculi in the hepatocytes in the centrilobular area.

◆ **Liver biopsy** in cases with extrahepatic cholestasis shows more marked changes of cholestasis **(Fig. 27.3, B)**. Since the obstruction is in the extrahepatic bile ducts, there is progressive retrograde extension of bile stasis into intrahepatic duct system. This results in dilatation of bile ducts and rupture of canaliculi with extravasation of bile producing *bile lakes*. Since bile is toxic, the regions of bile lakes are surrounded by focal necrosis of hepatocytes. Stasis of bile predisposes to ascending bacterial infections with accumulation of polymorphs around the dilated ducts (ascending cholangitis). Eventually, there is proliferation of bile ducts and the appearance may mimic biliary cirrhosis (page 549).

NEONATAL JAUNDICE

Jaundice appears in neonates when the total serum bilirubin is more than 3 mg/dl. It may be the result of unconjugated or conjugated hyperbilirubinaemia; the former being more common. Important causes of neonatal jaundice are listed in **Table 27.3**. Some of these conditions are considered below, while others are discussed elsewhere in the relevant sections.

Hereditary Non-Haemolytic Hyperbilirubinaemia

Hereditary non-haemolytic hyperbilirubinaemias are a small group of uncommon familial disorders of bilirubin metabolism when haemolytic causes have been excluded. The commonest is Gilbert's syndrome; others are Crigler-Najjar syndrome, Dubin-Johnson syndrome, Rotor's syndrome, benign recurrent intrahepatic cholestasis and progressive familial intrahepatic cholestasis. The features common to all these conditions are presence of icterus but almost normal liver function tests and no well-defined morphologic changes except in Dubin-Johnson syndrome. Gilbert's syndrome and Crigler-Najjar syndrome are examples of *hereditary non-haemolytic unconjugated hyperbilirubinaemia*, whereas Dubin-Johnson syndrome, Rotor's syndrome and benign familial recurrent cholestasis are conditions with *hereditary conjugated hyperbilirubinaemia*.

Neonatal Hepatitis

Neonatal hepatitis, also termed giant cell hepatitis or neonatal hepatocellular cholestasis, is a general term used for the constant morphologic change seen in conjugated hyperbilirubinaemia as a result of known infectious and metabolic causes listed in **Table 27.3**, or may have an idiopathic etiology. 'Idiopathic' neonatal hepatitis is more common and accounts for 75% of cases. Though all the cases with either known etiologies or idiopathic type are grouped together under neonatal hepatitis, all of them are

Table 27.3	Causes of neonatal jaundice.
A.	UNCONJUGATED HYPERBILIRUBINAEMIA
1.	Physiologic and prematurity jaundice
2.	Haemolytic disease of the newborn and kernicterus (page 388)
3.	Congenital haemolytic disorders (page 389)
4.	Perinatal complications (e.g. haemorrhage, sepsis)
5.	Gilbert's syndrome
6.	Crigler-Najjar syndrome (type I and II)
B.	CONJUGATED HYPERBILIRUBINAEMIA
1.	Hereditary (Dubin-Johnson syndrome, Rotor's syndrome)
2.	Infections (e.g. hepatitis B, hepatitis C or non-A non-B hepatitis, rubella, coxsackievirus, cytomegalovirus, echovirus, herpes simplex, syphilis, toxoplasma, gram-negative sepsis)
3.	Metabolic (e.g. galactosaemia, alpha-1-antitrypsin deficiency, cystic fibrosis, Niemann-Pick disease)
4.	Idiopathic (neonatal hepatitis, congenital hepatic fibrosis)
5.	Biliary atresia (intrahepatic and extrahepatic)
6.	Reye's syndrome

not necessarily inflammatory conditions, thus belying their nomenclature as 'hepatitis'. The condition usually presents in the first week of birth with jaundice, bilirubinuria, pale stools and high serum alkaline phosphatase.

Biliary Atresias

Biliary atresias, also called as *infantile cholangiopathies,* are a group of intrauterine developmental abnormalities of the biliary system. Though they are often classified as congenital, the abnormality of development in most instances is extraneous infection during the intrauterine development or shortly after birth that brings about inflammatory destruction of the bile ducts. The condition may, therefore, have various grades of destruction ranging from complete absence of bile ducts termed *atresia,* to reduction in their number called *paucity of bile ducts.*

Depending upon the portion of biliary system involved, biliary atresias may be extrahepatic or intrahepatic.

Extrahepatic biliary atresia The extrahepatic bile ducts fail to develop normally so that in some cases the bile ducts are *absent* at birth, while in others the ducts may have been formed but start undergoing sclerosis in the perinatal period. It is common to have multiple defects and other congenital lesions. Extrahepatic biliary atresia is found in 1 per 10,000 livebirths. Cholestatic jaundice appears by the first week after birth. The baby has severe pruritus, pale stools, dark urine and elevated serum transaminases. In some cases, the condition is correctable by surgery, while in vast majority the atresia is not correctable and in such cases hepatic portoenterostomy (Kasai procedure) or hepatic transplantation must be considered. Death is usually due to intercurrent infection, liver failure, and bleeding due to vitamin K deficiency or oesophageal varices. Cirrhosis and ascites are late complications appearing within 2 years of age.

Intrahepatic biliary atresia Intrahepatic biliary atresia is characterised by biliary hypoplasia so that there is *paucity of bile ducts* rather than their complete absence. The condition probably has its origin in viral infection acquired during intrauterine period or in the neonatal period. Cholestatic jaundice usually appears within the first few days of birth and is characterised by high serum bile acids with associated pruritus, and hypercholesterolaemia with appearance of xanthomas by first year of life. Hepatic as well as urinary copper concentrations are elevated. In some cases, intrahepatic biliary atresia is related to α-1-antitrypsin deficiency.

Reye's Syndrome

Reye's syndrome is defined as an acute postviral syndrome of encephalopathy and fatty change in the viscera. The syndrome may follow almost any known viral disease but is most common after influenza A or B and varicella. Viral infection may act singly, but more often its effect is modified by certain exogenous factors such as by administration of salicylates, aflatoxins and insecticides. These effects cause mitochondrial injury and decreased activity of mitochondrial enzymes in the liver. This eventually leads to rise in blood ammonia and accumulation of triglycerides within hepatocytes.

The patients are generally children between 6 months and 15 years of age. Within a week after a viral illness, the child develops intractable vomiting and progressive neurological deterioration due to encephalopathy, eventually leading to stupor, coma and death. Characteristic laboratory findings are elevated blood ammonia, serum transaminases, bilirubin and prolonged prothrombin time.

> **GIST BOX 27.1 Jaundice**
>
> ❖ Jaundice is yellow pigmentation of the skin or sclerae by bilirubin.
> ❖ It is due to rise in bilirubin level in the blood (hyperbilirubinaemia) above normal (0.3-1.3 mg/dl).
> ❖ Normally, bilirubin formed in the body is transported and metabolised through the liver, and excreted through the intestines and kidneys.
> ❖ All forms of liver cell injury result in necrosis of liver cells in the hepatic lobule which may be *diffuse* (submassive to massive), *zonal* and *focal*. Zonal necrosis may pertain to respective zone: centrilobular (zone 1), midzonal (zone 2) and periportal (zone 3).
> ❖ Predominantly unconjugated hyperbilirubinaemia is due to increased production and decreased hepatic uptake and conjugation, while reduced excretion causes mainly conjugated hyperbilirubinaemia.
> ❖ Neonatal jaundice appears at serum bilirubin level of more than 3 mg/dl and is more often unconjugated hyperbilirubinaemia.
> ❖ Hereditary non-haemolytic hyperbilirubinaemias are familial disorders of bilirubin metabolism; most common is Gilbert's syndrome; others are Crigler-Najjar syndrome (type 1 and 2), and Dubin-Johnson syndrome. Gilbert's and Dubin-Johnson syndrome have excellent prognosis.
> ❖ Neonatal hepatitis or giant cell hepatitis is morphologic change seen in conjugated hyperbilirubinaemia as a result of known infectious and metabolic causes.
> ❖ Biliary atresias (intrahepatic and extrahepatic) are intrauterine developmental abnormalities of the biliary system.
> ❖ Reye's syndrome is an acute postviral syndrome of encephalopathy and fatty change in the viscera including liver.

VIRAL HEPATITIS

The term viral hepatitis is used to describe infection of the liver caused by hepatotropic viruses. Currently there are 5 main varieties of these viruses causing distinct types of viral hepatitis:

◆ *Hepatitis A virus (HAV),* causing a faecally-spread self-limiting disease.

◆ *Hepatitis B virus (HBV),* causing a parenterally transmitted disease that may become chronic.

Section VI: Selected Topics from Systemic Pathology

♦ *Hepatitis C virus (HCV)*, previously termed non-A, non-B (NANB) hepatitis virus involved chiefly in transfusion-related hepatitis.
♦ *Hepatitis delta virus (HDV)* which is sometimes associated as superinfection with hepatitis B infection.
♦ *Hepatitis E virus (HEV)*, causing water-borne infection.

While HBV is a DNA virus, all other human hepatitis viruses are RNA viruses.

Though a number of other viral diseases such as infection with Epstein-Barr virus (in infectious mononucleosis), arbovirus (in yellow fever), cytomegalovirus, herpes simplex and several others affect the liver but the changes produced by them are nonspecific; the term 'viral hepatitis' is strictly applied to infection of the liver by the hepatitis viruses.

ETIOLOGIC CLASSIFICATION

Based on the etiologic agent, viral hepatitis is currently classified into 5 etiologic types—hepatitis A, hepatitis B, hepatitis C, hepatitis D and hepatitis E. The contrasting features of major types are presented in Table 27.4.

Hepatitis A

Infection with HAV causes hepatitis A (infectious hepatitis). Hepatitis A is responsible for 20-25% of clinical hepatitis in the developing countries of the world but the incidence is much lower in the developed countries. Hepatitis A is usually a benign, self-limiting disease and has an incubation period of 15-45 days. The disease occurs in epidemic form as well as sporadically. It is almost exclusively spread by faeco-oral route. The spread is related to close personal contact such as in overcrowding, poor hygienic and sanitary conditions. Frozen and stored contaminated foods and water have been blamed in many epidemics. Most frequently affected age group is 5-14 years; adults are often infected by spread from children.

HEPATITIS A VIRUS (HAV) The etiologic agent for hepatitis A, HAV, is a small, 27 nm diameter, icosahedral non-enveloped, single-stranded RNA virus. Viral genome has been characterised but only a single serotype has been identified. HAV infection can be transmitted to primates and the virus

Table 27.4 Features of various types of hepatitis viruses.

	FEATURE	HEPATITIS A	HEPATITIS B	HEPATITIS C	HEPATITIS D	HEPATITIS E
1.	Agent	HAV	HBV	HCV	HDV	HEV
2.	Year identified	1973	1965	1989	1977	1980
3.	Viral particle	27 nm	42 nm	30-60 nm	35-37 nm	32-34 nm
4.	Genome	RNA, ss, linear	DNA, ss/ds	RNA, ss, linear circular	RNA, ss, circular	RNA, ss, linear
5.	Morphology	Icosahedral non-enveloped	Double-shelled, enveloped	Enveloped	Enveloped, replication defective	Icosahedral, non-enveloped
6.	Spread	Faeco-oral	Parenteral, close contact	Parenteral, close contact	Parenteral, close contact	Water-borne
7.	Incubation period	15-45 days	30-180 days	20-90 days	30-50 days (In superinfection)	15-60 days
8.	Antigen(s)	HAV	HBsAg HBcAg HBeAg HBxAg	HCV RNA C 100-3 C 33c NS5	HBsAg HDV	HEV
9.	Antibodies	anti-HAV	anti-HBs anti-HBc anti-HBe	anti-HCV	anti-HBs anti-HDV	anti-HEV
10.	Severity	Mild	Occasionally severe	Moderate	Occasionally severe	Mild
11.	Chronic hepatitis	None	Occasional	Common	Common	None
12.	Carrier state	None	<1%	<1%	1-10%	Unknown
13.	Hepatocellular carcinoma	No	+	+	±	None
14.	Prognosis	Excellent	Worse with age	Moderate	Acute good; chronic poor	Good

(ss= single-stranded; ss/ds= partially single-stranded partially double-stranded)

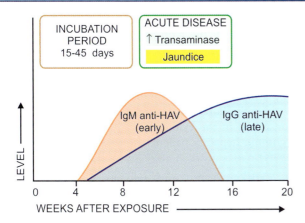

Figure 27.4 ▶ Sequence of appearance of antibodies to HAV.

can be cultivated *in vitro*. Inactivation of viral activity can be achieved by boiling for 1 minute, by ultraviolet radiation, or by contact with formaldehyde and chlorine. The virus is present in the liver cells, bile, stool and blood during the incubation period and in pre-icteric phase but viral shedding diminishes after the onset of jaundice. Chronic carriers have not been identified for HAV infection.

PATHOGENESIS Evidence that hepatitis caused by HAV has an immunologic basis comes from demonstration of following antibodies acting as serum markers for hepatitis A infection (Fig. 27.4):

1. *IgM anti-HAV antibody* appears in the serum at the onset of symptoms of acute hepatitis A.

2. *IgG anti-HAV antibody* is detected in the serum after acute illness and remains detectable indefinitely. It gives lifelong protective immunity against reinfection with HAV.

Hepatitis B

Hepatitis B (serum hepatitis) caused by HBV infection has a longer incubation period (30-180 days) and is transmitted parenterally such as in recipients of blood and blood products, intravenous drug addicts, patients treated by renal dialysis and hospital workers exposed to blood, and by intimate physical contact such as from mother to child and by sexual contact. The disease may occur at any age. HBV infection causes more severe form of illness that includes: acute hepatitis B, chronic hepatitis, progression to cirrhosis, fulminant hepatitis and an asymptomatic carrier stage. HBV plays some role in the development of hepatocellular carcinoma as discussed later.

HEPATITIS B VIRUS (HBV) The etiologic agent for hepatitis B, HBV, is a DNA virus which has been extensively studied. Electron microscopic studies on serum of patients infected with HBV show 3 forms of viral particles of 2 sizes: small (spheres and tubules/filaments) and large (spheres) as under:

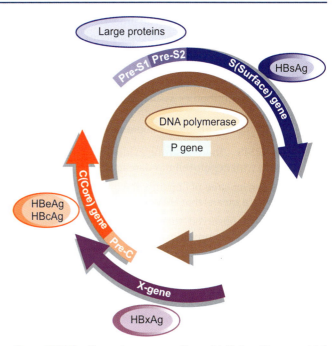

Figure 27.5 ▶ Genomic structure of hepatitis B virus (Dane particle).

i) *Small particles* are most numerous and exist in two forms— as 22 nm spheres, and as tubules 22 nm in diameter and 100 nm long. These are antigenically identical to envelope protein of HBV and represent excess of viral envelope protein referred to as hepatitis B surface antigen (HBsAg).

ii) *Large particles,* 42 nm in diameter, are double-shelled spherical particles, also called as *Dane particles*. These are about 100 to 1000 times less in number in serum compared to small 22 nm particles and represent intact virion of HBV.

The genomic structure of HBV is quite compact and complex. The HBV DNA consists of 4 overlapping genes which encode for multiple proteins (Fig. 27.5):

1. S gene codes for the surface envelope protein, hepatitis B surface antigen (HBsAg); this product is major protein. HBsAg is present on the outer surface of the large spherical particles as well as in small spherical and tubular structures. *Pre-S1 and pre-S2* regions of genome are upstream of S gene and code for pre-S gene protein products that includes receptor on the HBV surface and for hepatocyte membrane proteins. The protein product of S-gene plus adjacent pre-S2 region is the *middle protein*, while the protein products of pre-S1 plus pre-S2 regions is the *large protein*. Large protein coming from both pre-S proteins is rich in complete virions.

2. P gene is the largest and codes for DNA polymerase.

3. C gene codes for two nucleocapsid proteins, HBeAg and a core protein termed HBcAg.

4. X gene codes for HBxAg which is a small non-particulate protein. HbxAg has a role in transactivatiing the transcription of both viral and cellular genes. The processes transactivated by X-genes include signal-transduction pathways, increased replication of HBV DNA, replication of other viruses including HIV, enhanced susceptibility of HBV-infected hepatocytes to cytolytic T cells, and pro-apoptotic pathway. Expression of HBxAg and its antibodies associated with enhanced HBV DNA replication has been implicated in hepatocellular carcinoma in patients of chronic hepatitis.

PATHOGENESIS There is strong evidence linking immune pathogenesis with hepatocellular damage:

i) Since a carrier state of hepatitis B without hepatocellular damage exists, it means that HBV is not directly cytopathic.

ii) It has been observed that individuals with defect or deficiency of cellular immunity have more persistent hepatitis B disease instead of clearing HBV from their blood.

iii) In support of cell-mediated mechanism in hepatocellular damage by HBV comes from observation that viral antigens (in particular nucleocapsid proteins HbcAg and HbeAg) are attacked by host cytotoxic CD8+T lymphocytes.

iv) The host response of CD8+T lymphocytes by elaboration of antiviral cytokines is variable in different individuals and that determines whether an HBV-infected person recovers, develops mild or severe disease, or progresses to chronic disease.

Serologic and viral markers In support of immune pathogenesis is the demonstration of several immunological markers in the serum and in hepatocytes indicative of presence of HBV infection. These are as under **(Fig. 27.6)**:

1. **HBsAg** In 1965, Blumberg and colleagues in Philadelphia found a lipoprotein complex in the serum of a multiple-transfused haemophiliac of Australian aborigine which was subsequently shown by them to be associated with serum hepatitis. This antigen was termed *Australia antigen* by them (In 1977, Blumberg was awarded the Nobel prize for his discovery). The term Australia antigen is now used synonymous with hepatitis B surface antigen (HBsAg). HBsAg appears early in the blood after about 6 weeks of infection and its detection is an indicator of active HBV infection. It usually disappears in 3-6 months. Its persistence for more than 6 months implies a carrier state. HBsAg may also be demonstrated in the cytoplasm of hepatocytes of carriers and chronic hepatitis patients by *Orcein staining* (orange positivity).

2. **Anti-HBs** Specific antibody to HBsAg in serum called anti-HBs appears late, about 3 months after the onset. Anti-HBs response may be both IgM and IgG type. The prevalence rate of anti-HBs ranges from 10-15%. In these individuals it persists for life providing protection against reinfection with HBV.

3. **HBeAg** HBeAg derived from core protein is present transiently (3-6 weeks) during an acute attack. Its persistence beyond 10 weeks is indicative of development of chronic liver disease and carrier state.

4. **Anti-HBe** Antibody to HBeAg called anti-HBe appears after disappearance of HBeAg. Seroconversion from HBeAg to anti-HBe during acute stage of illness is a prognostic sign for resolution of infection.

5. **HBcAg** HBcAg derived from core protein cannot be detected in the blood. But HBcAg can be demonstrated in the nuclei of hepatocytes in carrier state and in chronic hepatitis patients by Orcein staining but not in the liver cells during acute stage.

6. **Anti-HBc** Antibody to HBcAg called anti-HBc can, however, be detected in the serum of acute hepatitis B patients during pre-icteric stage. In the initial period, it is IgM class antibody which persists for 4-6 months and is followed later by IgG anti-HBc. Thus, detection of high titre of IgM anti-HBc is indicative of recent acute HBV infection, while elevated level of IgG anti-HBc suggests HBV infection in the remote past.

7. **HBV-DNA** Detection of HBV-DNA by molecular hybridisation using the Southern blot technique is the most sensitive index of hepatitis B infection. It is present in pre-symptomatic phase and transiently during early acute stage.

Hepatitis D

Infection with delta virus (HDV) in the hepatocyte nuclei of HBsAg-positive patients is termed hepatitis D. HDV is a defective virus for which HBV is the helper. Thus, hepatitis D develops when there is concomitant hepatitis B infection. HDV infection and hepatitis B may be simultaneous *(co-infection),* or HDV may infect a chronic HBsAg carrier *(superinfection)* **(Fig. 27.7)**:

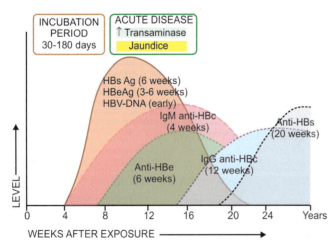

Figure 27.6 ▶ Sequence of serologic and viral markers in acute hepatitis B.

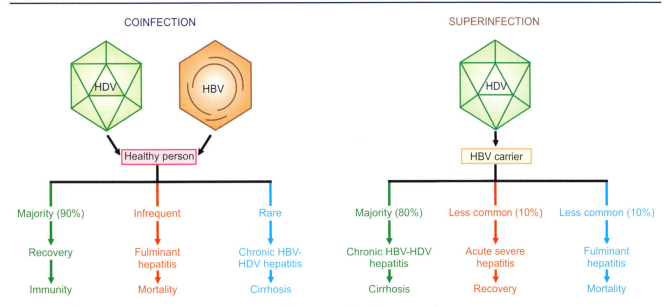

Figure 27.7 ▶ Consequences of coinfection *versus* superinfection in combined HDV-HBV infection.

◈ With **coinfection,** acute hepatitis D may range from mild to fulminant hepatitis but fulminant hepatitis is more likely in such simultaneous delta infection. Chronicity rarely develops in coinfection.

◈ With **superinfection** (incubation period 30-35 days), chronic HBV infection gets worsened indicated by appearance of severe and fulminant acute attacks, progression of carrier stage to chronic delta hepatitis or acceleration towards cirrhosis. Occurrence of hepatocellular carcinoma is, however, less common in HBsAg carriers with HDV infection.

HDV infection is worldwide in distribution though the incidence may vary in different countries. Endemic regions are Southern Europe, Middle-East, South India and parts of Africa. The high-risk individuals for HDV infection are the same as for HBV infection i.e. intravenous drug abusers, homosexuals, transfusion recipients, and health care workers.

HEPATITIS DELTA VIRUS (HDV) The etiologic agent, HDV, is a small single-stranded RNA particle with a diameter of 36 nm. It is double-shelled—the outer shell consists of HBsAg and the inner shell consists of delta antigen provided by a circular RNA strand. It is highly infectious and can induce hepatitis in any HBsAg-positive host. HDV replication and proliferation takes place within the nuclei of liver cells. Markers for HDV infection include the following:

1. *HDV identification* in the blood and in the liver cell nuclei.

2. *HDAg* detectable in the blood and on fixed liver tissue specimens.

3. *Anti-HD antibody* in acute hepatitis which is initially IgM type and later replaced by IgG type anti-HD antibody which persists for life to confer immunity against reinfection.

PATHOGENESIS HDV, unlike HBV, is thought to cause direct cytopathic effect on hepatocytes. However, there are examples of transmission of HDV infection from individuals who themselves have not suffered from any attack of hepatitis, suggesting that it may not be always cytopathic.

Hepatitis C

The diagnosis of this major category of hepatitis was earlier made after exclusion of infection with other known hepatitis viruses in those times and was initially designated non-A, non-B (NANB) hepatitis. However, now it has been characterised and is called hepatitis C.

Hepatitis C infection is acquired by blood transfusions, blood products, haemodialysis, parenteral drug abuse and accidental cuts and needle-pricks in health workers. About 90% of post-transfusion hepatitis is of hepatitis C type. About 1-2% of volunteer blood donors and up to 5% of professional blood donors are carriers of HCV. Hepatitis C has an incubation period of 20-90 days (mean 50 days). Clinically, acute HCV hepatitis is milder than HBV hepatitis but HCV has a higher rate of progression to chronic hepatitis than HBV. Persistence of infection and chronic hepatitis are the key features of HCV. Occurrence of cirrhosis after 5 to 10 years and progression to hepatocellular carcinoma are other late consequences of HCV infection. Currently, HCV is considered more important cause of chronic liver disease worldwide than HBV.

HEPATITIS C VIRUS (HCV) HCV is a single-stranded, enveloped RNA virus, having a diameter of 30-60 nm. HCV genome has about 3000 amino acids. The genomic

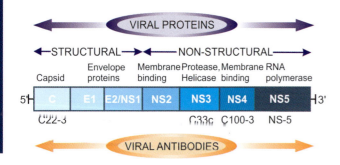

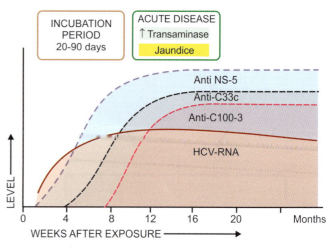

Figure 27.8 ▶ Diagrammatic structure of hepatitis C virus.

Figure 27.9 ▶ Sequence of serologic and viral markers of HCV infection.

organisation of HCV shows a 5′ terminal end, C (capsid) region and the envelope regions E1 and E2 in the exons **(Fig. 27.8)**.

The viral proteins result in corresponding serologic and virologic markers for HCV infection as under **(Fig. 27.9)**:

1. *Anti-HCV antibodies.* Three generations of anti-HCV IgG assays are available:
i) First generation antibodies are against C100-3 region proteins and appear 1 to 3 months after infection.
ii) Second generation antibodies are against C200 and C33c proteins and appear about one month earlier than the first generation.
iii) Third generation antibodies are against C22-3 and NS-5 region proteins and are detected even earlier.
2. *HCV-RNA.* HCV infection is, however, confirmed by HCV-RNA employing PCR technique which can be detected within a few days after exposure to HCV infection, much before appearance of anti-HCV and persists for the duration of HCV infection.

PATHOGENESIS HCV induces hepatocellular injury by cell-mediated immune mechanism is supported by the following:

i) It is possible that the host lymphoid cells are infected by HCV.
ii) HCV-activated CD4+ helper T lymphocytes stimulate CD8+ T lymphocytes via cytokines elaborated by CD4+ helper T cells.
iii) The stimulated CD8+T lymphocytes, in turn, elaborate antiviral cytokines against various HCV antigens.
iv) Further support to this T- cell mediated mechanism comes from the observation that immune response is stronger in those HCV-infected persons who recover than those who harbour chronic HCV infection.
v) There is some role of certain HLA alleles and innate immunity in rendering variable response by different hosts to HCV infection.
vi) Natural killer (NK) cells also seem to contribute to containment of HCV infection.
vii) In a subset of patients, there is crossreactivity between viral antigens of HCV and host autoantibodies to liver-kidney microsomal antigen (anti-LKM) which explains the association of autoimmune hepatitis and HCV hepatitis.

Hepatitis E

Hepatitis E is an enterically-transmitted virus, previously labelled as epidemic or enterically transmitted variant of non-A non-B hepatitis. The infection occurs in young or middle-aged individuals, primarily seen in India, other Asian countries, Africa and central America.

The infection is generally acquired by contamination of water supplies such as after monsoon flooding. However, compared with HAV, secondary person-to-person infection does not occur with HEV. Thus HEV has some common epidemiologic features with HAV. HEV infection has a particularly high mortality in pregnant women but is otherwise a self-limited disease and has not been associated with chronic liver disease.

HEPATITIS E VIRUS (HEV) HEV is a single-stranded 32-34 nm, icosahedral non-enveloped virus. The virus has been isolated from stools, bile and liver of infected persons. Serologic markers for HEV include the following:

1. Anti-HEV antibodies of both IgM and IgG class. Both fall rapidly after acute illness but routine serologic testing for HEV antibodies is not available.
2. HEV-RNA.

CLINICOPATHOLOGIC SPECTRUM

Among the various etiologic types of hepatitis, evidence linking HBV and HCV infection with the spectrum of clinico-pathologic changes is stronger than with other hepatotropic

viruses. The typical pathologic changes of hepatitis by major hepatotropic viruses are virtually similar. HAV and HEV, however, do not have a carrier stage nor cause chronic hepatitis. The various clinical patterns and pathologic consequences of different hepatotropic viruses can be considered under the following headings:
i) Carrier state
ii) Asymptomatic infection
iii) Acute hepatitis
iv) Chronic hepatitis
v) Fulminant hepatitis (Submassive to massive necrosis)

In addition, progression to cirrhosis and association with hepatocellular carcinoma are known to occur in certain types of hepatitis which are discussed separately later.

I. Carrier State

An asymptomatic individual without manifest disease, harbouring infection with hepatotropic virus and capable of transmitting it is called carrier state. There can be 2 types of carriers:
1. An *'asymptomatic healthy carrier'* who does not suffer from ill-effects of the virus infection but is capable of transmitting.
2. An *'asymptomatic carrier with chronic disease'* capable of transmitting the organisms.

As stated before, hepatitis A and E do not produce the carrier state. Hepatitis B is responsible for the largest number of carriers in the world, while concomitant infection with HDV more often causes progressive disease rather than an asymptomatic carrier state. There is geographic variation in incidence of HBV carrier state: while in normal population in US and western Europe it is less than 0.5%, its prevalence is much higher in Asian and tropical countries (5-20%). An estimated 2-3% of the general population are asymptomatic carriers of HCV. Data on HBV carrier state reveal role of 2 important factors rendering the individual more vulnerable to harbour the organisms—e*arly age at infection* and *impaired immunity*. Whereas approximately 10% of adults contracting hepatitis B infection develop carrier state, 90% of infected neonates fail to clear HBsAg from the serum within 6 months and become HBV carriers.

Clinical recognition of HBV carrier state is done by persistence of HBsAg in the serum of an infected person who fails to clear HBsAg from blood for more than 6 months. Concomitant infection of HDV with HBV depends upon the demonstration of anti-HD.

> **MORPHOLOGIC FEATURES** Carriers of HBV may or may not show changes on liver biopsy.
>
> ◆ *Healthy HBV carriers* may show no changes or minor hepatic change such as presence of finely granular, ground-glass, eosinophilic cytoplasm as evidence of HBsAg.
>
> ◆ *Asymptomatic carriers with chronic disease* may show changes of chronic hepatitis and even cirrhosis.

II. Asymptomatic Infection

These are cases who are detected incidentally to have infection with one of the hepatitis viruses as revealed by their raised serum transaminases or by detection of the presence of antibodies but are otherwise asymptomatic.

III. Acute Hepatitis

The most common consequence of all hepatotropic viruses is acute inflammatory involvement of the entire liver. In general, type A, B, C, D and E run similar clinical course and show identical pathologic findings.

Clinically, acute hepatitis is categorised into 4 phases: incubation period, pre-icteric phase, icteric phase and post-icteric phase.

1. **Incubation period** It varies among different hepatotropic viruses: for hepatitis A it is about 4 weeks (15-45 days); for hepatitis B the average is 10 weeks (30-180 days); for hepatitis D about 6 weeks (30-50 days); for hepatitis C the mean incubation period is about 7 weeks (20-90 days), and for hepatitis E it is 2-8 weeks (15-60 days). The patient remains asymptomatic during incubation period but the infectivity is highest during the last days of incubation period.

2. **Pre-icteric phase** This phase is marked by prodromal constitutional symptoms that include anorexia, nausea, vomiting, fatigue, malaise, distaste for smoking, arthralgia and headache. There may be low-grade fever preceding the onset of jaundice, especially in hepatitis A. The earliest laboratory evidence of hepatocellular injury in pre-icteric phase is the elevation of transaminases.

3. **Icteric phase** The prodromal period is heralded by the onset of clinical jaundice and the constitutional symptoms diminish. Other features include dark-coloured urine due to bilirubinuria, clay-coloured stools due to cholestasis, pruritus as a result of elevated serum bile acids, loss of weight and abdominal discomfort due to enlarged, tender liver. The diagnosis is based on deranged liver function tests (e.g. elevated levels of serum bilirubin, transaminases and alkaline phosphatase, prolonged prothrombin time and hyperglobulinaemia) and serologic detection of hepatitis antigens and antibodies.

4. **Post-icteric phase** The icteric phase lasting for about 1 to 4 weeks is usually followed by clinical and biochemical recovery in 2 to 12 weeks. The recovery phase is more prolonged in hepatitis B and hepatitis C. Up to 1% cases of acute hepatitis may develop severe form of the disease (fulminant hepatitis); and 5-10% of cases progress on to chronic hepatitis. Evolution into the carrier state (except in HAV and HEV infection) has already been described above.

> **MORPHOLOGIC FEATURES** *Grossly,* the liver is slightly enlarged, soft and greenish.
>
> *Histologically,* the changes are as follows (Fig. 27.10):

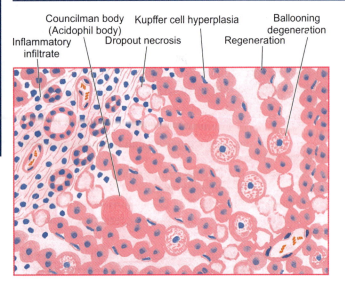
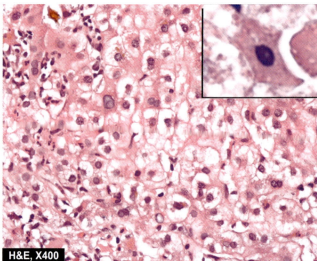

Figure 27.10 ▶ Acute viral hepatitis. The predominant histologic changes are: variable degree of necrosis of hepatocytes, most marked in zone 3 (centrilobular); and mononuclear cellular infiltrate in the lobule. Mild degree of liver cell necrosis is seen as ballooning degeneration while acidophilic Councilman bodies (inbox) are indicative of more severe liver cell injury.

1. Hepatocellular injury There may be variation in the degree of liver cell injury but it is most marked in zone 3 (centrilobular zone):

i) Mildly injured hepatocytes appear swollen with granular cytoplasm which tends to condense around the nucleus *(ballooning degeneration)*.

ii) Others show acidophilic degeneration in which the cytoplasm becomes intensely eosinophilic, the nucleus becomes small and pyknotic and is eventually extruded from the cell, leaving behind necrotic, acidophilic mass called *Councilman body* or *acidophil body* by the process of apoptosis.

iii) Another type of hepatocellular necrosis is *dropout necrosis* in which isolated or small clusters of hepatocytes undergo lysis.

iv) *Bridging necrosis* is a more severe form of hepatocellular injury in acute viral hepatitis and may progress to fulminant hepatitis or chronic hepatitis (discussed below). Bridging necrosis is characterised by bands of necrosis linking portal tracts to central hepatic veins, one central hepatic vein to another, or a portal tract to another tract.

2. Inflammatory infiltrate There is infiltration by mononuclear inflammatory cells, usually in the portal tracts, but may permeate into the lobules.

3. Kupffer cell hyperplasia There is reactive hyperplasia of Kupffer cells many of which contain phagocytosed cellular debris, bile pigment and lipofuscin granules.

4. Cholestasis Biliary stasis is usually not severe in viral hepatitis and may be present as intracytoplasmic bile pigment granules.

5. Regeneration As a result of necrosis of hepatocytes, there is lobular disarray. Surviving adjacent hepatocytes undergo regeneration and hyperplasia. If the necrosis causes collapse of reticulin framework of the lobule, healing by fibrosis follows, distorting the lobular architecture.

The above histologic changes apply to viral hepatitis by various types of hepatotropic viruses in general, and by HBV in particular. It is usually not possible to distinguish histologically between viral hepatitis of various etiologies, but the following morphologic features may help in giving an etiologic clue:

◆ **HAV hepatitis** is a panlobular involvement by heavy inflammatory infiltrate compared to other types.

◆ **HCV hepatitis** causes milder necrosis, with fatty change in hepatocytes, shows presence of lymphoid aggregates in the portal triads and degeneration of bile duct epithelium.

IV. Chronic Hepatitis

Chronic hepatitis is defined as continuing or relapsing hepatic disease for more than 6 months with symptoms along with biochemical, serologic and histopathologic evidence of inflammation and necrosis. Majority of cases of chronic hepatitis are the result of infection with hepatotropic viruses—hepatitis B, hepatitis C and combined hepatitis B and hepatitis D infection. However, some non-viral causes of chronic hepatitis include: Wilson's disease, α-1-antitrypsin deficiency, chronic alcoholism, drug-induced injury and autoimmune diseases. The last named gives rise to *autoimmune or lupoid hepatitis* which is characterised by positive serum autoantibodies (e.g. antinuclear, anti-smooth muscle and anti-mitochondrial) and a positive LE cell test but negative for serologic markers of viral hepatitis.

Until recent years, prediction of prognosis of chronic hepatitis used to be made on the basis of morphology which divided it into 2 main types—*chronic persistent* and *chronic active (aggressive) hepatitis*. A third form, *chronic lobular hepatitis* is distinguished separately by some as mild form of lobular inflammation without inflammation of portal tracts but these cases often recover completely. However, subsequent studies have revealed that morphologic subtypes do not necessarily correlate with prognosis since the disease is not essentially static but may vary from mild form to severe and *vice versa*. Besides, two other factors which determine the vulnerability of a patient of viral hepatitis to develop chronic hepatitis are: *impaired immunity* and *extremes of age* at which the infection is first contracted. Currently, therefore, chronic hepatitis is classified on the basis of etiology and hepatitis activity score (described below). The frequency and severity with which hepatotropic viruses cause chronic hepatitis varies with the organisms as under:

◆ *HCV* infection accounts for 40-60% cases of chronicity in adults. HCV infection is particularly associated with progressive form of chronic hepatitis that may evolve into cirrhosis.

◆ *HBV* causes chronic hepatitis in 90% of infected infants and in about 5% adult cases of hepatitis B.

◆ *HDV* superinfection on HBV carrier state may be responsible for chronic hepatitis in 10-40% cases.

◆ *HAV and HEV* do not produce chronic hepatitis.

MORPHOLOGIC FEATURES The pathologic features are common to both HBV and HCV infection and include the following lesions (Fig. 27.11):

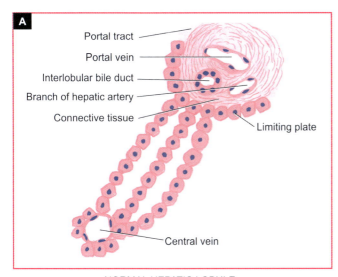
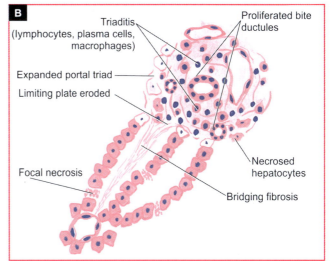
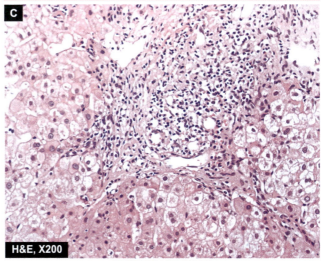

Figure 27.11 ▶ Chronic hepatitis. Diagrammatic representation of pathologic changes in chronic hepatitis (B) contrasted with normal morphology (A). Photomicrograph on right (C) shows stellate-shaped portal triad, with extension of fibrous spurs into lobules. The portal tract is expanded due to increased lymphomononuclear inflammatory cells which are seen to breach the limiting plate (i.e. hepatocytes at the interface of portal tract and lobule are destroyed).

1. Piecemeal necrosis Piecemeal necrosis is defined as periportal destruction of hepatocytes at the limiting plate (*piecemeal* = piece by piece). Its features in chronic hepatitis are as under:

i) Necrosed hepatocytes at the limiting plate in periportal zone.
ii) Interface hepatitis due to expanded portal tract by infiltration of lymphocytes, plasma cells and macrophages.
iii) Expanded portal tracts are often associated with proliferating bile ductules as a response to liver cell injury.

2. Portal tract lesions All forms of chronic hepatitis are characterised by variable degree of changes in the portal tract.

i) Inflammatory cell infiltration by lymphocytes, plasma cells and macrophages (triaditis).
ii) Proliferated bile ductules in the expanded portal tracts.
iii) Additionally, chronic hepatitis C may show lymphoid aggregates or follicles with reactive germinal centre and infiltration of inflammatory cells in the damaged bile duct epithelial cells.

3. Intralobular lesions Generally, the architecture of lobule is retained in mild to moderate chronic hepatitis.

i) There are focal areas of necrosis and inflammation within the hepatic parenchyma.
ii) Scattered acidophilic bodies in the lobule.
iii) Kupffer cell hyperplasia.
iv) More severe form of injury shows bridging necrosis (i.e. bands of necrosed hepatocytes that may bridge portal tract-to-central vein, central vein-to-central vein, and portal tract-to-portal tract).
v) Regenerative changes in hepatocytes in cases of persistent hepatocellular necrosis.
vi) Cases of chronic hepatitis C show moderate fatty change.
vii) Cases of chronic hepatitis B show scattered ground-glass hepatocytes indicative of abundance of HBsAg in the cytoplasm.

4. Bridging fibrosis The onset of fibrosis in chronic hepatitis from the area of interface hepatitis and bridging necrosis is a feature of irreversible damage.

i) At first, there is periportal fibrosis at the sites of interface hepatitis giving the portal tract stellate-shaped appearance.
ii) Progressive cases show bridging fibrosis connecting portal tract-to-portal tract or portal tract-to-central vein traversing the lobule.
iii) End-stage of chronic hepatitis is characterised by dense collagenous septa destroying lobular architecture and forming nodules resulting in postnecrotic cirrhosis.

As prognostic indicator of chronic hepatitis, a histologic grading of chronic hepatitis (ranging from none to minimal/mild to moderate and severe) was originally described by Knodell and Ishak. A combined histologic grade leads to hepatitis activity index (HAI) and takes into consideration *necroinflammatory activity* and *stage of fibrosis*.

CLINICAL FEATURES The clinical features of chronic hepatitis are quite variable ranging from mild disease to full-blown picture of cirrhosis.

i) Mild chronic hepatitis shows only slight but persistent elevation of transaminases ('transaminitis') with fatigue, malaise and loss of appetite.
ii) Other cases may show mild hepatomegaly, hepatic tenderness and mild splenomegaly.
iii) Laboratory findings may reveal prolonged prothrombin time, hyperbilirubinaemia, hyperglobulinaemia and markedly elevated alkaline phosphatase.
iv) Systemic features of circulating immune complexes due to HBV and HCV infection may produce features of immune complex vasculitis, glomerulonephritis and cryoglobulinaemia in a proportion of cases.

However, clinical features do not correlate with morphologic appearance of the liver biopsy. Some patients may have mild form of disease without progressing for several years while others may show rapid evolution into cirrhosis with its complications over a period of few years. Patients of long-standing HBV and HCV chronic infection are known to evolve into hepatocellular carcinoma.

V. Fulminant Hepatitis (Submassive to Massive Necrosis)

Fulminant hepatitis is the most severe form of acute hepatitis in which there is rapidly progressive hepatocellular failure. Two patterns are recognised—*submassive necrosis* having a less rapid course extending up to 3 months; and *massive necrosis* in which the liver failure is rapid and fulminant occurring in 2-3 weeks.

Fulminant hepatitis of either of the two varieties can occur from viral and non-viral etiologies:

◆ *Acute viral hepatitis* accounts for about half the cases, most often from HBV and HCV; less frequently from combined HBV-HDV and rarely from HAV. However, HEV infection is a serious complication in pregnant women. In addition, herpesvirus can also cause serious viral hepatitis.

◆ *Non-viral causes* include acute hepatitis due to drug toxicity (e.g. acetaminophen, non-steroidal anti-inflammatory drugs, isoniazid, halothane and anti-depressants), poisonings, hypoxic injury and massive infiltration of malignant tumours into the liver.

The patients present with features of hepatic failure with hepatic encephalopathy (page 558). The mortality rate is high if hepatic transplantation is not undertaken.

MORPHOLOGIC FEATURES *Grossly,* the liver is small and shrunken, often weighing 500-700 gm. The capsule is loose and wrinkled. The sectioned surface shows diffuse or random involvement of hepatic lobes. There are extensive areas of muddy-red and yellow necrosis (previously called *acute yellow atrophy)* and patches of green bile staining.

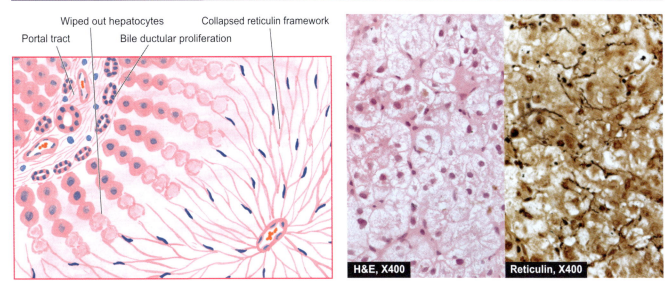

Figure 27.12 ▶ Fulminant hepatitis. There is wiping out of liver lobules with only collapsed reticulin framework left out in their place, highlighted by reticulin stain (right photomicrograph). There is no significant inflammation or fibrosis.

Histologically, two forms of fulminant necrosis are distinguished—submassive and massive necrosis **(Fig. 27.12)**.

i) In **submassive necrosis,** large groups of hepatocytes in zone 3 (centrilobular area) and zone 2 (mid zone) are wiped out leading to a collapsed reticulin framework. Regeneration in submassive necrosis is more orderly and may result in restoration of normal architecture.

ii) In **massive necrosis,** the entire liver lobules are necrotic. As a result of loss of hepatic parenchyma, all that is left is the collapsed and condensed reticulin framework and portal tracts with proliferated bile ductules plugged with bile. Inflammatory infiltrate is scanty. Regeneration, if it takes place, is disorderly forming irregular masses of hepatocytes. Fibrosis is generally not a feature of fulminant hepatitis.

The clinicopathologic course in two major forms of hepatitis, HBV and HCV, is summarised in **Fig. 27.13**.

IMMUNOPROPHYLAXIS AND HEPATITIS VACCINES

Best prophylaxis against the viral hepatitis remains prevention of its spread to the contacts after detection and identification of route by which infection is acquired such as from food or water contamination, sexual spread or parenteral spread. Of late, however, immunoprophylaxis and a few hepatitis vaccines have been developed and some more are under development. The principle underlying either of these two forms of prophylaxis is that the persons who develop good antibody response to the antigen of the hepatotropic virus following active infection are protected against the disease on reinfection. Thus, pre-testing of persons may be carried out so as to determine their antibody level. Immunoprophylaxis and hepatitis vaccination are unnecessary if the pre-testing for antibodies is positive.

1. Hepatitis A Passive immunisation with immune globulin as well as active immunisation with a killed vaccine are available.

2. Hepatitis B Earlier, only passive immunoprophylaxis with standard immune globulin was used. Later, active immunisation against HBsAg was introduced. Current recommendations include pre-exposure and post-exposure prophylaxis with recombinant hepatitis B vaccine:

◈ *Pre-exposure prophylaxis* is done for individuals at high-risk e.g. health care workers, haemodialysis patients and staff, haemophiliacs, intravenous drug users etc. Three intramuscular injections of hepatitis vaccine at 0, 1 and 6 months are recommended.

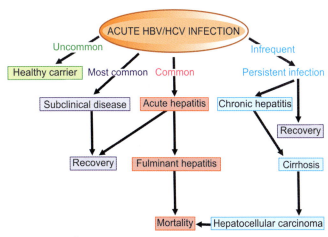

Figure 27.13 ▶ Clinicopathologic course of HBV and HCV infection.

◈ *Post-exposure prophylaxis* is carried out for unvaccinated persons exposed to HBV infection and includes prophylaxis with combination of hepatitis B immune globulin and hepatitis B vaccine.

3. **Hepatitis D** Hepatitis D infection can also be prevented by hepatitis B vaccine.

4. **Hepatitis C** Currently, hepatitis C vaccine has yet not been feasible though antibodies to HCV envelope have been developed.

5. **Hepatitis E** It is not certain whether immune globulin (like for HAV) prevents hepatitis E infection or not but a vaccine against HEV is yet to be developed.

| GIST BOX 27.2 | Viral Hepatitis |

- Viral hepatitis is infection of the liver caused by hepatotropic viruses. A, B, C, D and E.
- Hepatitis A is a faecally-spread self-limiting disease. Early, IgM and later IgG, antibodies appear in the blood.
- Hepatitis B is transmitted parenterally through blood and blood products. There are several immunological markers in the serum: HbsAg, anti-HBs, HbeAg, anti-Hbe, HbcAg, and anti-HBc.
- Hepatitis D develops with hepatitis B either as co-infection, or may infect an HBsAg carrier (superinfection).
- Hepatitis C infection is acquired by blood transfusions.
- Hepatitis E is an enterically-transmitted infection.
- Carrier state exists for hepatitis B and C only.
- Morphology of acute and fulminant hepatitis caused by different hepatotropic viruses is similar.
- Chronic hepatitis may occur in infection with hepatitis B, C and combined HBV-HDV.
- Immunoprophylaxis by a few hepatitis vaccines is done for high risk population.

CIRRHOSIS

Cirrhosis of the liver is one of the ten leading causes of death in the Western world. It represents the irreversible end-stage of several diffuse diseases causing hepatocellular injury and is characterised by the following 4 features:

1. It involves the entire liver.
2. The normal lobular architecture of hepatic parenchyma is disorganised.
3. There is formation of nodules separated from one another by irregular bands of fibrosis.
4. It occurs following hepatocellular necrosis of varying etiology so that there are alternate areas of necrosis and regenerative nodules. However, regenerative nodules are not essential for diagnosis of cirrhosis since biliary cirrhosis and cirrhosis in haemochromatosis have little regeneration.

PATHOGENESIS

Irrespective of the etiology, cirrhosis involves a combination of a few processes: hepatocellular necrosis, healing by fibrosis, formation of compensatory regenerative nodules and changes in vascular pattern of the hepatic parenchyma.

FIBROGENESIS Continued destruction of hepatocytes causes collapse of normal lobular hepatic parenchyma followed by fibrosis around necrotic liver cells. Fibrosis in the liver lobules may be portal-central, portal-portal, or both. The mechanism of fibrosis is by increased synthesis of type I and III collagen in the space of Disse. There is proliferation of fat-storing Ito cells underlying the sinusoidal epithelium which are transformed into myofibroblasts and fibrocytes. Besides collagen, two glycoproteins, fibronectin and laminin, are deposited in excessive amounts in area of liver cell damage. Stimulants for fibrosis are several growth factors (e.g. platelet-derived growth factor receptor-β, transforming growth factor-β, metalloproteineases), vasoactive factors, cytokines, lymphokines and chemokines released from lymphocytes, Kupffer cells, endothelial cells and hepatocytes.

REGENERATIVE NODULES The surviving hepatocytes act as stimulants for growth and proliferation of more hepatocytes under influence of growth factors. This compensatory proliferation of hepatocytes is restricted within fibrous nodules forming regenerative nodules.

VASCULAR REORGANISATION Due to damaged hepatic parenchyma and formation of fibrous nodules, the new vessels formed in the fibrous septa are connected to the vessels in the portal triad (i.e. branches of hepatic artery and portal vein) and then the blood is drained into hepatic vein. This way, the blood bypasses the hepatic parenchyma. Moreover, due to fibrous proliferation in the space of Disse, gaps in the hepatic sinusoids are closed which result in development of capillaries in the sinusoids (capillarisation of sinusoids).

CLASSIFICATION

Cirrhosis can be classified on the basis of morphology and etiology **(Table 27.5)**.

A. MORPHOLOGIC CLASSIFICATION There are 3 morphologic types of cirrhosis—micronodular, macronodular and mixed. Each of these forms may have an active and inactive form.

◈ An *active form* is characterised by continuing hepatocellular necrosis and inflammatory reaction, a process that closely resembles chronic hepatitis.

◈ An *inactive form*, on the other hand, has no evidence of continuing hepatocellular necrosis and has sharply-defined nodules of surviving hepatic parenchyma without any significant inflammation.

Chapter 27: Jaundice, Hepatitis and Cirrhosis

Table 27.5	Classification of cirrhosis.		
A.	MORPHOLOGIC	B.	ETIOLOGIC
I.	Micronodular (nodules less than 3 mm)	1.	Alcoholic cirrhosis (the most common, 60-70%)
II.	Macronodular (nodules more than 3 mm)	2.	Post-necrotic cirrhosis (10%)
		3.	Biliary cirrhosis (5-10%)
III.	Mixed	4.	Pigment cirrhosis in haemochromatosis (5%)
		5.	Cirrhosis in Wilson's disease
		6.	Cirrhosis in α-1-antitrypsin deficiency
		7.	Cardiac cirrhosis
		8.	Indian childhood cirrhosis (ICC)
		9.	Cirrhosis in autoimmune hepatitis
		10.	Cirrhosis in non-alcoholic steatohepatitis
		11.	Miscellaneous forms of cirrhosis (metabolic, infectious, GI, infiltrative) diseases
		12.	Cryptogenic cirrhosis

1. Micronodular cirrhosis In micronodular cirrhosis, the nodules are usually regular and small, *less than 3 mm* in diameter. There is diffuse involvement of all the hepatic lobules forming nodules by thick fibrous septa which may be portal-portal, portal-central, or both. The micronodular cirrhosis includes etiologic type of alcoholic cirrhosis (or nutritional cirrhosis or Laennec's cirrhosis) and represents impaired capacity for regrowth as seen in alcoholism, malnutrition, severe anaemia and old age.

2. Macronodular cirrhosis In this type, the nodules are of variable size and are generally *larger than 3 mm* in diameter. The pattern of involvement is more irregular than in micronodular cirrhosis, sparing some portal tracts and central veins, and more marked evidence of regeneration. Macronodular cirrhosis corresponds to post-necrotic (or post-hepatitis) cirrhosis of the etiologic classification.

3. Mixed cirrhosis In mixed type, some parts of the liver show micronodular appearance while other parts show macronodular pattern. All the portal tracts and central veins are not involved by fibrosis but instead some of them are spared. Mixed pattern is a kind of incomplete expression of micronodular cirrhosis.

B. ETIOLOGIC CLASSIFICATION Based on the etiologic agent for cirrhosis, various categories of cirrhosis are described as given in Table 27.5. Two of the major forms, alcoholic and post necrotic cirrhosis, are discussed below.

Alcoholic Liver Disease and Cirrhosis

Alcoholic liver disease is the term used to describe the spectrum of liver injury associated with acute and chronic alcoholism. There are three sequential stages in alcoholic liver disease: *alcoholic steatosis (fatty liver), alcoholic hepatitis* and *alcoholic cirrhosis.*

Before discussing the features of alcoholic liver disease and cirrhosis, a brief outline of ethanol metabolism is outlined below and is discussed earlier in Chapter 9 (page 88).

ETHANOL METABOLISM One gram of alcohol gives 7 calories. But alcohol cannot be stored in the body and must undergo obligatory oxidation, chiefly in the liver. Thus, these empty calories make no contribution to nutrition other than to give energy.

Ethanol after ingestion and absorption from the small bowel circulates through the liver where about 90% of it is oxidised to acetate by a *two-step enzymatic process* involving two enzymes: *alcohol dehydrogenase (ADH)* present in the cytosol, and *acetaldehyde dehydrogenase (ALDH)* in the mitochondria of hepatocytes (see Fig. 9.3). The remaining 10% of ethanol is oxidised elsewhere in the body.

First step: Ethanol is catabolised to acetaldehyde in the liver by the following three pathways, one major and two minor:
i) *In the cytosol,* by the major rate-limiting pathway of alcohol dehydrogenase (ADH).
ii) *In the smooth endoplasmic reticulum,* via microsomal P-450 oxidases (also called microsomal ethanol oxidising system, MEOS), where only part of ethanol is metabolised.
iii) *In the peroxisomes,* minor pathway via catalase such as H_2O_2.

Acetaldehyde is toxic and may cause membrane damage and cell necrosis. Simultaneously, the cofactor nicotinamide-adenine dinucleotide (NAD) which is a hydrogen acceptor, is reduced to NADH.

Second step: The second step occurs in the mitochondria where acetaldehyde is converted to acetate with ALDH acting as a co-enzyme. Most of the acetate on leaving the liver is finally oxidised to carbon dioxide and water, or converted by the citric acid cycle to other compounds including fatty acids. Simultaneously, the same cofactor, NAD, is reduced to NADH resulting in *increased NADH: NAD redox ratio* which is the basic biochemical alteration occurring during ethanol metabolism. A close estimate of NADH:NAD ratio is measured by the ratio of its oxidised and reduced metabolites in the form of *lactate-pyruvate ratio* and *β-hydroxy butyrate-acetoacetate ratio.*

RISK FACTORS FOR ALCOHOLIC LIVER DISEASE All those who indulge in alcohol abuse do not develop liver damage. The incidence of cirrhosis among alcoholics at autopsy is about 10-15%. Why some individuals are predisposed to alcoholic cirrhosis is not clearly known, but a few risk factors have been implicated. These are as under:

1. Drinking patterns Most epidemiologic studies have attributed alcoholic cirrhosis to chronic alcoholism. Available evidence suggests that chronic and excessive consumption of alcohol invariably leads to fatty liver in >90% of chronic alcoholics, progression to alcoholic hepatitis in 10-20% cases, and eventually to alcoholic cirrhosis in more than 10 years. It is generally agreed that continued daily imbibing of 60-80 gm of ethanol in any type of alcoholic beverage for at least 10 years is likely to result in alcoholic cirrhosis. Liver injury is related to the quantity of ethanol contained in alcoholic beverage consumed and its duration, but not related to the type of alcoholic beverage consumed. Ethanol content in an alcoholic beverage is given on the label of the container, but in general, it is about 4-6% in beer, 10-12% in wine, and about 40-50% in brandy, whisky and scotch. Intermittent drinking for long duration is less harmful since the liver is given chance to recover.

2. Gender Women have increased susceptibility to develop advanced alcoholic liver disease with much lesser alcohol intake (20-40 g/day). This gender difference in disease progression is unclear but is probably linked to effects of oestrogen.

3. Malnutrition Absolute or relative malnutrition of proteins and vitamins is regarded as a contributory factor in the evolution of cirrhosis. The combination of chronic alcohol ingestion and impaired nutrition leads to alcoholic liver disease and not malnutrition *per se*. It appears that calories derived from alcohol displace other nutrients leading to malnutrition and deficiency of vitamins in alcoholics. Additional factors contributing to malnutrition in alcoholics are chronic gastritis and pancreatitis. The evidence in favour of synergistic effect of malnutrition in chronic alcoholism comes from clinical and morphologic improvement in cases of alcoholic cirrhosis on treatment with protein-rich diets.

4. Infections Intercurrent bacterial infections are common in cirrhotic patients and may accelerate the course of the disease. Lesions similar to alcoholic cirrhosis may develop in non-alcoholic patients who have had viral infections in the past.

5. Genetic factors The rate of ethanol metabolism is under genetic control. It is chiefly related to altered rates of elimination of ethanol due to genetic polymorphism for the two main enzyme systems, MEOS (microsomal P-450 oxidases) and alcohol dehydrogenase (ADH). Various HLA histocompatibility types have been associated with susceptibility of different populations to alcoholic liver damage but no single genotype has been identified yet.

6. Hepatitis B and C infection Concurrent infection with either HBV or HCV is an important risk factor for progression of alcoholic liver disease. HBV or HCV infection in chronic alcoholic leads to development of alcoholic liver disease with much less alcohol consumption (20-50 g/day), disease progression at a younger age, having greater severity, and increased risk to develop cirrhosis and hepatocellular carcinoma, and overall poorer survival.

PATHOGENESIS Exact pathogenesis of alcoholic liver injury is yet unclear as to why only some chronic alcoholics develop the complete sequence of changes in the liver while others do not. However, knowledge and understanding of the ethanol metabolism has resulted in discarding the old concept of liver injury due to malnutrition. Instead, it is now known that ethanol and its metabolites are responsible for ill-effects on the liver in a susceptible chronic alcoholic having above-mentioned risk factors. Briefly, the biomedical and cellular pathogenesis due to chronic alcohol consumption culminating in morphologic lesions of alcoholic steatosis (fatty liver), alcoholic hepatitis and alcoholic cirrhosis can be explained as under and is schematically illustrated in **Fig. 27.14**:

1. Direct hepatotoxicity by ethanol There is evidence to suggest that ethanol ingestion for a period of 8-10 days regularly may cause direct hepatotoxic effect on the liver and produce fatty change. Ethanol is directly toxic to microtubules, mitochondria and membrane of hepatocytes.

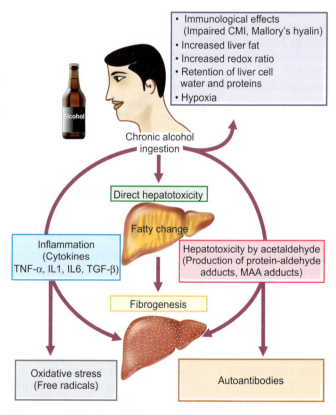

Figure 27.14 ▶ Pathogenesis of alcoholic liver disease.

2. Hepatotoxicity by ethanol metabolites The major hepatotoxic effects of ethanol are exerted by its metabolites, chiefly acetaldehyde. Acetaldehyde levels in blood are elevated in chronic alcoholics. Acetaldehyde produces hepatotoxicity by formation of two adducts:

i) *Production of protein-aldehyde adducts* which are extremely toxic and can cause cytoskeletal and membrane damage and bring about hepatocellular necrosis.

ii) *Formation of malon-di-aldehyde-acetaldehyde (MAA) adducts* which produce autoantibodies and initiate auto-immune response. Theses adducts have also a role in hepatic fibrogenesis due to peroxisome proliferator-activated receptor (PPAR)-γ on hepatocytes.

3. Oxidative stress Oxidation of ethanol by the cytochrome-450 oxidases (MEOS) leads to generation of free radicals which causes oxidative damage to the membranes and proteins.

4. Immunological mechanism Cell-mediated immunity is impaired in alcoholic liver disease. Ethanol causes direct immunologic attack on hepatocytes. In a proportion of cases, alcohol-related liver cell injury continues unabated despite cessation of alcohol consumption which is attributed to immunologic mechanisms. Immunological mechanism may also explain the genesis of Mallory's alcoholic hyalin though more favoured hypothesis for its origin is the aggregation of intermediate filaments of prekeratin type due to alcohol-induced disorganisation of cytoskeleton.

5. Inflammation Chronic ethanol ingestion is not only injurious to hepatocytes but also damages the intestinal cells. The injured intestinal cells elaborate endotoxins which release proinflammatory cytokines, chiefly tumour necrosis factor-α, IL-1, IL-6 and TGF-β. These cytokines and endotoxinaemia produce apoptosis and necrosis of hepatocytes and initiate inflammatory reaction in the alcohol-damaged liver.

6. Fibrogenesis Main event facilitating hepatic fibrogenesis is activation of stellate cells by various stimuli:
i) by damaged hepatocytes,
ii) by malon-di-aldehyde-acetaldehyde adducts,
iii) by activated Kupffer cells, and
iv) direct stimulation by acetaldehyde.

All forms of collagen are increased and there is increased transformation of fat-storing Ito cells into myofibroblasts and fibrocytes.

7. Increased redox ratio Marked increase in the NADH:NAD redox ratio in the hepatocytes results in increased redox ratio of lactate-pyruvate, leading to lactic acidosis. This altered redox potential has been implicated in a number of metabolic consequences such as in fatty liver, collagen formation, occurrence of gout, impaired gluconeogenesis and altered steroid metabolism.

8. Retention of liver cell water and proteins Alcohol is inhibitory to secretion of newly-synthesised proteins by the liver leading to their retention in the hepatocytes. Water is simultaneously retained in the cell in proportion to the protein and results in swelling of hepatocytes resulting in hepatomegaly in alcoholics.

9. Hypoxia Chronic ingestion of alcohol results in increased oxygen demand by the liver resulting in a hypoxic state which causes hepatocellular necrosis in centrilobular zone (zone 3). Redox changes are also more marked in zone 3.

10. Increased liver fat The origin of fat in the body was discussed in Chapter 6 (page 52). In chronic alcoholism, there is rise in the amount of fat available to the liver which could be from exogenous (dietary) sources, excess mobilisation from adipose tissue or increased lipid synthesis by the liver itself. This may account for lipid accumulation in the hepatocytes.

MORPHOLOGIC FEATURES Three types of morphologic lesions are described in alcoholic liver disease—alcoholic steatosis (fatty liver), alcoholic hepatitis and alcoholic cirrhosis.

1. ALCOHOLIC STEATOSIS (FATTY LIVER) The morphologic changes in fatty change in liver have already been described on page 53 and are briefly considered here.

Grossly, the liver is enlarged, yellow, greasy and firm with a smooth and glistening capsule.

Microscopically, the features consist of initial *microvesicular* droplets of fat in the hepatocyte cytoplasm followed by more common and pronounced feature of *macrovesicular* large droplets of fat displacing the nucleus to the periphery **(Fig. 27.15)**. *Fat cysts* may develop due to coalescence and rupture of fat-containing hepatocytes. Less often, *lipogranulomas* consisting of collection of lymphocytes, macrophages and some multinucleate giant cells may be found.

2. ALCOHOLIC HEPATITIS Alcoholic hepatitis develops acutely, usually following a bout of heavy drinking. Repeated episodes of alcoholic hepatitis superimposed on pre-existing fatty liver are almost certainly a forerunner of alcoholic cirrhosis.

Histologically, the features of alcoholic hepatitis are as follows **(Fig. 27.16)**:

i) Hepatocellular necrosis: Single or small clusters of hepatocytes, especially in the centrilobular area (zone 3), undergo ballooning degeneration and necrosis.

ii) Mallory bodies or alcoholic hyalin: These are eosinophilic, intracytoplasmic inclusions seen in perinuclear location within swollen and ballooned hepatocytes. They represent aggregates of cytoskeletal intermediate filaments (prekeratin). They can be best visualised with connective tissue stains like Masson's trichrome and chromophobe aniline blue, or by the use of immunoperoxidase methods. Mallory bodies are highly suggestive of, but not specific for, alcoholic hepatitis since Mallory bodies are also found in certain other conditions such as: primary biliary cirrhosis, Indian childhood cirrhosis, cholestatic syndromes, Wilson's disease, intestinal bypass surgery, focal nodular hyperplasia and hepatocellular carcinoma.

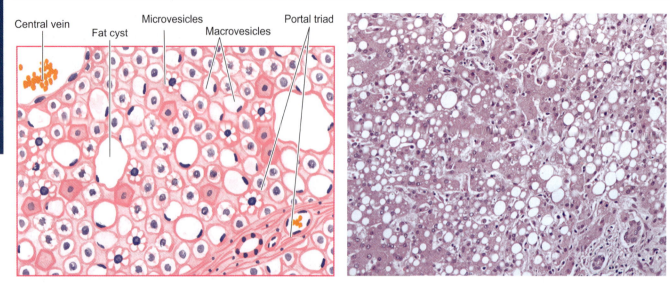

Figure 27.15 ▶ Fatty liver (alcoholic steatosis). Most of the hepatocytes are distended with large lipid vacuoles with peripherally displaced nuclei.

iii) Inflammatory response: The areas of hepatocellular necrosis and regions of Mallory bodies are associated with an inflammatory infiltrate, chiefly consisting of polymorphs and some scattered mononuclear cells. In more extensive necrosis, the inflammatory infiltrate is more widespread and may involve the entire lobule.

iv) Fibrosis: Most cases of alcoholic hepatitis are accompanied by pericellular and perivenular fibrosis, producing a web-like or chickenwire-like appearance. This is also termed as *creeping collagenosis*.

3. ALCOHOLIC CIRRHOSIS Alcoholic cirrhosis is the most common form of lesion, constituting 60-70% of all cases of cirrhosis. Several terms have been used for this type of cirrhosis such as *Laennec's cirrhosis, portal cirrhosis, hobnail cirrhosis, nutritional cirrhosis, diffuse cirrhosis* and *micronodular cirrhosis.*

Grossly, alcoholic cirrhosis classically begins as micronodular cirrhosis (nodules less than 3 mm diameter), the liver being large, fatty and weighing usually above 2 kg **(Fig. 27.17)**. Eventually over a span of years, the liver

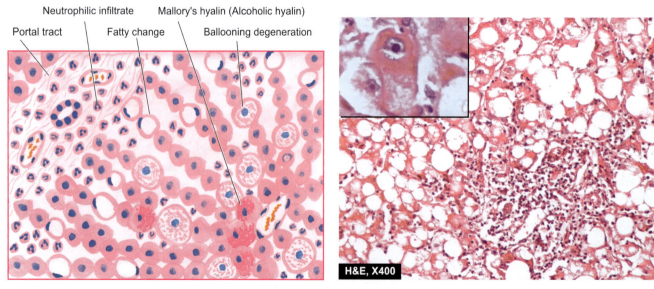

Figure 27.16 ▶ Alcoholic hepatitis. Liver cells show ballooning degeneration and necrosis with some containing Mallory's hyalin (Inbox). Fatty change and clusters of neutrophils are also present.

Chapter 27: Jaundice, Hepatitis and Cirrhosis

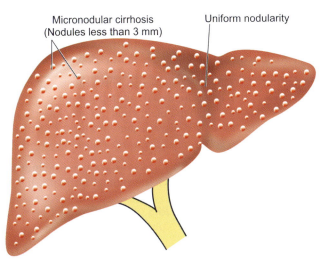
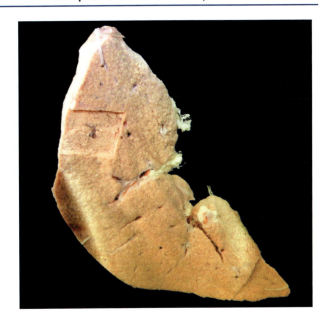

Figure 27.17 ▶ Alcoholic cirrhosis, showing the typical micronodular pattern in gross specimen. There is diffuse nodularity (nodules less than 3 mm diameter) on sectioned surface of the liver.

shrinks to less than 1 kg in weight, becomes non-fatty, having macronodular cirrhosis (nodules larger than 3 mm in diameter), resembling post-necrotic cirrhosis. The nodules of the liver due to their fat content are tawny-yellow, on the basis of which Laennec in 1818 introduced the term *cirrhosis* first of all (from Greek *kirrhos* = tawny). The surface of liver in alcoholic cirrhosis is studded with diffuse nodules which vary little in size, producing hobnail liver (because of the resemblance of the surface with the sole of an old-fashioned shoe having short nails with heavy heads). On cut section, spheroidal or angular nodules of fibrous septa are seen.

Microscopically, alcoholic cirrhosis is a progressive alcoholic liver disease. Its features include the following **(Fig. 27.18)**:

i) Nodular pattern: Normal lobular architecture is effaced in which central veins are hard to find and is replaced with nodule formation.

ii) Fibrous septa: The fibrous septa that divide the hepatic parenchyma into nodules are initially delicate and extend from central vein to portal regions, or portal tract to portal tract, or both. As the fibrous scarring increases with time, the fibrous septa become dense and more confluent.

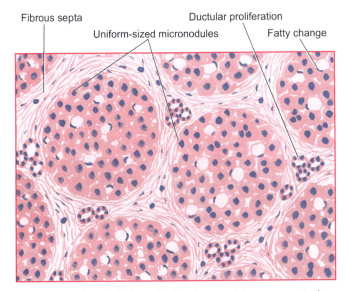
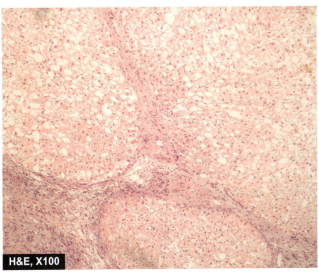

Figure 27.18 ▶ Alcoholic cirrhosis, microscopic appearance. It shows nearly uniform-sized micronodules, devoid of central veins and having thick fibrous septa dividing them. There is minimal inflammation and some reactive bile duct proliferation in the septa.

iii) Hepatic parenchyma: The hepatocytes in the islands of surviving parenchyma undergo slow proliferation forming regenerative nodules having disorganised masses of hepatocytes. The hepatic parenchyma within the nodules shows extensive fatty change early in the disease. But as the fibrous septa become more thick, the amount of fat in hepatocytes is reduced. Thus, there is an inverse relationship between the amount of fat and the amount of fibrous scarring in the nodules.

iv) Necrosis, inflammation and bile duct proliferation: The etiologic clue to diagnosis in the form of Mallory bodies is hard to find in a fully-developed alcoholic cirrhosis. The fibrous septa usually contain sparse infiltrate of mononuclear cells with some bile duct proliferation. Bile stasis and increased cytoplasmic haemosiderin deposits due to enhanced iron absorption in alcoholic cirrhosis are some other noticeable findings.

LABORATORY DIAGNOSIS The laboratory findings in the course of alcoholic liver disease may be quite variable and liver biopsy is necessary in doubtful cases. Progressive form of the disease, however, generally presents the following biochemical and haematological alterations:
1. Elevated transaminases; increase in SGOT (AST) is more than that of SGPT (ALT).
2. Rise in serum γ-glutamyl transpeptidase (γ-GT).
3. Elevation in serum alkaline phosphatase.
4. Hyperbilirubinaemia.
5. Hypoproteinaemia with reversal of albumin-globulin ratio.
6. Prolonged prothrombin time and partial thromboplastin time.
7. Anaemia.
8. Neutrophilic leucocytosis in alcoholic hepatitis and in secondary infections.

Post-necrotic Cirrhosis

Post-necrotic cirrhosis, also termed *post-hepatitic cirrhosis, macronodular cirrhosis* and *coarsely nodular cirrhosis,* is characterised by large and irregular nodules with broad bands of connective tissue and occurring most commonly after previous viral hepatitis.

ETIOLOGY Based on epidemiologic and serologic studies, the following factors have been implicated in the etiology of post-necrotic cirrhosis.

1. Viral hepatitis About 25% of patients give history of recent or remote attacks of acute viral hepatitis followed by chronic viral hepatitis. Most common association is with hepatitis B and C; hepatitis A is not known to evolve into cirrhosis. It is estimated that about 20% cases of HBV chronic hepatitis and about 20-30% cases of HCV chronic hepatitis progress to cirrhosis over 20-30 years.

2. Drugs and chemical hepatotoxins A small percentage of cases may have origin from toxicity due to chemicals and drugs such as phosphorus, carbon tetrachloride, mushroom poisoning, acetaminophen and α-methyl dopa.

3. Others Certain infections (e.g. brucellosis), parasitic infestations (e.g. clonorchiasis), metabolic diseases (e.g. Wilson's disease or hepatolenticular degeneration) and advanced alcoholic liver disease may produce a picture of post-necrotic cirrhosis.

4. Idiopathic After all these causes have been excluded, a group of cases remain in which the etiology is unknown.

MORPHOLOGIC FEATURES Typically, post-necrotic cirrhosis is macronodular type.

Grossly, the liver is usually small, weighing less than 1 kg, having distorted shape with irregular and coarse scars and nodules of varying size **(Fig. 27.19)**. Sectioned surface shows scars and nodules varying in diameter from 3 mm to a few centimeters.

Microscopically, the features are as follows **(Fig. 27.20)**:

1. Nodular pattern: The normal lobular architecture of hepatic parenchyma is mostly lost and is replaced by nodules larger than those in alcoholic cirrhosis. However, uninvolved portal tracts and central veins in the hepatic lobules can still be seen in some parts of surviving parenchyma.

2. Fibrous septa: The fibrous septa dividing the variable-sized nodules are generally thick.

3. Necrosis, inflammation and bile duct proliferation: Active liver cell necrosis is usually inconspicuous. Fibrous septa contain prominent mononuclear inflammatory cell infiltrate which may even form follicles, especially in cases following HCV chronic hepatitis. Often there is extensive proliferation of bile ductules derived from collapsed liver lobules.

4. Hepatic parenchyma: Liver cells vary considerably in size and multiple large nuclei are common in regenerative nodules. Fatty change may or may not be present in the hepatocytes.

CLINICAL FEATURES Post-necrotic cirrhosis is seen as frequent in women as in men, especially in the younger age group. Like in alcoholic cirrhosis, the patients may remain asymptomatic or may present with prominent signs and symptoms of chronic hepatitis. Splenomegaly and hypersplenism are other prominent features. The results of haematologic and liver function test are similar to those of alcoholic cirrhosis. Out of the various types of cirrhosis, post-necrotic cirrhosis, especially when related to hepatitis B and C virus infection in early life, is more frequently

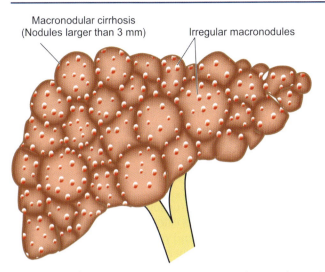
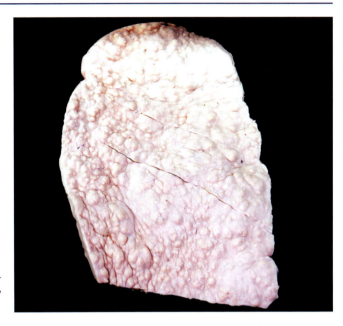

Figure 27.19 ▶ Post-necrotic cirrhosis, showing the typical irregular macronodular pattern (nodules larger than 3 mm diameter). Externally the liver is small, distorted and irregularly scarred.

associated with development of hepatocellular carcinoma later.

CLINICAL MANIFESTATIONS AND COMPLICATIONS OF CIRRHOSIS

The range of clinical features in cirrhosis varies widely, from an asymptomatic state to progressive liver failure and death. The onset of disease is insidious. In general, the features of cirrhosis are more marked in the alcoholic form than in other varieties. These include weakness, fatiguability, weight loss, anorexia, muscle wasting, and low-grade fever due to hepatocellular necrosis or some latent infection. Advanced cases develop a number of complications which are as follows:

1. *Portal hypertension* and its major effects such as ascites, splenomegaly and development of collaterals (e.g. oesophageal varices, spider naevi etc) as discussed below.
2. *Progressive hepatic failure* and its manifestations.
3. Development of *hepatocellular carcinoma*, more often in post-necrotic cirrhosis (HBV and HCV more often) than following alcoholic cirrhosis.
4. *Chronic relapsing pancreatitis*, especially in alcoholic liver disease.

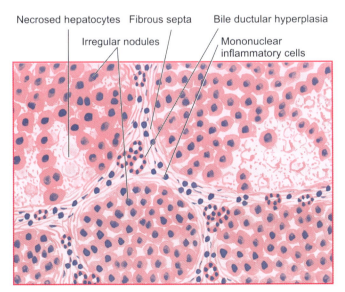
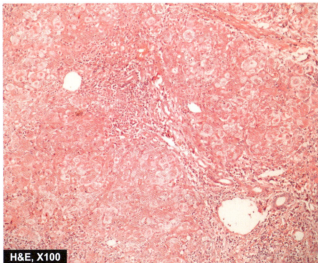

Figure 27.20 ▶ Post-necrotic cirrhosis. Fibrous septa dividing the hepatic parenchyma into nodules are thick and contain prominent mononuclear inflammatory cell infiltrate and bile ductular hyperplasia. A few intact hepatic lobules remain.

5. *Steatorrhoea* due to reduced hepatic bile secretion.
6. *Gallstones* usually of pigment type, are seen twice more frequently in patients with cirrhosis than in general population.
7. *Infections* are more frequent in patients with cirrhosis due to impaired phagocytic activity of reticuloendothelial system.
8. *Haematologic derangements* such as bleeding disorders and anaemia due to impaired hepatic synthesis of coagulation factors and hypoalbuminaemia are present.
9. *Cardiovascular complications* such as atherosclerosis of coronaries and aorta and myocardial infarction are more frequent in cirrhotic patients.
10. *Musculoskeletal abnormalities* like digital clubbing, hypertrophic osteoarthropathy and Dupuytren's contracture are more common in cirrhotic patients.
11. *Endocrine disorders* In males these consist of feminisation such as gynaecomastia, changes in pubic hair pattern, testicular atrophy and impotence, whereas in cirrhotic women amenorrhoea is a frequent abnormality.
12. *Hepatorenal syndrome* leading to renal failure may occur in late stages of cirrhosis.

The ultimate *causes of death* are hepatic coma, massive gastrointestinal haemorrhage from oesophageal varices (complication of portal hypertension), intercurrent infections, hepatorenal syndrome and development of hepatocellular carcinoma.

GIST BOX 27.3 | Cirrhosis

- Cirrhosis is a diffuse liver disease characterised by effacement of normal lobular architecture, formation of nodules separated by fibrous septa and alternate areas of hepatocellular necrosis and regenerative nodules.
- There are 3 morphologic types of cirrhosis—micronodular, macronodular and mixed.
- Based on etiology, major forms are alcoholic, postnectoric, biliary, and in haemochromatosis.
- Alcoholic cirrhosis evolves through preceding sequential stages of steatosis and alcoholic hepatitis.
- Most common etiologic factor for postnecrotic cirrhosis is preceding viral hepatitis with hepatitis B or C.
- A few variant forms are non-alcoholic fatty liver disease, cirrhosis in autoimmune hepatitis, non-cirrhostic portal fibrosis etc.
- Advanced cases of cirrhosis develop portal hypertension and its sequelae.

PORTAL HYPERTENSION

Increase in pressure in the portal system usually follows obstruction to the portal blood flow anywhere along its course. Portal veins have no valves and thus obstruction anywhere in the portal system raises pressure in all the veins proximal to the obstruction. However, unless proved otherwise, portal hypertension means obstruction to the portal blood flow by cirrhosis of the liver. The normal portal venous pressure is quite low (10-15 mm saline). Portal hypertension occurs when the portal pressure is above 30 mm saline. Measurement of *intrasplenic pressure* reflects pressure in the splenic vein; the *percutaneous transhepatic pressure* provides a measure of pressure in the main portal vein; and wedged hepatic *venous pressure represents sinusoidal pressure.* Measurement of these pressures helps in localising the site of obstruction and classifying the portal hypertension.

CLASSIFICATION

Based on the site of obstruction to portal venous blood flow, portal hypertension is categorised into 3 main types—*intrahepatic, posthepatic* and *prehepatic* **(Table 27.6)**. Rare cases of idiopathic portal hypertension showing non-cirrhotic portal fibrosis are encountered as discussed above.

1. Intrahepatic portal hypertension Cirrhosis is by far the commonest cause of portal hypertension. Other less frequent intrahepatic causes are metastatic tumours, non-cirrhotic nodular regenerative conditions, hepatic venous obstruction (Budd-Chiari syndrome), veno-occlusive disease, schistosomiasis, diffuse granulomatous diseases and extensive fatty change. In cirrhosis and other conditions, there is obstruction to the portal venous flow by fibrosis, thrombosis and pressure by regenerative nodules. About 30-60% patients of cirrhosis develop significant portal hypertension.

2. Posthepatic portal hypertension This is uncommon and results from obstruction to the blood flow through

Table 27.6	Major causes of portal hypertension.
A.	INTRAHEPATIC
	1. Cirrhosis
	2. Metastatic tumours
	3. Budd-Chiari syndrome
	4. Hepatic veno-occlusive disease
	5. Diffuse granulomatous diseases
	6. Extensive fatty change
B.	POSTHEPATIC
	1. Congestive heart failure
	2. Constrictive pericarditis
	3. Hepatic veno-occlusive disease
	4. Budd-Chiari syndrome
C.	PREHEPATIC
	1. Portal vein thrombosis
	2. Neoplastic obstruction of portal vein
	3. Myelofibrosis
	4. Congenital absence of portal vein

hepatic vein into inferior vena cava. The causes are neoplastic occlusion and thrombosis of the hepatic vein or of the inferior vena cava (including Budd-Chiari syndrome). Prolonged congestive heart failure and constrictive pericarditis may also cause portal hypertension by transmitting the elevated pressure through the hepatic vessels into the portal vein.

3. **Prehepatic portal hypertension** Blockage of portal flow before portal blood reaches the hepatic sinusoids results in prehepatic portal hypertension. Such conditions are thrombosis and neoplastic obstruction of the portal vein before it ramifies in the liver, myelofibrosis, and congenital absence of portal vein.

MAJOR SEQUELAE OF PORTAL HYPERTENSION

Irrespective of the mechanisms involved in the pathogenesis of portal hypertension, there are 4 major clinical consequences—*ascites, varices* (collateral channels or portosystemic shunts), *splenomegaly* and *hepatic encephalopathy* (Fig. 27.21).

1. Ascites

Ascites is the accumulation of excessive volume of fluid within the peritoneal cavity. It frequently accompanies cirrhosis and other diffuse liver diseases. The development of ascites is associated with haemodilution, oedema and decreased urinary output. Ascitic fluid is generally transudate with specific gravity of 1.010, protein content below 3 gm/dl and electrolyte concentrations like those of other extracellular fluids. It may contain a few mesothelial cells and mononuclear cells. Presence of neutrophils is suggestive of secondary infection and red blood cells in ascitic fluid points to disseminated intra-abdominal cancer. However, some cases of ascites may develop serious complication of *spontaneous bacterial peritonitis* characterised by spontaneous infection of the ascitic fluid without any intra-abdominal infection.

Pathogenesis The ascites becomes clinically detectable when more than 500 ml of fluid has accumulated in the peritoneal cavity. The mechanisms involved in its formation were discussed on page 232. Briefly, the systemic and local factors favouring ascites formation are as under (Fig. 27.22):

A. Systemic Factors:

i) *Decreased plasma colloid oncotic pressure* There is hypoalbuminaemia from impaired hepatic synthesis of plasma proteins including albumin, as well as from loss of albumin from the blood plasma into the peritoneal cavity. Hypoalbuminaemia, in turn, causes reduced plasma oncotic pressure and leads to loss of water into extravascular space.

ii) *Hyperaldosteronism* In cirrhosis, there is increased aldosterone secretion by the adrenal gland, probably due to reduced renal blood flow, and impaired hepatic metabolism and excretion of aldosterone.

iii) *Impaired renal excretion* Reduced renal blood flow and excessive release of antidiuretic hormone results in renal retention of sodium and water and impaired renal excretion.

B. Local Factors:

i) *Increased portal pressure* Portal venous pressure is not directly related to ascites formation but portal hypertension in combination with other factors contributes to the formation and localisation of the fluid retention in the peritoneal cavity.

ii) *Increased hepatic lymph formation* Obstruction of hepatic vein such as in Budd-Chiari syndrome and increased intra-sinusoidal pressure found in cirrhotic patients stimulates hepatic lymph formation that oozes through the surface of the liver.

2. Varices (Collateral Channels or Porto-systemic Shunts)

As a result of rise in portal venous pressure and obstruction in the portal circulation within or outside the liver, the blood tends to bypass the liver and return to the heart by development of porto-systemic collateral channels (or shunts or varices). These varices develop at sites where the systemic and portal circulations have common capillary beds. The principal sites are as under:

i) *Oesophageal varices:* The development of oesophago-gastric varices which is frequently manifested by massive

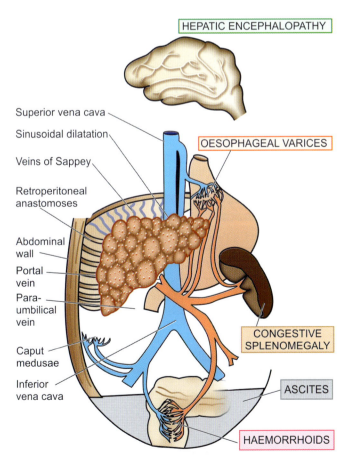

Figure 27.21 ▶ Major clinical consequences of portal hypertension.

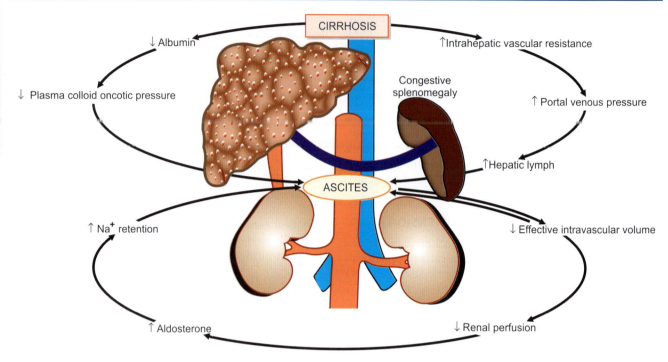

Figure 27.22 ▶ Mechanisms of ascites formation in cirrhosis.

haematemesis is the most important consequence of portal hypertension.

ii) Haemorrhoids: Development of collaterals between the superior, middle and inferior haemorrhoidal veins resulting in haemorrhoids is another common accompaniment. Bleeding from haemorrhoids is usually not as serious a complication as haematemesis from oesophageal varices.

iii) Caput medusae: Anastomoses between the portal and systemic veins may develop between the hilum of the liver and the umbilicus along the paraumbilical plexus of veins resulting in abdominal wall collaterals. These appear as dilated subcutaneous veins radiating from the umbilicus and are termed caput medusae (named after the snake-haired *Medusa*).

iv) Retroperitoneal anastomoses: In the retroperitoneum, portocaval anastomoses may be established through the veins of Retzius and the veins of Sappey.

3. Splenomegaly

The enlargement of the spleen in prolonged portal hypertension is called congestive splenomegaly. The spleen may weigh 500-1000 gm and is easily palpable. The spleen is larger in young people and in macronodular cirrhosis than in micronodular cirrhosis.

4. Hepatic Encephalopathy

Porto-systemic venous shunting may result in a complex metabolic and organic syndrome of the brain characterised by disturbed consciousness, neurologic signs and flapping tremors. Hepatic encephalopathy is particularly associated with advanced hepatocellular disease such as in cirrhosis.

| GIST BOX 27.4 | Portal Hypertension |

- Portal hypertension occurs when the portal pressure is above 30 mm saline (normal 10-15 mm saline).
- Based on the site of obstruction to portal venous blood flow, portal hypertension is categorised into intrahepatic (e.g. cirrhosis), posthepatic (e.g. CHF) and prehepatic (e.g. portal vein thrombosis).
- Major clinical consequences of portal hypertension are ascites, varices (collateral channels or portosystemic shunts), splenomegaly and hepatic encephalopathy.

28 Hypertension and its Consequences

SYSTEMIC HYPERTENSION

Hypertension is the term used to describe an elevation in blood pressure. The term hypertension is used with regard to raised pressure at three places—systemic (arterial), pulmonary and portal hypertension. However, when the term 'hypertension' is not prefixed with any word, it is implied to mean systemic hypertension.

Hypertension is a common disease in industrialised and developed countries and accounts for 6% of death worldwide. A persistent and sustained high blood pressure has damaging effects on the heart (e.g. hypertensive heart disease), brain (e.g. cerebrovascular accident or stroke) and kidneys (benign and malignant nephrosclerosis). Epidemiologic studies have revealed that with elevation in systolic and diastolic blood pressure above normal in adults, there is a continuous increased risk of cardiovascular disease, stroke and renal disease—cardiovascular risk doubles with every 20 mmHg increase in systolic and 10 mmHg increase in diastolic blood pressure above normal levels.

DEFINITION AND CLASSIFICATION

Criteria for normal blood pressure, prehypertension and hypertension (stage 1 and stage 2) have been laid by the National Institutes of Health (NIH), US **(Table 28.1)**. According to this criteria, normal cut-off values for systolic and diastolic blood pressure are taken as < 120 and < 80 mmHg respectively. As per this criteria, arterial or systemic hypertension in adults is defined clinically as persistent elevation of systolic blood pressure of 140-159 mmHg, or diastolic pressure of 90-99 mmHg as *stage 1 hypertension*, and corresponding values above 160 or above 100 mmHg as *stage 2 hypertension*. Cases falling between upper normal values for systolic and diastolic blood pressure (i.e. above 120/80 mmHg) and those for stage 1 hypertension (120-139/80-89 mmHg) are grouped under *prehypertension* requiring monitoring and follow-up. The diastolic pressure is often considered more significant. Since blood pressure varies with many factors such as age of the patient, exercise, emotional disturbances like fear and anxiety, it is important to measure blood pressure at least twice during two separate examinations under least stressful conditions.

Hypertension is generally classified into 2 types:

1. **Primary or essential hypertension** in which the cause of increase in blood pressure is unknown. Essential hypertension constitutes about 80-95% patients of hypertension.

2. **Secondary hypertension** in which the increase in blood pressure is caused by diseases of the kidneys, endocrines or some other organs. Secondary hypertension comprises remaining 5-20% cases of hypertension.

According to the clinical course, both essential and secondary hypertension may be benign or malignant.

◈ *Benign hypertension* is moderate elevation of blood pressure and the rise is slow over the years. About 90-95% patients of hypertension have benign hypertension.

◈ *Malignant hypertension* is marked and sudden increase of blood pressure to 200/140 mmHg or more in a known case of hypertension or in a previously normotensive individual; the patients develop papilloedema, retinal haemorrhages and hypertensive encephalopathy. Less than 5% of hypertensive patients develop malignant hypertension, life expectancy after diagnosis in these patients is generally less than 2 years if not treated effectively.

ETIOLOGY AND PATHOGENESIS

The etiology and pathogenesis of secondary hypertension that comprises less than 10% cases has been better understood, whereas the mechanism of essential hypertension, that constitutes about 90% of cases, remains largely obscure. In general, normal blood pressure is regulated by 2 haemo-dynamic forces—*cardiac output* and *total peripheral vascular resistance*. Factors which alter these two factors result in hypertension. The role of kidney in hypertension, particularly in secondary hypertension, by elaboration of renin and

Table 28.1 Clinical classification of hypertension*.

CATEGORY	SYSTOLIC (mmHg)	DIASTOLIC (mmHg)
Normal	< 120	and < 80
Prehypertension	120-139	or 80-89
Hypertension		
Stage 1	140-159	or 90-99
Stage 2	>160	or >100
Isolated systolic hypertension	≥140	and < 90
Malignant hypertension	> 200 (sudden onset)	≥ 140 (sudden onset)

*Chobanian et al, JAMA, 2003.

| Table 28.2 | Etiologic classification of hypertension. |

A. ESSENTIAL HYPERTENSION (90%)
  1. Genetic factors
  2. Racial and environmental factors
  3. Risk factors modifying the course
B. SECONDARY HYPERTENSION (10%)
  1. *Renal*
     i) Renovascular
     ii) Renal parenchymal diseases
  2. *Endocrine*
     i) Adrenocortical hyperfunction
     ii) Hypo- and hyperthyroidism
     iii) Hyperparathyroidism
     iv) Oral contraceptives
  3. *Coarctation of Aorta*
  4. *Neurogenic*

subsequent formation of angiotensin II, is well established (renin-angiotensin system).

With this background knowledge, we next turn to the mechanisms involved in the two forms of hypertension (Table 28.2).

Essential (Primary) Hypertension

By definition, the cause of essential hypertension is unknown but a number of factors are related to its development. These are as under:

1. Genetic factors The role of heredity in the etiology of essential hypertension has long been suspected. The evidences in support are the familial aggregation, occurrence of hypertension in twins, epidemiologic data, experimental animal studies and identification of hypertension susceptibility gene (angiotensinogen gene).

2. Racial and environmental factors Surveys in the US have revealed higher incidence of essential hypertension in African Americans than in whites. A number of environmental factors have been implicated in the development of hypertension including salt intake, obesity, skilled occupation, higher living standards and individuals under high stress.

3. Risk factors modifying the course of essential hypertension There is sufficient evidence to show that the course of essential hypertension that begins in middle life is modified by a number of factors. These are as under:

i) Age Younger the age at which hypertension is first noted but left untreated, lower the life expectancy.

ii) Sex Females with hypertension appear to do better than males.

iii) Atherosclerosis Accelerated atherosclerosis invariably accompanies essential hypertension. This could be due to contributory role of other independent factors like cigarette smoking, elevated serum cholesterol, glucose intolerance and obesity.

iv) Other risk factors Other factors which alter the prognosis in hypertension include: smoking, excess of alcohol intake, diabetes mellitus, persistently high diastolic pressure above normal and evidence of end-organ damage (i.e. heart, eyes, kidney and nervous system).

Pathogenesis in essential hypertension is explained by many theories. These are as under:
1. *High plasma level of catecholamines.*
2. *Increase in blood volume* i.e. arterial overfilling (volume hypertension) and arteriolar constriction (vasoconstrictor hypertension).
3. *Increased cardiac output.*
4. *Low-renin essential hypertension* found in approximately 20% patients due to altered responsiveness to renin release.
5. *High renin essential hypertension* seen in about 15% cases due to decreased adrenal responsiveness to angiotensin II.

Secondary Hypertension

Though much less common than essential hypertension, mechanisms underlying secondary hypertension with identifiable cause have been studied more extensively. Based on the etiology, these are described under four headings: renal hypertension, endocrine hypertension, hypertension associated with coarctation of aorta and neurogenic causes.

1. RENAL HYPERTENSION Hypertension produced by renal diseases is called renal hypertension. Renal hypertension is subdivided into 2 groups:

i) Renal vascular hypertension e.g. in occlusion of a major renal artery, pre-eclampsia, eclampsia, polyarteritis nodosa and fibromuscular dysplasia of renal artery.

ii) Renal parenchymal hypertension e.g. in various types of glomerulonephritis, pyelonephritis, interstitial nephritis, diabetic nephropathy, amyloidosis, polycystic kidney disease and renin-producing tumours.

In either case, renal hypertension can be produced by one of the following 3 inter-related pathogenetic mechanisms:

a) Activation of renin-angiotensin system Renin is a proteolytic enzyme produced and stored in the granules of the juxtaglomerular cells surrounding the afferent arterioles of glomerulus. The release of renin is stimulated by renal ischaemia, sympathetic nervous system stimulation, depressed sodium concentration, fluid depletion and decreased potassium intake. Released renin is transported through blood stream to the liver where it acts upon substrate angiotensinogen, an α_2-globulin synthesised in the liver, to form angiotensin I, a decapeptide. Angiotensin I is converted into angiotensin II, an octapeptide, by the action of convertase in the lungs. Angiotensin II is the most potent naturally-occurring vasoconstrictor substance and its pressor action is mainly attributed to peripheral arteriolar vasoconstriction. The other main effect of angiotensin II is to stimulate the

Chapter 28: Hypertension and its Consequences

iii) *Release of atriopeptin hormone* from atria of the heart in response to volume expansion. These peptides cause increased GFR and inhibit sodium reabsorption.

c) **Release of vasodepressor material** A number of vasodepressor materials and antihypertensives counterbalance the vasopressor effect of angiotensin II. These substances include: prostaglandins (PGE2, PGF2, PGA or medullin) released from interstitial cells of the medulla, urinary kallikrein-kinin system and platelet-activating factor.

2. **ENDOCRINE HYPERTENSION** A number of hormonal secretions may produce secondary hypertension as follows:

i) *Adrenal gland*—e.g. in primary aldosteronism, Cushing's syndrome, adrenal virilism and pheochromocytoma.

ii) *Thyroid gland*—e.g. in hypothyroidism, hyperthyroidism.

iii) *Parathyroid gland*—e.g. hypercalcaemia in hyperparathyroidism.

iv) *Oral contraceptives*—Oestrogen component in the oral contraceptives stimulates hepatic synthesis of renin substrate.

3. **COARCTATION OF AORTA** Coarctation of the aorta causes systolic hypertension in the upper part of the body due to constriction itself (page 478). Diastolic hypertension results from changes in circulation.

4. **NEUROGENIC** Psychogenic, polyneuritis, increased intracranial pressure and section of spinal cord are all uncommon causes of secondary hypertension.

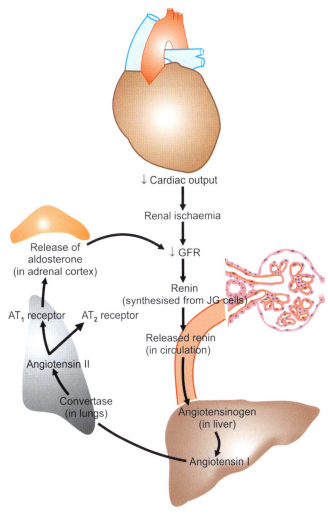

Figure 28.1 ▶ The renin-angiotensin mechanism.

adrenal cortex to secrete aldosterone via AT_1 receptor and thus promotes reabsorption of sodium and water.

Thus, the renin-angiotensin system is concerned mainly with 3 functions:

i) Control of blood pressure by altering plasma concentration of angiotensin II and aldosterone.

ii) Regulation of sodium and water content.

iii) Regulation of potassium balance.

The renin-angiotensin mechanism is summarised in **Fig. 28.1**.

b) **Sodium and water retention** Blood volume and cardiac output, both of which have a bearing on blood pressure, are regulated by blood level of sodium which is significant for maintaining extracellular fluid volume. Blood concentration of sodium is regulated by 3 mechanisms:

i) *Release of aldosterone* from activation of renin-angiotensin system, as already explained.

ii) *Reduction in GFR* due to reduced blood flow as occurs in reduced renal mass or renal artery stenosis. This results in proximal tubular reabsorption of sodium.

> **GIST BOX 28.1** | **Systemic Hypertension**
>
> ❖ Hypertension may be primary or essential hypertension in which the cause is unknown (about 90% cases) or secondary which is caused by diseases of the kidneys, endocrines or some other organs.
>
> ❖ Clinically, hypertension may be benign (moderate and slow elevation of blood pressure ≥ 90/140 mmHg) or malignant hypertension in which there is marked and sudden increase of blood pressure (≥ 200/140 mmHg) in a known case of hypertension.
>
> ❖ Main mechanisms of essential hypertension are activation of renin-angiotensin pathway while secondary hypertension may be due to endocrine, aortic coarctation or neurogenic causes.

CONSEQUENCES OF HYPERTENSION

Systemic hypertension causes major effects in following main organs—

1. Blood vessels —hypertensive arteriolosclerosis
2. Heart—hypertensive heart disease
3. Kidneys—nephrosclerosis
4. Nervous system—stroke
5. Eyes—hypertensive retinopathy
   These are briefly discussed below.

ARTERIOLOSCLEROSIS

Arteriolosclerosis is the term used to describe 3 morphologic forms of vascular disease affecting arterioles and small muscular arteries. These are: hyaline arteriolosclerosis, hyperplastic arteriolosclerosis and necrotising arteriolitis. All the three types are common in hypertension but may occur due to other causes as well.

Hyaline Arterioloscelosis

Hyaline sclerosis is a common arteriolar lesion that may be seen *physiologically* due to ageing, or may occur *pathologically* in benign nephrosclerosis in hypertensives and as a part of microangiopathy in diabetics.

MORPHOLOGIC CHANGES The visceral arterioles are particularly involved. The vascular walls are thickened and the lumina narrowed or even obliterated.

Microscopically, the thickened vessel wall shows structureless, eosinophilic, hyaline material in the intima and media (Fig. 28.2, A).

PATHOGENESIS The exact pathogenesis is not known. However, the following hypotheses have been proposed:
i) The lesions result most probably from *leakage of components of plasma* across the vascular endothelium. This is substantiated by the demonstration of immunoglobulins, complement, fibrin and lipids in the lesions. The permeability of the vessel wall is increased, due to haemodyanamic stress in hypertension and metabolic stress in diabetes, so that these plasma components leak out and get deposited in the vessel wall.
ii) An alternate possibility is that the lesions may be due to *immunologic reaction*.
iii) Some have considered it to be *normal ageing process* that is exaggerated in hypertension and diabetes mellitus.

Hyperplastic Arteriolosclerosis

The hyperplastic or proliferative type of arteriolosclerosis is a characteristic lesion of malignant hypertension; other causes include haemolytic-uraemic syndrome, scleroderma and toxaemia of pregnancy.

MORPHOLOGIC FEATURES The morphologic changes affect mainly the intima, especially of the interlobular arteries in the kidneys. Three types of intimal thickening may occur.

i) *Onion-skin lesion* consists of loosely-placed concentric layers of hyperplastic intimal smooth muscle cells like the bulb of an onion. The basement membrane is also thickened and reduplicated (Fig. 28.2, B).
ii) *Mucinous intimal thickening* is the deposition of amorphous ground substance, probably proteoglycans, with scanty cells.
iii) *Fibrous intimal thickening* is less common and consists of bundles of collagen, elastic fibres and hyaline deposits in the intima.

Severe intimal sclerosis results in narrowed or obliterated lumen. With time, the lesions become more and more fibrotic.

PATHOGENESIS The pathogenesis of hyperplastic intimal thickening is unclear. Probably, the changes result following endothelial injury from systemic hypertension, hypoxia or immunologic damage leading to increased permeability. A healing reaction occurs in the form of proliferation of smooth muscle cells with fibrosis.

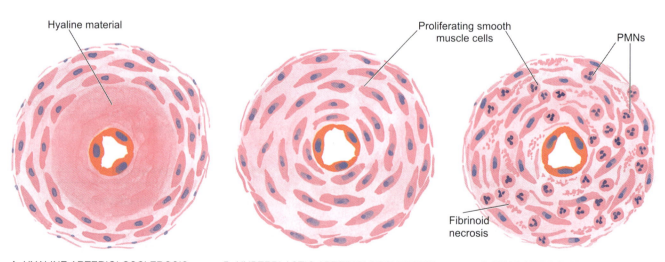

A, HYALINE ARTERIOLOSCLEROSIS   B, HYPERPLASTIC ARTERIOLOSCLEROSIS   C, NECROTISING ARTERIOLITIS

Figure 28.2 ▶ Diagrammatic representation of three forms of arteriolosclerosis, commonly seen in hypertension.

Necrotising Arteriolitis

In cases of severe hypertension and malignant hypertension, parts of small arteries and arterioles show changes of hyaline sclerosis and parts of these show necrosis, or necrosis may be superimposed on hyaline sclerosis. However, hyaline sclerosis may not be always present in the vessel wall.

MORPHOLOGIC FEATURES Besides the changes of hyaline sclerosis, the changes of necrotising arteriolitis include fibrinoid necrosis of vessel wall, acute inflammatory infiltrate of neutrophils in the adventitia. Oedema and haemorrhages often surround the affected vessels (Fig. 28.2, C).

PATHOGENESIS Since necrotising arteriolitis occurs in vessels in which there is sudden and great elevation of pressure, the changes are said to result from direct physical injury to the vessel wall.

HYPERTENSIVE HEART DISEASE

Hypertensive heart disease or hypertensive cardiomyopathy is the disease of the heart resulting from systemic hypertension of prolonged duration and manifesting by left ventricular hypertrophy. Even mild hypertension (blood pressure higher than 140/90 mmHg) of sufficient duration may induce hypertensive heart disease. It is the second most common form of heart disease after IHD. As already pointed out, hypertension predisposes to atherosclerosis. Therefore, most patients of hypertensive heart disease have advanced coronary atherosclerosis and may develop progressive IHD.

Amongst the causes of death in hypertensive patients, cardiac decompensation leading to CHF accounts for about one-third of the patients; other causes of death are IHD, cerebrovascular stroke, renal failure following arteriolar nephrosclerosis, dissecting aneurysm of the aorta and sudden cardiac death.

PATHOGENESIS Pathogenesis of left ventricular hypertrophy (LVH) which is most commonly caused by systemic hypertension is described here.

Stimulus to LVH is pressure overload in systemic hypertension. Both genetic and haemodynamic factors contribute to LVH. The stress of pressure on the ventricular wall causes increased production of myofilaments, myofibrils, other cell organelles and nuclear enlargement. Since the adult myocardial fibres do not divide, the fibres are hypertrophied. However, the sarcomeres may divide to increase the cell width.

LVH can be diagnosed by ECG. Aggressive control of hypertension can regress the left ventricular mass but which antihypertensive agents would do this, in addition to their role in controlling blood pressure, is not clearly known. Abnormalities of diastolic function in hypertension are more common in hypertension and is present in about one-third of patients with normal systolic function.

MORPHOLOGIC FEATURES **Grossly,** the most significant finding is marked hypertrophy of the heart, chiefly of the left ventricle (*see* Fig. 3.4). The weight of the heart increases to 500 gm or more (normal weight about 300 gm). The thickness of the left ventricular wall increases from its normal 13 to 15 mm up to 20 mm or more. The papillary muscles and trabeculae carneae are rounded and prominent. Initially, there is *concentric hypertrophy* of the left ventricle (without dilatation). But when decompensation and cardiac failure supervene, there is *eccentric hypertrophy* (with dilatation) with thinning of the ventricular wall and there may be dilatation and hypertrophy of right heart as well.

Microscopically, the features are not as prominent as gross appearance. The changes include enlargement and degeneration of myocardial fibres with focal areas of myocardial fibrosis. In advanced cases, there may be myocardial oedema and foci of necrosis in the myocardium.

NEPHROSCLEROSIS

Long term renal effects of hypertension appear in the form of nephrosclerosis—benign and malignant. An important and early clinical marker for renal injury from hypertension and risk factor for cardiovascular disease is *macroalbuminuria* (i.e. albuminuria > 150 mg/day or random urine albumin/creatinine ratio of >300 mg/gm creatinine), or *microalbuminuria* estimated by radioimmunoassay (i.e. microalbumin 30-300 mg/day or random urine microalbumin/creatinine ratio of 30-300 mg/gm creatinine).

Benign Nephrosclerosis

Benign nephrosclerosis is the term used to describe the kidney of benign phase of hypertension. Mild benign nephrosclerosis is the most common form of renal disease in persons over 60 years of age but its severity increases in the presence of hypertension and diabetes mellitus.

MORPHOLOGIC FEATURES **Grossly,** both the kidneys are affected equally and are reduced in size and weight, often weighing about 100 gm or less. The capsule is often adherent to the cortical surface. The surface of the kidney is finely granular and shows V-shaped areas of scarring. The cut surface shows firm kidney and narrowed cortex (Fig. 28.3).

Microscopically, there are primarily diffuse vascular changes which produce parenchymal changes secondarily as a result of ischaemia. The histologic changes are, thus, described as vascular and parenchymal (Fig. 28.4, A):

i) Vascular changes: Changes in blood vessels involve arterioles and arteries up to the size of arcuate arteries. There are 2 types of changes in these blood vessels:

a) *Hyaline arteriolosclerosis* that results in homogeneous and eosinophilic thickening of the wall of small blood vessels.

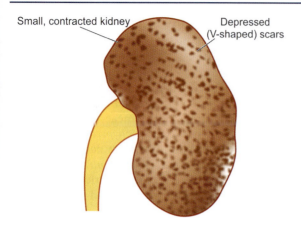
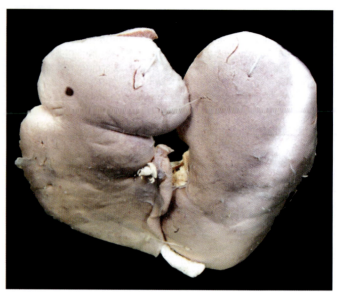

Figure 28.3 ▶ Small, contracted kidney in chronic hypertension (benign nephrosclerosis). The kidney is small and contracted. The capsule is adherent to the cortex and has granular depressed scars on the surface.

b) *Intimal thickening* due to proliferation of smooth muscle cells in the intima.

ii) **Parenchymal changes:** As a consequence of ischaemia, there is variable degree of atrophy of parenchyma. This includes: glomerular shrinkage, deposition of collagen in Bowman's space, periglomerular fibrosis, tubular atrophy and fine interstitial fibrosis.

CLINICAL FEATURES There is variable elevation of the blood pressure with headache, dizziness, palpitation and nervousness. Eye ground changes may be found but papilloedema is absent. Renal function tests and urine examination are normal in early stage. In long-standing cases, there may be mild proteinuria with some hyaline or granular casts. Rarely, renal failure and uraemia may occur.

Malignant Nephrosclerosis

Malignant nephrosclerosis is the form of renal disease that occurs in malignant or accelerated hypertension. Malignant nephrosclerosis is uncommon and usually occurs as a superimposed complication in 5% cases of pre-existing benign essential hypertension or in those having secondary hypertension with identifiable cause such as in chronic renal diseases. However, the pure form of disease also occurs, particularly at younger age with preponderance in males.

MORPHOLOGIC FEATURES *Grossly,* the appearance of the kidney varies. In a case of malignant hypertension superimposed on pre-existing benign nephrosclerosis, the kidneys are small in size, shrunken and reduced in weight and have finely granular surface. However, the kidneys of a patient who develops malignant hypertension in pure form are enlarged, oedematous and have petechial haemorrhages on the surface producing so called *'flea-bitten kidney'.* Cut surface shows red and yellow mottled appearance **(Fig. 28.5).**

Microscopically, most commonly the changes are superimposed on benign nephrosclerosis. These changes are as under **(Fig. 28.4, B):**

i) **Vascular changes** These are more severe and involve the arterioles. The two characteristic vascular changes seen are as under:

a) *Necrotising arteriolitis* develops on hyaline arteriolosclerosis. The vessel wall shows fibrinoid necrosis, a few acute inflammatory cells and small haemorrhages.

b) *Hyperplastic intimal sclerosis* or *onion skin proliferation* is characterised by concentric laminae of proliferated smooth muscle cells, collagen and basement membranes.

ii) **Ischaemic changes** The effects of vascular narrowing on the parenchyma include tubular loss, fine interstitial fibrosis and foci of infarction necrosis.

CLINICAL FEATURES The patients of malignant nephrosclerosis have malignant or accelerated hypertension with blood pressure of 200/140 mmHg or higher. Headache, dizziness and impaired vision are commonly found. The presence of papilloedema distinguishes malignant from benign phase of hypertension. The urine frequently shows microscopic haematuria and proteinuria. Renal function tests show deterioration during the course of the illness. Azotaemia (high BUN and serum creatinine) and uraemia develop soon if malignant hypertension is not treated aggressively. Approximately 90% of patients die within one

Chapter 28: Hypertension and its Consequences

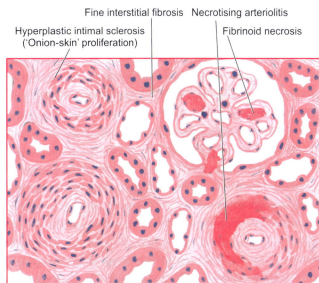

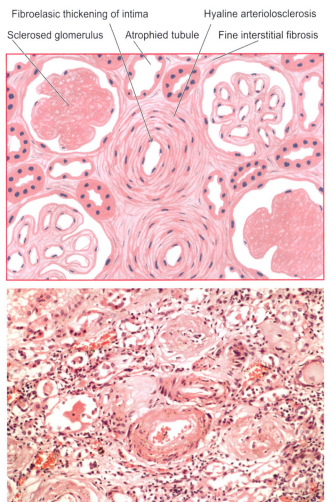

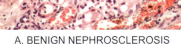

Figure 28.4 ▶ Microscopic changes in kidney in hypertension. A, *Benign nephrosclerosis*. The vascular changes are hyaline arteriolosclerosis and intimal thickening of small blood vessels in the glomerular tuft. The parenchymal changes include sclerosed glomeruli, tubular atrophy and fine interstitial fibrosis. B, *Malignant nephrosclerosis*. The vascular changes are necrotising arteriolitis and hyperplastic intimal sclerosis or onion-skin proliferation. The parenchymal changes are tubular loss, fine interstitial fibrosis and foci of infarction necrosis.

year from causes such as uraemia, congestive heart failure and cerebrovascular accidents.

STROKE (INTRACRANIAL HAEMORRHAGE)

Haemorrhage into the brain may be traumatic or non-traumatic (or spontaneous). There are two main types of spontaneous intracranial haemorrhage **(Fig. 28.6)**:
1. Intracerebral haemorrhage, which is usually of hypertensive origin.
2. Subarachnoid haemorrhage, which is commonly aneurysmal in origin.

In addition to hypertension and rupture of an aneurysm, other causes of spontaneous intracranial haemorrhage include haemorrhage into tumours, vascular malformations and haemorrhagic diathesis which produce mixed intracerebral and subarachnoid haemorrhage.

Intracerebral Haemorrhage

Spontaneous intracerebral haemorrhage occurs mostly in patients of hypertension. Most hypertensives over middle age have microaneurysms in very small cerebral arteries in the brain tissue. Rupture of one of the numerous microaneurysms is believed to be the cause of intracerebral haemorrhage. Unlike subarachnoid haemorrhage, it is not common to have recurrent intracerebral haemorrhages.

The common sites of hypertensive intracerebral haemorrhage are the region of the basal ganglia (particularly the putamen and the internal capsule), pons and the cerebellar

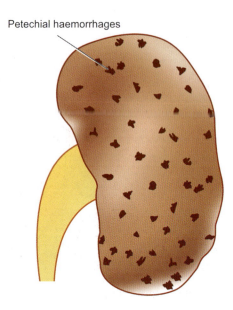

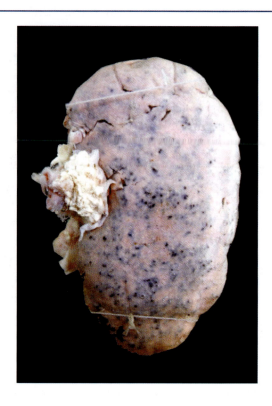

Figure 28.5 ▶ Malignant nephrosclerosis. The kidney is enlarged in size and weight. The cortex shows characteristic *'flea bitten kidney'* due to tiny petechial haemorrhages on the surface.

cortex. Clinically the onset is usually sudden with headache and loss of consciousness. Depending upon the location of the lesion, hemispheric, brainstem or cerebellar signs will be present. About 40% of patients die during the first 3-4 days of haemorrhage, mostly from haemorrhage into the ventricles. The survivors tend to have haematoma that separates the tissue planes which is followed by resolution and development of an *apoplectic cyst* accompanied by loss of function.

MORPHOLOGIC FEATURES *Grossly* and *microscopically*, the haemorrhage consists of dark mass of clotted blood replacing brain parenchyma. The borders of the lesion are sharply-defined and have a narrow rim of partially necrotic parenchyma. Small ring haemorrhages in the Virchow-Robin space in the border zone are commonly present. Ipsilateral ventricles are distorted and compressed and may contain blood in their lumina. Rarely, blood may rupture through the surface of the brain into the subarachnoid space. After a few weeks to months, the haematoma undergoes resolution with formation of a slit-like space called *apoplectic cyst* which contains yellowish fluid. Its margins are yellow-brown and have haemosiderin-laden macrophages and a reactive zone of fibrillary astrocytosis.

Subarachnoid Haemorrhage

Haemorrhage into the subarachnoid space is most commonly caused by rupture of an aneurysm, and rarely, rupture of a vascular malformation. Of the three types of aneurysms affecting the larger intracranial arteries—berry, mycotic and fusiform, berry aneurysms are most important and most common.

Berry aneurysms are saccular in appearance with rounded or lobulated bulge arising at the bifurcation of intracranial arteries and varying in size from 2 mm to 2 cm or more. They account for 95% of aneurysms which are liable to rupture. Berry aneurysms are rare in childhood but increase in frequency in young adults and middle life. They are, therefore,

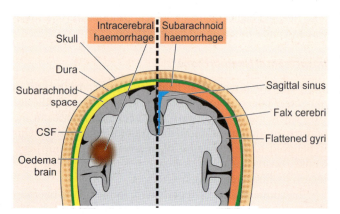

Figure 28.6 ▶ Two types of intracranial haemorrhage: intracerebral (left) and subarachnoid haemorrhage (right).

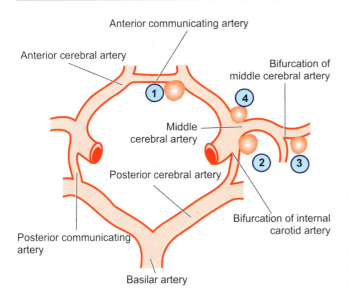

Figure 28.7 ▶ The circle of Willis showing principal sites of berry (saccular) aneurysms. The serial numbers indicate the frequency of involvement.

not congenital anomalies but develop over the years from developmental defect of the media of the arterial wall at the bifurcation of arteries forming thin-walled saccular bulges. Although most berry aneurysms are sporadic in occurrence, there is an increased incidence of their presence in association with congenital polycystic kidney disease and coarctation of the aorta. About a quarter of berry aneurysms are multiple.

In more than 85% cases of subarachnoid haemorrhage, the cause is massive and sudden bleeding from a berry aneurysm on or near the circle of Willis. The four most common sites of such aneurysms are as under (Fig. 28.7):
1. In relation to anterior communicating artery.
2. At the origin of the posterior communicating artery from the stem of the internal carotid artery.
3. At the first major bifurcation of the middle cerebral artery.
4. At the bifurcation of the internal carotid into the middle and anterior cerebral arteries.

The remaining 15% cases of subarachnoid haemorrhage are the result of rupture in the posterior circulation, vascular malformations and rupture of mycotic aneurysms that occurs in the setting of bacterial endocarditis. In all types of aneurysms, the rupture of thin-walled dilatation occurs in association with sudden rise in intravascular pressure but chronic hypertension does not appear to be a risk factor in their development or rupture.

Clinically, berry aneurysms remain asymptomatic prior to rupture. On rupture, they produce severe generalised headache of sudden onset which is frequently followed by unconsciousness and neurologic defects. Initial mortality from first rupture is about 20-25%. Survivors recover completely but frequently suffer from recurrent episodes of fresh bleeding.

MORPHOLOGIC FEATURES Rupture of a berry aneurysm frequently spreads haemorrhage throughout the subarachnoid space with rise in intracranial pressure and characteristic blood-stained CSF. An intracerebral haematoma may develop if the blood tracks into the brain parenchyma. The region of the brain supplied by the affected artery frequently shows infarction, partly attributed to vasospasm.

HYPERTENSIVE RETINOPATHY

In hypertensive retinopathy, the retinal arterioles are reduced in their diameter leading to retinal ischaemia. In acute severe hypertension as happens at the onset of malignant hypertension and in toxaemia of pregnancy, the vascular changes are in the form of spasms, while in chronic hypertension the changes are diffuse in the form of onion-skin thickening of the arteriolar walls with narrowing of the lumina.

Features of hypertensive retinopathy include the following (Fig. 28.8):
i) Variable degree of arteriolar narrowing due to arteriolosclerosis.
ii) 'Flame-shaped' haemorrhages in the retinal nerve fibre layer.
iii) Macular star i.e. exudates radiating from the centre of macula.
iv) Cotton-wool spots i.e. fluffy white bodies in the superficial layer of retina.
v) Microaneurysms.
vi) Arteriovenous nicking i.e. kinking of veins at sites where sclerotic arterioles cross veins.
vii) Hard exudates due to leakage of lipid and fluid into macula.

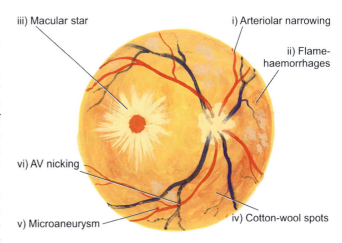

Figure 28.8 ▶ Ocular lesions in hypertension.

Hypertensive retinopathy is classified according to the severity of above lesions from grade I to IV. More serious and severe changes with poor prognosis occur in higher grades of hypertensive retinopathy. Malignant hypertension is characterised by necrotising arteriolitis and fibrinoid necrosis of retinal arterioles.

GIST BOX 28.2 — Consequences of Hypertension

- Systemic hypertension causes major effects in five main organs—blood vessels (arteriolosclerosis), heart (hypertensive heart disease), kidneys (benign and malignant nephrosclerosis), nervous system (stroke) and eye (hypertensive retinopathy).
- Arteriosclerosis is the term used for thickening and hardening of arterial wall.
- Hypertensive arteriolosclerosis affects arterioles and includes hyaline thickening, or hyperplastic or proliferative change or necrotising lesion.
- Hypertensive heart disease results from systemic hypertension of prolonged duration and manifests by left ventricular hypertrophy.
- Initially, there is *concentric hypertrophy* of the left ventricle (without dilatation). But when decompensation and cardiac failure supervene, there is *eccentric hypertrophy* (with dilatation).
- Benign nephrosclerosis is the term used to describe the kidney of benign phase of hypertension and is the most common form of renal disease in persons over 60 years of age.
- Malignant nephrosclerosis is less common but more severe form of renal disease that occurs in malignant or accelerated hypertension.
- Haemorrhage into the brain may be traumatic, non-traumatic, or spontaneous. There are two main types of spontaneous non-traumatic intracranial haemorrhage: intracerebral haemorrhage (usually of hypertensive origin) and subarachnoid haemorrhage (commonly aneurysmal in origin).
- Retinal capillary vessels are narrowed in hypertension causing ocular lesions due to retinal ischaemia.

29 Diabetes Mellitus and its Complications

NORMAL STRUCTURE OF ENDOCRINE PANCREAS

The human pancreas, though anatomically a single organ, histologically and functionally, has 2 distinct parts—the exocrine and endocrine. The endocrine pancreas consists of microscopic collections of cells called islets of Langerhans found scattered within the pancreatic lobules, as well as individual endocrine cells found in duct epithelium and among the acini. The total weight of endocrine pancreas in the adult, however, does not exceed 1-1.5 gm (total weight of pancreas 60-100 gm). The islet cell tissue is greatly concentrated in the tail than in the head or body of the pancreas. Islets possess no ductal system and they drain their secretory products directly into the circulation. Ultrastructurally and immunohistochemically, 4 *major* and 2 *minor* types of islet cells are distinguished, each type having its distinct secretory product and function. These are as follows:

A. Major cell types:

1. *Beta (β) or B cells* comprise about 70% of islet cells and secrete insulin, the defective response or deficient synthesis of which causes diabetes mellitus.

2. *Alpha (α) or A cells* comprise 20% of islet cells and secrete glucagon which induces hyperglycaemia.

3. *Delta (δ) or D cells* comprise 5-10% of islet cells and secrete somatostatin which suppresses both insulin and glucagon release.

4. *Pancreatic polypeptide (PP) cells or F cells* comprise 1-2% of islet cells and secrete pancreatic polypeptide having some gastrointestinal effects.

B. Minor cell types:

1. *D1 cells* elaborate vasoactive intestinal peptide (VIP) which induces glycogenolysis and hyperglycaemia and causes secretory diarrhoea by stimulation of gastrointestinal fluid secretion.

2. *Enterochromaffin cells* synthesise serotonin which in pancreatic tumours may induce carcinoid syndrome.

Major disease of endocrine pancreas is diabetes mellitus; others are uncommon islet cell tumours.

DIABETES MELLITUS

DEFINITION AND EPIDEMIOLOGY

As per the WHO, diabetes mellitus (DM) is defined as a heterogeneous metabolic disorder characterised by common feature of chronic hyperglycaemia with disturbance of carbohydrate, fat and protein metabolism. At this point, it is also important to understand another related term, *metabolic syndrome* (also called syndrome X or insulin resistance syndrome), consisting of a combination of metabolic abnormalities which increase the risk to develop diabetes mellitus and cardiovascular disease. Major features of metabolic syndrome are central obesity, hypertriglyceridaemia, low LDL cholesterol, hyperglycaemia and hypertension.

DM is a leading cause of morbidity and mortality world over. It is expected to continue as a major health problem owing to its serious complications, especially end-stage renal disease, IHD, gangrene of the lower extremities, and blindness in the adults. Top 5 countries with highest prevalence of DM are India, China, US, Indonesia and Japan. In India, its incidence is estimated at 7% of adult population (approximately 65 million affected people), largely due to genetic susceptibility combined with changing life style of low-activity high-calorie diet in the growing Indian middle class. The incidence is somewhat low in Africa. But prevalence of DM is expected to rise in developing countries of Asia and Africa due to urbanisation and associated obesity and increased body weight. The rise in prevalence is more for type 2 diabetes than for type 1. It is anticipated that by the year 2030 the number of diabetics globally will double from the present figure of 250 million.

CLASSIFICATION AND ETIOLOGY

The older classification systems dividing DM into primary (idiopathic) and secondary types, juvenile-onset and maturity onset types, and insulin-dependent (IDDM) and non-insulin dependent (NIDDM) types, have become obsolete and undergone major revision due to extensive understanding of etiology and pathogenesis of DM in recent times.

As outlined in Table 29.1, current classification of DM based on etiology divides it into two broad categories—type 1 and type 2; besides there are a few uncommon specific etiologic types, and gestational DM. American Diabetes Association (2007) has identified risk factors for type 2 DM listed in Table 29.2.

Brief comments on etiologic terminologies as contrasted with former nomenclatures of DM are as under:

TYPE 1 DM It constitutes about 10% cases of DM. It was previously termed as juvenile-onset diabetes (JOD) due to its

Table 29.1	Etiologic classification of diabetes mellitus (as per American Diabetes Association, 2007).
I.	TYPE 1 DIABETES MELLITUS (10%) (earlier called Insulin-dependent, or juvenile-onset diabetes) *Type IA DM:* Immune-mediated *Type IB DM:* Idiopathic
II.	TYPE 2 DIABETES MELLITUS (80%) (earlier called non-insulin-dependent, or maturity-onset diabetes)
III.	OTHER SPECIFIC TYPES OF DIABETES (10%) A. Genetic defect of β-cell function due to mutations in various enzymes (earlier called maturity-onset diabetes of the young or MODY) (e.g. hepatocyte nuclear transcription factor—HNF, glucokinase) B. Genetic defect in insulin action (e.g. type A insulin resistance) C. Diseases of exocrine pancreas (e.g. chronic pancreatitis, pancreatic tumours, post-pancreatectomy) D. Endocrinopathies (e.g. acromegaly, Cushing's syndrome, pheochromocytoma) E. Drug- or chemical-induced (e.g. steroids, thyroid hormone, thiazides, β-blockers etc) F. Infections (e.g. congenital rubella, cytomegalovirus) G. Uncommon forms of immune-mediated DM (stiff man syndrome, anti-insulin receptor antibodies) H. Other genetic syndromes (e.g. Down's syndrome, Klinefelter's syndrome, Turner's syndrome)
IV.	GESTATIONAL DIABETES MELLITUS (4%)

occurrence in younger age, and was called insulin-dependent DM (IDDM) because it was known that these patients have absolute requirement for insulin replacement as treatment. However, in the new classification, neither age nor insulin-dependence are considered as absolute criteria. Instead, based on underlying etiology, type 1 DM is further divided into 2 subtypes:

Table 29.2	Major risk factors for type 2 diabetes mellitus (ADA Recommendations, 2007).
1.	Family history of type 2 DM
2.	Obesity
3.	Habitual physical inactivity
4.	Race and ethnicity (Blacks, Asians, Pacific Islanders)
5.	Previous identification of impaired fasting glucose or impaired glucose tolerance
6.	History of gestational DM or delivery of baby heavier than 4 kg
7.	Hypertension
8.	Dyslipidaemia (HDL level < 35 mg/dl or triglycerides > 250 mg/dl)
9.	Polycystic ovary disease and acanthosis nigricans
10.	History of vascular disease

Subtype 1A (immune-mediated) DM characterised by autoimmune destruction of β-cells which usually leads to insulin deficiency.

Subtype 1B (idiopathic) DM characterised by insulin deficiency with tendency to develop ketosis but these patients are negative for autoimmune markers.

Though type 1 DM occurs commonly in patients under 30 years of age, autoimmune destruction of β-cells can occur at any age. In fact, 5-10% patients who develop DM above 30 years of age are of type 1A DM and hence the term JOD has become obsolete.

TYPE 2 DM This type comprises about 80% cases of DM. It was previously called maturity-onset diabetes, or non-insulin dependent diabetes mellitus (NIDDM) of obese and non-obese type.

Although type 2 DM predominantly affects older individuals, it is now known that it also occurs in obese adolescent children; hence the term MOD for it is inappropriate. Moreover, many type 2 DM patients also require insulin therapy to control hyperglycaemia or to prevent ketosis and thus are not truly non-insulin dependent contrary to its older nomenclature.

OTHER SPECIFIC ETIOLOGIC TYPES OF DM Besides the two main types, about 10% cases of DM have a known specific etiologic defect listed in Table 29.1. One important subtype in this group is *maturity-onset diabetes of the young (MODY)* which has autosomal dominant inheritance, early onset of hyperglycaemia and impaired insulin secretion.

GESTATIONAL DM About 4% pregnant women develop DM due to metabolic changes during pregnancy. Although they revert back to normal glycaemia after delivery, these women are prone to develop DM later in their life.

PATHOGENESIS

Depending upon etiology of DM, hyperglycaemia may result from the following:
- Reduced insulin secretion
- Decreased glucose use by the body
- Increased glucose production.

Pathogenesis of two main types of DM and its complications is distinct. In order to understand it properly, it is essential to first recall physiology of normal insulin synthesis and secretion.

Normal Insulin Metabolism

The major stimulus for both synthesis and release of insulin is glucose. The steps involved in biosynthesis, release and actions of insulin are as follows **(Fig. 29.1)**:

Synthesis Insulin is synthesised in the β-cells of pancreatic islets of Langerhans:
i) It is initially formed as *pre-proinsulin* which is single-chain 86-amino acid precursor polypeptide.

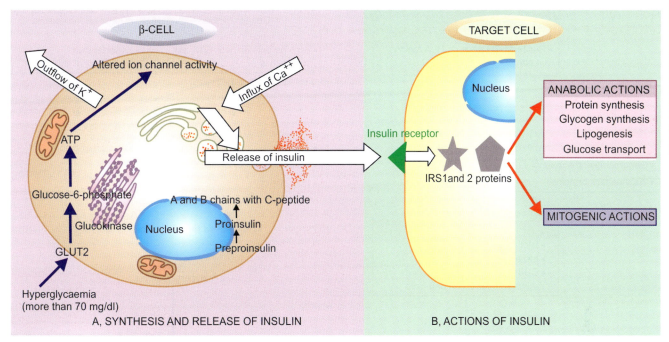

Figure 29.1 ▶ A, Pathway of normal insulin synthesis and release in β-cells of pancreatic islets. B, Chain of events in action of insulin on target cell.

ii) Subsequent proteolysis removes the amino terminal signal peptide, forming *proinsulin*.
iii) Further cleavage of proinsulin gives rise to *A (21 amino acids) and B (30 amino acids) chains* of insulin, linked together by connecting segment called *C-peptide*, all of which are stored in the secretory granules in the β-cells. As compared to A and B chains of insulin, C-peptide is less susceptible to degradation in the liver and is therefore used as a marker to distinguish endogenously synthesised and exogenously administered insulin.

For therapeutic purposes, *human insulin* is now produced by recombinant DNA technology.

Release Glucose is the key regulator of insulin secretion from β-cells by a series of steps:
i) Hyperglycaemia (glucose level more than 70 mg/dl or above 3.9 mmol/L) stimulates transport into β-cells of a *glucose transporter, GLUT2*. Other stimuli influencing insulin release include nutrients in the meal, ketones, amino acids etc.
ii) An islet transcription factor, *glucokinase*, causes glucose phosphorylation, and thus acts as a step for controlled release of glucose-regulated insulin secretion.
iii) Metabolism of glucose to glucose-6-phosphate by glycolysis generates *ATP*.
iv) Generation of ATP *alters the ion channel activity* on the membrane. It causes inhibition of ATP-sensitive K^+ channel on the cell membrane and opening up of calcium channel with resultant influx of calcium, which stimulates insulin release.

Action Half of insulin secreted from β-cells into portal vein is degraded in the liver while the remaining half enters the systemic circulation for action on the target cells:
i) Insulin from circulation binds to its receptor on the target cells. *Insulin receptor* has intrinsic tyrosine kinase activity.
ii) This, in turn, activates post-receptor intracellular signalling pathway molecules, *insulin receptor substrates (IRS) 1 and 2 proteins*, which initiate sequence of phosphorylation and dephosphorylation reactions.
iii) These reactions on the target cells are responsible for the main *mitogenic and anabolic actions of insulin*—glycogen synthesis, glucose transport, protein synthesis, lipogenesis.
iv) Besides the role of glucose in maintaining equilibrium of insulin release, *low insulin level in the fasting state* promotes hepatic gluconeogenesis and glycogenolysis, reduced glucose uptake by insulin-sensitive tissues and promotes mobilisation of stored precursors, so as to prevent hypoglycaemia.

Pathogenesis of Type 1 DM

The basic phenomenon in type 1 DM is destruction of β-cell mass, usually leading to absolute insulin deficiency. While type 1B DM remains idiopathic, pathogenesis of type 1A DM is immune-mediated and has been extensively studied. Currently, pathogenesis of type 1A DM is explained on the basis of 3 mutually-interlinked mechanisms: genetic susceptibility, autoimmunity, and certain environmental factors **(Fig. 29.2, A)**.

1. Genetic susceptibility Type 1A DM involves inheritance of multiple genes to confer susceptibility to the disorder:

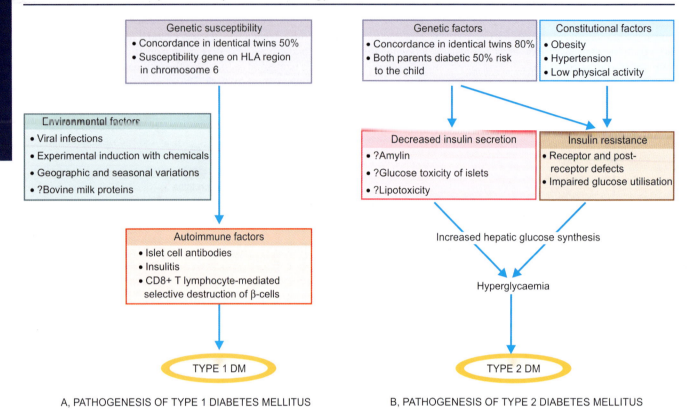

Figure 29.2 ▶ Schematic mechanisms involved in pathogenesis of two main types of diabetes mellitus.

i) It has been observed in *identical twins* that if one twin has type 1A DM, there is about 50% chance of the second twin developing it, but not all. This means that some additional modifying factors are involved in development of DM in these cases.

ii) About half the cases with genetic predisposition to type 1A DM have the *susceptibility gene* located in the HLA region of chromosome 6 (MHC class II region), particularly HLA DR3, HLA DR4 and HLA DQ locus.

2. Autoimmunity Studies on humans and animal models on type 1A DM have shown several immunologic abnormalities:

i) Presence of *islet cell antibodies* against GAD (glutamic acid decarboxylase), insulin etc, though their assay largely remains a research tool due to tedious method.

ii) Occurrence of lymphocytic infiltrate in and around the pancreatic islets termed *insulitis*. It chiefly consists of CD8+ T lymphocytes with variable number of CD4+ T lymphocytes and macrophages.

iii) *Selective destruction of β-cells* while other islet cell types (glucagon-producing alpha cells, somatostatin-producing delta cells, or polypeptide-forming PP cells) remain unaffected. This is mediated by T-cell mediated cytotoxicity or by apoptosis.

iv) Role of *T cell-mediated autoimmunity* is further supported by transfer of type 1A DM from diseased animal by infusing T lymphocytes to a healthy animal.

v) Association of type 1A DM with *other autoimmune diseases* in about 10-20% cases such as Graves' disease, Addison's disease, Hashimoto's thyroiditis, pernicious anaemia.

vi) Remission of type 1A DM in response to immuno-suppressive therapy such as administration of cyclosporin A.

3. Environmental factors Epidemiologic studies in type 1A DM suggest the involvement of certain environmental factors in its pathogenesis, though role of none of them has been conclusively proved. In fact, the trigger may precede the occurrence of the disease by several years. It appears that certain viral and dietary proteins share antigenic properties with human cell surface proteins and trigger the immune attack on β-cells by a process of molecular mimicry. These factors include the following:

i) *Certain viral infections* preceding the onset of disease e.g. mumps, measles, coxsackie B virus, cytomegalovirus and infectious mononucleosis.

ii) *Experimental induction* of type 1A DM with certain chemicals has been possible e.g. alloxan, streptozotocin and pentamidine.

iii) *Geographic and seasonal variations* in its incidence suggest some common environmental factors.
iv) Possible relationship of early exposure to *bovine milk proteins* and occurrence of autoimmune process in type 1A DM is being studied.

KEY POINTS Pathogenesis of type 1A DM can be summed up by interlinking the above three factors as under:
1. At birth, individuals with *genetic susceptibility* to this disorder have normal β-cell mass.
2. β-cells act as autoantigens and activate CD4+ T lymphocytes, bringing about immune destruction of pancreatic β-cells by *autoimmune phenomena* and takes months to years. Clinical features of diabetes manifest after more than 80% of β-cell mass has been destroyed.
3. The trigger for autoimmune process appears to be some *infectious or environmental factor* which specifically targets β-cells.

Pathogenesis of Type 2 DM

The basic metabolic defect in type 2 DM is either a delayed insulin secretion relative to glucose load *(impaired insulin secretion)*, or the peripheral tissues are unable to respond to insulin *(insulin resistance)*.

Type 2 DM is a heterogeneous disorder with a more complex etiology and is far more common than type 1, but much less is known about its pathogenesis. A number of factors have been implicated though, but HLA association and autoimmune phenomena are not implicated. These factors are as under **(Fig. 29.2, B)**:

1. **Genetic factors** Genetic component has a stronger basis for type 2 DM than type 1A DM. Although no definite and consistent genes have been identified, multifactorial inheritance is the most important factor in development of type 2 DM:
i) There is approximately 80% chance of developing diabetes in the other *identical twin* if one twin has the disease.
ii) A person with one parent having type 2 DM is at an increased risk of getting diabetes, but if *both parents* have type 2 DM the risk in the offspring rises to 40%.
2. **Constitutional factors** Certain environmental factors such as obesity, hypertension, and level of physical activity play contributory role and modulate the phenotyping of the disease.
3. **Insulin resistance** One of the most prominent metabolic features of type 2 DM is the lack of responsiveness of peripheral tissues to insulin, especially of the skeletal muscle and liver. Obesity, in particular, is strongly associated with insulin resistance and hence type 2 DM. Mechanism of hyperglycaemia in these cases is explained as under:
i) Resistance to action of insulin *impairs glucose utilisation* and hence hyperglycaemia.
ii) There is *increased hepatic synthesis* of glucose.
iii) *Hyperglycaemia in obesity* is related to high levels of free fatty acids and cytokines (e.g. TNF-α and adiponectin) affect peripheral tissue sensitivity to respond to insulin.

The precise underlying molecular defect responsible for insulin resistance in type 2 DM has yet not been fully identified. Currently, it is proposed that insulin resistance may be possibly due to one of the following defects:
a) Polymorphism in various *post-receptor intracellular signal pathway molecules*.
b) *Elevated free fatty acids* seen in obesity may contribute e.g. by impaired glucose utilisation in the skeletal muscle, by increased hepatic synthesis of glucose, and by impaired β-cell function.
c) *Insulin resistance syndrome* is a complex of clinical features occurring from insulin resistance and its resultant metabolic derangements that includes hyperglycaemia and compensatory hyperinsulinaemia. The clinical features are in the form of accelerated cardiovascular disease and may occur in both obese as well as non-obese type 2 DM patients. The features include: mild hypertension (related to endothelial dysfunction) and dyslipidaemia (characterised by reduced HDL level, increased triglycerides and LDL level).

4. **Impaired insulin secretion** In type 2 DM, insulin resistance and insulin secretion are interlinked:
i) Early in the course of disease, in response to insulin resistance there is compensatory increased secretion of insulin (*hyperinsulinaemia*) in an attempt to maintain normal blood glucose level.
ii) Eventually, however, there is *failure of β-cell function* to secrete adequate insulin, although there is some secretion of insulin i.e. cases of type 2 DM have mild to moderate deficiency of insulin (which is much less severe than that in type 1 DM) but not its total absence.

The exact genetic mechanism why there is a fall in insulin secretion in these cases is unclear. However, following possibilities are proposed:
a) Islet amyloid polypeptide (*amylin*) which forms fibrillar protein deposits in pancreatic islets in long-standing cases of type 2 DM may be responsible for impaired function of β-cells of islet cells.
b) Metabolic environment of chronic hyperglycaemia surrounding the islets *(glucose toxicity)* may paradoxically impair islet cell function.
c) Elevated free fatty acid levels (*lipotoxicity*) in these cases may worsen islet cell function.

5. **Increased hepatic glucose synthesis** One of the normal roles played by insulin is to promote hepatic storage of glucose as glycogen and suppress gluconeogenesis. In type 2 DM, as a part of insulin resistance by peripheral tissues, the liver also shows insulin resistance i.e. in spite of hyperinsulinaemia in the early stage of disease, gluconeogenesis in the liver is not suppressed. This results in increased hepatic synthesis of glucose which contributes to hyperglycaemia in these cases.

KEY POINTS In essence, hyperglycaemia in type 2 DM is not due to destruction of β-cells but is instead a failure of β-cells to meet the requirement of insulin in the body. Its pathogenesis can be summed up by interlinking the above factors as under:

1. Type 2 DM is a more *complex multifactorial disease*.
2. There is greater role of *genetic defect and heredity*.
3. Two main mechanisms for hyperglycaemia in type 2 DM—*insulin resistance and impaired insulin secretion*, are interlinked.
4. While *obesity* plays a role in pathogenesis of insulin resistance, impaired insulin secretion may be from many constitutional factors.
5. *Increased hepatic synthesis of glucose* in initial period of disease contributes to hyperglycaemia.

MORPHOLOGIC FEATURES IN PANCREATIC ISLETS

Morphologic changes in islets have been demonstrated in both types of diabetes, though the changes are more distinctive in type 1 DM:

1. **Insulitis:**

In type 1 DM, characteristically, in early stage there is lymphocytic infiltrate, mainly by T cells, in the islets which may be accompanied by a few macrophages and polymorphs. Diabetic infants born to diabetic mothers, however, have eosinophilic infiltrate in the islets.

In type 2 DM, there is no significant leucocytic infiltrate in the islets but there is variable degree of fibrous tissue in the islets.

2. **Islet cell mass:**

In type 1 DM, as the disease becomes chronic there is progressive depletion of β-cell mass, eventually resulting in total loss of pancreatic β-cells and its hyalinisation.

In type 2 DM, β-cell mass is either normal or mildly reduced. Infants of diabetic mothers, however, have hyperplasia and hypertrophy of islets as a compensatory response to maternal hyperglycaemia.

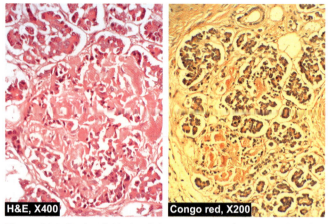

Figure 29.3 ▶ Amyloidosis of the pancreatic islet tissue. The islets are mostly replaced by structureless eosinophilic material which stains positively with Congo red.

3. **Amyloidosis:**

In type 1 DM, deposits of amyloid around islets are absent.

In type 2 DM, characteristically chronic long-standing cases show deposition of amyloid material, amylin, around the capillaries of the islets causing compression and atrophy of islet tissue **(Fig. 29.3)**.

β-cell degranulation:

In type 1 DM, EM shows degranulation of remaining β-cells of islets.

In type 2 DM, no such change is observed.

Table 29.3 Contrasting features of type 1 and type 2 diabetes mellitus.

	FEATURE	TYPE 1 DM	TYPE 2 DM
1.	Frequency	10-20%	80-90%
2.	Age at onset	Early (below 35 years)	Late (after 40 years)
3.	Type of onset	Abrupt and severe	Gradual and insidious
4.	Weight	Normal	Obese/non-obese
5.	HLA	Linked to HLA DR3, HLA DR4, HLA DQ	No HLA association
6.	Family history	< 20%	About 60%
7.	Genetic locus	Unknown	Chromosome 6
8.	Diabetes in identical twins	50% concordance	80% concordance
9.	Pathogenesis	Autoimmune destruction of β-cells	Insulin resistance, impaired insulin secretion
10.	Islet cell antibodies	Yes	No
11.	Blood insulin level	Decreased insulin	Normal or increased insulin
12.	Islet cell changes	Insulitis, β-cell depletion	No insulitis, later fibrosis of islets
13.	Amyloidosis	Infrequent	Common in chronic cases
14.	Clinical management	Insulin and diet	Diet, exercise, oral drugs, insulin
15.	Acute complications	Ketoacidosis	Hyperosmolar coma

CLINICAL FEATURES

It can be appreciated that hyperglycaemia in DM does not cause a single disease but is associated with numerous diseases and symptoms, especially due to complications. Two main types of DM can be distinguished clinically to the extent shown in **Table 29.3**. However, overlapping of clinical features occurs as regards the age of onset, duration of symptoms and family history. Pathophysiology in evolution of clinical features is schematically shown in **Fig. 29.4**.

Type 1 DM:
i) Patients of type 1 DM usually manifest at early age, generally below the age of 35.
ii) The onset of symptoms is often abrupt.
iii) At presentation, these patients have polyuria, polydipsia and polyphagia.
iv) The patients are not obese but have generally progressive loss of weight.
v) These patients are prone to develop metabolic complications such as ketoacidosis and hypoglycaemic episodes.

Type 2 DM:
i) This form of diabetes generally manifests in middle life or beyond, usually above the age of 40.
ii) The onset of symptoms in type 2 DM is slow and insidious.
iii) Generally, the patient is asymptomatic when the diagnosis is made on the basis of glucosuria or hyperglycaemia during physical examination, or may present with polyuria and polydipsia.
iv) The patients are frequently obese and have unexplained weakness and loss of weight.
v) Metabolic complications such as ketoacidosis are infrequent.

> **GIST BOX 29.1 | Diabetes Mellitus**
>
> ❖ Diabetes mellitus is a heterogeneous metabolic disorder characterised by common feature of chronic hyperglycaemia with disturbance of carbohydrate, fat and protein metabolism.
> ❖ Based on etiology, DM is classified into type 1 and 2.
> ❖ Type 1 occurs commonly in patients under 30 years of age and has autoimmune pathogenesis.
> ❖ Type 2 comprises about 80% cases of DM and predominantly affects older individuals and is complex multifactorial disease with greater role of genetic defect and heredity.

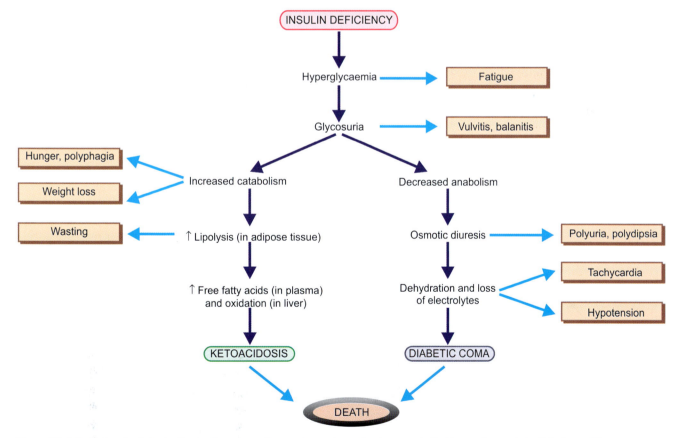

Figure 29.4 ▶ Pathophysiological basis of common signs and symptoms due to uncontrolled hyperglycaemia in diabetes mellitus.

COMPLICATIONS OF DIABETES

As a consequence of hyperglycaemia of diabetes, every tissue and organ of the body undergoes biochemical and structural alterations which account for the major complications in diabetics. which may be *acute metabolic* or *chronic systemic*.

Both types of diabetes mellitus may develop complications which are broadly divided into 2 major groups:

I. *Acute metabolic complications:* These include diabetic ketoacidosis, hyperosmolar nonketotic coma, and hypoglycaemia.

II. *Late systemic complications:* These are atherosclerosis, diabetic microangiopathy, diabetic nephropathy, diabetic neuropathy, diabetic retinopathy and infections.

PATHOGENESIS

It is now known that in both type 1 and 2 DM, *severity and chronicity of hyperglycaemia* forms the main pathogenetic mechanism for 'microvascular complications' (e.g. retinopathy, nephropathy, neuropathy); therefore control of blood glucose level constitutes the mainstay of treatment for minimising development of these complications. Long-standing cases of type 2 DM, however, in addition, frequently develop 'macrovascular complications' (e.g. atherosclerosis, coronary artery disease, peripheral vascular disease, cerebrovascular disease) which are more difficult to explain on the basis of hyperglycaemia alone.

The following biochemical mechanisms have been proposed to explain the development of complications of diabetes mellitus (Fig. 29.5, A):

1. **Non-enzymatic protein glycosylation** The free amino group of various body proteins binds by non-enzymatic mechanism to glucose; this process is called *glycosylation* and is directly proportionate to the severity of hyperglycaemia. Various body proteins undergoing chemical alterations in this way include haemoglobin, lens crystalline protein, and basement membrane of body cells. An example is the measurement of a fraction of haemoglobin called glycosylated haemoglobin (HbA_{1C}) as a test for monitoring glycaemic control in a diabetic patient during the preceding 90 to 120 days which is lifespan of red cells. Similarly, there is accumulation of labile and reversible glycosylation products

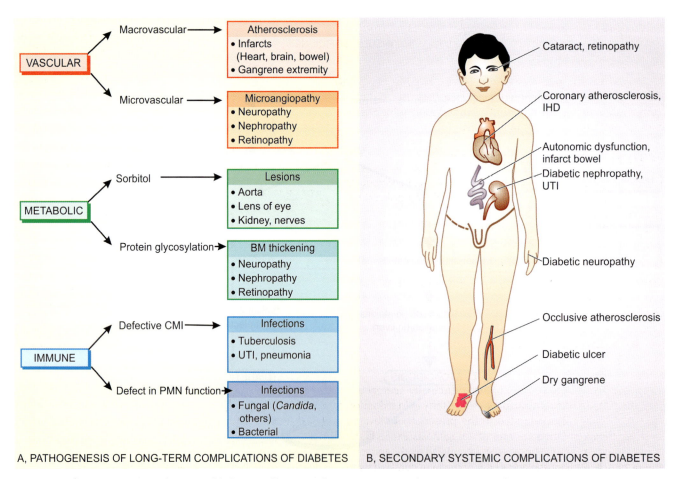

A, PATHOGENESIS OF LONG-TERM COMPLICATIONS OF DIABETES   B, SECONDARY SYSTEMIC COMPLICATIONS OF DIABETES

Figure 29.5 ▶ Long-term complications of diabetes mellitus. A, Pathogenesis. B, Secondary systemic complications.

on collagen and other tissues of the blood vessel wall which subsequently become stable and irreversible by chemical changes and form advanced glycosylation end-products (AGE). The AGEs bind to receptors on different cells and produce a variety of biologic and chemical changes e.g. thickening of vascular basement membrane in diabetes.

2. **Polyol pathway mechanism** This mechanism is responsible for producing lesions in the aorta, lens of the eye, kidney and peripheral nerves. These tissues have an enzyme, aldose reductase, that reacts with glucose to form sorbitol and fructose in the cells of the hyperglycaemic patient as under:

$$\text{Glucose} + \text{NADH} + \text{H}^+ \xrightarrow{\text{aldose reductase}} \text{Sorbitol} + \text{NAD}^+$$

$$\text{Sorbitol} + \text{NAD} \xrightarrow{\text{sorbitol dehydrogenase}} \text{Fructose} + \text{NADH} + \text{H}^+$$

Intracellular accumulation of sorbitol and fructose so produced results in entry of water inside the cell and consequent cellular swelling and cell damage. Also, intracellular accumulation of sorbitol causes intracellular deficiency of myoinositol which promotes injury to Schwann cells and retinal pericytes. These polyols result in disturbed processing of normal intermediary metabolites leading to complications of diabetes.

3. **Excessive oxygen free radicals** In hyperglycaemia, there is increased production of reactive oxygen free radicals from mitochondrial oxidative phosphorylation which may damage various target cells in diabetes.

ACUTE METABOLIC COMPLICATIONS

Metabolic complications develop acutely. While ketoacidosis and hypoglycaemic episodes are primarily complications of type 1 DM, hyperosmolar nonketotic coma is chiefly a complication of type 2 DM (also see **Fig. 29.4**).

1. *Diabetic ketoacidosis (DKA)*

Ketoacidosis is almost exclusively a complication of type 1 DM. It can develop in patients with severe insulin deficiency combined with glucagon excess. Failure to take insulin and exposure to stress are the usual precipitating causes. Severe lack of insulin causes lipolysis in the adipose tissues, resulting in release of free fatty acids into the plasma. These free fatty acids are taken up by the liver where they are oxidised through acetyl coenzyme-A to ketone bodies, principally acetoacetic acid and β-hydroxybutyric acid. Such free fatty acid oxidation to ketone bodies is accelerated in the presence of elevated level of glucagon. Once the rate of ketogenesis exceeds the rate at which the ketone bodies can be utilised by the muscles and other tissues, ketonaemia and ketonuria occur. If urinary excretion of ketone bodies is prevented due to dehydration, systemic metabolic ketoacidosis occurs. Clinically, the condition is characterised by anorexia, nausea, vomitings, deep and fast breathing, mental confusion and coma. Most patients of ketoacidosis recover.

2. *Hyperosmolar Hyperglycaemic Nonketotic Coma*

Hyperosmolar hyperglycaemic nonketotic coma (HHNC) is usually a complication of type 2 DM. It is caused by severe dehydration resulting from sustained hyperglycaemic diuresis. The loss of glucose in urine is so intense that the patient is unable to drink sufficient water to maintain urinary fluid loss. The usual clinical features of ketoacidosis are absent but prominent central nervous signs are present. Blood sugar is extremely high and plasma osmolality is high. Thrombotic and bleeding complications are frequent due to high viscosity of blood. The mortality rate in hyperosmolar nonketotic coma is high.

The contrasting features of diabetic ketoacidosis and hyperosmolar non-ketotic coma are summarised in **Table 29.4**.

3. *Hypoglycaemia*

Hypoglycaemic episode may develop in patients of type 1 DM. It may result from excessive administration of insulin, missing a meal, or due to stress. Hypoglycaemic episodes are harmful as they produce permanent brain damage, or may result in worsening of diabetic control and rebound hyperglycaemia, so called *Somogyi's effect*.

LATE SYSTEMIC COMPLICATIONS

A number of systemic complications may develop after a period of 15-20 years in either type of diabetes. Late

Table 29.4	Contrasting features of diabetic ketoacidosis (DKA) and hyperosmolar hyperglycaemic non-ketotic coma (HHNC).		
	LAB FINDINGS	DKA	HHNC
i.	Plasma glucose (mg/dL)	250-600	> 600
ii.	Plasma acetone	+	Less +
iii.	S. Na$^+$ (mEq/L)	Usually low	N, ↑ or low
iv.	S. K$^+$ (mEq/L)	N, ↑ or low	N or ↑
v.	S. phosphorus (mEq/L)	N or ↑	N or ↑
vi.	S. Mg^{++}	N or ↑	N or ↑
vii.	S. bicarbonate (mEq/L)	Usually <15	Usually >20
viii.	Blood pH	<7.30	> 7.30
ix.	S. osmolarity (mOsm/L)	<320	> 330
x.	S. lactate (mmol/L)	2-3	1-2
xi.	S. BUN (mg/dL)	Less ↑	Greater ↑
xii.	Plasma insulin	Low to 0	Some

complications are largely responsible for morbidity and premature mortality in diabetes mellitus. These complications are briefly outlined below (Fig. 29.5, B).

1. Atherosclerosis

Diabetes mellitus of both type 1 and type 2 accelerates the development of atherosclerosis. Consequently, atherosclerotic lesions appear earlier than in the general population, are more extensive, and are more often associated with complicated plaques such as ulceration, calcification and thrombosis (page 485). The cause for this accelerated atherosclerotic process is not known but possible contributory factors are hyperlipidaemia, reduced HDL levels (see metabolic syndrome on page 569), nonenzymatic glycosylation, increased platelet adhesiveness, obesity and associated hypertension in diabetes.

The possible ill-effects of accelerated atherosclerosis in diabetes are early onset of coronary artery disease, silent myocardial infarction, cerebral stroke and gangrene of the toes and feet. Gangrene of the lower extremities is 100 times more common in diabetics than in non-diabetics.

2. Diabetic Microangiopathy

Microangiopathy of diabetes is characterised by basement membrane thickening of small blood vessels and capillaries of different organs and tissues such as the skin, skeletal muscle, eye and kidney. Similar type of basement membrane-like material is also deposited in nonvascular tissues such as peripheral nerves, renal tubules and Bowman's capsule. The pathogenesis of diabetic microangiopathy as well as of peripheral neuropathy in diabetics is believed to be due to recurrent hyperglycaemia that causes *increased glycosylation* of haemoglobin and other proteins (e.g. collagen and basement membrane material) resulting in thickening of basement membrane.

3. Diabetic Nephropathy

Renal involvement is an important complication of diabetes mellitus. Chronic kidney disease with renal failure accounts for deaths in more than 10% of all diabetics. Renal complications are more severe, develop early and more frequently in type 1 (earlier called insulin-dependent) diabetes mellitus (30-40% cases) than in type 2 (earlier termed non-insulin-dependent) diabetics (about 20% cases). A variety of clinical syndromes are associated with diabetic nephropathy that includes asymptomatic proteinuria, nephrotic syndrome, progressive renal failure and hypertension. Cardiovascular disease is 40 times more common in patients of chronic kidney disease in diabetes mellitus than in non-diabetics and more diabetics die from cardiovascular complications than from uraemia.

MORPHOLOGIC FEATURES

Diabetic nephropathy encompasses 4 types of renal lesions in diabetes mellitus: diabetic glomerulosclerosis, vascular lesions, diabetic pyelonephritis and tubular lesions (Armanni-Ebstein lesions).

1. DIABETIC GLOMERULOSCLEROSIS Glomerular lesions in diabetes mellitus are particularly common and account for majority of abnormal findings referable to the kidney.

Pathogenesis of these lesions in diabetes mellitus is explained by following sequential changes: hyperglycaemia → glomerular hypertension → renal hyperperfusion → deposition of proteins in the mesangium → glomerulosclerosis → renal failure. In addition, cellular infiltration in renal lesions in diabetic glomerular lesions is due to growth factors, particularly transforming growth factor-β. Strict control of blood glucose level and control of systemic hypertension in these patients retards progression to diabetic nephropathy.

Glomerulosclerosis in diabetes may take one of the 2 forms: diffuse or nodular lesions:

i) Diffuse glomerulosclerosis Diffuse glomerular lesions are the most common. There is involvement of all parts of glomeruli. The pathologic changes consist of thickening of the GBM and diffuse increase in mesangial matrix with mild proliferation of mesangial cells. Various exudative lesions such as capsular hyaline drops and fibrin caps may also be present (Fig. 29.6, A) *Capsular drop* is an eosinophilic hyaline thickening of the parietal layer of Bowman's capsule and bulges into the glomerular space. *Fibrin cap* is homogeneous, brightly eosinophilic material appearing on the wall of a peripheral capillary of a lobule.

ii) Nodular glomerulosclerosis Nodular lesions of diabetic glomerulosclerosis are also called as *Kimmelstiel-Wilson (KW) lesions* or *intercapillary glomerulosclerosis*. These lesions are specific for type 1 diabetes (juvenile-onset diabetes) or islet cell antibody-positive diabetes mellitus. The pathologic changes consist of one or more nodules in a few or many glomeruli. *Nodule* is an ovoid or spherical, laminated, hyaline, acellular mass located within a lobule of the glomerulus. The nodules are surrounded peripherally by glomerular capillary loops which may have normal or thickened GBM (Fig. 29.6, B). The nodules are PAS-positive and contain lipid and fibrin. As the nodular lesions enlarge, they compress the glomerular capillaries and obliterate the glomerular tuft (Fig. 29.7). As a result of glomerular and arteriolar involvement, renal ischaemia occurs leading to tubular atrophy and interstitial fibrosis and results in grossly small, contracted kidney.

2. VASCULAR LESIONS *Atheroma* of renal arteries is very common and severe in diabetes mellitus. *Hyaline arteriolosclerosis* affecting the afferent and efferent

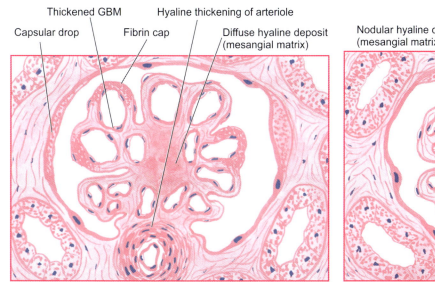
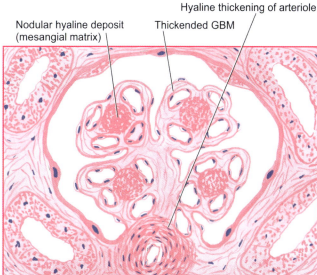

Figure 29.6 ▶ Diabetic glomerulosclerosis. *A, Diffuse lesions.* The characteristic features are diffuse involvement of the glomeruli showing thickening of the GBM and diffuse increase in the mesangial matrix with mild proliferation of mesangial cells and exudative lesions (fibrin caps and capsular drops). *B, Nodular lesion (Kimmelstiel-Wilson Lesion).* There are one or more hyaline nodules within the lobules of glomeruli, surrounded peripherally by glomerular capillaries with thickened walls.

arterioles of the glomeruli is also often severe in diabetes. These vascular lesions are responsible for renal ischaemia that results in tubular atrophy and interstitial fibrosis.

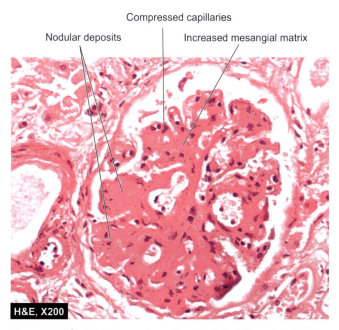

Figure 29.7 ▶ Diabetic nephropathy—nodular (Kimmelstiel-Wilson or KW) lesions.

3. DIABETIC PYELONEPHRITIS Poorly-controlled diabetics are particularly susceptible to bacterial infections. Papillary necrosis (necrotising papillitis) is an important complication of diabetes that may result in acute pyelonephritis. Chronic pyelonephritis is 10 to 20 times more common in diabetics than in others.

4. TUBULAR LESIONS (ARMANNI-EBSTEIN LESIONS) In untreated diabetics who have extremely high blood sugar level, the epithelial cells of the proximal convoluted tubules develop extensive glycogen deposits appearing as vacuoles. These are called Armanni-Ebstein lesions. The tubules return to normal on control of hyperglycaemic state.

4. Diabetic Neuropathy

Diabetic neuropathy may affect all parts of the nervous system but symmetric peripheral neuropathy is most characteristic. The basic pathologic changes are segmental demyelination, Schwann cell injury and axonal damage. The pathogenesis of neuropathy is not clear but it may be related to diffuse microangiopathy as already explained, or may be due to accumulation of sorbitol and fructose as a result of hyperglycaemia, leading to deficiency of myoinositol.

5. Diabetic Retinopathy

Diabetic retinopathy is an important cause of blindness. It is related to the degree and duration of glycaemic control. The condition develops in more than 60% of diabetics

15-20 years after the onset of disease, and in about 2% of diabetics causes blindness. Other ocular complications of diabetes include glaucoma, cataract and corneal disease. Most cases of diabetic retinopathy occur over the age of 50 years. The risk is greater in type 1 diabetes mellitus than in type 2 diabetes mellitus, although in clinical practice there are more patients of diabetic retinopathy due to type 2 diabetes mellitus because of its higher prevalence. Women are more prone to diabetes as well as diabetic retinopathy. Diabetic retinopathy is directly correlated with Kimmelstiel-Wilson nephropathy.

Histologically, two types of changes are described in diabetic retinopathy—background (non-proliferative) and proliferative retinopathy.

1. Background (non-proliferative) retinopathy This is the initial retinal capillary microangiopathy. The following changes are seen:

i) Basement membrane shows varying thickness due to increased synthesis of basement membrane substance.
ii) Degeneration of pericytes and some loss of endothelial cells are found.
iii) Capillary microaneurysms appear which may develop thrombi and get occluded.
iv) 'Waxy exudates' accumulate in the vicinity of micro-aneurysms especially in the elderly diabetics because of hyperlipidaemia.
v) 'Dot and blot haemorrhages' in the deeper layers of retina are produced due to diapedesis of erythrocytes.
vi) Soft 'cotton-wool spots' appear on the retina which are microinfarcts of nerve fibre layers. 'Scotomas' appear from degeneration of nerve fibres and ganglion cells.

2. Proliferative retinopathy (retinitis proliferans) After many years, retinopathy becomes proliferative. Severe ischaemia and chronic hypoxia for long period leads to secretion of angiogenic factor by retinal cells and results in the following changes:

i) Neovascularisation of the retina at the optic disc.
ii) Friability of newly-formed blood vessels causes them to bleed easily and results in vitreous haemorrhages.
iii) Proliferation of astrocytes and fibrous tissue around the new blood vessels.
iv) Fibrovascular and gliotic tissue contracts to cause retinal detachment and blindness.

In addition to the changes on retina, severe diabetes may cause diabetic iridopathy with formation of adhesions between iris and cornea (peripheral anterior synechiae) and between iris and lens (posterior synechiae). Diabetics also develop cataract of the lens at an earlier age than the general population.

The pathogenesis of blindness in diabetes mellitus is schematically outlined in Fig. 29.8.

6. Infections

Diabetics have enhanced susceptibility to various infections such as tuberculosis, pneumonias, pyelonephritis, otitis, carbuncles and diabetic ulcers. This could be due to various factors such as impaired leucocyte functions, reduced cellular immunity, poor blood supply due to vascular involvement and hyperglycaemia *per se*.

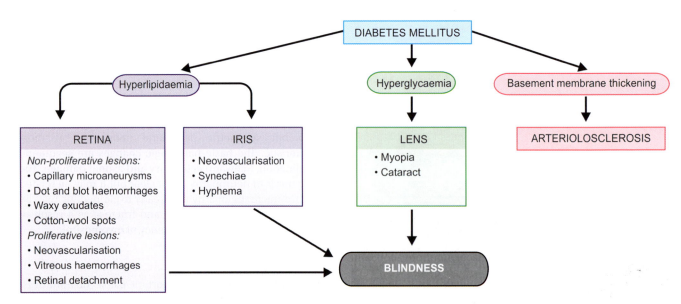

Figure 29.8 ▶ Schematic diagram showing the effects of diabetes mellitus on eye in causing blindness.

Chapter 29: Diabetes Mellitus and its Complications

GIST BOX 29.2 — Complications of Diabetes Mellitus

- Both types of DM may develop complications. These may be acute metabolic complications (e.g. diabetic ketoacidosis, hyperosmolar nonketotic coma, and hypoglycaemia) and late systemic complications (e.g. atherosclerosis, diabetic microangiopathy, diabetic nephropathy, diabetic neuropathy, diabetic retinopathy and infections).
- Diabetic nephropathy encompasses diabetic glomerulosclerosis, vascular lesions, diabetic pyelonephritis and tubular lesions.
- Symmetric neuropathy is most often neurologic complication of diabetes.
- Lesions of diabetic retinopathy may appear as background (non-proliferative) and proliferative lesions.
- Diabetics have enhanced susceptibility to various infections.

Table 29.5 Revised criteria for diagnosis of diabetes by oral GTT (as per American Diabetes Association, 2007).

PLASMA GLUCOSE VALUE*	DIAGNOSIS
FASTING (FOR > 8 HOURS) VALUE	
Below 100 mg/dl (< 5.6 mmol/L)	Normal fasting value
100-125 mg/dl (5.6-6.9 mmol/L)	Impaired fasting glucose (IFG)**
126 mg/dl (7.0 mmol/L) or more	Diabetes mellitus
TWO-HOUR AFTER 75 GM ORAL GLUCOSE LOAD	
< 140 mg/dl (< 7.8 mmol/L)	Normal post-prandial GTT
140-199 mg/dl (7.8-11.1 mmol/L)	Impaired post-prandial glucose tolerance (IGT)**
200 mg/dl (11.1 mmol/L) or more	Diabetes mellitus
RANDOM VALUE	
200 mg/dl (11.1 mmol/L) or more in a symptomatic patient	Diabetes mellitus

Note: * Plasma glucose values are 15% higher than whole blood glucose value.
** Individuals with IFG and IGT are at increased risk for development of type 2 DM later.

DIAGNOSIS OF DIABETES

Hyperglycaemia remains the fundamental basis for the diagnosis of diabetes mellitus. In *symptomatic cases*, the diagnosis is not a problem and can be confirmed by finding glucosuria and a random plasma glucose concentration above 200 mg/dl.

◆ The severity of clinical symptoms of polyuria and polydipsia is directly related to the degree of hyperglycaemia.
◆ In *asymptomatic cases*, when there is persistently elevated fasting plasma glucose level, diagnosis again poses no difficulty.
◆ The problem arises in asymptomatic patients who have normal fasting glucose level in the plasma but are suspected to have diabetes on other grounds and are thus subjected to oral glucose tolerance test (GTT). If abnormal GTT values are found, these subjects are said to have *'chemical diabetes'* **(Fig. 29.9)**. The American Diabetes Association (2007) has recommended definite diagnostic criteria for early diagnosis of diabetes mellitus **(Table 29.5)**.

The following investigations are helpful in establishing the diagnosis of diabetes mellitus:

I. URINE TESTING Urine tests are cheap and convenient but the diagnosis of diabetes cannot be based on urine testing

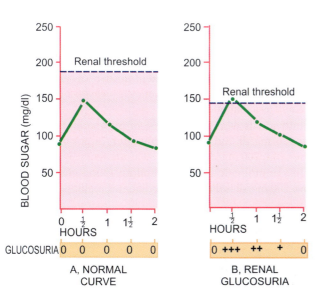
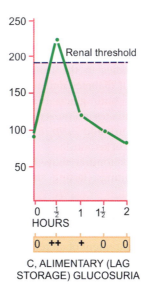
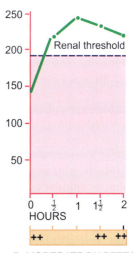

Figure 29.9 ▶ The glucose tolerance test, showing blood glucose curves (venous blood glucose) and glucosuria after 75 gm of oral glucose.

alone since there may be false-positives and false-negatives. They can be used in population screening surveys. Urine is tested for the presence of glucose and ketones.

1. Glucosuria *Benedict's qualitative test* detects any reducing substance in the urine and is not specific for glucose. More sensitive and glucose specific test is *dipstick* method based on enzyme-coated paper strip which turns purple when dipped in urine containing glucose.

The main disadvantage of relying on urinary glucose test alone is the individual variation in renal threshold. Thus, a diabetic patient may have a negative urinary glucose test and a nondiabetic individual with low renal threshold may have a positive urine test.

Besides diabetes mellitus, *glucosuria* may also occur in certain other conditions such as: renal glycosuria, alimentary (lag storage) glucosuria, many metabolic disorders, starvation and intracranial lesions (e.g. cerebral tumour, haemorrhage and head injury). However, two of these conditions—renal glucosuria and alimentary glucosuria, require further elaboration here.

◆ Renal glucosuria **(Fig. 29.9, B)**: Next to diabetes, the most common cause of glucosuria is the reduced renal threshold for glucose. In such cases although the blood glucose level is below 180 mg/dl (i.e. below normal renal threshold for glucose) but glucose still appears regularly and consistently in the urine due to lowered renal threshold.

Renal glucosuria is a benign condition unrelated to diabetes and runs in families and may occur temporarily in pregnancy without symptoms of diabetes.

◆ Alimentary (lag storage) glucosuria **(Fig. 29.9,C)**: A rapid and transitory rise in blood glucose level above the normal renal threshold may occur in some individuals after a meal. During this period, glucosuria is present. This type of response to meal is called 'lag storage curve' or more appropriately 'alimentary glucosuria'. A characteristic feature is that unusually high blood glucose level returns to normal 2 hours after meal.

2. Ketonuria Tests for ketone bodies in the urine are required for assessing the severity of diabetes and not for diagnosis of diabetes. However, if both glucosuria and ketonuria are present, diagnosis of diabetes is almost certain. *Rothera's test* (nitroprusside reaction) and *strip test* are conveniently performed for detection of ketonuria.

Besides uncontrolled diabetes, ketonuria may appear in individuals with prolonged vomitings, fasting state or exercising for long periods.

II. SINGLE BLOOD SUGAR ESTIMATION For diagnosis of diabetes, blood sugar determinations are absolutely necessary. *Folin-Wu method* of measurement of all reducing substances in the blood including glucose is now obsolete. Currently used are *O-toluidine, Somogyi-Nelson* and *glucose oxidase* methods. Whole blood or plasma may be used but *whole blood values are 15% lower than plasma values.*

A grossly elevated single determination of plasma glucose may be sufficient to make the diagnosis of diabetes. A *fasting plasma glucose value above 126 mg/dl (≥ 7 mmol/L) is certainly indicative of diabetes.* In other cases, oral GTT is performed.

III. SCREENING BY FASTING GLUCOSE TEST Fasting plasma glucose determination is a screening test for DM type 2. It is recommended that all individuals above 45 years of age must undergo screening fasting glucose test every 3-years, and relatively earlier if the person is overweight or at risk because of the following reasons:

i) Many of the cases meeting the current criteria of DM are asymptomatic and do not know that they have the disorder.
ii) Studies have shown that type 2 DM may be present for about 10 years before symptomatic disease appears.
iii) About half the cases of type 2 DM have some diabetes-related complication at the time of diagnosis.
iv) Course of the disease is favourably altered with treatment.

IV. ORAL GLUCOSE TOLERANCE TEST Oral GTT is performed principally for patients with borderline fasting plasma glucose value (i.e. between 100 and 140 mg/dl). The patient who is scheduled for oral GTT is instructed to eat a high carbohydrate diet for at least 3 days prior to the test and come after an overnight fast on the day of the test (for at least 8 hours). A fasting blood sugar sample is first drawn. Then 75 gm of glucose dissolved in 300 ml of water is given. Blood and urine specimen are collected at half-hourly intervals for at least 2 hours. Blood or plasma glucose content is measured and urine is tested for glucosuria to determine the approximate renal threshold for glucose. Venous whole blood concentrations are 15% lower than plasma glucose values.

Currently accepted criteria for diagnosis of DM (as per American Diabetes Association, 2007) are given in **Table 29.5**:

◆ Normal cut off value for fasting blood glucose level is considered as 100 mg/dl.

◆ Cases with fasting blood glucose value in range of 100-125 mg/dl are considered as *impaired fasting glucose tolerance (IGT);* these cases are at increased risk of developing diabetes later and therefore kept under observation for repeating the test. During pregnancy, however, a case of IGT is treated as a diabetic.

◆ Individuals with fasting value of plasma glucose higher than 126 mg/dl and 2-hour value after 75 gm oral glucose higher than 200 mg/dl are labelled as *diabetics* **(Fig. 29.9, D)**.

◆ In symptomatic case, the random blood glucose value above 200 mg/dl is diagnosed as diabetes mellitus.

V. OTHER TESTS A few other tests are sometimes performed in specific conditions in diabetics and for research purposes:

1. Glycosylated haemoglobin (HbA_{1C}) Measurement of blood glucose level in diabetics suffers from variation due to dietary intake of the previous day. Long-term objective assessment of degree of glycaemic control is better monitored by measurement of glycosylated haemoglobin (HbA_{1C}), a minor haemoglobin component present in normal persons (normal range 4-6%). This is because the non-enzymatic glycosylation of haemoglobin takes place over 90-120 days, lifespan of red blood cells. HbA_{1C} assay, therefore, gives an estimate of diabetic control and compliance for the preceding 3-4 months. This assay has the advantage over traditional blood glucose test that no dietary preparation or fasting is required. Increased HbA_{1C} value almost certainly means DM but normal value does not rule out IGT; thus the test is not used for making the diagnosis of DM. Moreover, since HbA_{1C} assay has a direct relation between poor control and development of complications, it is also a good measure of prediction of microvascular complications. Care must be taken in interpretation of the HbA_{1C} value because it varies with the assay method used and is affected by presence of haemoglobinopathies, anaemia, reticulocytosis, transfusions and uraemia.

2. **Glycated albumin** This is used to monitor degree of hyperglycaemia during previous 1-2 weeks when HbA_{1C} can not be used.

3. **Extended GTT** The oral GTT is extended to 3-4 hours for appearance of symptoms of hyperglycaemia. It is a useful test in cases of reactive hypoglycaemia of early diabetes.

4. **Intravenous GTT** This test is performed in persons who have intestinal malabsorption or in postgastrectomy cases.

5. **Cortisone-primed GTT** This provocative test is a useful investigative aid in cases of potential diabetics.

6. **Insulin assay** Plasma insulin can be measured by radioimmunoassay and ELISA technique. Plasma insulin deficiency is crucial for type 1 DM but is not essential for making the diagnosis of DM.

7. **Proinsulin assay** Proinsulin is included in immunoassay of insulin; normally it is ≤20% of total insulin.

8. **C-peptide assay** C-peptide is released in circulation during conversion of proinsulin to insulin in equimolar quantities to insulin; thus its levels correlate with insulin level in blood except in islet cell tumours and in obesity. This test is even more sensitive than insulin assay because its levels are not affected by insulin therapy.

9. **Islet autoantibodies** Glutamic acid decarboxylase and islet cell cytoplasmic antibodies may be used as a marker for type 1 DM.

10. **Screening for diabetes-associated complications** Besides making the diagnosis of DM based on the defined criteria, screening tests are done for DM-associated complications e.g. microalbuminuria, dyslipidaemia, thyroid dysfunction etc.

> **GIST BOX 29.3 | Diagnosis of Diabetes Mellitus**
>
> ❖ Diagnostic criteria have been developed, most important of which is blood glucose level: fasting value of plasma glucose higher than 126 mg/dl and 2-hour value after 75 gm oral glucose higher than 200 mg/dl are labelled as diabetics.
> ❖ Long term control of diabetes is best assessed by estimation of glycosylated haemoglobin (normal range below 6%).

30 Common Diseases of Bones, Cartilage and Joints

The skeleton consists of cartilage and bone. Cartilage has a role in growth and repair of bone, and in the adults forms the articular skeleton responsible for movement of joints. Bone is a specialised form of connective tissue which performs the function of providing mechanical support and is also a mineral reservoir for calcium homeostasis. There are 206 bones in the human body, and depending upon their size and shape may be long, flat, tubular etc.

NORMAL STRUCTURE OF SKELETON

BONES

Bones are divided into 2 components (Fig. 30.1):
◈ **Cortical or compact bone** comprises 80% of the skeleton and is the dense outer shell responsible for structural rigidity. It consists of haversian canals with blood vessels surrounded by concentric layers of mineralised collagen forming osteons which are joined together by cement lines.
◈ **Trabecular or cancellous bone** composes 20% of the skeleton and has trabeculae traversing the marrow space. Its main role is in mineral homeostasis.

HISTOLOGY Bone consists of large quantities of extracellular osteoid matrix which is loaded with calcium hydroxyapatite and relatively small number of bone cells which are of 3 main types: osteoblasts, osteocytes and osteoclasts.

1. Osteoblasts Osteoblasts are uninucleate cells found abundantly along the new bone-forming surfaces. They synthesise bone matrix. The serum levels of bone-related *alkaline phosphatase* (other being hepatic alkaline phosphatase) is a marker for osteoblastic activity. Its levels are raised at puberty during period of active bone growth and in pathologic conditions associated with high osteoblastic activity such as in fracture repair and Paget's disease of the bone.

2. Osteocytes Osteocytes are those osteoblasts which get incorporated into the bone matrix during its synthesis. Osteocytes are found within small spaces called lacunae lying in the bone matrix. The distribution of the osteocytic lacunae is a reliable parameter for distinguishing between woven and lamellar bone.
◈ *Woven bone* is immature and is rapidly deposited. It contains large number of closely-packed osteocytes and consists of irregular interlacing pattern of collagen fibre bundles in bone matrix. Woven bone is seen in foetal life and in children under 4 years of age.
◈ *Lamellar bone* differs from woven bone in having smaller and less numerous osteocytes and fine and parallel or lamellar sheets of collagen fibres. Lamellar bone usually replaces woven bone or pre-existing cartilage.

3. Osteoclasts Osteoclasts are large multinucleate cells of mononuclear-macrophage origin and are responsible for

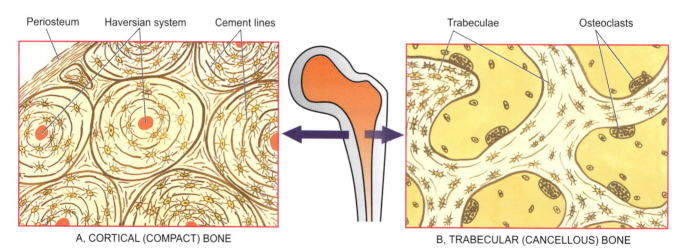

Figure 30.1 ▶ The normal structure of cortical (compact) bone (A) and trabecular (cancellous) bone (B) in transverse section. The cortical bone forming the outer shell shows concentric lamellae along with osteocytic lacunae surrounding central blood vessels, while the trabecular bone forming the marrow space shows trabeculae with osteoclastic activity at the margins.

bone resorption. The osteoclastic activity is determined by bone-related serum *acid phosphatase* levels (other being prostatic acid phosphatase). Osteoclasts are found along the endosteal surface of the cortical (compact) bone and the trabeculae of trabecular (cancellous) bone.

4. **Osteoid matrix** The osteoid matrix of bone consists of 90-95% of collagen type I and comprises nearly half of total body's collagen. Virtually whole of body's hydroxyproline and hydroxylysine reside in the bone. The architecture of bone collagen reflects the rate of its synthesis and may be woven or lamellar, as described above.

BONE FORMATION AND RESORPTION Bone is not a static tissue but its formation and resorption are taking place during period of growth as well as in adult life. Bone deposition is the result of osteoblasts while bone resorption is the function of osteoclasts. Bone formation may take place directly from collagen called *membranous ossification* seen in certain flat bones, or may occur through an intermediate stage of cartilage termed *endochondral ossification* found in metaphysis of long bones. In either case, firstly an uncalcified osteoid matrix is formed by osteoblasts which is then mineralised in 12-15 days. This delay in mineralisation results in formation of about 15 μm thick osteoid seams at calcification fronts (About > 1 μm of matrix osteoid is formed daily). Uncalcified osteoid appears eosinophilic in H & E stains and does not stain with von Kossa reaction, while mineralised osteoid is basophilic in appearance and stains black with von Kossa reaction (a stain for calcium). Areas of active bone resorption have scalloped edges of bone surface called Howship's lacunae and contain multinucleated osteoclasts. In this way, osteoblastic formation and osteoclastic resorption continue to take place into adult life in a balanced way termed *bone modelling*. There is important role of vitamin D_1, parathyroid hormone and calcitonin in calcium metabolism.

CARTILAGE

Unlike bone, the cartilage lacks blood vessels, lymphatics and nerves. It may have focal areas of calcification. Cartilage consists of 2 components: cartilage matrix and chondrocytes.

Cartilage matrix Like bone, cartilage too consists of organic and inorganic material. Inorganic material of cartilage is calcium hydroxyapatite similar to that in bone matrix but the organic material of the cartilage is distinct from the bone. It consists of very high content of water (80%) and remaining 20% consists of type II collagen and proteoglycans. High water content of cartilage matrix is responsible for function of articular cartilage and lubrication. Proteoglycans are macromolecules having proteins complexed with polysaccharides termed glycosaminoglycans. Cartilage glycosaminoglycans consist of chondroitin sulfate and keratan sulfate, the former being most abundant comprising 55-90% of cartilage matrix varying on the age of the cartilage.

Chondrocytes Primitive mesenchymal cells which form bone cells from chondroblasts which give rise to chondrocytes. However, calcified cartilage is removed by the osteoclasts.

Depending upon location and structural composition, cartilage is of 3 types:

1. *Hyaline cartilage* is the basic cartilaginous tissue comprising articular cartilage of joints, cartilage in the growth plates of developing bones, costochondral cartilage, cartilage in the trachea, bronchi and larynx and the nasal cartilage. Hyaline cartilage is the type found in most cartilage-forming tumours and in the fracture callus.

2. *Fibrocartilage* is a hyaline cartilage that contains more abundant type II collagen fibres. It is found in annulus fibrosus of intervertebral disc, menisci, insertions of joint capsules, ligament and tendons. Fibrocartilage may also be found in some cartilage-forming tumours and in the fracture callus.

3. *Elastic cartilage* is hyaline cartilage that contains abundant elastin. Elastic cartilage is found in the pinna of ears, epiglottis and arytenoid cartilage of the larynx.

Diseases of skeletal system include infection (osteomyelitis), disordered growth and development (skeletal dysplasias), metabolic and endocrine derangements, and tumours and tumour-like conditions.

> **GIST BOX 30.1** **Normal Structure of Bone and Cartilage**
>
> ❖ Bone is composed of cortical or compact bone (80%) which is the dense outer shell, and trabecular or cancellous bone (20%) which has trabeculae traversing the marrow space.
> ❖ Bone consists of extracellular osteoid matrix and bone cells (osteoblasts, osteocytes and osteoclasts).
> ❖ Cartilage consists of cartilage matrix and chondrocytes and lacks blood vessels, lymphatics and nerves. It may have focal areas of calcification.

INFECTION, NECROSIS, FRACTURE HEALING

OSTEOMYELITIS

An infection of the bone is termed osteomyelitis (myelo = marrow). A number of systemic infectious diseases may spread to the bone such as enteric fever, actinomycosis, mycetoma (madura foot), syphilis, tuberculosis and brucellosis. However, two of the conditions which produce significant pathologic lesions in the bone, namely pyogenic osteomyelitis and tuberculous osteomyelitis, are described below.

Pyogenic Osteomyelitis

Pyogenic or suppurative osteomyelitis is usually caused by bacterial infection and rarely by fungi. The profile of patients in developing and developed countries is different:

- In the developing countries of the world, it may occur by haematogenous route, most commonly in the long bones of infants and young children (5-15 years of age) (called haematogenous osteomyelitis).
- On the other hand, in the developed world, where institution of antibiotics is early and prompt, haematogenous spread of infection to the bone is uncommon; instead, direct extension of infection from the adjacent area, frequently involving the jaws and skull, is more common mode of spread.
- Bacterial osteomyelitis may be a complication at all ages in patients with compound fractures, surgical procedures involving prosthesis or implants, gangrene of a limb in diabetics, debilitation and immunosuppression.

Though any etiologic agent may cause osteomyelitis, *Staphylococcus aureus* is implicated in a vast majority of cases. Less frequently, other organisms such as streptococci, *Escherichia coli, Pseudomonas, Klebsiella* and anaerobes are involved. Mixed infections are common in post-traumatic cases of osteomyelitis. There may be transient bacteraemia preceding the development of osteomyelitis so that blood cultures may be positive.

Clinically, the child with acute haematogenous osteomyelitis has painful and tender limb. Fever, malaise and leucocytosis generally accompany the bony lesion. Radiologic examination confirms the bony destruction.

Occasionally, osteomyelitis remains undiscovered until it becomes chronic. Draining sinus tracts may form which may occasionally be the site for development of squamous carcinoma. Persistence, neglect and chronicity of osteomyelitis over a longer period of time may lead to development of amyloidosis.

MORPHOLOGIC FEATURES Depending upon the duration, osteomyelitis may be *acute, subacute* or *chronic*. The basic pathologic changes in any stage of osteomyelitis are: suppuration, ischaemic necrosis, healing by fibrosis and bony repair. The *sequence of pathologic changes* is as under (Fig. 30.2):

1. The infection begins in the metaphyseal end of the *marrow cavity* which is largely occupied by *pus*. At this stage, microscopy reveals congestion, oedema and an exudate of neutrophils.

2. The tension in the marrow cavity is increased due to pus and results in spread of infection along the marrow cavity, into the endosteum, and into the haversian and Volkmann's canal, causing *periosteitis*.

3. The infection may reach the subperiosteal space forming *subperiosteal abscesses*. It may penetrate through the cortex creating draining skin sinus tracts (Fig. 30.3).

4. Combination of suppuration and impaired blood supply to the cortical bone results in erosion, thinning and infarction necrosis of the cortex called *sequestrum*.

5. With passage of time, there is formation of new bone beneath the periosteum present over the infected bone. This forms an encasing sheath around the necrosed bone and is known as *involucrum*. Involucrum has irregular surface and has perforations through which discharging sinus tracts pass.

6. Long continued neo-osteogenesis gives rise to dense sclerotic pattern of osteomyelitis called *chronic sclerosing nonsuppurative osteomyelitis of Garré*.

7. Occasionally, acute osteomyelitis may be contained to a localised area and walled off by fibrous tissue and granulation tissue. This is termed *Brodie's abscess*.

8. In *vertebral pyogenic osteomyelitis*, infection begins from the disc (discitis) and spreads to involve the vertebral bodies (Fig. 30.4, A).

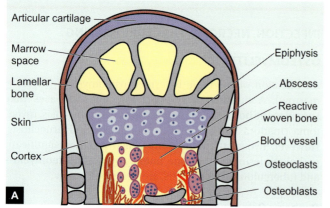
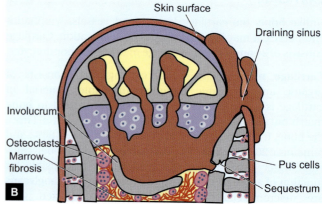

Figure 30.2 ▶ Pathogenesis of pyogenic osteomyelitis. A, The process begins as a focus of microabscess in a vascular loop in the marrow which expands to stimulate resorption of adjacent bony trabeculae. Simultaneously, there is beginning of reactive woven bone formation by the periosteum. B, The abscess expands further causing necrosis of the cortex called sequestrum. The formation of viable new reactive bone surrounding the sequestrum is called involucrum. The extension of infection into the joint space, epiphysis and the skin produces a draining sinus.

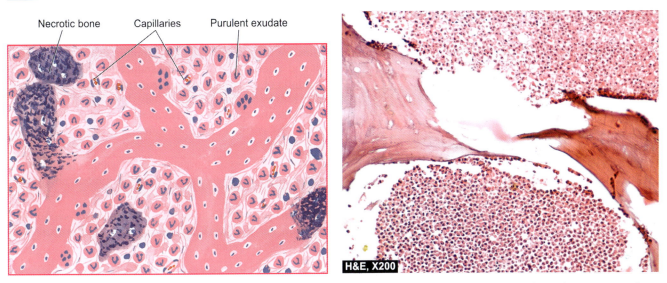

Figure 30.3 ▶ Chronic suppurative osteomyelitis. Histologic appearance shows necrotic bone and extensive purulent inflammatory exudate.

COMPLICATIONS Osteomyelitis may result in the following complications:
1. Septicaemia.
2. Acute bacterial arthritis.
3. Pathologic fractures.
4. Development of squamous cell carcinoma in long-standing cases.
5. Secondary amyloidosis in long-standing cases.
6. Vertebral osteomyelitis may cause vertebral collapse with paravertebral abscess, epidural abscess, cord compression and neurologic deficits.

Tuberculous Osteomyelitis

Tuberculous osteomyelitis, though rare in developed countries, continues to be a common condition in underdeveloped and developing countries of the world. The tubercle bacilli, *M. tuberculosis*, reach the bone marrow and synovium most commonly by haematogenous dissemination from infection elsewhere, usually from the lungs, and infrequently by direct extension from the pulmonary or gastrointestinal tuberculosis (page 141). The disease affects adolescents and young adults more often. Most frequently involved are the spine and bones of extremities.

MORPHOLOGIC FEATURES The bone lesions in tuberculosis have the same general histological appearance as in tuberculosis elsewhere and consist of central caseation necrosis surrounded by tuberculous granulation tissue and fragments of necrotic bone (Fig. 30.5). The tuberculous lesions appear as a focus of bone destruction and replacement of the affected tissue by caseous material and formation of multiple discharging sinuses through the soft tissues and skin. Involvement of joint spaces and

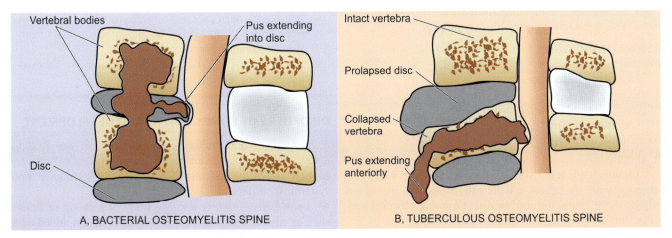

Figure 30.4 ▶ Osteomyelitis of the vertebral body.

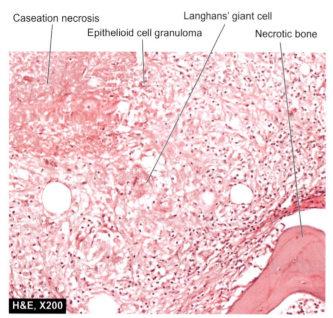

Figure 30.5 ▶ Tuberculous osteomyelitis. There are epithelioid cell granulomas with minute areas of caseation necrosis and surrounded by Langhans' giant cells. Pieces of necrotic bone are also seen.

intervertebral disc are frequent. Tuberculosis of the spine, *Pott's disease,* often commences in the vertebral body and may be associated with compression fractures and destruction of intervertebral discs, producing permanent damage and paraplegia. Extension of caseous material along with pus from the lumbar vertebrae to the sheaths of psoas muscle produces *psoas abscess* or *lumbar cold abscess* **(Fig. 30.4, B)**. The cold abscess may burst through the skin and form sinus. Long-standing cases may develop systemic amyloidosis.

AVASCULAR NECROSIS (OSTEONECROSIS)

Avascular necrosis of the bones or osteonecrosis results from ischaemia. It is a relatively common condition.

ETIOPATHOGENESIS   Some of the common causes are as follows:
1. Fracture or dislocation
2. Sickle cell disease
3. Corticosteroid administration
4. Radiation therapy
5. Chronic alcoholism
6. Idiopathic

The mechanism of osteonecrosis in many cases remains obscure, while in others it is by interruption in the blood supply to the bones induced by direct trauma, compression, or thromboembolic obstruction.

MORPHOLOGIC FEATURES There are pathological fractures of the involved bone due to infarcts. Most common sites are the ones where the disruption in blood supply is at end-arterial circulation. The infarcts mainly involve the medulla of the long bone in the diaphysis. This is because the nutrient arteries supply blood to sinusoids of the medulla and the inner cortex after penetrating the cortex, while the cortex is relatively unaffected due to collateral circulation.

Grossly, the lesional area shows a wedge-shaped area of infarction in the subchondral bone under the convex surface of the joint.

Microscopically, the infracted medulla shows saponified marrow fat. The overlying cartilage and the cortex of the long bones are relatively unaffected.

Long-term sequelae of osteonecrosis include occurrence of malignant tumours in this location such as osteosarcoma, malignant fibrous histiocytoma and fibrosarcoma etc.

FRACTURE HEALING

Fracture of the bone initiates a series of tissue changes which eventually lead to restoration of normal structure and function of the affected bone. Fracture of a bone is commonly associated with injury to the soft tissues. The various types of fractures and their mechanism of healing are discussed along with healing of specialised tissues in Chapter 12 (page 161).

> **GIST BOX 30.2** | **Infection, Necrosis, Fracture Healing**
>
> ❖ Suppurative or pyogenic osteomyelitis is usually caused by bacterial infection and rarely by fungi. It may be by haematogenous route or by direct spread of infection.
> ❖ Tuberculous osteomyelitis continues to be a common condition in developing countries of the world, either by haematogenous spread or by direct spread from adjacent focus.
> ❖ Avascular necrosis or osteonecrosis results from ischaemia and may occur be idiopathic or result from steroid administration, alcoholism etc.
> ❖ Healing of fractures occurs by callus formation, either as a primary or secondary union.

DISORDERS OF BONE GROWTH AND DEVELOPMENT

A number of abnormalities of the skeleton are due to disordered bone growth and development and are collectively termed *skeletal dysplasias.* These include both local and systemic disorders.

◆ *Local defects* involve a single bone or a group of bones such as: absence or presence in diminished form, fused with neighbouring bones (e.g. syndactyly), and formation of extra bones (e.g. supernumerary ribs).

◆ However, more importantly, skeletal dysplasias include *systemic disorders* involving particular epiphyseal growth plate. These include: achondroplasia (disorder of chondroblasts), osteogenesis imperfecta (disorder of osteoblasts), osteopetrosis (disorder of osteoclasts) and foetal rickets (disorder of mineralisation).

ACHONDROPLASIA

Achondroplasia is an autosomal dominant genetic abnormality. There is selective interference with normal endochondral ossification at the level of epiphyseal cartilaginous growth plates of long bones. Thus, the long bones are abnormally short but the skull grows normally leading to relatively large skull. Achondroplasia is the commonest cause of dwarfism.

OSTEOGENESIS IMPERFECTA

Osteogenesis imperfecta is an autosomal dominant or recessive disorder of synthesis of type I collagen that constitutes 90-95% of bone matrix. The disorder, thus, involves not only the skeleton but other extra-skeletal tissues as well containing type I collagen such as sclera, eyes, joints, ligaments, teeth and skin. The skeletal manifestations of osteogenesis imperfecta are due to defective osteoblasts which normally synthesise type I collagen. This results in thin or non-existent cortices and irregular trabeculae *(too little bone)* so that the bones are very fragile and liable to multiple fractures. The growth plate cartilage is, however, normal. The condition may be evident at birth (osteogenesis imperfecta congenita) when it is more severe, or may appear during adolescence (osteogenesis imperfecta tarda) which is a less incapacitating form. Extra-skeletal lesions of osteogenesis imperfecta include blue and translucent sclerae, hearing loss due to bony abnormalities of the middle and inner ear, and imperfect teeth.

OSTEOPETROSIS

Osteopetrosis, also called *marble bone disease,* is an autosomal dominant or recessive disorder of increased skeletal mass or osteosclerosis caused by a hereditary defect in osteoclast function. The condition may appear in 2 forms: autosomal recessive (malignant infantile form) and autosomal dominant (benign adult form). Failure of normal osteoclast function of bone resorption coupled with continued bone formation and endochondral ossification results in net overgrowth of calcified dense bone *(too much bone)* which occupies most of the available marrow space. Despite increased density of the bone, there is poor structural support so that the skeleton is susceptible to fractures. Besides the skeletal abnormalities, the infantile malignant form is characterised by effects of marrow obliteration such as anaemia, neutropenia, thrombocytopenia, hepatosplenomegaly with extramedullary haematopoiesis, hydrocephalus and neurologic involvement with consequent deafness, optic atrophy and blindness. Metabolically, hypocalcaemia occurs due to defective osteoclast function.

Histologically, the number of osteoclasts is increased which have dysplastic, bizarre and irregular nuclei and are dysfunctional.

GIST BOX 30.3 | Skeletal Dysplasias

❖ Disordered bone growth and development cause skeletal dysplasias which may be as local or systemic defects.
❖ Achondroplasia is form of dwarfism in which there is selective interference with normal endochondral ossification at the level of epiphyseal cartilaginous growth plates of long bones.
❖ Osteogenesis imperfecta is an autosomal dominant or recessive disorder of synthesis of type I collagen involving the skeleton (too little bone) and extra-skeletal tissues.
❖ Osteopetrosis or marble bone disease, is an autosomal disorder of increased skeletal mass (too much bone) caused by a hereditary defect in osteoclast function.

METABOLIC AND ENDOCRINE BONE DISEASES

A large number of metabolic and endocrine disorders produce generalised skeletal disorders. These include the following:

1. **Osteoporosis**—Resulting from quantitative reduction in otherwise normal bone.

2. **Osteomalacia and rickets**—Characterised by qualitative abnormality in the form of impaired bone mineralisation due to deficiency of vitamin D in adults and children respectively (page 99).

3. **Scurvy**—Caused by deficiency of vitamin C resulting in subperiosteal haemorrhages (page 102).

4. **Hyperparathyroidism**—Leading to osteitis fibrosa cystica.

5. **Pituitary dysfunctions**—Hyperpituitarism causing gigantism and acromegaly and hypopituitarism resulting in dwarfism.

6. **Thyroid dysfunctions**—Hyperthyroidism causing osteoporosis and hypothyroidism leading to cretinism.

7. **Renal osteodystrophy**—Occurring in chronic renal failure and resulting in features of osteitis fibrosa cystica, osteomalacia and areas of osteosclerosis.

8. **Skeletal fluorosis**—Occurring due to excess of sodium fluoride content in the soil and water in an area.

While some of the conditions listed above have been discussed in earlier chapters, a few common examples are considered below.

OSTEOPOROSIS

Osteoporosis or osteopenia is a common clinical syndrome involving multiple bones in which there is quantitative reduction of bone tissue mass but the bone tissue mass is otherwise normal. This reduction in bone mass results in fragile skeleton associated with increased risk of fractures and consequent pain and deformity. The condition is particularly common in elderly people and more frequent in postmenopausal women. The condition may remain asymptomatic or may cause only backache. However, more extensive involvement is associated with fractures, particularly of distal radius, femoral neck and vertebral bodies. Osteoporosis may be difficult to distinguish radiologically from other osteopenias such as osteomalacia, osteogenesis imperfecta, osteitis fibrosa of hyperparathyroidism, renal osteodystrophy and multiple myeloma. Radiologic evidence becomes apparent only after more than 30% of bone mass has been lost. Levels of serum calcium, inorganic phosphorus and alkaline phosphatase are usually within normal limits.

Many non-invasive techniques are now available for measurement of bone mass e.g. DEXA and SEXA scans (dual-energy and single-energy X-ray absorptiometry), quantitative CT and ultrasound.

PATHOGENESIS Osteoporosis is conventionally classified into 2 major groups: primary and secondary.

◈ **Primary osteoporosis** results primarily from osteopenia without an underlying disease or medication. Primary osteoporosis is further subdivided into 2 types: *idiopathic type* found in the young and juveniles and is less frequent, and *involutional type* seen in postmenopausal women and ageing individuals and is more common. The exact mechanism of primary osteoporosis is not known but there is a suggestion that it is the result of an excessive osteoclastic resorption and slow bone formation. A number of risk factors have been attributed to cause this imbalance between bone resorption and bone formation. These include the following:
1. *Genetic factors*—more marked in whites and Asians than blacks.
2. *Sex*—more frequent in females than in males.
3. *Reduced physical activity*—as in old age.
4. *Deficiency of sex hormones*—oestrogen deficiency in women as in postmenopausal osteoporosis and androgen deficiency in men.
5. *Combined deficiency of calcitonin and oestrogen.*
6. *Hyperparathyroidism.*
7. *Deficiency of vitamin D.*
8. *Local factors*—which may stimulate osteoclastic resorption or slow osteoblastic bone formation.

◈ **Secondary osteoporosis** is attributed to a number of factors and conditions (e.g. immobilisation, chronic anaemia, acromegaly, hepatic disease, hyperparathyroidism, hypogonadism, thyrotoxicosis and starvation), or as an effect of medication (e.g. hypercortisonism, administration of anticonvulsant drugs and large dose of heparin).

MORPHOLOGIC FEATURES Except disuse or immobilisation osteoporosis which is localised to the affected limb, other forms of osteoporosis have systemic skeletal distribution. Most commonly encountered osteoporotic fractures are: vertebral crush fracture, femoral neck fracture and wrist fracture. There is enlargement of the medullary cavity and thinning of the cortex.

Histologically, osteoporosis may be active or inactive type.

◈ **Active osteoporosis** is characterised by increased bone resorption and formation i.e. *accelerated turnover*. There is an increase in the number of osteoclasts with increased resorptive surface as well as increased quantity of osteoid with increased osteoblastic surfaces. The width of osteoid seams is normal.

◈ **Inactive osteoporosis** has the features of minimal bone formation and reduced resorptive activity i.e. *reduced turnover*. Histological changes of inactive osteoporosis include decreased number of osteoclasts with decreased resorptive surfaces, and normal or reduced amount of osteoid with decreased osteoblastic surface. The width of osteoid seams is usually reduced or may be normal.

OSTEITIS FIBROSA CYSTICA

Hyperparathyroidism of primary or secondary type results in oversecretion of parathyroid hormone which causes increased osteoclastic resorption of the bone. Severe and prolonged hyperparathyroidism results in osteitis fibrosa cystica. The lesion is generally induced as a manifestation of primary hyperparathyroidism, and less frequently, as a result of secondary hyperparathyroidism such as in chronic renal failure (renal osteodystrophy).

The clinical manifestations of bone disease in hyperparathyroidism are its susceptibility to fracture, skeletal deformities, joint pains and dysfunctions as a result of deranged weight bearing. The bony changes may disappear after cure of primary hyperparathyroidism such as removal of functioning adenoma. The chief biochemical abnormality of excessive parathyroid hormone is hypercalcaemia, hypophosphataemia and hypercalciuria.

MORPHOLOGIC FEATURES The bone lesions of primary hyperparathyroidism affect the long bones more severely and may range from minor degree of generalised bone rarefaction to prominent areas of bone destruction with cyst formation or brown tumours.

Grossly, there are focal areas of erosion of cortical bone and loss of lamina dura at the roots of teeth.

Histologically, the following sequential changes appear over a period of time:

i) Earliest change is *demineralisation* and *increased bone resorption* beginning at the subperiosteal and endosteal surface of the cortex and then spreading to the trabecular bone.

ii) There is replacement of bone and bone marrow by fibrosis coupled with increased number of bizarre osteoclasts at the surfaces of moth-eaten trabeculae and cortex *(osteitis fibrosa)*.

iii) As a result of increased resorption, microfractures and microhaemorrhages occur in the marrow cavity leading to development of cysts *(osteitis fibrosa cystica)*.

iv) Haemosiderin-laden macrophages and multinucleate giant cells appear at the areas of haemorrhages producing an appearance termed *'brown tumour'* or *'reparative giant cell granuloma of hyperparathyroidism'* requiring differentiation from giant cell tumour or osteoclastoma (page 603). However, the so-called brown tumours, unlike osteoclastoma, are not true tumours but instead regress or disappear on surgical removal of hyperplastic or adenomatous parathyroid tissue.

RENAL OSTEODYSTROPHY (METABOLIC BONE DISEASE)

Renal osteodystrophy is a loosely used term that encompasses a number of skeletal abnormalities appearing in cases of chronic kidney disease and in patients treated by dialysis for several years. Renal osteodystrophy is more common in children than in adults. Clinical symptoms of bone disease in advanced renal failure appear in less than 10% of patients but radiologic and histologic changes are observed in fairly large proportion of cases.

PATHOGENESIS Renal osteodystrophy involves two main events: *hyperphosphataemia* and *hypocalcaemia* which, in turn, leads to parathormone elaboration and resultant osteoclastic activity and major lesions of renal osteodystrophy—osteomalacia (rickets in children), secondary hyperparathyroidism, osteitis fibrosa cystica, osteosclerosis and metastatic calcification.

The mechanisms underlying renal osteodystrophy are schematically illustrated in **Fig. 30.6** and briefly outlined below:

1. **Hyperphosphataemia** In chronic kidney disease, there is impaired renal excretion of phosphate, causing phosphate retention and hyperphosphataemia. Hyperphosphataemia, in turn, causes hypocalcaemia which is responsible for secondary hyperparathyroidism.

2. **Hypocalcaemia** Hypocalcaemia may also result from the following:

◈ Due to renal dysfunction, there is decreased conversion of vitamin D metabolite 25(OH) cholecalciferol to its active form 1,25 (OH)$_2$ cholecalciferol.

◈ Reduced intestinal absorption of calcium.

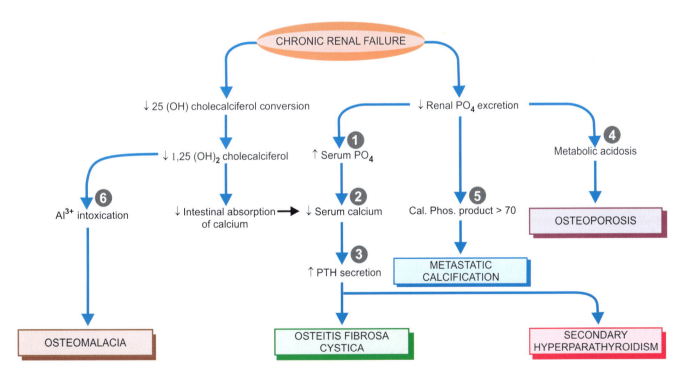

Figure 30.6 ▶ Pathogenesis of renal osteodystrophy in chronic renal failure. Circled serial numbers in the graphic representation correspond to the sequence described in the text under pathogenesis.

3. **Parathormone secretion** Hypocalcaemia stimulates secretion of parathormone, eventually leading to secondary hyperparathyroidism which, in turn, causes increased osteoclastic activity.

4. **Metabolic acidosis** As a result of decreased renal function, acidosis sets in which may cause osteoporosis and bone decalcification.

5. **Calcium phosphorus product > 70** When the product of biochemical value of calcium and phosphate is higher than 70, metastatic calcification may occur at extraosseous sites.

6. **Dialysis-related metabolic bone disease** Long-term dialysis employing use of aluminium-containing dialysate is currently considered to be a major cause of metabolic bone lesions. Aluminium interferes with deposition of calcium hydroxyapatite in bone and results in osteomalacia, secondary hyperparathyroidism and osteitis fibrosa cystica. In addition, accumulation of β_2-microglobulin amyloid in such cases causes dialysis-related amyloidosis (page 62).

MORPHOLOGIC FEATURES The following skeletal lesions can be identified in renal osteodystrophy:

1. *Mixed osteomalacia-osteitis fibrosa* is the most common manifestation of renal osteodystrophy resulting from disordered vitamin D metabolism and secondary hyperparathyroidism.
2. *Pure osteitis fibrosa* results from metabolic complications of secondary hyperparathyroidism.
3. *Pure osteomalacia* of renal osteodystrophy is attributed to aluminium toxicity.
4. *Renal rickets* resembling the changes seen in children with nutritional rickets with widened osteoid seams may occur (page 99).
5. *Osteosclerosis* is characterised by enhanced bone density in the upper and lower margins of vertebrae.
6. *Metastatic calcification* is seen at extraosseous sites such as in medium-sized blood vessels, periarticular tissues, myocardium, eyes, lungs and gastric mucosa (page 50).

SKELETAL FLUOROSIS

Fluorosis of bones occurs due to high sodium fluoride content in soil and water consumed by people in some geographic areas and is termed endemic fluorosis. Such endemic regions exist in some tropical and subtropical areas; in India it exists in some parts of Punjab and Andhra Pradesh. The condition affects farmers who consume drinking water from wells. Non-endemic fluorosis results from occupational exposure in manufacturing industries of aluminium, magnesium, and superphosphate.

PATHOGENESIS In fluorosis, fluoride replaces calcium as the mineral in the bone and gets deposited without any regulatory control. This results in heavily mineralised bones which are thicker and denser but are otherwise weak and deformed (just as in osteopetrosis). In addition, there are also deposits of fluoride in soft tissues, particularly as nodules in the interosseous membrane. The patient develops skeletal deformities and mottling of teeth.

MORPHOLOGIC FEATURES *Grossly*, the long bones and vertebrae develop nodular swellings which are present both inside the bones and on the surface.

Microscopically, these nodules are composed of heavily mineralised irregular osteoid admixed with fluoride which requires confirmation chemically.

PAGET'S DISEASE OF BONE (OSTEITIS DEFORMANS)

Paget's disease of bone or osteitis deformans was first described by Sir James Paget in 1877. Paget's disease of bone is an osteolytic and osteosclerotic bone disease of uncertain etiology involving one (monostotic) or more bones (polyostotic). The condition affects predominantly males over the age of 50 years. Though the etiology remains obscure, following factors have been implicated:

1. There has been some evidence that osteitis deformans is a form of *slow-virus infection* by paramyxovirus (e.g. respiratory syncytial virus, measles) in osteoclasts. However, the virus has not been cultured from the osteoclasts of Paget's disease.
2. Autosomal dominant inheritance and *genetic susceptibility* have been proposed on the basis of observation of 7-10 fold higher prevalence of disease in first-degree relatives. The susceptibility gene located on chromosome 18q encodes for a member of tumour necrosis factor called *RANK* (receptor activator of nuclear factor κB).

Clinically, the *monostotic form* of the disease may remain asymptomatic and the lesion is discovered incidentally or on radiologic examination. *Polyostotic form,* however, is more widespread and may produce pain, fractures, skeletal deformities, and occasionally, sarcomatous transformation. Typically, there is marked elevation of serum alkaline phosphatase and normal to high serum calcium level.

MORPHOLOGIC FEATURES Monostotic Paget's disease involves most frequently: tibia, pelvis, femur, skull and vertebra, while the order of involvement in polyostotic Paget's disease is: vertebrae, pelvis, femur, skull, sacrum and tibia. Three sequential stages are identified in Paget's disease:

1. Initial osteolytic stage: This stage is characterised by areas of osteoclastic resorption produced by increased number of large osteoclasts.

2. Mixed osteolytic-osteoblastic stage: In this stage, there is imbalance between osteoblastic laying down of new bone and osteoclastic resorption so that mineralisation of the newly-laid matrix lags behind, resulting in development of characteristic *mosaic pattern* or *jigsaw puzzle appearance* of osteoid seams or cement lines. The narrow space between the trabeculae and cortex is filled with collagen which gradually becomes less vascular.

3. Quiescent osteosclerotic stage: After many years, excessive bone formation results and thus the bone becomes more compact and dense producing osteosclerosis. However, newly-formed bone is poorly mineralised, soft and susceptible to fractures. Radiologically, this stage produces characteristic *cotton-wool appearance* of the affected bone.

> **GIST BOX 30.4 — Metabolic and Endocrine Bone Diseases and Paget's Disease**
>
> - Osteoporosis or osteopenia is a common clinical condition involving multiple bones in which there is quantitative reduction of bone tissue mass resulting in fragile skeleton associated with increased risk of fractures.
> - Severe and prolonged hyperparathyroidism results in osteitis fibrosa cystica.
> - Renal osteodystrophy is appearance of skeletal abnormalities appearing in cases of chronic kidney disease. It involves hyperphosphataemia and hypocalcaemia.
> - Skeletal fluorosis is due to consumption of high sodium fluoride content present in soil and water. In this, fluoride replaces calcium as the mineral in the bone and gets deposited without any regulatory control.
> - Paget's disease of bone or osteitis deformans is an osteolytic and osteosclerotic bone disease of uncertain etiology involving one (monostotic) or more bones (polyostotic).

TUMOUR-LIKE LESIONS OF BONE

In the context of bones, several non-neoplastic conditions resemble true neoplasms and have to be distinguished from them clinically, radiologically and morphologically. Table 30.1 gives a list of such tumour-like lesions. A few common conditions are described below.

FIBROUS DYSPLASIA

Fibrous dysplasia is not an uncommon tumour-like lesion of the bone. It is a benign condition, possibly of developmental origin, characterised by the presence of localised area of replacement of bone by fibrous connective tissue with a characteristic whorled pattern and containing trabeculae of woven bone. Radiologically, the typical focus of fibrous dysplasia has well-demarcated ground-glass appearance.

Three types of fibrous dysplasia are distinguished—monostotic, polyostotic, and Albright syndrome. The spectrum of phenotype of the disease is due to activating mutation in *GNAS1* gene, which encodes for α-subunits of the stimulatory G-protein, $G_{S\alpha}$.

◈ **Monostotic fibrous dysplasia** Monostotic fibrous dysplasia affects a solitary bone and is the most common type, comprising about 70% of all cases. The condition affects either sex and most patients are between 20 and 30 years of age. The bones most often affected, in descending order of frequency are: ribs, craniofacial bones (especially maxilla), femur, tibia and humerus. The condition generally remains asymptomatic and is discovered incidentally, but infrequently may produce tumour-like enlargement of the affected bone.

◈ **Polyostotic fibrous dysplasia** Polyostotic form of fibrous dysplasia affecting several bones constitutes about 25% of all cases. Both sexes are affected equally but the lesions appear at a relatively earlier age than the monostotic form. Most frequently affected bones are: craniofacial, ribs, vertebrae and long bones of the limbs. Approximately a quarter of cases with polyostotic form have more than half of the skeleton involved by disease. The lesions may affect one side of the body or may be distributed segmentally in a limb. Spontaneous fractures and skeletal deformities occur in childhood polyostotic form of the disease.

◈ **Albright syndrome** Also called McCune-Albright syndrome, this is a form of polyostotic fibrous dysplasia associated with endocrine dysfunctions and accounts for less than 5% of all cases. Unlike monostotic and polyostotic varieties, Albright syndrome is more common in females. The syndrome is characterised by polyostotic bone lesions, skin pigmentation *(café-au-lait* macular spots) and sexual precocity, and infrequently other endocrinopathies.

MORPHOLOGIC FEATURES All forms of fibrous dysplasia have an identical pathologic appearance.

Grossly, the lesions appear as sharply-demarcated, localised defects measuring 2-5 cm in diameter, present within the cancellous bone, having thin and smooth overlying cortex. The epiphyseal cartilages are generally spared in the monostotic form but involved in the polyostotic form of disease. Cut section of the lesion shows replacement of normal cancellous bone of the marrow cavity by gritty, grey-pink, rubbery soft tissue which may have areas of haemorrhages, myxoid change and cyst formation.

Histologically, the lesions of fibrous dysplasia have characteristic benign-looking fibroblastic tissue arranged in a loose, whorled pattern in which there are irregular and curved trabeculae of woven (non-lamellar) bone in the form fish-hook appearance or Chinese letter shapes.

Table 30.1	Classification of tumour-like lesions of bone.
1.	Fibrous dysplasia
2.	Fibrous cortical defect (metaphyseal fibrous defect, non-ossifying fibroma)
3.	Solitary bone cyst (simple or unicameral bone cyst)
4.	Aneurysmal bone cyst
5.	Ganglion cyst of bone (intraosseous ganglion)
6.	Brown tumour of hyperparathyroidism (reparative granuloma) (page 591)
7.	Langerhans' cell histiocytosis (Histiocytosis-X) (page 462)

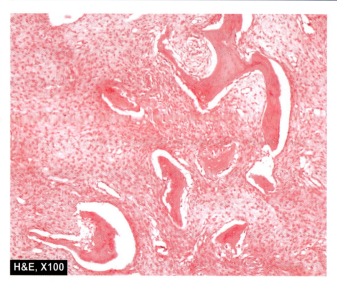

Figure 30.7 ▶ Fibrous dysplasia of the bone. The bony trabeculae have fish-hook appearance (or Chinese-letter appearance) surrounded by fibrous tissue. The osteoblastic rimming of the bony trabeculae are characteristically absent.

Characteristically, there are no osteoblasts rimming then trabeculae of the bone, suggesting a maturation defect in the bone (Fig. 30.7). Rarely, malignant change may occur in fibrous dysplasia, most often an osteogenic sarcoma.

FIBROUS CORTICAL DEFECT (METAPHYSEAL FIBROUS DEFECT, NON-OSSIFYING FIBROMA)

Fibrous cortical defect or metaphyseal fibrous defect is a rather common benign tumour-like lesion occurring in the metaphyseal cortex of long bones in children. Most commonly involved bones are upper or lower end of tibia or lower end of femur. The lesion is generally solitary but rarely there may be multiple and bilaterally symmetrical defects. Radiologically, the lesion is eccentrically located in the metaphysis and has a sharply-delimited border. The pathogenesis of fibrous cortical defect is unknown. Possibly, it arises as a result of some developmental defect at the epiphyseal plate, or could be a tumour of histiocytic origin because of close resemblance to fibrohistiocytic tumours (page 339).

Clinically, fibrous cortical defect causes no symptoms and is usually discovered accidentally when X-ray of the region is done for some other reason.

MORPHOLOGIC FEATURES **Grossly,** the lesion is generally small, less than 4 cm in diameter, granular and brown. Larger lesion (5-10 cm) occurring usually in response to trauma is referred to as *non-ossifying fibroma*.

Microscopically, fibrous cortical defect consists of cellular masses of fibrous tissue showing storiform pattern. There are numerous multinucleate osteoclast-like giant cells, haemosiderin-laden macrophages and foamy cells; hence the lesion is also termed histiocytic xanthogranuloma or fibrous xanthoma of bone.

SOLITARY (SIMPLE, UNICAMERAL) BONE CYST

Solitary, simple or unicameral bone cyst is a benign condition occurring in children and adolescents, most frequently located in the metaphyses at the upper end of humerus and femur. The cyst expands the bone causing thinning of the overlying cortex. Possibly, the lesion arises due to local disorder of bone growth and development. Clinically, solitary bone cyst may remain asymptomatic or may cause pain and fracture.

MORPHOLOGIC FEATURES **Grossly,** simple cyst of the bone is generally unilocular with smooth inner surface. The cavity is filled with clear fluid.

Histologically, the cyst wall consists of thin collagenous tissue having scattered osteoclast giant cells and newly formed reactive bony trabeculae. Fracture alters the appearance and produces sanguineous fluid in the cavity, and haemorrhages, haemosiderin deposits and macrophages in the cyst wall.

ANEURYSMAL BONE CYST

Aneurysmal bone cyst, true to its name, is an expanding osteolytic lesion filled with blood *(aneurysm* = dilatation, distension). The condition is seen more commonly in young patients under 30 years of age. Most frequently involved bones are shafts of metaphyses of long bones or the vertebral column. The radiographic appearance shows characteristic ballooned-out expansile lesion underneath the periosteum. Clinically, the aneurysmal bone cyst may enlarge over a period of years and produce pain, tenderness and pathologic fracture.

The pathogenesis is not clear but it has been suggested by some authors that the condition probably arises from persistent local alteration in haemodynamics. 17p13 translocation has been identified in these cases.

MORPHOLOGIC FEATURES **Grossly,** the lesion consists of a large haemorrhagic mass covered over by thinned out reactive bone (Fig. 30.8).

Histologically, the cyst consists of blood-filled aneurysmal spaces of variable size, some of which are endothelium-lined. The spaces are separated by connective tissue septa containing osteoid tissue, numerous osteoclast-like multinucleate giant cells and trabeculae of bone (Fig. 30.9). The condition has to be distinguished histologically from giant cell tumour or osteoclastoma (page 603) and telangiectatic osteosarcoma (page 599).

Chapter 30: Common Diseases of Bones, Cartilage and Joints

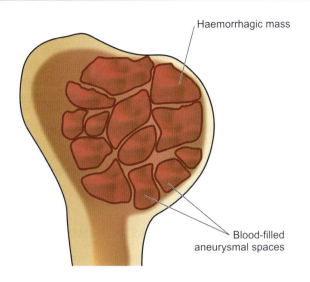

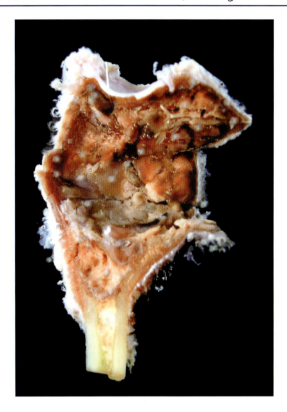

Figure 30.8 ▶ Aneurysmal bone cyst, ulna. The end of the long bone is expanded due to a cyst. The inner wall of the cyst is tan and haemorrhagic.

GIST BOX 30.5 | Tumour-like Lesions of Bone

- Fibrous dysplasia is a benign condition having presence of localised area of replacement of bone by fibrous connective tissue with a characteristic whorled pattern. It is of three types—monostotic, polyostotic, and Albright syndrome.
- Fibrous cortical defect or metaphyseal fibrous defect occurs in the metaphyseal cortex of long bones in children, most commonly on upper or lower end of tibia or lower end of femur and resembles fibrohistiocytic tumours.
- Solitary, simple or unicameral bone cyst is a benign condition occurring in children and adolescents,

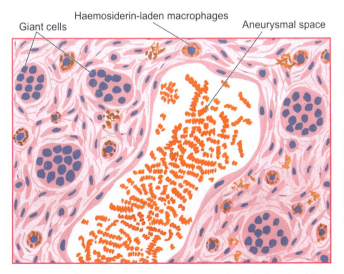

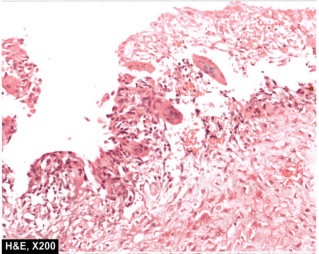

Figure 30.9 ▶ Aneurysmal bone cyst. Histologic hallmark of lesion is presence of aneurysmal spaces filled with blood, partly lined by endothelium and separated by connective tissue septa containing osteoclast-like giant cells along the wall of vascular spaces.

- frequently located in the metaphyses at the upper end of humerus and femur.
- ❖ Aneurysmal bone cyst is an expanding osteolytic lesion filled with blood and requires distinction from giant cell tumour of bone.

TUMOURS OF BONE AND CARTILAGE

Bone and cartilage tumours, commonly called together as bone tumours, are comparatively infrequent but they are clinically quite significant since some of them are highly malignant. Bone tumours may be primary or metastatic. Since histogenesis of some bone tumours is obscure, the WHO has recommended a widely accepted classification of primary bone tumours based on both histogenesis and histologic criteria. Table 30.2 lists the various types of bone tumours arising from different tissue components—osseous and non-osseous, indigenous to the bone. However, in the following discussion, only osseous bone tumours are considered, while non-osseous bone tumours are described elsewhere in the book. The anatomic origin of common primary bone tumours is illustrated in Fig. 30.10.

It may be mentioned here that the diagnosis of any bone lesion is established by a combination of clinical, radiological and pathological examination, supplemented by biochemical and haematological investigations wherever necessary. These include: serum levels of calcium, phosphorus, alkaline phosphatase and acid phosphatase. Specific investigations like plasma and urinary proteins and the bone marrow examination in case of myeloma, urinary catecholamines in metastatic neuroblastoma and haematologic profile in lymphoma and leukaemic involvement of the bone, are of considerable help.

BONE-FORMING (OSTEOBLASTIC) TUMOURS

Bone-forming or osteoblastic group of bone tumours are characterised by the common property of synthesis of osteoid or bone, or both, directly by the tumour cells (osteogenesis). Formation of reactive bone and endochondral ossification should not be construed as osteogenesis. Benign bone-forming tumours include: osteoma, osteoid osteoma

Table 30.2 Classification of primary bone and cartilage tumours.

	HISTOLOGIC DERIVATION	BENIGN	MALIGNANT
A.	OSSEOUS TUMOURS		
I.	Bone-forming (osteogenic, osteoblastic) tumours	Osteoma (40-50 yrs) Osteoid osteoma (20-30 yrs) Osteoblastoma (20-30 yrs)	Classic osteosarcoma (10-20 yrs) Surface osteosarcoma (50-60 yrs)
II.	Cartilage-forming (chondrogenic) tumours	Enchondroma (20-50 yrs) Osteochondroma (20-50 yrs) (Osteocartilaginous exostosis) Chondroblastoma (10-20 yrs) Chondromyxoid fibroma (20-30 yrs)	Chondrosarcoma (40-60 yrs)
III.	Haematopoietic (marrow) tumours	—	Myeloma (50-60 yrs) Lymphoplasmacytic lymphoma (50-60 yrs)
IV.	Unknown	Giant cell tumour (20-40 yrs) (osteoclastoma)	Malignant giant cell tumour (30-50 yrs) Ewing's sarcoma (5-20 yrs) Adamantinoma of long bones
V.	Notochordal tumour	—	Chordoma (40-50 yrs)
B.	NON-OSSEOUS TUMOURS		
I.	Vascular tumours	Haemangioma	Haemangioendothelioma Haemangiopericytoma Angiosarcoma
II.	Fibrogenic tumours	Non-ossifying fibroma (metaphyseal fibrous defect)	Fibrosarcoma
III.	Neurogenic tumours	Neurilemmoma and neurofibroma	Neurofibrosarcoma
IV.	Lipogenic tumours	Lipoma	Liposarcoma
V.	Histiocytic tumours	Fibrous histiocytoma	Malignant fibrous histiocytoma

Figures in brackets indicate common age of occurrence.

and osteoblastoma, while the malignant counterpart is osteosarcoma (osteogenic sarcoma).

Osteoma

An osteoma is a rare benign, slow-growing lesion, regarded by some as a hamartoma rather than a true neoplasm. Similar lesions may occur following trauma, subperiosteal haematoma or local inflammation. Osteoma is almost exclusively restricted to flat bones of the skull and face. It may grow into paranasal sinuses or protrude into the orbit. An osteoma may form a component of Gardner's syndrome. Radiologic appearance is of a dense ivory-like bony mass.

Microscopically, the lesion is composed of well-differentiated mature lamellar bony trabeculae separated by fibrovascular tissue.

Osteoid Osteoma and Osteoblastoma

Osteoid osteoma and osteoblastoma (or giant osteoid osteoma) are closely related benign tumours occurring in children and young adults. Osteoid osteoma is more common than osteoblastoma. There are no clear-cut histologic criteria to distinguish the two. The distinction between them is based on clinical features, size and radiographic appearance.

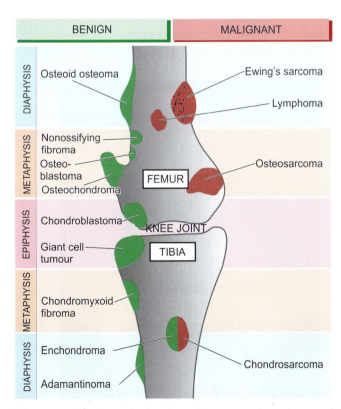

Figure 30.10 ▶ Anatomic locations of common primary bone and cartilage tumours.

◆ **Osteoid osteoma** is small (usually less than 1 cm) tumour located in the cortex of a long bone, associated characteristically with noctural pain. The tumour is clearly demarcated having surrounding zone of reactive bone formation which radiographically appears as a small radiolucent central focus or nidus surrounded by dense sclerotic bone. The pain is possibly due to increased elaboration of prostaglandin E2 by proliferating osteoblasts.

◆ **Osteoblastoma,** on the other hand, is larger in size (usually more than 1 cm), painless, located in the medulla, commonly in the vertebrae, ribs, ilium and long bones, and there is absence of reactive bone formation.

Histologically, the distinction between osteoid osteoma and osteoblastoma is not obvious. In either case, the lesion consists of trabeculae of osteoid, rimmed by osteoblasts and separated by highly vascularised connective tissue stroma. Later, some of the trabeculae are mineralised and calcified.

Osteosarcoma

Osteosarcoma or osteogenic sarcoma is the most common primary malignant tumour of the bone. The tumour is characterised by *formation of osteoid or bone, or both, directly by sarcoma cells.* The tumour is thought to arise from primitive osteoblast-forming mesenchyme. Depending upon their locations within the bone, osteosarcomas are classified into 2 main categories: central (medullary or classic) and surface (parosteal and periosteal).

Central (Medullary) Osteosarcoma

This is the more common and classic type and is generally referred to as 'osteosarcoma' if not specified. The tumour occurs in young patients between the age of 10 and 20 years. Males are affected more frequently than females. The tumour arises in the metaphysis of long bones. Most common sites, in descending order of frequency, are: the lower end of femur and upper end of tibia (i.e. around knee joint about 60%); the upper end of humerus (10%); pelvis and the upper end of femur (i.e. around hip joint about 15%); and less often in jaw bones, vertebrae and skull. Rarely, an osteosarcoma may occur in extraskeletal soft tissues.

Based upon the pathogenesis, osteosarcoma is divided into 2 types: primary and secondary.

◆ *Primary osteosarcoma* is more common and occurs in the absence of any known underlying disease. Its etiology is unknown but there is an evidence linking this form of osteosarcoma with genetic factors (e.g. hereditary mutation of chromosome 13 in common with retinoblastoma locus), period of active bone growth (occurrence of the tumour in younger age), and with certain environmental influences (e.g. radiation, oncogenic virus). Cases of hereditary retinoblastoma have a very high prevalence risk of development of osteosarcoma implicating *RB* gene in their pathogenesis. About 20% sporadic osteosarcomas show mutation in *p53* tumour suppressor gene; some have overexpression of *MDM2* gene and mutation in *cyclin D1, p16* and *CDK4*.

❖ *Secondary osteosarcoma,* on the other hand, develops following pre-existing bone disease e.g. Paget's disease of bone, fibrous dysplasia, multiple osteochondromas, chronic osteomyelitis, infarcts and fractures of bone. The tumour has a more aggressive behaviour than the primary osteosarcoma.

Medullary osteosarcoma is a highly malignant tumour. The tumour arises centrally in the metaphysis, extends longitudinally for variable distance into the medullary cavity, expands laterally on either side breaking through the cortex and lifting the periosteum. If the periosteum is breached, the tumour grows relentlessly into the surrounding soft tissues. The only tissue which is able to stop its spread, *albeit* temporarily, is the cartilage of epiphyseal plate. The radiographic appearance is quite distinctive: characteristic *'sunburst pattern'* due to osteogenesis within the tumour and presence of *Codman's triangle* formed at the angle between the elevated periosteum and underlying surface of the cortex.

Clinically, the usual osteosarcoma presents with pain, tenderness and an obvious swelling of affected extremity. Serum alkaline phosphatase level is generally raised but calcium and phosphorus levels are normal. The tumour metastasises rapidly and widely to distant sites by haematogenous route and disseminates commonly to the lungs, other bones, brain and various other sites.

MORPHOLOGIC FEATURES *Grossly,* the tumour appears as a grey-white, bulky mass at the metaphyseal end of a long bone of the extremity. The articular end of the bone is generally uninvolved in initial stage. Codman's triangle, though identified radiologically, may be obvious on macroscopic examination **(Fig. 30.11)**. Cut surface of the tumour is grey-white with areas of haemorrhages and necrotic bone. Tumours which form abundance of osteoid, bone and cartilage may have hard, gritty and mucoid areas. *Histologically,* osteosarcoma shows considerable variation in pattern from case-to-case and even within a tumour from one area to the other. However, the following two features characterise all classic forms of osteosarcomas **(Fig. 30.12)**:

1. Sarcoma cells The tumour cells of osteosarcomas are undifferentiated mesenchymal stromal cells which show marked pleomorphism and polymorphism i.e. variation in size as well as shape. The tumour cells may have various shapes such as spindled, round, oval and polygonal and bizarre tumour giant cells. The tumour cells have variable size and show hyperchromatism and atypical mitoses. Histochemically, these tumour cells are positive for alkaline phosphatase. Immunohistochemically, sarcoma cells of osteosarcoma express vimentin, osteocalcin, osteonectin and type I collagen.

2. Osteogenesis The anaplastic sarcoma cells form osteoid matrix and bone directly; this is found interspersed in the areas of tumour cells. In addition to osteoid and bone, the tumour cells may produce cartilage, fibrous tissue or myxoid tissue.

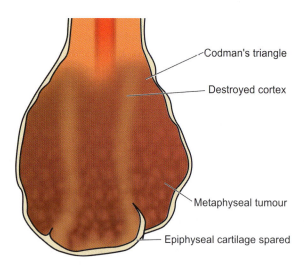
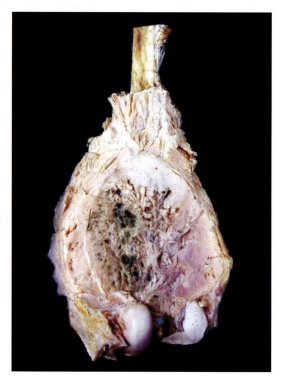

Figure 30.11 ▶ Osteosarcoma. The lower end of the femur shows a bulky expanded tumour in the region of metaphysis sparing the epiphyseal cartilage. Sectioned surface of the tumour shows lifting of the periosteum by the tumour and eroded cortical bone. The tumour is grey-white with areas of haemorrhage and necrosis.

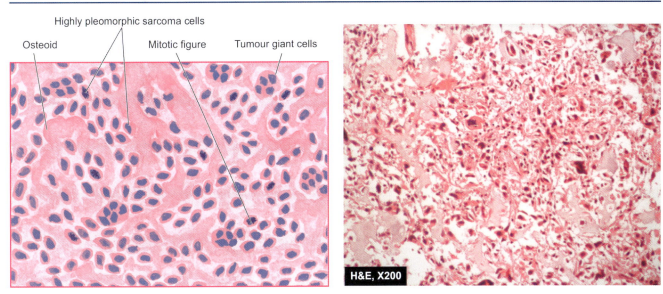

Figure 30.12 ▶ Osteosarcoma. Hallmarks of microscopic picture of the usual osteosarcoma are the sarcoma cells characterised by variation in size and shape of tumour cells, bizarre mitosis and multinucleate tumour giant cells, and osteogenesis i.e. production of osteoid matrix and bone directly by the tumour cells.

VARIANTS A few histologic variants of the classic osteosarcoma have been described as under:

1. Telangiectatic osteosarcoma The tumour in this variant presents with pathological fractures. The tumour has large, cavernous, dilated vascular channels. This variant has a more aggressive course.

2. Small cell osteosarcoma This variant has small, uniform tumour cells just like the tumour cells of Ewing's sarcoma or lymphoma but osteogenesis by these tumour cells is the distinguishing feature.

3. Fibrohistiocytic osteosarcoma This variant resembles malignant fibrous histiocytoma but having osteogenesis by the tumour cells.

4. Anaplastic osteosarcoma In this variant, the tumour has so marked anaplasia that it may resemble any other type of pleomorphic sarcoma and is identified by the presence of osteoid formed directly by the tumour cells.

5. Well-differentiated osteosarcoma Although generally classic form of osteosarcoma is a highly malignant tumour, rarely a well-differentiated variant having minimal cytologic atypia resembling parosteal osteosarcoma may be seen.

Surface Osteosarcoma

About 5% of osteosarcomas occur on the surface of bone and are slow-growing tumours compared to medullary osteosarcomas. Surface osteosarcoma includes 2 variants: parosteal and periosteal.

Parosteal or juxtacortical osteosarcoma is an uncommon form of slow-growing osteosarcoma having its origin from the metaphysis on the external surface of the bone (*parosteal* or *juxtacortical* means outer to cortex). The tumour should be distinguished from the more common medullary osteosarcoma because of its better prognosis and different presentation. The tumour occurs in older age group (3rd to 4th decade), has no sex predilection and is slow growing. Its common locations are metaphysis of long bones, most frequently lower end of the femur and upper end of the humerus. X-ray examination usually reveals a dense bony mass attached to the outer cortex of the affected long bone.

Grossly, the tumour is lobulated and circumscribed, calcified mass in the subperiosteal location.

Microscopically, the features which characterise the usual osteosarcoma (sarcomatous stroma and production of neoplastic osteoid and bone) are present, but the tumour shows a high degree of structural differentiation, and there are generally well-formed bony trabeculae. These features account for distinctly better prognosis in these cases.

Periosteal osteosarcoma is a rarer form of osteosarcoma than parosteal type and arises between the cortex and the overlying periosteum. Its common location is the diaphysis of the tibia or the femur. It occurs in young adults (average age 25 years).

Microscopically, periosteal osteosarcoma has cartilaginous differentiation and higher degree of anaplasia than that seen in parosteal osteosarcoma but lower grade than conventional osteosarcoma i.e. it is an intermediate grade sarcoma.

Section VI: Selected Topics from Systemic Pathology

Table 30.3 Contrasting features of central (medullary) and surface (parosteal and periosteal) osteosarcoma.

	FEATURE	CENTRAL (MEDULLARY)	SURFACE (PAROSTEAL AND PERIOSTEAL)
1.	Age	10-20 years	Older patients
2.	Sex	More common in males	No sex predilection
3.	Anatomic site	Metaphysis	Metaphysis/diaphysis
4.	Location	Femur (lower end), tibia (upper end), humerus (upper end), around hip	Femur (lower-end), humerus (upper end)
5.	Pathogenesis	Primary: genetic factors (mutations in *Rb* gene, *p53*, *MDM2*) Secondary: Paget's disease, fibrous dysplasia	Parosteal: Arises outer to cortex Periosteal: Arises between cortex and periosteum
6.	Behaviour	Highly malignant	Slow growing
7.	G/A	Bulky, necrotic, forms Codman's triangle	Smaller, well-formed bone present
8.	M/E	i. Sarcomas cells: Polymorphic and pleomorphic ii. Osteoid formation	i. Parosteal: Fibrous stromal cells with subtle atypia ii. Periosteal: High grade iii. Both form bony trabeculae
9.	Histologic types	Telangiectatic, small cell, fibrohistiocystic, well-differentiated, anaplastic	Parosteal (juxta cortical), periosteal
10.	Spread and prognosis	Haematogenous spread, prognosis poor	Recurrences common, may metastasise, prognosis generally good, better for parosteal than periosteal

Table 30.3 sums up the contrasting features of central (medullary) and surface (parosteal and periosteal) osteosarcomas.

CARTILAGE-FORMING (CHONDROBLASTIC) TUMOURS

The tumours which are composed of frank cartilage or derived from cartilage-forming cells are included in this group. This group comprises benign lesions like osteocartilaginous exostoses (osteochondromas), enchondroma, chondroblastoma and chondromyxoid fibroma, and a malignant counterpart, chondrosarcoma.

Osteocartilaginous Exostoses (Osteochondromas)

Osteocartilaginous exostoses or osteochondromas are the commonest of benign cartilage-forming lesions. Though designated and discussed with neoplasms, exostosis or osteochondroma is not a true tumour but is regarded as a disorder of growth and development. It may occur as a *'solitary sporadic exostosis'* or there may be *'multiple hereditary exostoses.'* Hereditary forms are due to germline muatation in *EXT1 or EXT2* gene while sporadic type is due to mutated *EXT1* only.

Exostoses arise from metaphyses of long bones as exophytic lesions, most commonly lower femur and upper tibia (i.e. around knee) and upper humerus but may also be found in other bones such as the scapula or ilium. They are discovered most commonly in late childhood or adolescence and are more frequent in males. They may remain asymptomatic and discovered as an incidental radiographic finding or may produce obvious deformity. Both solitary and multiple exostoses may undergo transformation into chondrosarcoma but the risk is much greater with multiple hereditary exostoses.

MORPHOLOGIC FEATURES *Grossly*, osteochondromas have a broad or narrow base (i.e. may be either sessile or pedunculated) which is continuous with the cortical bone. They protrude exophytically as mushroom-shaped, cartilage-capped lesions enclosing well-formed cortical bone and marrow **(Fig. 30.13)**.

Microscopically, they are composed of outer cap composed of mature cartilage resembling epiphyseal cartilage and the inner mature lamellar bone and bone marrow **(Fig. 30.14)**.

Enchondroma

Enchondroma is the term used for the benign cartilage-forming tumour that develops centrally within the interior of the affected bone, while chondroma refers to the peripheral development of lesion similar to osteochondromas. Enchondromas may occur singly or they may be multiple, forming a non-hereditary disorder called *enchondromatosis* or *Ollier's disease*. The coexistence of multiple enchondromas with multiple soft tissue haemangiomas constitutes a familial syndrome called *Maffucci's syndrome.*

Most common locations for enchondromas are short tubular bones of the hands and feet, and less commonly, they

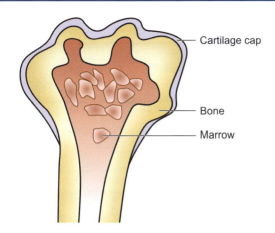
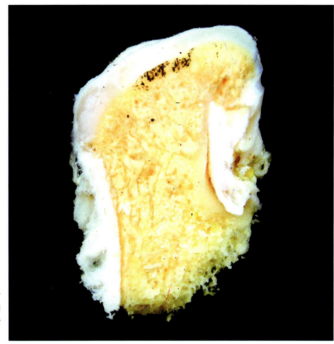

Figure 30.13 ▶ Osteochondroma (osteocartilaginous exostosis), upper end humerus. The amputated head of the long bone shows mushroom-shaped elevated nodular areas. These nodules have cartilaginous caps and inner osseous tissue.

involve the ribs or the long bones. They may appear at any age and in either sex. Enchondromas, like osteochondromas, may remain asymptomatic or may cause pain and pathologic fractures. X-ray reveals a radiolucent, lobulated tumour mass with spotty calcification. Malignant transformation of solitary enchondroma is rare but multiple enchondromas may develop into chondrosarcoma.

MORPHOLOGIC FEATURES *Grossly*, the enchondroma is lobulated, bluish-grey, translucent, cartilaginous mass lying within the medullary cavity.

Histologically, the tumour has characteristic lobulated appearance. The lobules are composed of normal adult hyaline cartilage separated by vascularised fibrous stroma. Foci of calcification may be evident within the tumour. Enchondroma is distinguished from chondrosarcoma by the absence of invasion into surrounding tissues and lack of cellular features of malignancy.

Chondroblastoma

Chondroblastoma is a relatively rare benign tumour arising from the epiphysis of long bones adjacent to the epiphyseal cartilage plate. Most commonly affected bones are upper tibia and lower femur (i.e. about knee) and upper humerus. The tumour usually occurs in patients under 20 years of age with male preponderance (male-female ratio 2:1). The radiographic appearance is of a sharply-circumscribed, lytic lesion with multiple small foci of calcification. Chondroblastoma may be asymptomatic, or may produce local pain, tenderness and discomfort. The behaviour of the tumour is benign though it may recur locally after curettage.

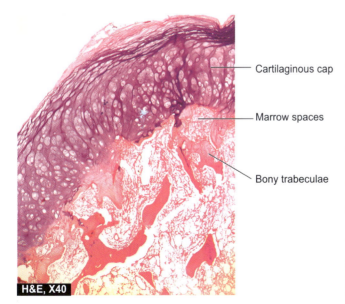

Figure 30.14 ▶ Osteochondroma. The overlying cap shows mature cartilage cells covering the underlying mature lamellar bone containing marrow spaces.

MORPHOLOGIC FEATURES *Grossly*, chondroblastoma is a well-defined mass, up to 5 cm in diameter, lying in the epiphysis. The tumour is surrounded by thin capsule of dense sclerotic bone. Cut surface reveals a soft chondroid tumour with foci of haemorrhages, necrosis and calcification.

Histologically, the tumour is highly cellular and is composed of small, round to polygonal mononuclear cells resembling chondroblasts and has multinucleate osteoclast-like giant cells. There are small areas of cartilaginous intercellular matrix and focal calcification.

Chondromyxoid Fibroma

Chondromyxoid fibroma is an uncommon benign tumour of cartilaginous origin arising in the metaphysis of long bones. Most common locations are upper end of tibia and lower end of femur i.e. around the knee joint. Majority of tumours appear in 2nd to 3rd decades of life with male preponderance. Radiographically, the tumour appears as a sharply-outlined radiolucent area with foci of calcification and expansion of affected end of the bone. The lesion may be asymptomatic, or may cause pain, swelling and discomfort in the affected joint. The lesions may recur after curettage. Thus, there are many similarities with chondroblastoma.

MORPHOLOGIC FEATURES Grossly, chondromyxoid fibroma is sharply-demarcated, grey-white lobulated mass, not exceeding 5 cm in diameter, lying in the metaphysis. The tumour is often surrounded by a layer of dense sclerotic bone. Cut surface of the tumour is soft to firm and lobulated but calcification within the tumour is not as common as with other cartilage-forming tumours.

Histologically, the tumour has essentially lobulated pattern. The lobules are separated by fibrous tissue and variable number of osteoclast-like giant cells. The lobules themselves are composed of immature cartilage consisting of spindle-shaped or stellate cells with abundant myxoid or chondroid intercellular matrix.

In view of close histogenetic relationship between chondromyxoid fibroma and chondroblastoma, occasional tumours show a combination of histological features of both.

Chondrosarcoma

Chondrosarcoma is a malignant tumour of chondroblasts. In frequency, it is next in frequency to osteosarcoma but is relatively slow-growing and thus has a much better prognosis than that of osteosarcoma. Two types of chondrosarcoma are distinguished: *central* and *peripheral.*

◆ **Central chondrosarcoma** is more common and arises within the medullary cavity of diaphysis or metaphysis. This type of chondrosarcoma is generally primary i.e. occurs *de novo.*

◆ **Peripheral chondrosarcoma** arises in the cortex or periosteum of metaphysis. It may be primary or secondary occurring on a pre-existing benign cartilaginous tumour such as osteocartilaginous exostoses (osteochondromas), multiple enchondromatosis, and rarely, chondroblastoma.

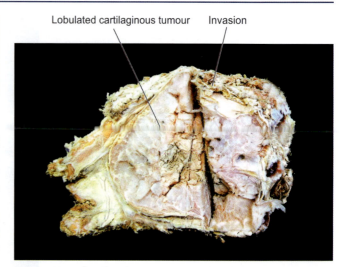

Figure 30.15 ▶ Chondrosarcoma, scapula. The bone is expanded externally due to a gelatinous tumour. Sectioned surface shows lobulated mass with bluish cartilaginous hue infiltrating the soft tissues.

Both forms of chondrosarcoma usually occur in patients between 3rd and 6th decades of life with slight male preponderance. In contrast to benign cartilaginous tumours, majority of chondrosarcomas are found more often in the central skeleton (i.e. in the pelvis, ribs and shoulders); sometimes around the knee joint. Radiologic appearance is of hugely expansile and osteolytic growth with foci of calcification. Clinically, the tumour is slow-growing and comes to attention because of pain and gradual enlargement over the years. Lower grades of the tumour recur following surgical removal but higher grades cause metastatic dissemination, commonly to the lungs, liver, kidney and brain.

MORPHOLOGIC FEATURES Grossly, chondrosarcoma may vary in size from a few centimeters to extremely large and lobulated masses of firm consistency. Cut section of the tumour shows translucent, bluish-white, gelatinous or myxoid appearance with foci of ossification (Fig. 30.15).

Histologically, the two hallmarks of chondrosarcoma are: invasive character and formation of lobules of anaplastic cartilage cells. These tumour cells show cellular features of malignancy such as hyperchromatism, pleomorphism, two or more cells in the lacunae and tumour giant cells (Fig. 30.16). However, sometimes distinction between a well-differentiated chondrosarcoma and a benign chondroma may be difficult and in such cases location, clinical features and radiological appearance are often helpful.

Rare variants of chondrosarcoma are mesenchymal chondrosarcoma, dedifferentiated chondrosarcoma and clear cell chondrosarcoma.

Chapter 30: Common Diseases of Bones, Cartilage and Joints

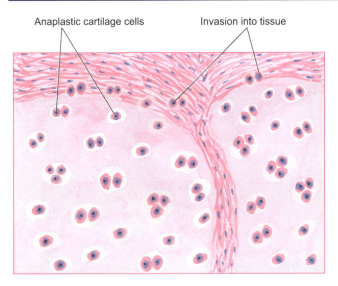
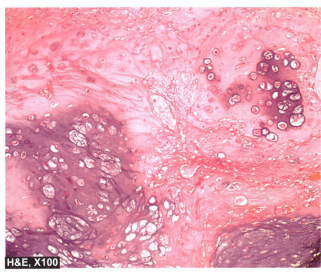

Figure 30.16 ▶ Chondrosarcoma. Histologic features include invasion of the tumour into adjacent soft tissues and cytologic characteristics of malignancy in the tumour cells.

GIANT CELL TUMOUR (OSTEOCLASTOMA)

Giant cell tumour or osteoclastoma is a distinctive neoplasm with uncertain histogenesis and hence classified separately. The tumour arises in the epiphysis of long bones close to the articular cartilage. Most common sites of involvement are lower end of femur and upper end of tibia (i.e. about the knee), lower end of radius and upper end of fibula. Giant cell tumour occurs in patients between 20 and 40 years of age with no sex predilection. Clinical features at presentation include pain, especially on weight-bearing and movement, noticeable swelling and pathological fracture. Radiologically, giant cell tumour appears as a large, lobulated and osteolytic lesion at the end of an expanded long bone with characteristic *'soap bubble'* appearance.

MORPHOLOGIC FEATURES **Grossly,** giant cell tumour is eccentrically located in the epiphyseal end of a long bone which is expanded. The tumour is well-circumscribed, dark-tan and covered by a thin shell of subperiosteal bone. Cut surface of the tumour is characteristically haemorrhagic, necrotic, and honey-combed due to focal areas of cystic degeneration (Fig. 30.17).

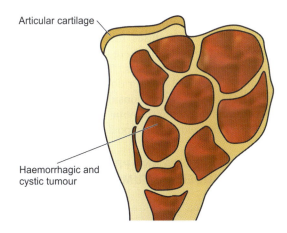
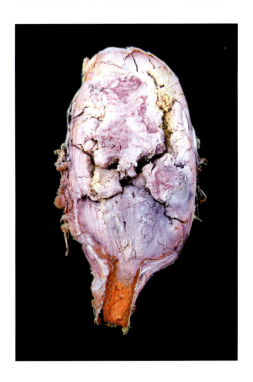

Figure 30.17 ▶ Giant cell tumour (osteoclastoma). The end of the long bone is expanded in the region of epiphysis. Sectioned surface shows circumscribed, dark tan, haemorrhagic and necrotic tumour.

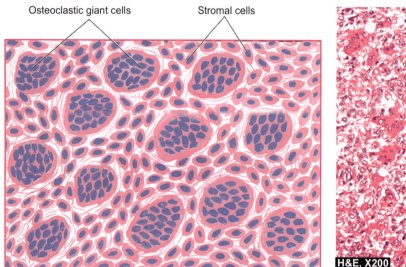 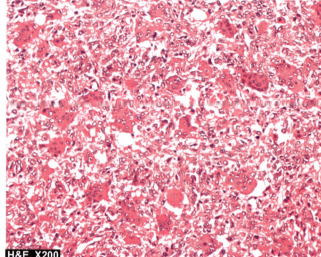

Figure 30.18 ▶ Osteoclastoma. Microscopy reveals osteoclast-like multinucleate giant cells which are regularly distributed among the mononuclear stromal cells.

Histologically, the hallmark features of giant cell tumour are the presence of large number of multinucleate osteoclast-like giant cells regularly scattered throughout the stromal mononuclear cells (Fig. 30.18):

1. Giant cells often contain as many as 100 benign nuclei and have many similarities to normal osteoclasts. These cells have very high acid phosphatase activity.

2. Stromal cells are mononuclear cells and are the real tumour cells and their histologic appearance determines the biologic behaviour of the tumour. Typically, they are uniform, plump, spindle-shaped or round to oval cells with numerous mitotic figures.

3. Other features of the stroma include its scanty collagen content, rich vascularity, areas of haemorrhages and presence of macrophages.

Giant cell tumour of the bone has certain peculiarities which deserve further elaboration. These are: its *cell of origin,* its *differentiation from other giant cell lesions* and its *biologic behaviour.*

CELL OF ORIGIN Though designated as giant cell tumour or osteoclastoma, the actual tumour cells are round to spindled mononuclear cells while proliferated osteoclastic giant cells are seen as background cells. Histogenesis of stromal cells is uncertain but possibly they are of mesenchymal origin. Molecular profiling of giant cell tumour suggests that *RANK* (receptor activator of nuclear factor κB), a physiologic growth factor for osteoclastic proliferation, is expressed in stromal cells. Giant osteoclastic cells are believed to be formed by *RANK/RANKL* signaling pathway.

OTHER GIANT CELL LESIONS This peculiar tumour with above description is named 'giant cell tumour' but giant cells are present in several other benign tumours and tumour-like lesions from which the giant cell tumour is to be distinguished. These *benign giant cell lesions* are: chondroblastoma, brown tumour of hyperparathyroidism, reparative giant cell granuloma, aneurysmal bone cyst, simple bone cyst and metaphyseal fibrous defect (non-ossifying fibroma).

BIOLOGIC BEHAVIOUR Giant cell tumours are best described as aggressive and recurrent tumours. About 40 to 60% of them recur after curettage, sometimes after a few decades of initial resection. Approximately 4% cases result in distant metastases, mainly to lungs. Metastases are histologically benign and there is usually history of repeated curettages and recurrences. Thus attempts at histologic grading of giant cell tumour do not always yield satisfactory results. One of the factors considered significant in malignant transformation of this tumour is the role of radiotherapy resulting in development of post-radiation bone sarcoma.

EWING'S SARCOMA AND PRIMITIVE NEUROECTODERMAL TUMOUR (ES/PNET)

Ewing's sarcoma (ES) is a highly malignant small round cell tumour occurring in patients between the age of 5 and 20 years with predilection for occurrence in females. Since its first description by James Ewing in 1921, histogenesis of this tumour has been a debatable issue. At different times, the possibilities suggested for the cell of origin have been endothelial, pericytic, bone marrow, osteoblastic, and mesenchymal; currently it is settled for its origin from

primitive neuroectodermal cells. Now, Ewing's sarcoma includes 3 variants:
i) classic (skeletal) Ewing's sarcoma;
ii) soft tissue Ewing's sarcoma; and
iii) primitive neuroectodermal tumour (PNET).

The three are linked together by a common neuroectodermal origin and by a common cytogenetic translocation abnormality t(11; 22) (q24; q12). This suggests a phenotypic spectrum in these conditions varying from undifferentiated Ewing's sarcoma to PNET positive for rosettes and neural markers (neuron-specific enolase, S-100). However, PNET ultimately has a worse prognosis.

The skeletal Ewing's sarcoma arises in the medullary canal of diaphysis or metaphysis. The common sites are shafts and metaphysis of long bones, particularly femur, tibia, humerus and fibula, although some flat bones such as pelvis and scapula may also be involved.

Clinical features include pain, tenderness and swelling of the affected area accompanied by fever, leucocytosis and elevated ESR. These signs and symptoms may lead to an erroneous clinical diagnosis of osteomyelitis. However, X-ray examination reveals a predominantly osteolytic lesion with patchy subperiosteal reactive bone formation producing characteristic *'onion-skin'* radiographic appearance.

MORPHOLOGIC FEATURES *Grossly*, Ewing's sarcoma is typically located in the medullary cavity and produces expansion of the affected diaphysis (shaft) or metaphysis, often extending into the adjacent soft tissues. The tumour tissue is characteristically grey-white, soft and friable (Fig. 30.19).

Histologically, Ewing's tumour is a member of *small round cell tumours* which includes other tumours such as: PNET, neuroblastoma, embryonal rhabdomyosarcoma, lymphoma-leukaemias, and metastatic small cell carcinoma. Ewing's tumour shows the following histologic characteristics (Fig. 30.20):

1. Pattern The tumour is divided by fibrous septa into irregular lobules of closely-packed tumour cells. These tumour cells are characteristically arranged around capillaries forming *pseudorosettes.*

2. Tumour cells The individual tumour cells comprising the lobules are small and uniform resembling lymphocytes and have ill-defined cytoplasmic outlines, scanty cytoplasm and round nuclei having 'salt and pepper' chromatin and frequent mitoses. Based on these cytological features the tumour is also called *round cell tumour* or *small blue cell tumour.* The cytoplasm contains glycogen that stains with periodic acid-Schiff (PAS) reaction. A consistently expressed cell surface marker by tumour cells of ES/PNET group is CD99 which is a product of *MIC-2* gene located on X and Y chromosome.

3. Other features The tumour is richly vascularised and lacks the intercellular network of reticulin fibres. There may be areas of necrosis and acute inflammatory cell infiltration. Focal areas of reactive bone formation may be present.

Ewing's sarcoma metastasises early by haematogenous route to the lungs, liver, other bones and brain. Involvement of other bones has prompted a suggestion of *multicentric origin* of Ewing's sarcoma. The prognosis of Ewing's sarcoma used to

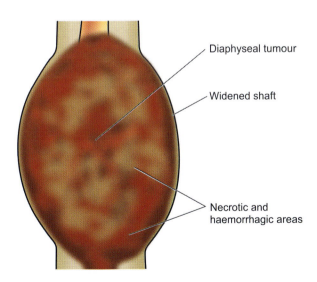
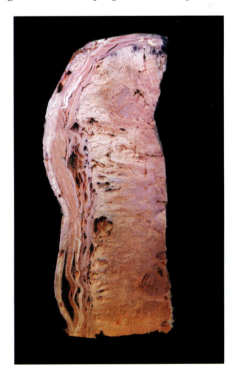

Figure 30.19 ▶ Ewing's sarcoma. The tumour is largely extending into soft tissues including the skeletal muscle. Cut surface of the tumour is grey-white, cystic, soft and friable.

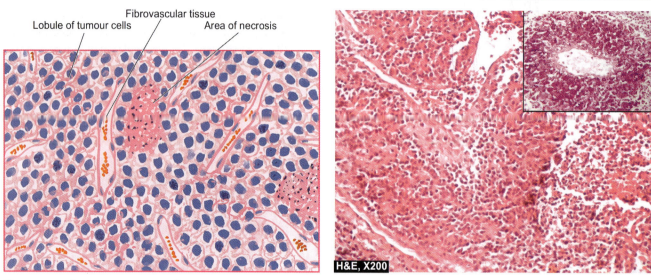

Figure 30.20 ▶ Ewing's sarcoma. Characteristic microscopic features are irregular lobules of uniform small tumour cells with indistinct cytoplasmic outlines which are separated by fibrous tissue septa having rich vascularity. Areas of necrosis and inflammatory infiltrate are also included. Inbox in the right photomicrograph shows PAS positive tumour cells in perivascular location.

be dismal (5-year survival rate less than 10%). But currently, use of combined regimen consisting of radiotherapy and systemic chemotherapy has improved the outcome greatly (5-year survival rate 40-80%).

CHORDOMA

Chordoma is a slow-growing malignant tumour arising from remnants of notochord. Notochord is the primitive axial skeleton which subsequently develops into the spine. Normally, remnants of notochord are represented by notochordal or physaliphorous (*physalis* = bubble, *phorous* = bearing) cells present in the nucleus pulposus and a few clumps within the vertebral bodies. Chordomas thus occur in the axial skeleton, particularly sacrum and coccyx (50%), spheno-occipital region (35%), and less often in the spine (15%). Chordoma is usually found in patients over the age of 40 years with no sex predilection. Radiographically, the tumour usually appears as an osteolytic lesion. Symptoms of spinal cord compression may be present. The tumour grows slowly and infiltrates adjacent structures but metastases develop rarely. Recurrences after local excision are frequent and the tumour almost invariably proves fatal.

MORPHOLOGIC FEATURES *Grossly,* the tumour is soft, lobulated, translucent and gelatinous with areas of haemorrhages.

Microscopically, chordoma is composed of highly vacuolated physaliphorous cells surrounded by a sea of intercellular mucoid material **(Fig. 30.21)**. Histologic differentiation between chordoma and chondrosarcoma or mucin-secreting carcinoma may sometimes be difficult and is facilitated by positive cytokeratin and S-100 immunostaining in the former.

METASTATIC BONE TUMOURS

Metastases to the skeleton are more frequent than the primary bone tumours. Metastatic bone tumours are exceeded in frequency by only 2 other organs—lungs and liver. Most skeletal metastases are derived from haematogenous spread.

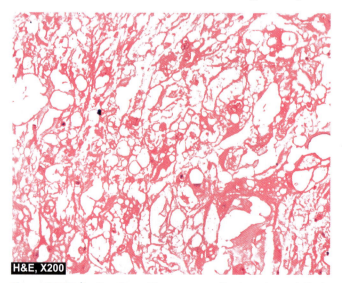

Figure 30.21 ▶ Chordoma. The tumour cells are quite variable in size having characteristic bubbly cytoplasm (physaliphorous cells) and anisonucleocytosis. The background is myxoid.

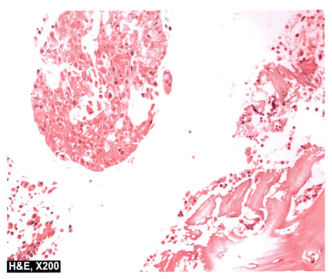

Figure 30.22 ▶ Osseous deposits from carcinoma breast.

Bony metastases of carcinomas predominate over the sarcomas (page 275). Some of the common *carcinomas* metastasising to the bones are from: breast, prostate, lung, kidney, stomach, thyroid, cervix, body of uterus, urinary bladder, testis, melanoma and neuroblastoma of adrenal gland. Examples of *sarcomas* which may metastasise to the bone are: embryonal and alveolar rhabdomyosarcoma, Ewing's sarcoma and osteosarcoma.

Skeletal metastases may be single or multiple. Most commonly involved bones are: the spine, pelvis, femur, skull, ribs and humerus. Usual radiographic appearance is of an *osteolytic* lesion. *Osteoblastic* bone metastases occur in cancer of the prostate, carcinoid tumour and small cell carcinoma of lung.

Metastatic bone tumours generally reproduce the microscopic picture of primary tumour **(Fig. 30.22)**. Many a times, evidence of skeletal metastases is the first clinical manifestation of an occult primary cancer in the body.

| GIST BOX 30.6 | Tumours of Bone and Cartilage |

- Primary bone tumours are classified on the basis of histogenesis and histologic criteria and include osseous and non-osseous tumours. Each of these may be benign or malignant.
- Benign bone-forming osseous tumours are osteoma, osteoid osteoma and osteoblastoma.
- Osteosarcoma is the common malignant bone-forming tumour. The classic form (medullary osteosarcoma) occurs in young patients between the age of 10 and 20 years, arising in the metaphysis. Most common site is around the knee joint and is a highly malignant tumour. Surface osteosarcomas include parosteal and periosteal type, occur in older age group than classic osteosarcoma and have a better prognosis.
- Osteochondromas are the commonest of benign cartilage-forming lesions. Others are enchondroma, chondroblastoma and chondromyxoid fibroma.
- Chondrosarcoma occurs in 4th to 6th decade, is seen more often in central skeleton and is a slow growing malignant tumour.
- Giant cell tumour is an aggressive and recurrent tumour arising in epiphysis, often occurring in young adults.
- Ewing's sarcoma occurs in the age group of 5-20 years, and arises in diaphysis. It is a malignant small round cell tumour.
- Metastatic bone tumours are more common and may arise from various carcinomas and some sarcomas.

DISEASES OF JOINTS

NOMRAL STRUCTURE OF JOINTS

The joints are of 2 types—*diarthrodial or synovial joints* with a joint cavity, and *synarthrodial or nonsynovial joints* without a joint cavity. Most of the diseases of joints affect diarthrodial or synovial joints. In diarthrodial joints, the ends of two bones are held together by joint capsule with ligaments and tendons inserted at the outer surface of the capsule. The articular surfaces of bones are covered by hyaline cartilage which is thicker in weight-bearing areas than in nonweight-bearing areas. The joint space is lined by synovial membrane or synovium which forms synovial fluid that lubricates the joint during movements. The synovium may be smooth or thrown into numerous folds and villi. The synovial membrane is composed of inner layer of 1-4 cell thick synoviocytes and outer layer of loose vascular connective tissue. On electron microscopy, two types of synoviocytes are distinguished: type A and type B. *Type A* synoviocytes are more numerous and are related to macrophages and produce degradative enzymes, while *type B* synthesise hyaluronic acid.

Diseases of joints are numerous and joints are also involved in several systemic disorders. In the following discussion, only those joint diseases which are morphologically significant are described. Synovial tumours are discussed in the next chapter together with other soft tissue tumours.

DEGENERATIVE JOINT DISEASE (OSTEOARTHRITIS)

Osteoarthritis (OA), also called osteoarthrosis or degenerative joint disease (DJD), is the most common form of chronic disorder of synovial joints. It is characterised by progressive degenerative changes in the articular cartilages over the years, particularly in weight-bearing joints.

TYPES AND PATHOGENESIS OA occurs in 2 clinical forms—primary and secondary.

◈ **Primary OA** occurs in the elderly, more commonly in women than in men. The process begins by the end of 4th decade and then progressively and steadily increases producing clinical symptoms. Little is known about the etiology and pathogenesis of primary OA. The condition may be regarded as a reward of longevity. Probably, wear and tear with repeated minor trauma, heredity, obesity, ageing *per se*, all contribute to focal degenerative changes in the articular cartilage of the joints. Genetic factors favouring susceptibility to develop OA have been observed; genetic mutations in proteins which regulate the cartilage growth have been identified e.g. *FRZB* gene.

◆ **Secondary OA** may appear at any age and is the result of any previous wear and tear phenomena involving the joint such as previous injury, fracture, inflammation, loose bodies and congenital dislocation of the hip.

The molecular mechanism of damage to cartilage in OA appears to be the breakdown of collagen type II, probably by IL-1, TNF and nitric oxide.

MORPHOLOGIC FEATURES As mentioned above, the weight-bearing joints such as hips, knee and vertebrae are most commonly involved but interphalangeal joints of fingers may also be affected. The pathologic changes occur in the articular cartilages, adjacent bones and synovium (Fig. 30.23):

1. Articular cartilages The regressive changes are most marked in the weight-bearing regions of articular cartilages. Initially, there is loss of cartilaginous matrix (proteoglycans) resulting in progressive loss of normal metachromasia. This is followed by focal loss of chondrocytes, and at other places, proliferation of chondrocytes forming clusters. Further progression of the process causes loosening, flaking and fissuring of the articular cartilage resulting in breaking off of pieces of cartilage exposing subchondral bone. Radiologically, this progressive loss of cartilage is apparent as narrowed joint space.

2. Bone The denuded subchondral bone appears like polished ivory. There is death of superficial osteocytes and increased osteoclastic activity causing rarefaction, microcyst formation and occasionally microfractures of the subjacent bone. These changes result in remodelling of bone and changes in the shape of joint surface leading to flattening and mushroom-like appearance of the articular end of the bone. The margins of the joints respond to cartilage damage by *osteophyte* or *spur formation*. These are cartilaginous outgrowths at the joint margins which later get ossified. Osteophytes give the appearance of lipping of the affected joint. Loosened and fragmented osteophytes may form free 'joint mice' or loose bodies.

3. Synovium. Initially, there are no pathologic changes in the synovium but in advanced cases there is low-grade chronic synovitis and villous hypertrophy. There may be some amount of synovial effusion associated with chronic synovitis.

The manifestations of OA are most conspicuous in large joints such as hips, knee and back. However, the

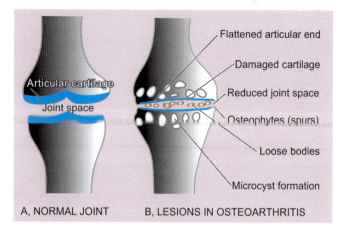

Figure 30.23 ▶ Fully-developed lesions in osteoarthritis (B), contrasted with appearance of a normal joint (A).

pattern of joint involvement may be related to the type of physical activity such as ballet-dancers' toes, karate fingers etc. Minor degree of OA may remain asymptomatic. In symptomatic cases, clinical manifestations are joint stiffness, diminished mobility, discomfort and pain. The symptoms are more prominent on waking up from bed in the morning. Degenerative changes in the interphalangeal joints lead to hard bony and painless enlargements in the form of nodules at the base of terminal phalanx called *Heberden's nodes*. These nodes are more common in females and heredity seems to play a role. In the spine, osteophytes of OA may cause compression of cervical and lumbar nerve root with pain, muscle spasms and neurologic abnormalities.

INFLAMMATORY JOINT DISEASES

Rheumatoid Arthritis

Rheumatoid arthritis (RA) is a chronic multisystem disease of unknown cause. Though the most prominent manifestation of RA is inflammatory arthritis of the peripheral joints, usually with a symmetrical distribution, its systemic manifestations include haematologic, pulmonary, neurological and cardio-vascular abnormalities.

RA is a common disease having peak incidence in 3rd to 4th decades of life, with 3-5 times higher preponderance in females. The condition has high association with HLA-DR4 and HLA-DR1 and familial aggregation. This association is particularly marked in those RA cases who have cyclic citrullinated polypeptide (CCP) antibodies. The onset of disease is insidious, beginning with prodrome of fatigue, weakness, joint stiffness, vague arthralgias and myalgias. This is followed by pain and swelling of joints usually in symmetrical fashion, especially involving joints of hands, wrists and feet. Unlike migratory polyarthritis of rheumatic fever, RA usually persists in the involved joint. Approximately 20% of patients develop rheumatoid nodules located over the extensor surfaces of the elbows and fingers. Extra-articular manifestations infrequently produce symptoms, but when present complicate the diagnosis.

ETIOPATHOGENESIS Present concept on etiology and pathogenesis proposes that RA occurs in an *immunogenetically predisposed individual to the effect of microbial agents acting as trigger antigen*. The role of *superantigens* which are produced by several microorganisms with capacity to bind to HLA-DR molecules (MHC-II region) has also emerged.

I. Immunologic derangements A number of observations in patients and experimental animals indicate the role of immune processes, particularly autoimmune phenomenon, in the development of RA (page 216). These include the following:

1. Detection of circulating autoantibody called rheumatoid factor (RF) against Fc portion of autologous IgG in about 80% cases of RA. RF antibodies are heterogeneous and consist of IgM and IgG class.
2. The presence of antigen-antibody complexes (IgG-RF complexes) in the circulation as well as in the synovial fluid.
3. The presence of other autoantibodies such as antinuclear factor (ANF), antibodies to collagen type II, and antibodies to cytoskeleton.
4. Antigenicity of proteoglycans of human articular cartilage.
5. The presence of γ-globulin, particularly IgG and IgM, in the synovial fluid.
6. Association of RA with amyloidosis.
7. Activation of cell-mediated immunity as observed by presence of numerous inflammatory cells in the synovium, chiefly CD4+ T lymphocytes and some macrophages.

II. Trigger events Though the above hypothesis of a possible role of autoimmunity in the etiology and pathogenesis of RA is generally widely accepted, controversy continues as regards the trigger events which initiate the destruction of articular cartilage. Various possibilities which have been suggested are as follows:

1. The existence of an infectious agent such as mycoplasma, Epstein-Barr virus (EBV), cytomegalovirus (CMV) or rubella virus, either locally in the synovial fluid or systemic infection some time prior to the attack of RA.
2. The possible role of HLA-DR4 and HLA-DR1 in initiation of immunologic damage.

The proposed events in **immunopathogenesis** of RA are as under **(Fig. 30.24)**:

i) In response to antigenic exposure (e.g. infectious agent) in a genetically predisposed individual (HLA-DR), *CD4+ T-cells* are activated.
ii) These cells elaborate *cytokines*, the important ones being tumour necrosis factor (TNF)-α, interferon (IF)-γ, interleukin (IL)-1 and IL-6.
iii) These cytokines *activate* endothelial cells, B lymphocytes and macrophages.
iv) Activation of B-cells releases IgM antibody against IgG (i.e. anti-IgG); this molecule is termed *rheumatoid factor (RF)*.

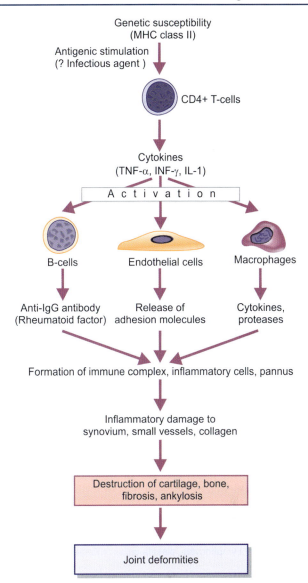

Figure 30.24 ▶ Pathogenesis of rheumatoid arthritis.

v) IgG and IgM immune complexes trigger *inflammatory damage* to the synovium, small blood vessels and collagen.
vi) Activated endothelial cells express *adhesion molecules* which stimulate collection of inflammatory cells.
vii) Activation of macrophages releases more cytokines which cause damage to joint tissues and vascularisation of cartilage termed *pannus formation*.
viii) Eventually damage and destruction of bone and cartilage are followed by *fibrosis* and *ankylosis* producing joint deformities.

LABORATORY FINDINGS These include following investigations:

i) About 80% of cases are seropositive for *RA factor*. However, RA factor titres are elevated in certain

unrelated diseases too such as in viral hepatitis, cirrhosis, sarcoidosis and leprosy.
  ii) *HLA-DR4 and HLA-DR1* association in familial cases.
  iii) *Anti-CCP antibodies* for evaluation of association of RA factor with HLA.
  iv) Other laboratory findings include mild normocytic and normochromic anaemia, elevated ESR, mild leucocytosis and hypergammaglobulinaemia.
  v) Advanced cases show characteristic radiologic abnormalities such as narrowing of joint space and ulnar deviation of the fingers and radial deviation of the wrist.

MORPHOLOGIC FEATURES The predominant pathologic lesions are found in the joints and tendons, and less often, extra-articular lesions are encountered.

ARTICULAR LESIONS RA involves first the small joints of hands and feet and then symmetrically affects the joints of wrists, elbows, ankles and knees. The proximal interphalangeal and metacarpophalangeal joints are affected most severely. Frequently cervical spine is involved but lumbar spine is spared.

Histologically, the characteristic feature is diffuse proliferative synovitis with formation of pannus. The microscopic changes are as under **(Fig. 30.25)**:
1. Numerous folds of large villi of synovium.
2. Marked thickening of the synovial membrane due to oedema, congestion and multilayering of synoviocytes.
3. Intense inflammatory cell infiltrate in the synovial membrane with predominance of lymphocytes, plasma cells and some macrophages, at places forming lymphoid follicles.
4. Foci of fibrinoid necrosis and fibrin deposition.

The pannus progressively destroys the underlying cartilage and subchondral bone. This invasion of pannus results in demineralisation and cystic resorption of underlying bone. Later, fibrous adhesions or even bony ankylosis may unite the two opposing joint surfaces. In addition, persistent inflammation causes weakening and even rupture of the tendons.

EXTRA-ARTICULAR LESIONS Nonspecific inflammatory changes are seen in the blood vessels (acute vasculitis), lungs, pleura, pericardium, myocardium, lymph nodes, peripheral nerves and eyes. But one of the characteristic extra-articular manifestation of RA is occurrence of rheumatoid nodules in the skin. *Rheumatoid nodules* are particularly found in the subcutaneous tissue over pressure points such as the elbows, occiput and sacrum. The centre of these nodules consists of an area of fibrinoid necrosis and cellular debris, surrounded by several layers of palisading large epithelioid cells, and peripherally there are numerous lymphocytes, plasma cells and macrophages. Similar nodules may be found in the lung parenchyma, pleura, heart valves, myocardium and other internal organs.

There are a few *variant forms* of RA:

1. Juvenile RA found in adolescent patients under 16 years of age is characterised by acute onset of fever and predominant involvement of knees and ankles. Pathologic changes are similar but RF is rarely present.

2. Felty's syndrome consists of polyarticular RA associated with splenomegaly and hypersplenism and consequent haematologic derangements.

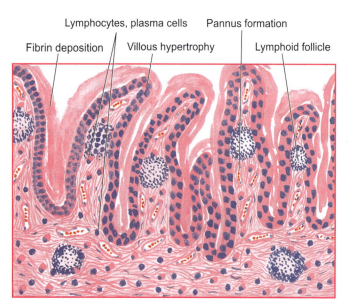
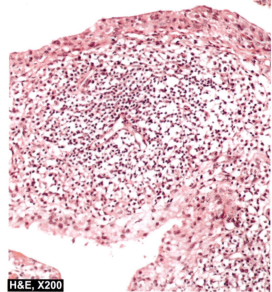

Figure 30.25 ▶ Rheumatoid arthritis. The characteristic histologic features are villous hypertrophy of the synovium and marked mononuclear inflammatory cell infiltrate in synovial membrane with formation of lymphoid follicles at places.

3. Ankylosing spondylitis or rheumatoid spondylitis is rheumatoid involvement of the spine, particularly sacroiliac joints, in young male patients. The condition has a strong HLA-B27 association and may have associated inflammatory diseases such as inflammatory bowel disease, anterior uveitis and Reiter's syndrome.

Suppurative Arthritis

Infectious or suppurative arthritis is invariably an acute inflammatory involvement of the joint. Bacteria usually reach the joint space from the bloodstream but other routes of infection by direct contamination of an open wound or lymphatic spread may also occur. Immunocompromised and debilitated patients are increasingly susceptible to suppurative arthritis. The common causative organisms are gonococci, meningococci, pneumococci, staphylococci, streptococci, *H. influenzae* and gram-negative bacilli. Clinically, the patients present with manifestations of any local infection such as redness, swelling, pain and joint effusion. Constitutional symptoms such as fever, neutrophilic leucocytosis and raised ESR are generally associated.

MORPHOLOGIC FEATURES The haematogenous infectious joint involvement is more often monoarticular rather than polyarticular. The large joints of lower extremities such as the knee, hip and ankle, shoulder and sternoclavicular joints are particularly favoured sites. The process begins with hyperaemia, synovial swelling and infiltration by polymorphonuclear and mononuclear leucocytes along with development of effusion in the joint space. There may be formation of inflammatory granulation tissue and onset of fibrous adhesions between the opposing articular surfaces resulting in permanent ankylosis.

Tuberculous Arthritis

Tuberculous infection of the joints results most commonly from haematogenous dissemination of the organisms from pulmonary or other focus of infection (page 141). Another route of infection is direct spread from tuberculous osteomyelitis close to the joint. Uncommon in the West, the disease is seen not infrequently in developing countries more commonly in children and also in adults.

MORPHOLOGIC FEATURES Tuberculous involvement of the joints is usually monoarticular type but tends to be more destructive than the suppurative arthritis. Most commonly involved sites are the spine, hip joint and knees, and less often other joints are affected. Tuberculosis of the spine is termed *Pott's disease* or *tuberculous spondylitis*.

Grossly, the affected articular surface shows deposition of grey-yellow exudate and occasionally tubercles are present. The joint space may contain tiny grey-white loose bodies and excessive amount of fluid.

Histologically, the synovium is studded with solitary or confluent caseating tubercles. The underlying articular cartilage and bone may be involved by extension of tuberculous granulation tissue and cause necrosis *(caries)*.

GOUT AND GOUTY ARTHRITIS

Gout is a disorder of purine metabolism manifested by the following features, occurring singly or in combination:
1. Increased serum uric acid concentration *(hyperuricaemia)*.
2. Recurrent attacks of characteristic type of acute arthritis in which crystals of *monosodium urate monohydrate* may be demonstrable in the leucocytes present in the synovial fluid.
3. Aggregated deposits of monosodium urate monohydrate *(tophi)* in and around the joints of the extremities.
4. *Renal disease* involving interstitial tissue and blood vessels.
5. Uric acid *nephrolithiasis.*

The disease usually begins in 3rd decade of life and affects men more often than women. A family history of gout is present in a fairly large proportion of cases indicating role of inheritance in hyperuricaemia. Clinically, the natural history of gout comprises 4 stages: asymptomatic hyperuricaemia, acute gouty arthritis, asymptomatic intervals of intercritical periods, and chronic tophaceous stage. In addition, gout nephropathy and urate nephrolithiasis may occur.

TYPES AND PATHOGENESIS The fundamental biochemical hallmark of gout is *hyperuricaemia.* A serum uric acid level in excess of 7 mg/dl, which represents the upper limit of solubility of monosodium urate in serum at 37°C at blood pH, is associated with increased risk of development of gout. Thus, *pathogenesis of gout is pathogenesis of hyperuricaemia.*

Hyperuricaemia and gout may be classified into 2 types: *metabolic* and *renal,* each of which may be *primary* or *secondary.* Primary refers to cases in which the underlying biochemical defect causing hyperuricaemia is not known, while secondary denotes cases with known causes of hyperuricaemia.

1. Hyperuricaemia of metabolic origin This group comprises about 10% cases of gout which are characterised by overproduction of uric acid. There is either an accelerated rate of purine biosynthesis *de novo,* or an increased turnover of nucleic acids. The causes of *primary metabolic gout* include a number of specific enzyme defects in purine metabolism which may be either of unknown cause or are inborn errors of metabolism. The *secondary metabolic gout* is due to either increased purine biosynthesis or a deficiency of glucose-6-phosphatase.

2. Hyperuricaemia of renal origin About 90% cases of gout are the result of reduced renal excretion of uric acid. Altered renal excretion could be due to reduced glomerular filtration of uric acid, enhanced tubular reabsorption or decreased secretion. The causes of gout of renal origin include diuretic therapy, drug-induced (e.g. aspirin, pyrazinamide, nicotinic acid, ethambutol and ethanol), adrenal insufficiency, starvation, diabetic ketosis, and disorders of parathyroid and thyroid. Renal disease *per se* rarely causes secondary hyperuricaemia such as in polycystic kidney disease and leads to urate nephropathy.

MORPHOLOGIC FEATURES The pathologic manifestations of gout include: acute gouty arthritis, chronic tophaceous arthritis, tophi in soft tissues, and renal lesions as under:

1. Acute gouty arthritis This stage is characterised by acute synovitis triggered by precipitation of sufficient amount of needle-shaped crystals of monosodium urate from serum or synovial fluid. There is joint effusion containing numerous polymorphs, macrophages and microcrystals of urates. The mechanism of acute inflammation appears to include phagocytosis of crystals by leucocytes, activation of the kallikrein system, activation of the complement system and urate-mediated disruption of lysosomes within the leucocytes leading to release of lysosomal products in the joint effusion. Initially, there is monoarticular involvement accompanied with intense pain, but later it becomes polyarticular along with constitutional symptoms like fever. Acute gouty arthritis is predominantly a disease of lower extremities, affecting most commonly *great toe*. Other joints affected, in order of decreasing frequency, are: the instep, ankles, heels, knees, wrists, fingers and elbows.

2. Chronic tophaceous arthritis Recurrent attacks of acute gouty arthritis lead to progressive evolution into chronic arthritis. The deposits of urate encrust the articular cartilage. There is synovial proliferation, pannus formation and progressive destruction of articular cartilage and subchondral bone. Deposits of urates in the form of tophi may be found in the periarticular tissues.

3. Tophi in soft tissue A *tophus* (meaning 'a porous stone') is a mass of urates measuring a few millimeters to a few centimeters in diameter. Tophi may be located in the periarticular tissues as well as subcutaneously such as on the hands and feet. Tophi are surrounded by inflammatory reaction consisting of macrophages, lymphocytes, fibroblasts and foreign body giant cells (Fig. 30.26).

4. Renal lesions Chronic gouty arthritis frequently involves the kidneys. Three types of renal lesions are described in the kidneys: acute urate nephropathy, chronic urate nephropathy and uric acid nephrolithiasis.

i) *Acute urate nephropathy* is attributed to the intratubular deposition of monosodium urate crystals resulting in acute obstructive uropathy.

ii) *Chronic urate nephropathy* refers to the deposition of urate crystals in the renal interstitial tissue.

iii) *Uric acid nephrolithiasis* is related to hyperuricaemia resulting in hyperuric aciduria.

PIGMENTED VILLONODULAR SYNOVITIS AND TENOSYNOVIAL GIANT CELL TUMOUR (NODULAR TENOSYNOVITIS)

The terms 'pigmented villonodular synovitis' and 'nodular tenosynovitis' represent diffuse and localised forms respectively of the same underlying process. The localised form of lesion is also termed *xanthofibroma* or *benign synovioma*. When the giant cells are numerous in localised tenosynovitis, the condition is called *giant cell tumour of tendon sheath*.

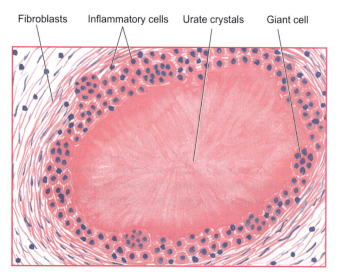
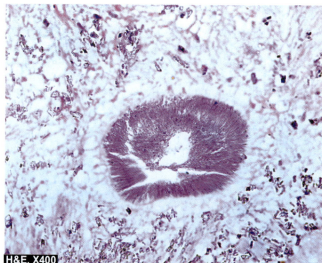

Figure 30.26 ▶ A gouty tophus, showing central aggregates of urate crystals surrounded by inflammatory cells, fibroblasts and occasional giant cells.

The origin and histogenesis of these conditions are unknown. They were initially regarded as inflammatory in origin and hence the name synovitis. But currently cytogenetic studies have shown clonal proliferation of cells indicating that these lesions are neoplastic. Clinically, they present with pain, swelling and limitation of movement of the affected joint and may be easily mistaken for rheumatoid or infective arthritis. The lesions are adequately treated by excision but recurrences are common.

MORPHOLOGIC FEATURES Though the two conditions have many morphologic similarities, they are best described separately.

◈ **Giant cell tumour of tendon sheath (Nodular tenosynovitis)** The localised nodular tenosynovitis is seen most commonly in the tendons of fingers.

Grossly, it takes the form of a solitary, circumscribed, pedunculated, small and lobulated nodule, measuring less than 2 cm in diameter. It is closely attached to and sometimes grooved by the underlying tendon. On section, the lesion is yellowish-brown.

Histologically, it is well encapsulated and is composed of sheets of small oval to spindle-shaped cells, foamy xanthoma cells, scattered multinucleate giant cells and irregular bundles of collagen. Many of the spindle-shaped cells are haemosiderin-laden (Fig. 30.27).

◈ **Pigmented villonodular tenosynovitis** This is a diffuse form of synovial overgrowth seen most commonly in the knee and hip.

Grossly, the synovium has characteristic sponge-like reddish-brown or tan appearance with intermingled elongated villous projections and solid nodules.

Histologically, the changes are modified by recurrent injury. The enlarged villi are covered by hyperplastic synovium and abundant subsynovial infiltrate of lymphocytes, plasma cells and macrophages, many of which are lipid-laden and haemosiderin-laden. Multinucleate giant cells are scattered in these areas.

CYST OF GANGLION

A ganglion is a small, round or ovoid, movable, subcutaneous cystic swelling of synovium. The most common location is dorsum of wrist but may be found on the dorsal surface of foot near the ankle. Histogenesis of the ganglion is disputed. It may be the result of herniated synovium, embryologically displaced synovial tissue, or post-traumatic degeneration of connective tissue.

MORPHOLOGIC FEATURES *Grossly,* a ganglion is a small cyst filled with clear mucinous fluid. It may or may not communicate with the joint cavity or tendon where it is located.

Microscopically, the cyst has a wall composed of dense or oedematous connective tissue which is sometimes lined by synovial cells but more often has indistinct lining (Fig. 30.28).

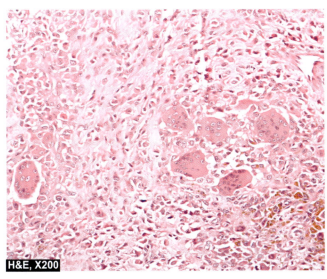

Figure 30.27 ▶ Tenosynovial giant cell tumour. The tumour shows infiltrate of small oval to spindled histiocytes with numerous interspersed multinucleate giant cells lying in a background of fibrous tissue.

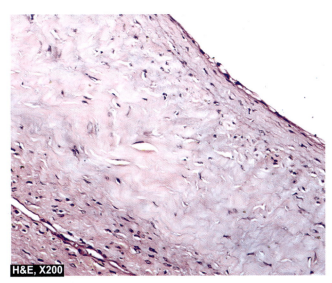

Figure 30.28 ▶ Cyst of ganglion. The cyst wall is composed of dense connective tissue lined internally by flattened lining. The cyst wall shows myxoid degeneration.

BURSITIS

Inflammation of bursa is termed bursitis. Bursae are synovial-lined sacs found over bony prominences. Bursitis occurs following mechanical trauma or inflammation. It may result following a single injury such as *olecranon bursitis* and *prepatellar bursitis*, but is more often due to repeated injuries from excessive pressure such as in *housemaid's knee* or *tennis elbow*.

MORPHOLOGIC FEATURES **Grossly,** the bursal sac is thick-walled and may contain watery, mucoid or granular brown material.

Histologically, the bursal wall is composed of dense fibrous tissue lined by inflammatory granulation tissue. The wall is infiltrated by lymphocytes, plasma cells and macrophages and may show focal calcium deposits.

GIST BOX 30.7 | Diseases of Joints

- Osteoarthritis or degenerative joint disease is chronic disorder of synovial joints characterised by progressive degenerative changes in the articular cartilages over the years.
- Rheumatoid arthritis is a chronic multisystem disease of unknown cause occurring in 3rd to 4th decade of life commonly in women. It occurs in immunogenetically predisposed individual to the effect of some microbial infection as trigger event.
- Suppurative arthritis is an acute inflammatory involvement of the joint by bacteria, usually from the bloodstream.
- Gout is a disorder of purine metabolism manifested by hyperuricaemia, recurrent attacks of characteristic acute arthritis, deposits of tophi in and around the joints, and in some cases uric acid nephrolithiasis.
- Pigmented villonodular synovitis and nodular tenosynovitis are diffuse and localised form respectively of the same underlying process. When the giant cells are numerous in localised tenosynovitis, the condition is called giant cell tumour of tendon sheath.
- A ganglion is a small, round or ovoid, movable, subcutaneous cystic swelling due to degeneration of synovium.
- Bursal cyst or bursitis is inflammation of the sac-like synovial tissue.

Index

In the following index, letter *t* after page number denotes table on that page while the letter *f* refers to figure.

A

AA protein, 62
ABL-BCR gene, 290, 432
Abscess, 126
    apical, 522
    Brodie's, 586
    cold, 137, 588
    psoas, 588
    pyaemic, 127
    pyogenic, 126
    subperiosteal, 586
    stitch, 158
Absolute values, 363
Acanthocytosis, 367
Accumulations, intracellular, 52-60
Acid phosphatase, 585
Acid-base balance, 223, 233
Acid-fast staining, 134, 145
Acidophil body, 42, 544
Acinic cell tumour, salivary, 531
Acquired immunodeficiency syndrome (AIDS), 204-11
Actinomycosis, 151-2
Activated partial thromboplastin time (APTT), 403
Acute inflammation, *details under* inflammation, acute, 107-28
Acute phase reactant proteins, 121
Acute transforming viruses, 308
Adamantinoma, 524
Adaptations, cellular, 18-26
Addison's disease, 55
Addisonian anaemia, 384
Adenoameloblastoma, 524
Adenocarcinoma, salivary gland, 531
Adenomatus polyposis coli, 282, 293
Adenoid cystic carcinoma, 531
Adenolymphoma, 529
Adenoma, 267*t*
    colorectal, 321-4
    monomorphic, 529
    pleomorphic, 528-9
    salivary, 528-9
Adenoviruses, 308
ADH, 227-8
Adhesion molecules, 13-4
Adipose tissue, tumours of, 341-3
Adult T cell leukaemia-lymphoma (ATLL), 309, 444*t*, 457
Aeroembolism, 257

Aflatoxin B, 298*t*, 300
Agenesis, 73
Ageing, cellular, 16-7
AL protein, 62
Albinism, 56
Albright syndrome, 593
Alcoholic liver disease, 52, 549-54
Alcoholism, 88-90, 549
Aldosterone, 227, 561
Alkaline phosphatase, 535, 584
Alkaptonuria, 56
Alpha1-antitrypsin deficiency, cirrhosis in, 549*t*
Alpha-foetoprotein (AFP), 318-9
Altitude, high, oedema, 231
Alzheimer's disease, amyloid in, 62
Ameloblastoma, 524
Ames' test, 301
Aminotransferase, 539, 542, 543
Amniotic fluid embolism, 258
Amoebiasis, 188-9
Amyloidosis, 61-72
    primary *versus* secondary, 66*t*
    stains for, 68
Anaemia of blood loss, 396-7
Anaemia of chronic disorders, 376-7
Anaemia, aplastic, 397-8
Anaemia, Cooley's, 395
Anaemia, Fanconi's, 397
Anaemia, general considerations, 364-8
    classification of, 367-8
    clinical features of, 364-5
    investigations of, 365-7
    pathophysiology of, 364
Anaemia, haemolytic, 385-97
    acquired (extracorpuscular), 386-9
    autoimmune (AIHA), 387-8
    classification of, 385*t*
    hereditary (intracorpuscular), 389-97
Anaemia, haemorrhagic, 396
Anaemia, hypochromic, 368-77
    laboratory diagnosis, 372-4
Anaemia, iron deficiency, 368-74
Anaemia, Mediterranean, 395
Anaemia, megaloblastic, 378-85
Anaemia, microcytic hypochromic, 368-74
Anaemia, myelophthisic, 398
Anaemia, normocytic and normochromic, 368, 377
Anaemia, pernicious, 384
Anaemia, sideroblastic, 374-6

Anaphylactic reaction, 211-2
Anaphylatoxins, 116
Anaplasia, 271
Anasarca, 226
Anencephaly, 74
Aneuploidy, 75
Aneurysmal bone cyst, 594-5
Angina pectoris, 490-1
Angiogenesis, 157, 273, 294-5
Angiosarcoma, 349-50
Angiotensin, 227, 472*f*
Anisocytosis, 271, 365
Anisonucleosis, 271
Anitschkow cells, 502
Ann Arbor staging, 449*t*
Annexin V, 42
Antibody, definition of, 195
Antibody-dependent cell-mediated cytotoxicity (ADCC), 312
Anti-oncogenes, 292*t*
Antigen, definition of, 195
Antigen-antibody complex, definition of, 195
Antiglobulin test, 386
Antinuclear antibodies (ANAs), 217
Antioxidants, 34
Antithrombotic factors, 247
Aphthae, 514-5
Apical abscess, 522
Apical granuloma, 522
APLA, 250, 412
Aplasia, 73
Apoptosis, 42-5
    in cancer, 294
    versus necrosis, 45*t*
Apoptotic bodies, 44*f*
Appendicitis, acute, 126-7
Arachidonic acid metabolites, 116-7
Argyria, 59
Ariboflavinosis, 104
Arrhythmias, 497
Arteriolosclerosis,
    hypertensive, 562
Arthritis,
    gouty, 611-2
    in Reiter's, 220
    in RHD, 500, 505
    rheumatoid, 608-11
    suppurative, 611
    tuberculous, 611
Arthus reaction, 202

Aschoff cells, 501-2
Aschoff nodules, 501-2
Ascites, 232-3, 557
Ascorbic acid, 102-3
Aspergillosis, 181
Aspiration, bone marrow, 358-9
Aspirin therapy, in platelet functions, 409
Asteroid bodies, 153, 154f
Atheroma, 484-6
Athcrosclerosis, 479-88
Atheromatous plaques, 484-7
    calcification in, 485
    complicated, 485
Atherosclerosis, 479-88
Atopic reaction, 211
ATP, cellular, 29, 31
Atrophy, 18-20
Atrophy, brown, heart, 59
Atypical lymphocytes, 426f
Atypical mycobacteria, 134
Auer rods, 438f
Australia antigen, 540
Autocoids, 116
Autohaemolysis test, 386
Autoimmune diseases, 215-21
    pathogenesis of, 215-6
Autolysis, 38-9
Autophagy, 45
Autopsy pathology, 8
Autosomal disorders, 78
Axial flow, 110, 250f
Axonal degeneration, 163

B

Bacteraemia, 127
Bacterial diseases, 168-80
Bacterial endocarditis, 507-11
Bacterial index (BI), in leprosy, 145
Bactericidal mechanisms, 113-4
Balance, acid base, 223
    water and electrolyte, 222-3
Ballooning degeneration, 544
Banding techniques, 75
Bantu's siderosis, 58
Barr body, 74f
Basal cell carcinoma, 326-7
Basophilia, 424, 433
    punctate, 366
Basophilic stippling, 366
Basophils, 123, 199, 424
B-cells, 197
    versus T cells, 198t
BCG vaccination, 135
BCL, 43, 294
Bedsores, 47
Bence Jones' proteins, 64f, 461
Benedict's test, 582
Beriberi, 104
Bernard-Soulier syndrome, 408

Berry aneurysms, 566-7
Beta carotene, 97
Beta fibrillosis, 62
Beta-amyloid protein, 62, 66
Beta -microglobulin, 563
Betel nut cancer, 283, 517
Bile acids (salts), 535
Bile lakes, 536f
Bile plugs, 536f
Biliary atresia, 537
Bilirubin, 58, 532
    conjugated versus unconjugated, 533
Bilirubin metabolism, 532-3
Biopsy, surgical, 7, 315
Biotin, 105
Birefringence, 61, 68, 70f, 71f
Bitot's spots, 99f
Bittner milk factor, 309
Blackwater fever, 190, 389
Blast crisis in CML, 433
Blastomas, 284
Blastomycosis, 182
Bleeding disorders, (also see under
    haemorrhagic diatheses), 400-14
Bleeding time, 402
Blindness, night, 97
Blood smear examination, 365-7
Blood volume, 222, 240
Blots, western, 210
Boeck's sarcoid, 153-4
Boil, 127
Bone, diseases of, 584-607
    cysts, 594-5
    lamellar, 584
    metastatic tumours in, 606-7
    normal structure of, 584-5
    tumour-like lesions of, 593-6
    tumours of, 596-607
    woven, 584
Bone marrow examination, 358-60
Botryoid rhabdomyosarcoma, 343-4
Botulism, 179
Boyd, William, 6
Boyden's chamber experiment, 112f
BRCA gene, 293
Bread and butter appearance, 505
Brodie's abscess, 586
Broncho-(lobular) pneumonia, 175-6
    versus lobar pneumonia, 176t
Bronchogenic carcinoma, 87, 300
Brown atrophy, heart, 59
Brown induration, lung, 236-7
Brown tumour of
    hyperparathyroidism, 591
Buccal smear, 74
Buffer system, 223-4
Burkitt's lymphoma, 455, 307
Burr cells, 367
Bursitis, 614
Button-hole appearance, 503

C

Cachexia, cancer, 313
Cadherins, 13
Caduceus, 3
Café-au-lait spots, 55, 283
Caissons disease, 257
Calcification, pathologic, 48-51
    dystrophic, 48-50
    dystrophic versus metastatic, 51t
    metastatic, 48, 50
Calcinosis cutis, 50
Calcitriol, 99
Calcospherites, 49
Calculus, gum, 522
Callus formation, 161-2
Cancer cervix, invasive, 283, 305-6
Cancer, definition of, 265
    diagnosis of, 315-20
    grading of, 280
    hallmarks of, 287-96
    immunology of, 311-3
    molecular basis of, 287-96
    staging of, 280-1
Cancrum oris, 515
Canker sores, 514-5
Candidiasis, 182-3
Carbon monoxide poisoning, 91
Carbuncle, 127
Carcinoembryonic antigen (CEA), 319
Carcinogens, 296-310
    biologic, 301-10
    chemical, 298t
    initiator, 299-300
    physical, 301-3
    promoter, 300
    viral, 301-10
Carcinogenesis, 296-310
    biologic, 301-10
    chemical, 296-301
    hormonal, 285
    physical, 301-3
    viral, 301-10
Carcinoma, acinic cell, 531
Carcinoma, adenoid cystic, 531
Carcinoma, basal cell, 326-7
Carcinoma, cervix, 25f, 283, 305-6
Carcinoma, definition of, 265
Carcinoma, lung, 87, 283
Carcinoma, mucoepidermoid, 529-30
Carcinoma, nasopharyngeal, 307-8
Carcinoma, oral cavity, 518-20
Carcinoma, skin, 324-9
Carcinoma, squamous cell, 324-6
Carcinoma, stomach, 331f
Carcinoma, transitional cell, 329-31
Carcinoma, urinary bladder, 329-31
Carcinoma in situ, 25, 284
    cervix, 24-6, 284
    oral cavity, 517-8

Cardiac markers, serum, 496-7
Cardiac oedema, 230
Cardiovascular interventions, 512-3
Caries, dental, 521-22
Caries, spine, 587-8
Carrier state, hepatitis, 543
Cartilage-forming tumours, 600-3
Cartilage, normal structure of, 585
Caseous necrosis, 40, 136
Castleman's disease, 417
Catenin, beta, 292t, 293
Cat-scratch disease, 184t, 177
Cell adhesion molecules (CAMs), 13-4
Cell ageing, 16-7
Cell cycle, 14-6
Cell death, 31, 38-51
Cell injury, etiology and pathogenesis of, 27-35
Cell membrane, 9-10
Cell structure, 9-14
Cell-mediated reaction, 215
Cellular adaptations, 18-26
Cellular swelling, 36-7
Cellulitis, 127
Cementomas, 525-6
Cementum, 520
Centrilobular haemorrhagic necrosis, 237, 533
Cerebral infarction, 40
Cerebral malaria, 190
Cerebral oedema, 232
Cervical intraepithelial neoplasia (CIN), 25, 284
Chancre, 150
Chemical carcinogenesis, 296-301
Chemical carcinogens, 298t
Chemical injury, 34
Chemical mediators of inflammation, 114-21
Chemokines, 14
Chemotaxis, 112
Chickenpox, 187
Chikungunya, 185-6
Childhood tumours, 284, 82-4
Chloroma, 437
Cholestasis, 535
Choline, 105-6
Chondroblastoma, 601-2
Chondroma, 600-1
Chondromyxoid fibroma, 602
Chondrosarcoma, 602-3
Chordoma, 606
Chorea minor, 505
Choristoma, 266
Christmas disease, 410
Chromatin, sex,
Chromosomes, 9, 74
Chronic inflammation, (*also see under* inflammation), 129-54
Chronic ischaemic heart disease, 498-9

Chronic lymphocytic leukaemia (CLL), 453-4
Chronic myeloid leukaemia (CML), 432-4
 blastic phase in, 433
Chronic venous congestion (CVC), 236-9
 kidney, 239
 liver, 237
 lungs, 236-7
 spleen, 237-8
Chutta cancer, 300
Cicatrisation, 157
Circle of Willis, 567f
Cirrhosis, liver, 548-6
 alcoholic, 549-54
 classification of, 549t
 macronodular, 549,554
 micronodular, 549, 552
 pathogenesis of, 548
 post-necrotic, 554
Clefts, facial, 514
Clostridial disease, 178-9
Clotting system, 248-9, 403
Cloudy swelling, 36
Coagulation disorders, 409-13
Coagulation system, 248-9, 403
Coagulation tests, 403-4
Coagulative necrosis, 39, 260-4
Coccidioidomycosis, 182
Codman's triangle, 598
Cold abscess, 137, 588
Cold agglutinin disease, 387
Collagen, 160
Collagen diseases, 215-21
Colliquative necrosis, 40
Colony-stimulating factor, 358
Coma, non-ketotic, 577
Complement system, 120
Complicated plaques, 485
Conchoid bodies, 153-4
Condyloma acuminatum, 305
Congenital heart disease, 474-9
Congestion, chronic venous, 236-9
Congestive heart failure (CHF), 470-4
Congestive splenomegaly, 237-8, 464
Congo red, 61, 68, 69f, 70f, 71f
Conjugated *versus* unconjugated bilirubin, 533t
Consolidation, 171-5
Consumptive coagulopathy, 412
Contractures, 159-60
Coombs' test, 386
Cor bovinum, 104
Cord factor, 135
Coronary artery disease (CAD), (*also see under* IHD), 488-500
Coronary syndromes, acute, 490
Councilman (acidophil) body, 42, 544
Craniotabes, 101f
Crigler-Najjar syndrome, 536
Cryptococcosis, 182

Cyanmethaemoglobin method, 365
Cyanocobalamin, 105, 378
Cyclo-oxygenase pathway, 116-7
Cylindroma, salivary gland, 531
Cysticercosis, 191-2
Cysts,
 apical, 522
 bone, 594
 dentigerous, 522-3
 dermoid, 354-6, 516, 524
 echinococcal, 192-3
 epidermal, 159
 eruption, 523
 gingival, 523
 hydatid, 192-3
 implantation, 159
 jaw, 522t
 nasopalatine, 523
 odontogenic, 522t
 primordial, 523
 radicular, 522
Cytochemistry, 436t, 316
 acute leukaemias, 438
Cytogenetics, 74-7
Cytokines, 13-4, 117-9
Cytology, diagnostic, 8, 316
Cytometry, flow, 319
Cytoskeleton, 11
Cytosol, structure of, 11-2
Cytotoxic reaction, 212-3

D

Dane particle, 539
Debridement, 159
Decompression sickness, 257-8
Defibrination syndromes, 412-3
Deficiency diseases, nutritional, 93-7
Degenerations, 36-8
Degenerative joint disease (DJD), 607-8
Dehydration, 233
Delayed hypersensitivity, 135, 215
Deletions, chromosomal, 76
Dengue fever, 185
Dentin, 520
Denver classification, 10
Dependent oedema, 30
Dermatofibrosarcoma protuberans, 339-40
Dermatomyositis-polymyositis, 220
Desmoid tumours, 338
Desmoplasia, 274
Desmosomes, 13
Desmoplastic small round cell tumour, 353
Developmental defects, 73-4
Devil's pinches, 405
Diabetes mellitus, 569-83
Diabetic ketosis, 577, 582
Diabetic microangiopathy, 578
Diabetic nephropathy, 578-9
Diabetic neuropathy, 579

Diabetic retinopathy, 579-80
Diagnosis of cancer, 315-20
Dialysis-related bone disease, 62, 66, 592
Diapedesis, 112, 239
Diet and cancer, 106
Differentiation, neoplastic cells, 271
Disease, definition of, 1
Disseminated intravascular coagulation (DIC), 412-3
Divers' palsy, 257-8
DNA oncogenic viruses, 305-8
DNA, structure of, 11f
Dohle bodies, 422f
Downey cells, 426
Down's syndrome, 75
Drepanocytes, 367
Dressler's syndrome, 498
Dropsy, 226
Drumstick appendage, 74f
Dry gangrene, 46
    versus wet, 48t
Dry tap, 360, 398
Dubin Johnson syndrome, 56, 536
Dupuytren's contracture, 159
Dysentery, amoebic, 189
    bacillary, 170
Dyslipidaemia, 480
Dysplasia, 23-4
    cervical, 24-5
    developmental, 73
    fibrous, 593-4
    oral cavity, 517-8
    versus metaplasia, 24t
Dysraphic anomalies, 73
Dystrophic calcification, 48, 49-50

E

Ecchymoses, 239
Echinococcosis, 192-3
Ectopic hormone production, 313-5
Electrolytes, 223
Electron microscopy, 6, 318
Electrophoresis in myeloma, 462f
Elephantiasis, 227
Elliptocytosis, 367, 390
Embden-Meyerhof pathway, 362, 390
Embolism, 253-9
    air, 257
    amniotic fluid, 258
    fat, 256
    gas, 256-8
    pulmonary, 254-5
    systemic, 255-6
Embolus, 253
Embryomas, 83t, 266, 284
Emigration, leucocytic, 112
Enamel, 520
Enchondroma, 600-1
Encrustation hypothesis, 482

Endocarditis,
    bacterial (infective), 507-11
    non-bacterial, 507
    rheumatic, 502-4
Endoplasmic reticulum, 12
Enteric fever, 168-70
Enterocolitis, 179
    ischaemic, 47
    necrotising, 179
Eosinophilia, 123, 199, 424
Environmental pollution, 85-8
Eosinophilic granuloma, 463
Eosinophils, 123, 199, 424
Epidermodysplasia verruciformis, 305
Epidermoid carcinoma, 324-6, 531
Epithelioid cells, 40, 136
Epstein-Barr virus, 306-7
Epulis, 515-6
Erythema marginatum, 505
Erythema nodosum leprosum (ENL), 148
Erythroblast, 360-1
Erythroblastosis foetalis, 388
Erythrocytic sedimentation rate (ESR), 367
Erythroid series, 360-1
Erythrophagocytosis, 169
Erythropoiesis, 360-1
Erythropoietin, 360
Ethanol, 88-91, 549-50
Euchromatin, 10
Eumycetoma, 182
Ewing's sarcoma, 604-6
Exanthemata, viral, 187
Exfoliative cytology, 6, 22-5, 316
Exostosis, osteocartilaginous, 600-1
Extracellular fluid compartment, 222
Exudate *versus* transudate, 226t

F

FAB classification, 442
    acute leukaemia, 436t
    lymphoid leukaemia, 442
    myelodysplastic syndrome, 439
Facial clefts, 514
Familial Mediterranean fever, 65t, 67
Familial polyposis coli syndrome, 282, 293
Fanconi's anaemia, 397
Fat necrosis, 40-1
Fat-soluble vitamins, 97-102
Fat stains, 54, 54f
Fatty change, 52-4
Fatty infiltration, stromal, 54
Fatty liver, 52-4
Fenton reaction, 33
Ferritin, 56, 374, 377
Ferroptosis, 45
Fever,
    enteric, 168-70
    dengue, 185
    viral haemorrhagic, 184-7
    yellow, 546-7

Fibril protein, 62-3
Fibrin-split products (FSP), 404, 413
Fibrinogen, 404
Fibrinoid necrosis, 41
Fibrinolysis, 404, 413
Fibrinolytic defects, 411-2
Fibrinolytic system, 119-20, 403f
    tests for, 404
Fibrohistiocytic tumours, 339-41
Fibroma, 336
    ameloblastic, 525
    cementifying, 525
    chondromyxoid, 602
    non-ossifying, 594
    oral mucosa, 517
    soft tissue, 336
Fibromatosis, 337-8
Fibronectin, 160
Fibrosarcoma, 338-9
Fibrous cortical defect, 594
Fibrous dysplasia of bone, 593-4
FIGLU test, 383
Filariasis, 190-1, 227
Fish-mouth appearance, 503
Fite-Faraco staining, 145
Flavanoids, 106
Flea-bitten kidney, 566f
Flow cytometry, 319
Flu, 186-7
    bird, 186
    swine, 186-7
Fluid compartments, 222
Fluorosis, skeletal, 592
Focal necrosis, liver, 533
Folate, 105, 378
Follicular hyperplasia, lymph node, 417
Folliculitis, 177
Food poisoning, 179
Fordyce's granules, 514
Fracture healing, 161-3
Free radicals, 32-4, 119
Frozen section, 7, 316
Fungal diseases, 180-4
Fungal stains, 167t
Furuncle, 177

G

Gamma glutamyl transpeptidase (γ-GT), 535
Gamna-Gandy bodies, 238
Ganglion cyst, 613
Gangrene, 46-8
    Dry *versus* wet, 48t
    gas, 48
Gap junctions, 13
Gastric carcinoma, 331f
Gastroenteropathy, haemorrhagic, 47, 245, 261
Gaucher's disease, 80-1

Genetic diseases, 73-81
Ghon's complex, 137
Giant cell lesions of bone, 604
Giant cell tumour of bone, 603-4
Giant cells, 124
Gibbs-Donnan equilibrium, 223
Gingivitis, 522
Globi, 145f
Glomus tumour (glomangioma), 348
Glossitis, 514
Glucose tolerance test (GTT), 582
Glucose 6-phosphate dehydrogenase (G6PD) deficiency, 391
Glucosuria, 582
    alimentary (lag storage), 581f, 582
    renal, 581f, 582
Glycogen stains, 55, 316t
Glycogen storage diseases, 79-81
Glycosaminoglycans (GAGs), 63, 160
Glycosylated haemoglobin (HbA$_{1C}$), 582-3
Golgi apparatus, 12
Grading of tumours, 280
Granulation tissue formation, 156-7
Granulocytes, 122-3, 199, 421-3
Granuloma, 130-1
    apical, 522
    eosinophilic, 463
    pyogenicum, 348, 516
    reparative, 591
    sarcoid, 153-4
Granulomatous inflammation, 130-54
    actinomycosis, 151-2
    leprosy, 144-9
    sarcoidosis, 153-4
    syphilis, 149-51
    tuberculosis, 132-44
Granulopoiesis, 418-20
Growth, adaptive disorder of, 18-26
Growth factors in neoplasia, 268-9
Gum hypertrophy, 437, 522
Gumma, 150

H

Haemangioma, 346-7
    granulation tissue type, 348
    mouth, 348, 517
Haematin, 58
Haematogenous spread of tumours, 276-7
Haematopoiesis, 357-8
Haemochromatosis, 58
Haemodialysis-associated amyloid, 62, 66-7
Haemodynamic disorders, 235-64
Haemoglobin, 56, 362-3
Haemoglobinopathies, 391-6
Haemolysis, general features of, 385-6
Haemolytic anaemia, (also see under anaemia, haemolytic), 385-97
Haemolytic disease of newborn (HDN), 388
Haemolytic uraemic syndrome, 405, 408

Haemophilia, 409-10
    A, 409-10
    B, 410
Haemoprotein-derived pigments, 56-8
Haemorrhage, 239
    intracerebral, 565-6
    intracranial, 565-7
    subarachnoid, 566-7
Haemorrhagic diatheses (bleeding disorders), 404-14
Haemorrhagic disease of newborn (HDN), 388
Haemorrhagic fevers, viral, 184-6
Haemorrhagic gastroenteropathy, 47, 245, 261
Haemosiderin, 56-8
Haemosiderosis, 57-8
Haemostasis, screening tests of, 401-4
Haemostasis, vascular, 401-2, 404-5
Haemostatic function, tests for, 401-44
Hageman factor, 119
Hairy cell leukaemia, 456
Hamartoma, 82, 266
Hand-Schüller-Christian disease, 463
Hapten, 195
Hay fever, 212
Hb Barts' hydrops foetalis, 394
HbH disease, 394
HBsAg, 539, 540
HDL, 62, 480
Healing, 155-64
    fracture, 161-3
Health, definition of, 1
Heart failure, 470-4
Heart failure cells, 237
Heat-shock protein (HSP), 14
Heinz bodies, 391
Helicobacter pylori, 303
Henoch-Schönlein's purpura, 405
Hepadnaviruses, 308
Hepar lobatum, 150f
Hepatisation, lung, 171-3
Hepatitis, viral, 537-48
    acute, 543-4
    autoimmune, 544-5
    carrier state of, 543
    chronic, 544-5
    classification of, 538
    clinicopathologic spectrum of, 542-7
    contrasting features of, 538f
    fulminant, 546-7
    lupoid, 544-5
    massive to submassive, 546-7
Herpes simplex virus, 187, 306-7
Herpes zoster, 187
Hess capillary test, 402
Heterochromatin, 10
Heterogeneity of cancer, 295
Heterophile antibody, 426

Hexose-monophosphate (HMP) shunt, 362, 390
Hippocrates, 3
Histamine, 115-6, 123, 199, 424
Histiocytes, 123-4, 198, 462
    cardiac, 502
Histiocytoma, malignant fibrous, 340-1
Histiocytosis-X (Langerhans' cell histiocytosis), 462-3
Histochemistry, 316
Histocompatibility leucocyte antigens (HLA), 200-1
HIV, structure of, 204
    infection, *see under* AIDS, 204-11
HLA system, 200-1
Hodgkin's disease, 445-50
    versus non-Hodgkin's lymphoma, 450t
Homeostasis, 222-24
Homogentisic acid, 56
Hormonal carcinogenesis, 285
Human herpes virus (HHV), 307, 350-1
Human immunodeficiency virus (HIV), 204-11
Human papilloma virus (HPV), 25f, 305-6
Human T cell lymphotropic virus (HTLV), 204, 309
Hyaline, alcoholic, 36, 551
Hyaline change, 36-7
Hyaline membrane, 232
Hybridisation, *in situ,* 8, 319
Hydatid cyst, 192-3
Hydrolytic enzymes, 31, 32t, 40
Hydropic change, 36
Hydrops foetalis, 388, 394
Hydrostatic pressure, 224
Hydroxytryptamine (HT), 115-6
Hyperaemia, 235-9
    active, 235-6
    passive, 236-9
Hyperbilirubinaemia, 58, 533-5
Hypercholesterolaemia, 54, 480
Hyperchromatism, 271
Hypercoagulability of blood, 250, 412
Hyperlipidaemia, 54, 480
Hyperosmolar non-ketotic coma, 577
Hyperparathyroidism, 591, 589
Hyperphosphataemia, 591
Hyperpigmentation, 55-6
Hyperplasia, 21-2
Hypersensitivity reactions, 211-5
Hypertension, portal, 556-8
Hypertension, systemic, 559-68
Hypertensive heart disease, 563
Hypertensive nephropthay, 563-5
Hypertensive retinopathy, 567
Hypertrophy, 20
Hyperviscosity syndrome, 461
Hypervitaminosis A, 98
Hypervitaminosis D, 101
Hypocalcaemia, 591

Hypochromasia, 366, 368, 373
Hypoglycaemia, 577
Hypopigmentation, 56
Hypoplasia, 73
Hypoprothrombinaemia, 102, 404
Hypoxic cell injury, 28-34
    irreversible, 31-2
    reversible, 29-30

I

Idiopathic (immune) thrombocytopenic purpura (ITP), 406-8
Immunity, normal, 195, 200
    diseases of, 203-221
Immunodeficiency syndrome, acquired, (AIDS), 203-11
Immunohistochemistry, 317-8
Immunologic tissue injury, 211-5
Immunology of cancer, 311-3
Immunotherapy, 313
Impaired glucose tolerance (IGT), 581t
Inborn errors of metabolism, 78-81
Infarction, 39, 260
Infarcts, 260-4
    brain, 40, 565-6
    heart, 490-500
    intestine, 47
    kidney, 39, 262-3
    laminar, 491
    liver, 264
    lung, 262
    myocardial, 490-500
    spleen, 263
Infectious agents, 166-94
    bacteria, 169t
    factors relating to, 167
    fungi, 180t
    identification of, 167t
    parasites, 188t
    viruses, 184t
Infectious mononucleosis, 424-7
Infestations, 188-93
Infiltrations, 36, 54
Inflammation, acute, 107-28
Inflammation, chronic, 129-54
    granulomatous, 130-54
Inflammatory cells, 122-5, 196-9, 421-4
Inflammatory response, factors determining, 125
Influenza, 186-7
Inheritance, autosomal, 77
In situ hybridisation, 8, 319
Insulin metabolism, 570-1
Integrins, 13
Interferon, 13, 119
Interleukin, 13, 117-9
Intermediate filaments, 11
Internal environment, 222-4
Interphase, 15f

Intracellular accumulations, 52-60
    of fat, 52-4
    of glycogen, 54-5
    of proteins, 54
Intracellular fluid compartment, 222
Intracerebral haemorrhage, 565-6
Intracranial haemorrhage, 565-7
Intravascular haemolysis, 387
    versus extravascular, 387t
Intrinsic factor (IF), 384
Inversions, chromosomal, 75
Involucrum, 586
Ionising radiation, 34-5, 302-3
Iron cycle, 369f
Iron metabolism, 368-71
Irreversible cell injury, 31-4
    morphology of, 36-51
Ischaemia, 28-34, 39, 260
Ischaemic bowel disease, 47, 245, 261
Ischaemic brain damage, 40, 566
Ischaemic heart disease (IHD), 488-500
Islet cell changes in diabetes, 574

J

Jamshidi needle, 359
Janeway's spots, 511
Jaundice, 58, 533-5
Jaw, lumpy, 152
    cysts of, 522t
Joints, diseases of, 607-14
Junctions, intercellular, 12-3

K

Kallikrein, 120f
Kangri cancer, 300, 325
Kaposi's sarcoma, 307, 350-1
Karyolysis, 39f
Karyorrhexis, 39f
Karyotypic abnormalities, 74-7
Karyotyping, 75
Keloid, 159
Keratomalacia, 97
Keratosis, smokers', 517
Kerley lines, 231
Kernicterus, 58, 535
Ketoacidosis, diabetic, 577
Ketonuria, 582
Kidney,
    CVC, 239
    flea-bitten, 566f
    infarcts, 39, 262-3
    shock, 245
Killing, bacterial, 113-4
Kinin system, 119
Klinefelter syndrome, 75
Koch's bacillus, 133
Koch's phenomenon, 135
Kupffer cells, 123

Kviem test, 153
Kwashiorkor, 95-6

L

Lactic dehydrogenase (LDH), 497
Laennec's cirrhosis, 552
Langerhans' cell histiocytosis (LCH), 462-4
Langhans' giant cells, 41f, 124, 136
LE cell phenomenon, 218
Leiomyoma, 37, 345-6
Leiomyosarcoma, 346
Lentigo, 56
Lepra reaction, 148
Lepromin test, 146
Leprosy, 144-9
Leptocytosis, 367
Letterer-Siwe disease, 463
Leucocytes in health and disease, 418-24
    reactive proliferations, 421-28
Leucocyte alkaline phosphatase (LAP), 427, 434
Leucoderma, 56
Leukaemias, 428
    acute lymphoblastic (ALL), 442t, 444t, 450-2
    acute myeloid (AML), 436-9
    AML *versus* ALL, 452t
    chronic lymphocytic (CLL), 429
    chronic myeloid (CML), 432-4
    etiology of, 429-30
    pathogenesis of, 430-1
Leukaemoid reaction, 427
    versus CML, 428t
Leukoedema, 514
Leukoplakia, oral, 517-8
Leukotrienes, 117
Lewis experiment, 112
Lichen planus, 514
Lines of Zahn, 251
Linitis plastica, 274, 332
Lipofuscin, 58-9
Lipogranuloma, 54
Lipoma, 341-2
Lipooxygenase pathway, 117
Lipoproteins, 480
Liposarcoma, 342-3
Lipoxins, 117
Liver, diseases of, 532-58
    coagulation disorders, 411
    CVC, 237
    fatty change, 52-3
    metastasis in, 237
Liver cell necrosis, types of, 532-3
    bridging, 546
    piecemeal, 546
Lobar pneumonia, 171-4
Lukes-Collins classification, 441

Lung,
    cancer, 87, 283
    CVC, 236
    oedema, 230-2
    shock, 245
    tuberculosis, 137-42
Lupus erythematosus, 217-8
Lupus nephritis, 219*t*
Lymph nodes,
    Metastatic tumours, 275-6, 457-8
    structure of, 415-6
Lymphadenitis, reactive, 416-8
Lymphangioma, 348
Lymphangitis, 227
Lymphatic obstruction, 227
Lymphatic spread of tumours, 275-6
Lymphoblast, 420
Lymphoblast *versus* myeloblast, 421*t*
Lymphocytes, 123, 196-8, 423
    atypical, 426
    T *versus* B, 198*t*
Lymphocytosis, 423
Lymphoedema, 227
Lymphogranuloma venereum, 169*t*
Lymphoid hyperplasia, 417-8
    angiofollicular, 417
Lymphoid series, 421-2
Lymphomas, malignant, 441-64
    B-cell neoplasms, 450-6
    Burkitt's, 455
    classification of, 444*t*
    contrasting features of, 450*t*
    cutaneous T cell, 457
    Hodgkin's, 445-50
    non-Hodgkin's (NHL), 450-64
    T-cell neoplasms, 457
Lymphopenia, 423
Lysosomal storage diseases, 78-81
Lysosomes, 12

M

M-band, 461-2
MacCallum's patch, 504
Macrocytes, 378, 381
Macroglossia, 514
Macrophages, alveolar, 237
Madura foot, 182
Maffucci's syndrome, 600
Major histocompatibility complex, 200-1
Malaria, 189-90
Malignant melanoma, 327-9
Mallory hyaline, 36, 551
Mantoux test, 135
Marasmus, 95-6
Margination, 250
Markers in hepatitis B, 540
Mast cells, 123, 199, 424
Matrix, extracellular, 160
M. avium-intracellulare, 134

Mediators of inflammation, 114-21
Megakaryocyte, 400
Megaloblasts, 378, 382
Melanin, 55, 324, 327
Melanoma, 327-9
Membrane attack complex (MAC), 120
Membrane damage, 31
MEN syndrome, 283
Mendelian disorders, 77-8
Metachromasia, 68
Metamyelocyte, 419
Metaphyseal fibrous defect, 594
Metaplasia, 22-3
    versus dysplasia, 24*t*
Metastasis, 275-80
    haematogenous, 276-7
    lymphatic, 275-6
    mechanisms of, 278-80
    retrograde, 275
    skip, 275
Metastatic calcification, 48-51
    versus dystrophic, 51*t*
Microarrays, cDNA, 320
Microcytes, 365, 373
Microfilaments, 11
Microfilaria, 190-2
Microglossia, 514
Microorganisms, identification of, 167*t*
MicroRNA, 295-6
Microtubules, 11
Mikulicz syndrome, 527
Milk-alkali syndrome, 50
Mitochondria, 11
Mitotic figures, 271-2
Mitral stenosis and insufficiency, 503, 506
Mitsuda reaction, 146
Mixed salivary tumour, 528-9
    malignant, 530-1
MMTV, 309
Molecular basis, cancer, 287-96
Molecular pathology, 8
Mönckeberg's arteriosclerosis, 49
Moniliasis, 182
Monoblast, 420
Monoclonal gammopathy,
    of undetermined significance (MGUS), 461-2
Monoclonal hypothesis, 286, 482
Monocyte-macrophage series, 123-4, 198, 420
Monocytes, 123, 198, 420, 423
Monocytosis, 424
Mononuclear phagocyte system, 123-4, 198, 420*f*
Mononucleosis cells, 426
Monosomy, 75
Morphometry, 320
Mucocele, 516
Mucoepidermoid carcinoma, 529-30
Mucoid degeneration, 38

Mucopolysaccharidoses, 79*t*
Multifactorial inheritance, 78
Multiple myeloma, 458-61
Mumps, 526
Mutagenicity (Ames') test, 301
Mutations, 76, 287
Mutator gene, 295
Mycetoma, 182
Mycobacteria, atypical, 134
Mycobacterium, avium intracellulare, 134
Mycobacterium leprae, 145
Mycobacterium tuberculosis, 133-4
Mycosis, fungoides, 457
Mycosis, superficial, 183
Myelin figures, 30*f*
Myeloblast, 418-9
Myeloblast *versus* lymphoblast, 421*t*
Myelocyte, 419
Myelodysplastic syndrome (MDS), 439-41
Myelofibrosis, 398
Myelogram, 359
Myeloid series, 418-20
Myeloma, 458-61
    kidney, 460-1
Myeloma cells, 460
Myeloproliferative diseases, 432-6
Myoblastoma, granular cell, 353
Myocardial infarction, 491-8
Myocardial ischaemia, non-infarct effects of, 490, 498-9
Myxoedema, 226, 233
Myxoma, odontogenic, 525

N

Naevi, naevocellular, 324
Natural killer (NK) cells, 198
Necrosis, 38-41
    versus apoptosis, 45*t*
Necroptosis, 44
Necrotising papillitis, 579
Negri bodies, 187
Neoplasia, (*also see under* tumours), 265-356
    characteristics of, 267-75
    classification of, 265-7
    clinical aspects of, 313-20
    definition of, 265
    diagnosis of, 315-20
    epidemiology of, 282-5
    etiology of, 282-310
    immunology of, 311-3
    incidence of, 282
    intraepithelial, 25, 284
    pathogenesis of, 285-310
Neoplastic cells, 271-3
Nephritic syndrome, 229
Nephritic *versus* nephritic oedema, 229*t*
Nephropathy,
    diabetic, 578-9
    myeloma, 460

Nephrosclerosis, 578-9
Nephrotic syndrome, 229
Neurofibromatosis, 284
Neurosyphilis, 151
Neutropenia, 422
Neutrophil alkaline phosphatase (NAP), 427, 434
Neutrophilia, 422
Neutrophils, 122-3, 199, 421-3
    toxic granules in, 422
    vacuoles in, 422
Niacin, 104-5
Niemann-Pick disease, 81
Nitric oxide mechanism, 33, 114
Nitrogen gas, 257
Noma, 515
Non-Hodgkin's lymphoma (NHL), 450-64
    versus Hodgkins' disease, 450*t*
Non-ossifying fibroma, 594
Normoblastaemia, 386, 395
Normoblasts, 360-1
Nuclear sexing, 74
Nucleocytoplasmic ratio, 271
Nucleotides, 10
Nucleus, structure of, 9-12
Nutmeg liver, 237
Nutritional disorders, 93-106

O

Obesity, 94-5
Odontogenic, 522
    cysts, 522-3
    tumours, 524-6
Odontomas, 525
Oedema, 225-33
    cardiac, 230
    cerebral, 232
    hepatic, 232-3
    nephritic *versus* nephritic, 229*t*
    nutritional, 96*t*, 226
    pulmonary, 230-2
    renal, 229
Oestrogen, in cancer, 285
Ollier's disease, 600
Oncofoetal antigens, 318
Oncogenes, 287-91
    versus antioncogenes, 294*t*
Oncogenesis, *(also see under*
    carcinogenesis), 296-310
Oncogenic viruses, 303-310
    DNA, 305-8
    RNA, 308-9
Oncomirs, 295-6
Oncotic pressure, 224
Opportunistic infections, 166, 208*f*
Opsonins, 113
Oral soft tissues, 514-20
    developmental anomalies of, 514
    inflammatory conditions of, 514-5

    mucocutaneous lesions of, 514
    normal structure of, 514
    tumours of, 515-20
    white lesions of, 517-8
Organelles, 11-2
Osler's nodes, 511
Osler-Weber-Rendu disease, 405
Osmolality, 223
Osmolarity, 223
Osmotic fragility, 386, 390, 395
Osmotic pressure, 224
Ossification, 585
Osteitis deformans, 592-3
Osteitis fibrosa cystica, 590
Osteoarthritis, 607-8
Osteoblastic tumours, 596-600
Osteoblastoma, 597
Osteochondroma, 600
Osteoclastoma, 603-4
Osteodystrophy renal, 591
Osteogenesis imperfecta, 589
Osteoid osteoma, 597
Osteoma, 597
Osteomalacia, 101, 589
Osteomyelitis, 585-8
    pyogenic, 585-7
    tuberculous, 587-8
Osteoporosis, 590
Osteosarcoma, 597-600
Ovalocytosis, 367
Overhydration, 233
Oxygen-derived radicals, 32-4, 119

P

P-component, 62, 64*f*
Paediatric diseases, 82-4
Paget's disease, 592-3
Pancarditis, rheumatic, 502-5
Pancytopenia, 397-8
Papilloma, 321-2
    Mucocutaneous, 321, 517
    urothelial, 321
Papovaviruses, 305-6
Pappenheimer bodies, 374
Paraneoplastic syndrome (PNS), 313-5
Paraproteinaemias, 458-64
Parasitic diseases, 188-93
Parasitism, 166
Paroxysmal nocturnal haemoglobinuria (PNH), 389
Partial thromboplastin time with kaolin (PTTK), 403
Pathology, definition of, 1
    evolution of, 2-7
Paul-Bunnel test, 426
Pavementing, 250
Pelger-Huet anomaly, 422*f*
Pellagra, 104-5
Pemphigoid, 514

Pemphigus, 514
Periodontal disease, 522
Permeability factors, 114-20
Permeability, vascular, 109-10
Pertussis, 175-6
p53 gene, 43*f*, 292
pH of blood, 223
Phagocytes, 112
Phagocytosis, 112-4
Philadelphia chromosome, 290, 432
Phlebothrombosis, 251
Phosphatidyl serine, 42
Physical injury, 34-5
Pigments, 55-60
    malarial, 58
    wear and tear, 58
Plaques, atheromatous, 484-5
Plasma cells,
    disorders of, 458-62
Plasmacytoma, localised, 461
Plasmacytosis, reactive, 460
Platelets, 248, 400
Pleomorphic adenoma, salivary gland, 528-9
Pleomorphic sarcoma, 340-1
Pleomorphism, 271
Pneumonias, 170-5
    broncho (lobular), 175-6
    caseous, 140
    lobar, 170-4
    lobar *versus* broncho, 176*t*
    Pneumocystis jirovecii, 180-1, 209
Poikilocytosis, 365-6
Polychromasia, 366
Polycyclic hydrocarbons, 298*t*, 300
Polycythaemia vera, 434-5
Polymorphonuclear neutrophils (PMN), 122-3, 199, 421
Polyploidy, 75
Porphyrins, 58
Portal hypertension, 556-8
Post-myocardial infarction syndrome, 498
Pott's disease, 588
Poxviruses, 187, 308
Predisposing factors in tumours, 282-4
Pregnancy tumour, 348, 516
Premalignant lesions, 284-5
Pressure gradients, 224
Primary complex, 137
Primitive neuroectodermal tumour (PNET), 604-6
Procallus, 161-2
Prostacyclin, 116
Prostaglandins, 116-7
Protein-energy malnutrition (PEM), 95-6
Proteinuria, 226, 460
Proteoglycans, 63, 160
Prothrombin time, 403-4, 414*t*
Prussian blue reaction, 57*f*, 373, 376, 382
Psammoma bodies, 49

Pseudocartilage, 528
Ptyalism, 526
Pulmonary tuberculosis, (*see under* tuberculosis), 137-42
Pulpitis, 521-2
Punctate basophilia, 366
Pure red cell aplasia, 399
Purpuras, 239, 405-8
    Henoch-Schönlein, 405
    immune thrombocytopenic (ITP), 406-8
    thrombotic thrombocytopenic (TTP), 408
Pus, 127
Pyaemia, 128
Pyridoxine (vitamin B_6), 105
Pyroptosis, 44-5

Q

Quick's one stage method, 386
Quinacrine banding, 75

R

Rabies, 187
Radiation carcinogenesis, 301-3
Radicals, free, 32-4, 119
Radiolysis, 34
Ranula, 516
Rappaport classification, 441
Rb gene, 291-2
REAL classification, 442-3
Receptors, cell membrane, 14, 296*f*
Red blood cell, 361
Red line response, 108*f*
Reed-Sternberg (RS) cell, 445-6
Reiter's syndrome, 220
Rejection, transplant, 201-2
Regeneration, 155-6, 164-5
Renin-angiotensin-aldosterone mechanism, 227-8, 560-1
Repair, 155-7
Reperfusion injury, 32-4
Response-to-injury hypothesis, 482-3
Reticulocyte, 361
Reticuloendothelial system (RES), 123-4, 198, 420
Retinopathy,
    diabetic, 579-80
    hypertensive, 567-8
Retroviruses, 304, 308
Reye's syndrome, 52, 537
Rhabdomyoma, 343
Rhabdomyosarcoma, 343
Rheumatoid arthritis, 608-11
Rheumatic fever and RHD, 500-6
Rhinosporidiosis, 183
Riboflavin, 104
Rickets, 100-1
Ridley-Jopling classification, 146

RNA oncogenic viruses, 304, 308
Rodent ulcer, 326-7
Rye classification, 445

S

Salivary glands, diseases of, 526-31
Sarcoidosis, 153-4
Sarcoma, 265
    Alveolar soft part, 352-3
    botryoides, 343
    clear cell, 353
    epithelioid, 353
    Kaposi's, 350-1
    pleomorphic, 340
    synovial, 352
Scar, hypertrophic, 159
Schaumann bodies, 153
Schilling test, 383
Schistocytosis, 366
Scirrhous tumours, 274
Scurvy, 102-3
Selectins, 13
Sequestrum, 586
Serotonin, 116
Severe acute respiratory syndrome (SARS), 186
Sezary syndrome, 457
Shift-to-left, myeloid, 422-3
Shigellosis, 170
Shingles, 187
Shock, 240-6
Sialadenitis, 526-7
Sialorrhoea, 526
Sickle syndromes, 391-3
Sideroblasts, 374-5
Siderocytes, 374
Sinus histiocytosis, 417-8
Sjogren's syndrome, 220
Smoking, tobacco, 86-8
Sodium and water retention, mechanisms of, 228
Soft tissue tumours, 334-53
Sorbitol mechanism, 577
Spectrin, 390
Spherocytosis, 390-1
Spinal cord defects, 73
Spleen, diseases of, 464-6
Splenectomy, effects of, 465
Spread of tumours, 275-80
Squamous cell carcinoma, 324-9, 518-20
Squamous intraepithlial lesion (SIL), 24
Staging of tumours, 280-1, 336
Staphylococcal infections, 177-8
Steatosis, 52-4
Stem cells, haematopoietic, 357-8
Stomatitis, 514-5
Storage diseases, 78-81
Streptococcal infections, 178
Stress proteins, 14, 16

Stroke, 565-7
Sulfur granules, 152
Suppuration, 127
Syphilis, 149-51
Systemic lupus erythematosus (SLE), 217-8

T

Target cell, 366*f*
Tartar, 522
Teeth, diseases of, 520-6
Telomere, 16, 294
Teratomas, 353-6
Tetanus, 179
Thalassaemias, 393-8
Thiamine, 103-4
Thrombocytopenias, 405-8
Thrombocytosis, 408, 435-6
Thromboembolism, 254-5
Thrombogenesis, 247-50
Thrombogenic theory, 482
Thrombolytic therapy, 495
Thrombopoiesis, 400-1
Thrombosis, 247-53
Thrombotic thrombocytopenic purpura (TTP), 408
Thrombus, 247
    Antemortem *versus* post-mortem, 252
    Arterial *versus* venous, 251*t*
Thrush, oral, 182, 515
Tobacco smoking, 86-8
TORCH complex, 193-4
Tourniquet test, 402
Toxic granules, in neutrophils, 422
Transcoelomic spread, 277-8
Transitional cell carcinoma, 321
Transudate *versus* exudate, 226*t*
Trephine biopsy, 359-60
Triple response, 107
Troponins, cardiac, 497
Tubercle, 136
Tubercle bacilli, 133-4
Tuberculin test, 135-6
Tuberculosis, 132-42
    primary, 137-8
    pulmonary, 137-42
    intestinal, 143
Tumour lysis syndrome, 313
Tumour markers, serum, 318-9
Tumours (*also see under* neoplasia), 265-56
    Benign *versus* malignant, 268*t*
    characteristics of, 267-75
    classification of, 267*t*
    diagnosis of, 315-20
    epidemiology of, 282-5
    etiology and pathogenesis of, 282-310
    grading of, 280
    metastasis of, 275-80
    specific tumours, 321-56

spread of, 275-80
staging of, 280
Turner's syndrome, 75
Typhoid fever, 168-70

U

Ubiquitin, 14, 10
UICC staging, 280
Ulcer, 126
    aphthous, 514-5
    rodent, 326-7
Ultraviolet light, 301-2
Union, wounds, 157-61
    primary *versus* secondary, 159*t*
Urinary tract infection (UTI), 169*t*
Urine testing, 581-2

V

Varicella-zoster infection, 187
Vascular permeability, 109-10
Vascular tumours, 346-51
Villonodular synovitis, 612-3

Viral infections, 184*t*, 184-8
Viral hepatitis, (*also see under* hepatitis, viral), 537-48
Viral oncogenesis, 303-10
Virchow cells, 147
Virchow, Rudolf, 5
Viruses, oncogenic, 305-9
    DNA, 305-8
    RNA, 308-9
Vitamins, disorders of, 97-106
Von Gierke's disease, 80
von Recklinghausen disease, 284
von Willebrand's disease, 410-1

W

Warthin's tumour, 529
Warts, 305
Water, total body, 222
Wear and tear pigment, 58-9
White blood cells, diseases of, 415-464
White lesions, oral cavity, 517-8
Whooping cough, 175-6
Working formulation for clinical usage, 442

Wound, 157-61
    Contraction of, 160
    healing of, 157-9
    strength, 160
Woven bone callus, 162

X

X-chromosome, 74
Xeroderma pigmentosum, 295
Xerostomia, 526
X-linked disorders, 78

Y

Y-chromosome, 78
Yellow atrophy, acute, 185, 546
Yellow fever, 185

Z

Zahn, lines of, 252*f*
Zenker's degeneration, 36
Ziehl-Neelsen staining, 134, 145
Zonal necrosis, liver, 533
Zoster virus infection, 187